Pharmacology and the Nursing Process

Third Edition

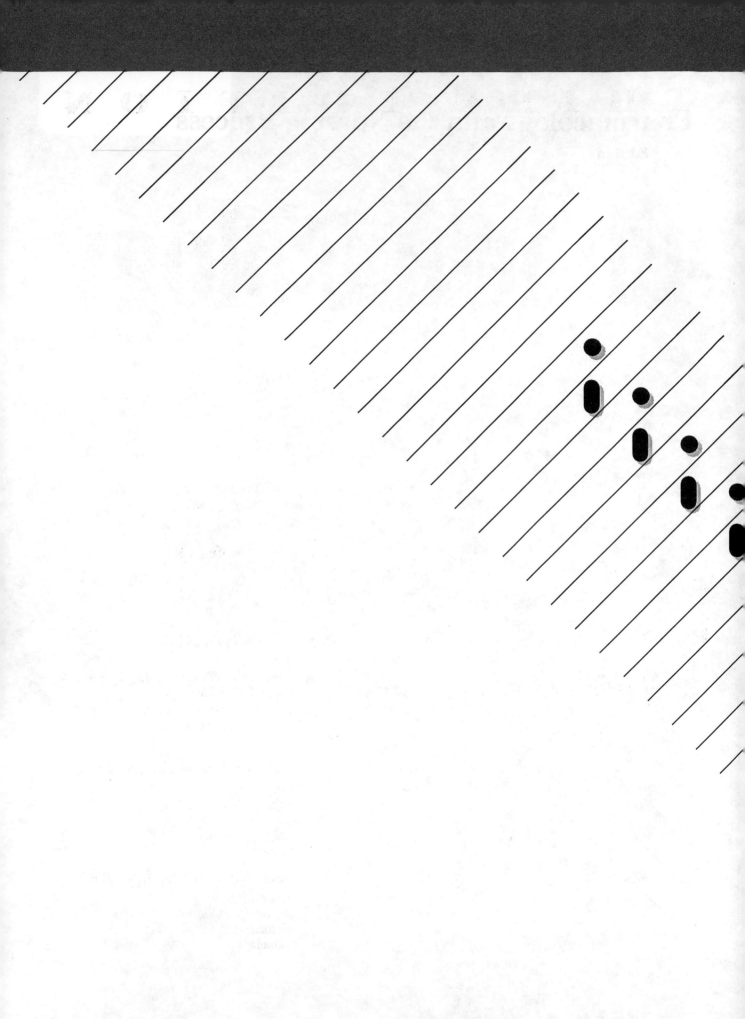

THIRD EDITION

Pharmacology
and the
Nursing
Process

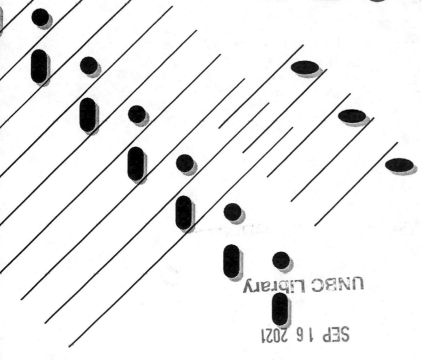

G.E. Johnson, Ph.D.

Professor
Department of Pharmacology
Faculty of Medicine
University of Saskatchewan
Saskatoon, Saskatchewan
Canada

Kathryn J. Hannah, R.N., Ph.D.

Professor
Faculty of Nursing
University of Calgary
Calgary, Alberta
Canada

Sheila Rankin Zerr, R.N., M.Ed.

School of Nursing
University of Victoria
Victoria, British Columbia
Canada

W.B. Saunders

The Curtis Centre
Independence Square West
Philadelphia, PA 19106

W.B. Saunders Company Canada Limited
55 Horner Avenue
Toronto, Ontario M8Z 4X6

Pharmacology and the Nursing Process

Third Edition

ISBN 0-920513-08-5
Copyright © 1992 by W.B. Saunders Company Canada
Limited.

Canadian Cataloguing in Publication Data

Johnson, G.E. (Gordon E.)
    Pharmacology and the nursing process

3rd ed.
Includes bibliographical references and index.
ISBN 0-920513-08-5

1. Pharmacology. 2. Drugs. 3. Nursing.
I. Hannah, Kathryn J. (Kathryn Jane), 1944- .
II. Zerr, Sheila Rankin. III. Title.

RM300.J6 1992   615'.1'024613
C92-094139-4

Design/illustrations/desktop publishing:
Blair Kerrigan/Glyphics

Editing/production coordination:
Francine Geraci

Printed in Canada at Webcom Limited

Last digit is print number: 9 8 7 6 5 4 3 2 1

Dedication

We would like to dedicate this book to three individuals who together have contributed greatly to its completion. First, to our respective spouses, Mary-Jane Johnson and Ray Zerr, we would like to say thank you. Writing a text can strain any relationship. The fact that we are still happily married, and the book is finished, is more a reflection of the maturity of our long-time companions than our skills as writers. In addition, G.E.J. would like to acknowledge the assistance of his wife Mary-Jane, who typed the manuscript and read the proofs. Finally, we must say thank you to Francine Geraci, our editor, who laboured long hours to ensure the successful completion of this work. It is hoped that our relationship with Francine will continue in years to follow.

Preface

Nursing education is a continual process. Beginning when the neophyte first enters Nursing School or College, it continues long after graduation. Recognizing this point, we have attempted to meet the needs of nurses at all levels of education who are interested in learning about the use of drugs. Obviously, some chapters will appeal more to people at one educational stage than another. Undergraduate students will find the material pertaining to the systematic study of drugs, such as autonomic pharmacology, of great interest. Staff nurses, charged with the daily care of the ill, may be more interested in the less didactic chapters that discuss the use of drugs in the treatment of a specific condition, such as bronchial asthma. Regardless of the particular appeal of one chapter versus another, we hope that all readers will appreciate our approach to the study of pharmacology.

Pharmacology is not the study of individual drugs. Rather, it involves an understanding of the interaction between drugs and the physiological, psychological and pathological processes occurring in the body. Therefore, we have discussed the physiology and pathology of the organ systems concerned before presenting the drugs. It is only by following this system that nurses will understand the actions of the drugs currently being used and be prepared for new drugs when they appear on the market.

The title, *Pharmacology and the Nursing Process,* was selected because it reflects our approach to the use of drugs. Following the prescription of a drug by a physician, nurses must assess the patient, administer the drug, evaluate its effects, and instruct the patient and/or family in all matters related to the use of the drug. Accordingly, the nursing process associated with each drug, or groups of drugs, is presented in both the body of the text and then summarized in the tables that accompany each chapter.

This book is not a comprehensive text on drug therapy. It provides a synopsis of the topic, together with a list of recommended readings at the end of each chapter. If more detailed information is required, nurses should consult more extensive texts. These include *AMA Drug Evaluations* and the *Compendium of Pharmaceuticals and Specialties.* Both are excellent sources of information.

Table of Contents

List of Tables

List of Figures

A Statement on Drug Doses

This text contains numerous drug dosages. Unless otherwise stated, these doses are intended for the average adult patient. Pediatric and geriatric doses have been provided when available. Although every effort has been made to ensure that the doses listed are correct, nurses must check with the latest information from the manufacturer if any doubt exists concerning the dosage of a drug. In order to reduce the size of the book, it has been necessary to abbreviate many measurements and terms. The table opposite will assist the nurse with regard to quantities and abbreviations.

Abbreviations used in this book

1 gram (g)	=	1000 milligrams (mg)
1 milligram (mg)	=	1000 micrograms (μg)
1 microgram (μg)	=	1000 nanograms (ng)
IU	=	International Units
prn	=	when required
stat	=	immediately
od	=	once daily
bid	=	twice daily
tid	=	three times daily
qid	=	four times daily
qod	=	every other day
qh	=	every hour
hs	=	at bedtime
q4h	=	every four hours
q6h	=	every six hours
q8h	=	every eight hours
ac	=	before meals
pc	=	after meals
ATC	=	around the clock
PO	=	by mouth
NPO	=	nothing by mouth
pt	=	patient
tx	=	treatment, therapy
hx	=	history
s/s	=	signs and symptoms

SECTION 1

General Principles of Pharmacology

Section 1 introduces the reader to the meaning of the word drug and the general principles underlying the use of drugs. The section is divided into three chapters. The first discusses the physical and chemical properties of drugs and their influence on drug absorption. In Chapter 1 we also present the various routes by which drugs may be administered. Chapter 2 describes the distribution of drugs throughout the body and their elimination, primarily by metabolism in the liver and/or excretion by the kidneys. We also take this opportunity to discuss the nature of the interaction of drugs with their receptors. Chapter 3 presents the general principles of nursing responsibilities related to drug use. It contains a brief review of the nursing process and a discussion of its application when drugs are given. Although Section 1 contains little information on any one group of drugs or the treatment of any disease, it forms the core of this book with direct links to all other chapters. The general principles of pharmacology, outlining as they do drug absorption, distribution and metabolism, as well as responsibilities of the nurse when drugs are given, can be applied to all subsequent sections of the book.

CHAPTER 1

Routes of Administration and Drug Absorption

Teaching Objectives
Following completion of this chapter, the reader should be able to:
1. Define the words drug and pharmacology.
2. Divide drugs into their two major chemical classes and describe the two forms in which they exist.
3. State the relative lipid and water solubilities of the ionized and nonionized drug molecules and the significance of these solubilities to drug diffusion in the body.
4. Discuss the effect of pH on the ratio of ionized/nonionized drug molecules for acids and bases.
5. List the parenteral routes for drug administration and discuss the relative advantages and disadvantages of each route.
6. List the oral dosage forms for drugs and discuss the relative merits of each type of formulation.
7. Discuss drug absorption from the gastrointestinal tract, explaining which types of drugs may be absorbed from the stomach and/or intestine and the relative rates of drug absorption from these sites.
8. Discuss the various factors that may influence drug absorption from the gastrointestinal tract.
9. Explain the rationale for the sublingual administration of drugs and the types of drugs that may be administered by this route.
10. Explain the rationale for the rectal administration of drugs and the problems that may be encountered when this route is used.
11. Discuss the term bioavailability.

A drug is a chemical that alters body functions. Pharmacology is the study of the effects of drugs on the body. Some chemicals are readily classified as drugs; others are not so easily recognized. For example, morphine and penicillin are known to everyone as drugs. However, how would you classify airplane glue? Is it a drug? The answer to that question depends on the manner in which the glue is used. If it is used to hold pieces of wood or plastic together, airplane glue is not a drug. If, on the other hand, it is inhaled by someone to alter brain function, airplane glue is a drug because it is used to modify physiological activity.

Physical and Chemical Properties of Drugs

Most drugs are either weak acids or weak bases. In solution in the body, they exist in both ionized and nonionized forms. The ionized form of a drug is usually water soluble, or lipid insoluble, and does not diffuse readily throughout the body. The nonionized form is less water soluble and more lipid soluble. It is more likely to diffuse across the lipid membranes of the body (Figure 1).

Figure 1
Diffusion of a drug across a lipid membrane.

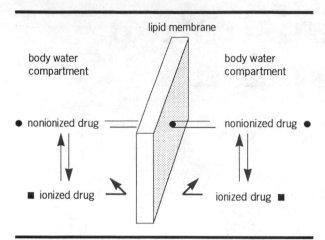

The percentage of drug found in the ionized and nonionized forms is determined, in part, by the pH of the body fluids. Consider the example of salicylic acid. It exists in the body both as the nonionized form, salicylic acid, and its ionized component, salicylate.

$$\text{Salicylic acid} \underset{}{\overset{}{\rightleftharpoons}} \text{H}^+ + \text{Salicylate}$$
nonionized ⟶ ionized

Making the solution more acidic has the effect of adding hydrogen ions (H^+). This drives the equation to the left and increases the ratio of salicylic acid/salicylate. From this example, it is possible to derive a general principle. The nonionized fraction of an acidic drug increases when the pH is reduced. An increase in pH has the effect of increasing the ionized, and decreasing the nonionized, fractions of acidic drugs.

The reverse is true for basic drugs. Raising the pH has the effect of removing hydrogen ions (H^+) from the environment.

$$\text{Morphine} - \text{H}^+ \rightleftharpoons \text{Morphine} + \text{H}^+$$
ionized ⟶ nonionized

This drives the reaction to the right side of the equation and increases the percentage of a basic drug, morphine in this case, found in nonionized form. The general rule can be stated that increasing the pH increases the nonionized, and decreases the ionized, fractions of basic drugs. Reducing the pH has the opposite effect. It decreases the morphine/morphine – H^+ ratio. The significance of this will become apparent when we discuss drug absorption, distribution and renal excretion.

Routes of Drug Administration

Drugs may be injected, ingested, inhaled or insufflated. In addition, they may be applied on the skin or instilled in the ear, nose or eye. Drugs may be used for their local effects or for their systemic actions. The following pages will discuss the absorption of drugs following their parenteral, oral or rectal administration.

Parenteral Administration

Intravenous Injection and Infusion

Drug absorption is immediate via the intravenous route. The advantages of this route of administration include immediate effect, predictable blood levels and rapid modification of dose. This is the preferred route of administration of medications to patients in shock. Intravenous administration is, however, a double-edged sword. Although the effect of the drug is very rapid, an incorrect calculation of the dose can lead to immediate toxicity.

Drugs should not be injected rapidly when they are given intravenously. When they are given as intravenous injections, the rapid injection of any drug leads to high concentrations reaching the heart. Regardless of the pharmacological properties of the drug, this can be dangerous because the presentation of a relatively large amount of any osmotically active material to the heart can lead to arrhythmias. It is advisable to give an intravenous injection slowly. By doing so the administered drug can be diluted in the blood. This will reduce the possibility of high concentrations reaching the heart and altering myocardial function.

Also of concern is the rapid intravenous infusion of a drug that has been diluted in a large volume of fluid. This situation can create problems associated with fluid volume (see Chapter 18).

Intramuscular Injection

Drugs given in solution are usually absorbed rapidly from muscle, in ten to thirty minutes. The blood flow to the muscle mass is usually adequate to guarantee rapid absorption. Drugs administered in suspension are usually absorbed slowly and are intended to produce a sustained effect. The rate-limiting factor in the absorption of a drug from a suspension, or depot-type product, is its slow dissolution by the body fluids in the muscle. Once the drug is dissolved it is rapidly absorbed and carried away in the circulation.

Subcutaneous Injection

The subcutaneous route of administration usually provides for reliable and rapid action. It is usually more acceptable for self-administration than intramuscular injection. However, irritant drugs often cause too much pain when injected subcutaneously. They are normally administered intramuscularly. In addition, usually only relatively small volumes of fluid can be tolerated by subcutaneous injection. Larger volumes are usually injected intramuscularly. A subcutaneous injection is not advised in shock because the reduced state of the peripheral circulation may severely decrease the rate of drug absorption.

Intradermal Injection

Intradermal injections are usually used when a local effect is desired, as in local anesthetics or testing for sensitivity (e.g., tuberculin testing or allergy testing). Injections are made into the dermis.

Oral Administration

Oral Dosage Forms

Most drugs are given orally. This is the easiest route of administration. Drugs can be administered in solutions, suspensions, capsules, compressed tablets, coated tablets and sustained-release tablets and capsules. The type of formulation used may determine the rate and extent of drug absorption. Generally speaking, drugs are not as well absorbed from solid dosage forms, i.e., tablets or capsules, as from liquid formulations.

Solutions, in which drugs are dissolved in a liquid, are usually absorbed quickly. **Suspensions**, in which drug particles are mixed with but not dissolved in a liquid, are absorbed more slowly because the drug must be dissolved in the gastrointestinal tract before it is absorbed.

Gelatin capsules, in which the drug is encased in a capsule made of gelatin, usually disintegrate rapidly in the stomach. Thereafter, the drug must be dispersed in the stomach and/or intestine and dissolved before absorption can occur. Soft gelatin capsules often contain drugs in solution or suspension. Following the disintegration of the capsule in the stomach, the drug is rapidly absorbed.

Compressed tablets are manufactured under considerable pressure. These tablets must disinte-

Figure 2
Schematic representation of the relationship between a solid drug in the lumen and the absorption process.

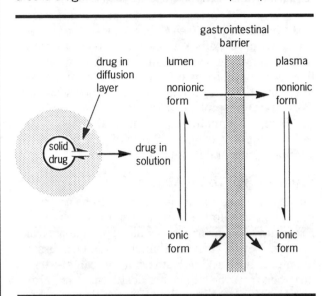

From: D. J. Jallow and B. B. Brodie, "Mechanisms of Drug Absorption and Drug Solution." In: *Bioavailability of Drugs*, ed. B. B. Brodie and W. M. Heller. S. Karger, 1972. Reproduced with permission.

grate in the gastrointestinal tract before the drug can be dispersed and dissolved.

Coated tablets, covered with wax, may present a greater problem to drug absorption than the ordinary compressed tablet. Before the tablet can disintegrate, the gastric juices must penetrate the wax coating. If the tablet stays in the stomach for thirty to sixty minutes, it should disintegrate. Where doubt exists about drug absorption from a compressed or coated tablet, a liquid formulation should be used. This is usually the pediatric product that tastes acceptable enough for even an adult to swallow.

Enteric-coated tablets are used to protect the drug from the stomach or vice versa. The coating placed on the tablet is acid resistant and the tablet does not disintegrate in the stomach. Disintegration occurs when the drug reaches the duodenum. Aspirin irritates the stomach. To protect the gastric mucosa from it, aspirin can be incorporated into an enteric-coated tablet. Erythromycin is destroyed by gastric acid. It is protected from the stomach by giving it in an enteric-coated tablet.

Sustained-release tablets and capsules are intended to release the drug over a period of several hours. The purpose of using this type of formulation is to decrease the number of times a day a patient must take a medication, reduce fluctuations in drug levels in the body, and maintain therapeutic concentrations of the drug in the body for longer periods of time. Not all drugs benefit from being incorporated in sustained-release products. Drugs with short half-lives (see Chapter 2), such as theophylline, benefit from sustained-release formulations. By way of contrast, drugs with long half-lives do not require sustained-release formulations to prolong their durations of action. Their long half-lives guarantee prolonged effects.

Figure 2 summarizes schematically the relationship between a solid drug in the gastrointestinal lumen and its absorption.

Sites of Oral Drug Absorption

Acidic drugs are mainly nonionized in the gastric juices and therefore absorbed from the stomach. Examples of acidic drugs include aspirin and barbiturates. Drugs, such as ethanol, that do not dissociate into ionized and nonionized forms can also be absorbed from the stomach. Most basic drugs are highly ionized in the acidic pH of the stomach and are not absorbed. Confusion as to which drugs are basic may be eliminated by remembering that the generic names of most basic drugs end with the letters "amine" or "ine". Thus amphetamine, meperidine, codeine and chlorpromazine are bases and will not be absorbed from the stomach.

Once in the intestine the concentration of the nonionized form of a basic drug increases and absorption occurs. Drug absorption occurs mainly in the duodenum, but can also take place in the jejunum and ileum. Acidic drugs can also be absorbed from the small bowel. Although they are mainly ionized in the intestine, there is usually sufficient nonionized drug to permit absorption. Once some of the nonionized acidic drug is absorbed, more will switch from the ionized to nonionized form in the intestinal lumen to maintain the ionized/nonionized ratio constant. The newly formed nonionized drug molecules are then absorbed. Most drugs are absorbed poorly from the large intestine.

As shown in Figure 3, the surface of the small intestine contains many folds (plicae circulares) and projections (microvilli and villi) that provide a much larger surface for drug absorption than is afforded by the gastric mucosa. These evolutionary adaptations have resulted in the typical adult having an intestinal surface area that is roughly equivalent to that of a doubles tennis court. As a result, for drugs that can be absorbed from both the stomach and small intestine, notably acids and chemicals that do not dissociate, drug absorption proceeds faster from the intestine.

Figure 3
Electron micrographs of the plicae circulares, villi and microvilli of the intestine.

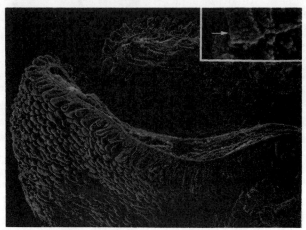

Courtesy of Dr. Richard S. Hannah, Department of Anatomy, Faculty of Medicine, University of Calgary.

Ethanol can be used to illustrate this principle. Most nurses are well aware of the effects of this libacious liquid when consumed on an empty stomach. Its immediate effects are most profound as it is passed quickly from the stomach into the duodenum, from whence it is rapidly absorbed. If consumed with food, ethanol is retained in the stomach because the pyloric sphincter closes in response to the presence of the food. Taken under these conditions the effects of ethanol are not so dramatic because it is absorbed more slowly through the gastric mucosa.

Factors Influencing Drug Absorption After Oral Administration

The stability of drugs in the stomach can play a major role in the percentage of an oral dose of a drug that is absorbed. Some drugs are not stable in acid and are rapidly destroyed in the gastric juices. Penicillin G and erythromycin are two examples. In the case of penicillin G, the drug is taken on an empty stomach to speed its transfer to the duodenum. As mentioned before, érythromycin is usually given in an enteric-coated tablet to protect it from the gastric secretions.

Food in the stomach can alter drug absorption. As described before, most basic drugs are absorbed only from the intestine. Even acidic drugs, which can be absorbed from the stomach, are more rapidly absorbed from the intestine. The presence of food in the stomach will increase the time a drug is held there and, as a result, reduce its rate of absorption. Drugs that are unstable in acid should not be taken with food. The longer they are retained in the stomach the greater the amount that will be destroyed. On the other hand, drugs that irritate the stomach and are stable in an acidic pH are best taken with meals. The presence of food will decrease irritation of the gastric mucosa and improve patient compliance.

First-pass metabolism can significantly reduce the percentage of an oral dose reaching the systemic circulation. Some drugs are very rapidly destroyed in the liver on their first pass through this organ in the portal circulation. As a result, only a small percentage of the amount absorbed manages to escape the metabolic activity of the liver and reach the heart to be distributed throughout the body. Propranolol is an example of this type of drug. It is almost completely absorbed from the intestine but only ten to twenty per cent of the dose passes through the liver unmetabolized.

Sublingual Administration

Sublingual administration may be an alternative to the oral route if a drug is either destroyed in the stomach or completely inactivated as it passes through the liver for the first time. Drugs may also be considered for sublingual administration if the patient is vomiting. To be effective sublingually, a drug must be absorbed very quickly. Otherwise, its presence in the mouth will result in the accumulation of saliva that must be swallowed, carrying with it the drug. It is also imperative that a drug not be irritating if it is to be held under the tongue. Few drugs satisfy these criteria.

Nitrates, such as nitroglycerin, are given sublingually to circumvent extensive first-pass inactivation (see Chapter 2) that occurs if they are given orally. Ergotamine can be given sublingually to treat migraine headaches. The drug can produce nausea and vomiting which are often already present as a result of the migraine headache. For this reason ergotamine is more effective if taken sublingually. Otherwise, patients who swallow ergotamine tablets for the treatment of migraine headaches often have the opportunity to see the drug for a second time as it passes their teeth in the reverse direction.

Rectal Administration

Drugs may be given rectally for either a local or a systemic effect. Little will be said at this time about the local use, except to mention that a variety of anti-inflammatory substances and local anesthet-ics are inserted or squirted into the rectum to soothe inflamed tissues and/or freeze hemorrhoids.

Drugs can be given rectally when it is difficult, if not impossible, to administer them orally. The case of migraine headaches with accompanying nausea and vomiting was mentioned before. Ergotamine can be given in suppository form in this situation. Young children or babies may be unable to swallow a drug. Rectal administration is advisable in these cases. Some drugs may be absorbed more slowly from a suppository and provide a benefit for several hours. It is not uncommon for these agents to be given by suppository before retiring in the evening. Two examples of this use are aminophylline suppositories for the treatment of bronchial asthma and indomethacin suppositories for arthritis.

Drug absorption from suppositories is erratic. The rate-limiting factor in absorption appears to be extracting the drug from the suppository mass and its subsequent solubilization in the rectal or colonic secretions. Once dissolved, drugs are absorbed in relation to the lipid solubility of the nonionized component.

Bioavailability

Bioavailability refers to the quantity of drug that is absorbed from the site of administration and distributed via the systemic circulation to the tissues of the body. Bioavailability following oral administration is reduced by two factors — incomplete absorption and/or first-pass metabolism. Incomplete absorption occurs when some of the drug never enters the circulatory system and thus is never available to the site of action. First-pass metabolism occurs after drug absorption when drugs are carried through the liver in the portal circulation. Some drugs are extensively metabolized during this initial transport through the liver, and this first-pass effect significantly reduces their bioavailability.

Drug bioavailability is usually studied by comparing the concentration of the drug measured in blood or plasma following oral administration with the concentration of drug in the blood or plasma following intravenous administration. When the blood or plasma concentrations of the drug are plotted over a period of many hours or days, a curve is obtained for each route of administration. The values obtained after intravenous administration are taken as representing 100% absorption and the concentrations measured following ingestion are compared against them to determine the bioavailability of the oral dosage form.

The advent of generic drugs has given additional interest to bioavailability. With several suppliers of any one drug it may be important to compare the relative bioavailability of each formulation. In this case, the study would involve two or more formulations of the same drug given orally.

Further Reading

Benet, Leslie Z. and Sheiner, Lewis B. (1990). "Pharmacokinetics: The Dynamics of Drug Absorption, Distribution and Elimination." In: *Goodman and Gilman's The Pharmacological Basis of Therapeutics,* 8th ed. (pp. 3-32), ed. Alfred Goodman Gilman, Theodore W. Rall, Alan S. Nies and Palmer Taylor. New York: Pergamon.

Okine, L.K.N. and Gram, T.E. (1986). "Drug Absorption and Distribution." In: *Modern Pharmacology,* 2nd ed. (pp. 21-40), ed. Charles R. Craig and Robert E. Stitzel. Boston: Little, Brown.

C H A P T E R   2

Drug Distribution and Elimination

Teaching Objectives

Following completion of this chapter, the reader should be able to:

1. Discuss the importance of tissue perfusion, plasma protein binding and lipid solubility in determining drug distribution.
2. Explain the consequence of plasma protein binding on drug elimination.
3. Define the expression blood-brain barrier and explain its significance.
4. Describe drug diffusion across the placenta.
5. Discuss the factors influencing the blood levels of drugs.
6. List the major routes of drug elimination.
7. Discuss the influence of filtration, secretion and reabsorption on the renal excretion of drugs.
8. Explain the term renal clearance and its relationship to the need to adjust the dose of a drug in a patient with renal impairment.
9. Discuss the abilities of the young and old to eliminate drugs through the kidneys.
10. Discuss biotransformation, explaining the purpose of drug metabolism.
11. Describe the influence of age, genetics, environmental chemicals and other drugs on biotransformation.
12. Describe briefly biliary excretion and the significance of enterohepatic recirculation.
13. Define the expression pharmacokinetics.
14. Explain the term half-life.
15. Explain the meaning of the expression steady state and differentiate between a loading dose and a maintenance dose.
16. Describe drug receptors and the difference between a drug with affinity for a receptor and intrinsic activity and a drug with affinity and no intrinsic activity.

Drug Distribution

Chapter 1 discussed drug absorption. Following absorption, drugs are distributed throughout the body. Three factors control drug distribution. They are tissue perfusion, plasma protein binding and lipid solubility.

Drug molecules are picked up in the circulation and carried throughout the body. **Tissue perfusion** plays an important part in the initial distribution of a drug because the more richly perfused organs receive most of the drug molecules. Once presented to the tissues most drugs must leave the blood if they are to have an effect. Their ability to do so may be limited by **plasma protein binding**. Drug molecules bound to plasma albumin cannot diffuse into the interstitial water and are, at that moment, pharmacologically inert. Only unbound molecules can leave the blood to exert an effect in the tissues.

Once in interstitial water some drug molecules may cross cell membranes. Their ability to do so depends on their **lipid solubility**. Lipid-soluble drugs cross cell membranes easily. Water-soluble drugs experience greater difficulty. As a result, lipid-soluble or nonionized drug molecules are distributed throughout the total body water. Water-soluble or ionized molecules usually are restricted in their distribution to the plasma and interstitial water compartments, which together make up the extracellular water compartment.

With this brief discussion as a background, we will now consider in greater detail the factors controlling drug distribution, beginning with tissue perfusion.

Tissue Perfusion

Organs richly perfused with blood receive more drug initially than tissues with a relatively poor blood flow. This is illustrated in Figure 4. Liver and muscle, as well as heart, kidneys, brain and adrenals, are richly perfused with blood and as a result receive more drug than poorly perfused fat or bone during the initial distribution of the drug in the body. Even thiopental, a very fat-soluble drug, cannot be found in high concentration in adipose tissue during the first thirty minutes after its absorption. Thereafter, however, its concentration in fat continues to climb and eventually exceeds the levels in the more richly perfused tissues. This is explained by the fact that thiopental is retained by fat. Acting like a sponge, fat takes up most of the drug brought to it in the circulation. As a result, thiopental is removed from the richly perfused tissues, for which it has little affinity, and concentrated in fat.

Figure 4
Distribution of thiopental in the dog. Note the high levels found initially in the liver and muscle and the subsequent redistribution to fat.

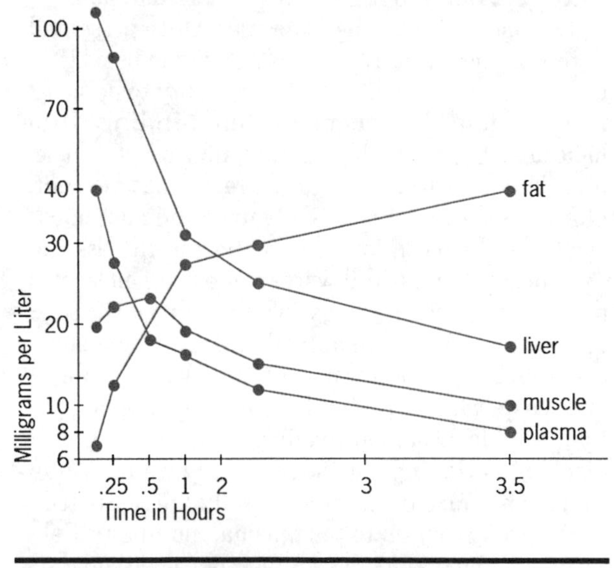

From: B. B. Brodie, "Distribution and Fate of Drugs: Therapeutic Implications." In: *Absorption and Distribution of Drugs*, ed. T.B. Binns. E. & S. Livingstone, 1964. Reproduced with permission.

From this example, it is possible to derive a principle. Drugs are distributed initially to those tissues that are richly perfused. Thereafter, a redistribution occurs with the drugs accumulating in tissues for which they have affinity. Thiopental

was used as an example of a fat-soluble drug accumulating in adipose tissue. But fat is not the only tissue that can retain a drug. Any tissue that has an affinity for a particular drug can retain it in high concentrations. A further example is the binding of tetracycline antibiotics in bone and teeth. These antibiotics bind to calcium and, as a result, are found in high concentrations in bones and teeth.

Plasma Protein Binding

Effect of Plasma Protein Binding on Drug Distribution

Under normal circumstances the plasma proteins do not leave the vascular system and drugs bound to them are denied access to the tissues. Phenylbutazone, warfarin and salicylate are 98% bound to albumin. If the total plasma level of phenylbutazone is 10 µg/mL, 9.8 µg/mL are bound to albumin and 0.2 µg/mL are free in solution in the plasma (Figure 5). Only drug molecules free in solution diffuse through the capillary endothelium and equilibrate between the plasma water and the interstitial water.

Unless the capacity of the plasma proteins to bind a drug is saturated, the ratio of bound/free drug remains constant. As the free level of a drug falls, due to metabolism and/or renal excretion, more drug leaves the albumin to become free in the plasma before diffusing out of the vascular system.

Figure 5
Schematic representation of the diffusion of a drug that is 98% bound to plasma proteins across a capillary.

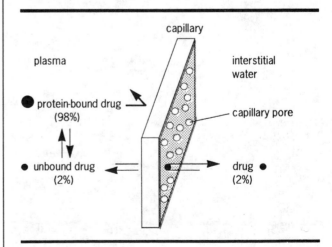

Effect of Plasma Protein Binding on Drug Elimination

Plasma protein binding often reduces the rate of drug elimination. Under normal conditions, plasma proteins are not filtered by renal glomeruli and drugs eliminated by glomerular filtration have longer half-lives if they are bound to plasma albumin. Likewise, many drugs eliminated by liver metabolism will have longer half-lives in the body if they are bound to plasma proteins because they cannot easily diffuse into the liver to be metabolized.

There are, of course, always exceptions to the basic rule that plasma protein binding reduces the rate of drug elimination. Drugs secreted by the renal tubules or rapidly metabolized in the liver are not influenced by plasma protein binding. Whereas it is true that only free molecules are secreted, tubular secretion proceeds so rapidly that new molecules quickly dissociate from plasma proteins to maintain the ratio bound/free constant. The newly freed molecules are themselves then secreted. For the same reason, rapidly metabolized drugs are not affected by plasma protein binding.

Saturation of Plasma Protein Binding Sites with Drugs

Plasma contains a finite concentration of albumin. If enough drug is given, it is possible to occupy all the binding sites on albumin and thereby saturate the plasma proteins. When this occurs, the free level of drug in the plasma will increase suddenly. In this event the pharmacological activity of the drug increases as more molecules diffuse into the tissues. Nurses will be aware that disease can affect plasma protein concentrations. Patients with cirrhosis, for example, can have lower plasma protein concentrations and are more likely to experience the consequences of saturation of plasma protein binding sites with drugs.

Elderly patients may also have lower plasma albumin. Saturation of protein binding sites and increased concentrations of free drug are more likely in this age group. If this happens, the elderly patient will experience an increased drug effect.

Drugs can compete for the available plasma protein binding sites. For example, warfarin and salicylate are both bound extensively to plasma albumin. If a patient, previously stabilized on warfarin, is given ASA, bleeding may occur because the salicylate displaces some warfarin from its binding sites on plasma albumin. As a result, more warfarin is able to enter the liver, where it blocks prothrombin synthesis, thereby decreasing the clotting mechanism of the blood.

Blood-Brain Barrier

To summarize the information presented so far, drugs are carried throughout the body in the blood. Richly perfused tissues receive more drug initially than organs with poorer blood supply. Thereafter, drugs may redistribute in accordance with their affinities for particular tissues. Plasma protein binding prevents a drug from leaving the blood vessels. Drug molecules that are not bound to plasma proteins can leave the blood vessels and enter the interstitial water of all tissues — with one exception, the brain.

The distribution of drugs into the brain is unique. Brain capillary endothelial cells differ from most other areas of the body by the absence of pores. In addition, glial connective tissue, called astrocytes, is attached closely to the basement membrane of the capillary endothelium. Together these structural modifications are referred to as the **blood-brain barrier**. Ionized molecules are practically excluded from entering the brain. Nonionized molecules, not bound to plasma proteins, enter the brain easily.

The rate at which a drug enters the brain is determined largely by the percentage of the drug nonionized in the blood and the lipid solubility (partition coefficient) of the nonionized molecules. Thiopental and phenobarbital have the same ratio of ionized/nonionized drug molecules in the plasma. Thiopental enters the brain very quickly and phenobarbital more slowly. This is because the lipid solubility of nonionized thiopental molecules is much greater than the lipid solubility of nonionized phenobarbital molecules. Stated simply, drugs with significant lipid solubility cross the blood-brain barrier easily; drugs that are poorly soluble in fat experience considerable difficulty entering the brain.

Drug Diffusion across the Placenta

The mature placenta contains a network of maternal blood sinuses that interface with villi that carry the fetal capillaries. The membranes that separate the fetal capillary blood from maternal blood resemble membranes elsewhere in the body. Lipid-soluble drugs diffuse readily from the maternal to the fetal circulation. Water-soluble molecules experience greater difficulty. However, if taken for a sufficient period of time, most drugs, regardless of their physical or chemical properties, will cross the placenta. It is important to emphasize that, in contradistinction to the blood-brain barrier, there is no placental barrier to the diffusion of drugs. Some drugs cross more easily than others, but almost any drug will be able to gain access to the developing fetus. Only drugs with very high molecular weights, such as insulin or heparin, will not cross the placenta.

Factors Influencing the Blood Levels of Drugs

Several factors influence the blood level of a drug. First, obviously, is the dose of the drug. Higher doses produce higher blood levels. Second is the bioavailability of a drug. If two drugs are given in identical doses to the same individual, the one with the greater bioavailability will produce the higher blood concentrations.

Volume of distribution is also an important factor in influencing the blood level of a drug. If one drug is distributed throughout the total body water, it will have a lower concentration in the blood than an equivalent dose of a drug that is distributed only in the extracellular fluid. Drugs bound to plasma proteins will have higher blood levels than drugs not bound to albumin.

Big patients have larger body water compartments than small patients. As a result, equal doses of any drug will produce higher blood levels in the smaller individual. Rotund patients, with large fat deposits, will provide better repositories of lipid-soluble drugs than will thin patients. Because fat drains drug from the blood, short fat individuals will show lower plasma concentrations of lipid-soluble drugs than long thin patients of the same body mass/weight.

Finally, the elimination rate of drugs influences significantly the concentration of drugs in the blood. If a drug is eliminated quickly, its plasma concentration will fall rapidly. The major routes of drug elimination are **renal excretion, hepatic metabolism** and **biliary excretion.** These will be discussed below.

Nurses will be aware that considerable importance is often given to measuring the concentrations of a drug in plasma or serum. The reason for this is not so much to determine the actual concentration of the drug in these specimens but rather to use these values as a reflection of the concentration of the drug in the appropriate tissue. It is very important, for example, to know the concentration of digoxin in the heart. However, for obvious reasons one cannot take a sample of heart tissue for analysis. Instead, one draws a blood sample and measures the concentration of digoxin in the serum, on the assumption that the concentration in the serum is in equilibrium with the concentration in the heart and therefore reflects the level of drug in cardiac muscle.

The plasma or serum concentration of a drug can best be thought of as a "window" to look at the level of a drug in the affected tissue. If the concentration of the drug in the serum is low, then its concentration in the tissue will also be low, and little effect will be seen. On the other hand, if the concentration of drug in serum is high, its level will also be high in the tissue concerned, and drug-induced toxicities may be seen. After considerable work it has been possible to establish serum concentrations for many drugs that correlate with safe and effective levels of these compounds in the tissues concerned. For digoxin, serum levels range from 0.5 – 2 nanograms/mL (1.0 – 2.6 nanomoles/L). Concentrations below 0.5 nanograms/mL (1.0 nanomoles/L) usually do not increase cardiac function. Levels above 2 nanograms/mL (2.6 nanomoles/L) can be expected to produce cardiac and other toxicities. The range between the minimum effective level and maximum tolerated level is referred to as the **therapeutic window.**

In the United States it is common practice to report serum or plasma levels of drugs in micrograms or nanograms of drug per milliliter of fluid. In Canada and many other parts of the world serum levels are routinely reported in Standard International Units (SI Units) which present the concentration of drug in millimoles, micromoles, or nanomoles of drug per liter of fluid. In this text both systems are used, with the serum or plasma levels of a drug reported first in micrograms or nanograms per milliliter, followed (in brackets) by its concentration in SI units.

Drug Elimination

Renal Excretion

Filtration, Secretion and Reabsorption

The kidney is a major organ for the elimination of drugs. It can filter, secrete and reabsorb drugs (Figure 6). All drugs not bound to plasma proteins can be filtered through the renal glomeruli. Thereafter, some of the filtered drug may be reabsorbed from the tubular lumen back into the blood perfusing the nephron. The extent of reabsorption depends on the overall lipid solubility of the filtered drug molecules. If the drug is almost entirely in its nonionized form, reabsorption will be significant. On the other hand, if the drug molecules are mainly in their ionized form, reabsorption will be minimal.

Figure 6
Diagrammatic representation of the excretion of drugs by the kidney.

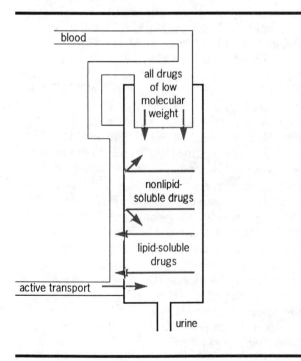

From: B. B. Brodie, "Distribution and Fate of Drugs: Therapeutic Implications." In: *Absorption and Distribution of Drugs*, ed. T.B. Binns. E. & S. Livingstone, 1964. Reproduced with permission.

The ratio of the ionized/nonionized drug molecules depends on the pH of the renal tubular fluid. Changes in the pH of urine may have a marked effect on the ability of the kidney to reabsorb a drug. For example, sodium bicarbonate, given to a patient poisoned with salicylate, will raise the pH in the tubular fluid and increase the percentage of drug molecules ionized. This will reduce tubular reabsorption and increase the renal excretion of the drug.

By way of contrast, if an individual takes sodium bicarbonate with the basic drug amphetamine, he may well get a longer "trip" for his money. By raising the pH in the tubular lumen, sodium bicarbonate increases the percentage of drug molecules in the nonionized form and the amount of drug reabsorbed into the systemic circulation. To decrease the reabsorption of amphetamine and other basic drugs, one must acidify the developing urine with a drug such as ammonium chloride or ascorbic acid, thereby increasing the amount of drug in the ionized form.

The renal tubular secretion of drugs, or their metabolites, is an active process. Drugs that are secreted are taken from the blood by the tubular cells and transported into the lumen of the kidney tubules. As mentioned earlier, this can happen very quickly, and drugs that undergo extensive renal tubular secretion are usually eliminated quickly from the body. Penicillin, for example, is secreted rapidly by the renal tubular cells and has a half-life in the body of one-half hour to an hour.

The kidney has two separate secretory mechanisms. One will secrete only acids and the other only bases. For each system there is a transport maximum. When this is exceeded, tubular secretion can no longer eliminate increased amounts of drugs brought to the kidney and their concentrations in the body suddenly increase.

Competition can exist between drugs for the same secretory mechanism. Two acidic drugs that are secreted may compete with each other for active transport into the tubular lumen. A similar competition can be noted between various basic drugs for tubular secretion. Acidic and basic drugs do not compete with each other.

The ability of drugs to compete with one another may be used clinically. Ampicillin is a semisynthetic penicillin that is secreted rapidly by the kidney. Its uses include the treatment of gonorrhea. Probenecid, like ampicillin, is also an acid and it, too, undergoes tubular secretion. When both drugs are present in the kidney they will compete for tubular secretion. Venereal disease clinics often dispense probenecid together with ampicillin because it will decrease the tubular secretion of the antibiotic and increase both its half-life in the body and its efficacy against the gonococcus.

Renal Clearance

The capacity of the kidney to excrete a drug can be expressed as a renal clearance value. This is obtained by dividing the amount of drug excreted in the urine by its plasma concentration. For example, if drug A has a plasma level of 1.5 nanograms per milliliter and the kidney excretes 180 nanograms per minute, the renal clearance of drug A is 180/1.5 = 120 mL/min. This is the volume of plasma that contains the amount of drug excreted. In theory, in this example 120 mL of plasma were cleared of drug A every minute.

The renal clearance value is helpful in determining what happens when a drug reaches the kidney. The renal glomeruli filter 120 mL of plasma every minute. Thus, it may be stated on the basis of a renal clearance value of 120 mL/min that drug A is filtered through the renal glomeruli and no net reabsorption has occurred as it passes down the renal tubules. The expression "net reabsorption" is used because it is always possible that some of the drug is reabsorbed, but this quantity is equalled by the amount that is secreted.

If a drug has a renal clearance value considerably below 120 mL/min, it means that the drug is either not filtered well as it passes through the renal glomeruli or it is filtered and extensively reabsorbed in the tubules. The only factor that stops a drug from being filtered is plasma protein binding.

Renal clearance values in excess of 120 mL/min indicate that the drug undergoes filtration and tubular secretion. The renal plasma flow is 600 mL/min. Penicillin has a renal clearance value of about 600 mL/min. This means that all drug molecules carried to the kidney in the blood are eliminated.

Drugs with high renal clearance values depend heavily on the kidney for their elimination from the body. If, for example, a drug has a renal clearance value of 120 mL/min or more, the kidney is an important organ for its elimination. This drug will accumulate if normal doses are given repeatedly to an individual with kidney failure. Drugs with low renal clearance values must be eliminated by other means, usually liver metabolism. It is not necessary to modify their doses in patients with renal impairment. However, the dose may need to be reduced if the patient has a liver disorder because a diseased liver may be unable to eliminate drugs (see following section, Biotransformation).

Newborns have immature kidneys. As a result, they cannot excrete drugs as rapidly as babies a few months old. Aminoglycoside antibiotics (e.g., gentamicin, tobramycin) and digoxin are among the drugs eliminated more slowly by the neonate. As a result, newborns must receive lower doses of these drugs to prevent their accumulation in the body to toxic levels.

Elderly patients may also demonstrate varying degrees of renal impairment. As a person ages, renal blood flow falls, reduced glomerular filtration becomes apparent, and a decreased capacity to secrete chemicals occurs. To compensate for these changes, elderly patients must receive lower doses of many drugs that are eliminated by the kidneys. Failure to do so can result in overdose.

Biotransformation

Many drugs are changed chemically in the body. This process is called biotransformation. It is also referred to as metabolism. (In this book, the terms biotransformation and metabolism will be used interchangeably.) Most tissues have the capacity to metabolize drugs. The liver is the major organ involved in drug metabolism, with the lungs, kidneys, intestinal mucosa and placenta also playing a role for certain compounds.

Lipophilic drugs, that is, those that are fat soluble, cannot be eliminated by the kidney. After being filtered they are reabsorbed into the blood. In response to the inability of the kidney to eliminate lipophilic agents (including endogenous materials such as steroids) the body evolved a system of enzymes to metabolize these chemicals. Drug metabolism or biotransformation involves the conversion of lipophilic chemicals into compounds with increased water solubility, thereby facilitating their elimination by the kidneys.

Drug metabolism does not invariably inactivate a drug. True, most drugs have their actions terminated when they are changed chemically. However, some are activated and still others undergo no change in activity when metabolized. Drug metabolism is best thought of as a polarization process during which fat-soluble drugs are made more polar or water soluble.

Several factors can influence the rate of drug metabolism. Age is one. Neonates have a reduced capacity to metabolize drugs. Chloramphenicol, for example, has a half-life of four hours in the adult and twenty-six hours in the neonate. Failure to recognize this point in the 1950s resulted in the accumulation of lethal concentrations of the drug in many premature infants.

Elderly patients may also experience difficulty

in metabolizing drugs. Benzodiazepines are frequently used by the elderly. These drugs may have longer half-lives in older patients compared to younger ones. This is one reason the standard dose of a benzodiazepine for a patient over 65 is only one-half the amount recommended for younger adults. Other drugs that are metabolized more slowly in the elderly include the antidepressants imipramine, desipramine and amitriptyline. Reference will made in subsequent chapters of this book to the reduced capacity of the elderly to metabolize specific groups of drugs.

Genetic factors also control drug metabolism. Identical twins often metabolize drugs at identical rates. Fraternal twins metabolize drugs at different rates. Reference is made in Chapter 66 to the fact that genetic control of drug metabolism has been observed for the acetylation of the antitubercular drug isoniazid. The capacity for rapid acetylation of this drug occurs in families as a Mendelian dominant. Dicoumarol (an anticoagulant), phenylbutazone (a nonsteroidal anti-inflammatory) and nortriptyline (an antidepressant) are three other drugs whose metabolism has been shown to be controlled by genetic factors. Their rates of metabolism are determined by multifactorial inheritance. This means that three or more genes contribute to their control. Identical twins metabolize these drugs at identical rates.

The activity of drug-metabolizing enzymes can be increased or decreased by the administration of certain drugs and by exposure to various chemicals in the environment. Phenobarbital can increase the metabolism of several drugs, including warfarin (an anticoagulant) and phenytoin (an antiepileptic). Competitive inhibition between drugs for metabolizing enzymes is less readily found. However, dicoumarol can inhibit the metabolism of phenytoin. These are but two examples of the many interactions possible between drugs and their metabolizing enzymes. Nurses are encouraged to review the information provided in the Drug Interaction columns in the tables accompanying Chapters 4 to 71 for specific information relating to this form of interaction.

Biliary Excretion

Some drugs, or their metabolites, are removed from the plasma by the liver and secreted into the bile, before being passed into the duodenum. The concentrations of these drugs may be several hundred times higher in the bile than in plasma.

Little is known of the means by which the liver secretes drugs into the bile or why it selects some drugs and neglects others.

Once passed into the intestines in the bile, some drugs, or their metabolites, are reabsorbed into the blood. This is called **enterohepatic recirculation.** Anyone who has taken phenolphthalein, the active ingredient in Ex Lax and many other laxatives, has experienced the consequence of enterohepatic recirculation. Phenolphthalein acts as a laxative because it irritates the colon. When the drug is taken, its desired effect is seen within twelve to sixteen hours. However, unbeknownst to the patient, some of the phenolphthalein is absorbed into the circulatory system. Following glucuronide conjugation in the liver, the drug is returned to the intestinal tract in the bile. Upon reaching the depths of the intestinal tract the glucuronide is cleaved from the parent drug by bacterial enzymes, freeing the phenolphthalein to work its wonders again. After the second bout of catharsis patients may think that they are rid of the effects of the drug. This may not be the case. Some phenolphthalein may be absorbed from the colon and the entire process repeated. The moral of the story is don't put away the running shoes because the effects of phenolphthalein may be seen, in ever-decreasing intensity, every twelve to sixteen hours for several days.

Pharmacokinetics

The expression pharmacokinetics refers to the dynamics of drug absorption, distribution and elimination. From this description it will appear obvious to the reader that most of the information provided in Chapters 1 and 2 can be classified under the term pharmacokinetics. The study of pharmacokinetics has taken on increasing importance over the years with the realization that the intensity of drug action is most frequently related to the concentration of the drug at the site of action. As we have discussed drug absorption, distribution and elimination, the factors that control the concentration of a drug at its site of action, only two additional topics relating to pharmacokinetics remain to be discussed. These are **half-life** and **steady state.**

Half-Life

Pharmacologists routinely determine the plasma or serum levels of drugs. This is done because these measures reflect the levels found in the circulating blood. Chemically, it is easier to measure a drug in the plasma or serum than in blood. Immediately following intravenous injection of a drug, blood levels of the drug fall dramatically. Figure 7 plots the serum concentrations of ampicillin in the four hours immediately following its injection. The initial fall in blood levels results from its distribution out of the vascular system and into the various body compartments. If a drug is extensively bound to plasma proteins, its ability to leave the blood will be reduced and the initial fall in plasma or serum levels will be minimal.

Figure 7

Serum concentrations of ampicillin following intravenous injection of 500 mg of the drug.

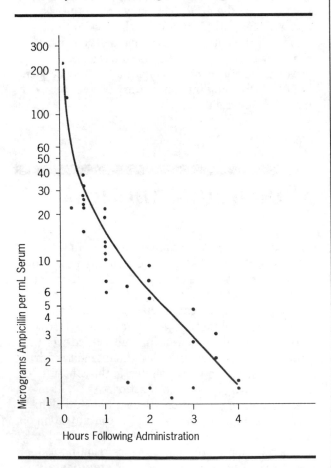

From: J. E. Perry and A. L. Leblanc (1967), Transfer of ampicillin across the human placenta. Tex. *Rep. Biol. Med. 25* :547-557. Reproduced with permission.

The second phase in the blood concentration – time curve reflects the rate at which the drug is eliminated from the body. In the case of ampicillin, the second phase becomes apparent about one hour after administration. It is possible to calculate the half-life of a drug in the body from the slope of the second phase. Using the ampicillin example, readers are asked to pick any concentration during the second phase of the curve and measure the time taken for that level to drop by one-half. That time is the half-life of the drug. In the case of ampicillin, it is about one hour.

Steady State

Drugs are often administered on a regular basis for long periods of time. During the first few doses of a drug its concentration in the body usually increases. Taking tetracycline as an example, we can see that if the dose of 500 mg is given every eight hours (tetracycline has a half-life of eight hours) the level of the drug will rise quickly at first and then gradually plateau (Table 1). Eventually, the amount of drug lost will equal the quantity ingested and the level in the body will remain constant. When this happens a condition of steady state is reached. From Table 1 it can be seen that ten doses of the drug are required before the quantity entering the body equals the amount lost. However, it is also apparent that the increases in the amount found in the body are very small when the last few doses are administered. From a practical point of view, a drug given repeatedly will reach steady state within a time period of five half-lives. In the case of tetracycline, this is forty hours.

The 500 mg dose of tetracycline is called a **maintenance dose** and from the example presented in Table 1 it is apparent that steady state can be achieved by repeatedly administering the maintenance dose. However, this requires time. It is possible to reach the level desired in the body quickly by giving in one dose the amount desired in the body. In the case of tetracycline this is 1000 mg and is referred to as a **loading dose**. If 1000 mg of tetracycline is given as the first dose, 500 mg will remain in the body at the end of eight hours. At this time the 500 mg lost can be replaced by administering this amount. The loading dose – maintenance dose regimen has the advantage of producing the desired levels in the body immediately.

Table 1
Accumulation of tetracycline in the body when doses of 500 mg are given every eight hours.

Dose Administered Every 8 h	Amount in Body Immediately After Taking Latest Dose	Amount Lost from Body During 8 h After Latest Dose	Amount Remaining in Body at the End of Each 8 h Period
500 mg (0)	500 mg	250 mg	250 mg
500 mg (8)	750 mg	375 mg	375 mg
500 mg (16)	875 mg	437.5 mg	437.5 mg
500 mg (24)	937.5 mg	468.75 mg	468.75 mg
500 mg (32)	968.75 mg	484.4 mg	484.4 mg
500 mg (40)	984.4 mg	492.2 mg	492.2 mg
500 mg (48)	992.2 mg	496.1 mg	496.1 mg
500 mg (56)	996.1 mg	498.5 mg	498.5 mg
500 mg (64)	998.5 mg	499.2 mg	499.2 mg
500 mg (72)	999.5 mg	499.75 mg	499.75 mg

( ) indicates hours since starting therapy.

Drug Receptors

Most drug effects are the result of the interaction of the drug with drug receptors. A drug receptor is a specialized macromolecule located on a cell membrane or within a cell. The drug receptor combines with a drug to produce the drug's characteristic biological effects. Although the exact nature of each drug receptor is not known, it is recognized that each type of receptor shows an amazing degree of specificity for the drug or drugs with which it unites. For example, narcotic receptors in the brain show an affinity for both natural and synthetic narcotics. They will not unite with other drugs such as aspirin, which also relieve pain.

Attention will be directed throughout this book to specific types of drug receptors. At this point it will suffice to indicate the general nature of drug-receptor interactions. A drug may have affinity for a receptor and, once attached to the receptor, may stimulate it to produce a response. The ability of a drug to stimulate a receptor is called **intrinsic activity.** Drugs that stimulate receptors possess both affinity for a receptor and intrinsic activity, and are called **agonists.**

Drugs that have affinity for a receptor but no intrinsic activity are called **antagonists.** These agents will occupy a receptor but not stimulate it. During the time they occupy the receptor they block any chemical that might stimulate it from binding to the receptor. Antagonists, therefore, prevent effects from occurring. They may be used to block the effects of other drugs or to prevent endogenous chemicals from working. Sympathetic beta antagonists (beta blockers) are widely used in medicine. Propranolol is the best known. It has affinity for a beta receptor but no intrinsic activity. Consequently, this drug blocks the beta receptors in the heart, preventing the endogenous chemicals released by the sympathetic nerves and adrenals from stimulating these receptors. As a result, the heart rate slows.

Not all drug effects are mediated by drug receptors. For example, antacids given for the treatment of gastric or duodenal ulcers neutralize gastric acid. Cathartics, which work either by irritating the bowel or by drawing water from the blood into the feces by osmosis, are not interacting with specific receptors. Other examples of a similar nature could be cited. It will become apparent later in this book which drug effects depend on drug-receptor interactions.

Further Reading

Benet, Leslie Z. and Sheiner, Lewis B. (1990). "Pharmacokinetics: The Dynamics of Drug Absorption, Distribution and Elimination." In: *Goodman and Gilman's The Pharmacological Basis of Therapeutics,* 8th ed. (pp. 3-32), ed. Alfred Goodman Gilman, Theodore W. Rall, Alan S. Nies and Palmer Taylor. New York: Pergamon.

Boreus, L.O. (1985). "Principles of Pediatric Pharmacology." In: *Monographs in Clinical Pharmacology 6* :60. New York: Churchill Livingston.

Gram, T. E. (1986). "Metabolism of Drugs." In: *Modern Pharmacology,* 2nd ed. (pp. 41-64), ed. Charles R. Craig and Robert E. Stitzel. Boston: Little, Brown.

Okine, L.K.N. and Gram, T. E. (1986). "Drug Absorption and Distribution." In: *Modern Pharmacology* , 2nd ed. (pp. 21-40), ed. Charles R. Craig and Robert E. Stitzel. Boston: Little, Brown.

Pucino, F., Beck, C. L., Seifert, R. L., Strommen, G. L., Sheldon, P. A. and Silbergleit, I.L. (1985). Pharmacogenetics. *Pharmacotherapy 5* : 314-326.

Roberts, Robert J. (1984). "Pharmacologic Principles in Therapeutics in Infants." In: *Drug Therapy in Infants*. Philadelphia: W. B. Saunders.

Stitzel, R.E. (1986). "Excretion of Drugs." In: *Modern Pharmacology,* 2nd ed. (pp. 65-74), ed. Charles R. Craig and Robert E. Stitzel. Boston: Little, Brown.

C H A P T E R   3

The Relationship between Nursing and Pharmacology

by Kathryn J. Hannah, R.N., Ph.D. and
Maureen Osis, R.N., M.N.,
edited by Sheila Rankin Zerr, R.N., M.Ed.

Teaching Objectives

Following completion of this chapter, the reader will be able to:

1. Describe the application of principles of pharmacology in the nursing management of patients receiving drug therapy.
2. Assess the biophysical and psychosocial aspects of the patient receiving drug therapy to arrive at a nursing diagnosis.
3. Describe the intervention phase of the nursing process during nursing management of patients receiving drug therapy.
4. Understand the importance of nonpharmaceutical nursing interventions to enhance the therapeutic effectiveness of medications.
5. Describe the nursing responsibilities associated with the evaluation component of the nursing process in the care of patients receiving drug therapy.
6. Describe the nursing responsibilities for patient teaching associated with the intervention component of the nursing process in the care of patients receiving drug therapy.

One of the main premises in this book is that the practice of professional nursing is based on use of the **nursing process**. The nursing process provides a logical, rational approach to patient situations. Murchison et al. (1982) suggest that the nursing process

> … offers a structure through which the nurse … identifies patient/client priorities and mobilizes available resources to provide optimum care. It is action oriented, yet its most telling feature is judgment, for in professional practice there are no ready solutions to problems.

Figure 8 summarizes the essential elements and relationships of the nursing process.

Figure 8
Essential elements and relationships of the nursing process.

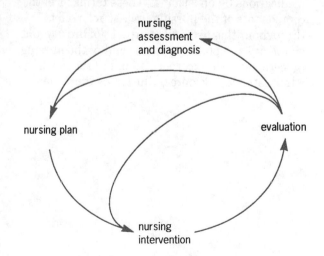

Historically, physicians were responsible for diagnosing, prescribing, preparing and administering medications to patients. With the increase in knowledge and the rise of the era of specialization came the development of the health care team. Specifically with regard to pharmacology, the current practice in health care institutions in the developed countries is that the physician diagnoses the illness and prescribes medications which the pharmacist dispenses and the nurse administers. Thus, the administration of medications has become a medically delegated nursing task. Expectations of society and increasing nursing expertise have expanded that role even further. The role of the nurse in drug therapy has evolved from one of safe calculation and administration to one of participatory collaboration. Today, the professional nurse is expected to contribute to the design, implementation and evaluation of the patient's drug regimen.

As stated earlier, one of the primary assumptions upon which this book is based is that all nursing activities are performed within the context of the nursing process. Within this context, administration of medications is a nursing intervention rather than merely an isolated task or act. In the sequence of the nursing process, nursing interventions are preceded by assessment/planning and followed by evaluation. The nursing assessment and evaluation related to the administration of medications almost invariably precipitates other nursing interventions classified as patient teaching or health education. Throughout this book we use the terms **assessment, administration, evaluation** and **teaching** to indicate the implications for nursing care associated with the prescription of medications by physicians. These terms form the components of the nursing process referred to throughout this text. For purposes of brevity and simplicity, the planning component of the nursing process has been incorporated under the heading, administration. Figure 9 illustrates these ideas.

Use of the Nursing Process in the Management of Drug Therapy

Assessment

Information Gathering

The term assessment refers to nursing observations conducted prior to the administration of a prescribed medication to a patient. The major goal of nursing assessment is to identify factors that might affect the safety and effectiveness of drug treatment. Assessment includes gathering biophysical and psychosocial data known to be associated with patients' responses to the prescribed drug. It requires a synthesis of knowledge of principles from pharmacology, physiology and pathophysiology. It also considers the patient's ability and willingness to participate in the treatment plan, that is, compliance.

The assessment phase is initiated by considering the completeness of the drug order. A physician's order for a drug must be clearly legible and complete. It must specify the full name of the drug, the dose (amount) to be administered, as well as the route and time (or frequency) of administration. Nurses are expected to be familiar with the usual dosage range and frequency of administration for medications that they administer. Ordinarily, nursing units have a pharmacologic reference book readily available to the nursing staff. The dispensing pharmacist is another willing and competent resource for obtaining information about usual dosage ranges and frequency of administration. If in doubt, consult the prescribing physican.

It is essential that the nurse administering a medication to a patient understand the goal of the drug therapy. The nurse must understand *why* the patient is receiving a particular drug. This is particularly important when drugs are ordered **p.r.n.** (*pro re nata*), or as necessary; that is, when administration is at the discretion of the nurse. Furthermore, it is impossible to evaluate the therapeutic effectiveness of a drug if the desired outcome is not known. Similarly, supportive nursing interventions to promote the desired outcome of drug therapy and/or enhance compliance depend on the nurse's understanding the rationale for use of the

Figure 9
Nursing management of drug therapy.

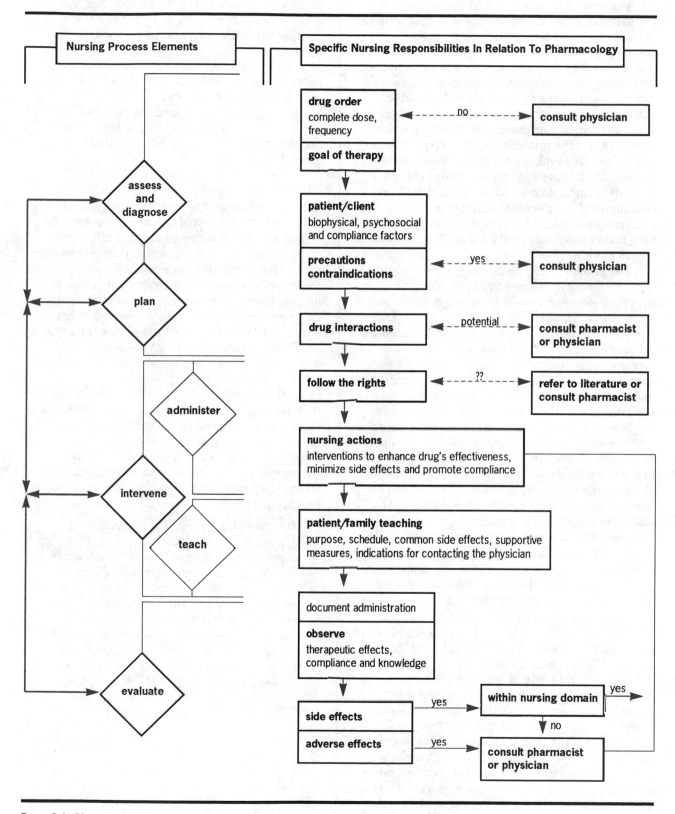

From: Osis, Maureen (1984), unpublished manuscript. Adapted with the consent of the author.

medication. Do not make assumptions; if the goal of therapy is unclear, consult the physician.

The nursing assessment includes a review of the patient's medical history for evidence of physical or emotional conditions that contraindicate the administration of the medication. Previous use of and response to the prescribed drug provide important information for predicting potential allergy, hypersensitivity or undesirable nontherapeutic outcomes. It is not the nurse's responsibility to know all medical contraindications to drug treatment. This is the primary responsibility of the prescriber. However, nurses should know major contraindications of drug classifications and should recognize information pertinent to the drug being administered. In the event that a patient reveals previously undisclosed or pertinent new information, the nurse should communicate that information to the physician.

The patient's drug history and current drug regimen are reviewed, usually in consultation with the physician or pharmacist, for drugs that might interact in a negative or synergistic fashion. Both prescription and nonprescription (over-the-counter) drugs must be considered. Again, it is not a nursing responsibility to know all possible interactions among drugs. Understanding the basic principles and well-known, clinically significant interactions is the general expectation.

Simultaneously, the patient's current physical status is thoroughly assessed in order to provide baseline measures against which to evaluate the patient's response to the medication and, in the case of p.r.n. orders, to determine the patient's need for the medication. Body mass/weight is a factor that often influences the drug dosage for a particular patient. Similarly, liver and kidney function and certain diseases can alter the absorption or excretion rates of drugs. These may require adjustments in administration techniques, frequency or amount of dosage. Age is another important factor in determining an individual's response to a medication. This book addresses primarily the response of young and middle-aged adult patients to drug therapy. Pediatric and elderly patients respond differently to medications for a variety of reasons. Nurses working with these patients should refer to specialized sources for specific information about dosages and frequency of administration.

Equally important is nursing assessment of the patient's emotional, psychological and social status. Cultural attitudes towards and beliefs about drugs influence patients' decisions to accept (comply with) a treatment plan. Drug taking is a psychosocial phenomenon as well as a biophysical experience.

This information has relevance in the design of patient teaching plans. In some situations, the therapeutic intent (goal of treatment) is alteration of the patient's emotional or psychological status. In other circumstances, altered emotional or psychological status is an undesirable adverse effect of a prescribed medication. In either case, it is important to have established baseline observations prior to initiating treatment.

Finally, the patient's understanding of the medication, its purpose and effects are assessed. This information forms the basis for the development of the teaching plan.

Nursing Diagnosis

Although the concept of nursing diagnosis is becoming more widely accepted among nurses, the standardization of terms used for labelling and defining nursing diagnoses are still under development. Nurses now acknowledge that the final element of the assessment component of the nursing process is to make a concluding statement or hypothesis about the data gathered during the nursing assessment in the form of a nursing diagnosis. These statements or conclusions must fall within the realm of nursing practice.

Clinical Example

A 57-year-old patient with essential hypertension is treated with a diuretic and antihypertensive drug. She is experiencing dizzy spells and weakness when she gets out of bed or stands up after sitting. Knowing that orthostatic hypotension is an adverse effect of the drug, the nurse generates the following nursing diagnosis:

Potential injury related to orthostatic hypotension associated with drug therapy. Interventions based on this nursing diagnosis will have the goal of promoting patient safety. They might include such activities as teaching the patient how to change position slowly or providing assistance or supervision when she moves about her room or unit. In addition, the nurse will discuss the observations with the physician in order to promote evaluation of the drug treatment.

Intervention

Planning

Nurses plan for the administration of medications on the basis of the information gained during patient assessment, knowledge of the pharmacology of the drugs involved, understanding of the patient's condition, and the nursing diagnosis. Adequate planning is necessary to ensure that drug therapy is effective with minimal risk to the patient. Planning will also identify those nondrug actions which nurses initiate to enhance the potential benefits of drug therapy. These nursing interventions include supportive actions as well as anticipatory and preventive measures used to promote the effectiveness of the drug, minimize side effects, promote patient safety or enhance compliance.

Administration

Traditionally, administration has been given the greatest priority in the nursing management of drug therapy. Nurses placed great emphasis on the task of giving drugs and "getting the pills out on time." The actual administration of medications to the patients by the nurse is a medically delegated nursing intervention performed under the legal direction and supervision of a physician. The nurse is morally and legally responsible and accountable for providing the correct drug at the designated time interval via the prescribed route in the correct amount to the right patient. These are sometimes referred to as the "rights" of giving medications. The rights of drug administration include:

- right patient
- right drug
- right dose
- right route
- right time
- right technique
- right approach.

The first five rights are self-explanatory. The last two rights might be unfamiliar to readers. Technique refers to correct use of psychomotor skills appropriate to the prescribed route of administration (for example, maintenance of medical asepsis with oral medications, or using aluminum foil to cover the bag containing an intravenous solution known to deteriorate when exposed to light). Approach refers to the interpersonal and psychosocial skills associated with preparing a patient for the administration of a medication (for example, the preparation of a child to receive an injection). Approach also refers to the skills used by the nurse

in implementing the patient teaching plan.

The rights of medication administration provide a framework or check list for use in reducing the incidence of medication errors. The American Society of Hospital Pharmacists defines a medication error as:

> The administration of the wrong medication or dose of medication, drug, diagnostic agent, or treatment requiring the use of such agents to the wrong patient or at the wrong time or the failure to administer such agents at the specified time or in the manner prescribed or normally considered as acceptable practice.

The literature indicates that the average rate of medication error in institutions is approximately eleven per cent. Fortunately, not all of these errors cause harm to the patient, but the incidence of harm to patients resulting from medication error could be as high as six per cent. The most frequent types of medication error by all categories of health professionals are related to failure to follow policy or procedure (72%). Examples include improper verification of the order, inaccurately reading the label, failure to check patient's armband, and calculation errors. Additional errors are caused by communications problems (21%), such as use of improper or nonstandard abbreviations, incomplete or illegible orders or failure to verify verbal orders.

The psychomotor skills involved in the preparation and administration of medications via the various routes are beyond the scope of this book. Readers should consult specialized texts on these topics; examples are included in the Further Reading section at the end of this chapter. However, unique features of the administration of specific drugs will be included as appropriate throughout the text.

Patient Teaching

Instructing the patient and family regarding the drug treatment is a shared responsibility of the nurse, the pharmacist and the physician. All three professionals must collaborate to complement, supplement and validate the information provided by the others to patients. Patient teaching by nurses in relation to pharmacology is designed to provide individuals with information and explanations about the medications that have been prescribed for them. Patient teaching promotes patient independence by facilitating self-administration of the medication and self-evaluation of its therapeutic effectiveness and adverse effects. By alerting the patient to potentially hazardous situations, nurses can promote patient safety — for example, explaining the dangers of drinking alcohol while on diazepam or driving while taking antihistamines. Increased understanding will help the patient in choosing to comply with the prescribed drug regime. The literature on compliance indicates the controversy surrounding the term. When defined as an outcome, compliance is a measurement of self-medication behavior or of ability to adhere to a personal goal, for example, to exercise daily. When discussed as a process, compliance becomes a controversial issue associated with coercion, power struggles and blame. Although other terms have been suggested, such as adherence or therapeutic alliance, none of these terms guarantees the context in which we use the term, that is, a cooperative and mutually trusting relationship between care giver and patient. A major goal of patient teaching in drug therapy is to ensure safe compliance, that is, adherence to the therapeutic plan provided within the therapeutic patient/physician/nurse relationship.

The purpose in this text is to identify the information content that should be communicated to patients about individual drugs. The techniques and strategies of patient education are subjects for other authors to address. Selected references on patient teaching are included in the Further Reading section at the end of this chapter.

Evaluation

Nurses are required by law to document the administration of all medications in the patient's clinical record. For quality patient care, this minimum legal requirement should be augmented with documentation of the nurse's evaluation of the patient following the administration of the medication. Evaluation in this text is used to refer to the nursing observations conducted following the administration of a prescribed medication to a patient. Nursing evaluation of a patent who has received a drug has two objectives. The first is to determine drug efficacy. The nurse must note the patient's progress towards the expected goals of the drug therapy. This is usually determined by evaluating the patient for therapeutic effects of the drug and comparing the findings to the baseline established during nursing assessment prior to the administration of the medication. Communication of the nurse's findings from this evaluation is of invaluable assistance to the physician in regulating the type and amount of subsequent medication that the patient receives.

The second objective is to observe the patient for evidence of drug-induced adverse effects. Often pharmacologists (scientists who develop drugs and study their pharmacological effects) state that the frequency of adverse effects from a particular drug is statistically very low. Patients do not like to think of themselves as statistics! As far as the patient is concerned, it is all or nothing — either an adverse effect of the drug is experienced or it is not. No one can be 1% pregnant or 49% dead. Therefore, low frequency of occurrence for an adverse effect of a drug is no excuse for reduced vigilance in nursing evaluation.

Obviously, in clinical practice, nurses must set priorities for the use of their time. The intensity of the observation of a patient for drug-induced adverse effects is related to the risk that the drug presents. This risk is a function of several factors. In determining the portion of their time allocated to the evaluation of a particular patient for adverse effects, nurses must consider the severity of the adverse effects, the statistical frequency of occurrence, the length of time the drug has been studied, its half-life in the body, the number of previous times it has been administered to the patient, and the nature of the illness being treated. In addition, nurses must consider the patients' general physiological and/or psychological condition, including medical history and age, which might predispose them to increased risk of drug-induced adverse effects.

Thus, a patient receiving a first administration of a new and highly potent drug with a long half-life and a high incidence of adverse effects will be the subject of intense nursing evaluation. On the other hand, a patient receiving a well-known drug, having a low incidence of innocuous adverse effects and a short half-life, for the one-hundredth time will be the subject of correspondingly less intense, but no less rigorous, nursing evaluation. The alert nurse should identify adverse responses early to avoid serious consequence.

Pharmacology and the Nursing Process

The nursing management of drug therapy is a significant role and requires the application of complex knowledge from a variety of sources. Nurses must accept accountability for their performance. Society and the law expect nurses to perform to a reasonable standard consistent with that of other nurses with similar education and experience. In order for nurses to fulfill their responsibilities within the nursing process for management of drug therapy, they must have a thorough understanding of the pharmacology of the drugs being administered. Knowledge of the pharmacological properties of drugs provides the nurse with the information necessary to make decisions related to nursing management of drug therapy. Nurses use this knowledge of pharmacology to guide their assessment of patients, to plan and carry out the administration of medications, to focus their evaluation of patients following drug treatment and to identify areas of emphasis for patient teaching.

Our knowledge of pharmacology is constantly changing and new drugs are continually being developed. Nurses who try to memorize all the details of all available drugs will rapidly sink in a sea of minutiae. The authors suggest that readers learn basic information about major classifications of the drugs used most commonly in their own clinical setting. Learn one drug in the group very well; then, relate others in the same classification to the drug already learned. Nurses should be prepared to consult reliable sources of drug information, such as specialized text books, pharmacists and pharmacologists, physicians, or other nurses who are more familiar with use of a particular drug classification. Nurses who repeatedly use the same systematic approach to study new drugs find that they learn the new material easier and retain it longer. Figure 9 is intended for this purpose. Finally, readers should take advantage of all opportunities to participate in continuing education seminars on this topic.

Further Reading

Boggs, P. et al. (1988). Nurses' drug knowledge. *Western Journal of Nursing Research 10* (1):84-93.

Carr, D.S. (1989). New strategies for avoiding medication errors. *Nursing 19* (8): 38-46.

Cohen, M.R. (1991). Avoiding errors caused by drug suffixes. *Nursing 21* (2): 48-49.

Oseasohn, C., Graveley, E.A. and Hudepohl, N.C. (1989). Issues in medication compliance research. *Canadian Journal of Nursing Research 21* (4): 35-43.

Registered Nurses Association of British Columbia (1989). Telephone orders. *RNABC News 21* (4): 11-12

Trainor, P.A. (1988). Over-the-counter drugs: Count them in. *Geriatric Nursing 9* (5): 298-299.

SECTION 2

Autonomic Nervous System Pharmacology and Neuromuscular Blocking Drugs

The pharmacology of the autonomic nervous system
was selected for presentation early in this book
because drugs that affect the autonomic nervous
system influence many areas of the body.
Autonomic pharmacology forms the basis for the
understanding of the effects of drugs on many
systems. For example, it would be most difficult to
discuss cardiovascular pharmacology or gastrointestinal pharmacology without first understanding
the importance of autonomic nervous system innervation to these systems and the manner in which
drugs may tamper with it. Somatic nerves are not
part of the autonomic nervous system. The means
by which drugs may influence the transmission of
impulses from somatic nerves to skeletal muscles is
discussed in this section because of the similarities
between autonomic pharmacology and the pharmacology of drugs affecting motor end-plate function.

CHAPTER 4

Introduction to the Neurochemical Transmission of Autonomic and Somatic Nerves

Teaching Objectives

Following completion of this chapter, the reader should be able to:
1. Discuss the functions of the parasympathetic and sympathetic divisions of the autonomic nervous system with relation to smooth muscle, cardiac muscle and glandular activity.
2. Describe the synthesis, release and action of the neurotransmitters secreted at ganglionic and neuromuscular synapses as well as the mechanisms by which the body terminates the actions of the transmitters.
3. List and discuss the different types of cholinergic and adrenergic receptors in the body.

Divisions of the Autonomic Nervous System

The autonomic nervous system innervates smooth muscles, cardiac muscle and glands. It has also been called the involuntary or visceral nervous system. The autonomic nervous system consists of two divisions, called sympathetic and parasympathetic. These divisions have certain common anatomical characteristics:
1. They originate within the central nervous system.
2. Their activities and integration are controlled from within the brain.
3. Each sympathetic and parasympathetic nerve contains a preganglionic neuron, whose cell of origin lies within the central nervous system, and a postganglionic neuron, whose cell of origin lies within one of the ganglia outside the central nervous system. The two neurons synapse at a ganglion.

The Sympathetic Division of the Autonomic Nervous System

The preganglionic sympathetic nerves leave the spinal cord from the first thoracic to the second lumbar segments. Once outside the spinal cord, the preganglionic fibers synapse with their postganglionic nerves at ganglia located in three major areas of the body. Most preganglionic sympathetic nerves travel to ganglia that lie in two chains, one on each side of the vertebral column. These are called the vertebral or paravertebral ganglia. Some preganglionic sympathetic nerves travel to the abdominal cavity where they meet their postganglionic counterparts at prevertebral ganglia. The prevertebral ganglia are the celiac, superior mesenteric, inferior mesenteric, and aorticorenal ganglia. Finally, a few prevertebral sympathetic nerves run to the urinary bladder and rectum where they synapse with the postganglionic fibers. The ganglia that provide the meeting place for these pre- and postganglionic fibers and which lie near the organs innervated are called terminal ganglia. Functionally, paravertebral, prevertebral and terminal ganglia are identical. They have the same neurotransmitter and the same receptors and they are all affected in the same way by drugs.

Stimulation of the sympathetic division of the autonomic nervous system, usually referred to simply as the sympathetic nervous system, prepares the body to meet situations of mild to severe stress. Standing can be considered a very mild stress. In this position blood must be returned to the heart against the pull of gravity. To meet this situation the sympathetic nerves to veins are stimulated and the blood vessels constrict, returning blood to the heart. During conditions of more acute stress, such as a final examination, stimulation of the sympathetic nervous system increases heart rate, cardiac output and intermediary metabolism, dilates the bronchioles and redistributes blood from the gastrointestinal tract to the skeletal muscles. Obviously, defecation is not desired at that moment. Therefore, sympathetic nervous system stimulation reduces peristalsis. Fatigue is common in patients receiving sympathetic blocking drugs, particularly if they are stressed and cannot generate the increase in cardiac output and intermediary metabolism required to meet the needs of the body.

The Parasympathetic Division of the Autonomic Nervous System

Most parasympathetic preganglionic fibers originate in the midbrain or medulla oblongata areas of the brain. After leaving the central nervous system, they travel directly to the organs innervated where they meet their postganglionic nerves at ganglia that are found close to or within the organs.

A few preganglionic parasympathetic nerves leave the central nervous system from the sacral portion of the spinal cord. They too synapse with the postganglionic nerves in ganglia that are close to or within the innervated organs. All parasympathetic ganglia are identical with respect to the neurotransmitter released, receptors stimulated and reaction to drugs.

If it may be said that sympathetic stimulation prepares the body to meet stress, the parasympathetic division carries on many of the mundane day-to-day activities. Parasympathetic stimulation increases the flow of saliva and promotes peristalsis. The use of a parasympathomimetic drug leaves patients drowning in their own saliva and not daring to venture more than a few meters from the nearest washroom. Parasympathetic stimulation also constricts the pupil in the presence of bright light and allows the ciliary body to accommodate the lens for near vision. Stimulation of the parasympathetic vagus nerve slows heart rate.

Interaction between the Sympathetic and Parasympathetic Divisions of the Autonomic Nervous System

As was mentioned before, the autonomic nervous system innervates blood vessels, the heart, glands and smooth muscle. Many organs receive nervous supply from both the sympathetic and parasympathetic divisions. These include the heart, bronchi, gastrointestinal tract, sex organs and bladder. Some organs are innervated by only one division. These include sweat glands, piloerector muscles and arterioles, which receive only sympathetic innervation.

In general, if an organ is innervated by both the sympathetic and parasympathetic divisions, their actions are **antagonistic**. For example, sympathetic stimulation increases heart rate and force of contraction while parasympathetic stimulation produces bradycardia. Sympathetic activation dilates the pupil; parasympathetic constricts it.

In a few organs their actions are not antagonistic. Both sympathetic and parasympathetic stimulation produce saliva. Parasympathetic activation of the salivary glands, such as occurs upon the stimulus of the smell of food, causes the secretion of a copious amount of thin watery saliva. Students exposed to the rigors of oral examinations know only too well the consequences of the sympathetic stimulation of the salivary glands. A thick mucalogenous saliva is produced, with the result that candidates may be lucky if they can unstick their tongues from the roofs of their mouths.

Special attention must be paid to the innervation of the arterioles and veins. These vessels are innervated mainly by the sympathetic nervous system. As a result, the contractile state is determined by the extent of the sympathetic stimulation at any moment. Increased sympathetic activity produces both a rise in peripheral resistance, due to constriction of the arterioles, and an increase in venous return to the heart, as a result of vasoconstriction in the veins. Drugs that block sympathetic nervous system innervation of these vessels produce both a decrease in peripheral resistance, due to a dilatation of the arterioles, and postural hypotension, as a result of vasodilatation in the veins. When the patient stands, blood cannot be returned to the heart because the veins cannot constrict. With the sudden decrease in venous return to the heart, the amount of blood pumped to the brain is reduced dramatically and the patient may faint.

Neurotransmitters

Chemical Transmission of Impulses

Nerve impulses are transmitted across synapses by chemicals (Figure 10). In the ganglia of both parasympathetic and sympathetic nerves, the chemical neurotransmitter is **acetylcholine.** When an impulse reaches the end of a preganglionic nerve, acetylcholine is released and crosses the ganglionic synapse to stimulate the postganglionic neuron.

Acetylcholine is also the neurotransmitter released by all postganglionic parasympathetic nerves. In this case it is responsible for the stimulation of innervated tissue. A few postganglionic sympathetic nerves also release acetylcholine. The most notable example of this is the sympathetic innervation of sweat glands.

Somatic nerves release acetylcholine which stimulates the motor end-plates of skeletal muscles. Nerves that release acetylcholine are called **cholinergic.**

Figure 10
Chemical transmission of impulses.

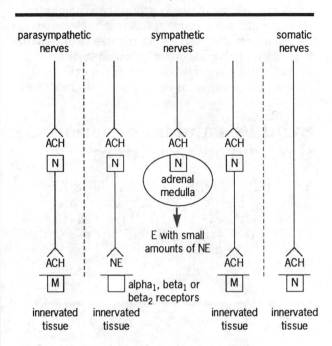

ACH = acetylcholine; NE = norepinephrine; E = epinephrine; N = nicotinic receptors; M = muscarinic receptors.

Sympathetic stimulation is mediated by the chemicals epinephrine and norepinephrine. (In many parts of the world, epinephrine and norepinephrine are called adrenaline and noradrenaline, respectively.) Functions mediated by epinephrine and/or norepinephrine are called **adrenergic.** It is important to recognize the physiological functions of each chemical. Epinephrine is an emergency hormone and is released by adrenal medullae in response to stress. It increases heart rate and force of contraction, shunts blood from the gastrointestinal tract, where it is not needed during stress, to the skeletal muscles, where it is required. Epinephrine also dilates the bronchioles and increases intermediary metabolism. In other words, it prepares individuals for either fight or flight, depending on their preference (flight is safer; if caught, you can always fight).

Norepinephrine is not usually considered a hormone, although small amounts may be secreted by the adrenal medullae. Instead, norepinephrine should be considered a neurotransmitter, released by the very great majority of postganglionic sympathetic nerves. Its physiological function is to assist in routine cardiovascular control. It is responsible for control of vascular tone. Increased norepinephrine release by the appropriate nerves will constrict arterioles and increase peripheral resistance. As mentioned earlier, the simple act of standing up increases norepinephrine release from nerves innervating veins. This causes vasoconstriction and promotes adequate venous return to the heart. Norepinephrine released by the cardiac sympathetic accelerator nerves increases heart rate.

Synthesis and Inactivation of the Neurotransmitters

Acetylcholine is synthesized within nerves from choline and acetylcoenzyme A by the enzyme choline acetylase (Figure 11). It is stored intraneuronally within vesicles until such time as a wave of

Figure 11
Synthesis of acetylcholine.

$$CH_3 - \overset{\overset{O}{\|}}{C} - CoA \quad + \quad HO - CH_2 - CH_2 - \overset{+}{N} \overset{- CH_3}{\underset{- CH_3}{\overset{- CH_3}{}}}$$

acetyl CoA   choline

choline acetylase

$$CH_3 - \overset{\overset{O}{\|}}{C} - O - CH_2 - CH_2 - \overset{+}{N} \overset{- CH_3}{\underset{- CH_3}{\overset{- CH_3}{}}}$$

acetylcholine

depolarization releases it. The enzyme **acetylcholinesterase,** also formed within cholinergic nerves, rapidly inactivates acetylcholine, once it has been released, by hydrolyzing it to acetic acid and choline (Figure 12).

Acetylcholinesterase, or true cholinesterase as it is sometimes called, should not be confused with pseudocholinesterase. The latter enzyme is found in the serum and is therefore also called **serum cholinesterase.** Whereas it can also hydrolyze acetylcholine, its specificity is not limited to this chemical. Serum cholinesterase can inactivate a number of drugs containing ester groups, including procaine and succinylcholine.

The synthesis of norepinephrine and epinephrine is more complex (see Figure 13). The precursor of these chemicals is the amino acid

Figure 12
Inactivation of acetylcholine.

$$CH_3 - \overset{\overset{O}{\|}}{C} - O - CH_2 - CH_2 - \overset{+}{N} \overset{- CH_3}{\underset{- CH_3}{\overset{- CH_3}{}}}$$

acetylcholine

acetylcholinesterase

$$CH_3 - \overset{\overset{O}{\|}}{C} - OH + HOCH_2 - CH_2 - \overset{+}{N} \overset{- CH_3}{\underset{- CH_3}{\overset{- CH_3}{}}}$$

acetic acid   choline

Figure 13
Synthesis of norepinephrine and epinephrine.

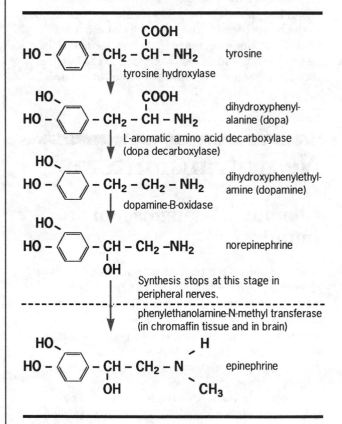

tyrosine. Tyrosine is first converted to dopa (dihydroxyphenylalanine) and then to dopamine (dihydroxyphenylethylamine). Dopamine is subsequently metabolized to norepinephrine, within sympathetic nerves, or norepinephrine and epinephrine, within chromaffin tissue and the brain. The rate-limiting step in the formation of epinephrine and norepinephrine involves the epinephrine and norepinephrine involves the conversion of tyrosine to dopa. Once formed, both epinephrine and norepinephrine are stored in small particles called **granules.** Their release occurs when the adrenal medullae or sympathetic nerves are stimulated.

Epinephrine, norepinephrine and dopamine are often called the **catecholamines.** When doctors order a catecholamine analysis of blood or urine, they are attempting to determine the extent of sympathetic nervous system activity as a prelude to diagnosing the cause of a disease. For example, in a very small number of people hypertension (high blood pressure) may be caused by a tumor of the chromaffin tissue. The adrenal medullae are the major sites of chromaffin tissue in the body. A tumor of chromaffin tissue is called a **pheochromocytoma.** Patients so afflicted will have very high concentrations of epinephrine, and possibly also norepinephrine, in their blood and urine.

The inactivation of epinephrine and norepinephrine once they have been released has been the subject of considerable research. It is now known that norepinephrine, released by sympathetic postganglionic fibers, is removed from innervated tissue by neuronal reuptake and diffusion away in the blood. These are the main means by which the effects of released norepinephrine are terminated. Small amounts of the released neurotransmitters are inactivated by the enzymes catechol-O-methyl transferase and monoamine oxidase.

Epinephrine is secreted into the blood and carried throughout the body. Its effects on any particular tissue may be terminated by diffusion away in the blood or uptake into sympathetic nerves innervating the organ concerned. Similar to norepinephrine, epinephrine may, in part, be inactivated by monoamine oxidase and catechol-O-methyl transferase. Enzymatic inactivation may be a more important means of terminating epinephrine's effects because it is carried in blood throughout the body and will have a greater opportunity to encounter the inactivating enzymes.

Autonomic Receptors

Cholinergic Receptors

Following their release, acetylcholine, epinephrine and norepinephrine stimulate autonomic receptors on or in the tissues affected (Figure 10). In the case of acetylcholine the cholinergic receptors are classified as **nicotinic** or **muscarinic.** This division goes back many decades to the time when it was demonstrated that small doses of nicotine stimulated cholinergic receptors in both sympathetic and parasympathetic ganglia, giving rise to the term nicotinic receptors. It was also determined at that time that nicotine did not stimulate the organs innervated by parasympathetic nerves. The cholinergic receptors in these tissues were called muscarinic because they were stimulated by small amounts of the chemical muscarine, obtained from mushrooms. Muscarine did not stimulate autonomic ganglia. This was the first evidence that the cholinergic receptors in ganglia are not identical to those found in innervated tissues.

Skeletal muscles have cholinergic receptors that are stimulated by acetylcholine released from somatic nerves. These receptors also are stimulated by low doses of nicotine and are classified as nicotinic. It would be convenient, at this point, if we could state that cholinergic receptors in the ganglia and on skeletal muscle are identical because they both are stimulated by nicotine. However, Nature is never that kind to the suffering student. On the contrary, there is evidence that the nicotinic receptors in ganglia are not identical to the nicotinic receptors in skeletal muscle.

Ganglionic blockers are drugs that competitively prevent acetylcholine from uniting with ganglionic nicotinic receptors. These drugs, in usual therapeutic doses, do not stop acetylcholine, released by somatic nerves, from stimulating the nicotinic receptors on skeletal muscle. Neuromuscular blockers, such as tubocurarine, block competitively nicotinic receptors at the motor end-plate. In normal therapeutic doses they do not block the ganglia. If the nicotinic receptors on skeletal muscle were identical to those in the ganglia, tubocurarine should block both. By the same token, ganglionic blockers should also paralyze skeletal muscles. The fact that ganglionic blockers affect only ganglia, and tubocurarine only skeletal muscles, indicates that the two groups of nicotinic receptors are not identical.

Adrenergic Receptors

Epinephrine and norepinephrine stimulate adrenergic receptors. It has been known for many years that epinephrine can cause either an excitation or an inhibition of smooth muscle contraction. For example, it constricts the blood vessels in the peritoneal area and dilates those in skeletal muscle. To explain these disparate actions, the existence of two types of adrenergic receptors, called **alpha** and **beta,** were proposed. Stimulation of the alpha receptors on blood vessels produces vasoconstriction. Beta receptor stimulation causes vasodilatation.

To fulfill its function as an emergency hormone, epinephrine must stimulate both types of receptors at the same time. This is essential if it is to redistribute blood in the body, moving it from areas not involved in the body's response to stress and shifting it to tissues responsible for meeting emergency situations. Epinephrine accomplishes this by constricting blood vessels (alpha stimulation) supplying the gastrointestinal tract and dilating (beta stimulation) those perfusing skeletal muscles.

The bronchodilatation produced by epinephrine is also a beta receptor mediated response.

The general rule may be stated that alpha receptor stimulation produces excitation and beta receptor stimulation causes inhibition. The exception to this rule can be found in the heart. In this tissue the chronotropic and inotropic effects of epinephrine are mediated by the beta receptors. Drugs that are only beta stimulants increase heart rate and force of contraction, and drugs that block beta receptors decrease heart rate. Alpha stimulants usually slow the heart beat.

Norepinephrine can also stimulate both alpha and beta receptors. It is, however, a far more effective alpha stimulant. This is consistent with its physiological role to maintain normal vascular tone. The degree of vasoconstriction under resting conditions is determined by the quantity of norepinephrine released by sympathetic nerves. When relatively large amounts are secreted, alpha receptors are stimulated and the blood vessels involved constrict. A decrease in norepinephrine release allows the vessels to relax.

Norepinephrine, released by the cardiac accelerator nerves, stimulates the beta receptors to increase heart rate and force of contraction. This is one of the few areas of the body where the beta receptor stimulant effects of norepinephrine can be seen.

Not all beta receptors are identical. The beta receptors in the heart differ from those in other parts of the body. Accordingly, the receptors in the heart are designated as **beta₁** and those in other parts of the body as **beta₂**. Drugs have been synthesized that are capable of stimulating more selectively beta₂ receptors. They are used to treat bronchial asthma. Their advantage over previous agents that stimulate both beta₁ and beta₂ receptors is that the newer drugs will dilate the bronchioles without producing a marked tachycardia.

Finally, a new form of the alpha receptor has been found. It has been known for some time that the secretion of large amounts of norepinephrine reduces the subsequent release of this neurotransmitter. Recent work has suggested the presence of a receptor on the nerve ending. When norepinephrine, which has been released by the nerve, stimulates this presynaptic receptor on the outside of the nerve membrane it reduces the subsequent secretion of the neurotransmitter. The new receptor has been designated **alpha₂**. It differs from the alpha receptor previously described, and now called **alpha₁,** in two ways. Alpha₁ receptors are located in the tissue innervated. Alpha₂ receptors are found on the nerve membrane itself. Stimulation of alpha₁ receptors causes smooth muscle excitation. Stimulation of alpha₂ receptors reduces the subsequent secretion of norepinephrine.

A moment of quiet contemplation reviewing Figure 10 and Table 2 will indicate the possibility of tampering selectively with one or another aspect of autonomic function. The subsequent pages in this section will discuss the pharmacology and nursing process related to drugs that influence one or more of these sites.

Further Reading

Fleming, William W. (1986). "Adrenergic and Cholinergic Neurotransmission." In: *Modern Pharmacology,* 2nd ed. (pp. 149-157), ed. Charles R. Craig and Robert E. Stitzel. Boston: Little, Brown.

Lefkowitz, Robert J., Hoffman, Brian B. and Taylor, Palmer (1990). "Neurohumoral Transmission: The Autonomic and Somatic Motor Nervous Systems." In: *Goodman and Gilman's The Pharmacological Basis of Therapeutics,* 8th ed. (pp. 84-121), ed. Alfred Goodman Gilman, Theodore W. Rall, Alan S. Nies and Palmer Taylor. New York: Pergamon.

Robinson, Robert L. (1986). "Introduction to the Autonomic Nervous System." In: *Modern Pharmacology,* 2nd ed. (pp. 137-148), ed. Charles R. Craig and Robert E. Stitzel. Boston: Little, Brown.

Table 2
Neurochemical transmission of autonomic and somatic nerves.

Chemical	Classification	Source	Type of Receptor	Action	Means of Terminating Effect
Acetylcholine	Neurotransmitter	Ganglia of both parasympathetic and sympathetic nerves	Nicotinic	Stimulates postganglionic neurons.	Acetylcholinesterase
		Postganglionic parasympathetic neurons	Muscarinic	Stimulates innervated tissues.	Acetylcholinesterase
		Some postganglionic sympathetic neurons	Muscarinic	Stimulates some sympathetically innervated tissues.	Acetylcholinesterase
		Somatic nerves	Nicotinic	Motor end-plate stimulation of skeletal muscles	Acetylcholinesterase
Epinephrine (adrenaline)	Hormone	Adrenal medulla	Alpha$_1$ adrenergic	Vasoconstriction	Uptake into sympathetic postganglionic nerves; monoamine oxidase; catechol-O-methyl transferase
			Beta$_1$ adrenergic	Increases heart rate and force of cardiac contraction.	
			Beta$_2$ adrenergic	Vasodilatation and bronchodilatation	
Norepinephrine (noradrenaline)	Neurotransmitter	Postganglionic sympathetic nerves	Alpha$_1$ adrenergic	Vasoconstriction (arterioles and veins)	Reuptake into nerve; diffusion away in blood; monoamine oxidase; catechol-O-methyl transferase
			Beta$_1$ adrenergic	Increases heart rate and force of cardiac contraction.	

CHAPTER 5

Cholinergic Drugs

Cholinergic drugs mimic the effects of acetylcholine. They may act directly, by stimulating muscarinic or nicotinic receptors, or indirectly, by inhibiting the enzyme acetylcholinesterase, thereby allowing acetylcholine to accumulate around the receptors.

Acetylcholine itself is not suitable for use as a drug. It cannot be given orally; it is rapidly destroyed by both acetylcholinesterase and pseudo-cholinesterase; and its action is nonspecific, affecting both nicotinic and muscarinic receptors. Ideally, cholinergic drugs should rectify these obvious sins of acetylcholine and, to a degree, they do. Some cholinergic drugs can be given orally. They all have longer durations of action than acetylcholine and some specificity for either the nicotinic or muscarinic receptors.

Directly Acting Cholinergic Drugs

Mechanism of Action and Pharmacologic Effects

The directly acting cholinergics stimulate muscarinic receptors. In some cases they also stimulate nicotinic receptors. Their pharmacological effects include salivation, secretion of sweat, vasodilatation, bronchiolar constriction, increased gastrointestinal activity, gastric acid secretion and increased urinary bladder tone.

The effects of these drugs on the cardiovascular system are complex. They stimulate the muscarinic receptors in the heart to produce bradycardia. This action may be offset by a reflex increase in sympathetic stimulation to the heart because of the peripheral vasodilatation produced by muscarinic stimulation.

The most commonly used directly acting cholinergics are carbamylcholine (Carbachol), bethanechol (Urecholine) and pilocarpine (Isopto Carpine).

Therapeutic Uses

Carbamylcholine and bethanechol stimulate muscarinic, and to some extent nicotinic, receptors. They are given orally or parenterally for the treatment of postoperative intestinal atony or urinary retention.

Pilocarpine and carbamylcholine are instilled in the eye to produce miosis by stimulating the muscarinic receptors on the circular muscle of the iris. The resulting increase in the drainage of aqueous humor through the Canals of Schlemm lowers the intraocular pressure, thereby aiding in the treatment of glaucoma (see Chapter 37). Both drugs can also be used to produce miosis during ocular surgery.

Adverse Effects

When given systemically, these drugs stimulate muscarinic receptors throughout the body. As a result their adverse effects include sweating, abdominal cramps, salivation, flushing of the skin, asthmatic attacks, headache and a fall in blood pressure.

Bethanechol and carbamylcholine are contraindicated in patients with bronchial asthma, peptic ulcers, pronounced bradycardia or hypotension, vasomotor instability, coronary artery disease, epilepsy and parkinsonism. Many of these contraindications require little comment. For obvious reasons, a drug that constricts bronchioles, increases gastric acid secretion, slows the heart and dilates blood vessels is contraindicated in the above conditions. It is perhaps less obvious why these drugs are contraindicated in parkinsonism. Patients with parkinsonism have a relatively large amount of acetylcholine in the brain, compared to their levels of dopamine. It is this imbalance of acetylcholine relative to dopamine in brain basal ganglia that is responsible for the problems in muscle movement. Administering a cholinergic drug to a parkinsonian patient accentuates the imbalance and worsens the disease.

Nursing Process: Systemic Uses

Assessment
Prior to the initial systemic administration of a directly acting cholinergic drug, the nurse should review the patient history for evidence of asthma, peptic ulcers, hypotension, vasomotor instability, coronary artery disease, epilepsy or parkinsonism. If any of these conditions are documented, the order should be verified. Vital signs must be recorded as a baseline for measurements taken after the medication has been given.

Administration
Carbamylcholine and bethanechol should be administered subcutaneously. Intravenous or intramuscular injections should not be undertaken because of the high risk of adverse effects due to rapid absorption. Because the onset of action following subcutaneous injection is usually five to fifteen minutes, either a bed pan should be at hand or an obstacle-free route for rapid bathroom access planned! Oral doses should be administered on an empty stomach to reduce the incidence of nausea and vomiting.

Evaluation
All patients receiving systemic treatment with a directly acting cholinergic drug should be observed for flushing of the skin, headache, sudden drop in blood pressure, decreased pulse rate, and alterations in the rate, depth or rhythm of respiration. These signs may indicate impending toxicity (**cholinergic crisis**). Intramuscular or intravenous atropine (0.6 – 1.2 mg is the adult dose) should be kept on hand. Nurses should also be alert for abdominal cramps and asthmatic attacks.

The effectiveness of bethanechol or carbamylcholine in postoperative urinary retention can be evaluated by measuring the patient's urinary output. Occasionally, catheterization is ordered following voiding to determine the quantity of residual urine.

Nursing Process: Local Use

Assessment
Nursing responsibilities related to the assessment of patients prior to the local administration of carbamylcholine or pilocarpine are the same as those discussed for systemic treatment.

Administration
These drugs should be instilled in the lower conjunctival sac and the canaliculi and nasal-lacrimal ducts immediately compressed against the

bridge of the nose. This will prevent excess medication from draining with the tears into the nasopharynx. Pilocarpine is light sensitive. It should be stored in a light-resistant container.

Evaluation
Evaluation of the effect of either pilocarpine or carbamylcholine instilled in the eye is conducted by measuring the intraocular pressure with a tonometer. This is generally done by a physician or under the direction of a physician. Patients should be evaluated for the warning signs of a cholinergic crisis.

Teaching
Patients should be warned about the dangers of driving or working with dangerous tools (power saws, lathes, grinders, etc.) immediately following the instillation of either drug because carbamylcholine and pilocarpine can blur vision and impair the ability of the eye to focus.

Indirectly Acting Cholinergic Drugs (Cholinesterase Inhibitors)

Mechanism of Action and Pharmacologic Effects

The indirectly acting cholinergic drugs inhibit acetylcholinesterase. They are called cholinesterase inhibitors or **anticholinesterases.** By inhibiting the inactivation of acetylcholine they increase cholinergic stimulation. Cholinesterase inhibitors may be divided into the reversibly and irreversibly acting drugs. The effects of the former last a few hours, the latter several days or weeks.

The reversibly acting cholinesterase inhibitors include physostigmine (Eserine, Antilirium), demecarium (Humorsol), neostigmine (Prostigmin), pyridostigmine (Mestinon), ambenonium (Mytelase) and edrophonium (Tensilon). Isoflurophate (DFP, Floropryl) and echothiophate (Echodide, Phospholine Iodide) are two of the more commonly used irreversibly acting cholinesterase inhibitors. A spin-off from the war gas industry, irreversibly acting cholinesterase inhibitors were developed to

poison people. Long after the war buffs lost interest in them, these agents remain as valuable drugs in the treatment of disease.

The pharmacologic effects of the cholinesterase inhibitors are similar to those listed for the directly acting cholinergics. They include a generalized parasympathomimetic action, including salivation, increased gastrointestinal activity and urinary bladder tone, as well as vasodilatation and increased sweating.

Therapeutic Uses

Cholinesterase inhibitors are used for their effects on the eye, the skeletal muscles and the gastrointestinal and urinary tracts. Instilled in the eye, the inhibition of acetylcholinesterase in the iris increases parasympathetic stimulation of the circular muscle, producing miosis. The resulting increase in the drainage of aqueous humor through the Canals of Schlemm lowers intraocular pressure and is valuable in the treatment of glaucoma (see Chapter 37). The drugs used most frequently to treat glaucoma are physostigmine, demecarium, isoflurophate and echothiophate.

The systemic administration of a cholinesterase inhibitor can have a dramatic effect on skeletal muscle function. The inhibition of acetylcholinesterase increases acetylcholine stimulation of nicotinic receptors on the motor end-plates of skeletal muscle.

Pyridostigmine, neostigmine and ambenonium have been used to great advantage in the treatment of myasthenia gravis, a disease characterized by decreased neuromuscular transmission, together with weakness and fatigability of skeletal muscles (see Chapter 56). Myasthenia gravis is caused by an autoimmune response to the nicotinic receptors on motor end-plates. Antibodies are formed that reduce the number of receptors. Cholinesterase inhibitors increase acetylcholine concentration around nicotinic receptors on skeletal muscle. They are used to increase skeletal muscle strength in patients with myasthenia gravis.

In addition to their ability to increase acetylcholine concentration, both neostigmine and pyridostigmine directly stimulate skeletal muscle nicotinic receptors. Experiments performed with denervated tissue, in which there is neither acetylcholine nor acetylcholinesterase, have shown that the drugs can stimulate skeletal muscle. Obviously, this direct action complements their anticholinesterase effects in the treatment of the myasthenic patient.

Neostigmine is also used after surgery to reverse the skeletal muscle paralysis produced by tubocurarine and other drugs with similar actions. Tubocurarine is a competitive blocker of nicotinic receptors on skeletal muscle. Its effects can be reversed by increasing acetylcholine concentration in the vicinity of the receptors.

Neostigmine can be employed for the treatment of postoperative intestinal atony or urinary retention. The rationale for its use is the same as presented for the directly acting cholinergics.

One additional use of an anticholinesterase drug deserves attention. Parenteral physostigmine (Antilirium) can be used to treat patients poisoned with anticholinergics or tricyclic antidepressants. The latter group has extensive anticholinergic properties. Physostigmine is used in preference to neostigmine or pyridostigmine because it will cross the blood-brain barrier and can, therefore, antagonize both the central and peripheral toxicities of the anticholinergics and antidepressants. Neostigmine or pyridostigmine do not cross the blood-brain barrier and are ineffective in combatting the action of anticholinergics or antidepressants within the brain.

Adverse Effects

The adverse effects of cholinesterase inhibitors result from an accumulation of acetylcholine throughout the body, producing a generalized stimulation of all cholinergic receptors. Obviously, the intensity of these effects is much greater when the drugs are administered systemically than when they are instilled in the eye. In spite of this comment, many patients have experienced systemic adverse effects when irreversibly acting agents have been applied to the eye.

It is beyond the scope of this book to list all the effects of a cholinergic crisis. However, muscarinic stimulation produces miosis, ocular pain, bronchoconstriction, increased bronchial secretion, salivation, abdominal cramps and diarrhea.

The consequences of excessive nicotinic stimulation include skeletal muscle paralysis. If large doses are used, sufficient acetylcholine may accumulate around skeletal muscle receptors to produce a depolarizing block of the motor end-plates. This effect requires an explanation. In the normal course of neuromuscular transmission, acetylcholine is released. It stimulates nicotinic receptors and depolarizes motor end-plates. The beginning of muscle contraction occurs. However, the contraction of muscles requires many waves of depolarization. For this to happen, acetylcholine must first be destroyed to allow motor end-plates to repolarize so that they can accept the next impulse. If large doses of a cholinesterase inhibitor are used,

acetylcholine is not metabolized and repolarization does not take place. Successive waves of depolarization cannot occur and muscular paralysis ensues.

High doses of cholinesterase inhibitors can affect the central nervous system to produce slurred speech, ataxia, confusion, convulsions and paralysis of the respiratory center. If untreated, the patient will die from respiratory failure.

The treatment of a cholinergic crisis involves the use of large doses of atropine, a competitive blocker of muscarinic receptors. However, atropine does not affect nicotinic receptors on skeletal muscle. If these are paralyzed, it may be necessary to ventilate the patient. If the patient has absorbed an irreversibly acting cholinesterase inhibitor it may be possible to reactivate the enzyme by administering the drug pralidoxime (PAM). This chemical may remove the irreversible inhibitor from the cholinesterase enzyme.

Although we have concentrated on the toxicities of the cholinesterase inhibitors that are used as drugs, nurses should be aware that many individuals are poisoned by anticholinesterases used as insecticides. Two popular insecticides that are irreversibly acting cholinesterase inhibitors are malathion and parathion. They may be swallowed or accidentally absorbed through the skin or lungs.

Nursing Process: Reversible Anticholinesterases

Assessment

Nursing assessment depends largely on the route by which the cholinesterase inhibitor is administered and the purpose for which is it used. The nursing process related to the systemic administration of physostigmine (Antilirium) as an antidote for anticholinergic or antidepressant poisoning is essentially the same as previously described for the directly acting cholinergics.

Prior to the administration of neostigmine, pyridostigmine or ambenonium for the treatment of myasthenia gravis, nurses should investigate the patient's history for asthma, peptic ulcers, bradycardia, hypotension, vasomotor instability, coronary artery disease, epilepsy and parkinsonism. Before each administration the nurse should check the patient's pulse, respiration and blood pressure. In the event of a fall in the pulse rate below 80 beats per minute, a progressive change in the rate, depth or rhythm of respiration, or a decrease in blood pressure, the drug should be withheld and the physician notified.

Administration

Nurses should pay particular attention to the patient during the intravenous administration of physostigmine because of its rapid onset of action. Following administration of the drug, nurses should check the patient's vital signs and level of consciousness every fifteen minutes. Atropine sulfate must be kept on hand for possible use if overdosage with physostigmine leads to a cholinergic crisis. Physostigmine has a short duration of action and the patient must be guarded against a return of the effects of the anticholinergic or antidepressant.

The adverse gastrointestinal effects of oral neostigmine may be reduced by giving the drug in combination with meals or milk.

Evaluation

Following administration of neostigmine, pyridostigmine or ambenonium for myasthenia gravis, nurses should determine the drug's effect on muscle strength. This will assist in establishing optimal dosage for the individual patient. The optimal dosage is often established by trial and error for each patient and objective nursing evaluation is essential to this process.

Teaching

Patient teaching should emphasize the importance of taking the designated drug regularly, observing its effects, and reporting these to the physician. The patient and family must be able to differentiate between the effects of an overdose and an underdose of the drug. Describing some of the effects of a cholinergic crisis should help in this regard.

Physostigmine is often applied to the eye to treat glaucoma. When used in this manner the nursing process is the same as for pilocarpine since the result of the administration of either drug is the same.

Nursing Process: Irreversible Anticholinesterases

Assessment

The irreversible inhibitors of cholinesterase can be very toxic drugs. They are intended only for local application to the eye. Prior to the administration of isoflurophate or echothiophate, measurements of the intraocular pressure should be taken either by, or under the direction of, a physician. Additional initial assessment should include vital signs as a baseline for comparison with postadministration evaluation.

Administration

The initial instillation should be performed by a physician because of the need to monitor intraocular pressure due to the risk of transient paradoxical increases in pressure. Subsequent administrations are best given at bedtime (**h.s.**, or *hora somni*) in order to minimize the effects of the visual disturbances that often accompany use of these medications, especially in the early phases of treatment. Ointments should be instilled in the lower conjunctival sac and the excess blotted from the eyelid to prevent contact dermatitis. These medications may deteriorate when placed in contact with moisture. Therefore, nurses must guard against touching the tube to the conjunctiva. Never wash the tube with water.

Teaching

Patients should be instructed on the proper technique of administration, the importance of regular contact with the physician, and the signs of impending cholinergic crisis. Because of the transient visual disturbances that often accompany use of these medications, patients should be reminded of the principles of safe mobility (for example, holding hand railings on stairs, removing small area rugs, ensuring well-lighted passageways that are free of obstacles). Patients using these medications should also be cautioned against driving at night because of reduced visual perception in poor lighting conditions, and advised to wear a Medic Alert ID for drugs taken.

Further Reading

Colasanti, Brenda K. (1986). "Directly Acting Cholinomimetics." In: *Modern Pharmacology,* 2nd ed. (pp. 193-199), ed. C.R. Craig and R.E. Stitzel. Boston: Little, Brown.

Hoover, Donald B. (1986). "Cholinesterases and Cholinesterase Inhibitors." In: *Modern Pharmacology,* 2nd ed. (pp. 200-212), ed. C.R. Craig and R.E. Stitzel. Boston: Little, Brown.

Taylor, Palmer (1990). "Anticholinesterase Agents." In: *Goodman and Gilman's The Pharmacological Basis of Therapeutics,* 8th ed. (pp. 131-149), ed. A. Goodman Gilman, T.W. Rall, A.S. Nies and P. Taylor. New York: Pergamon.

Taylor, Palmer (1990). "Cholinergic Agents." In: *Goodman and Gilman's The Pharmacological Basis of Therapeutics,* 8th ed. (pp. 122-130), ed. A. Goodman Gilman, T.W. Rall, A.S. Nies and P. Taylor. New York: Pergamon.

Table 3
Cholinergic drugs.

Generic Name (Trade Name)	Use (Dose)	Action	Adverse Effects	Drug Interactions	Nursing Process
Pharmacologic Classification: Directly Acting Cholinergics					
Bethanechol (Urecholine)	Relief of postoperative intestinal atony or urinary retent'n (**Oral:** 10-50 mg tid or qid)	Stim. of muscarinic receptors in intestine and urinary bladder	Vasodilatat'n, incr. gastric secret'n, GI peristalsis, bronchiolar constrict'n, bradycardia		**Assess:** Pt for hx asthma, bradycardia, hypotens'n, vasomotor instability. Establish baseline VS. **Administer:** Orally, on empty stomach to reduce nausea and vomiting. Parenteral - SC only to slow absorpt'n. **Evaluate:** Effectiveness, flushing, headache, hypotens'n, asthmatic attacks, bradycardia, altered respirat'n.
Carbamylcholine (Carbachol)	**Systemically:** As for bethanechol (**Oral:** 1-4 mg; **SC:** 0.25-0.5 mg)	**Systemic:** As for bethanechol	**Systemic:** As for bethanechol		
	Ophthalmic: Tx of primary open-angle glaucoma (**Instill:** 1 drop of 0.75-3% solut'n q8h)	**Ophthalmic:** Stim. of muscarinic receptors on circular muscles in iris to produce miosis and incr. drainage of aqueous humor	**Ophthalmic:** Local irritat'n, ciliary spasm, allergic reactions, miosis, poor night vision		**Assess:** As above **Administer:** From light-resistant containers, into lower conjunctival sac; compress lacrimal duct against bridge of nose to prevent absorpt'n of excess into nasopharynx. **Teach:** To avoid driving following administrat'n.
Pilocarpine (Adsorbocarpine, Akarpin, Isopto Carpine, Pilocar, Pilocel)	Miotic of choice in tx of primary open-angle glaucoma (**Instill:** Initially, 1 drop 1-2% solut'n q4-8h. Primary angle-closure glaucoma, initially 1-2% drops, frequently, until angle opens and pressure decreases)	Stim. of muscarinic receptors on circular muscles in iris to produce miosis	As for ophthalmic carbamylcholine		
Pharmacologic Classification: Indirectly Acting Cholinergics (Reversibly Acting Anticholinesterases)					
Physostigmine - eserine (Miocel, Isopto P-ES)	Tx of primary open-angle glaucoma (**Instill:** 1 drop 0.25% sol'n q4-6h, or ointment hs)	Inhibit'n of acetylcholinesterase, producing ciliary muscle contract'n w. miosis and incr. drainage of aqueous humor	Hyperemia of conjunctiva and iris		As for pilocarpine

Drug	Uses	Action	Side effects/Adverse reactions	Nursing considerations
Physostigmine (Antilirium)	To counteract CNS toxicity caused by anticholinergic activity (**IM/IV:** 0.5-4 mg)	Rapid diffus'n across blood-brain barrier to block CNS effects of anticholinergics	As for directly acting cholinergics	**Assess:** As for directly acting cholinergics **Administer:** IV w. special attent'n to rate of administrat'n, w. atropine (0.6-1.2 mg) available. **Evaluate:** VS and LOC q15 min beginning 1 h after administrat'n.
Neostigmine (Prostigmine)	Tx of myasthenia gravis (**Oral:** Adults - initially, 15 mg q3-4h. Children - 2 mg/kg/day in divided doses prn. **IM/SC:** Adults - 0.5 mg. Children/infants - 0.01-0.04 mg/kg q2-3h. **IV:** 1 mg in 100 mL saline, infused at a rate of 25 mL/h)	Inhibit'n of acetylcholinesterase, producing incr. stim. of nicotinic receptors on skeletal muscle motor end-plates	Nausea, vomiting, abdominal cramps, incr. peristalsis, salivat'n, bronchial secret'n, miosis, diaphoresis, bradycardia, hypotens'n, muscle cramps, fasciculat'ns, weakness See Table 56	**Assess:** As for directly acting cholinergics; If pulse below 80; progr. change in rate, depth, rhythm of respirat'ns; or decr. in BP, notify physician. **Administer:** Orally w. food to reduce adverse GI effects. **Evaluate:** Effect on muscle strength to assist in establishing optimal dose. **Teach:** Importance of taking drug regularly, reporting effect of drug to physician.
Pyridostigmine (Mestinon, Regonol)	Tx of myasthenia gravis (**Oral:** Adults - initially, 60-120 mg q3-4h. Children - 7 mg/kg/day in divided doses. **IM/IV:** Adults - approx. 1/30th oral dose; newborn infants of myasthenic mothers, 0.05-0.15 mg/kg)	As for neostigmine	As for neostigmine See Table 56	
Ambenonium (Mytelase)	Tx of myasthenia gravis (**Oral:** Adults - initially, 5 mg tid or qid; incr. as required. Dosage should be adjusted at intervals of 1-2 days to avoid accumulat'n. Children - initially, 0.3 mg/kg/day in divided doses; incr. prn to 1.5 mg/kg/day in divided doses)	As for neostigmine	As for neostigmine See Table 56	As for neostigmine

Pharmacologic Classification: Indirectly Acting Cholinergics (Irreversibly Acting Anticholinesterases)

Drug	Uses	Action	Side effects/Adverse reactions	Nursing considerations
Demecarium bromide (Humorsol)	Tx of primary open-angle glaucoma and other chronic glaucomas (**Instill:** 1 drop q12-48h)	Inhibit'n of acetylcholinesterase, producing ciliary muscle contract'n, long-acting miosis, and incr. drainage of aqueous humor	Cataracts, spasm of accommodat'n, systemic cholinergic effects, iris cysts	**Assess:** Intraocular pressure (by physician), baseline VS. **Administer:** Initially by physician, due to need to monitor intraocular pressure w. tonometer in light of paradoxic incr. in intraocular pressure w. first doses. Instill hs to reduce effects of visual disturbances. Instill in lower conjunctival sac;

Generic Name (Trade Name)	Use (Dose)	Action	Adverse Effects	Drug Interactions	Nursing Process
Echothiophate iodide (Echodide, Phospholine)	As for demecarium (**Instill:** 1 drop of 0.03-0.06% solut'n q12-48h)	As for demecarium	As for demecarium	**Procaine:** Isoflurophate, echothiophate reduce pseudocholinesterase activity, slowing hydrolysis of procaine. **Succinylcholine:** Pseudocholinesterase metabolizes succinylcholine. Echothiophate, isoflurophate incr. duration of action of succinylcholine.	blot excess to prevent contact dermatitis. Keep ointments dry; do not contact eye or wash tip of tube; store liquids in light-resistant containers. **Teach:** Symptoms of cholinergic crisis; proper technique to self-administrat'n; principles of safe mobility. Emphasize no night driving.
Isoflurophate (DFP, Floropryl)	As for demecarium (**Instill:** 1/4-inch ointment strip applied q8-72h)	As for demecarium	As for demecarium	As for echothiophate	As above

CHAPTER 6

Anticholinergic Drugs and Ganglionic Blocking Drugs

Teaching Objectives
Following completion of this chapter, the reader should be able to:
1. Describe the mechanism of action of anticholinergic drugs.
2. Describe and explain the effects of anticholinergic drugs on body functions.
3. Explain the therapeutic uses of atropine and its adverse effects.
4. Identify the nursing process related to the administration of atropine.
5. Discuss the difference between the effects of atropine and those of scopolamine (hyoscine).
6. Discuss the nursing evaluation related to the administration of atropine and of scopolamine.
7. Discuss atropine-like cycloplegics and mydriatics.
8. Discuss atropine-like antispasmodics.
9. Discuss atropine-like antiasthmatics.
10. Describe the nursing process related to the use of each major group of atropine-like drugs.
11. Describe the mechanism of action and effects of ganglionic blockers and explain why these drugs are rarely used in medicine today.

Anticholinergic Drugs

Anticholinergic drugs block stimulation of cholinergic receptors by acetylcholine. They are also referred to as **cholinergic blocking drugs.** Since acetylcholine is the neurotransmitter at autonomic ganglia, postganglionic cholinergic neuromuscular junctions and somatic motor end-plates, it would be logical to assume, on the basis of their name, that anticholinergic drugs block all types of cholinergic receptors. However, in its usual context the expression means only the competitive blockade of muscarinic receptors. In this book anticholinergic drugs can be taken to mean **antimuscarinic agents.**

Anticholinergics are best studied by discussing atropine first. It is the standard drug in this category and the chemical against which all other agents should be compared. If nurses understand the actions of atropine, they will have little difficulty incorporating newer anticholinergics into their therapeutic armamentaria.

Atropine

Mechanism of Action and Pharmacological Effects

Atropine is obtained from the belladonna plant. It combines reversibly with muscarinic receptors, preventing acetylcholine from stimulating them. Atropine blocks muscarinic receptors throughout the body. This includes all receptors innervated by parasympathetic postganglionic nerves and those few muscarinic receptors that receive innervation from cholinergic sympathetic nerves. The blocking of muscarinic receptors is competitive in nature and can be overcome if large amounts of acetylcholine accumulate around the receptors. Thus, it is possible to reverse the effects of atropine by administering a cholinesterase inhibitor.

If nurses understand the actions of parasympathetic nerves, they will have no difficulty remembering atropine's effects. Parasympathetic stimulation decreases heart rate; increases respiratory tract, salivary gland and gastric secretion; stimulates motor activity in the stomach, duodenum, jejunum, ileum and colon; constricts the pupil; and enables the eye to accommodate for near vision. Sympathetic cholinergic stimulation increases the secretion of sweat.

The cholinergic block induced by atropine produces exactly the opposite effects. It increases heart rate, decreases the secretions of the respiratory tract, salivary and sweat glands, reduces gastric secretion and motor activity of the stomach, duodenum, jejunum, ileum and colon, dilates the pupil and produces a paralysis of accommodation for near vision (cycloplegia).

Not all cholinergic functions are equally susceptible to the blocking actions of atropine. Secretions of the sweat, salivary and respiratory tract glands are most easily depressed. Larger systemic doses are required to produce dilatation of the pupil (mydriasis), cycloplegia and inhibition of vagal tone to the heart. Still higher doses of atropine are needed to inhibit parasympathetic activity to the gastrointestinal tract, ureter and urinary bladder. A reduction in gastric secretion requires the highest doses of atropine, and there is some suggestion that it is impossible to obtain this effect with normal therapeutic quantities.

Therapeutic Uses

One of the major uses of atropine has been to modify gastrointestinal function. Prior to the introduction of the histamine$_2$ blocker cimetidine (Tagamet), atropine and atropine-like drugs were widely used in the management of peptic ulcers (see Chapter 22). They were used alone and in combination with antacids and central nervous system depressants. Many of these products had only minimal effect. As mentioned before, very high doses of atropine, and most atropine-like drugs, must be used to inhibit gastric acid secretion and reduce gastrointestinal motility.

Atropine is well established as a component of preanesthetic medications. It is used because of its ability to inhibit the secretions of the salivary glands and the respiratory tract. Scopolamine (hyoscine) is also derived from belladonna. It mimics the peripheral effects of atropine but has a greater effect on the brain, producing considerable drowsiness, euphoria and amnesia. Scopolamine can also cause fatigue and sleep and is used as one component of preanesthetic medication.

Atropine can be used to treat bradycardia and syncope caused by a hyperactive carotid sinus reflex. In this condition even a small increase in blood pressure stimulates the carotid sinus pressor receptors to slow the heart reflexly by increasing vagal stimulation. As a result of the abrupt fall in heart rate, patients may faint. Atropine blocks muscarinic receptors on the heart and prevents the action of the vagus nerve. It can also assist in the treatment of A-V conduction disturbances caused by increased vagal activity.

The use of atropine to treat the toxicities of the cholinesterase inhibitors is discussed in Chapter 5. Patients treated with neostigmine, pyridostigmine or ambenonium for myasthenia gravis sometimes also receive atropine, or an atropine-like drug, to minimize the consequence of acetylcholine accumulation around muscarinic receptors. However, neither atropine nor any other anticholinergic drug should be routinely incorporated into the patient's therapeutic regimen. Masking the signs of increased muscarinic stimulation may lead to cholinergic crisis.

Atropine and scopolamine are effective in preventing motion sickness. The mechanism of this effect is not clear. However, there is little doubt that humans will spend considerably less time bent over in the washroom on ocean cruises if they premedicate with atropine or scopolamine. The scopolamine-impregnated disc, known either as Transderm-SCOP or Transderm-V, can be stuck behind the ear. Scopolamine is absorbed through the skin over a period of thirty-six to forty-eight hours. Patients often receive considerable protection from motion sickness if they use the product.

Adverse Effects

The adverse effects of atropine result from its ability to diminish or block most cholinergic functions in the body. These have already been listed in the paragraph dealing with the drug's pharmacological effects. Obviously, a desired effect for one patient may be an adverse effect for another. For example, if atropine is used to decrease the flow of saliva, its adverse effects include cycloplegia, mydriasis, tachycardia, decreased gastrointestinal and urinary bladder activity and a reduction in sweat production. On the other hand, if the drug is given to reduce vagal effects on the heart, an increase in heart rate is the desired, and not an adverse, effect. In that case, dry mouth joins the other actions of atropine as an adverse effect. The major difference between atropine and scopolamine is the ability of the latter agent to produce a marked central nervous system depression.

Nursing Process

Assessment

Prior to the administration of atropine or scopolamine, nurses must check the patient's history for documentation of glaucoma, hypertension, coronary artery disease, chronic gastrointestinal conditions, asthma or pulmonary disease. With respect to glaucoma, the mydriasis produced by atropine reduces aqueous humor drainage, increasing intraocular pressure. Giving it to a patient who already suffers from glaucoma can have disastrous consequences. Atropine increases heart rate and patients who suffer from hypertension or coronary artery disease should not receive a drug that produces tachycardia unless it is absolutely necessary.

Physical assessment should focus on the patient's cardiovascular status. Baseline measures of vital signs should be carefully documented, particularly the cardiovascular parameters.

Administration

Atropine should be administered only from a light-resistant (brown glass or opaque plastic) container since it is altered by exposure to light. When atropine or scopolamine are administered as part of a preanesthetic medication, the patient should remain in bed and the nurse must raise the side rails to prevent falls.

Evaluation

Atropine blocks salivation. Patients often consume large amounts of fluids, just to wet their mouths. As a result, their urine volumes may increase two-to three-fold and urinary electrolytes may be affected by the large volumes voided. Nurses caring for patients on long-term atropine therapy should evaluate their patients' electrolyte status and fluid balance regularly.

Teaching

Patients who are receiving long-term atropine therapy should be warned of the drug's adverse effects but advised not to discontinue taking the drug abruptly. Members of the family should also be alerted to the indicators of the drug's toxicity.

Atropine-like Mydriatics and Cycloplegics

Atropine is an effective mydriatic and cycloplegic. It does, however, have a long duration of action. Patients would obviously not be impressed if they were forced to walk around for a day or more unable to accommodate for near vision and with one or both pupils the size of small bowling balls just because a physician needed to produce mydriasis for a short period of time.

Synthetic or semisynthetic anticholinergics, such as cyclopentolate (Cyclogyl) and homatropine, may be substituted for atropine when a shorter duration of action is desired (see Chapter 36). The drugs are used to produce mydriasis in order to allow for a thorough retinal examination. They are also used to treat iritis, iridocyclitis, keratitis and choroiditis. The cycloplegic effects are desirable for accurate measurement of refractive errors.

Nursing Process

The nursing process is the same for these drugs as for the ophthalmic use of atropine.

Assessment

As mentioned before, mydriatics reduce the drainage of the aqueous humor and are contraindicated in patients who are predisposed to narrow-angle glaucoma. Their use in this condition may lead to an abrupt increase in the intraocular pressure and attack of acute glaucoma.

Administration

When instilled in the eye these drugs should be placed in the lower conjunctival sac and followed by compression of the nasal-lacrimal duct for one minute to prevent systemic absorption.

Atropine-like Antispasmodics

Many synthetic and semisynthetic anticholinergics have been placed on the market for the treatment of peptic ulcers and intestinal spasms (see Chapter 22). The drugs are claimed to be more effective than atropine and produce a lower incidence of systemic adverse effects. To a degree these claims may be justified. Most of the drugs are less readily absorbed from the intestinal tract than atropine and do not cross the blood-brain barrier as readily as atropine. This should reduce their systemic and central nervous system adverse effects.

It is beyond the scope of this book to discuss all

atropine substitutes. Some of the more popular ones include the semisynthetic drug homatropine methyl bromide and the synthetic compounds propantheline (Probanthine), glycopyrrolate (Robinul), isopropamide (Darbid) and oxyphenonium (Antrenyl). Attention should be drawn to pirenzepine (Gastrozepin). This anticholinergic effectively inhibits gastric acid secretion. It is effective in treating peptic ulcers and has minimal additional effects.

Nursing Process

Nurses should remember that these drugs are essentially atropine-like in their effects. They also have the same adverse effects and contraindications. Therefore, the nursing processes are also the some as those for atropine.

Atropine-like Antiasthmatics

Ipratropium bromide (Atrovent Inhaler) is an anticholinergic drug that is administered by inhalation. By blocking the action of the vagus competitively, it dilates bronchioles, reduces mucus secretion and decreases edema. Ipratropium is poorly absorbed and has few systemic effects. It is a less effective bronchodilator than inhaled $beta_2$ stimulants. The action of ipratropium and its role in the treatment of asthma is discussed in more detail in Chapter 32.

Nursing Process

Assessment
It is important to assess the patient for palpitations. If they become severe, it may be necessary to consider altering drug therapy.

Administration
Store ipratropium at room temperature. Have items such as hard candy, frequent drinks and gum on hand to relieve dry mouth.

Evaluation
Evaluate the patient for therapeutic response and the ability to breathe adequately. Also evaluate for long-term tolerance.

Teaching
Nurses should caution the patient that compliance to the number of inhalations per twenty-four hours is necessary to eliminate the chance of drug overdose.

Ganglionic Blocking Drugs

Ganglionic blockers competitively inhibit acetylcholine from stimulating the nicotinic receptors in the autonomic ganglia. They are rarely used today because they indiscriminately block both the sympathetic and parasympathetic nervous systems. Historically, their use has been to inhibit sympathetic function and thereby lower blood pressure. However, the fact that they also prevent parasympathetic function has given them an unacceptable level of toxicity. In addition, the rapid fall in blood pressure produced by ganglionic blockers can be dangerous to patients with coronary or cerebrovascular insufficiency.

Ganglionic blockers are used occasionally during surgery to produce a rapid and controlled fall in blood pressure. This is done to reduce blood loss during surgery.

Hexamethonium (the original drug introduced in the early 1950s), mecamylamine (Inversine), chlorisondamine (Ecolid) and trimethapan (Arfonad) are ganglionic blockers currently available for use. The differences between these agents and the nursing process related to them will not be discussed, as it is unlikely that most nurses will be charged with the clinical management of patients treated with any of them.

Further Reading

Brown, Joan Heller (1990). "Atropine, Scopolamine and Related Antimuscarinic Drugs." In: *Goodman and Gilman's The Pharmacological Basis of Therapeutics,* 8th ed. (pp. 150-165), ed. Alfred Goodman Gilman, Theodore W. Rall, Alan S. Nies and Palmer Taylor. New York: Pergamon.

Hoover, D. B. (1986). "Muscarinic Blocking Drugs." In: *Modern Pharmacology,* 2nd ed. (pp. 213-225), ed. Charles R. Craig and Robert E. Stitzel. Boston: Little, Brown.

Taylor, Palmer (1990). "Agents Acting at the Neuromuscular Junction and Autonomic Ganglia." In: *Goodman and Gilman's The Pharmacological Basis of Therapeutics,* 8th ed. (pp. 166-186), ed. Alfred Goodman Gilman, Theodore W. Rall, Alan S. Nies and Palmer Taylor. New York: Pergamon.

Table 4
Anticholinergic drugs.

Pharmacologic Classification: Anticholinergic Drugs — Antimuscarinic Drugs

Generic Name (Trade Name)	Use (Dose)	Action	Adverse Effects	Drug Interactions	Nursing Process
Atropine	**Preoperative:** To inhibit salivary and respiratory secret'n; prevent anesthetic depress'n of CV system (**SC/IM/IV:** 0.4-0.6 mg approx. 0.5 h preop)	Competitive blocking of acetylcholine stim. of muscarinic receptors	Tachycardia, bronchial plugs, decr. GI motility, mydriasis, cycloplegia, dry flushed skin, urinary retention		**Assess:** Hx of glaucoma, hypertens'n, coronary artery disease, chronic GI conditions, asthma or pulmonary disease. VS. **Administer:** From light-resistant container. Ophthalmic: Compress canaliculi and nasal-lacrimal duct for 1 min. **Evaluate:** Effectiveness for purpose given; atropine toxicity; fluid balance and electrolyte status prn for pts on long-term therapy.
	Bradycardia and syncope due to hyperactive carotid sinus reflex (**Oral/parenteral:** 0.4-0.6 mg q4-6h)	Competitive blocking of vagal impulses to the heart; incr. heart rate	Decr. GI motility, mydriasis, cycloplegia, dry flushed skin, urinary retention		
	Ophthalmic: For refract'n and to treat uveitis or iritis (**Topically:** 0.125-3% solut'n or ointment. For additional details on usage refer to Table 36)	Competitive blocking of parasympathetic fibers to iris and ciliary body leads to mydriasis and cycloplegia	**Local:** Acute angle-closure glaucoma, contact dermatitis, allergic conjunctivitis, posterior synechiae. **Systemic:** See above		
	To counteract toxicity caused by cholinesterase inhibitors (**SC/IM/IV:** As above)	As above	As above		As above
Scopolamine (Hyoscine)	**Preoperative:** To induce drowsiness, fatigue, sleep, euphoria, amnesia; to decr. respiratory and salivary secret'ns (**Oral:** 0.5-1 mg. **SC/IM:** 0.3-0.6 mg)	As for atropine, w. addit'nal CNS depress'n	As for atropine		As for atropine

CHAPTER 7

Adrenergic Drugs

Adrenergic drugs stimulate either alpha$_1$, beta$_1$ or beta$_2$ receptors or all three. These drugs mimic, at least in part, the effects of sympathetic nervous system stimulation. Adrenergic drugs are best studied by reviewing first the actions of epinephrine, levarterenol (norepinephrine) and isoproterenol, because all newer compounds have been designed to mimic some of the actions of these three.

Epinephrine (Adrenalin)

Mechanism of Action and Pharmacological Effects

Epinephrine is an emergency hormone, released by the adrenal medullae in times of stress. The chemical is known as adrenaline in many parts of the world. Adrenalin (without the e on the end) is a trade name. Epinephrine stimulates alpha$_1$, beta$_1$ and beta$_2$ receptors. When epinephrine is secreted by the adrenals it increases heart rate and force of contraction (beta$_1$); dilates bronchioles (beta$_2$); and redistributes blood in the body by constricting the blood vessels in the peritoneal cavity (alpha$_1$) and dilating those in skeletal muscle, myocardium and liver (beta$_2$). Other effects of epinephrine include a contraction of the radial muscles in the iris (alpha$_1$) and a constriction of the blood vessels in the skin (also alpha$_1$).

Nurses often see the last-named effects — dilatation of the pupils and constriction of the blood vessels in the skin. Patients about to receive a needle or undergo some other stressful procedure are "all eyes" and have a complexion that closely resembles stripped whitefish. This is simply a manifestation of the patient's fight-or-flight mechanism and should not overly concern the nurse.

Epinephrine also increases the respiratory rate and tidal volume, thereby reducing alveolar carbon dioxide. This effect, together with the increase in cardiac output, improves tissue oxygenation. At the same time, epinephrine increases the concentrations of glucose, lactate and free fatty acids in the blood. All are necessary if the stimulated tissues are to receive the metabolic materials to meet their increased needs.

The effects of injected epinephrine may differ from those observed when the chemical is released from the adrenals. This difference is due to the fact that the quantities injected may exceed the amounts normally secreted by the adrenals. If epinephrine is infused at a rate that approximates the physiological release ($10 - 30$ µg/min), heart rate and cardiac output increase and blood is shunted according to the route outlined above.

If, however, epinephrine is infused in supra-physiological amounts, it produces a generalized alpha$_1$-mediated effect on blood vessels. All blood vessels in the body will constrict. Although the heart rate may increase initially, it will later decrease, and bradycardia will ensue in response to the increase in blood pressure. Remember that the purpose of the pressor receptors in the carotid sinus and aortic arch is to protect the body from excessive increases in blood pressure. When stimulated by an increase in blood pressure, such as would be produced by an epinephrine-induced increase in peripheral resistance, the carotid sinus and aortic arch receptors reflexly slow the heart by stimulating the parasympathetic vagus nerve. Blood pressure then falls in response to the decrease in cardiac output.

Therapeutic Uses

Epinephrine cannot be given orally because it is inactivated in the gastrointestinal tract. It is usually administered intramuscularly or subcutaneously. Occasionally epinephrine is given by inhalation to produce bronchodilatation.

The therapeutic uses of epinephrine are based on its actions on the cardiovascular system and bronchioles. By stimulating beta$_2$ receptors, epinephrine dilates bronchioles. Because of its potency and rapid onset of action, epinephrine can be used to treat status asthmaticus, an emergency situation. It has also been used in the past on a chronic basis to treat bronchial asthma. However, more selective beta$_2$ stimulant drugs are available, and these have largely replaced inhalation epinephrine for this indication (see Chapter 32).

Epinephrine may be injected to treat acute hypersensitivity or anaphylactic reactions. The release of histamine in these conditions constricts bronchioles and dilates blood vessels. Epinephrine

is the drug of choice because its pharmacological effects are opposite to those of histamine. It dilates the bronchioles constricted by histamine and constricts the blood vessels dilated by histamine.

Anyone who has enjoyed a visit to the dentist may remember the cardiac palpitations experienced shortly after the local anesthetic was injected. These effects are due to the absorption of epinephrine from the local anesthetic-epinephrine mixture. Epinephrine is routinely added to solutions of local anesthetics as a vasoconstrictor to keep the local anesthetic local for as long a period as possible.

Epinephrine is also the Hollywood drug of salvation. Administered routinely in the movies or on television, it invariably restarts even the deadest of hearts. Alas, in true life its effects are not usually so predictable. Rare is the still heart that springs back to life after a spurt of epinephrine. However, epinephrine is used in attempts to restore cardiac rhythm in patients following cardiac arrest.

Adverse Effects

The adverse effects of epinephrine resemble a very acute case of stage fright. These include fear, anxiety, tenseness, restlessness and a throbbing headache — effects often experienced by performers before going on stage. Once in front of the audience, tremor, weakness, pallor, respiratory difficulties and palpitations take over. This may seem a cavalier way to view the adverse effects or toxicities of epinephrine, but by thinking of them in this way all but the coolest individual will remember them by association.

The inadvertent intravenous injection of a large dose of epinephrine can cause cerebral hemorrhage and cardiac arrhythmias. The cerebral hemorrhage results from the abrupt increase in blood pressure.

Nursing Process

Assessment
Pending confirmation from the physician, the initial dose of epinephrine should be withheld from patients who are pregnant or who report a history of glaucoma, cardiovascular, circulatory or cerebrovascular disease, prostatic hypertrophy, diabetes mellitus or hyperthyroidism. The patient's current drug profile should also be reviewed for use of tricyclic antidepressants, antidiabetic drugs, antihistamines, beta blockers, or l-thyroxine. Drug interactions may occur when these drugs are taken concurrently with epinephrine. Baseline measurements should include blood pressure, rate and rhythm of pulse and the color and temperature of the patient's extremities. These can be compared

with the same parameters measured after epinephrine administration.

Administration

Epinephrine is light sensitive and should be kept in light-proof containers. It is a very potent drug; that is, the strength and power of the drug is such that a small amount has a very dramatic, major effect. This high potency leaves no room for administration error and therefore a tuberculin syringe should be used. Nurses should aspirate from the injection site to ensure that the needle has not entered a blood vessel. Remember, epinephrine is highly potent to the extent that it can be life threatening if inadvertently given intravenously. If long-term administration is required, the injection sites should be rotated to prevent tissue necrosis. According to one authority, the injection site should be massaged after administration.

Evaluation

Following epinephrine administration, nurses should monitor the patient's response. Particular attention should be paid to the early detection of epinephrine-induced toxicities. Blood pressure should be taken and recorded at frequent intervals. If the decision is taken to inject epinephrine intravenously, the nurse should measure the blood pressure constantly until it stabilizes and at five-minute intervals thereafter.

Accurate recording of the urinary output will detect urinary retention. If it occurs, appropriate treatment must be taken.

The patient's posture, frequency of changes in position, and respiratory rate will often provide early indications of anxiety. Feelings of anxiety and tension that are disproportionate to the situation may reflect excessive doses of epinephrine.

Teaching

Patient teaching is essential if epinephrine is prescribed for self-medication. The patient should be instructed to sit or lie prior to using the medication in order to prevent falls resulting from dizziness. Patients should be taught to store epinephrine in a cool dark place and discard discolored (pinkish) solutions. Instruction in the proper use of the delivery vehicle (aerosol, nebulizer, individual metered-dose unit) is essential. All patients should be taught to use only the minimum number of puffs to provide relief from respiratory problems. Depending on the product used, the usual dose is one or two puffs. If repeated doses are necessary, they should be separated by an interval of at least two minutes. Both the patient and a responsible member of the family should be instructed in the symptoms of toxicity and in the proper method for counting the pulse rate. Patients and their families should also be aware that if respiratory distress is not relieved after twenty minutes, immediate medical assistance should be sought.

Norepinephrine; Noradrenaline; Levarterenol (Levophed)

Mechanism of Action and Pharmacological Effects

Norepinephrine (also known as noradrenaline and levarterenol) must feel much like a younger child at school who is always compared to an older sibling. Although sharing some characteristics with epinephrine, norepinephrine is not able to do everything epinephrine can. This only stands to reason. Norepinephrine is not an emergency hormone. It should, therefore, not be expected to shunt blood from one part of the body to another, increase respiration or stimulate intermediary metabolism. Rather, it is a neurotransmitter, primarily responsible for cardiovascular control.

Norepinephrine is a potent $alpha_1$ stimulant, affecting both arterioles and veins. It has little activity on $beta_2$ receptors. The release of norepinephrine throughout the body constricts arterioles and increases peripheral resistance. One manifestation of norepinephrine-induced arteriolar constriction is a reduction in blood flow through skeletal muscles. This is in contrast to the increase in skeletal muscle blood flow produced by the $beta_2$-stimulating actions of epinephrine.

As mentioned above, norepinephrine constricts veins. The simple act of standing releases norepinephrine from nerves innervating these vessels. The ensuing vasoconstriction prevents blood from accumulating in the lower extremities of the body and ensures adequate venous return to the heart.

Like epinephrine, norepinephrine stimulates $beta_1$ receptors in the heart. The release of norepinephrine by the sympathetic cardiac accelerator nerves increases heart rate. On the other hand, the infusion of norepinephrine slows the heart. In this situation, the $alpha_1$-mediated increase in peripheral resistance reflexly stimulates the parasympathetic vagus nerves. The increase in parasympathetic stimulation to the heart more than offsets the direct $beta_1$-stimulant effects of the drug.

Therapeutic Uses

Similar to epinephrine, norepinephrine cannot be given orally. It is injected intravenously for the maintenance of blood pressure in acute hypotensive states, surgical and nonsurgical trauma, central vasomotor depression and hemorrhage (see Chapter 15).

Adverse Effects

Norepinephrine can produce bradycardia, as a result of the increase in peripheral resistance. The consequences of an overdosage are similar to those of epinephrine. They include hypertension, headaches and severely decreased blood flow producing renal or hepatic failure. Local tissue necrosis may occur at the injection site.

Nursing Process

The nursing responsibilities related to norepinephrine are similar to those for epinephrine.

Assessment
Patient assessment prior to the injection of norepinephrine is identical to that required before epinephrine administration. It includes a review of the patient's history for glaucoma, cardiovascular, circulatory, or cerebrovascular disease, prostatic hypertrophy, diabetes mellitus, hyperthyroidism or pregnancy. Baseline blood pressure, pulse rate and rhythm should be established, and the skin color and temperature of the extremities should be recorded. Because drug interactions are possible, the patient's drug history should be reviewed for concurrent use of amphetamines, tricyclic antidepressants, guanethidine, or methyldopa.

Administration
Norepinephrine is administered intravenously and only by a physician. Nurses may be called upon to prepare the equipment necessary for administration and to monitor the patient carefully during administration. The medication should be stored in a light-resistant container until required, in order to prevent its oxidation. Norepinephrine is diluted in solutions of dextrose in water or saline, rather than saline alone, also to prevent oxidation. Infusion is via a piggyback, double-bottle administration setup, preferably with an infusion pump attached, to ensure the accuracy of the dosage. Under no circumstances should norepinephrine be administered using the same parenteral solution or tubing as heparin, since they are physically incompatible. Similarly, whole blood or plasma should not be administered via the same tubing setup as norepinephrine.

Evaluation
Nursing evaluation related to norepinephrine is the same as for epinephrine: continuous monitoring of blood pressure and pulse; observation of fluid intake and output and color of skin; and a notation of mentation. Special attention should be directed to the monitoring of fluid intake and output of patients receiving norepinephrine. This provides an accurate surrogate measure of renal blood flow, which is important because renal failure is a potential adverse effect of norepinephrine. The infusion site should be observed closely for evidence of extravasation that can result in ischemia and tissue sloughing.

Isoproterenol (Isuprel)

Mechanism of Action and Pharmacological Effects

Isoproterenol is a potent stimulant of $beta_1$ and $beta_2$ receptors. It increases both heart rate and force of contraction, a $beta_1$-mediated effect, while decreasing peripheral resistance and blood pressure, a $beta_2$ response. Isoproterenol also dilates the bronchioles as a result of its ability to stimulate $beta_2$ receptors.

Therapeutic Uses

Isoproterenol can be used to treat bronchial asthma but has three major drawbacks. First, it cannot be given orally. Although oral and sublingual products are on the market, their effects are very unpredictable. Therefore, isoproterenol is usually given by inhalation for the treatment of asthma. Second, it stimulates both $beta_1$ and $beta_2$ receptors. As a result, it usually produces both bronchodilatation along with annoying tachycardia. Finally, isoproterenol has a short duration of action of two to three hours. Newer adrenergic bronchodilators, such as albuterol/salbutamol, terbutaline and fenoterol circumvent these problems. They have a more selective action on $beta_2$ receptors, may be administered both orally and by inhalation, and have a longer duration of action than isoproterenol.

Isoproterenol is also available in a parenteral dosage form. Given by injection isoproterenol is used for the prevention or treatment of (1) Adams-Stokes syndrome and other episodes of heart block, except when caused by ventricular tachycardia or fibrillation, (2) cardiac arrest, (3) carotid sinus hypersensitivity, (4) ventricular arrhythmias, especially certain types of ventricular tachycardia and fibrillation, (5) laryngobronchospasm during anesthesia and (6) as adjunctive therapy in shock.

The cardiac effects are due to the beta$_1$ stimulation produced by isoproterenol. The use of the drug to modify cardiac function has decreased over the past two decades.

Adverse Effects

The adverse effects of isoproterenol are predictable. Excessive sympathetic beta receptor stimulation leads to tachycardia, palpitation, nervousness, nausea and vomiting. Other adverse effects are headache, flushing of the skin, tremor, dizziness, weakness, precordial distress or anginal-type pain. Again, these effects can be accounted for by the vasodilatation and cardiac stimulation produced by the drug.

Nursing Process

Assessment
Prior to the first administration of isoproterenol, the patient's history should be examined in the same fashion as for epinephrine. Documentation of the following should be sought: current pregnancy; glaucoma; cardiovascular, circulatory, or cerebrovascular disease; prostatism; diabetes mellitus; or hyperthyroidism. In addition, nurses should review the patients' current drug regimen for concurrent use of tricyclic antidepressents and beta blockers. If any of these conditions are present, the physician should be consulted. It is imperative that physical assessment of the patient establish baseline measures of vital signs.

Administration
The administration of isoproterenol is most commonly achieved using a metered nebulizer. The patient should be instructed to insert the mouthpiece between his teeth and close his lips around it. He should be instructed to exhale completely through his nose. This is then followed by simultaneously inhaling through the mouth and releasing the dose of medication from the nebulizer. The patient should hold his breath for as long as possible and then exhale slowly.

Evaluation
Nursing evaluation related to the patient's self-administration of isoproterenol should include monitoring the frequency of use, effectiveness of the medication on the bronchioles, as well as blood pressure and pulse.

Teaching
The most important aspect of patient teaching is the proper method of self-administration and use of the nebulizer. Many patients, including long-time users of nebulizers, use them incorrectly. It will enhance the nurse's teaching and the patient's understanding to use well-developed visual education materials. Make sure to observe the patient's use of the nebulizer.

Patients should be advised that pink sputum and saliva can occur following the use of isoproterenol. They should also be instructed regarding the necessity of keeping the nebulizer clean. The patient and responsible family members should all be aware that failure of the medication to relieve respiratory difficulty or the necessity of more than three doses in a twenty-four hour period are indications of the need to seek immediate medical attention. Nurses should also ensure that patients and their families know how to take pulse rates and that they are aware of the symptoms of adverse effects of isoproterenol. Nurses should caution patients against overconfidence with this medication. Patients must be instructed to seek medical treatment quickly if use of the medication does not provide adequate relief.

Ephedrine

Ephedrine is not a new adrenergic drug. Prior to its introduction in North America in 1924, ephedrine had been used for about 2000 years in China. It is an alpha$_1$, beta$_1$ and beta$_2$ stimulant and can also produce central nervous system excitation.

Oral ephedrine is used alone and in combination with theophylline as a bronchodilator. Because it is a less effective bronchodilator and also increases heart rate, ephedrine has largely been replaced by beta$_2$ stimulants, such as albuterol/salbutamol, fenoterol and terbutaline. In addition, ephedrine produces unwanted vasoconstriction and central nervous system stimulation.

Use is made of the alpha$_1$ stimulant properties of ephedrine in various cold remedies to constrict blood vessels in the nose and reduce tissue swelling. It may be given orally or instilled locally when its nasal vasoconstrictor action is desired.

Nursing Process

The nursing process related to the use of ephedrine is identical to that discussed for epinephrine. The only difference is the need to assess the potential for drug interaction with guanethidine and monoamine oxidase inhibitors.

Dopamine (Dopastat, Intropin, Revimine) and Dobutamine (Dobutrex)

Mechanism of Action and Pharmacological Effects

Dopamine and dobutamine are newer adrenergic agents with major cardiovascular effects. They are discussed together because they share many pharmacological effects and the nursing process related to their use is the same. Dopamine is the precursor of norepinephrine as well as a transmitter in its own right within the brain. When injected as a drug, dopamine stimulates the beta$_1$ receptors in the heart to increase both heart rate and stroke volume. It produces a smaller increase in heart rate than isoproterenol. In contrast to the pure alpha$_1$ stimulants, which increase peripheral resistance, and the beta$_2$ stimulants, which decrease peripheral resistance, dopamine, in low to intermediate therapeutic doses, has no effect on peripheral resistance. A significant effect of dopamine is its ability to increase the glomerular filtration rate, renal blood flow and sodium excretion. This has been attributed to the presence of specific dopamine receptors on the kidney blood vessels.

Dobutamine stimulates beta$_1$ receptors in the heart. It is claimed to produce a greater increase in contractile force than in heart rate. Dobutamine does not stimulate the dopamine receptors on the renal vasculature and, as a result, does not produce renal vasodilation, increase the glomerular filtration or sodium excretion. The major advantage of dobutamine over the other sympathomimetics with beta stimulating properties is its apparent ability to increase cardiac output with minimal effects on heart rate. As a result, the increase in oxygen requirements for the heart are not so great as might have been predicted on the basis of the jump in cardiac output.

Therapeutic Use

Both dopamine and dobutamine must be given by injection. They have fleeting actions and their effects stop within minutes of completing the infusion. Dopamine is used in the treatment of shock patients (see Chapter 15) who are experiencing decreased renal function and normal, or low, peripheral resistance. In these patients the increase in cardiac output and glomerular filtration rate produced by dopamine will provide great benefit. Patients with chronic refractory heart failure may also respond to dopamine treatment (see Chapter 10).

Patients suffering from acute congestive heart failure often benefit from an increase in cardiac output and a decrease in the pulmonary wedge pressure produced by dobutamine (see Chapter 10). The pulmonary wedge pressure is a reflection of the capacity of the left ventricle to accept blood coming back from the lungs. In congestive heart failure, it increases because the heart cannot pump all the blood that should be returned in the pulmonary vessels. Patients who have just undergone cardiopulmonary bypass operations will also benefit from dobutamine.

Adverse Effects

Dopamine and dobutamine produce tachycardia, anginal pain, arrhythmias, headache and hypertension. Nausea and vomiting may also be seen. As mentioned before, low to medium therapeutic doses of dopamine increase renal blood flow. High doses of the drug stimulate alpha$_1$ receptors on the renal blood vessels and produce vasoconstriction.

Nursing Process

Assessment
Nursing assessment includes examining the patient's history for evidence of tachycardia, ventricular fibrillation, a current pregnancy, diabetes mellitus or hypothermia. The patient's blood pressure and pulses (both apical and peripheral), as well as the color and temperature of the extremities, should be recorded prior to the first administration of either of these two drugs. Because the potential for drug interaction exists, nurses should also be alert for concurrent use of dopamine and dobutamine with tricyclic antidepressants, diuretics, halogenated hydrocarbon anesthetics, monoamine oxidase inhibitors and sympathomimetics.

Administration
Only freshly mixed dilutions should be administered. The patency of the intravenous tubing and catheter should be ensured at all times and the infusion site observed for evidence of extravasation that can cause tissue necrosis. An infusion pump should be used to facilitate precise regulation of the flow rate.

Evaluation
Constant nursing evaluation of the patient is essential because of the potency of these drugs. The patient's blood pressure, pulses, color, peripheral limb temperatures, urinary output and level of mental activity should be observed and recorded at frequent and regular intervals. Measurement of

fluid intake and output is imperative for those patients who are receiving dopamine. These measures serve as indicators of renal blood flow.

Phenylephrine (Neosynephrine)

Phenylephrine is an adrenergic drug with major cardiovascular effects. It stimulates alpha$_1$ receptors. When given orally, subcutaneously or intravenously it raises both systolic and diastolic blood pressure. As might be expected, the increase in peripheral resistance produces reflex bradycardia by stimulating the vagus nerves. Phenylephrine can be used systemically to increase blood pressure in hypotensive conditions. It is also used to dilate the pupils. Its greatest use is as a nasal vasoconstrictor in cold preparations. In this situation, it is taken orally, together with an antihistamine and an analgesic, or instilled locally in the nose as drops or mist.

Metaproterenol/Orciprenaline (Alupent), Albuterol/ Salbutamol (Proventil, Ventolin), Terbutaline (Brethine, Bricanyl), Fenoterol (Berotec), Procaterol (Pro-Air)

These newer adrenergic bronchodilators were previously discussed (see Therapeutic Uses of isoproterenol, earlier in this chapter). They have the following advantages over isoproterenol:
1. They stimulate preferentially beta$_2$ receptors.
2. They may be given orally, as well as by inhalation.
3. They have longer durations of action than isoproterenol.

The availability of the beta$_2$ stimulants has drastically reduced the use of isoproterenol and ephedrine.

In spite of their relative selectivity for beta$_2$ receptors, these drugs can produce palpitations, tachycardia, nervousness and tremor. The tachycardia reflects the fact that, in higher doses, the drugs stimulate beta$_1$ receptors. Other side effects, which can also be attributed to their sympathomimetic actions, are nausea and vomiting.

It is difficult to predict beforehand which drug will best suit a particular patient. If one agent fails to produce adequate bronchodilatation, or produces unacceptable toxicities, another drug should be tried. The nursing process for patients receiving these drugs is the same as that previously described for isoproterenol.

Further Reading

Hoffman, Brian B. and Lefkowitz, Robert J. (1991). "Catecholamines and Sympathomimetic Drugs." In: *Goodman and Gilman's The Pharmacological Basis of Therapeutics,* 8th ed. (pp. 187-220), ed. Alfred Goodman Gilman, Theodore W. Rall, Alan S. Nies and Palmer Taylor. New York: Pergamon.

Robinson, Robert L. (1986). "Adenomimetic Drugs." In: *Modern Pharmacology,* 2nd ed. (pp. 158-173), ed. Charles R. Craig and Robert S. Stitzel. Boston: Little, Brown.

Table 5
Adrenergic drugs.

Generic Name (Trade Name)	Use (Dose)	Action	Adverse Effects	Drug Interactions	Nursing Process
Pharmacologic Classification: Adrenergic Drugs					
Epinephrine/adrenaline (Adrenalin, Primatene Mist, Medihaler-Epi, Vaponephrin)	Parenteral tx for emergencies, status asthmaticus (**IM/SC:** Adults - 0.2-0.5 mL 1/1000 solut'n. Children - 0.01 mL/kg to max. of 0.5 mL SC, repeated q4h prn) Inhalat'n for systemic relief of bronchospasm and mucus secret'ns (**Inhalat'n:** Us. 2 puffs of Primatene Mist, Medihaler-Epi or Vaponephrin q4h. If no relief after initial tx, repeat in 5 min)	Bronchodilat'n due to beta$_2$ stimulat'n, incr. respiratory rate and tidal volume, reduced alveolar CO_2 concentrat'ns, reduced mucosal congest'n due to vasoconstrict'n of bronchiolar blood vessels	Fear, anxiety, tenseness, restlessness, headache, tremor, pallor, incr. intraocular pressure, respiratory difficulties, palpitat'ns, tachycardia, incr. cardiac output, hypertens'n, urinary retent'n, altered metabolism. Rapid IV infus'n of large doses can cause cerebral vascular accidents and/or cardiac arrhythmia.	**Antidepressants, tricyclic:** May incr. several-fold the pressor responses to epinephrine. **Antidiabetic drugs:** Epinephrine increases blood glucose levels. **Antihistamines:** Effects potentiated by some antihistamines. **Beta blockers:** Pts receiving beta blockers show an exaggerated alpha$_1$ (vasoconstrictor) response to epinephrine. This can produce hypertens'n and reflex vagal-induced bradycardia. **I-Thyroxine:** Effects potentiated by I-thyroxine.	**Assess:** For pt hx of glaucoma; CV, circulatory or cerebrovascular disease; prostatic hypertrophy; diabetes mellitus; hyperthyroidism; pregnancy. Establish baseline BP, rate and rhythm of pulse, color and temp. of extremities. Check for potential drug interact'ns. **Administer:** Parentally, from a light-resistant vial, using a tuberculin syringe; aspirate carefully; use SC route preferentially; rotate sites. **Evaluate:** BP and pulse carefully, esp. when IV route used; urine output, mental activity, color. **Teach** (rel. to inhalat'n): Use only number of doses nec. to achieve relief; wait 2 min bet. doses; symptoms of side effects; sit or lie down to use; discard discolored solut'ns; count pulse rate.
Epinephrine/adrenaline (Adrenalin)	In local anesthetics to extend durat'n of effect (**Parenteral:** 1:100 000 to 1:200 000 solut'n w. anesthetic)	Alpha$_1$ receptor stimulat'n produces vasoconstrict'n to reduce blood flow and therefore slows removal of local anesthetic from tissues.	As above	As above	As above
Epinephrine/adrenaline (Adrenalin)	Acute hypersensitivity react'ns and anaphylactic shock (**SC/IM:** Adults - Initially, 0.5 mL of 1:1000 solut'n, repeated q5min. Children - 0.01 mL/kg, max. 0.3 mL)	Bronchodilat'n and vasoconstrict'n due to stim. of beta$_2$ and alpha$_1$ receptors, respectively	As above	As above	As above
Epinephrine/adrenaline (Adrenalin)	Cardiac resuscitat'n (**IV or intracardiac:** 0.5 mL diluted to 10 mL with NaCl)	Beta$_1$ myocardial stimulat'n incr. myocardial contractility and ventricular irritability.	As above	As above	As above

Drug	Uses / Dosage	Action	Side Effects	Nursing Considerations
Norepinephrine/ noradrenaline/ levarterenol (Levophed)	Acute hypotens'n (shock) due to trauma, myocardial infarct, bacteremia, anaphylaxis (**IV:** Adults - 0.03-0.15 μg/kg/min)	Vasoconstrict'n due to stim. of alpha₁ receptors	Headache, restlessness, anxiety, weakness, pallor, dizziness, tremor, precordial pain, palpitat'ns, respiratory distress, convuls'ns, cerebral hemorrhage and bradycardia	**Amphetamine:** May incr. the pressor response to IV levarterenol. **Antidepressants, tricyclic:** May incr. several-fold the pressor response to levarterenol. Give IV levarterenol only with great caution. **Guanethidine:** Incr. response to levarterenol. Administer levarterenol very cautiously. **Methyldopa:** Can incr. and prolong pressor effect of levarterenol. Pts on methyldopa should be given levarterenol cautiously, beginning w. small doses.	**Assess:** As for epinephrine. **Administer:** From light-resistant storage container; in dextrose solut'n via piggyback double-bag IV administrat'n setup; do not use same parenteral solut'n or tubing to administer whole blood, plasma or heparin; most accurate administrat'n is achieved using an infus'n pump. **Evaluate:** As for epinephrine, particularly fluid intake/output; observe for symptoms of overdose (photophobia, headache, blurred vision, vomiting, palpitation, chest pain, arrhythmia); check infus'n site for extravasat'n, which can result in ischemia and tissue sloughing.
Dopamine (Dopastat, Intropin, Revimine)	To incr. cardiac output and improve renal blood flow in shock due to myocardial infarct, sepsis, trauma, as well as in acute renal failure, open heart surgery and chronic congestive heart failure (**IV:** 2-5 μg/kg/min, to max. 20-50 μg/kg/min for seriously ill pts)	Stim. of beta₁ receptors in the heart to incr. both heart rate and stroke volume. Low to intermediate doses have no effect on peripheral resistance. Stimulates specific dopamine receptors on renal blood vessels to incr. GFR, renal blood flow and Na excret'n.	Tachycardia, angina, cardiac arrhythmias, headache, hypertens'n, nausea, vomiting. High doses cause vasoconstrict'n of renal blood vessels.	**Antidepressants, tricyclic:** Pressor response to dopamine may be potentiated by TCAs. **Diuretics:** Dopamine should be used extra cautiously concurrently w. diuretics because it may produce an additive or potentiating effect. **Halogenated hydrocarbon anesthetics:** Incr. cardiac autonomic irritability and sensitize the myocardium to dopamine's action. Dopamine should be used w. extreme caution in these pts. **MAOIs:** Reduce rate of dopamine inactivat'n. Reduce starting dose of dopamine to at least 10% of usual dose. **Sympathomimetics:** Use dopamine cautiously in pts receiving sympathomimetics concomitantly. **Assess:** Pt hx of tachycardia, ventricular fibrillat'n, pregnancy, diabetes, hypothermia; establish baseline BP, pulses, color and temp. of extremities. Check for potential drug interact'ns. **Administer:** Freshly mixed dilut'n through patent IV, avoiding extravasat'n, which can cause necrosis; provide constant nsg observat'n. **Evaluate:** BP, pulses (apical and peripheral), color and temp. of extremities, urinary output, mentation.

Generic Name (Trade Name)	Use (Dose)	Action	Adverse Effects	Drug Interactions	Nursing Process
Dobutamine (Dobutrex)	Tx of cardiac decompensat'n due to depressed contractility from organic heart disease or surgical procedures **(IV:** *For congestive heart failure,* 2.5-10 µg/kg/min; *for hypotens'n and shock,* 8-24 µg/kg/min)	Stimulates beta$_1$ receptors in heart, incr. cardiac output w. minimal effects on heart rate. Does not produce renal vasodilatat'n, incr. GFR or Na excret'n.	Tachycardia, angina, cardiac arrhythmias, headache, hypertens'n, nausea, vomiting	As for dopamine	As for dopamine
Isoproterenol (Isuprel, Vapo-Iso, Medihaler-Iso)	Symptomatic relief of bronchospasm in asthma and other chronic bronchopulmonary disorders in which bronchospasm is a complicating factor **(Inhalat'n:** 1-2 puffs from preset nebulizing unit, max. 8x/day for adults) To treat low output states caused by myocardial failure (excluding pts w. coronary artery disease), cardiac surgery, pericardial compress'n, bacteremic shock and bradyarrhythmias **(SC/IM:** 200 µg. **IV:** 20 µg. **IV infus'n:** Containing 1 mg in 200 mL of 5% glucose at a rate of 1 mL [5 µg]/min. **Intracardiac:** 20 µg [0.1 mL 1:5000 solut'n])	Bronchodilatat'n and vasodilatat'n due to stim. of beta$_2$ receptors in the bronchioles and arterioles; myocardial stimulat'n due to beta$_1$ effects	Refractory bronchospasm, tachycardia, cardiac arrhythmias, cardiac arrest, decr. BP, headache, nausea, palpitat'ns, tremor, insomnia	**Antidepressants, tricyclic:** TCA and isoproterenol produce cumulative effects. **Beta blockers:** Can inhibit the actions of isoproterenol.	**Assess:** As for epinephrine. **Administer:** From metered nebulizer by instructing pt to insert mouthpiece bet. teeth, close lips around mouthpiece, exhale through nose, simultaneously inhale through mouth, release dose from nebulizer, hold breath for as long as possible, then exhale slowly. IV as for norepinephrine. **Evaluate:** BP and pulse; effectiveness. **Teach:** That pink saliva and sputum may occur; to contact physician if no relief or if more than 3 doses/24 h; cleanliness of nebulizer; symptoms of adverse effects; to count pulse rate; to carry nebulizer at all times. Caution pts against overconfidence w. this medicat'n for asthma. Pts must be instructed to seek medical tx quickly if use of the medicat'n does not provide adequate relief.

CHAPTER 8

Antiadrenergic Drugs

Teaching Objectives

Following completion of this chapter, the reader should be able to:

1. Identify the therapeutic uses of antiadrenergic drugs.
2. Describe the mechanism of action by which drugs may block sympathetic nervous system function.
3. Describe the effects of alpha$_1$ blockers, discuss their therapeutic uses and identify the related nursing process.
4. Describe the pharmacologic effects of propranolol and compare the action of the newer beta blockers with that of propranolol.
5. List the therapeutic uses of beta blockers, explain their toxicities and identify the associated nursing process.
6. Describe the pharmacologic effects, therapeutic uses, adverse effects and nursing actions related to the use of labetalol.
7. Explain the basis for the term adrenergic neuron blocker.
8. Describe the general pharmacologic effects and discuss briefly the uses, adverse effects and nursing process for reserpine, guanethidine and guanadrel.
9. Describe the general pharmacologic effects and discuss briefly the uses, adverse effects and nursing processes for the central sympathetic inhibitors methyldopa and clonidine.

Antiadrenergic drugs are used to block, in whole or in part, the sympathetic nervous system. The pharmacological effects they produce are due to the degree to which they decrease adrenergic functions. They are used in the treatment of hypertension, cardiac arrhythmias, angina pectoris and migraine headaches, to mention but four disorders. The pharmacology and the nursing process related to use of antiadrenergic drugs will be discussed in the present chapter. Their clinical value in the treatment of specific conditions will be discussed in greater detail in other sections of this book.

Antiadrenergic drugs are divided into adrenergic receptor blockers, adrenergic neuron blockers and central sympathetic inhibitors. The first group blocks either alpha$_1$ or beta adrenergic receptors. Adrenergic neuron blockers inhibit the release of norepinephrine from sympathetic postganglionic neurons. Central sympathetic inhibitors act within the brain to reduce sympathetic function. These groups differ significantly in their pharmacologic effects. Adrenergic neuron blockers and central sympathetic inhibitors reduce most sympathetically mediated functions. Alpha and beta blockers, on the other hand, prevent only those activities mediated by their respective receptors.

Alpha$_1$ Receptor Blockers

Phenoxybenzamine (Dibenzyline), Phentolamine (Regitine, Rogitine), Prazosin (Minipress), Terazosin (Hytrin)

Mechanism of Action and Pharmacologic Effects

Alpha$_1$ receptor blockers, more commonly called alpha blockers, include phenoxybenzamine (Dibenzyline), phentolamine (Regitine, Rogitine), prazosin (Minipress) and terazosin (Hytrin). These drugs prevent norepinephrine from stimulating alpha$_1$ receptors.

The effects they produce depend, to a great extent, on the degree of sympathetic tone existing prior to the administration of the blocker. For example, an alpha$_1$ receptor blocker will prevent sympathetic stimulation of blood vessels. Given to a recumbent subject, it will have minimal effect on blood pressure because in a reclining person the sympathetic nerves release little norepinephrine. If, however, an alpha$_1$ blocker is given to a standing patient, the blood pressure may fall dramatically because the erect body depends on norepinephrine to constrict blood vessels and maintain venous return. The vasodilatation produces a commensurate increase in heart rate.

Therapeutic Uses

Phentolamine and phenoxybenzamine were originally developed to treat essential hypertension. However, the reflex tachycardia accompanying their use offsets, to a major degree, the antihypertensive effects of the vasodilatation.

Phentolamine is used in the diagnosis of a pheochromocytoma. This is a tumor of chromaffin tissue that secretes large amounts of epinephrine and/or norepinephrine. A patient with a pheochromocytoma has bouts of severe hypertension, sweating, cardiac palpitations and other manifestations of sympathetic activity. The ability of phentolamine to produce a rapid fall in blood pressure is taken as a positive test for the present of a tumor (Regitine or Rogitine test). The availability of methods to measure epinephrine and norepinephrine concen-

trations in urine and plasma has reduced the need to use the phentolamine test.

Prazosin and terazosin are useful in treating high blood pressure (see Chapter 14). Although heart rate can increase, the tachycardia resulting from their use is not as great as would normally be expected from the drugs' ability to dilate arterioles. This is because prazosin and terazosin block only alpha$_1$ receptors and, in contradistinction to phenoxybenzamine and phentolamine, do not block alpha$_2$ receptors.

Patients with peripheral vascular disease, such as Raynaud's syndrome, may be treated with an alpha$_1$ blocker (see Chapter 13). Phenoxybenzamine has been reported to relieve vasospasm and the sensitivity to cold experienced by patients with this condition.

Adverse Effects

The adverse effects of blocking alpha$_1$ receptors include postural hypotension and reflex tachycardia. Nasal stuffiness is another consequence of vasodilatation. Blocking alpha$_1$ receptors in the iris produces parasympathetic predominance and constriction of the pupil (miosis).

Nursing Process

Assessment
Prazosin is a popular drug for the treatment of hypertension. Nurses should assess the patient's history for documentation of chronic renal failure, current pregnancy or lactation before beginning treatment. Physical assessment of patients by nursing personnel must focus on establishing baseline measures of vital signs.

In assessing patients who are on continuing prazosin therapy, nurses should determine compliance and identify patient teaching needs related to this drug.

Terazosin is a more recent introduction into the list of drugs approved from the treatment of hypertension. Its place in therapy has yet to be established. At this point the nursing process associated with its use should be considered similar to that involving the administration of prazosin.

Administration
Prazosin should be administered with food and/or milk to control the rate of absorption and reduce the possibility of dizziness from postural hypotension.

Evaluation
The initial few days of treatment with prazosin or terazosin are the most important in evaluating the patient's response to this medication. Severe postu-

ral hypotension is most often encountered during this time. Nurses should observe the patient for any evidence of syncope with sudden loss of consciousness after the initial dose of the drug, or after an increase in dose or the addition of another antihypertensive drug to the therapeutic regimen.

Teaching
The single most important factor related to prazosin or terazosin therapy is patient compliance, that is, the patient's willingness to take the prescribed medication. Prazosin's unpleasant adverse effects (dry mouth, nasal stuffiness and, occasionally, impotence) contribute to a poor record of consistent drug use. For terazosin the most frequently reported adverse effects that led to stopping the drug were dizziness, asthenia and headache. Nurses should play a very important role in teaching patients about their drug. This will include supporting patients through their initial period by assisting them to accommodate to the effects of either drug. In spite of this support some patients cannot, or will not, tolerate prazosin's effects. In this case, nurses should help them explain their problems to the physician. Requesting another drug is a much better alternative to simply stopping the medication and dropping out of the treatment program.

Four to six weeks may be required before the full antihypertensive effects of prazosin are seen. The patient should be instructed to move from the recumbent to the standing position slowly with a stop in the sitting position. This should reduce the dizziness that results from postural hypotension when the patient stands. Patients should also be instructed to lie down quickly if they feel dizzy.

Patients should be warned against driving, using power tools, or working around heavy manufacturing equipment, particularly during the initial period of treatment, during dosage adjustment, or during the addition of another antihypertensive medication to the treatment program. The antihypertensive effects of prazosin may be intensified if patients take over-the-counter cold, cough or allergy medications. Patients should be taught to seek medical advice before any of these products are taken.

Beta Blockers

1. Non-Selective Beta Receptor Blockers

Propranolol (Inderal)

Mechanism of Action and Pharmacologic Effects

The introduction of beta blockers in the 1960s represented a major therapeutic advance. Propranolol was the first beta blocker accepted in most countries of the world. Propranolol blocks the ability of epinephrine and norepinephrine to stimulate the $beta_1$ and $beta_2$ receptors (Table 6).

Table 6
Distribution of beta receptors.

Organ	Receptor Type	Effects of Stimulation
Heart	$Beta_1$	Increase in heart rate
	$Beta_1$	Increase in cardiac contractility
	$Beta_1$	Acceleration of A-V conduction
Bronchi	$Beta_2$	Dilatation
Arterioles	$Beta_2$	Dilatation
Kidney	$Beta_1$	Release of renin
Metabolism	$Beta_2$	Increase in blood sugar
	$Beta_1$	Increase in free fatty acids

Propranolol produces major effects on the cardiovascular system. Similar to $alpha_1$ receptor blockers, the consequences of propranolol treatment are determined by the degree of sympathetic stimulation that existed prior to drug treatment. In the resting individual with low sympathetic drive, propranolol has little effect on the heart. However, in the stressed or exercising human, whose myocardial function depends heavily on sympathetic stimulation, propranolol reduces or prevents the usual increase in heart rate, A-V conduction, force of contraction and cardiac output.

Propranolol lowers blood pressure. Part of this action is due to a decrease in cardiac output. The drug also reduces sympathetic nervous system activity in the brain, and this may play a role in its antihypertensive effects. In addition, propranolol decreases renin release by the kidney, and this may also be a factor in the fall in blood pressure.

Beta$_2$ receptors mediate adrenergic bronchodilatation. Propranolol blocks this effect and should not be given to asthmatic patients. If propranolol is given to the asthmatic individual, bronchiolar constriction occurs, the forced expiratory volume in one second (FEV$_1$) falls, and the patient is placed in jeopardy.

Propranolol can have marked effects on intermediary metabolism. Sympathetic stimulation increases plasma free fatty acid levels. Propranolol blocks this effect. The drug also has major effects on carbohydrate metabolism and should be used with caution in insulin-dependent diabetics. Following the injection of insulin the blood sugar falls. This triggers the release of epinephrine whose hyperglycemic effects offset, in part, the action of insulin. The resulting blood sugar is a balance between the hypoglycemic action of insulin and the hyperglycemic effects of the released epinephrine. If a diabetic patient is treated with propranolol, the effects of insulin are greater because the beta blocker decreases the effects of the released epinephrine.

Pharmacokinetics

Propranolol is usually administered orally. It is completely absorbed but subject to extensive first-pass metabolism. Only twenty to thirty per cent of the oral dose survives hepatic metabolism to reach the systemic circulation. In addition, there is considerable person-to-person variability in the extent of first-pass metabolism. This is one factor that accounts for the wide range of doses required to treat patients. Patients who require larger doses may inactivate a higher percentage of the absorbed drug during first pass through the liver. It is not uncommon to find patients managed adequately for angina pectoris on as little as 80 mg daily, whereas others may need 320 mg of the drug for the same condition.

Therapeutic Uses

Propranolol is used to prevent angina pectoris attacks (see Chapter 12). By reducing sympathetic stimulation to the heart, the drug decreases the oxygen requirements of the myocardium, protecting the patient with chronic stable angina.

Propranolol is also used to treat essential hypertension (see Chapter 14). Its mechanism of action in reducing blood pressure has been described above.

Because propranolol reduces sympathetic stimulation of the atria and A-V node, it is a valuable drug in the treatment of adrenergically

induced supraventricular arrhythmias (see Chapter 11). Propranolol is also of value in reducing mortality in patients who have suffered a myocardial infarct.

Propranolol is also used to prevent migraine headaches (see Chapter 55). Although its mechanism of action in this condition is still not clear, chronic propranolol use reduces the incidence of vascular headaches.

Obviously, propranolol is an ideal drug for the patient with a pheochromocytoma. However, this condition is very rare and most nurses may never encounter it.

Adverse Effects

Bradycardia and congestive heart failure are the most obvious adverse effects of propranolol. Nature did not provide humans with sympathetic innervation of the heart just so pharmacologists could block it with propranolol (or any other beta blocker, for that matter). A complete block of sympathetic impulses to the heart runs the risk of reducing heart rate and cardiac output to the point where heart failure ensues.

A block of beta$_2$ receptors in the bronchioles can produce bronchoconstriction in an asthmatic patient.

The other adverse effects of propranolol are not so easily explained. They include nausea, vomiting, constipation or diarrhea. Central nervous system effects are depression, disturbed sleep and nightmares. These effects, more often than any of the others, are the reasons given by patients for stopping or wanting to stop taking propranolol. Allergic reactions to propranolol include rash, fever and purpura.

Nursing Process

The pharmacological properties, therapeutic uses and adverse effects presented previously provide the rationale for the nursing process activated when propranolol is prescribed.

Assessment

In collaboration with the physician and pharmacist, the nurse should review the patient's history for evidence of any contraindications to use of propranolol. Specifically, these include: congestive heart failure, bradycardia, heart block, asthma, obstructive lung disease, diabetes or myasthenia gravis. Propranolol should be used with caution by patients with hay fever, liver or kidney disease. If the patient is pregnant or lactating, the drug should be withheld until the physician is contacted.

Nurses should discuss the patient's drug history with the pharmacist to determine potential drug interactions. Interactions can occur with antidiabetic agents, atropine, digitalis glycosides, epinephrine or levodopa. The use of psychotropic medication in conjunction with propranolol is not recommended because of the potential adverse mood-altering effects of the beta blocker. In addition, if the patient has received a monoamine oxidase inhibitor in the two weeks preceding the prescription, the physician should be contacted before the nurse administers the medication.

Nursing assessment must provide baseline measurements of blood pressure; rate and rhythm of respirations; color, warmth and peripheral pulses in the extremities. If these assessment parameters fall outside the range of normal, this information should be discussed with the physician before the drug is administered. This is an important factor in patient safety because of the physiologic effects of propranolol on cardiac and respiratory function. The results of this assessment will also be used for comparative purposes later following administration of the drug.

Administration
Propranolol should be administered from an airtight, light-resistant container. If given on a four-times-daily basis, it should be given before meals and at bedtime to facilitate absorption from the patient's empty stomach.

Evaluation
Nursing evaluation of the patient's response should focus on assessing the efficacy of propranolol in order to assist in determining the appropriate dose for the individual patient. Nurses should also concentrate on the early identification of adverse effects. To this end, the following observations should be made and recorded regularly: apical-radial pulse, fluid intake and output, daily body mass/weight, blood pressure, respirations, circulation of the extremities (including color, warmth, blanching of the skin, and peripheral pulses). Diabetics should be observed for evidence of hypoglycemia and insulin shock. If propranolol is administered intravenously, the patient's electrocardiogram should be monitored closely.

Teaching
Patients and their families should be taught to observe responses to physical and psychological stress. They should also be encouraged to develop a schedule of activity that is tailored to the individual needs of each person. Patients formerly used to intense activity in sports, for example, should be cautioned that effort of this nature may produce profound fatigue. The sudden withdrawal of propranolol can result in a rapid increase in heart rate. Patients and their families should be alerted to the danger of myocardial infarction or arrhythmias if the drug is discontinued abruptly. It is essential to have sufficient quantities of propranolol on hand at all times so that sudden accidental withdrawal of the drug will not occur.

Propranolol is often used to alter blood pressure. Accordingly, patients should be discouraged from smoking, drinking alcohol and using over-the-counter medications for colds, coughs or allergies. In addition to an antihistamine, which compounds the problems of central nervous system depression produced by propranolol, cold preparations contain an alpha$_1$ receptor stimulant that constricts blood vessels and offsets much of the antihypertensive effect of propranolol.

Because propranolol can produce drowsiness, patients should avoid driving, using power tools, or working with industrial machinery during the time the proper dosage is being established. During the period of dosage selection, while patients are learning to adjust both physically and mentally to the effects of propranolol, they should be instructed to move slowly from the recumbent to the standing position. Although propranolol does not normally cause postural hypotension, this precaution will minimize any possibility of dizziness. Finally, the patient and the family should be instructed to seek immediate medical attention if any of the signs and symptoms of adverse effects appear.

Timolol (Blocadren) and Nadolol (Corgard)

Timolol and nadolol are two beta blockers with properties similar to those of propranolol. Timolol has been shown to reduce the likelihood of death if administered to patients after a myocardial infarct. In this respect it appears to have the same benefit as propranolol.

Nadolol has a longer half-life than propranolol and timolol. It is more water soluble than propranolol and less likely to enter the brain to produce central nervous system effects.

Both timolol and nadolol are usually prescribed for the treatment of angina pectoris and hypertension. Their pharmacological properties, adverse effects and nursing process are the same as those explained for propranolol.

2. Cardioselective Beta Blockers

Acebutolol (Monitan, Sectral), Atenolol (Tenormin) and Metoprolol (Betaloc, Lopresor, Lopressor)

Acebutolol, atenolol and metoprolol are called cardioselective, suggesting that the only receptors blocked are those in the heart. This is not true. Although they do block more easily the receptors in the heart, these drugs can diminish $beta_2$ receptor effects in the bronchioles and blood vessels if sufficiently high doses are used. To understand the differences between nonselective and cardioselective beta blockers, nurses are referred to Table 7. Acebutolol differs pharmacodynamically from atenolol and metoprolol. The latter two are competitive inhibitors of $beta_1$ receptors. Acebutolol, on the other hand, is a partial agonist, affecting $beta_1$ receptors. The mechanism of action of partial-agonist beta blockers is explained below.

Attention has been focused on the reduced ability of the cardioselective drugs to block beta receptors in bronchioles. None of these drugs should be used in the asthmatic patient. These patients depend greatly on sympathetic activity to maintain their airways, and any degree of bronchoconstriction will place them at risk.

There are a few situations in which the cardioselective beta blockers are preferred over propranolol. They are better drugs in the diabetic patient receiving insulin because they do not reduce the epinephrine-induced effects on blood glucose as much as propranolol.

Acebutolol, atenolol and metoprolol may also be better than the nonselective beta blockers in their effects on peripheral circulation. During periods of stress, propranolol, timolol and nadolol may increase peripheral resistance. This occurs because of the release of epinephrine which, in the face of a $beta_2$ block, produces a generalized $alpha_1$ vascular stimulation. A patient, after waiting anxiously in

Table 7
Differences between groups of beta blockers.

	Nonselective	Cardioselective	Partial Agonist
Heart rate and force of contraction ($beta_1$)	Decrease both rate and force of contraction	Decrease both rate and force of contraction	Decrease both rate and force of contraction. Fall in resting heart rate is less with this group of beta blockers because of their partial-agonist activity.
Peripheral resistance ($beta_2$)	Increases, owing to the fact that $alpha_1$ receptors can act unopposed because $beta_2$ receptors are blocked	Little effect because $beta_2$ receptors are not blocked by cardioselective beta blockers.	May produce a slight decrease because of the $beta_2$-agonist properties.
Renin release ($beta_1$)	Decreased release	Decreased release	Decreased release
Bronchioles ($beta_2$)	Bronchoconstriction in asthmatics	Less bronchoconstriction in asthmatics but cardioselective beta blockers are not recommended for asthmatics.	Asthmatics have a reduced capacity to dilate bronchioles if a partial-agonist beta blocker is used.
Glucose metabolism ($beta_2$)	Reduced hyperglycemic response to epinephrine. Use caution in diabetes because insulin can produce increased hypoglycemia if it is given to a patient on a nonselective beta blocker.	Little effect	Reduced response to epinephrine because partial-agonist beta blockers are not as potent $beta_2$ stimulants as endogenously released epinephrine.

the doctor's office, may show an abnormally elevated diastolic pressure because of the effects of released epinephrine on the alpha$_1$ receptors. Theoretically at least, this effect should not be seen in patients who receive a cardioselective beta blocker because the epinephrine released is free to stimulate both alpha$_1$ and beta$_2$ receptors, with the effects of one offsetting those of the other.

Atenolol and acebutolol are water-soluble beta blockers. They are eliminated by renal excretion and have longer half-lives than other beta blockers, with the exception of nadolol. As a result, atenolol can be administered once a day and acebutolol twice daily. Their water solubility also reduces entry into the brain, and this may be accompanied by fewer CNS adverse effects.

Cardioselective beta blockers have the same basic clinical indications and adverse effects as propranolol. Because of this, and because the pharmacological properties of these drugs will be presented in subsequent chapters dealing with the treatment of angina and hypertension, it is appropriate to end this discussion and move on to the last group of beta blockers.

3. Beta Blockers with Intrinsic Sympathetic Activity (ISA) – Partial- Agonist Beta Blockers

Acebutolol (Monitan, Sectral), Oxprenolol (Trasicor) and Pindolol (Visken)

Acebutolol, oxprenolol and pindolol are not true beta blockers. In contrast to the drugs previously mentioned in this section, such as propranolol and metoprolol, which attach to beta receptors and block them, acebutolol, oxprenolol and pindolol have affinity for the receptors and, once attached, stimulate them. However, because their intrinsic sympathetic activity (ISA) is much less than that of either epinephrine or norepinephrine, the degree of beta stimulation is less when acebutolol, oxprenolol or pindolol occupies the receptor in place of the normal mediators epinephrine and norepinephrine. These drugs are sometimes called **partial agonists,** a term that reflects their limited ability to stimulate adrenergic receptors.

Acebutolol differs from oxprenolol and pindolol because it is a cardioselective partial agonist,

affecting only beta$_1$ receptors. It is for this reason that it was also presented above under the topic of cardio-selective beta blockers. Oxprenolol and pindolol act on both beta$_1$ and beta$_2$ receptors.

Partial agonists do not reduce the resting heart rate as much as other beta blockers because their intrinsic sympathetic activity ensures some degree of sympathetic stimulation. During times of stress, however, when an increase in heart rate and cardiac output are required to meet the needs of the body, patients given a partial agonist still have a diminished myocardial function when compared to untreated subjects.

It is also claimed that beta blockers with ISA can stimulate the beta$_2$ receptors to produce bronchodilatation and vasodilatation in the resting patient. The clinical significance of this fact is not obvious. Partial agonists may also dilate peripheral blood vessels, and this can reduce coldness and intermittent claudication. Most beta blockers can increase serum cholesterol. The clinical significance of this is not clear. However, beta blockers with ISA or partial-agonist activity may be preferred in patients with high serum cholesterol because they usually do not increase blood lipids.

Acebutolol, oxprenolol and pindolol are effective in the treatment of angina pectoris and hypertension. Their pharmacological properties, adverse effects and nursing process are similar to those for the other beta blockers.

Alpha and Beta Blockers

Labetalol (Trandate)

Mechanism of Action and Pharmacological Effects

Labetalol blocks both alpha and beta receptors. Although it is more potent as a beta blocker, its antihypertensive effects are due primarily to alpha$_1$ receptor antagonism, resulting in a decrease in peripheral resistance. The reflex tachycardia normally seen with arteriolar dilatation is prevented by the partial beta blockade. Heart rate usually does not slow when labetalol is administered. Presumably the increase in sympathetic stimulation, secondary to vasodilatation, compensates partially for the beta blockade.

Therapeutic Uses

Labetalol is used in the treatment of essential hypertension (see also Chapter 14). Although some authorities may recommend the drug for initial therapy, most physicians prefer to add it to existing therapeutic regimens if the need arises.

Adverse Effects

The most serious reported adverse effects of labetalol are severe postural hypotension, jaundice and bronchospasm. Nausea and vomiting may also be experienced with the drug.

Nursing Process

Assessment

Prior to administering the initial dose of labetalol, nurses should review the patient's history for asthma, chronic obstructive pulmonary disease (COPD), cardiovascular or liver disease, and diabetes mellitus. In the presence of any of these conditions the medication should be withheld pending consultation with the prescribing physician. In addition, nurses must establish baseline measures of the patient's blood pressure and pulse in both lying and standing positions for later use in determining the efficacy of the medication.

Administration

When administered orally, labetalol should either follow a meal or be accompanied by food. When the route of administration is intravenous, the patient should be lying down during and for three hours after receiving the medication. The use of an infusion pump or other similar device for accurate measurement of intravenous administration is highly recommended.

Evaluation

Blood pressure measurements both lying and standing are compared to the baseline measures in order to determine the effectiveness of the drug.

Teaching

Patient teaching associated with labetalol revolves around its antihypertensive effect. Therefore the nurse should implement the same teaching measures as those previously identified for propranolol.

Adrenergic Neuron Blockers

Mechanism of Action and Pharmacological Effects

These drugs derive their name from their ability to inhibit the formation, storage or release of norepinephrine from postganglionic sympathetic nerve endings. They do not block adrenergic receptors. The consequences of administering an adrenergic neuron blocker are more devastating than either alpha$_1$ or beta blockers because it abolishes all sympathetic function, not merely those activities mediated by one receptor or another.

Adrenergic neuron blockers lower blood pressure by reducing peripheral resistance and decreasing cardiac output. Peripheral resistance decreases because the drugs inhibit sympathetic function in the arterioles. Cardiac output falls as a result of dilatation of the veins and reduction in venous return. The consequences of venodilatation are not limited solely to a decrease in cardiac output. The inability of the veins to constrict when an individual stands allows blood to pool in the lower extremities of the body, producing postural or orthostatic hypotension.

The decrease in cardiac output and blood pressure reduces renal blood flow. This causes a retention of body fluids as less blood is filtered and a higher percentage of the glomerular filtrate is reabsorbed. The resulting increase in blood and extracellular fluid volume diminishes the hypotensive effects of the drugs.

The sympathetic nervous system is antagonistic to the actions of the parasympathetic nervous system in the gastrointestinal tract. Under normal conditions the stimulant effects of the latter are offset, in part, by the inhibitory actions of the former. A reduction in sympathetic outpourings, as produced by adrenergic neuron blockers, leads to parasympathetic dominance. This causes increased gastrointestinal motility and diarrhea.

The patient treated with one of these drugs may be a sad sight. Upon standing quickly, because of peristaltic urges, he or she may suffer an acute attack of postural hypotension and faint. In male patients, adrenergic neuron blockers inhibit erection and ejaculation. This situation can be stressful for both the patient and his sexual partner. It may be most difficult to convince either of them that the patient is in better shape than he has been in years because his diastolic pressure has been reduced!

In view of this catastrophic picture, it seems a little mundane to mention that patients receiving adrenergic neuron blockers often complain of a stuffy nose. This effect is due to vasodilatation of the blood vessels perfusing the mucous membranes of the nasopharynx.

Reserpine (Serpasil)

Mechanism of Action and Pharmacological Effects

Reserpine was originally obtained from the plant *Rauwolfia serpentina* (hence the trade name Serpasil). It is now chemically synthesized. Reserpine depletes sympathetic nerve endings of their supply of norepinephrine and as a result depresses sympathetic functions both within the brain and peripheral tissues. It produces sedation and depression as well as a reduction in cardiac output and postural hypotension. Reserpine also depletes dopamine stores in the brain and produces extrapyramidal, or parkinsonian, effects.

Therapeutic Uses

Reserpine was the first adrenergic neuron blocker introduced into patient care. Initially, it was marketed as a tranquilizer and then later as an antihypertensive. It has been largely replaced for both indications by newer drugs. The majority of patients on reserpine are older and have been receiving the drug for many years for the treatment of hypertension. There appears to be no justification for starting patients on reserpine today.

Adverse Effects

The adverse effects of reserpine are directly attributable to the depletion of norepinephrine and inhibition of sympathetic nervous system activity. The drug can produce a marked depression in the patient's mood. It often causes bradycardia and postural hypotension. Nasal congestion is common. The inhibition of sympathetic activity in the gastrointestinal tract allows the parasympathetic nervous system to act unopposed. As a result, reserpine treatment produces increased gastric secretion, nausea, vomiting, anorexia, aggravation of peptic ulcer or ulcerative colitis, increased intestinal motility and diarrhea. Impotence or decreased libido are also consequences of reserpine's use.

Nursing Process

Assessment

Nursing assessment prior to the administration of reserpine should include examination of the patient's history for evidence of episodes of depression, peptic ulcer, ulcerative colitis, epilepsy, chronic obstructive lung disease, renal disease, cardiac or cerebral vascular atherosclerosis, or cardiac arrhythmias. The presence of any of these conditions should be brought to the attention of the attending physician. Similarly, a family history of cancer of the breast should be reported prior to the administration of the initial dose.

Baseline readings of the patient's blood pressure and pulse must be established, in order to evaluate the patient's response to the medication. The patient's dietary habits and body mass/weight should also be documented before the first administration of reserpine. Reserpine often causes alteration in sleeping patterns and nightmares. Therefore, nurses should question patients about their normal sleep patterns because the appearance of nightmares often precedes depression.

Administration

Reserpine should be administered only from airtight, light-resistant containers. It should be taken with meals or milk to minimize gastric irritation. However, if nausea accompanies the administration of reserpine, give the drug after meals with nothing to eat or drink for two or three hours.

Evaluation

Patient evaluation following its administration should include supine and standing blood pressures, apical and radial pulses two hours after oral treatment, evaluation of the psychological status, intake and output of fluids, edema and daily weight gain. The last-mentioned parameters are important because reserpine can cause water retention and edema, and, for reasons that are not clear, it often increases appetite and weight gain.

Teaching

Patients should be told that the full therapeutic effect of the medication might not be experienced for up to three weeks following the initial dose. The patient should also be cautioned about the possibility of postural hypotension and advised to change positions slowly, avoid driving and working with heavy machinery or power tools. Sex counselling should be offered to those patients who experience impotence as a result of taking the drug.

Guanethidine (Ismelin)

Guanethidine has been used for more than twenty years for the treatment of hypertension. It reduces the levels of norepinephrine in sympathetic nerve endings. As a result, guanethidine reduces venous return and decreases both heart rate and cardiac output. Consistent with these effects, guanethidine reduces kidney perfusion, with the result that salt and water are retained.

The major adverse effects of guanethidine are those described for adrenergic blockers in general. Guanethidine does not cross the blood-brain barrier, and the central nervous system effects reported for reserpine are not encountered with guanethidine. Patients treated with guanethidine should not be given a tricyclic or tetracyclic antidepressant because these drugs prevent the effect of guanethidine on sympathetic nerve endings.

The nursing process initiated by the prescription of guanethidine is the same as that for reserpine, with the exception that actions related to the central nervous system do not apply because guanethidine does not enter the brain.

Guanadrel (Hylorel)

The mechanism of action and hemodynamic effects of guanadrel are similar to those of guanethidine. It has a more rapid onset and shorter duration of antihypertensive action than guanethidine. Guanadrel is as effective as guanethidine, but is less likely to cause morning orthostatic hypotension, diarrhea or impaired erection/ejaculation. In other other regards, it seems similar to guanethidine. The nursing process related to the use of guanadrel is similar to that for guanethidine.

Central Sympathetic Inhibitors

Central sympathetic inhibitors act within the brain to impair sympathetic centers. They are used primarily to lower blood pressure. The use of clonidine and methyldopa in the treatment of hypertension is described in more detail in Chapter 14.

Clonidine (Catapres)

Clonidine is a potent antihypertensive drug. It is claimed to lower blood pressure by stimulating the $alpha_2$ receptors in the brain. Stated simply, this means that by stimulating these receptors on the sympathetic nerves in the brain, clonidine prevents the neurons from releasing norepinephrine. This inhibits sympathetic centers in the brain, with the result that peripheral sympathetic nerves, which depend on stimulation from the central sympathetic centers, are also blocked.

Clonidine can produce postural hypotension, but its effects are not pronounced. It often produces a dry mouth and sedation. These effects can be severe. Impotence occurs occasionally. Treatment with clonidine will lead to the retention of sodium, chloride and water. Similar to guanethidine, tricyclic and tetracyclic antidepressants should not be given to patients receiving clonidine, as they can diminish or abolish the actions of the drug.

The nursing process associated with the prescription of clonidine is the same as that described for reserpine. Patients should be informed that the drug must be taken regularly. Stopping the drug for a day or two can cause a marked rebound hypertensive response. Patients should be advised to contact their physician immediately in the event that they develop a temporary illness, such as flu or gastrointestinal upset, that prevents them from taking their medication.

Methyldopa (Aldomet)

Methyldopa is a very popular antihypertensive. Its mechanism of action is not clear. At the present time it is believed to reduce sympathetic nervous system function by inhibiting the sympathetic centers in the brain. The drug is usually preferred to guanethidine because it often does not produce significant postural hypotension. If postural hypotension does occur, it is not as severe as after guanethidine. Methyldopa decreases peripheral resistance and this accounts, at least in part, for the fall in blood pressure. Its effects on cardiac output are still disputed. Some studies report a fall in cardiac output that correlates with the decrease in blood pressure, while other investigations report no effect on cardiac output.

The adverse effects of methyldopa include sedation, postural hypotension, edema and impotence. These can be attributed to sympathetic blockade. Other adverse reactions are not so easily explained. They include drug fever, hepatic dysfunction, hemolytic anemia and lactation (in either sex). These occur only rarely. A problem for the clinical chemist is the fact that up to twenty-five per cent of patients taking 1000 mg of methyldopa daily for six months or more develop a positive direct Coombs' test. This has no clinical significance but it makes cross-matching blood difficult.

The nursing process related to the care of patients receiving methyldopa is identical to that presented for reserpine.

Further Reading

Hoffman, Brian B. and Lefkowitz, Robert J. (1990). "Adrenergic Receptor Antagonists." In: *Goodman and Gilman's The Pharmacological Basis of Therapeutics,* 8th ed. (pp. 221-243), ed. Alfred Goodman Gilman, Theodore W. Rall, Alan S. Nies and Palmer Taylor. New York: Pergamon.

Westfall, David P. (1986). "Adrenoceptor Antagonists." In: *Modern Pharmacology,* 2nd ed. (pp. 174-192), ed. Charles R. Craig and Robert E. Stitzel. Boston: Little, Brown.

Table 8
Antiadrenergic drugs.

Generic Name (Trade Name)	Use (Dose)	Action	Adverse Effects	Drug Interactions	Nursing Process
Pharmacologic Classification: Alpha₁ Receptor Blockers					
Phentolamine (Regitine, Rogitine)	Dx and management of pheochromocytoma (**Oral:** 50 mg 4-6x daily. **IV/IM:** 5 mg)	Inhibit'n of sympathetic alpha₁ stimulat'n. Effects depend on sympathetic tone at time of administrat'n.	Reflex tachycardia, postural hypotens'n, nasal congest'n, GI hypermotility, inhibit'n erect'n/ejaculat'n		**Assess:** For pt hx of gastritis, peptic ulcer, coronary artery disease, pregnancy. Establish baseline VS. **Administer:** With pt in supine position. **Evaluate:** BP and pulse q2min until stabilized.
Prazosin (Minipress)	Tx of hypertens'n (**Oral:** Highly individualized. Build up dose gradually. Max. 1 mg given hs [w. instruct'ns that pt remain in bed for several hours], followed by 1 mg bid; incr. to tid prn. This dose may be incr. gradually to 20 mg/day prn. Children - 0.1 mg/kg/day)	Decr. peripheral resistance by blocking alpha₁ receptors.	Reflex tachycardia, postural hypotens'n, nasal congest'n, GI hypermotility, impotence (painful erect'n), fluid retent'n, weakness, dizziness, headache, palpitat'ns, lethargy	**Antihypertensive drugs:** Reduce dose of other antihypertensive agents and initiate prazosin at 0.5 mg bid or tid. When adding another antihypertensive agent to pre-existing prazosin tx, reduce prazosin dose to 1-2 mg bid or tid and retitrate. **Diuretics:** Reduce dose of the diuretic to maint. level for that agent and initiate prazosin at 0.5 mg bid or tid. Gradually incr. prazosin dosage prn.	**Assess:** For pt hx of chronic renal failure, pregnancy, lactat'n; establish BP and weight. Check for potential drug interact'ns. **Administer:** With food and/or milk. **Evaluate:** Drug effectiveness (decr. in BP); adverse effects. Following inital dose, incr. in dosage or addit'n of other antihypertensives, watch for syncope w. sudden unconsciousness. 4-6 weeks may be required for full therapeutic effect to be observed. **Teach:** To move from recumbent to standing position slowly w. stop in sitting position before rising; to lie down quickly if dizzy, faint or weak; not to drive a vehicle, operate power tools or work around heavy machinery until dosage is established and indiv. responses identified; to seek medical advice before taking OTC medicat'ns for colds, coughs or allergies; to seek sex counselling for impotence.
Terazosin (Hytrin)	Tx of hypertens'n (**Oral:** 1 mg hs initially. Slowly incr. dose to achieve desired effect. Us. dose range is 1-5 mg 1x/day. Some pts may benefit from doses up to 20 mg/day)	As for prazosin	Syncope, dizziness, headache, asthenia, somnolence, nasal congest'n, palpitat'ns, occ. impotence		
Pharmacologic Classification: Nonselective Beta Blockers					
Propranolol (Inderal)	Tx of hypertens'n, prophylaxis of angina pectoris, tx and prevent'n of cardiac arrhythmia,	Blocks both beta₁ and beta₂ receptors. Effects depend on	Bronchoconstrict'n in asthmatics; potentiates effect of insulin;	*Reference is made to propranolol, but drug interact'ns apply to all beta blockers.*	**Assess:** For pt hx of CHF, bradycardia, heart block, asthma, hay fever, COPD, liver or kidney disease, diabetes,

Drug	Action / Uses / Dosage	Action	Side Effects	Drug Interactions	Nursing Implications
(propranolol, cont'd)	prevent'n of migraine headaches (**Oral:** *For hypertens'n*, 40 mg bid, incr. prn to 80 or 160 mg bid. *For angina pectoris*, initially, 10-20 mg tid or qid. Incr. gradually prn. Most pts require 160-240 mg daily. *For cardiac arrhythmias*, adults - 10-80 mg tid or qid. **IV:** 0.1-0.15 mg/kg given in increments of 0.5-0.75 mg q1-2min)	level of sympathetic nervous activity. Decr. heart rate, ventricular systolic pressure, myocardial contractility and cardiac output. Reduces coronary blood flow and oxygen consumpt'n, lowers BP, reduces sinus rate, slows A-V conduct'n, decr. spontaneous rate of ectopic pacemakers.	asystole, A-V block, bradycardia, heart failure, nausea, vomiting, constipat'n, diarrhea, depress'n, sleep disturbances and allergic react'ns	**Antidiabetic agents:** Propranolol and other beta$_1$ and beta$_2$ blockers reduce rebound of blood glucose following insulin-induced hypoglycemia. Cardioselective beta blockers less likely to have this effect. Nonselective beta blockers will have same interact'n with oral hypoglycemics. Beta blockers may prevent signs of hypoglycemia (sweating, tachycardia). **Atropine** (and other anticholinergics): May prevent bradycardia produced by propranolol. **Digitalis glycosides:** Positive inotropic action of digitalis may be reduced by propranolol's negative inotropic effect. Propranolol and digitalis are additive in depressing A-V conduct'n. Use propranolol with caution in pts on digitalis preparat'ns who develop bradycardia. **Epinephrine:** In pts receiving propranolol, epinephrine can incr. BP; less likely with acebutolol, atenolol and metoprolol. **Levodopa:** Propranolol may antagonize both hypotensive and intropic effects of levodopa.	myasthenia gravis; check potential drug interact'ns, incl. use of MAOIs within preceding 2 weeks; record apical/radial pules (rate and rhythm), BP, respirat'ns (incl. color, warmth, blanching effect and peripheral pulses) as baseline. **Administer:** From airtight, light-resistant containers; ac and hs in order to facilitate absorpt'n of medicat'n from stomach into circulatory system. **Evaluate:** Apical/radial pulses, fluid intake/output, daily weight, BP, respirat'ns, circulat'n of extremities for indicat'ns of adverse effects and to assist physician in establishing best indiv. dose; monitor diabetic pts for hypoglycemia and insulin shock; monitor ECG of pts receiving IV propranolol. **Teach:** Family and pt to observe responses to physical/psychological stress and to develop an individually appropriate pace/amount of activity; importance of avoiding abrupt withdrawal of drug because of danger of myocardial infarct or arrhythmias; to avoid alcohol, smoking and OTC medicat'ns for colds, coughs or allergies because of potential effects on BP; caution to avoid driving vehicles, using machinery during regulation of dosage; instruct pt to move from recumbent to standing position slowly w. stop in sitting position before rising to feet; pt and family to seek medical attent'n if s/s of adverse effects occur.
Nadolol (Corgard)	Tx of hypertens'n, prophylaxis of angina pectoris (**Oral:** *For hypertens'n*, adults - initially, 80 mg 1x daily, incr. weekly prn. Max. daily dose 320 mg. *For angina pectoris*, 40 mg 1x daily, incr. gradually by 40-80 mg increments at 3-7 day intervals prn)	As for propranolol	As for propranolol	As for propranolol	
Timolol (Blocadren)	Tx of hypertens'n, prophylaxis of angina pectoris. For tx of glaucoma, refer to Table 56 (**Oral:** *For hypertens'n*, adults - in pts already receiving other antihypertensives, initially 5-10 mg bid; incr. prn q2weeks by 5 mg bid. Max. daily dose 60 mg. If used alone, initially 10 mg bid; incr. prn. *For angina pectoris*, initially 5 mg bid or tid. Incr. gradually at intervals of more than 3 days. Max. daily dose 45 mg)	As for propranolol	As for propranolol	As for propranolol	

Pharmacologic Classification: Cardioselective Beta Blockers

Drug	Uses / Dosage	Action	Side Effects	Drug Interactions	Nursing Implications
Acebutolol (Monitan, Sectral)	Tx of hypertens'n, prophylaxis of angina pectoris (**Oral:** *For hypertens'n*, initially 100 mg bid. If nec., incr. after 1 week	Partial agonist w. preferential effects on beta$_1$ receptors.	As for propranolol	As for propranolol	As for propranolol

Generic Name (Trade Name)	Use (Dose)	Action	Adverse Effects	Drug Interactions	Nursing Process
	to 200 mg bid. In some cases, daily dosage may need further increments of 100 mg bid at intervals of < than 2 weeks, up to a max. of 400 mg bid. Maint. dose, 400-800 mg daily. For angina pectoris, initially 200 mg bid, incr. prn to max. of 300 mg bid)				
Atenolol (Tenormin)	Tx of hypertens'n, prophylaxis of angina pectoris (**Oral:** For hypertens'n, adults - initially, 50 mg 1x/day; incr. within 1-2 weeks to 100 mg 1x/day prn. For angina pectoris, adults - initially, 50 mg 1x/day; incr. to 100 mg 1x/day prn)	Partial agonist w. preferential effects on beta$_1$ receptors.	As for propranolol	As for propranolol	As for propranolol
Metoprolol (Betaloc, Lopresor, Lopressor)	Tx of hypertens'n, prophylaxis of angina pectoris (**Oral:** For hypertens'n, adults - initially, 50 mg bid; incr. to 100 mg bid prn. Us. maint. dose, 100-200 mg/day. For angina pectoris, initially, 50 mg bid; incr. to 100 mg bid prn)	As for atenolol	As for propranolol	As for propranolol	As for propranolol

Pharmacologic Classification: Beta Blockers with Intrinsic Sympathetic Activity (ISA) — Partial-Agonist Beta Blockers

Generic Name (Trade Name)	Use (Dose)	Action	Adverse Effects	Drug Interactions	Nursing Process
Acebutolol (Monitan, Sectral)	Tx of hypertens'n, prophylaxis of angina pectoris (**Oral:** For hypertens'n, initially 100 mg bid. If nec., incr. after 1 week to 200 mg bid. In some cases, daily dosage may need further increments of 100 mg bid at intervals of < than 2 weeks, up to a max. of 400 mg bid. Maint. dose, 400-800 mg daily. For	Partial agonist w. preferential effects on beta$_1$ receptors.	As for propranolol	As for propranolol	As for propranolol

Drug	Use/Dosage	Action	Side Effects	Interactions	Nursing Considerations
Oxprenolol (Trasicor)	*angina pectoris*, initially 200 mg bid, incr. prn to max. of 300 mg bid) Tx of hypertens'n (**Oral:** Adult - initially, 20 mg tid; followed w. incr. of 60 mg/day q2-3weeks prn. Us. range is 120-320 mg/day. Max. 480 mg/day)	Weak beta agonist that competes w. epinephrine and norepinephrine at receptor sites, resulting in reduct'n in beta-mediated responses.	As for propranolol	As for propranolol	As for propranolol
Pindolol (Visken)	Tx of hypertens'n, prophylaxis of angina pectoris (**Oral:** *For hypertens'n*, adults - initially, 5 mg bid; incr. after 1-2 weeks by a 10-mg daily increment in 2 equal doses. Max. 15 mg bid. *For angina pectoris*, adults - initially, 5 mg tid w. meals; incr. gradually prn. Us. maint. dose, 15-40 mg/day)	As for oxprenolol	As for propranolol	As for propranolol	As for propranolol

Pharmacologic Classification: Alpha and Beta Blockers

Drug	Use/Dosage	Action	Side Effects	Interactions	Nursing Considerations
Labetalol (Trandate, Normodyne)	Tx of hypertens'n, us. in combinat'n w. other medicat'ns (**Oral:** Initially, 100 mg bid; maint. dose, 200-400 mg bid. **IV:** Initially, 20 mg given by slow inject'n over 2 min; addit'nal inject'n of 40-80 mg can be given at 10-min intervals until desired effect is attained, or a total dose of 300 mg has been administered)	Blocks alpha$_1$ and beta receptors. Antihypertensive effect due to alpha$_1$ receptor antagonism, resulting in decr. peripheral resistance	Severe postural hypotens'n, jaundice, bronchospasm, nausea and vomiting	**Antidiabetics:** May have more prolonged activity if labetalol is used concomitantly. **Antihypertensives:** Increase the hypotensive actions of labetalol. **Cimetidine:** Increases bioavailability of labetalol. **Halothane:** Increases hypotensive effects of labetalol. **Nitroglycerin:** Adds to hypotensive effects of labetalol.	**Assess:** For pt hx of asthma, COPD, CV disease, liver disease, diabetes mellitus. Establish baseline BP and pulse both lying and standing. **Administer:** Orally, w. food; IV with pt supine during and for 3 h following, pref. using infus'n pump. **Evaluate:** BP and pulse both lying and standing; fluid intake/output; daily weight; for pedal edema. **Teach:** As for propranolol.

Pharmacologic Classification: Adrenergic Neuron Blockers

Drug	Use/Dosage	Action	Side Effects	Interactions	Nursing Considerations
Reserpine (Serpasil)	Tx of hypertens'n (**Oral:** Adults not receiving other antihypertensive agents, initially 500 µg daily for 1-2 weeks. Maint. dose, 100-250 µg daily. Administer w. food, meals or milk)	Inhibits format'n, storage and release of norepinephrine from postganglionic sympathetic nerve endings; vasodilatat'n,	Nasal congest'n, postural hypotens'n, incr. blood and extracellular fluid volume, diarrhea, male impotence, decr.	**Guanethidine:** Concurrent use of guanethidine and reserpine may cause bradycardia, mental depress'n, postural hypotens'n. **Levodopa:** Reserpine depletes dopamine; avoid in levodopa-	**Assess:** Family hx of breast cancer, pt hx of depress'n, peptic ulcer, ulcerative colitis, epilepsy, COPD, renal disease, cardiac or cerebrovascular atherosclerosis; cardiac arrhythmias; pregnancy or lactat'n. Establish baseline levels of BP

Generic Name (Trade Name)	Use (Dose)	Action	Adverse Effects	Drug Interactions	Nursing Process
		decr. heart rate, cardiac output and BP.	libido, sedat'n, depress'n, suicide, extrapyramidal side effects	treated pts. **Methotrimeprazine:** Can produce orthostatic hypotens'n and gen'l decr. in BP. Its effects may be additive with reserpine. **MAOIs:** MAOI plus reserpine may cause excitat'n and hypertens'n. Avoid MAOI use.	and pulse, sleep patterns, dietary habits, weight. **Administer:** From airtight and light-resistant container, w. meals or milk to minimize gastric irritation; if nausea accompanies administrat'n, give following meals w. NPO for 2-3 h after taking medicat'n. **Evaluate:** Supine and standing BP and pulse 2 h after oral administrat'n; mental status; fluid intake/output; edema; daily weight. **Teach:** Family and pt to observe for s/s of adverse effects; that therapeutic effect might not be fully achieved for up to 3 weeks following initiat'n of medicat'n and might continue for as long as 4 weeks after withdrawal of medicat'n; to take precautions related to postural hypotens'n.
Guanethidine (Ismelin)	Tx of hypertens'n (**Oral:** Adults - intially, 10 mg daily. Maint. dose us. 25-50 mg daily. Children - initially, 0.2 mg/kg/day; incr. by the same amount q7-10days prn)	Reduces venous return, heart rate and cardiac output. Does not cross blood-brain barrier.	Reduces kidney perfusion, salt and fluid retention; as for reserpine, except for CNS effects.	**Amphetamines, tricyclic antidepressants, ephedrine, methylphenidate and phenothiazines:** These drugs antagonize the adrenergic neuron blockade produced by guanethidine. **Antidiabetic agents:** Guanethidine possesses antidiabetic activity. Watch closely for altered hypoglycemic effects. **Ethanol:** Vasodilatat'n enhances orthostatic hypotens'n of guanethidine. **Levarterenol (norepinephrine):** Guanethidine enhances the pressor effects of norepinephrine. Administer norepinephrine cautiously. **MAOIs:** May antagonize antihypertensive effects of guanethidine. Watch pts for excessive sympathomimetic activity upon initiat'n of guanethidine tx. **Phenylephrine:** Is probably more potent in pts receiving guanethidine. Use topical or systemic phenylephrine with caution.	
Guanadrel (Hylorel)	Tx of hypertens'n (**Oral:** Initially, 10 mg/day; us. maint. dose, 25-75 mg daily)	As for guanethidine	As for guanethidine, but less morning orthostatic hypotens'n, less diarrhea, less impairment of erect'n/ejaculat'n		

Pharmacologic Classification: Central Sympathetic Inhibitors

Drug	Uses and Dosage	Action	Side Effects	Drug Interactions	Nursing Implications
Clonidine (Catapres)	Tx of hypertens'n, migraine headaches and dysmenorrhea (**Oral:** *For hypertens'n,* adults - initially, 0.1 mg daily hs for several weeks, followed by 0.1 mg bid. Dosage may be incr. gradually by 0.1-0.2 mg. For maintenance, us. 0.2-0.8 mg daily in divided am'ts)	Alpha$_2$ stimulat'n, decr. central sympathetic secret'n, produces decr. BP	Sedat'n, dry mouth, fluid retent'n, weight gain, dizziness, headache; dryness, itching or burning of the eyes; corneal ulcerat'n (rare), nocturnal unrest, nausea, euphoria, constipat'n, impotence (rare), agitat'n upon withdrawal of tx	**Antidepressants, tricyclic:** May antagonize clonidine's antihypertensive effects. **Beta blockers:** Tx w. a beta$_1$ and beta$_2$ blocker may exaggerate vasoconstrictor response when clonidine tx is withdrawn. Withdraw beta blocker before stopping clonidine. **Levodopa:** Clonidine may inhibit antiparkinsonian activity of levodopa.	As for reserpine.
Methyldopa (Aldomet)	Tx of hypertens'n (**Oral:** Adults - initially, 250 mg hs; incr. to 250 mg bid after 1 week. Thereafter, incr. dose gradually until BP is controlled. Us. daily maint. dose, 500 mg - 2 g in 2-4 doses. Children - initially, 10 mg/kg/day in 2-4 doses; incr. or decr. until an adequate response is achieved. Max. 65 mg/kg or 3 g daily, whichever is less. **IV:** Adults - 250-500 mg q6h. Max. 1 g q6h. Children - 20-40 mg/kg/day divided into 4 doses)	Reduced sympathetic nerve function in the CNS	Sedat'n, postural hypotens'n, edema, impotence, drug fever, hepatic dysfunction, hemolytic anemia, lactat'n. Others as for reserpine	**Beta blockers:** Pts receiving methyldopa and a beta blocker should be monitored for hypertensive episodes if there is likelihood of catecholamine release produced by such factors as physiologic stress, cholinesterase inhibit'n or administrat'n of indirect sympathomimetics. **Haloperidol:** With methyldopa, may prolong adverse psychiatric symptoms. **Levarterenol (norepinephrine):** A slight incr. in the pressor response to levarterenol has been seen following methyldopa tx.	As for reserpine.

Neuromuscular Blocking Drugs

Teaching Objectives

Following completion of this chapter, the reader should be able to:

1. Describe the mechanisms of action of competitive and noncompetitive, or depolarizing, neuromuscular blocking drugs.
2. Discuss the pharmacologic effects, therapeutic uses and nursing processes related to the use of tubocurarine, atracurium, gallamine and pancuronium.
3. Discuss the pharmacologic effects, therapeutic uses and nursing processes related to the use of succinylcholine.
4. Describe the use of cholinesterase inhibitors in reversing the effects of competitive neuromuscular blocking drugs.

Acetylcholine released from somatic nerves stimulates nicotinic receptors on motor end-plates to contract skeletal muscles. Because nicotinic receptors on skeletal muscle are not identical to nicotinic receptors in autonomic ganglia, it is possible to block skeletal muscle function without altering autonomic activities. The drugs discussed in this chapter are used to block skeletal neuromuscular transmission. They can be divided, on the basis of their mechanisms of action, into competitive and noncompetitive (or depolarizing) blockers.

Competitive Blockers

Tubocurarine

Mechanism of Action and Pharmacologic Effects

Tubocurarine is the best-known competitive blocker of the actions of acetylcholine on skeletal muscle nicotinic receptors. South American Indians recognized the ability of tubocurarine to paralyze skeletal muscles hundreds of years ago and utilized the drug, a naturally occurring chemical obtained from the curare plant, as their drug of choice for dispatching adversaries. Delivered with considerable velocity on the end of an arrow, tubocurarine served these people well. The unlucky foe, on the receiving end of the arrow, found it most difficult to flee as his legs soon became paralyzed. Shortly thereafter respiration failed, as both the intercostal and diaphragmatic muscles succumbed to the effects of the drug.

Anesthetists make use of the same property of the drug to relax skeletal muscles during surgery.

However, in contradistinction to the natives of South America, anesthetists do not stand around the curarized individual while respiration becomes ever more feeble. In the clinical situation, patients receiving tubocurarine are artificially ventilated until the drug's effects subside.

Tubocurarine also releases histamine from mast cells. This may account for the bronchospasm, hypotension and excessive bronchial and salivary secretion that can accompany use of the drug. Heparin, also stored in mast cells, is released by tubocurarine, causing decreased blood coagulability.

Therapeutic Uses

The primary indication for neuromuscular blockers, such as tubocurarine, is as adjuvant drugs in surgical anesthesia. They relax skeletal muscles and reduce the concentration of anesthetic required, thereby decreasing the risk of cardiovascular and respiratory depression. Muscular relaxation can be used to assist in the alignment of a fracture or the relocation of a dislocated joint.

The actions of tubocurarine can be terminated by administering a cholinesterase inhibitor, such as neostigmine. The increase in acetylcholine concentration around nicotinic receptors overcomes the effects of competitive blockers. However, acetylcholine also accumulates around muscarinic receptors. To prevent muscarinic stimulation, an anticholinergic, such as atropine, can also be given.

Nursing Process

Assessment

The pharmacologic effects and potential for adverse reactions provide the rationale for the nursing actions related to the use of tubocurarine. Nursing assessment should consider the patient's history. The presence of renal, liver, circulatory or respiratory disease must be recognized because of the possibility of adverse effects on the circulatory or respiratory systems resulting from the use of tubocurarine. The existence of allergies and/or bronchial asthma must be documented very carefully because of the ability of tubocurarine to release histamine from mast cells.

Baseline body temperature must be measured because tubocurarine may cause malignant hyperthermia, especially in the presence of diazepam (Valium). Pre-existing electrolyte imbalance in combination with the administration of tubocurarine can contribute to circulatory collapse. Nursing assessment must establish baseline vital signs, including temperature, pulse, respirations and blood pressure, in order to provide a basis of comparison for evaluation following drug administration.

Administration

Tubocurarine is administered only by an anesthetist because of the need to intubate the patient.

Evaluation

Once the drug has been administered, nursing evaluation should focus on early identification of adverse effects. Specifically, vital signs (temperature, pulse, respirations and blood pressure) should be monitored every fifteen minutes for the first hour following administration, and every hour thereafter for four hours, until twenty-four hours have elapsed. A comparison of these measurements with the patient's previous norms will provide early evidence of adverse effects. Measuring the patient's fluid intake and output will permit determination of fluid retention. The patient's bowel sounds should be monitored and the first bowel movement noted as an indication that normal gastrointestinal motility has returned.

Atracurium Besylate (Tracrium), Gallamine Triethiodide (Flaxedil) and Pancuronium Bromide (Pavulon)

These drugs are also competitive blockers of acetylcholine on nicotinic skeletal muscle receptors. Pancuronium is used extensively. It is about five times more potent than tubocurarine and has little histamine-releasing action. Nursing processes related to these drugs are the same as those identified for tubocurarine.

Depolarizing or Noncompetitive Blockers

Succinylcholine Chloride (Anectine, Quelicin, Sucostrin, Sux-Cert)

Mechanism of Action and Pharmacologic Effects

Succinylcholine depolarizes nicotinic receptors on motor end-plates, producing muscle fasciculations. In this regard it is similar to the initial actions of acetylcholine. In the case of acetylcholine, however, the neurotransmitter is metabolized, allowing the end-plate to repolarize before it is subsequently depolarized by the next series of acetylcholine molecules. It is a series of depolarization-repolarization cycles that is responsible for purposeful muscle movement. If the motor end-plate cannot repolarize, the cycle is broken and purposeful muscle action is prevented.

This is what happens when succinylcholine is administered. Although it is metabolized rapidly by pseudocholinesterase to succinic acid and choline, its rate of inactivation is considerably slower than acetylcholine's. Because of this, it remains attached to nicotinic receptors, preventing motor end-plate repolarization and paralyzing muscles. However, as stated before, succinylcholine is inactivated rapidly. Therefore, it must be given by continuous intravenous drip if prolonged muscular relaxation is required. Some individuals have an atypical pseudocholinesterase, incapable of metabolizing succinylcholine. If the drug is given to these patients, it will have a prolonged duration of action.

Therapeutic Uses

Succinylcholine chloride is used in surgery as a skeletal muscle relaxant. Its effects cannot be reversed by the injection of an anticholinesterase. As explained in Chapter 5, the accumulation of large amounts of acetylcholine can, in itself, lead to a depolarizing block. Bearing in mind that succinylcholine is inactivated by pseudo-cholinesterase, the injection of an anticholinesterase, such as neostigmine, that inhibits both acetylcholinesterase and pseudo-cholinesterase, will not only allow acetylcholine to accumulate but will also reduce the rate at which succinylcholine is metabolized. These effects combine to increase the duration of the depolarization block.

Nursing Process

Although the mechanisms of action of competitive and depolarizing blockers differ, the consequences of their administration to patients are much the same. Therefore, the nursing processess for depolarizing neuromuscular blockers are the same as those for tubocurarine.

Further Reading

Buck, Marcia L. and Reed, Michael D. (1990). Use of nondepolarizing neuromuscular blocking agents in mechanically ventilated patients. *Clinical Pharmacy 10* : 32-48.

Taylor, Palmer (1990). "Agents Acting at the Neuromuscular and Autonomic Ganglia." In: *Goodman and Gilman's The Pharmacological Basis of Therapeutics,* 8th ed. (pp. 166- 186), ed. Alfred Goodman Gilman, Theodore W. Rall, Alan S. Nies and Palmer Taylor. New York: Pergamon.

Volle, R.L. (1986). "Drugs that Affect Neuromuscular Transmission." In: *Modern Pharmacology,* 2nd ed. (pp. 234-244), ed. Charles R. Craig and Robert E. Stitzel. Boston: Little, Brown.

Table 9
Neuromuscular blocking drugs.

Generic Name (Trade Name)	Use (Dose)	Action	Adverse Effects	Drug Interactions	Nursing Process
Pharmacologic Classification: Competitive Blockers					
Tubocurarine	Adjunct in anesthesia, shock tx and manipulat'n; in small doses, in dx of myasthenia gravis (**IV:** Adults and children - 0.2-0.5 mg/kg initially, followed by 0.04-0.1 mg/kg. Infants up to 1 month - 0.3 mg/kg initially, followed by 0.1 mg/kg)	Competitive blocking of acetylcholine action on skeletal muscle nicotinic receptors	Prolonged apnea, release of histamine and accompanying allergic responses, bronchospasm, hypotens'n, excessive bronchial and salivary secret'ns	**Beta blockers:** Propranolol may incr. the neuromuscular blocking activity of tubocurarine. **Magnesium salts:** Can incr. activity of neuromuscular blockers. **Methotrimeprazine:** Prolongs curare effects. **Narcotics:** Incr. neuromuscular blockade. **IV procaine:** May intensify or resemble action of curare. **Potassium:** Deplet'n increases sensitivity to neuromuscular blockers. **Quinidine:** Potentiates both competitive and depolarizing muscle relaxants.	**Assess:** Pt hx of renal, liver, circulatory or respiratory disease, allergies, hyperthermia, electrolyte imbalance; establish baseline VS. **Administer:** Only by anesthetist or physician. **Evaluate:** VS (temp., BP, pulse, respira'ns) for 24 h following administrat'n, fluid intake/output for 24 h following administrat'n.
Atracurium besylate (Tracrium)	Muscle relaxant during gen'l anesthesia (**IV:** Initially, 0.4-0.5 mg/kg; subsequent doses, 0.08-0.1 mg/kg. If given after succinylcholine-assisted intubat'n, 0.3-0.4 mg/kg is recommended initially)	As for tubocurarine	Decreased BP, tachycardia, bradycardia, urticaria and bronchospasm	As for tubocurarine	As for tubocurarine
Gallamine triethiodide (Flaxedil)	Muscle relaxant during surgery (**IV:** Adults and children - 1 mg/kg initially, followed by 0.3-0.5 mg/kg. Infants up to 1 month - initially 1 mg/kg, followed by doses of 0.5 mg/kg)	As for tubocurarine	As for tubocurarine, plus moderate incr. in BP and changes in ventricular rhythm	As for tubocurarine	As for tubocurarine
Pancuronium bromide (Pavulon)	Muscle relaxant during surgery (**IV:** Adults and children - initially, 0.04-0.1 mg/kg; for intubat'n, 0.1 mg/kg; subsequently, 0.01-0.02 mg/kg repeated prn [us. q20-40min])	As for tubocurarine	As for tubocurarine; however, pancuronium does not block ganglia or release histamine.	As for tubocurarine	As for tubocurarine

Pharmacologic Classification: Noncompetitive (Depolarizing) Blockers

Succinylcholine chloride (Anectine, Quelicin, Sucostrin, Sux-cert)

Adjunct to anesthesia to induce skeletal muscle relaxat'n. May be used to reduce intensity of muscle contract'ns of pharmacologically or electrically induced convuls'ns (**IV:** Adults - initially, 0.3-1.5 mg/kg; subsequent doses, 0.01-0.05 mg/kg. For continuous infus'n, a 0.1% (1 mg/mL) or 0.2% (2 mg/mL) solut'n is administered at an av. rate of 2.5-7.5 mg/min. Reduce dose to maintain paralysis in pregnant women. Infants - 2 mg/kg. Children - 1 mg/kg. Continuous infus'n of succinylcholine is not recommended for neonates and young children. **IM:** Infants, 4 mg/kg; children, 2-3 mg/kg, not to exceed a total dose of 150 mg)

Depolarizat'n of nicotinic receptors on the motor end-plate resulting in initial muscle fascicula'n followed by muscle paralysis

Profound and prolonged muscular relaxat'n, respiratory depress'n, bradycardia, tachycardia, hypertens'n, hypotens'n, cardiac arrest, arrhythmias

Aminoglycosides: Potentiate action of succinylcholine.
Cyclophosphamide: May decr. plasma pseudocholinesterase levels and prolong action of succinylcholine.
Digitalis: Succinylcholine may potentiate both conduct'n and incr. ventricular irritability.
Echothiophate: Prolonged use can reduce systemic pseudocholinesterase activity, leading to prolonged apnea.
Lithium carbonate: May prolong succinylcholine apnea.
Magnesium salts: Can incr. succinylcholine muscle relaxat'n.
MAOIs: May decr. plasma pseudocholinesterase.
Narcotics: Incr. neuromuscular blockade.
Procaine: Can inhibit metabolism of succinylcholine.
Quinidine: Potentiates action of succinylcholine.

As for tubocurarine

S E C T I O N   3

Cardiovascular Pharmacology

Section 3 deals with cardiovascular pharmacology. Beginning with a discussion of drugs used for the treatment of congestive heart failure, it proceeds through antiarrhythmic drugs, antianginal drugs, drugs for the treatment of peripheral and cerebral vascular disorders, antihypertensive drugs and antihypotensive drugs. The importance of these drugs cannot be overstated. Without them, countless millions would either die or have their lifestyles severely hampered by conditions such as congestive heart failure, supraventricular and ventricular arrhythmias, angina pectoris, hypertension, and hypotension or shock. The importance of the material presented in Section 2 will become apparent in the current section. A complete discussion of cardiovascular pharmacology and an understanding of the related nursing process require a good knowledge of autonomic physiology, pharmacology and related nursing measures. The reader is encouraged to refer back to the relevant chapters in Section 2 if difficulty is encountered in understanding the rationale underlying either the autonomic implications of drugs or the associated nursing process discussed in this section of the book.

CHAPTER 10

Drugs for the Treatment of Congestive Heart Failure

Teaching Objectives

Following completion of this chapter, the reader should be able to:

1. Describe the fundamental defect in low-output congestive heart failure and the consequences of this defect on heart size, sympathetic stimulation and the production of edema.
2. List the types of drugs used to treat congestive heart failure.
3. Discuss the mechanism of action, therapeutic uses, adverse effects and nursing process for diuretics in the treatment of congestive heart failure.
4. Describe the actions, therapeutic uses, adverse effects and nursing process of nitrates used in the treatment of congestive heart failure.
5. Discuss the mechanism of action, pharmacological effects, therapeutic uses, adverse effects and nursing process related to the use of the angiotensin-converting enzyme inhibitors captopril and enalapril in the treatment of congestive heart failure.
6. Explain the rationale for the use of nitroprusside in congestive heart failure, together with its adverse effects and related nursing process.
7. Describe the major actions, therapeutic uses and adverse effects of digoxin, together with the nursing process associated with its administration.
8. Discuss the pharmacological effects, therapeutic uses, adverse effects and nursing process related to the use of the inotropic drugs amrinone, dobutamine and dopamine in the treatment of congestive heart failure.
9. Present an approach to the treatment of congestive heart failure.

Congestive Heart Failure

Congestive heart failure occurs when the heart fails to pump enough blood to meet the needs of tissues. It can be divided into low-output and high-output failure. Low-output failure results when cardiac output drops owing to a decrease in myocardial contractility. This chapter will concentrate on drugs for the treatment of low-output failure. In high-output failure, cardiac output may be in the high normal range or even higher but is still too low to meet the needs of the body. It is caused by conditions such as hyperthyroidism, anemia, Paget's disease and beriberi. Because high-output failure is addressed by treating the specific metabolic condition leading to the failure, it will not be subject to discussion in this chapter.

Congestive heart failure can also be divided into left-sided and right-sided failure. If the difficulty is left-sided failure, the heart is unable to pump blood returned from the lungs. As a result, pulmonary congestion occurs, bringing with it dyspnea and orthopnea. If the difficulty is right-sided failure, the heart is unable to accommodate blood returned to it via the systemic veins. Orthopnea and paroxysmal nocturnal dyspnea are less common but systemic venous congestion occurs, leading to ankle edema, congestive hepatomegaly and systemic venous distention.

The differentiation between left-sided and right-sided heart failure is somewhat fallacious because their symptoms often overlap. For example, subjects with left-sided failure may experience edema and patients with right-sided failure often suffer from exertional dyspnea.

Figure 14
Diagrammatic representation of the effects of a decrease in myocardial contractility with the development of congestive heart failure.

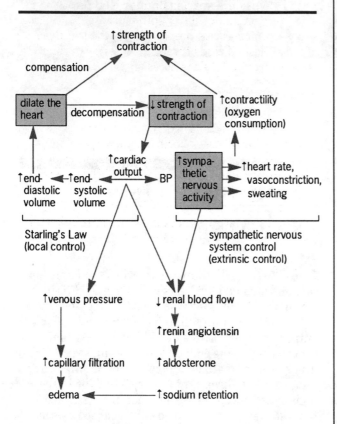

As mentioned before, the contractility of the heart is reduced in low-output failure. Contractility is defined as the force with which the heart contracts for any given fiber length. Initially, decreased contractility of the heart may not be evident because of two compensatory mechanisms. These are an increase in both heart size and sympathetic nervous system activity. They are depicted in Figure 14.

The increase in heart size can be understood when it is recognized that a decrease in myocardial contractility, stroke volume and cardiac output produces an increase in end-systolic end-diastolic volumes. To compensate for these phenomena the heart dilates. The larger heart allows for an increase in force of contraction, offsetting for a time the initial defect in myocardial contractility.

The increase in sympathetic stimulation has two major effects on the patient bordering on congestive heart failure. First, norepinephrine, released by the cardiac accelerator nerves, increases heart rate and myocardial contractility. For a period of time the elevated sympathetic tone helps to maintain cardiac output within normal limits. Second, the elevated sympathetic stimulation produces a generalized vasoconstriction and this, too, assists in the maintenance of blood pressure. Unfortunately, it also reduces tissue perfusion. Other consequences of the increased sympathetic stimulation include an increased release of renin and angiotensin. This effect is counterproductive because it promotes salt and water retention and edema formation (see below).

Eventually, as myocardial contractility continues to deteriorate, the compensatory mechanisms are insufficient to maintain cardiac output. At this point congestive heart failure occurs. A major consequence of the heart failure is the production of edema. Figure 14 describes the forward and backward flow theories to explain the occurrence of edema. According to the **forward flow theory,** the decrease in cardiac output results in a diminished renal blood flow. This leads to an increased release of renin and angiotensin by the kidney. Angiotensin, in turn, triggers the secretion of aldosterone from the adrenal cortex. Aldosterone promotes sodium, chloride and water retention.

The **backward flow theory** states that venous pressure increases, owing to the inability of the heart to accommodate venous blood returned to it. The increased pressure in the veins causes a commensurate increase in venule and capillary hydrostatic pressure, with the result that fluid is extruded from capillaries into the tissues. It is likely that alterations in both forward and backward flows account for edema in most patients.

The preceding may be summarized by stating that:
1. Heart failure occurs when the heart does not pump enough blood to meet the needs of the tissues.
2. Low cardiac output leads to congestion, dyspnea and edema.
3. The compensating mechanisms in heart failure are:
   a. Enlarged heart.
   b. Increased release of renin, resulting in increased angiotensin II and aldosterone secretion.
      • Angiotensin II constricts renal vessels.
      • Aldosterone promotes salt and water retention.
   c. Increased sympathetic stimulation.
      • Stimulation of beta$_1$ receptors in the heart increases heart rate.
      • Stimulation of alpha$_1$ receptors on blood vessels increases peripheral resistance and venous return.

4. The consequences of the compensating mechanisms include increased:
   a. Blood volume.
   b. Venoconstriction (preload).
   c. Systemic vascular resistance (afterload).

Drug Treatment of Heart Failure

Congestive heart failure may be treated by drugs that (1) decrease preload (diuretics and nitrates), (2) reduce afterload (angiotensin-converting enzyme inhibitors), or (3) increase myocardial contractility (inotropic drugs). **Preload** refers to the cardiac filling pressure or venous return to the right side of the heart. **Afterload** is the systemic vascular resistance against which the heart must pump to circulate blood throughout the body.

Drugs that Decrease Preload

Diuretics

Mechanism of Action and Pharmacologic Effects

The pharmacologic actions of these drugs is presented in detail in Chapter 16. At this time it is sufficient to point out that by increasing sodium chloride and water excretion, diuretics decrease blood volume and lower cardiac filling pressure. As a result, pulmonary congestion and peripheral edema are reduced.

Therapeutic Uses

Diuretics are first-line agents for all grades of cardiac failure when sinus rhythm is present. They are usually sufficient alone in mild heart failure. When the patient is afflicted with more severe failure diuretics are usually given with other drugs, such as a vasodilator and/or digoxin. When symptoms are mild, the less potent thiazides or chlorthalidone may suffice. In more severe cases, a loop diuretic, such as furosemide, may be required.

Potassium loss is a common problem encountered with thiazides, chlorthalidone and loop diuretics. This can be reduced by combining these drugs with a potassium-sparing diuretic, such as triamterene, amiloride, or spironolactone, or adding a potassium chloride preparation to the therapeutic regimen. In all cases careful monitoring of fluid and electrolyte levels is necessary.

Adverse Effects

Diuretics, particularly loop diuretics, frequently produce side effects. Elderly patients are especially at risk. The adverse effects include hypovolemia, reduced renal perfusion, increased blood urea, hyponatremia and hypokalemia. Mild to moderate hypokalemia can potentiate digoxin toxicity. Other adverse effects of diuretics, which include hyperglycemia, hypercalcemia, magnesium depletion and hyperlipidemia, are discussed in Chapter 16.

Nursing Process

The nursing process for diuretics used to treat heart failure is the same as that described for edema and hypertension in Chapter 16. Special emphasis should be placed on observing patients for changes in cardiac function, i.e., measuring fluid intake and output, daily body mass/weight, respiratory function, blood pressure and electrolyte balance (particularly hypokalemia).

Nitrates

Mechanism of Action, Pharmacologic Effects and Therapeutic Uses

Nitrates dilate veins and decrease cardiac filling pressure. This can reduce congestion. Oral isosorbide dinitrate (Isordil, Sorbitrate) is a venodilator with a duration of action of four to six hours. The drug increases exercise tolerance and may have a minor role in treatment of congestive heart failure.

Adverse Effects

Headache and hypotension are the most common adverse effects of isosorbide dinitrate. The chronic use of any nitrate can lead to the development of tolerance. If the drug is then withdrawn, rebound vasoconstriction can occur.

Nursing Process

The nursing process related to the use of nitrates is presented in Chapter 12.

Drugs that Decrease Afterload

Angiotensin-Converting Enzyme Inhibitors (ACE Inhibitors) — Captopril (Capoten) and Enalapril (Vasotec)

Mechanism of Action and Pharmacologic Effects

Drugs that dilate precapillary resistance vessels (arterioles) are called **vasodilators**. By dilating precapillary resistance vessels, vasodilators reduce systemic vascular resistance. In the face of a reduced systemic vascular resistance, afterload falls and cardiac output increases.

Myocardial failure increases renin secretion. Renin is converted to angiotensin I which, in turn, is changed to angiotensin II by the angiotensin-converting enzyme (ACE). Angiotensin II has two major effects. It constricts blood vessels and increases aldosterone secretion. Captopril and enalapril are ACE inhibitors. They block the conversion of angiotensin I to angiotensin II and dilate arterioles and veins, reducing respectively afterload and preload. In addition, by decreasing aldosterone secretion, ACE inhibitors reduce blood volume, further contributing to their ability to decrease preload.

Therapeutic Uses

The therapeutic value of ACE inhibitors can be attributed to their actions on both veins and arterioles. Venodilatation leads to a decrease in both right- and left-sided filling pressures. Arteriolar dilatation decreases peripheral resistance, leading to a reduction in afterload on the heart. The consequences of these effects is an improvement in cardiac output. ACE inhibitors are effective in chronic congestive heart failure. Blood pressure often falls initially, but usually returns to a value not significantly below the pretreatment level, if the patient was not hypertensive.

The effects of ACE inhibitors depend on the patient's salt balance. Sodium depletion activates the renin-angiotensin system and increases ACE inhibitor activity. Patients on high-dose diuretic therapy are most likely to experience a severe fall in blood pressure following the first dose(s) of the drugs. As a result, it is often recommended that diuretic therapy be stopped a few days before starting an ACE inhibitor to minimize the initial hypotensive effects of the drugs.

Enalapril must be converted in the liver to its active metabolite, enalaprilate. It has a longer duration of action than captopril and may often be given once daily. However, its long duration of action may compromise renal function, leading to the retention of sodium and water.

Adverse Effects

ACE inhibitors are usually safe in normal doses. Hypotension can be produced by either drug. ACE inhibitors can also cause reversible deterioration of renal function in patients with pre-existing chronic renal disease or renal artery stenosis.

Captopril's adverse effects include taste loss, proteinuria, dermatologic reactions and neutropenia. Doses of 150 mg per day, or less, produce fewer adverse effects. Pre-existing renal disease increases captopril-induced adverse effects. Enalapril can cause hirsutism, pruritus and rash, in addition to the hypotension referred to before.

Nursing Process

Assessment
Patients should be carefully evaluated for evidence of prior renal or hematologic abnormalities that might contraindicate use of these medications. Baseline measures of blood pressure and pulse should be established. Nurses should also expect that the physician will order electrolytes, white blood counts and urinary function tests.

Administration
Absorption of captopril is best when it is taken on an empty stomach. Therefore, it is best administered one hour before meals. The absorption of enalapril is not affected by food.

Evaluation
Nurses caring for patients receiving either of these drugs should monitor the patient's blood pressure and pulse rate. Patients should also be evaluated for possible symptoms of congestive heart failure. These include edema, dyspnea and wet rales. Laboratory reports of proteinuria or depressed white cell counts should be drawn to the attention of the physician. Nurses should be alert for indicators of neutropenia or agranulocytosis. These include unexplained fever, unusual or prolonged fatigue, sore throat or easy bruising and bleeding. Patients should also be monitored for possible

allergic reactions, which include rash, pruritus and urticaria.

Teaching
Patients should be taught that such symptoms as fever of undetermined origin, excessive fatigue, sore mouth or throat, increased bruising or bleeding tendencies may indicate agranulocytosis and should be reported to the physician at once. They should also be told not to discontinue drug therapy abruptly. Nurses should instruct patients not to use over-the-counter products unless directed by a physician.

Nitroprusside (Nipride)

Mechanism of Action and Pharmacologic Effects
Nitroprusside relaxes both arterial and venous smooth muscle, decreasing arterial impedance and venous pooling, respectively. Systemic and pulmonary vascular resistance fall, right ventricular filling pressure decreases, and cardiac output increases when nitroprusside is used. In addition, the drug reduces pulmonary-capillary wedge pressure in patients with congestive heart failure.

Therapeutic Uses
Administered intravenously, nitroprusside is one of the most widely used drugs for the immediate reduction of systemic vascular resistance in patients with congestive heart failure. Arterial and pulmonary arterial end-diastolic or pulmonary-capillary wedge pressure should be monitored constantly, along with frequent estimates of cardiac output, to determine changes in systemic vascular resistance. Drug dosage should be adjusted to maintain a left ventricular filling pressure of 15 – 18 mm Hg without producing a marked fall in arterial pressure. Nitroprusside should be stopped if arterial pressure decreases markedly before left ventricular filling pressure falls or cardiac output increases. If hypotension complicates severe congestive heart failure during myocardial infarction, nitroprusside should be combined with a potent inotropic drug such as dobutamine. An adequate arterial pressure must be maintained in patients with an acute myocardial infarction to sustain the coronary perfusion pressure and prevent increasing myocardial ischemia.

Nitroprusside should not be stopped quickly. If it is discontinued abruptly, patients may experience rebound increases in systemic vascular resistance and a decrease in cardiac output.

Adverse Effects
Nitroprusside can cause flushing, headache, hypotension, nausea, vomiting, anorexia, muscle spasms, skin rash and mental changes. Prolonged use can result in pulmonary shunting of blood, hypoxia, methemoglobinemia and increased blood levels of thiocyanate and cyanide.

Nursing Process
Assessment
Nurses should check the patient's history for documentation of liver or kidney disease, hypothyroidism or hyponatremia. In the presence of these conditions, nurses should be prepared to provide particularly stringent evaluation and monitoring to patients receiving this medication. Baseline measures of blood pressure, pulse and body mass/weight must be established prior to administering nitroprusside.

Administration
This medication is administered only intravenously. It must be stored in light-resistant containers at room temperature and always be freshly mixed and used within four hours. Immediately after mixing, it should be wrapped in foil to prevent deterioration caused by exposure to light. Reconstituted solutions should have a faint brownish tinge; strongly colored solutions should be discarded. Because of the potency of the medication and its adverse effects, intravenous infusions are best regulated using an infusion pump or similar control device. Other drugs should not be added to a nitroprusside infusion.

Evaluation
Patient response is determined by monitoring cardiac output, blood pressure, edema, daily body mass/weight, fluid intake and output, and arterial and pulmonary arterial end-diastolic or pulmonary-capillary wedge pressure.

Inotropic Drugs

Digoxin (Lanoxin)

Mechanism of Action and Pharmacologic Effects

The word digitalis is used to refer to a family of drugs, the cardiac glycosides. Included in this group are digoxin, digitoxin and deslanoside. The major sources of digitalis drugs are the plants *Digitalis purpurea* and *Digitalis lanata*. These drugs are called glycosides because they contain sugar molecules attached to a steroid nucleus. The steroid component of each cardiac glycoside is called the **aglycone fraction** of the drug.

All digitalis drugs have the same basic actions in the body. They differ only in the routes by which they may be administered, the rates at which they are eliminated from the body and the doses that are required for the treatment of patients. Digoxin is the drug used almost exclusively in North America; therefore, discussion will be restricted to its properties.

The major action of digoxin is to increase heart contractility. Its mechanism of action is still not completely understood. Digoxin is not alone in its ability to increase myocardial contractility. Many other drugs, notably the beta₁ stimulants, have the same effect. However, digoxin and the other cardiac glycosides are unique in their ability to increase contractility without elevating the oxygen requirements of the myocardium. It is this property that sets cardiac glycosides apart from other cardiac stimulants.

As a result of a digoxin-induced increase in myocardial contractility, heart size and heart rate decrease in the patient with congestive heart failure. This is to be expected because the increase in both heart size and heart rate were present only as compensatory mechanisms to assist the organ to meet the blood flow needs of the tissues. Once digoxin improves contractility, and end-systolic and end-diastolic volumes decrease, the stimulus to cardiac enlargement disappears and the heart returns to a more normal size.

Similarly, the improved cardiac output of the digitalized heart removes the need for increased sympathetic stimulation. Vagal (parasympathetic) tone increases and the heart slows. Tissue perfusion is also improved because the reduction in sympathetic stimulation to the arterioles (precapillary resistance vessels) allows these vessels to dilate. Edema is reduced or eliminated because the improved cardiac output increases kidney perfusion and/or reduces pre-existing venous congestion.

Digoxin also influences the electrical activities of the heart. As mentioned before, digitalis glycosides decrease sympathetic stimulation to the heart and return normal vagal activity to the sinoatrial (S-A) and atrioventricular (A-V) nodes. This reduces impulse formation in the S-A node and decreases the conduction of electrical activity between the atria and ventricles. In higher therapeutic doses digoxin also has a direct depressant effect on A-V conduction.

The delay in A-V conduction benefits the patient with atrial flutter or fibrillation. By reducing the speed at which impulses are transmitted to the ventricles, the ventricular rate of contraction is reduced. This allows more time for these chambers to fill, and cardiac efficiency is improved.

Not all electrical changes produced in the heart by digoxin benefit the patient. The drug can produce an increase in conductivity and a decrease in the refractory period in the atria. As a result, atrial flutter can be converted to atrial fibrillation. Greater toxic significance is attached to the actions of digoxin on the electrical activity of the ventricles. The drug reduces the resting potential of Purkinje cells and increases their automaticity while decreasing their refractory periods. When these actions are combined with a decrease in A-V conduction so that normal impulses from the atria have difficulty reaching the ventricles, the stage is set for one or more Purkinje cells to serve as ectopic pacemakers. This is seen with toxic doses of the drug.

Pharmacokinetics

Digoxin can be given intravenously or orally. Its action is relatively rapid, beginning within five to thirty minutes after intravenous injection and one to two hours after ingestion. Digoxin is excreted unchanged in the urine and has a half-life of about 1.5 days in patients with normal renal function. Digoxin's clearance varies directly with creatinine clearance, and its dosage must be reduced in proportion to a decrease in creatinine clearance. Elderly patients should be given reduced maintenance dosages of digoxin.

Two basic methods may be used to reach steady-state levels of digoxin in a patient. In the first method the patient may be "digitalized" by giving an oral loading dose of 1 – 1.5 mg of digoxin divided over the first day of treatment (see Table 11). This is then followed by a maintenance dose of 0.125 – 0.5 mg daily. This method is used if there is an urgent need to digitalize the patient rapidly. If necessary, digitalization can be accomplished even faster by giving 0.5 – 1 mg of digoxin intravenously, in place of the oral loading dose. The second method of digitalization involves giving the patient a maintenance dose of 0.125 – 0.5 mg daily. Full digitalization will be obtained using the maintenance dose method in approximately one week. Many physicians prefer the second procedure because it is safer, with less risk of overdose.

The toxic levels of digoxin are only two to three times higher than its therapeutically effective concentrations. In view of this, methods have been developed to measure the concentrations of the cardiac glycosides in the serum of patients. Most hospital laboratories have a rapid radioimmunoassay method for the measurement of serum digoxin. The therapeutic window usually falls between 0.5 – 2.0 nanograms/mL (1.0 – 2.6 nmol/L). The development of the radioimmunoassay for digoxin has been a great help in managing patients. As the serum levels of digoxin approach 2.0 nanograms/mL (2.6 nmol/L), the physician is alerted to possible toxicities. Concentrations below 0.5 nanograms of digoxin per mL (1.0 nmol/L) of serum are usually ineffective. However, nurses should be aware that these values are only aids in the clinical management of the individual, and must be taken in context with the condition of the patient. Several clinical conditions, such as hypokalemia, hypothyroidism, age and myocardial infarction, can increase the actions of digoxin on the heart. In the final analysis, the physician's clinical judgment must serve as the basis for patient management.

Therapeutic Uses

Congestive heart failure is the major indication for the use of digoxin. The increased myocardial contractility improves cardiac output and tissue perfusion and reduces venous congestion. Patients with congestive heart failure due to coronary heart disease, hypertensive heart disease, aortic stenosis, aortic insufficiency, mitral insufficiency or congenital heart disease with left-to-right shunts respond better to digoxin than those with congestive heart failure due to cardiomyopathy or cor pulmonale.

Diuretics complement digoxin because they reduce blood volume and venous congestion. However, care must be taken to prevent hypokalemia. It is usually necessary to use a potassium-sparing diuretic with the thiazide, chlorthalidone, metolazone or loop diuretic, or to supplement the patient's diet with potassium.

The role, and success, of digoxin (or any other digitalis glycoside) in the treatment of cardiac disorders can be divided into those conditions involving

arrhythmias and those in which the patient has a normal sinus rhythm. In the former, digoxin is still often considered to be a useful drug. In the latter, its place is challenged.

The role of digoxin in the treatment of patients with cardiac failure and atrial fibrillation is still accepted. By slowing the ventricular rate, digoxin allows more time for filling. This action, combined with its inotropic effects, improves cardiac output and provides patients with significant clinical benefit.

Because of its ability to increase A-V conduction time, digoxin is widely used in the treatment of supraventricular tachyarrhythmias. The most common use for the drug is the treatment of atrial fibrillation with a rapid ventricular response. By the same token, atrial flutter can also be managed by digoxin to produce a ventricular rate of 70 – 100 beats per minute. Paroxysmal supraventricular tachycardia can also be treated with digoxin, provided that it can be established that digoxin is not the cause of the arrhythmia. Digoxin can often be successful in interrupting the re-entrant circuit in the Wolff-Parkinson-White syndrome. However, it is contraindicated in patients in whom the syndrome is associated with atrial fibrillation.

As suggested earlier, digoxin's role in patients with sinus rhythm is controversial. Most studies suggest that digoxin's inotropic effect persists during chronic therapy, but it has been difficult to demonstrate the clinical usefulness of the drug. Whether or not digoxin provides significant additional benefit to the patient in sinus rhythm over that produced by diuretic therapy is uncertain. There is no evidence that digoxin improves long-term survival in patients with cardiac failure. Because of its toxicities and the recent introduction of ACE inhibitors in the treatment of heart failure, the use of digoxin in patients with heart failure and normal sinus rhythm may well fall to third-line therapy, behind diuretics and ACE inhibitors.

Adverse Effects

The adverse effects of digoxin may be divided into those involving the heart and those occurring in other tissues. The toxic effects on the heart are due to alterations in electrical activity. Digoxin can affect the atria, the A-V conduction system or the ventricles. Within the atria digoxin can cause a marked sinus bradycardia, due to withdrawal of sympathetic stimulation and reinsertion of parasympathetic (vagal) activity. In addition, digoxin can affect atrial rhythm. As a result of an increase in automaticity, premature beats or paroxysmal or nonparoxysmal atrial tachycardia may be seen. Mention has already been made of the fact that digoxin may convert atrial flutter to atrial fibrillation.

The effects of digoxin on A-V conduction have been discussed. The impediment to the conduction of impulses from the atria to the ventricles may be either a beneficial or a toxic effect, depending on the condition of the patient. Obviously, patients with atrial flutter or fibrillation will benefit from some degree of A-V block. However, a complete heart block is a sign of impending digitalis intoxication. At this point, accelerated A-V junctional rhythms may be produced because of the ability of high levels of digoxin to increase the automaticity of this tissue. A-V junctional tachycardia can occur.

The most common ventricular rhythm disturbance caused by digitalis is premature ventricular depolarizations. These appear as coupled beats (**bigeminy**), with an ectopic beat following immediately upon the normal beat. This can lead to trigeminy, ventricular tachycardia and ventricular fibrillation.

The toxic effects of digoxin on the heart are seen more often when high concentrations of the drug are present. However, they can also occur with normal, or even low levels of the drug, depending on the clinical condition of the patient. Tolerance to digoxin is reduced in old age, renal insufficiency or hypothyroidism and following acute myocardial infarction, among other conditions. Patients who fall into one or more of these categories may experience toxic reactions to digoxin with relatively low doses or concentrations of the drug. In addition, hyperkalemia can increase the A-V block produced by digoxin, and hypokalemia can enhance the increase in automaticity of an ectopic pacemaker.

It is apparent from the discussion that digoxin can produce just about any kind of arrhythmia imaginable. Table 10 lists the frequency of various kinds of arrhythmias in patients bothered with digitalis-induced cardiac arrhythmias.

Physicians treat digoxin-induced tachyarrhythmias by first withdrawing the drug. Depending on the degree of intoxication, this may be all the treatment required. If potassium levels are low, potassium chloride may be given in divided doses totaling 50 – 80 mEq for adults (5 – 8 mEq/h), provided renal function is adequate. When correction of the arrhythmia is urgent, and the serum potassium concentration is low or normal, potassium is administered intravenously in 5% dextrose in water. A total of 40 – 100 mEq (30 mEq/500 mL) at a rate of 20 mEq/h may be given unless limited by pain due to local irritation. Additional amounts may be

given if the arrhythmia is uncontrolled and the potassiumn well tolerated. Electrocardiographic monitoring is indicated to avoid potassium toxicity (e.g., peak of T-waves). Children must be given reduced doses of potassium chloride. Nurses are referred to detailed information on specific products for pediatric doses of potassium.

Potassium should not be used and may be dangerous for severe or complete heart block due to digoxin, not related to any tachycardia. The electrocardiogram should be observed continuously so that the infusion may be stopped promptly when the desired effect is achieved.

Other agents that have been used in the treatment of digoxin intoxication include lidocaine, phenytoin, quinidine, procainamide and beta blockers. The three last-mentioned agents should be used with caution when A-V block is a component of digoxin intoxication because they may exaggerate this arrhythmic property.

Purified digoxin-specific antibody fragments (Fab fragments) bind with digoxin and the resulting complex is excreted by the kidney. This approach to treating digoxin toxicity appears to be highly effective.

Table 10
Frequency of arrhythmias in digitalis intoxication.

Arrhythmia	Percentage of Various Arrhythmias in Patients with Digitalis-Induced Cardiac Arrhythmias
Ventricular premature beats	33%
Ventricular tachycardia	8%
Nonparoxysmal A-V junctional tachycardia	17%
A-V junctional escape rhythms	12%
Atrial tachycardia with block	10%
Second- and third-degree A-V block	18%
S-A block with sinus arrest	2%

From: David H. Huffman (1976), Clinical use of digitalis glycosides. *Am. J. Hosp. Pharm. 33* :179-185. Reproduced with permission.

The adverse effects of digoxin on tissues other than the heart involve primarily the gastrointestinal tract. Anorexia, nausea and vomiting represent some of the earliest signs of digitalis poisoning. Abdominal discomfort and diarrhea may also be seen. Neurological effects, including headache, fatigue, malaise and drowsiness, may be produced by digitalis. In addition, vision may also be blurred in some patients.

Nursing Process

Assessment

The range between the therapeutic and toxic concentrations of digoxin is narrow. As a result of this fact and the uniqueness of individual responses, nurses should review a patient's history for evidence of renal insufficiency, hypothyroidism, recent myocardial infarct, electrolyte imbalance, pulmonary disease, hypoxia, myocarditis or Adams-Stokes syndrome prior to the administration of the drug. Physical assessment of the patient by the nurse prior to the first dose of digoxin should focus on establishing the patient's age, body mass/weight, baseline measures of the apical and radial pulse rate, rhythm and quality, and electrolyte concentrations.

Administration

Digoxin should be administered with, or immediately following, meals in order to reduce gastric irritation. Nurses should take the patient's pulse for one minute before every administration of digoxin. If the radial pulse is less than 60 beats per minute, the apical pulse should be taken for one minute. If the apical pulse is also less than 60 beats per minute, if its rhythm or quality is changed, or if the serum electrolyte levels are low or have declined from previous levels, the dose should be withheld and the physician contacted.

Evaluation

Both patients undergoing digitalization and those on maintenance doses of digoxin should be observed carefully for signs of drug effectiveness to assist in dosage regulation. These indicators include improved rate, rhythm and quality of pulses with accompanying improvement in color; decreased dyspnea; improved tolerance to moderate physical activity; fewer chest rales; reduced frequency of productive cough; diuresis as indicated by increased proportion of urinary output in relation to fluid intake; weight loss; and decreased peripheral edema.

Digoxin toxicity is increased in the presence of hypokalemia. Therefore, nursing evaluation of the patient must emphasize observing for the physical or behavioral signs of hypokalemia. Obviously, low serum electrolyte levels indicate potential or impending hypokalemia. Other early indicators of low serum potassium levels are anorexia, weakness, lethargy, irritability, mental confusion, flaccid paralysis, shallow respirations and constipation.

Finally, nursing evaluation of patients who are receiving digoxin should stress observation for early evidence of digitalis toxicity, as indicated by such signs and symptoms as anorexia, lethargy, irritability, insomnia, visual disturbances, disorientation, hallucinations, anxiety, dizziness, palpitations, precordial pain and difficulty in swallowing ("lump in throat").

Teaching

Both patients and their families should be instructed in the maintenance regimen, including the proper dose, precautions relating to digoxin administration, the time to take the drug and the importance of taking it regularly. The patient's family should be taught the behavioral and physical indicators of adverse effects and of hypokalemia. They should also be advised to avoid over-the-counter medications and antacids because of possible adverse drug interactions. In addition, nurses must emphasize the importance of contacting the physician should any of these symptoms appear.

Amrinone (Inocor)

Mechanism of Action and Pharmacologic Effects

Amrinone is a potent inotropic vasodilator. It increases myocardial contractility, even after full doses of digoxin, and reduces left and right ventricular filling pressures and pulmonary-capillary wedge pressure. The drug improves resting and exercise hemodynamics, increases left ventricular ejection fraction and improves exercise capacity.

Therapeutic Uses

Amrinone has been used in patients with severe chronic congestive heart failure not adequately controlled by digoxin, diuretics, antiarrhythmic drugs and vasodilators. In patients with atrial fibrillation or flutter, digoxin should be administered concomitantly to control possible enhanced A-V conduction induced by amrinone. In such cases, and in patients with multifocal or runs of premature ventricular contractions, careful dose titration and close electrocardiographic monitoring is advisable during intravenous therapy. The potential for arrhythmia, present in congestive heart failure, may be increased by amrinone.

Adverse Effects

Administration of amrinone has reduced platelet counts to 100 000 platelets/mm^3 in 2.4% of patients. Blood platelet counts should be determined before and during amrinone therapy. Clinically significant lowering of platelet counts ($\leq$ 50 000 platelets/mm^3)

warrants discontinuation of amrinone therapy. Amrinone has been reported to produce fever and nephrogenic diabetes insipidus. Hepatotoxicity has occurred rarely.

Nursing Process

Assessment

Prior to the administration of amrinone, nurses should review the patient's history for evidence of previous hypersensitivity or allergic reaction to either amrinone or to bisulfites. They should also enquire as to the existence of renal or hepatic disease, since amrinone should be used with caution in patients having these conditions. Patients should also be examined for the symptoms of either hypokalemia or dehydration. In the presence of these conditions the physician who prescribed the medication should be consulted. In addition, the nurse caring for the patient should establish baseline measurements of blood pressure and body mass/weight to be used later in determining drug efficacy.

Administration

When administered orally, amrinone should be given with meals to reduce nausea and vomiting often associated with its use. Intravenous solutions should be stored at room temperature in light-resistant containers. Only intravenous solutions that are clear yellow should be used; discolored solutions or ones containing precipitates should be discarded. *Amrinone should not be diluted for intravenous infusion with solutions containing glucose or dextrose because of chemical reactions that occur over a twenty-four hour period.* All diluted solutions of amrinone should be discarded after twenty-four hours.

Evaluation

The patient's body mass/weight and blood pressure should be taken daily and compared against the baseline measurements as an indicator of drug efficacy. Fluid intake and output should be monitored because diuresis, which often occurs with improved cardiac output, can lead to hypokalemia and the associated risk of adverse effects such as arrhythmias. Hemodynamic indicators of drug efficacy are increased cardiac output and decreased pulmonary wedge pressure. Other patient measures indicating drug efficacy include: reduced dyspnea, orthopnea, paroxysmal nocturnal dyspnea, fatigue, and edema; reduced or stabilized weight; and increased exercise tolerance.

Nurses caring for patients receiving this medication should expect that the physician will order laboratory tests to facilitate early detection of adverse effects. Platelet counts, liver enzymes, serum electrolytes and renal function studies are all regularly used for this purpose.

Dobutamine (Dobutrex) and Dopamine (Intropin, Revimine)

Mechanism of Action and Pharmacologic Effects

Dobutamine stimulates beta$_1$ receptors in the heart. In contrast to other sympathomimetics, it increases cardiac output with minimal effects on heart rate, thereby reducing myocardial oxygen requirements. Dobutamine does not produce renal vasodilation, or increase glomerular filtration or sodium excretion.

Dopamine also stimulates the beta$_1$ receptors in the heart to increase both heart rate and stroke volume. In low to intermediate doses, it has no effect on peripheral resistance. The drug stimulates specific dopamine receptors on renal blood vessels to increase the glomerular filtration rate, renal blood flow and sodium excretion.

Therapeutic Uses

Intravenous dobutamine is used for short-term therapy to increase cardiac output in patients with severe chronic cardiac failure. In patients who have atrial fibrillation with rapid ventricular response, digoxin should be used prior to starting dobutamine therapy. Because dobutamine facilitates A-V conduction, patients with atrial fibrillation are at risk of developing rapid ventricular response.

Dopamine increases cardiac output and glomerular filtration and is of great help to shocked patients experiencing decreased renal function and normal or low peripheral resistance. Dopamine is also used in patients with cardiogenic or bacteremic shock or with chronic refractory heart failure.

Adverse Effects

Dopamine and dobutamine's adverse effects include tachycardia, anginal pain, arrhythmias, headache and hypertension. Nausea and vomiting may also be seen. Dopamine may produce a lower incidence of these effects. Although low to medium doses of dopamine increase renal blood flow, high doses stimulate alpha$_1$ receptors on the renal blood vessels and produce vasoconstriction.

Nursing Process

The nursing process related to the use of these two drugs was discussed in detail in Chapter 7. It will only be summarized here and in the table at the end of this chapter.

Assessment

Nursing assessment includes examining the patient's history and current drug use profile for contraindications, and establishing baseline measures of physiological indicators to determine later drug efficacy.

Administration

Only freshly mixed intravenous solutions should be administered. The patency of the intravenous tubing and catheter should be ensured at all times and the infusion site observed for evidence of extravasation that can cause tissue necrosis.

Evaluation

Evaluation should provide constant monitoring of the patient because of the potency of these drugs. Emphasis should be placed on frequent observation and recording of the patient's blood pressure, pulses, color, peripheral limb temperatures, urinary output and level of mental activity. Measurement of fluid intake and output is imperative to provide early indicators of adverse renal effects.

Approach to the Treatment of Congestive Heart Failure

A diuretic, to reduce preload, should be the first form of drug therapy. Usually, the drug selected is hydrochlorothiazide, given in the morning or twice daily. If a stronger drug is required for more severe disease or in patients with renal insufficiency, furosemide is the agent of choice. The potassium-sparing diuretics spironolactone, triamterene or amiloride may be combined with the primary diuretic to reduce the risk of hypokalemia. If another drug is required to reduce preload further, isosorbide dinitrate may be given (40 mg four times daily).

If the symptoms of heart failure are not controlled adequately with diuretic therapy, either digoxin or an ACE inhibitor may be added. There appears to be little doubt as to the efficacy of digoxin in patients with atrial fibrillation. However, the role of the drug in patients with normal sinus rhythm is being questioned. Although digoxin may affect favorably twenty-five per cent of patients in sinus rhythm, significant toxicity has been seen in twelve per cent of inpatients and significant cardiac toxicity in nine per cent.

ACE inhibitors are particularly useful additions to diuretic therapy because they reduce both hyponatremia and urinary potassium loss. If an ACE inhibitor is used, however, the patient should not receive a potassium-sparing diuretic or potassium supplements. Failure to heed this advice can lead to significant hyperkalemia. Care should also be taken in starting an ACE inhibitor in patients previously receiving diuretic therapy. The physician may wish to reduce the dose of the diuretic or stop it two to three days before beginning ACE inhibitor treatment. In addition, it is recommended that the patient receive low doses of the ACE inhibitor initially (e.g., 6.25 mg or 12.5 mg of captopril daily). After the patient has demonstrated the ability to tolerate these doses, the physician can gradually increase the dose of the ACE inhibitor selected to meet the individual needs of the patient.

The treatment of heart failure due to outflow obstruction is more complicated, because small reductions in ventricular filling pressures and aortic impedance can cause a major decrease in cardiac output. As a result, diuretics should be used with greater caution and afterload reduction is generally contraindicated. Furthermore, digoxin can worsen outflow obstruction in hypertrophic cardiomyopathy. Despite the lack of good data to support its efficacy, propranolol is generally used to reduce the number of anginal attacks and decrease syncope. Calcium channel blockers (nifedipine and verapamil) may offer another alternative. Nifedipine and propranolol reduce left ventricular outflow gradient.

Acute heart failure is a medical emergency and is treated by drugs that decrease preload, reduce afterload and increase myocardial contractility. Parenteral furosemide is used to reduce preload in the treatment of acute heart failure associated with increased left ventricular end-diastolic pressure. Nitroprusside can be used to decrease afterload. Nitroprusside has been successful in the treatment of acute left ventricular failure due to hypertension. It decreases both peripheral resistance and pulmonary congestion.

As suggested earlier, the efficacy of digoxin to treat patients with acute heart failure and normal sinus rhythm is questionable. Dopamine and dobutamine are adrenergic drugs widely used for the patient with low cardiac output when left ventricular end-diastolic pressure is normal or increased. Low doses of dopamine (5 µg/kg/min) increase cardiac output and preserve renal blood flow, while producing only a small increase in peripheral resistance. Dobutamine is particularly valuable in treating heart failure without hypotension. If hypotension is present, dopamine may be preferred.

The place of amrinone must still be established. Although this drug is an effective inotrope, it can cause serious adverse effects (see earlier discussion).

Further Reading

ACE inhibitors for congestive heart failure (1988). *The Medical Letter 30* :97-98.

Brogden, R. N., Todd, P. A. and Sorkin, E. M. (1988). Captopril. An update of its pharmacodynamic and pharmacokinetic properties, and therapeutic use in hypertension and congestive heart failure. *Drugs 36* :540-600.

Jessup, M. (1989). Angiotensin-converting enzyme inhibitors: Are there significant clinical differences? *J. Amer. Coll. Cardiol. 13* :1248-1250.

Krukemyer, J. J. (1990). Use of ß-adrenergic blocking agents in congestive heart failure. *Clinical Pharmacy 9* :853-863.

Lees, K. R. (1988). Angiotensin-converting enzyme inhibitors. *Rational Drug Therapy 22* (9) [Sept.].

Porterfield, L.M. et al. (1990). How digoxin interacts with other drugs: A practical guide. *Nursing 20* (2): 65–72.

McMurray, J., Lang, C. C., MacLean, D. D., McDevitt, G. G. and Struthers, A. D. (1989). A survey of current use of angiotensin-converting enzyme inhibitors by Scottish physicians in the treatment of chronic cardiac failure. *Scottish Medical Journal 34* :425-427.

Ogilvie, R. I. (1987). Digoxin — When and how to use it. *Medicine North America 5* (Jan.):925-932.

Shocken, D. D. and Holloway, J. D. (1988). Vasodilators in the management of congestive heart failure. *Rational Drug Therapy 22* (April):1-7.

Todd, P. A. and Heel, R. C. (1986). Enalapril. A review of its pharmacodynamic and pharmacokinetic properties, and therapeutic use in hypertension and congestive heart failure. *Drugs 31* :198-248.

Table 11
Drugs for the treatment of congestive heart failure.

Generic Name (Trade Name)	Use (Dose)	Action	Adverse Effects	Drug Interactions	Nursing Process
Pharmacologic Classification: Thiazide and Thiazide-like Diuretics That Decrease Preload					
Hydrochlorothiazide (Esidrix, Hydro-Diuril)	Tx of congestive heart failure (**Oral:** Adults - 25-200 mg/day initially; maint. 25-100 mg/day. Children - 2 mg/kg/day in 2 divided doses)	Incr. renal excret'n of Na and Cl, w. an accompanying volume of H_2O, resulting in decr. blood volume and decr. preload	Hypovolemia, hypokalemia, hyponatremia, hyperglycemia, hyperuricemia, renal colic, hematuria, crystalluria, hypersensitivity, pancreatitis, jaundice, hepatic coma, gout	**ACE inhibitors:** When used together w. a diuretic, can produce postural hypoten's'n. Avoid by stopping the diuretic before starting w. low doses of ACE inhibitor. Thereafter, try reintroducing the diuretic and incr. dose of ACE inhibitor. **Corticosteroids:** Diuretics potentiate K-lowering effects of corticosteroids. **Digoxin:** Reduct'n in plasma K produced by diuretics incr. risk of digoxin toxicity. Incr. sensitivity to digoxin appears related to rate of fall in plasma K and ratio of extracellular/intracellular concentrat'n. **Insulin & oral hypoglycemics:** Diuretics can incr. blood sugar, necessitating higher doses of insulin or oral hypoglycemics. **Lithium:** Diuretics can incr. plasma Li levels and Li-induced toxicities. **Nonsteroidal anti-inflammatory drugs (NSAIDs):** May inhibit natriuretic response to diuretics, offsetting their benefit in tx of heart failure.	**Assess:** Hx for contraindicat'n (incl. kidney/liver disease, low serum K or Na levels, chronic respiratory disease), establish baseline BP and weight, document site and extent of edema. Check daily weight, fluid intake/output for fluid loss. **Administer:** Pref. in early a.m. **Evaluate:** Efficacy of medicat'n (daily weight, fluid intake/output, BP); for evidence of adv. effects. Check rate, depth, rhythm of respirat'ns and effect of exert'n. **Teach:** Expected outcome of medicat'n (diuresis); not to consume licorice or alcohol while on thiazide diuretics; to eat foods rich in K. Advise pt to avoid sudden posture changes and to wear sunscreen.
Chlorthalidone (Hygroton)	Tx of congestive heart failure (**Oral:** Adults - 50-100 mg/day)	As for hydrochlorothiazide	As for hydrochlorothiazide		
Metolazone (Zaroxolyn)	Tx of congestive heart failure (**Oral:** Adults - 2.5-10 mg/day)	As for hydrochlorothiazide	As for hydrochlorothiazide		
Pharmacologic Classification: Loop Diuretics That Decrease Preload					
Furosemide (Lasix)	Tx of congestive heart failure (**IV:** Adults - 40 mg. **Oral:** Adults - 40-80 mg; max. 200 mg)	Inhibits reabsorpt'n of Na and Cl in ascending limb of Henle's loop; reduces hypertonicity of renal medulla and impairs concentrating ability of collecting ducts. Decr. preload.	Hypovolemia, electrolyte imbalance (see thiazide diuretics), gout, deafness, fluid deplet'n, dermatitis		
Ethacrynic acid (Edecrin)	Tx of congestive heart failure (**IV:** Adults - 50 mg (0.5-1 mg/kg). **Oral:** Begin w. 50 mg 1x/daily pc and incr. gradually by 50 mg/day, if nec., to 150-200 mg daily over 4 days. Children - initially, 25 mg; incr. by 25-mg increments until a satisfactory response is obtained)	As for furosemide	As for furosemide		

Generic Name (Trade Name)	Use (Dose)	Action	Adverse Effects	Drug Interactions	Nursing Process
Pharmacologic Classification: Vasodilator That Decreases Preload					
Isosorbide dinitrate (Isordil, Sorbitrate)	Tx of congestive heart failure (**Oral:** Up to 40 mg qid)	Dilates arterioles and veins, reducing peripheral resistence and left ventr. filling pressure, resulting in incr. cardiac output.	Incr. heart rate, headache, postural hypotens'n (dizziness, weakness)	**Ethanol:** Hypotens'n may occur following combined use of ethanol and a nitrate. Pts receiving nitrates should take ethanol cautiously.	**Evaluate:** Efficacy, tolerance. Observe for daily change in cardiac and respiratory funct'n, fluid intake/output, weight, BP, electrolyte balance. **Teach:** S/s of adv. effects; proper storage and administrat'n; danger of consuming alcohol w. nitrates.
Pharmacologic Classification: Vasodilators That Decrease Afterload					
Captopril (Capoten)	Tx of congestive heart failure (**Oral:** Adults - initially, 25 mg tid. In volume-depleted or hyponatremic pts, init. dose should be 6.25-12.5 mg tid. Dosage may be titrated upward to 50 mg tid. Children - 5-10 mg/kg/day in 4 divided doses)	Inhibits convers'n of angiotensin I to angiotensin II, reducing vasoconstrict'n and decr. aldosterone secret'n.	Poss. nephrotoxicity, neutropenia/agranulocytosis reported, skin rashes, angioedema, gastric irritat'n, nausea, vomiting, dysgeusia	**Antihypertensive agents:** ACE inhibitor effect will be incr. by antihypertensive agents that cause renin release. **Beta blockers:** Incr. antihypertensive effect of ACE inhibitors. **Diuretics:** Pts on diuretics, esp. those recently beginning this tx as well as those on severe dietary salt restrict'n or dialysis, may experience a sharp reduct'n in BP within first hours after receiving init. dose of ACE inhibitor. **K-sparing diuretics:** Used w. ACE inhibitors, may lead to incr. in serum K.	**Assess:** For hx of renal or hematologic abnormalities. **Administer:** 1 h ac. **Evaluate:** BP, heart rate, protein in urine, WC count. **Teach:** S/s of impending neutropenia/agranulocytosis.
Enalapril (Vasotec)	Tx of congestive heart failure (**Oral:** Adults - 5-10 mg od or bid)	As for captopril	Hypotens'n, hirsutism, pruritus, rash		As for captopril, also: **Evaluate:** For heart failure, edema, wet rales. **Teach:** Pt not to take OTC drugs without physician's orders.
Nitroprusside (Nipride)	Tx of hypertensive crisis, congestive heart failure and myocardial infarct (**Infus'n:** Start at lower dosage range, 0.5 µg/kg/min, and adjust in increments of 0.2 µg/kg/min, us. q5min until desired effect is obtained)	Relaxes both arterial and venous smooth muscle, decr. arterial impedance and venous pooling.	Nausea, vomiting, palpitat'ns, muscle twitching, restlessness, sweating. Thiocyanate may accumulate during prolonged tx, particularly in renal insufficiency. Fatalities have occurred due to cyanide accumulat'n.		**Administer:** Only IV freshly mixed from light-resistant containers; wrap reconstituted solut'n in foil during administrat'n; use infus'n pump to control rate. **Evaluate:** BP, pulse, fluid intake/output, arterial and pulmonary arterial end-diastolic or pulmonary wedge pressures, cardiac output.

Pharmacologic Classification: Inotropic Drugs

Digoxin (Lanoxin)

Tx of congestive heart failure and supraventricular arrhythmias (**Parenteral digitalizat'n:** *10 yrs. and over* - 0.25-0.5 mg IV, then 0.25 mg q4-6h prn to max. 1.0 mg. **Total pediatric IV doses:** In divided am'ts at 6-h intervals. *Premature infants* - 0.015-0.025 mg/kg; *full-term newborns* - 0.02-0.03 mg/kg; *1 mo.-2 yrs.* - 0.03-0.05 mg/kg; *2-5 yrs.* - 0.025-0.035 mg/kg; *5-10 yrs.* - 0.015-0.03 mg/kg. **IV maintenance:** 20-30% of oral loading dose in premature infants and 25-30% of oral loading dose in full-term infants and children. **Oral digitalizat'n, rapid:** Adults - 0.5-0.75 mg, then 0.25-0.5 mg q6-8h prn [total 0.75-1.5 mg]. **Oral maintenance:** Adults - 0.125-0.5 mg/day; elderly - 0.125-0.25 mg/day. **Oral digitalizat'n:** Total pediatric doses - give in divided am'ts at 6-h intervals. *Premature infants* - 0.02-0.03 mg/kg. *Full-term newborns* - 0.025-0.035 mg/kg; *1 mo.-2 yrs.* - 0.035-0.06 mg/kg; *2-5 yrs.* - 0.03-0.04 mg/kg; *5-10 yrs.* - 0.02-0.035 mg/kg; *over 10 yrs.* - 0.01-0.015 mg/kg. **Oral maintenance:** *Premature infants* - 20-30% of loading dose/day; *full-term infants and children* - 25-35% of oral loading dose/day)

Incr. cardiac contractility without incr. myocardial O₂ requirements; decr. sympathetic cardiac stimulat'n resulting in slower heart rate, incr. cardiac output and reduced heart size.

Cardiac: Sinus bradycardia, atrial tachycardia, atrial fibrillat'n, AV block, A-V junct'nal tachycardia, bigemy, trigemy, ventr. tachycardia, ventr. fibrillat'n **GI:** anorexia, nausea, vomiting, abdominal pain, diarrhea **CNS:** headache, fatigue, malaise, drowsiness, blurred vision

Amiloride: This K-sparing diuretic incr. serum digoxin concentrat'n.

Amiodarone: Incr. digoxin serum concentrat'n.

Ca: Digitalis preparat'ns have similar effects to Ca on the myocardium. Parenteral Ca has been reported to precipitate cardiac arrhythmias in pts receiving digitalis products.

Diuretics: With the except'n of K-sparing diuretics, all can cause K deficiencies and incr. digitalis toxicity.

Metoclopramide: May decr. digoxin absorpt'n from GI tract.

Propafenone: Incr. serum digoxin concentrat'n.

Quinidine: Can incr. serum digoxin levels. Also been reported to incr. digoxin's half-life in the body.

Rifampin: Can decr. serum digoxin concentrat'n.

Sympathomimetics: Concomitant use with digoxin incr. possibility of cardiac arrhythmias.

Verapamil: Incr. serum digoxin levels.

Assess: Pt hx for renal insufficiency, hypothyroidism, acute myocardial infarct, electrolyte imbalance, pulmonary disease, hypoxia, myocarditis, Adams-Stokes syndrome. Establish pt's age; apical/radial pulse rates, rhythm, quality; serum electrolytes; weight.

Administer: If apical pulse is less than 60 beats/min, if rhythm or quality of pulse changes, or if serum electrolyte levels are low, withhold medicat'n and contact physician. Administer w. meals to reduce gastric irritat'n. Check label extra carefully when preparing medicat'n.

Evaluate: Observe indicators of drug effectiveness (improved rate, rhythm, quality of pulses; decr. dyspnea; improved exercise tolerance; fewer chest rales; reduced frequency of prod. cough; decr. peripheral edema). Monitor fluid intake/output for diuresis; weigh daily during digitalizat'n for weight loss.

Teach: Maintenance regimen. How and when to take pulse. What physical and behavioral indicators should precipitate contacting physician. Avoid OTC drugs and antacids because of possible adv. drug interact'ns.

Generic Name (Trade Name)	Use (Dose)	Action	Adverse Effects	Drug Interactions	Nursing Process
Amrinone (Inocor)	Tx of severe congestive heart failure despite digitalis and diuretic tx (**IV: Adults** - Initially, 0.75 mg/kg bolus over 2-3 min. Maintenance, infuse at a rate of 5-10 µg/kg/min. If needed, 0.75 mg/kg may be given 30 min after initiat'n of tx. Maintain infus'n at approx. 5-10 µg/kg/min such that total daily dose (incl. boluses) does not exceed 10 mg/kg. Amrinone administrat'n is not recommended for a period over 24 h unless potential benefits clearly outweigh risks of longer tx)	Potent inotropic-vasodilator. Incr. myocardial contractility, reduces left and right ventr. filling pressures and pulmonary-capillary wedge pressure.	Thrombocytopenia, fever and nephrogenic diabetes insipidus	**Disopyramide:** And amrinone should be administered together w. caution until clinical experience is available.	**Assess:** Pt hx for hypersensitivity to amrinone or to bisulfites; renal or hepatic disease; hypokalemia, dehydration. Establish baseline BP and weight. **Administer:** IV solut'ns only if clear yellow. Do not dilute w. glucose or dextrose solut'n; use diluted within 24 h; store in light-resistant containers at room temp. **Evaluate:** Fluid intake/output; daily weight; hemodynamic parameters; pt perceptions of drug efficacy; lab. values for platelets, liver enzymes, serum electrolytes, renal fuction studies. Allergic or hypersensitivity react'ns.
Dopamine (Dopastat, Intropin, Revimine)	Tx of shock w. related renal shutdown or chronic refractory congestive heart failure (**IV only:** Must be diluted before administrat'n. 1-5 µg/kg/min; may be incr'd to 50 µg/kg/min for seriously ill pts)	Stim. beta₁ receptors to incr. heart rate and stroke volume. Stim. dopamine receptors on renal blood vessels to incr. GFR, renal blood flow, Na excret'n.	Tachycardia, angina, cardiac arrhythmias, headache, hypertens'n, nausea, vomiting. High doses cause vasoconstrict'n of renal blood vessels.	*Interactions also apply to dobutamine.* **Antidepressants, tricyclic:** May potentiate pressor response to dopamine. **Diuretics:** Use dopamine cautiously concurrently; may cause an additive or potentiating effect. **Halogenated anesthetics:** Incr. cardiac autonomic irritability and sensitize myocardium to dopamine's action. Use dopamine w. extreme caution in these pts. **Monoamine oxidase inhibitors (MAOIs):** Reduce rate of dopamine inactivat'n. Reduce starting dose of dopamine in these pts to at least 10% of us. dose. **Sympathomimetics:** Use dopamine cautiously in pts receiving sympathomimetics concomitantly.	**Assess:** Pt hx of tachycardia, ventr. fibrillat'n, pregnancy, diabetes, hypothermia; establish baseline BP, pulse (apical/peripheral), color and temp. of extremities. **Administer:** Freshly mixed dilut'n through patent IV; avoid extravasat'n which can cause necrosis; provide constant nsg observat'n. **Evaluate:** BP, pulse (apical/peripheral), color and temp. of extremities, urinary output, mental'n.
Dobutamine (Dobutrex)	Acute congestive heart failure or after cardiac surgery in which parenteral tx is required for inotropic support (**IV only:** Not for direct inject'n. Dilute according to manufacturer's direct'n. Us. reconstituted w. sterile H₂O or 5% dextrose by adding 10-20 mL diluent to 250 mg dobutamine. Dosage determined by pt response; ordinarily, 2.5-10 µg/kg/min)	Stim. beta₁ receptors. Incr. cardiac output w. minimal effects on heart rate. Does not produce renal vasodilatat'n or incr. GFR or Na excret'n.	As for dopamine		

CHAPTER 11

Antiarrhythmic Drugs

Etiology of Cardiac Arrhythmias

Cardiac arrhythmias are caused by disorders of rate, rhythm, origin or conduction within the heart. They may be produced by drugs, such as digoxin, or by cardiac disease. It has been estimated that between eighty and ninety per cent of patients with myocardial infarcts have cardiac arrhythmias at some time during their hospital management. The significance of this becomes apparent when it is recognized that death following an infarct usually results from ventricular arrhythmias.

Disorders of Impulse Formation

Cardiac tachyarrhythmias are the result of disorders of impulse formation and/or impulse conduction. With regard to the former, the heart has many cells that possess the potential to act as pacemakers. These cells, found in specialized conducting systems, such as the A-V node, the A-V bundle and the Purkinje network in the ventricles, depolarize spontaneously. This is the property of **automaticity.**

Although possessing the potential to act as **ectopic pacemakers,** these latent pacemakers do not usually trigger heart beats. The S-A node is the most rapidly depolarizing tissue in the heart. Under normal circumstances it serves as the site for impulse formation. Once the S-A node reaches its threshold it sends an electrical wave throughout the heart, depolarizing all latent pacemakers before they have a chance to act as sites of impulse formation. If, however, the normal S-A pacemaker node is damaged, or the rate at which its impulses are conducted throughout the heart is reduced, a formerly latent pacemaker may reach its threshold potential and fire before a depolarization wave sweeps over it from the S-A node. If this happens, it becomes an ectopic site for impulse formation.

Disorders of Impulse Conduction

Disorders of impulse conduction are more often the cause of cardiac arrhythmias. A-V blocks or bundle branch blocks are obvious causes of abnormal heart rhythms and need little explanation. It is more difficult to explain the etiology of paroxysmal atrial tachycardia, A-V nodal tachycardias, and ventricular tachycardias because they depend on the complex condition known as re-entry. Reference to Figure 15 may assist in the explanation.

Figure 15
Diagrammatic representation of the phenomenon of re-entry.

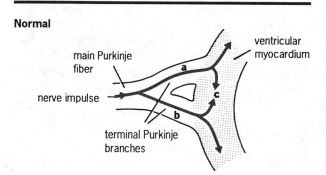

Normal

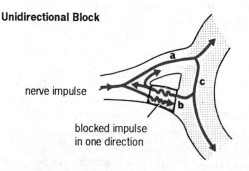

Unidirectional Block

If a localized area of the heart is damaged by a myocardial infarct, the transmission of impulses along a portion of a normal conducting system may be blocked in one direction. In Figure 15, impulse transmission is blocked unidirectionally along pathway (b). As a result, the impulse that travels

along (a) and (c) is allowed to come up (b) in a retrograde manner and re-enter (a) in the manner shown. This results in an extra heart beat. If it happens at several sites it can produce severe tachyarrhythmia leading to fibrillation.

Antiarrhythmic Drugs

Cardiac tachyarrhythmias can be treated by either (1) reducing the rate at which ectopic pacemakers depolarize or (2) modifying the conduction defects that lead to re-entry arrhythmias. Quinidine, procainamide, propranolol and phenytoin act by the first mechanism. These drugs decrease the rate of firing of ectopic pacemakers. As explained below, these drugs also modify impulse conduction.

Re-entry mediated ectopic rhythms can be altered either by increasing conductivity in the damaged tissue, in effect overcoming the block, or by decreasing further the conduction velocity, thereby converting a unidirectional block to a bidirectional one. Lidocaine and phenytoin are claimed to increase conductivity through damaged tissue. Quinidine, procainamide and propranolol have the opposite effect. By decreasing conductivity, they convert a unidirectional block into a bidirectional one. A bidirectional block is depicted in Figure 16.

Figure 16
Diagrammatic representation of a bidirectional block.

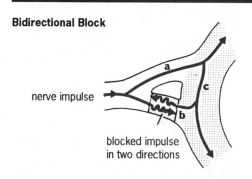

Bidirectional Block

With the exception of digoxin, antiarrhythmic drugs can be placed in one of four categories (see below). As the inotropic properties of digoxin have been described in Chapter 10, only its antiarrhythmic effects will be described at this time.

Digoxin (Lanoxin)

Mechanism of Action, Pharmacologic Effects and Therapeutic Uses

The complex actions of digoxin and the other cardiac glycosides have been explained in Chapter 10. As an antiarrhythmic drug, digoxin lengthens A-V nodal conduction time and functional refractory period. Many cardiologists consider digoxin the drug of choice to slow the ventricular response in patients with atrial fibrillation or flutter. Patients with stable, chronic atrial fibrillation usually respond better to digoxin than patients with unstable, acute atrial fibrillation. If digoxin proves unsatisfactory alone, it may be combined with propranolol or verapamil.

Generally, digoxin is contraindicated or given very cautiously in the presence of type I A-V block. Digoxin should also not be used as the only drug in Wolff-Parkinson-White patients because it can increase the ventricular response to atrial fibrillation or flutter.

Classes of Antiarrhythmic Drugs

Class IA (Quinidine, Procainamide, Disopyramide)

Mechanism of Action and Pharmacologic Effects

Quinidine, procainamide and disopyramide reduce the maximal rate of depolarization. They increase the threshold for excitation, depress conduction velocity and prolong the effective refractory period in the atrial, His-bundle, and ventricular conducting systems.

Therapeutic Uses and Adverse Effects

Quinidine is used to treat both atrial and ventricular arrhythmias. It has been used to maintain sinus rhythm after cardioversion in supraventricular arrhythmias. Quinidine is also often used with digoxin to treat atrial fibrillation. Because quinidine has an atropinic action, it increases A-V conduction. Digoxin, on the other hand, decreases A-V conduction. By combining the two drugs the physician can slow the atria with quinidine and

reduce A-V conduction with digoxin.

Quinidine's toxicities are usually dose related. At plasma concentrations above 8 µg/mL the direct depressant effects on A-V conduction appear and the QRS complex widens. As the concentration rises, S-A block or arrest, high-grade A-V block, ventricular arrhythmias or asystole may occur. These effects can also be produced by small amounts of quinidine in individuals allergic to the drug, or patients with congestive heart failure or renal impairment. The other adverse effects of quinidine include diarrhea, nausea and vomiting, headache, vertigo, palpitations, tinnitus and visual disturbances.

Procainamide (Pronestyl, Procan) has essentially the same therapeutic effects and clinical indications as quinidine. In contrast to quinidine, procainamide has little atropinic action. It is used mainly for the treatment of ventricular arrhythmias. Procainamide is also employed in the treatment of atrial fibrillation and paroxysmal supraventricular tachycardias. Effective therapeutic blood levels of procainamide lie between 4 – 8 µg/mL. Hypersensitivity to procainamide is an absolute contraindication to its use. In this connection, cross-sensitivity to procaine and related drugs must be borne in mind. Procainamide should not be administered to patients with complete A-V heart block. It is also contraindicated in cases of second-degree and third-degree A-V block unless an electric pacemaker is operative. Procainamide may also be contraindicated in patients with myasthenia gravis.

Procainamide may cause less anorexia, nausea and vomiting than quinidine. A reversible lupus erythematosus-like syndrome may result from its use. Both procainamide and its active metabolite N-acetylprocainamide are eliminated by the kidneys and will accumulate in patients with renal impairment unless lower doses are given. Unless the serum concentrations of procainamide can be measured, it is better not to use the drug in end-stage renal failure. Granulocytopenia may follow the use of procainamide.

Disopyramide (Norpace, Rythmodan) has actions similar to those of quinidine. Some clinicians believe it should be reserved for patients who are not in heart failure and who cannot tolerate quinidine or procainamide. Disopyramide is eliminated by both hepatic metabolism and renal excretion. Its dosage should be reduced in patients with liver or kidney impairment. Disopyramide is contraindicated in the presence of shock, renal failure, severe intraventricular conduction defects, pre-existing second- and third-degree A-V block (if no pacemaker is present) or known hypersensitivity to the drug. The drug should not be used in the presence of uncompensated or inadequately compensated congestive heart failure because it can worsen heart failure. Severe hypotension has been observed after administration of isopyramide, usually in patients with primary myocardial disease (cardiomyopathy) and in patients with inadequately compensated congestive heart failure or advanced myocardial disease with low-output state.

Other adverse effects of disopyramide include heart block, ventricular fibrillation and tachyarrhythmias. Its pronounced anticholinergic effects are often marked, and the drug is contraindicated in most patients with glaucoma or in patients in whom urinary retention is present. Treatment must often be stopped because of urinary retention.

Nursing Process — Quinidine

Assessment

Quinidine is contraindicated in patients with a previous hypersensitivity (either to quinidine or any cinchona derivative), complete heart block, hypotension, extensive myocardial damage, bacterial endocarditis, hyperthyroidism, digitalis toxicity, bundle branch block, congestive heart failure, extensive cardiac hypertrophy, kidney or liver disease, chronic respiratory disease or myasthenia gravis.

Before administering quinidine nurses should determine baseline values for all vital signs. At this time nurses should also review the patient's history for any contraindications to the medication that may inadvertently have been overlooked.

The nursing assessment should always include consideration of the potential interactions of a newly prescribed drug with those a patient is currently taking. The interaction of quinidine and digoxin has already been discussed. Consultation and collaboration with the pharmacist will assist the nurse to identify other potential interactions. Some patients show an idiosyncratic reaction to quinidine. The danger of this can be minimized by administering a 200-mg test dose and evaluating the patient's response before proceeding to give the remainder of the prescribed quantity.

Administration

Nurses must be particularly careful in preparing this medication for administration. Quinidine must *not* be confused with quinidine salts (i.e., quinidine gluconate, quinidine sulfate); these are not interchangeable as they contain varying amounts of anhydrous quinidine alkaloid. Quinidine should be given with meals to reduce gastric irritation. On the infrequent occasions when quinidine is adminis-

tered parenterally, it should be given only if it is a clear, colorless solution. Solutions that are brown should be discarded, since this indicates that the drug has crystallized as a result of exposure to light.

Evaluation

Nurses should evaluate the patient's response to quinidine. During the initial period of treatment the patient's cardiac response is best monitored by the use of a continuous electrocardiogram. Prolonged P-R intervals, absence of P-waves, and/or a heart rate over 120 beats per minute should be reported immediately to the physician. In the absence of electrocardiogram monitoring, the patient's apical pulse should be counted for one full minute every hour and the pulse rate, rhythm and quality noted. Blood pressure should be measured at hourly intervals during the initial stages of quinidine use; this can be reduced to daily readings once the patient is placed on a prophylactic maintenance dose.

Other vital signs should be monitored every two hours during the intensive early use of quinidine. Respiratory difficulty and hyperthermia are the early signs of toxicity. Quinidine may produce prolonged diuresis or diarrhea. Therefore, the intake and output of fluids should be recorded, together with the serum electrolytes.

In addition, nurses must be alert for early indications of hypersensitivity reactions. These might appear as prolonged hyperthermia, anaphylaxis, thrombocytopenia, respiratory distress resembling asthma and vascular collapse. Nurses should also be alert for the other adverse effects of quinidine, such as arterial embolism, hypotension, prolonged nausea, vomiting or diarrhea, cardiotoxicity (S-A block, A-V block, ventricular arrhythmias, asystole) and cinchonism (headache, vertigo, palpitations, tinnitus, hearing and visual disturbances, gastrointestinal disturbances, confusion, delirium, pyschosis).

Teaching

Patients should be instructed in the correct dose of quinidine and the frequency of administration at home. Without causing alarm, inform both patient and family of the early signs of cardiotoxicity to quinidine.

Nursing Process — Procainamide

The nursing process for procainamide is identical to that for quinidine. During intravenous administration, patients should be kept in a recumbent position and their blood pressure monitored constantly. Intravenous solutions that have turned dark amber or are otherwise discolored should be discarded. In addition to the patient evaluation suggested following the administration of quinidine, patients who are receiving procainamide should be observed for polyarthralgia, arthritis, pleuritic pain, fever, myalgia and skin lesions. These symptoms suggest reversible drug-induced lupus erythematosus. When procainamide is injected intramuscularly, nurses must be sure to aspirate to avoid intravascular administration. Patient teaching related to the use of procainamide is identical to that presented in relation to the use of quinidine.

Nursing Process — Disopyramide

The nursing process for disopyramide is identical to that for quinidine. Attention should be paid to the drug's anticholinergic effects (see Chapter 6). Patients should be assessed for the possibility of renal failure or glaucoma. Disopyramide is a newer drug than either quinidine or procainamide. Its safety has not been established in pregnancy. Therefore, female patients of childbearing age should be assessed to determine whether they are pregnant. Mothers should not nurse infants while taking disopyramide. The possibility that the anticholinergic effects may lead to urinary retention or constipation makes it mandatory that fluid intake and output be evaluated.

Class IB (Lidocaine, Mexiletine, Phenytoin, Tocainide)

Mechanism of Action and Pharmacologic Effects

Similar to the drugs in Class IA, lidocaine, tocainide and mexiletine decrease conduction. However, in contrast to the Class IA drugs which lengthen the effective refractory period in the atrial, His-bundle, and ventricular conducting systems, Class IB agents lengthen the effective refractory period only in the ventricular conducting system. As a result, Class IB drugs can not be used to treat atrial arrhythmias.

Therapeutic Uses and Adverse Effects

Lidocaine (Xylocaine) depresses automaticity in the ventricles. It has little effect on the atria and in usual doses does not depress myocardial contractility. It is used for the immediate control of ventricular premature extrasystoles and ventricular tachycardia. Ventricular arrhythmias secondary to cardiac surgery, cardiac catheterization, acute myocardial infarction and electrical conversion are treated with lidocaine. Although phenytoin is preferred, lidocaine can be used to treat digitalis-induced arrhythmias. Lidocaine is contraindicated in patients with known hypersensitivity to local anesthetics of the amide type, Adams-Stokes syndrome, or severe degrees of S-A, A-V or intraventricular block. It should be used with caution in patients with bradycardia or severe digoxin intoxication. Constant electrocardiographic monitoring is essential for the proper administration of lidocaine. Signs of excess depression of cardiac contractility, such as prolongation of P-R interval and QRS complex, with an aggravation of arrhythmias, should lead to prompt cessation of the intravenous injection.

Lidocaine's major toxicities involve the central nervous and cardiovascular systems. Patients may experience drowsiness, paresthesias, muscle twitching, convulsions, coma, respiratory depression and depressed myocardial contractility. Lidocaine is rapidly metabolized. Patients with hepatic insufficiency and individuals over the age of seventy should, as a rule, receive half to two-thirds the usual loading dose, and lower than normal maintenance doses.

The serum therapeutic window for lidocaine is 1 – 5 µg/mL (4.3 – 21.3 µmol/L). Serum levels below 1 µg/mL (4.3 µmol/L) are usually ineffective. Lidocaine concentrations in serum above 5 µg/mL (21.3 µmol/L) usually herald the start of central nervous system depression, stimulation or seizures.

Mexiletine (Mexitil) is similar in structure and activity to lidocaine. Given orally, mexiletine is used to treat or prevent ventricular ectopy and tachycardia. The drug is also used to suppress ventricular arrhythmias in survivors of acute myocardial infarction following therapy with lidocaine. Mexiletine may be as effective as procainamide and better tolerated. It appears to be less effective in patients with long-standing refractory ventricular arrhythmias. The concomitant use of propranolol may allow for a lower dose of mexiletine and better arrhythmia control.

Mexiletine's cardiovascular toxicities include sinus bradycardia or tachycardia, atrial fibrillation, hypotension, dyspnea and ventricular tachyarrhythmias, including *torsade de pointes*. Mexiletine is contraindicated in the presence of second- or third-degree A-V block in the absence of a pacemaker. It is also contraindicated in cardiogenic shock. Mexiletine should be used with caution in patients with hypotension or congestive heart failure because of its potential for depression of myocardial contractility. Caution should also be exercised when mexiletine is used in patients with severe first-degree A-V block or intraventricular conduction abnormalities. If the drug is given to a patient with the sick sinus syndrome, severe bradycardia and prolongation of sinus node recovery time may occur. Patients with severe bradyarrhythmias should not be given mexiletine. The extracardiac adverse reactions attributed to mexiletine include nausea, vomiting, malaise, dizziness, tremor, diplopia, paresthesias, confusion and ataxia.

Phenytoin (Dilantin) depresses spontaneous atrial and ventricular automaticity without altering intraventricular conduction. Phenytoin may also increase conduction through damaged Purkinje fibers. The drug is used mainly to reverse digitalis-induced arrhythmias.

The adverse effects of phenytoin include fatigue, dizziness, ataxia, nausea, vomiting, pruritus and rashes. If the drug is given rapidly intravenously, it can cause slowing of the heart rate, myocardial depression, hypotension, reduction in A-V conduction and (very occasionally) cardiac arrest. Phenytoin is contraindicated in sinus bradycardia, S-A block, second- and third-degree A-V block and Adams-Stokes syndrome.

Tocainide (Tonocard) is structurally related to lidocaine and has electrophysiologic properties similar to the latter drug. In therapeutic doses tocainide decreases the effective refractory period of the atrium, A-V node and right ventricle without affecting A-V conduction. Tocainide does not alter heart rate. Peripheral and pulmonary vascular resistance may increase slightly. Given orally, tocainide is initially effective in about sixty per cent of patients with ventricular arrhythmias that have proven refractive to quinidine, procainamide, disopyramide or propranolol. If tocainide is not effective when used alone, success in the treatment of ventricular arrhythmias may be attained by combining it with quinidine, disopyramide or propranolol. Tocainide is contraindicated in patients with a known hypersensitivity to local anesthetics of the amide type and in patients with second- or third-degree A-V block in the absence of a pacemaker.

Nausea and tremor are the most common adverse effects of tocainide. It can also cause anorexia, vomiting, abdominal pain and constipation. Tocainide's other adverse effects include dizziness, lightheadedness, confusion, anxiety and paresthesias. Congestive heart failure, conduction disturbances and ventricular arrhythmias can occur with tocainide, but are not common. Reports of hematological disorders (including leukopenia, agranulocytosis, bone marrow depression, hypoplastic anemia and thrombocytopenia) with tocainide have caused concern.

Nursing Process — Lidocaine

Assessment
Nursing responsibilities related to the use of lidocaine begin with the assessment of the patient's history for evidence of such contraindications as previous hypersensitivity to the drug, Adams-Stokes syndrome, hepatic disease and congestive heart failure. Also, the nursing assessment must include the establishment of baseline measurements for all vital signs.

Administration
For the treatment of cardiac arrhythmias, lidocaine is administered only intravenously. It should never be added to blood transfusion assemblies. Nurses must monitor blood pressure continuously for possible fluctuations.

Evaluation
Patient evaluation following the administration of lidocaine should focus on early detection of central nervous system effects that indicate developing toxicity. These include dizziness, restlessness, apprehension, euphoria, drowsiness, paresthesias, visual or auditory disturbances, confusion and disorientation, muscle twitching, difficulty in breathing, convulsions and respiratory arrest. Therapeutic effects should be constantly monitored using an electrocardiogram. Infusions of lidocaine should be discontinued as soon as cardiac rhythm has been stabilized or as soon as adverse effects are demonstrated.

Nursing Process — Mexiletine

Nursing measures related to the use of mexiletine are essentially the same as those identified below in relation to tocainide. The following points require additional emphasis.

Assessment
Establish baseline measures of pulse and blood pressure for later comparison in determining drug efficacy and/or adverse effects.

Administration
Oral administration with food or milk will reduce the possiblity of gastric distress. Intravenous administration should occur only in facilities equipped to provide continuous cardiac monitoring, cardiopulmonary resuscitation and cardioversion.

Evaluation

Observe for evidence of bradycardia; specifically, apical pulse rate below 60 beats per minute, light-headedness, syncope and dizziness. Patients should also be observed for postural hypotension. Adverse effects on the central nervous system are exhibited as intention tremors, nystagmus, blurred vision, dizziness, ataxia, confusion and nausea.

Teaching

Patients should be taught to request assistance with ambulation during the period when drug dosage is being stabilized. Patients on maintenance dosages should be taught to take their own pulses and should be advised to seek medical attention if bradycardia occurs.

Nursing Process — Phenytoin

Refer to Table 12 and Chapter 51.

Nursing Process — Tocainide

Assessment

Tocainide is contraindicated in individuals who are hypersensitive to it or to local anesthetics of the amide type. The drug is also contraindicated in second- or third-degree A-V block, hypokalemia, myasthenia gravis or pregnancy. Therefore, the nurse should review the patient's history for the presence of any of these conditions prior to administering this medication. The presence of renal or hepatic disease should signal the need for particularly careful evaluation of the patient following the administration of tocainide. A baseline electrocardiogram should be taken and baseline blood pressure established before treatment with this medication is initiated.

Administration

Oral administration of tocainide with food or milk will reduce gastric distress and slow absorption. Slower absorption will decrease the likelihood of peak concentrations and the accompanying risk of toxicity.

Evaluation

Drug efficacy is monitored by apical pulse rate and rhythm, fluctuations in blood pressure, electrocardiogram and laboratory tests of serum concentrations. Patients' pulse rate and rhythm should be monitored for evidence of bradycardia. Fluid intake and output should be measured so that disturbances indicating adverse renal effects can be noted early. Chest pain, dyspnea on exertion, wheezing and cough, in the absence of fever, indicate pulmonary fibrosis, which is a serious adverse

respiratory effect. Patients should also be observed for evidence of blood dyscrasias as indicated by an increased tendency to bruising, unusual bleeding, fever, chills and sore throat.

Teaching

Patients should be instructed as to the importance of having laboratory tests performed when ordered by the physician. They should also be taught the cardiovascular, respiratory, renal and hematologic indicators of adverse effects as indicated above in the evaluation section. Patients should also be advised that tocainide may cause dizziness, fine tremors, and drowsiness; therefore, caution should be exercised in driving or using power equipment.

Class IC (Encainide, Flecainide, Propafenone)

Mechanism of Action and Pharmacologic Effects

Drugs in Class IC depress the rate of rise of the membrane action potential. They have minimal effects on the duration of the membrane action potential and the effective refractory period of ventricular myocardial cells.

Therapeutic Uses and Adverse Effects

Encainide (Enkaid), when administered intravenously, slows conduction in the His-Purkinje system, without a major effect on conduction or refractoriness in other parts of the conduction system. Given orally, it slows conduction in the A-V node, His-Purkinje system and accessory pathways. In addition, oral encainide increases the refractoriness of atrial, ventricular and accessory pathways. The differences in effects between oral and intravenous therapy reflect the formation of active metabolites following ingestion. Encainide is used to treat ventricular arrhythmias that, in the judgment of the physician, are life threatening. Because of its proarrhythmic effects, encainide should be reserved for patients in whom, in the opinion of the physician, the benefits outweigh the risks.

Encainide's adverse effects include worsening of ventricular arrhythmias and an aggravation of sinus node disorders. Other effects of the drug are dizziness, headache, blurred vision, paresthesias and gastrointestinal disturbances.

Flecainide acetate (Tambocor) depresses sinus node automaticity, prolongs conduction, particularly in the His-Purkinje system and ventricles, and increases ventricular refractoriness.

Flecainide is indicated for the treatment of documented ventricular arrhythmias, such as sustained ventricular tachycardia, that are judged life threatening. Because of the proarrhythmic effects of flecainide, its use should be reserved for patients in whom the benefits of treatment are believed to outweigh the risks. Flecainide is not recommended in patients with less severe ventricular arrhythmias, even if the patients are symptomatic. Unless a pacemaker is present to sustain rhythm, flecainide is contraindicated in patients with second- or third-degree A-V block or in those with bifascicular or trifascicular bundle branch block. It is also contraindicated in the presence of cardiogenic shock.

Administered orally, flecainide is absorbed quickly. Peak plasma levels are attained in three hours. Its bioavailability is not affected by food. When given in multiple doses, the drug has a half-life of twenty hours. Its half-life is increased in patients with congestive heart failure or renal failure.

The adverse effects of flecainide include blurred vision and dizziness. Flecainide may also cause headache, nausea, fatigue, nervousness, tremor and paresthesias. It has also been reported to produce QT prolongation with subsequent ventricular tachycardia.

Propafenone (Rythmol) slows atrial, ventricular, A-V node, His-Purkinje and accessory pathway conduction. The drug should have the same restricted indications and contraindications as other Class IC drugs, such as flecainide. Propafenone is contraindicated in the presence of severe or uncontrolled congestive heart failure; cardiogenic shock; S-A, A-V, and intraventricular disorders of impulse conduction and sinus node dysfunction in the absence of an artificial pacemaker; severe bradycardia (less than 50 beats per minute); marked hypotension; severe obstructive pulmonary disease; severe disorders of electrolyte balance; and severe hepatic failure.

Propafenone's adverse effects include a worsening of congestive heart failure, A-V and intraventricular conduction disturbances and ventricular arrhythmias. The drug can also cause nausea, diarrhea, constipation, paresthesias and taste disturbances.

Nursing Process

The nursing process related to the use of encainide, flecainide and propafenone are the same as those discussed above for use of tocainide. In addition, the lung fields of encainide patients should be observed closely. Possible bilateral rales in conges-

tive heart failure patients on encainide should also be monitored. The dose of flecainide should be reduced as soon as the dysrhythmia is controlled. Nurses are advised to check propafenone package inserts for administration directions.

Class II (Beta Blockers — Propranolol)

Mechanism of Action and Pharmacologic Effects

Propranolol (Inderal) is the beta blocker used most extensively as an antiarrhythmic drug. Other beta blockers that could be used as antiarrhythmic drugs include atenolol, metoprolol and timolol. At this time, in the interests of space, attention will be focused only on propranolol. However, many of the general comments made about the properties and uses of propranolol can be applied to the other beta blockers.

By blocking $beta_1$ receptors in the heart, beta blockers reduce cardiac output, diminish myocardial oxygen requirements and prevent cardiac arrhythmias, particularly those caused by increased sympathetic activity. The cardiac effects of beta blockade include bradycardia, a decrease in contractility, an increase in A-V conduction time and a reduction in automaticity.

Therapeutic Uses and Adverse Effects

Beta blocker treatment is best suited for catecholamine-induced arrhythmias. Propranolol is also used to treat atrial flutter and fibrillation, paroxysmal atrial tachycardia and digitalis-induced arrhythmias.

The major adverse effects of the drug are bradycardia, congestive heart failure, cardiac arrest (in patients with A-V block) and bronchospasm. Propranolol can precipitate congestive heart failure in patients with heart disease. It is contraindicated in bronchospasm, including bronchial asthma, and allergic rhinitis during the pollen season; sinus bradycardia and greater than first-degree block; cardiogenic shock; right ventricular failure secondary to pulmonary hypertension; and congestive heart failure, unless the failure is secondary to a tachyarrhythmia treatable with propranolol. Chronic occlusive peripheral vascular disease is a relative contraindication to the use of propranolol.

Nursing Process

The nursing processes related to propranolol's use are detailed in Chapter 8 and summarized in Table 12 at the end of this chapter.

Class III (Amiodarone)

Mechanism of Action and Pharmacologic Effects

Class III drugs increase the refractory period of the atria, A-V node, ventricles, His-Purkinje system and bypass tracts. Amiodarone (Cordarone) also depresses sinus node automaticity and slows conduction in the atria, A-V node, His-Purkinje system and ventricles. The prominent effect seen after acute intravenous administration of amiodarone is slow conduction and prolonged refractoriness of the A-V node. The drug may also have a marked negative inotropic effect following acute intravenous administration.

Therapeutic Uses and Adverse Effects

Amiodarone is used to treat life-threatening ventricular and supraventricular arrhythmias that are refractory to other antiarrhythmic drugs. The oral form of the drug is often successful in suppressing recurrence of ventricular tachycardia or fibrillation. Unfortunately, its severe adverse effects limit amiodarone's usefulness in some patients.

The drug may be used to prevent the recurrence of atrial flutter and fibrillation and A-V nodal re-entrant tachycardia. Amiodarone is also very useful in patients with reciprocating tachycardia or atrial flutter and fibrillation associated with the Wolff-Parkinson-White syndrome. This effect can be attributed to the ability of the drug to prolong refractoriness in both the A-V node and accessory pathways, in addition to slowing A-V nodal conduction.

Supraventricular and ventricular arrhythmias in patients with hypertrophic cardiomyopathy may also be treated with amiodarone. The drug may also control episodes of tachycardia in patients with a syndrome of bradycardia-tachycardia. However, because amiodarone may exacerbate bradycardia, a permanent pacemaker should be in place.

Unfortunately, amiodarone can also be a most toxic drug. It can cause anorexia, nausea, vomiting, abdominal pain and constipation. Other effects include headache, weakness, myalgia, tremor, ataxia, paresthesias, depression, insomnia, nightmares and hallucinations. Peripheral neuropathy, accompanied by histologic changes in nerve fibers, can also occur. Amiodarone can cause photosensitivity reactions.

Its effects on the cardiovascular system include myocardial depression, hypotension, S-A block, A-V block, ventricular arrhythmias, fatal congestive heart failure, cardiogenic shock and cardiac arrest.

Hypersensitivity pneumonia and pulmonary fibrosis have developed in some patients taking amiodarone. Elevated serum creatinine levels have been reported in patients taking this drug.

Amiodarone is contraindicated in severe sinus node dysfunctions, sinus bradycardia, and second- and third-degree A-V block. It is also contraindicated in patients with episodes of bradycardia sufficient to cause syncope, unless used in conjunction with a pacemaker. Amiodarone's contraindications include acute hepatitis. The drug should not be used in patients showing radiographic evidence of pulmonary interstitial abnormalities.

Nursing Process

Assessment
The nurse should review the patient's history for evidence of goiter, Hashimoto's thyroiditis, previous heart block problems, and for liver and kidney function status. Laboratory evaluation for electrolytes should be checked before administration. Baseline values for the electrocardiogram, fluid intake and output ratio and vital signs should be established before administration.

Administration
Vital signs and blood pressure should be checked continuously during administration. Reduce dosage slowly with electrocardiogram monitoring.

Evaluation
Monitor patients for alteration in central nervous system, thyroid and pulmonary functions throughout drug administration. Cardiac rate should be noted. Nurses should also observe respiration rate, rhythm and character, and evaluate patients for chest pain. If changes in any of these parameters occur, contact the physician for directions regarding possible discontinuation of the drug.

Teaching
Teach both patient and family all aspects of drug action and side effects. Also inform them of the need to notify the physician immediately if side effects occur. Although sun discoloration is usually reversible, nurses should caution patients to stay out of the sun and advise them to use sunscreen and dark glassess.

Class IV — Calcium Channel Blockers (Verapamil)

Mechanism of Action and Pharmacologic Effects

Calcium channel blockers selectively inhibit the slow channel calcium ion transport into cardiac tissue. This slow inward current links myocardial excitation to contraction and control of energy storage and utilization. The pacemaker cells of the S-A node and cells in the proximal region of the A-V node are depolarized primarily by the calcium current. Blocking the calcium channel has the effect of depressing A-V conduction.

Therapeutic Uses and Adverse Effects

Verapamil (Calan, Isoptin) is highly effective for the treatment and prevention of supraventricular tachycardias and re-entrant tachycardias that use the A-V node as part of their re-entrant circuits. The drug can also decrease the ventricular response to atrial flutter or fibrillation. It has little effect on ventricular arrhythmias. Its effects are more predictable following parenteral administration. Taken orally, a large percentage of the drug is inactivated during its first pass through the liver.

Because of verapamil's negative inotropic effect, it is contraindicated in patients with poorly compensated congestive heart failure, unless the failure is complicated by or caused by dysrhythmia. If verapamil is used in such patients, they must be digitalized prior to treatment. Contraindications to the use of verapamil also include acute myocardial infarction, cardiogenic shock, severe hypotension, second- or third-degree A-V block, sick sinus syndrome and marked bradycardia.

The incidence of adverse effects from verapamil is nine per cent, lower than for most other antiarrhythmic drugs. The most common adverse effect following intravenous administration is a transient and mild fall in arterial blood pressure. There have been reports of serious adverse effects, including hypotension, bradycardia and, on rare occasions, ventricular asystole. Oral verapamil almost invariably causes constipation. Nausea, vomiting, lightheadedness, headache, flushing, nervousness, rashes and pruritus also may occur following oral treatment.

Nursing Process

Assessment

A baseline electrocardiogram as well as laboratory evaluation of renal and hepatic function should be established before treatment with this medication is initiated. In addition, baseline measurements of blood pressure and pulse should be documented. The presence of renal or hepatic disease should signal the need for particularly careful evaluation of the patient following the administration of verapamil. The patient's current drug regimen should be reviewed for procainamide or quinidine therapy, which are contraindicated for concurrent use with verapamil. The nurse should also check the patient's history for any of the following conditions which contraindicate the use of verapamil: severe hypotension, cardiogenic shock, cardiomegaly, digitalis toxicity, A-V block, severe congestive heart failure or pregnancy.

Administration

Parenteral treatment with this medication should be initiated only in facilities equipped to provide continuous cardiac monitoring, cardiopulmonary resuscitation and cardioversion. Administer only intravenous solutions that are clear and colorless and are stored in light-resistant containers at room temperature.

Evaluation

Blood pressure and pulse should be monitored prior to each dose to determine drug efficacy and provide early indication of adverse effects or toxicity. During the administration of verapamil, evaluate the effects of the drug on blood pressure and dysrhythmias.

Teaching

Ensure that the patient and a responsible care giver are aware of the indicators of drug efficacy, adverse effects and toxicity. Teach patients how to take their pulse before taking the drug and the importance of recording or graphing their observations. Driving or the use of power equipment are not advisable during the early phase of treatment with verapamil because of the risk of lightheadedness or dizziness. Patients should also be advised to change position slowly to avoid dizziness.

Caffeine intake should be reduced because it might interfere with the calcium-blocking effects of verapamil. For the same reason, patients should be counselled not to use over-the-counter medications, which might contain caffeine or theophylline, without consulting their physician.

Further Reading

Campbell, R.W.F. (1988). Assessment of the risk-benefit ratio for antiarrhythmic drug use. *Drugs 36* :6l6-632.

Drugs for cardiac arrhythmias. (1989). *The Medical Letter 31* :35-40.

Drugs for cardiac arrhythmias: New warning. (1989). *The Medical Letter 31* :48.

Garrat, C., Ward, D. E. and Camm, A. J. (1989). Lesson from the cardiac arrhythmia suppression trial. Death increased in patients given encainide and flecainide. *Brit. Med. J. 299* :805-806.

Klein, H. O. and Kaplinsky, E. (1986). Digitalis and verapamil in atrial fibrillation and flutter. Is verapamil now the preferred agent? *Drugs 31* :185-197.

Morganroth, J. (1987). New antiarrhythmic agents: Mexiletine, tocainide, encainide, flecainide and amiodarone. *Rational Drug Therapy 21* (4):1-6.

Nestico, P. R., Morganroth, J. and Horowitz, L. N. (1988). New antiarrhythmic drugs. *Drugs 35* :286-319.

Rotmensch, H. H., Rotmensch, S. and Elkayam, U. (1987). Management of cardiac arrhythmias during pregnancy. Current concept. *Drugs 33* :623-633.

Treatment of cardiac arrhythmias. Drugs of choice. (1989). *The Medical Letter 31* :5-17.

Woosley, R. L. (1987). Mesiletine and tocainide: A profile of two lidocaine analogues. *Rational Drug Therapy 21* (3):1-7.

Table 12
Antiarrhythmic drugs.

Pharmacologic Classification: Class 1A Antiarrhythmic Drugs — Digoxin — Refer to Table 11

Generic Name (Trade Name)	Use (Dose)	Action	Adverse Effects	Drug Interactions	Nursing Process
Quinidine	Maint. normal sinus rhythm following countershock; prevent premature ventr. extrasystoles or paroxysmal ventr. tachycardia; prevent paroxysmal supraventr. tachycardia or supraventr. premature contract'ns **(Oral:** Adults - Give test dose of 200 mg quinidine sulfate initially to determine poss. hypersensitivity. In absence of hypersensitivity, 200-400 mg may be taken q4-6h. A loading dose of 400-1000 mg can be used to produce effective serum levels rapidly. Children - 6 mg/kg q4-6h. *Time-release quinidine gluconate:* Adults - 324-972 mg q8-12h)	Depresses automaticity, retards conductivity and prolongs refractory period in heart. Lower doses incr. A-V conductivity.	Severe cardiotoxicity, diarrhea, nausea, vomiting, cinchonism, hypotens'n, arterial embolism, hypersensitivity react'ns	**Anticholinergic drugs:** Have additive anticholinergic effects w. quinidine. **Anticoagulants, oral:** Have incr. activity in the presence of quinidine, which depresses prothrombin format'n, inhibits synthesis of vitamin K-sensitive clotting factors. **Cimetidine:** May decr. metabolism of quinidine, thereby reducing its rate of eliminat'n. **Digoxin:** Serum levels can be incr. by quinidine which reduces the renal and nonrenal clearance of digoxin. GI disturbances and ventr. arrhythmias have occurred as a result of this interact'n. The dose of digoxin should be reduced by 50% before starting quinidine tx. Pts receiving both drugs should be monitored carefully, particularly during initial 5 days of combined tx. If quinidine is discontinued, pts should be monitored for underdigitalizat'n. **Neuromuscular blocking drugs:** Should be used cautiously w. quinidine because of additive effects. **Nifedipine:** May incr. serum quinidine concentrat'n and cause hypotens'n. **Phenobarbital and phenytoin:** May incr. metabolism of quinidine, thereby increasing its eliminat'n.	**Assess:** Pt hx for contraindicat'ns, establish digitalizat'n status, test for idiosyncratic response to quinidine, establish baseline measurements for all VS. **Administer:** Orally w. meals; parenteral solut'n that is clear and colorless. **Evaluate:** Effectiveness of tx using ECG monitor; hourly observat'n of apical pulse, BP; respirat'ns and temp. q2h; fluid intake/output; for early evidence of hypersensitivity, arterial embolism, GI disturbances, cardiotoxicity, cinchonism. **Teach:** Correct dose and frequency for home administrat'n; s/s that should precipitate medical contact. Provide aids to facilitate pt compliance.

Drug	Use / Dosage	Side Effects	Interactions	Nursing Considerations
Procainamide (Pronestyl, Procan)	Tx of ventr. extrasystoles, ventr. tachycardia, cardiac arrhythmias associated w. anesthesia and surgery, atrial fibrillat'n and paroxysmal atrial tachycardia that cannot be controlled by other measures (**Oral:** Adults - initially, 250-500 mg q3-6h. 1 g can be given as a loading dose to produce effective serum levels quickly. Children - 50 mg/kg/day in 4-6 divided doses. *Time-release preparat'n:* Adults - 1 g q6h or 50 mg/kg/day in divided doses at 6-h intervals)	As for quinidine	**Procainamide, propranolol:** Effects may be additive to those of quinidine. **Potassium:** Hyperkalemia incr., and hypokalemia decr., activity of quinidine. **Rifampin:** May incr. metabolism of quinidine, thereby incr. its eliminat'n.	**Assess:** As for quinidine. **Administer:** IV solut'ns w. pt recumbent and constant monitoring of BP. Discard solut'ns that are dark amber or otherwise discolored. **Evaluate:** As for quinidine, for s/s of drug-induced lupus erythematosus. **Teach:** As for quinidine.
		As for quinidine, except for cinchonism; also, reversible systemic lupus erythematosus-like syndrome	**Antihypertensive agents:** Additive hypotensive effect may be seen w. concomitant procainamide use. **Beta blockers:** Prior administrat'n of procainamide in pts w. acute myocardial infarct may potentiate cardiac depressant action of beta-blocking drugs. **Cholinergic drugs:** Procainamide has anticholinergic activity and may antagonize cholinergic drugs.	
Disopyramide (Norpace, Rythmodan)	Episodes of ventr. tachycardia and premature ventr. contract'ns (**Oral:** Adults - us. daily dose, 400-800 mg given in 4 divided doses. Use smaller doses in pts w. small stature, hepatic insufficiency, cardiomyopathy or cardiac decompensat'n. *Time-release preparat'n:* 300 mg q12h. Do not use the time-release preparat'n in pts w. severe renal insufficiency, cardiomyopathy or cardiac decompensat'n)	As for quinidine	**Antiarrhythmic drugs:** Disopyramide should be used w. great care in pts receiving other antiarrhythmic agents such as quinidine or procainamide and/or propranolol. Their concomitant use should be reserved for pts w. life-threatening arrhythmias. **Beta blockers:** Have additive negative inotropic effects w. disopyramide.	**Assess:** As for quinidine; pt hx of renal failure, glaucoma or current pregnancy. **Evaluate:** As for quinidine. **Teach:** As for quinidine.
		Bradycardia, shortness of breath, chest pain, lightheadedness, heart block, CV collapse, paradoxical ventr. tachycardia or ventr. fibrillat'n, fatigue, muscle weakness, dizziness, headache		

Generic Name (Trade Name)	Use (Dose)	Action	Adverse Effects	Drug Interactions	Nursing Process

Pharmacologic Classification: Class IB Antiarrhythmic Drugs

Generic Name (Trade Name)	Use (Dose)	Action	Adverse Effects	Drug Interactions	Nursing Process
Lidocaine (Xylocaine)	Ventr. tachycardia following cardiac surgery or catheterizat'n, acute myocardial infarct, electrical convers'n, and digitalis-induced arrythmias (**IV:** For ventr. arrhythmias: A loading dose of 50-100 mg over 2-3 min. This dose can be repeated in 5 min. Alternatively, 1-2 addit'nal doses of 25-50 mg may be administered at 5-10 min intervals; max. dose, 300 mg in a 1-h period. Following administrat'n of loading dose, lidocaine can be used at a rate of 1-4 mg/min. For prophylaxis after acute myocardial infarct: A loading dose of 200 mg, given as 4 [50-mg] inject'ns 5 min apart, or 20 mg/min infused for 10 min. Each bolus should be given slowly. Simultaneously w. the loading dose, an infus'n is started at a rate of 3 mg/min. The infus'n should be continued for 24-36 h or until a dx of acute myocardial infarct is excluded)	Depresses automaticity in ventricles. Has little effect on atria. In us. doses, does not depress myocardial contractility.	Drowsiness, paresthesias, muscle twitching, convuls'ns, coma, respiratory depress'n, depressed myocardial contractility.	**Beta blockers:** May decr. cardiac output and hepatic blood flow, thereby reducing lidocaine clearance. **Cimetidine:** May decr. lidocaine clearance.	**Assess:** Pt hx of hepatic disease, CHF, Adams-Stokes syndrome, heart block; establish baseline VS. **Administer:** IV only. **Evaluate:** Tx effect using ECG monitoring; for addit'nal CNS effects; for respiratory depress'n.
Mexiletine HCl (Mexitil)	Orally, to prevent or treat ventr. ectopy and tachycardia (**Oral:** Adults - initially, 200 mg q8h. If nec. for rapid effect, a loading dose of 400 mg may be administered, followed by a 200-mg dose in 8 h. Thereafter, dose may be incr. or decr. by 50 mg or 100 mg. Us. maint. dose, 200-300 mg q8h. Max. 1.2 g/day)	Structurally related to lidocaine; has similar electrophysiological properties. Depresses automaticity in ventricles, has little effect on atria. Does not depress sinus node funct'n except in pts w. sick sinus syndrome. Does not depress A-V conduct'n in pts w. normal A-V conduct'n. A-V	Sinus bradycardia or tachycardia, atrial fibrillat'n, A-V dissociat'n, hypotens'n, dyspnea, ventr. tachyarrhythmias. Avoid in pts w. severe bradyarrhythmias, nausea, vomiting, dizziness, tremor, diplopia, dysarthria, paresthesias, confus'n and ataxia.	**Metaclopramide:** May incr. rate of absorpt'n of mexiletine. **Narcotics:** Can slow rate of absorpt'n of mexiletine. **Phenytoin, rifampin:** Can induce drug-metabolizing enzymes and decr. half-life of mexiletine.	As for tocainide, plus: **Assess:** Establish baseline BP, pulse. **Administer:** Orally with food or milk; IV in coronary ICU only. **Evaluate:** For bradycardia, postural hypotens'n, adv. effects. **Teach:** Need for assistance w. ambulat'n; to take own pulse; to seek medical attent'n if bradycardia ensues.

Drug	Uses and Dosage	Action	Side Effects/Adverse Reactions	Drug Interactions	Nursing Considerations
Phenytoin (Dilantin)	Tx of digitalis-induced ventr. arrhythmia (**Oral:** Adults - 1 g on first day; then 300-600 mg on days 2 and 3. Maint. dose, 300-400 mg daily in 1-4 divided doses. Children - Initially, 10-15 mg/kg in 2-3 doses over 24 h. Maint. dose, 5-10 mg/kg/day in 2-3 doses)	Depresses spontaneous atrial and ventr. automaticity without altering intraventr. conduct'n. Incr. conduct'n through damaged Purkinje fibers. conduct'n may be incr. in pts w. pre-existing conduct'n disturbances.	Fatigue, dizziness, ataxia, nausea, vomiting, pruritus and rashes. Rapid IV infus'n causes bradycardia, myocardial depress'n, hypotens'n, reduced A-V conduct'n, cardiac arrest.	**Antidepressants, tricyclic:** In high doses, may precipitate seizures; dosage of phenytoin may have to be adjusted accordingly. **Metabolism:** Phenytoin metabolism may be incr. significantly by use of barbiturates, and its metabolism may be decr. by concomitant administrat'n of coumarin anticoagulants, chloramphenicol, disulfiram, phenylbutazone and isoniazid.	**Assess:** Pt hx for asthma, allergies, kidney or liver disease, alcohol abuse, heart block, bradycardia, hypotens'n; establish VS. **Administer:** Prepare IV solut'n w. diluent supplied by manufacturer; use only clear solut'ns. Complete dissolut'n requires approx. 10 min. Follow IV inject'n w. normal saline; use immed. after reconstitut'n. Do *not* add to IV solut'ns in glass bottles; *never* add to running IV. Give oral doses w. meals. **Evaluate:** BP, pulse, respirat'n; for adv. CNS effects; for hepatoxicity; for hematological toxicity; for folic acid and vitamin D deficiency.
Tocainide HCl (Tonocard)	Tx of ventr. arrhythmias resistant to quinidine, procainamide, disopyramide or propranolol (**Oral:** Adults - initially, 400 mg q8h. Us. maint. dose, 1.2-1.8 g/day in 3 doses)	Electrophysiological properties sim. to lidocaine. Decr. refractory period of atrium, A-V node, and right ventricle without affecting A-V conduct'n. Does not alter heart rate.	Nausea, tremor, anorexia, vomiting, abdominal pain, constipat'n, dizziness, lightheadedness, confus'n, anxiety, paresthesias, leukopenia, agranulocytosis, bone marrow depress'n, hypoplastic anemia, thrombocytopenia		**Assess:** Pt hx of hypersensitivity to local anesthetics, A-V block, hypokalemia, myasthenia gravis, pregnancy, renal or hepatic disease. Establish baseline BP. **Administer:** Orally with food. **Evaluate:** Apical pulse rate and rhythm, ECG, fluid intake/output, respiratory status; for blood dyscrasias. **Teach:** Importance of having lab. tests; indicators of adv. effects; to use caution if driving or running power equipment.

Pharmacologic Classification: Class IC Antiarrhythmic Drugs

Drug	Uses and Dosage	Action	Side Effects/Adverse Reactions	Drug Interactions	Nursing Considerations
Encainide (Enkaid)	Tx of life-threatening ventr. arrythmias (**Oral:** Adults - 75-300 mg/day, given in 3 divided doses)	Slows conduct'n in A-V node, His-Purkinje system and accessory pathways.	Worsening of ventr. arrhythmias and aggravat'n of sinus node disorders. Dizziness, headache, blurred vision, paresthesias, GI disturbances		**Assess:** Cardiac status, BP, fluid intake/output. Check GI status for bowel pattern and no. of stools; respiratory status, w. pulmonary funct'n tests and lung fields, as rales may occur in CHF pts. Stop drug w. incr. respirat'n or pulse. **Administer:** Pts on doses of 200 mg/day or more should be hospitalized.

Generic Name (Trade Name)	Use (Dose)	Action	Adverse Effects	Drug Interactions	Nursing Process
					Evaluate: For tx response, cardiac status, respiratory rate and rhythm, drug toxicity. **Teach:** Warn pt of risk of incr. drug dosage on his own.
Flecainide acetate (Tambocor)	Suppress'n of ventr. ectopy and tachycardia **(Oral:** Adults - start tx in hospital w. rhythm monitoring. Initially, 100 mg q12h. Incr. by 50 mg bid q4 days prn. Max. dose, 400 mg/day. *In pts w. a hx of congestive heart failure or myocardial dysfunction,* initially, no more than 100 mg q12h. Incr. cautiously by 50 mg bid, q4 days. Max. dose, 200 mg q12h. *In pts w. severe renal impairment* (creatinine clearance of 35 mL/min/1.73m^2 or less), initially 50-100 mg 1x daily)	Prolongs conduct'n and incr. ventr. refractoriness.	Dizziness, vis. disturbances, headache, nausea, dyspnea, new or worsened arrythmia, chest pain, new or worsened CHF, edema, syncope, conduct'n disturbances, tachycardia, angina pectoris	**Digoxin:** Serum levels may incr. when flecainide is administered. **Propranolol:** Plus flecainide may lead to a slight incr. in plasma levels of both drugs.	As for tocainide (see above).
Propafenone (Rythmol)	For suppress'n of the following ventr. arrhythmias, occurring singly or in combinat'n: episodes of ventr. tachycardia; premature (ectopic) ventr. contract'ns, such as premature ventr. beats of unifocal or multifocal origin; couplets; R-on-T phenomenon, when of suff. severity to require tx **(Oral:** Initially, 150 mg q8h. Incr. q3-4 days to 300 mg q12h. Max. dose, 300 mg q8h. In those pts in whom widening of QRS complex or prolongat'n of P-R interval occurs, reduce dose. *In pts w. mild to moderate hepatic insufficiency,* start w. 150 mg 1x daily. Dosage may be incr. at a min. of 4-day intervals to	Slows atrial, ventr., A-V node, His-Purkinje and accessory pathway conduct'n.	Worsening of CHF; A-V, intraventr. conduct'n disturbances and ventr. arrhythmias. Nausea, diarrhea, constipat'n, paresthesias and dysgeusia	**Digoxin:** Serum levels incr. if propafenone is administered.	**Assess:** Before tx, assess for contraindicat'ns: CHF; cardiogenic shock; S-A, A-V, intraventr. disorders; severe bradycardia; marked hypoten'sn; severe pulmonary or hepatic pathology. **Administer:** Continuous cardiac monitoring is recommended during initiat'n of tx. Give drug w. food to reduce adverse GI react'ns. **Teach:** Necessity of frequent ECG monitoring if drug given w. digoxin, as propafenone incr. serum digoxin levels.

150 mg bid, then to 150 mg q8h, and prn to 300 mg q12h. *In elderly pts, effective dose may be lower)*

Pharmacologic Classification: Class II Antiarrhythmic Drugs — Beta Blockers

Drug	Action	Dose	Side Effects	Drug Interactions	Nursing Process
Propranolol (Inderal)	Beta blocker; decr. heart rate, ventr. systolic pressure, myocardial contractility, cardiac output, coronary blood flow and O$_2$ consumpt'n, and BP. Reduces sinus rate. Slows A-V conduct'n and spontaneous rate of ectopic pacemakers.	Tx of cardiac arrhythmias (**Oral:** Adults - 10-30 mg tid or qid. Children - 0.5-4 mg/kg/day in 4 divided doses. **IV:** Adults - 0.1-0.15 mg/kg, administered in increments of 0.5-0.75 mg q1-2min. Children - 0.01-0.15 mg/kg over 3-5 min. Monitor the ECG and BP continuously in all pts receiving IV propranolol. Use lower doses, or avoid using the drug entirely, where there is a risk of myocardial depress'n)	Bronchoconstrict'n in asthmatics; potentiates effect of insulin; asystole, A-V block, bradycardia, heart failure, nausea, vomiting, constipat'n, depress'n, sleep disturbances, allergic react'ns	*For drug interact'ns rel. to the use of propranolol, refer to Tables 8 and 15.*	*For nsg process rel. to the use of propranolol, refer to Tables 8 and 15.*

Pharmacologic Classification: Class III Antiarrhythmic Drugs

Drug	Action	Dose	Side Effects	Drug Interactions	Nursing Process
Amiodarone (Cordarone)	Incr. refractory period of the atria, A-V node, ventricles, His-Purkinje system and bypass tracts. Depresses sinus node automaticity and slows conduct'n in atria, A-V node, His-Purkinje system and ventricles. Prominent effect after IV administrat'n is slow conduct'n and prolonged refractoriness of A-V node. May also have a marked negative inotropic effect following IV administrat'n.	Tx of life-threatening ventr. and supraventr. arrhythmias that are refractory to other antiarrhythmic drugs. Oral form of the drug is often successful in suppressing recurrence of ventr. tachycardia or fibrillat'n (**Oral:** Adults - *For refractory ventr. arrhythmias* - 800 mg - 1.6 g od initially, followed by 600-800 mg od after 1-2 weeks and then 400-600 mg od. Then use smallest dose possible. *For supraventr. arrhythmias* - 600 mg/day in 3 divided doses for 1 week, followed by 200-400 mg daily. After this, use lowest dose possible. *For bradycardia-tachycardia syndrome (w. a pacemaker in place)* - initially, 200 mg bid, followed by 200-600 mg daily. Children - 3-20	Anorexia, nausea, vomiting, abdominal pain, constipat'n, headache, weakness, myalgia, tremor, ataxia, paresthesias, depress'n, insomnia, nightmares, hallucinat'ns, photosensitivity react'ns, myocardial depress'n, hypotens'n, S-A block, A-V block, ventr. arrhythmias, fatal CHF, cardiogenic shock, cardiac arrest, hypersensitivity pneumonia and pulmonary fibrosis, elevated serum creatinine	**Anticoagulants, oral** (such as warfarin): Have their effects incr. by amiodarone. Reduce dose of the anticoagulant by 50% during concomitant tx with amiodarone. **Digoxin, quinidine, procainamide and phenytoin:** Can have their serum levels and effects incr. by amiodarone. **Digoxin, beta blockers and verapamil:** Can cause symptomatic bradycardia or sinus arrest if given w. amiodarone. **Disopyramide, quinidine, mexiletine or propafenone:** Plus amiodarone, have caused ventr. arrhythmias (torsade de pointes). **Hypokalemia:** May incr. the risk of amiodarone-induced ventr. arrhythmias.	**Assess:** Pt hx of goiter, Hashimoto's thyroiditis, heart block. Liver and kidney funct'n; baseline ECG; lab. test for electrolytes; VS, fluid intake/output status. **Administer:** Monitor VS and BP continuously during administrat'n. Reduce dose slowly with ECG monitoring. **Evaluate:** CNS, thyroid, pulmonary and cardiac funct'n. If changes occur, contact physician for direct'ns regarding discontinuing tx. **Teach:** Pt and family all aspects of drug action, side effects. Caution pts to keep out of the sun.

Generic Name (Trade Name)	Use (Dose)	Action	Adverse Effects	Drug Interactions	Nursing Process

Pharmacologic Classification: Class IV Antiarrhythmic Drug — Calcium Channel Blocker

Generic Name (Trade Name)	Use (Dose)	Action	Adverse Effects	Drug Interactions	Nursing Process
Verapamil (Isoptin, Calan)	mg/kg/day) Tx of paroxysmal supraventr. tachycardia, atrial fibrillat'n, atrial flutter (**IV:** Adults - 5-10 mg administered over 2 min [3 min for elderly pts]. If nec., give addit'nal 10 mg in 30 min. For maint. tx, infus'ns of 0.005 mg/kg/min have been used. Infants up to 1 yr. - 0.1-0.2 mg/kg over 2 min, repeated prn in 30 min. Children 1-15 yrs. - 0.1-0.3 mg/kg, repeated prn in 30 min. Do not exceed 10 mg as a single dose. **Oral:** Adults - 240-480 mg daily in 3-4 divided doses)	Calcium channel blocker; depresses A-V conduct'n.	Hypotens'n and bradycardia associated w. IV use, constipat'n w. oral use. Transient asystole, hypotens'n, development or worsening of heart failure, development of rhythm disturbances including A-V block and ventr. dysrhythmias, stenocardia (angina), flushing, peripheral and pulmonary edema, dizziness, headache, fatigue, excitat'n, vertigo, syncope, tremor	**Antihypertensive drugs:** In pts on antihypertensive drugs, the addit'nal hypotensive effect of verapamil should be taken into considerat'n. **Beta blockers:** Generally, verapamil should not be given to pts receiving beta blockers. However, in exceptional cases when (in the physician's opinion) concomitant use is essential, such use should be instituted gradually in a hospital under careful supervis'n. **Digoxin:** Plasma levels may be incr. by verapamil.	**Assess:** Baseline ECG; lab. tests for renal and hepatic funct'n; BP and pulse; current drug profile for use of digitalis, procainamide or quinidine; check hx for severe hypotens'n, cardiogenic shock, cardiomegaly, digitalis toxicity, A-V block, severe CHF or pregnancy. **Administer:** Initiate in coronary ICU only; IV only if solut'n is clear and colorless. **Evaluate:** BP and pulse; use of nitroglycerin. **Teach:** Indicators of adv. effects, efficacy, toxicity; to avoid driving, using power equipment; to reduce caffeine intake; not to take OTC medicat'ns without medical advice; strict adherence to exercise regime.

CHAPTER 12

Antianginal Drugs

Teaching Objectives

Following completion of this chapter, the reader
should be able to:
1. Explain the etiology of angina pectoris.
2. State the therapeutic goals in the treatment of
   angina pectoris.
3. Explain the possible pharmacologic means of
   attaining these goals.
4. List the groups of drugs used to treat angina
   pectoris, explain their mechanisms of action,
   pharmacologic effects, therapeutic uses and
   adverse effects.
5. Describe the nursing process in the use of the
   above drugs.

Etiology of Angina Pectoris

Angina pectoris is a syndrome of paroxysmal left-sided chest pain. It is produced when the oxygen requirements of the heart exceed the oxygen supply. Angina pectoris is a problem of regional ischemia. Not all areas of the heart are anoxic. The heart, more than other tissues, is particularly prone to the development of regional ischemia. Considering its resting metabolic rate, it is the most underperfused organ in the body. Unlike other tissues that extract approximately 25% of the oxygen provided in arterial blood, the heart removes 75% of the oxygen perfusing coronary vessels. In contrast to other tissues, such as the skeletal muscles, in which a major increase in oxygen requirement can be satisfied by increasing both blood flow and the percentage of oxygen extracted from the blood, the heart must depend almost entirely on a significant increase in myocardial perfusion.

Angina pectoris may be divided into stable, unstable and variant angina. In **stable angina** the cause of the problem is a reduction of blood flow to a particular area of the heart as a result of atherosclerosis. When the heart is required to work harder, regional ischemia develops. Patients who suffer from stable angina pectoris experience attacks when they are exposed to exercise, cold temperatures, cigaret smoke and excitement (including, alas, sexual excitement). Eating diverts blood flow to the gastrointestinal tract, away from the coronary blood vessels, and it too can precipitate an attack. These attacks often begin suddenly and stop abruptly.

Unstable angina is an intermediate syndrome

between stable angina pectoris (in which the myocardial blood supply is temporarily inadequate, but there is no tissue death) and myocardial infarction (which is characterized by death of myocardial tissue). The term unstable angina cannot be used to label a specific clinical entity. Rather, it represents another pattern of presentation in the spectrum of coronary artery disease and may be added to the problems of a patient with stable exertional angina pectoris. Patients may range from having normal coronary anatomy to severe three-vessel involvement. Unstable angina may also represent the first manifestation of symptomatic ischemic heart disease. Its characteristics may include discrete episodes of severe ischemic chest pain that can occur at rest. Unstable angina will not be discussed further in this chapter. Drug therapy for unstable angina involves the use of nitrates and beta blockers.

Variant, or vasospastic, angina is not caused by a fixed atherosclerotic narrowing of the vessel lumen but rather results from a coronary artery spasm. It often occurs when the patient is resting.

Drug Treatment of Angina Pectoris

Drugs can overcome the regional oxygen debt in angina pectoris either by increasing oxygen supply to ischemic areas or by decreasing myocardial oxygen requirements. It is, however, difficult for drugs to effect an increase in oxygen supply in stable angina by relaxing coronary precapillary resistance vessels (arterioles). The presence of atherosclerosis prevents many of these vessels from dilating. As a result, patients with stable angina are usually helped by drugs such as nitrates or beta blockers, which decrease the oxygen requirements of the myocardium.

Variant angina, on the other hand, is best treated with a drug that increases oxygen supply to the areas of anoxia. Because this form of angina is caused by a coronary artery spasm and not by atherosclerosis, it responds to treatment with drugs that dilate the constricted blood vessels.

Whereas it is true that drugs that decrease the oxygen requirement of the heart are best suited to treat stable angina, and compounds that prevent

coronary vasospasm are better in variant angina, many patients suffer from a mixture of stable and vasospastic angina pectoris and benefit from both types of therapy. These persons will, therefore, be treated with a combination of nitrate, which reduces the oxygen requirements of the heart, and a calcium channel blocker, which dilates coronary vessels and increases oxygen supply.

Drugs for the Treatment of Stable Angina Pectoris

Nitrates

Mechanism of Action and Pharmacologic Effects

The exact mechanism of action of nitrates is still unclear. However, the drugs interact with nitrate receptors on vascular smooth muscle. Nitrate receptors contain sulfhydryl groups, which reduce nitrate to nitrite ions. The resulting formation of nitrite ions may stimulate the cyclic guanosine monophosphate (cGMP) formation to relax smooth muscle.

Nitrates owe their effect in angina primarily to their ability to dilate capacitance vessels (veins) throughout the body. The oxygen requirements of the heart are determined, at least in part, by the degree to which it is stretched as it fills in diastole. The greater the venous filling pressure (preload), the higher will be the intramyocardial tension and the greater the oxygen requirements. By dilating capacitance vessels, nitrates reduce the rate of venous return, decrease left ventricular volume and intramyocardial tension, and diminish myocardial oxygen requirements.

An indirect result of venodilatation may be an increased oxygen delivery to the subendocardium. Blood flow to the subendocardium occurs primarily in diastole. Therefore, the reduction in left ventricular end-diastolic pressure induced by a nitrate reduces extravascular compression around the subendocardial vessels and favors a redistribution of coronary blood flow in this area. This effect of nitrates on the distribution of coronary flow is important because the subendocardium is particularly vulnerable to ischemia during acute attacks.

Nitrates also relax the large epicardial arteries and can improve regional myocardial blood flow to ischemic areas. They have little effect on intramyocardial resistance vessels. In patients with coronary artery disease, nitrates dilate both normal and diseased coronary arteries and collateral vessels and thus improve regional distribution of myocardial blood flow, even though the overall coronary blood flow may decrease because of the fall in central aortic pressure.

At higher doses, nitrates dilate peripheral precapillary resistance vessels (arterioles) to decrease peripheral resistance (afterload). This reduction in ventricular outflow resistance also decreases the oxygen requirements of the myocardium. The decrease in peripheral resistance can lead to a compensatory increase in heart rate that is counterproductive because it increases the oxygen requirements of the heart. Fortunately, the increased oxygen demand created by tachycardia is not sufficient to override the beneficial effects of nitrates.

Therapeutic Uses

Various nitrate preparations that differ in therapeutic aims and effectiveness are available. Nitrates are taken to prevent or to terminate anginal attacks. Nitroglycerin, absorbed from the mouth, is the drug of choice to stop the pain of angina pectoris. Sublingual tablets will usually relieve pain within two minutes; their duration of action is approximately thirty minutes. Alternatively, nitroglycerin spray (Nitrolingual) can be used under or on the tongue. This form of the drug is most popular and effective and may eventually replace sublingual tablets. If the patient can anticipate a situation that will stress the heart, nitroglycerin, placed under the tongue or sprayed on or under the tongue, can also prevent an attack of angina pectoris. However, its short duration of action makes this use of nitroglycerin impractical for chronic prophylactic use.

Nitroglycerin is also used chronically to prevent attacks. When applied to the skin as an ointment (Nitro-Bid; Nitrol, Nitrong; Nitrostat) or as patches (Transderm Nitro; Nitrodisc), nitroglycerin is absorbed through the stratum corneum. Because tolerance develops rapidly to the patches if they are applied on a twenty-four-hour basis, they should be applied for only twelve hours per day. Used this way, they provide effective long-term prophylaxis without the development of tolerance. Recipients of intermittent nitroglycerin therapy usually receive concomitant calcium channel blockers or beta blockers, or both, which reduce the risk of ischemic

episodes during the nitrate-free period.

Isosorbide dinitrate (Isordil, Sorbitrate), pentaerythrityl tetranitrate (Peritrate) and erythrityl tetranitrate (Cardilate) were introduced to provide prophylaxis against angina pectoris. Some investigators feel that the only compound with demonstrated efficacy is isosorbide dinitrate, which may be taken orally or sublingually. Unfortunately, tolerance may also develop to isosorbide dinitrate. If this occurs, intermittent therapy may be warranted.

Adverse Effects

Headache, the most commonly encountered adverse effect of the nitrates, is attributable to vasodilatation of blood vessels in the scalp. The other adverse effects are dizziness and weakness, which may be attributed to postural hypotension produced when the drugs dilate capacitance vessels and allow blood to pool in the veins.

As already noted, tolerance to nitrates may develop. If this happens, the drug should be discontinued for a time until the responsiveness of the blood vessels returns.

Nursing Process

Administration
Nitroglycerin is usually self-administered, even in the hospital. Therefore, the nurse must monitor the number of tablets used and replenish the supply. Nitroglycerin tends to deteriorate when exposed to air, light or heat. Even being carried too close to the body (for example, inside a suit pocket) is sufficient to cause deterioration. Therefore, the nurse must emphasize proper storage of the medication in a tightly sealed, dark container kept in a cool place. Nurses should assume that nitroglycerin tablets become ineffective three to six months after the bottle has been opened. The nurse should be aware of the special precautions necessary when administering nitroglycerin patches to the skin. The sites should be carefully cleaned before and after application, and close observation for skin reactions is advised. Read the drug package insert instructions carefully before administration. Apply on body surfaces free of hair and rotate sites with each application.

Teaching
The primary nursing responsibility is patient teaching. Nurses should caution patients to keep the nitroglycerin tablet under the tongue until it is completely dissolved. No saliva should be swallowed until the tablet is dissolved. Patients should be told that they can repeat the dosage every

five minutes. However, if no relief is experienced following the third repetition (i.e., fifteen minutes after the first dose), the patient should seek medical attention.

Patients should also be warned of the adverse effects of nitrate therapy, particularly the hypotensive effects, and instructed to rest for a short time after taking sublingual nitroglycerin. Cessation of activity will reduce the danger of accidents due to dizziness, induced by postural hypotension. In addition, resting will also reduce the oxygen requirements of the heart. A cool cloth to the forehead will sometimes relieve or reduce the headache. The patient can be advised that sublingual nitroglycerin may be taken before stressful activities such as exercise or sexual activity. Alcohol should not be consumed by people using nitrates because of the danger of syncope.

Beta Blockers

Mechanism of Action and Pharmacologic Effects

The pharmacology of beta blockers is presented in Chapter 8 and is summarized in Table 13 at the end of this chapter. At this time it will suffice to discuss only their clinical usefulness in the treatment of angina pectoris. Drugs such as propranolol (Inderal), timolol (Blocadren), nadolol (Corgard), metoprolol (Betaloc, Lopresor, Lopressor), atenolol (Tenormin), acebutolol (Monitan, Sectral), and pindolol (Visken) block the beta adrenergic receptors in the heart. In response to the decrease in sympathetic nervous system stimulation of the heart, heart rate decreases, myocardial contractility falls, and the oxygen requirements of the heart diminish.

Therapeutic Use

Beta blockers form the mainstay of prophylactic treatment of chronic stable angina pectoris. They are often used with other drugs such as isosorbide dinitrate, when it is believed that the combined agents may achieve better results than either drug given alone. Furthermore, beta blockers prevent the reflex tachycardia that often accompanies nitrate therapy. Obviously, beta blockers are contraindicated in the patient with congestive heart failure or bronchial asthma. They are also contraindicated in sinus bradycardia, heart block greater than first degree, cardiogenic shock, and right ventricular failure secondary to pulmonary hypertension, unless the failure is due to a tachyarrhythmia treatable with the beta blocker.

However, beta blockers are ideal drugs for patients suffering from both hypertension and angina pectoris.

Adverse Effects

The major adverse effects of beta blockers result from inhibition of the sympathetic nervous system innervation of the heart. Heart rate and cardiac output fall as the cardiac sympathetic nerves are blocked. This may predispose the borderline patient to congestive heart failure. As mentioned earlier, beta blockers are contraindicated in these individuals. The other adverse effects of beta blockers are presented in detail in Chapter 8.

Nursing Process

Assessment

In view of the adverse effects of beta blockers, the primary nursing responsibility is assessment. Prior to administering the first dose, the nurse must ensure that the patient has no history of either congestive heart failure or asthma. Subsequent administration of the drug during hospitalization should be preceded by nursing assessment of the patient's blood pressure, heart and respiratory rates. If hypotension, bradycardia, shortness of breath or peripheral edema occur, the drug should be withheld until the physician is contacted.

Administration

Usually, beta blockers are best administered with food.

Evaluation

Two hours following the first administration of a beta blocker, the nurse should measure the patient's blood pressure and heart rate. Apical/radial pulses should be taken before administration and the physician notified if significant changes are seen or a pulse rate of less than 60 beats per minute is noted. A significant drop in blood pressure or heart rate should be reported to the physician immediately.

Teaching

Patients should be taught to self-evaluate for adverse effects and be advised to keep adequate supplies of the beta blocker on hand at all times. Abrupt withdrawal of the medication has been known to precipitate rebound ischemia, even to the extreme of myocardial infarction. Other nursing measures related to beta blockers are considered in Chapter 8 and summarized in Table 13 at the end of this chapter.

Drugs for the Treatment of Variant Angina Pectoris

Calcium Channel Blockers

Mechanism of Action and Pharmacologic Effects

Vasoconstriction depends upon the entry of small amounts of calcium into the vascular smooth muscle. The calcium enters the muscle cell through a special channel designed for it — the so-called calcium channel. Verapamil (Isoptin, Calan), nifedipine (Adalat, Procardia), nicardipine (Cardene) and diltiazem (Cardizem) block this entry of calcium into the vascular muscle and, as a result, prevent vasoconstriction.

All four drugs are effective to the same extent in dilating the coronary vessels. In spite of the fact that all have essentially the same mechanism of action, they differ from each other in some important respects. Nifedipine and nicardipine are similar pharmacologically and produce the greatest dilatation of peripheral vasculature. As a result of their ability to decrease peripheral resistance, nifedipine and nicardipine reflexly increase heart rate. Verapamil and diltiazem also dilate peripheral blood vessels and decrease peripheral resistance. However, these drugs depress the myocardium, and this action prevents the reflex tachycardia that would normally be expected of a vasodilator. Verapamil prolongs A-V conduction time and is also used as an artiarrhythmic (see Chapter 11). Diltiazen has less effect on A-V conduction than verapamil and is not used as an antiarrhythmic.

Therapeutic Uses

All four drugs can be used prophylactically in patients with variant angina because they will dilate the constricted blood vessels in the heart. These drugs are also used to treat angina of effort (stable angina). In this case their beneficial effects may be attributable to both reduced myocardial oxygen demand (perhaps secondary to decreased peripheral resistance) and improved myocardial perfusion.

The calcium channel blockers can be combined with nitrates in patients with a mixture of vasospastic and coronary occlusive angina. Verapamil has the greatest depressant effect on myocardial function and cannot be combined with a beta blocker. Diltiazem can also depress the myocardium and it, too, should not be given with a beta blocker. Nifedipine and nicardipine can be taken with a beta blocker in patients with a combination of variant and stable angina pectoris.

The four drugs differ significantly with respect to their effects on myocardial contractility, cardiac conduction and peripheral circulation. Verapamil has the greatest depressant effect on A-V conduction. Nifedipine and nicardipine are the most potent peripheral vasodilators. They have little or no depressant effect on S-A or A-V nodal function. Rather, because the drugs dilate arterioles they can cause reflex tachycardia. Because of this effect, nifedipine and nicardipine are safer than verapamil or diltiazem in patients with left ventricular dysfunction and, as explained before, they are the preferred calcium channel blockers in patients taking beta blockers.

On the other side of the coin, the reflex tachycardia of nifedipine and nicardipine can occasionally cause an exacerbation of anginal symptoms. This contrasts with the mild bradycardia produced by verapamil and diltiazem, which aids the patient with angina.

Adverse Effects

Diltiazem's most common adverse effects are nausea, swelling/edema, arrhythmia (A-V block, bradycardia, tachycardia and sinus arrest), headache, rash and fatigue. Diltiazem should be avoided in patients with sick sinus syndrome.

The most common adverse effects of nifedipine and nicardipine result from their vasodilating action. These include headache, dizziness, lightheadedness and giddiness, flushing and heat sensation, peripheral edema and hypotension. Nifedipine can also cause nausea, vomiting and gastrointestinal distress.

Adverse reactions to verapamil include bradycardia, transient asystole, hypotension, development or worsening of heart failure and development of rhythm disturbances, including A-V block and ventricular dysrhythmias, flushing, peripheral edema and pulmonary edema. Central nervous system effects involve dizziness, headache, fatigue, excitation, vertigo, syncope and tremor. Constipation, nausea, vomiting and gastrointestinal complaints are the most common adverse effects seen after oral administration. A smaller percentage of patients may experience bronchospasm and dyspnea, which are more prevalent following parenteral administration of verapamil.

Nursing Process

Assessment

Nurses should ensure that the cardiac workup and laboratory evaluation of renal and hepatic function ordered by the physician have been completed before treatment with any of the calcium channel blockers is initiated. In addition, nursing assessment of the patient should establish baseline measures of blood pressure and pulse. A patient history of renal or hepatic disease signals the need for particularly careful evaluation of the patient following the administration of these medications. The patient's current drug regimen and history should be reviewed for contraindications to the use of verapamil and other calcium channel blockers (see Chapter 11 for details).

The teratogenic potential of nifedipine and diltiazem must always be borne in mind, and nurses must inquire whether the patient is pregnant (or has plans to become pregnant).

Administration

Parenteral treatment with verapamil should be initiated only in facilities equipped to provide continuous cardiac monitoring, cardiopulmonary resuscitation and cardioversion. Administer only intravenous solutions of verapamil that are clear and colorless and have been stored in light-resistant containers at room temperature.

Nifedipine capsules should be stored at room temperature in light-resistant containers. They should also be protected from moisture and high humidity.

Diltiazem should be administered before meals and at bedtime. Patients who have trouble swallowing tablets may have one crushed and administered in a small amount of beverage.

Evaluation

Blood pressure and pulse should be monitored prior to each dose of verapamil to determine drug efficacy and provide early indication of adverse effects or toxicity. Monitor nitroglycerin use as an indicator of drug efficacy.

Teaching

Ensure that the patient and a responsible care giver are aware of the indicators of drug efficacy, adverse effects and toxicity. Driving or the use of power equipment is not advisable during the early phase of treatment with verapamil because of the risk of lightheadedness or dizziness. Patients should also be advised to change position slowly to avoid dizziness.

Caffeine intake, either in coffee or over-the-counter drugs, should be reduced because it might interfere with the calcium-blocking effects of verapamil. Strict adherence to the prescribed exercise regime is important because the absence of angina in patients being treated with verapamil is not an indicator of increased exercise tolerance.

Patients should be informed that nifedipine and nicardipine may increase heart rate. They should also be warned that abrupt cessation of either drug may cause chest pain, increased angina, myocardial infarction or dysrhythmias. It goes without saying that patients requiring treatment with calcium channel blockers should not smoke. Smoking decreases drug efficacy and increases adverse cardiac effects.

Further Reading

Amtorp, O. and Ryden, L. (1987). New aspects of nitrates. *Drugs 33* (Suppl. 4):1-152.

Flaherty, J. T. (1989). Nitrate tolerance: A review of the evidence. *Drugs 37* :523-550.

Frishman, W. H. and Ryden, L. (1989). Symposium on patient preference in antianginal therapy. *Drugs 38* (Suppl. 2):1-91.

Frye, R.L., Gibbons, R.J., Shaff, H.V., Vlietstra, R. E., Gersh, B.J. et al. (1989). Treatment of coronary artery disease. *J. Amer. Coll. Cardiol. 13* :957-968.

Gladstone, P.S.J. and Ogilvie, R. I. (1988). Cardiovascular pharmacology. Nitrate tolerance: Facts, fiction and practical pointers. *Current Cardiology 3* (Sept.):22-26.

Gleeson, B. (1991). Teaching your patient about his antianginal drugs. *Nursing 21* (2) : 65-72

Higginson, L. (1989). Single agent selection in angina. *Perspectives in Cardiology 5* (5):23-29.

Reichek, N. (1989). Intermittent nitrate therapy in angina pectoris. *European Heart J. 10* (Suppl. A):7-10.

Scriabine, A. (1987). Current and potential indications for Ca^{2+} antagonists. *Rational Drug Therapy 21* (9):1-5.

Singh, B. N., Nademanee, K. and Josephson, M. A. (1986). Newer concepts in the pathogenesis of myocardial ischemia: Implications for the evaluation of antianginal therapy. *Drugs 32* : 1-14.

Soward, A. L., Vanhaleweyk, G.L.J. and Serruys, P. W. (1986). The hemodynamic effects of nifedipine, verapamil and diltiazem in patients with coronary artery disease: A review. *Drugs 32* : 66-101.

Table 13
Antianginal drugs.

Pharmacologic Classification: Peripheral Vasodilators

Generic Name (Trade Name)	Use (Dose)	Action	Adverse Effects	Drug Interactions	Nursing Process
Nitroglycerin sublingual tablets	For acute attacks of angina pectoris (**Sublingual:** Initially, 0.15-0.6 mg)	Dilates veins and arterioles, causing reduced venous return and peripheral resistance, thereby decr. cardiac O_2 requirements.	Incr. heart rate, headache, postural hypotens'n (dizziness, weakness)	**Ethanol:** Pts receiving nitrates should take ethanol cautiously because hypotens'n may occur with combined use of the 2 drugs (both produce vasodilatat'n). **Nitrates, long-acting:** Administered chronically, can produce tolerance to nitroglycerin. This does not nec. mean that pts should not receive both types of nitrate products. However, if pts fail to respond well to sublingual nitroglycerin, nurses should consider the possibility that large doses of long-acting nitrates administered chronically may have resulted in tolerance to the effects of nitrate tx.	**Evaluate:** Drug effectiveness; frequency of use; evidence of tolerance. **Teach:** S/s of adv. effects; proper storage and administrat'n; danger of consuming alcohol and nitrates. To take drug before strenuous activity (exercise, sexual activity).
Lingual nitroglycerin aerosol (Nitrolingual)	(**Aerosol:** 1-2 doses of 0.4 mg sprayed into mouth or under tongue)	As for nitroglycerin sublingual tablets	As for nitroglycerin sublingual tablets		As for nitroglycerin sublingual tablets
Nitroglycerin ointment (Nitro-BID, Nitrol, Nitrong, Nitrostat)	For prophylaxis of ischemic heart pain (**Topical:** 0.5-4 inches of 2% ointment prn q3-8h. Rotate skin sites)	As for nitroglycerin sublingual tablets	As for nitroglycerin sublingual tablets		As for nitroglycerin sublingual tablets
Nitroglycerin patches (Nitrodisc, Transderm Nitro)	For prophylaxis of ischemic heart pain (**Patches:** Initially, patch that releases 0.2 mg/h, us. in a.m. If dose is tolerated, incr. prn to 0.3-0.4 mg/h. Daily patch-on period, 12-14 h)	As for nitroglycerin sublingual tablets	As for nitroglycerin sublingual tablets		As for nitroglycerin sublingual tablets
Nitroglycerin sustained-release tablets (Nitrong-SR); nitroglycerin sustained-release capsules (Nitrostat)	For prophylaxis of ischemic heart pain (**Tablet or capsule:** 1 tablet, containing 2.6 mg nitroglycerin, tid; 1 capsule, containing 2, 5, 6.5 or 9 mg nitroglycerin, bid or tid)	As for nitroglycerin sublingual tablets	As for nitroglycerin sublingual tablets	As for nitroglycerin sublingual tablets	As for nitroglycerin sublingual tablets
Isosorbide dinitrate (Isordil, Sorbitrate)	For prophylaxis of ischemic heart pain (**Sublingual:** 2.5-10 mg q2-4h for prophylaxis; may be supplemented by 5-10 mg prior to stressful situat'ns. **Oral:** 5-30 mg qid)	As for nitroglycerin sublingual tablets	As for nitroglycerin sublingual tablets	As for nitroglycerin sublingual tablets	As for nitroglycerin sublingual tablets

Generic Name (Trade Name)	Use (Dose)	Action	Adverse Effects	Drug Interactions	Nursing Process
Pharmacologic Classification: Beta Blockers					
Propranolol (Inderal)	For prophylaxis of angina pectoris (**Oral:** Adults - initially, 10-20 mg tid or qid. Incr. prn. Most require 160-240 mg/day. *Long-acting tablets:* Initially, 80 mg/day, incr. gradually at 3-7 day intervals)	Blocks both beta₁ and beta₂ receptors. Effects depend on level of sympathetic nervous activity. Decr. heart rate, ventr. systolic pressure, myocardial contractility and cardiac output.	Bronchoconstrict'n; potentiates effect of insulin; asystole, AV block, bradycardia, heart failure, nausea, vomiting, constipat'n, diarrhea, depress'n, sleep disturbances, allergic react'ns	*Reference is made to propranolol, but drug interact'ns apply to all beta blockers.* **Antiarrhythmic drugs** (disopyramide, lidocaine, tocainide and perhaps other Class I antiarrhythmics): Plus a beta blocker, can result in exagerat'n of unwanted effects of antiarrhythmic agents, as reflected	**Assess:** For pt thx of CHF, bradycardia, heart block, asthma, hay fever, COPD, liver or kidney disease, diabetes, myasthenia gravis; use of psychotropic medicat'n; pregnancy or lactat'n; use of MAOIs within preceding 2 weeks. Record apical/radial pulses (incl. rate, rhythm), BP, respirat'ns (incl. rate, rhythm), circulat'n of extremities (incl. color, warmth, blanching effect and peripheral pulses) as baseline for evaluating indiv. pt response.
Nadolol (Corgard)	As for propranolol (**Oral:** Adults - initially, 40 mg/day; incr. gradually by 40-80 mg increments at 3-7 day intervals. Max. dose, 240 mg/day)	Reduces coronary blood flow and O₂ consumpt'n. Lowers BP. Reduces sinus rate. Slows A-V conduct'n. Decr.	As for propranolol	in enhanced myocardial depress'n, hypotens'n, bradycardia, A-V blockade and asystole. **Antiasthmatics** (beta₂ stimulants, e.g., albuterol/ salbutamol, fenoterol,	**Administer:** From airtight, light-resistant containers; ac and hs in order to facilitate absorpt'n of medicat'n from stomach into the circulatory system.
Timolol (Blocadren)	As for propranolol (**Oral:** Adults - initially, 5 mg bid or tid. Incr. gradually at intervals of more than 3 days. Max dose, 45 mg/day)	spontaneous rate of ectopic pacemakers.	As for propranolol	terbutaline): Their bronchodilating action is antagonized by nonselective beta blockers, incl. those w. partial-agonist activity. Cardioselective beta blockers are less likely to affect the action of beta₂ stimulants.	**Evaluate:** Apical/radial pulses, fluid intake/output, daily weight, BP, respirat'n, circulat'n to extremities; for indicat'ns of adv. effects and to assist physician in establishing best indiv. dose; monitor diabetic pts for hypoglycemia and insulin shock; monitor ECG of pts receiving IV propranolol.
Atenolol (Tenormin)	As for propranolol (**Oral:** Adults - 50, 100 or 200 mg 1x daily)	Cardioselective beta₁ blocker	As for propranolol	**Antidiabetic agents:** Their actions are incr. by nonselective beta blockers, which reduce glycogen breakdown and delay the rise in blood glucose after insulin (or oral-hypoglycemic) tx. Further, nonselective beta	**Teach:** Pt and family to observe responses to physical and psychological stress and to develop an indiv. appropriate level, pace and am't of activity; importance of avoiding abrupt w'drawal of drug because of danger of
Metoprolol (Betaloc, Lopresor, Lopressor)	As for propranolol (**Oral:** Adults - 50 mg bid; incr. to 100 mg bid prn. *Sustained-release tablets,* 200 mg 1x daily)	Cardioselective beta₁ blocker	As for propranolol	blockers modify normal physiologic react'ns to hypoglycemia. In presence of a nonselective beta blocker, the hypoglycemic react'n is accompanied by bradycardia rather than tachycardia, and a	myocardial infarct or arrhythmias; to avoid alcohol, smoking and OTC medicat'ns for colds, coughs or allergies because of their potential effects on BP; to avoid driving vehicles, using power tools or working w. industrial machinery during regulat'n of dosage; to move
Pindolol (Visken)	As for propranolol (**Oral:** Adults - initially, 5 mg tid, w. meals; incr. gradually prn. Us. maint. dose, 15-40 mg/day)	Intrinsic sympathetic activity (weak beta₁ and beta₂ stimulants). Replaces endogenous epinephrine and/or norepinephrine, causing reduced beta stimulat'n.	As for propranolol	rise in diastolic BP as well as the us. systolic pressor response. **Atropine** (and other	from recumbent to standing position slowly w. a stop in sitting posit'n before rising to feet. Teach pt and family to

Drug	Action/Use	Dosage	Side Effects	Interactions	Nursing Considerations
Acebutolol (Monitan, Sectral)	Cardioselective beta blocker w. intrinsic sympathetic activity.	As for propranolol (**Oral:** Adults - initially, 200 mg bid; incr. after 2 weeks prn to a max. of 300 mg bid. In pts adequately controlled on 400 mg daily, a lower maint. dose of 100 mg bid may be tried)	As for propranolol	anticholinergics): May prevent bradycardia produced by beta blockers. **Clonidine:** Plus a beta blocker, can lead to a potentiat'n of the hypertensive response during clonidine w'drawal. **Digoxin:** Its positive inotropic actions may be reduced by the negative inotropic effect of a beta blocker. Beta blockers and digoxin are additive in depressing A-V conduct'n. *Use beta blockers w. caution in pts on digoxin who develop bradycardia.* **Epinephrine:** Can incr. BP in pts taking nonselective beta blockers. **Nifedipine:** Plus a beta blocker, can occ. provoke severe hypotens'n and overt heart failure in a susceptible pt w. poor myocardial reserve. **Prazosin:** And a beta blocker, can result in incr. postural hypotens'n after first dose of prazosin. **Sympathomimetics:** Plus a nonselective beta blocker, can result in hypertens'n when large doses of the sympathomimetic are used. **Verapamil:** Plus a beta blocker, can result in enhanced myocardial depress'n, hypotens'n, bradycardia, A-V blockade and asystole.	seek medical attent'n if s/s of adv. effects occur.

Pharmacologic Classification: Calcium Channel Blocker

Drug	Action/Use	Dosage	Side Effects	Interactions	Nursing Considerations
Diltiazem (Cardizem)	Blocks entry of Ca into myocardial blood vessels, producing vasodilatat'n and relief from vasospastic (variant) angina.	Prophylaxis of angina pectoris due to coronary artery spasm and management of chronic stable angina in pts who fail to respond to, or cannot tolerate, beta blockers and/or nitrates (**Oral:** Adults - intially, 30 mg qid ac; incr. gradually to max. of 360 mg daily)	Nausea, swelling/edema, arrhythmias, headache, rash, fatigue	**Beta blockers:** And diltiazem can lead to severe sinus bradycardia, hypotens'n and heart failure. **Nitroglycerin** (time-release): And diltiazem can produce exaggerated hypotens'n.	**Assess:** Baseline ECG, lab. tests for renal/hepatic funct'n; BP and pulse; current drug profile for use of digitalis, procainamide or quinidine; check hx for severe hypotens'n, cardiogenic shock, cardiomegaly, digitalis toxicity, A-V block, severe CHF or pregnancy. **Administer:** Parentally in coronary ICU only; orally ac and hs.

Generic Name (Trade Name)	Use (Dose)	Action	Adverse Effects	Drug Interactions	Nursing Process
					Evaluate: BP and pulse; use of nitroglycerin. **Teach:** S/s of adv. effects, efficacy, toxicity; to avoid driving and use of power equipment; not to take OTC drugs without medical advice; strict adherence to exercise regimen.
Nifedipine (Adalat, Procardia)	As for diltiazem (**Oral:** Initially, 10 mg tid. Us. effective range, 10-20 mg tid. Max. daily dose, 120 mg)	As for diltiazem on heart vessels. Nifedipine produces more profound peripheral vasodilat'n, resulting in greater fall in BP and greater reflex tachycardia.	Dizziness, lightheadedness, peripheral edema, nausea, weakness, headache, flushing, transient hypotens'n, pilpitat'ns, syncope	**Antihypertensives:** Nifedipine or nicardipine may potentiate effects of hypotensive agents. **Beta blockers:** Antihypertensive effect of beta blockers may be augmented by nifedipine or nicardipine's reduct'n of peripheral vascular resistance.	As for diltiazem, plus: **Administer:** From light-resistant containers stored at room temp.; protect from moisture.
Nicardipine (Cardene)	As for diltiazem (**Oral:** Adults - 20 mg tid initially; incr. after 3 days prn to 30 mg tid and then 40 mg tid. Pts w. impaired hepatic funct'n should start w. 20 mg bid)	As for diltiazem on heart vessels. Nicardipine is sim. to nifedipine in that it produces more profound peripheral vasodilatat'n than diltiazem, resulting in greater fall in BP and greater reflex tachycardia.	Headache, dizziness, lightheadedness, giddiness, flushing, heat sensat'n, peripheral edema and hypotens'n	As above	As for diltiazem, plus: **Teach:** Pt to limit caffeine consumpt'n and avoid OTC drugs unless directed by doctor. Notify physician of irreg. heart beat, SOB, swelling of hands/feet, dizziness, hypotens'n, nausea, constipat'n.
Verapamil (Calan, Isoptin)	As for diltiazem (**Oral:** Initially, 80 mg tid or qid; incr. to 120 mg tid or qid prn. Max. dose, 480 mg/day)	As for diltiazem on heart vessels. Verapamil also dilates systemic blood vessels and can lower BP. In addit'n, it depresses myocardium and prolongs A-V conduct'n time.	Transient asystole, hypotens'n, development or worsening of heart failure, rhythm disturbances, stenocardia (angina), flushing, peripheral and pulmonary edema, dizziness, headache, fatigue, excitat'n, vertigo, syncope, tremor, constipat'n	**Antihypertensives:** In pts using antihypertensive drugs, the addit'nal hypotensive effects of verapamil should be considered. **Beta blockers:** Should not be combined with verapamil. If concomitant use is considered essential, start tx gradually in hospital under careful supervis'n. **Digoxin:** Chronic oral administrat'n of verapamil has been reported to incr. plasma digoxin levels.	As for diltiazem, plus: **Administer:** IV only if solut'n is clear and colorless.

CHAPTER 13

Drugs Used in the Treatment of Peripheral and Cerebral Vascular Disorders

Teaching Objectives

Following completion of this chapter, the reader should be able to:

1. Discuss the etiology of vasospastic disorders.
2. List the types of drugs used to treat vasospastic disorders and explain their mechanisms of action.
3. Discuss the nursing process related to the use of drugs to treat vasospastic disorders.
4. Discuss the etiology of intermittent claudication.
5. Discuss the effects of ischemia on vasodilatation in normal and atherosclerotic blood vessels.
6. Discuss the effectiveness of drugs in the treatment of peripheral and cerebral vascular disorders.
7. Explain the mechanisms of action of these drugs.
8. Discuss the drug pentoxifylline, explaining its mechanism of action, therapeutic use and the nursing process related to its use.

Vasospastic Disorders

Vasospastic disorders result from a reduction in blood flow secondary to vasoconstriction. Regardless of whether vasoconstriction is precipitated by such factors as exposure to cold or emotional stress or occurs as a complication of collagen disease, arterial disease or other conditions, vasodilators may improve blood flow to ischemic areas, thereby providing relief. However, their usefulness is limited by two basic problems. First, they may decrease blood pressure, thereby reducing blood flow; second, they may dilate other vascular beds, thereby redirecting blood flow from the ischemic areas.

Drugs used to treat vasospastic disorders may (1) decrease central sympathetic tone (reserpine and methyldopa), (2) act on peripheral sympathetic nerve endings to reduce norepinephrine release (guanethidine), (3) block alpha$_1$ receptors on blood vessels (phenoxybenzamine), (4) stimulate beta$_2$ receptors on blood vessels (nylidrin), or (5) directly dilate blood vessels (calcium channel blockers and hydralazine). The pharmacology of reserpine, methyldopa and guanethidine has been discussed in Chapter 8 and need not be repeated here. By the same token, the pharmacology of calcium channel blockers is presented in Chapters 12 and 14; hydralazine is covered in Chapter 14. Thus, they will not be discussed now.

Phenoxybenzamine (Dibenzyline)

Phenoxybenzamine blocks alpha$_1$ receptors on blood vessels, dilating both arterioles and veins. Arteriolar dilatation decreases peripheral resistance. For this reason it may be useful in vasospastic disorders. However, the drug has no established value in chronic occlusive vascular disease. The decrease in peripheral resistance produced by phenoxybenzamine can produce troublesome reflex tachycardia. Venodilatation reduces venous return to the heart, causing postural hypotension. Other effects of phenoxybenzamine include nasal congestion, gastrointestinal hypermotility and inhibition of erection and ejaculation.

Nursing process should emphasize assessment of the patient for contraindications, including pregnancy or a history of renal failure. Patient evaluation and teaching should focus on the risk of postural hypotension associated with the use of this medication. Further details of the nursing process related to the use of phenoxybenzamine are contained in Chapter 8.

Nylidrin (Arlidin)

Nylidrin reputedly stimulates beta$_2$ receptors on blood vessels, thereby causing vasodilatation. It should be effective for the treatment of vasospastic disorders. However, there is little evidence to suggest that it is effective in Raynaud's phenomenon, cerebrovascular disorders, or other conditions such as circulatory disorders of the inner ear. Patients taking the drug may experience dizziness, tachycardia, hypotension, nausea and vomiting.

The nursing process associated with nylidrin should begin with assessment of the patient for recent myocardial infarct or untreated cardiac disease. Patient evaluation following administration of this medication emphasizes observation for evidence of drug efficacy.

Chronic Occlusive Peripheral Vascular Disease

Nurses are well aware of the term placebo. It is derived from the Latin and literally means "I will please". In practice, it is an inactive substance or preparation given to satisfy a patient's symbolic need for drug therapy. There are few, if any, deliberate placebo tablets or capsules on the North American market. However, most drugs used to relieve peripheral and cerebral vascular disorders come, in the minds of many, very close to being expensive placebos. There is little evidence that the great majority of these agents have any therapeutic value, other than setting the patient's mind at ease by allowing him to believe that he is receiving an active drug. If it were not for the fact that these drugs are extensively advertised and prescribed, one could argue that they should not be discussed in this book.

Skeletal muscle blood flow is reduced by atherosclerosis. When this happens, intermittent **claudication** (lameness) may occur. Patients may experience no pain at rest but once they have walked a short distance, the pain of ischemia may force them to stop. The muscles in the leg(s) receive, under these conditions, inadequate blood flow to satisfy their metabolic requirements. Nurses who peruse the professional journals are well aware of the touching photos showing old granddad interrupted in his walk through the woods, clutching his calf muscles in pain while concerned grandchildren look on in horror. The opposite side of the same advertisement shows the old fellow happily cantering beside the children through the forest after being established on a peripheral vasodilator.

These ads are misleading because, with the possible exception of pentoxifylline (see below), there is little evidence to suggest that any drug can help restore circulation to grandfather's aging muscles and alleviate his plight. Furthermore, there is no scientific reason to expect them to have this effect. Ischemia is a potent vasodilator. The products of anoxia and the increase in pCO_2 are effective vasodilators. This is the normal response of ischemic tissues in an attempt to increase blood flow. However, in the clinical situation pictured above, the blood vessels are often nondilatable because they are sclerotic and neither the products of anoxia nor vasodilator drugs will help.

It might be said that the drugs used to treat peripheral vascular disorders are caught in a "catch-22 situation". That is, if the normal products of ischemia work to dilate the blood vessels and increase skeletal muscle blood flow, then you don't need drugs. However, if the normal products of ischemia fail to increase skeletal muscle blood flow, drugs also won't be effective.

Some vasodilators are claimed to restore aging brain function to its previous state of competence. One product, Hydergine, has even been claimed to "add life to years" by both increasing blood flow and altering brain cell metabolism. Before endorsing such claims, one must realize that resistance in the cerebrovascular bed is also controlled by local autoregulation. A decrease in blood flow increases pCO_2 and produces local vasodilatation. No known drug can decrease cerebral vascular resistance as much as does an increase in arterial pCO_2. If the blood vessels will not dilate when pCO_2 rises, drug therapy will also prove ineffective.

The preceding discussion should not be interpreted to indicate that the drugs prescribed to treat peripheral and cerebral vascular disorders are completely without effect. This is not true. These drugs, regardless of their mechanism of action, can dilate those vessels which are still dilatable and unaffected by the products of ischemia. These are, of course, healthy blood vessels perfusing tissues that are not ischemic. In this we have a unique situation: drugs that work on healthy tissues, which don't require drug therapy, but fail in damaged areas, where some form of effective treatment would be desirable. There is another side to this story. By decreasing peripheral resistance in healthy parts of the body and not affecting it in damaged areas, vasodilators reduce the percentage of cardiac output perfusing the tissues of concern. This makes the situation even worse.

Little time will be spent discussing most of the drugs used to treat peripheral and cerebral vascular disorders or related nursing actions. They work either by stimulating beta receptors in the vascular bed or by directly relaxing arterioles. Nylidrin (Arlidin) is believed to be a beta$_2$ agonist. Isoxsuprine (Vasodilan) was originally thought of as a beta$_2$ stimulant. Current views consider it to be a direct vascular smooth muscle relaxant. Cyclandelate (Cyclospasmol) and tolazoline (Priscoline) are other vascular smooth muscle relaxants used.

Nursing Process

Nursing time with patients receiving these medications would best be spent assisting them to change their expectations of their bodies' ability to perform certain physical activities. Such patients should be assisted to plan, implement and maintain an altered lifestyle that reflects the physical limitations imposed on them by their medical condition.

Pentoxifylline (Trental)

Mechanism of Action and Pharmacologic Effects

Pentoxifylline is discussed separately because, in contrast to the other drugs previously mentioned, evidence can be found to support its clinical effectiveness. The primary actions of pentoxifylline include increased erythrocyte flexibility, reduced blood viscosity and improved microcirculatory flow and tissue perfusion. As a result, orally administered pentoxifylline improves the supply of oxygen to ischemic muscles of the limbs.

Therapeutic Uses

Pentoxifylline has been shown to be effective in the treatment of intermittent claudication. Most double-blind trials conducted in patients with moderate chronic obstructive arterial disease have demonstrated a significant improvement in walking performance in pentoxifylline-treated patients compared to those treated by placebo. In spite of these most encouraging results, it is still not clear if pentoxifylline will improve the walking distance attained through an exercise regimen or if it will help the severely limited patient who cannot walk fifty meters.

Adverse Effects

The most common adverse effects of pentoxifylline involve the gastrointestinal tract. Patients most often complain of nausea, vomiting, dyspepsia, abdominal discomfort and bloating. However, the approximately ten per cent incidence of adverse effects with pentoxifylline does not appear to exceed that reported in placebo-treated patients.

Nursing Process

Assessment
Patients should be assessed for hypersensitivity to xanthines (caffeine or theophylline) or untreated cardiac disease. The presence of these conditions contraindicates the use of pentoxifylline.

Administration

Absorption of this medication is prolonged by the presence of food in the stomach. Although this does not affect the amount of the drug eventually absorbed, serum levels are lower. Therefore, in order to regulate the dosage, pentoxifylline must be taken consistently on either an empty or a full stomach.

Evaluation

Drug efficacy is determined by patients' subjective reports of reduced pain and cramping of the muscles of the legs and feet, as well as increased tolerance of walking.

Teaching

Patients should be cautioned to take appropriate safety precautions in light of the possibility of drowsiness, blurred vision and dizziness. They should be advised to have their cardiovascular status checked by a physician before resuming active walking exercise. They should also be encouraged to decrease fats and cholesterol, increase exercise and decrease smoking to assist in correcting circulatory disease.

Further Reading

Coffman, J. D. (1979). Intermittent claudication and rest pain: Physiologic concepts and therapeutic approaches. *Pro. Cardiovasc. Dis. 22* (1):53-72.

Coffman, J. D. and Mannick, J. A. (1972). Failure of vasodilator drugs in arteriosclerosis obliterans. *Ann. Intern. Med. 76* :35-39.

Table 14
Drugs used in the treatment of peripheral and cerebral vascular disorders.

Pharmacologic Classification: Peripheral and Cerebral Vascular Drugs

Generic Name (Trade Name)	Use (Dose)	Action	Adverse Effects	Drug Interactions	Nursing Process
Cyclandelate (Cyclospasmol)	Adjunctive tx in occlusive and vasospastic diseases. *Efficacy questioned.* **(Oral:** 400-800 mg/day, in 2-4 divided doses. 1200-1600 mg/day may be given in 4 divided doses ac and hs for 2-4 weeks; then reduce gradually to us. dose)	Vascular smooth muscle relaxant.	GI distress (pyrosis, pain, eructat'n), mild flushing, headache, weakness, tachycardia		**Assess:** Baseline cardiac status, BP, pulse (rate, rhythm). **Administer:** With meals to reduce GI symptoms. **Evaluate:** For tx response — incr. temp. in limbs; incr. pulse volume; ability to walk without pain. **Teach:** Medicat'ns may need to be taken continuously. Tx is not a cure. Importance of changes in lifestyle (diet and exercise; quit smoking). Report weakness, headaches, incr. pulse. Avoid hazardous activities until drug effects stabilize, as dizziness may occur.
Dihydroergotoxine mesylate (Hydergine)	Tx of selected s/s of cerebral insufficiency in elderly pts (e.g., mood, depress'n, confus'n, unsociability, dizziness, impaired self-care). *Efficacy questioned.* **(Oral:** 1 tablet tid or qid w. food)	Claimed to incr. blood flow to brain, improve brain cell metabolism.	Nausea, vomiting, headache, dizziness, flushing, blurred vision, rashes, anorexia, nasal stuffiness, abdominal cramps		As for cyclandelate.
Isoxsuprine (Vasodilan)	For symptomatic relief in peripheral and cerebral vascular disorders. *Efficacy questioned.* **(Oral:** 10-20 mg tid or qid) *For management of premature labor, refer to Table 49.*	Vascular smooth muscle relaxant.	Mild tachycardia, palpitat'ns, tremor, nausea	**Anesthetics:** Used in surgery, may potentiate hypotensive effects. **Beta blockers:** Inhibit the action of isoxsuprine. **Corticosterioids:** Used concomitantly, induce pulmonary edema. **Sympathomimetics:** Are potentiated by isoxsuprine.	
Nylidrin (Arlidin)	Tx of mild to moderate s/s commonly associated w. organic mental disorders in elderly; Raynaud's phenomenon; cerebral vascular disorders. *Efficacy questioned.* **(Oral:** *For peripheral vascular disorders,* 12-48 mg/day in 3-4 divided doses. *For organic mental disorders,* 12-24 mg/day in 3-4 divided doses)	Reputedly stims. beta₂ receptors on blood vessels, thereby causing vasodilatat'n.	Trembling, nervousness, weakness, dizziness, palpitat'ns, nausea, vomiting, postural hypotens'n, allergic react'ns		**Assess:** For recent myocardial infarct or untreated cardiac disease. **Evaluate:** Drug efficacy on basis of pt percept'ns.

Generic Name (Trade Name)	Use (Dose)	Action	Adverse Effects	Drug Interactions	Nursing Process
Pentoxifylline (Trental)	Symptomatic tx of chronic occlusive peripheral vascular disorders of the extremities (**Oral:** Initially, 400 mg bid pc. Us. maint. dose, 400 mg bid or tid. Max. dose, 400 mg tid)	Relaxes peripheral blood vessels; improves flexibility of red blood cells.	Nausea, vomiting, abdominal discomfort, diarrhea, dizziness/lightheadedness, headache		**Assess:** For sensitivity to xanthines, untreated cardiac disease. **Administer:** At consistant time rel. to food intake. **Evaluate:** Pt percept'n of effect on pain, cramping. **Teach:** Necessity to decr. fats, cholesterol; to exercise and to quit smoking.
Phenoxybenzamine (Dibenzyline)	Peripheral arterial disorders in which neurogenic vasoconstrict'n is prominent. No established value in chronic occlusive peripheral vascular disease. (**Oral:** Initially, 10 mg/day; incr. by 10-mg am'ts at 4-day intervals prn. Maint. dose, 20-60 mg/day)	Alpha$_1$ adrenergic receptor blocker, resulting in vasodilatat'n of arterioles and veins.	Orthostatic hypotens'n, reflex tachycardia, nasal congest'n, GI disturbances (nausea, vomiting, diarrhea)		**Assess:** For pregnancy or hx of renal failure. **Evaluate/Teach:** Risk of postural hypotens'n.

CHAPTER 14

Antihypertensive Drugs

Teaching Objectives

Following completion of this chapter, the reader should be able to:

1. List the major determinants of blood pressure and the means by which drugs may lower blood pressure.
2. List the anatomical sites at which antihypertensives may work.
3. Discuss the mechanisms of action of antihypertensive drugs and the physiological factors that attenuate these actions.
4. Name the most important antihypertensive drugs acting at each anatomical site and describe their basic pharmacological properties.
5. Discuss the pharmacologic approach to the treatment of hypertension.
6. Describe the nursing process related to the use of each antihypertensive.

Hypertension

Hypertension is a major hazard to public health. Affecting the lives of millions, it is critically important in the pathogenesis of many cardiovascular diseases, including angina pectoris, acute myocardial infarction and congestive heart failure. Although the boundary between normotensive and hypertensive is subject to debate, many authorities consider that blood pressures above 140/90 increase significantly the risk of cardiovascular disease. The reduction of elevated blood pressures by drugs lowers the risk of many of the complications of cardiovascular disease.

The past thirty years have seen the introduction of many drugs capable of reducing elevated blood pressures. With so many drugs available, it is important to select a drug, or combination of drugs, that best meets the needs of individual patients. In this regard, it is not only important to treat a patient with a drug or drugs that lower his or her blood pressure, but equally vital to select the agent(s) that will improve the patient's quality of life.

This point must never be forgotten. Remember, essential hypertension is often symptomless. In the early stages of the disease it is the drug or drugs that make the patient feel ill or compromise his or her ability to carry out normal daily activities. If a drug is prescribed that disturbs the patient's quality of life, the patient may not only complain but may also fail to comply with the drug treatment.

Often it is not the patient who complains, but rather the spouse who must also endure the adverse effects of therapy. It is in this area that newer forms of treatment, such as the angiotensin-converting enzyme (ACE) inhibitors, have provided a definite advance. They lower blood pressure just as well as older forms of treatment but with fewer adverse effects than diuretics, beta blockers and central sympathetic inhibitors.

Cardiac output and peripheral resistance are the two major determinants of blood pressure. Drugs that lower blood pressure reduce cardiac output or peripheral resistance, or both. These drugs work at the following anatomic sites:

1. the kidneys, to increase salt and water loss and decrease blood volume (diuretics);
2. the arterioles, to decrease peripheral resistance (vasodilators);
3. the veins, to decrease venous return and reduce cardiac output (venodilators);
4. the heart, to reduce cardiac output (beta blockers);
5. the sympathetic centers in the brain, to decrease sympathetic stimulation of the heart and blood vessels (central sympathetic inhibitors).

This chapter will study the actions of antihypertensive drugs. Much of the pharmacology of these agents is discussed in Chapters 8 (antiadrenergic drugs) and 16 (diuretics). It is not necessary to repeat this material. This chapter will deal exclusively with the antihypertensive actions of these drugs.

Diuretics

Thiazides, Chlorthalidone and Metolazone

Mechanism of Action and Pharmacologic Effects

Thiazides, chlorthalidone (Hygroton) and metolazone (Zaroxolyn) increase salt and water elimination. Initially, in response to a decrease in circulating blood volume, cardiac output falls. Later, however, cardiac output increases to near normal. At this point, the drugs lower blood pressure by decreasing peripheral resistance. Two explanations can be offered for this decreased peripheral resistance. First, because the drugs increase body water loss and decrease blood volume, less blood is forced through arterioles. Second, in an action unrelated to their effects on the kidneys, the drugs directly dilate precapillary resistance vessels (arterioles). It

is this action that is primarily responsible for the antihypertensive effects of diuretics during chronic therapy.

Therapeutic Uses

Thiazides or chlorthalidone are often used first in treating hypertension. Few differences can be found between the many available thiazides. Hydrochlorothiazide (Hydrodiuril, Esidrix) is the most frequently used. Chlorthalidone and metolazone have effects similar to those of thiazides but have longer durations of action. For most patients metolazone offers no advantage over chlorthalidone and is more expensive.

Often either a thiazide or chlorthalidone may suffice alone in patients with mild hypertension. If a second drug is necessary, a beta blocker or an ACE inhibitor can be added.

To understand why either a diuretic plus a beta blocker, or a diuretic with an ACE inhibitor, is necessary, the nurse must recognize that the fall in blood pressure produced by diuretics triggers an increase in sympathetic nervous system activity. The increased sympathetic drive stimulates vasoconstrictor $alpha_1$ receptors and releases renal renin. The newly released renin is converted first to angiotensin I and then to angiotensin II, a potent vasoconstrictor. Angiotensin II also releases aldosterone, which increases salt and water retention by the kidneys.

The release of renin is mediated by beta receptors in the kidney. The use of a beta blocker with a diuretic will reduce the renal secretion of renin and increase the antihypertensive response of the patient. An alternative approach is to give an ACE inhibitor with the diuretic. By blocking the angiotensin-converting enzyme, ACE inhibitors reduce the conversion of angiotensin I to angiotensin II, thereby reducing the vasoconstriction produced by angiotensin II and decreasing aldosterone secretion and salt and water retention.

Adverse Effects

The adverse effects of the thiazides, chlorthalidone and metolazone are presented in detail in Chapter 16. It will suffice here to mention that hypokalemia, hyperglycemia, hyperuricemia and hyperlipidemia are the most frequently encountered adverse effects. Hypokalemia can be controlled by the concomitant administration of either a potassium salt, such as Slow-K or Micro-K Extencaps, or a potassium-sparing diuretic, such as triamterene (found in the product Dyazide, which contains both triamterene and hydrochlorothiazide), amiloride (supplied in Moduret, which provides both amiloride and hydrochlorothiazide), or spironolactone (provided in Aldactazide, which contains both spironolactone and hydrochlorothiazide).

Diuretics also increase plasma cholesterol and triglyceride levels, and this is a matter of concern. However, the hyperlipidemic effects of these drugs can be diminished by administering lower doses (25 mg of hydrochlorothiazide or 25 mg of chlorthalidone per day).

Nursing Process

Assessment

Prior to the administration of a thiazide, chlorthalidone or metolazone, the nurse should review the patient's history for contraindications to their use. These include kidney or liver disease, low serum potassium or sodium levels, chronic respiratory disease or pregnancy. If evidence of these exist, the nurse should consult with the physician. The nurse should also establish baseline body mass/weight and fluid intake and output prior to the administration of the diuretic. The presence and extent of peripheral edema should also be documented carefully to permit later comparison. Baseline vital signs should be obtained, with blood pressure taken in lying and standing postion.

Administration

Thiazides and chlorthalidone should be administered early in the morning. In this way, the effects of the drug will present themselves during the day. Patients will thus be allowed to slumber worry-free through the night without the danger that waves of urine may lap over the bladder. However, those patients whose lifestyles involve limited access to toilet facilities (e.g., crane operators, bus drivers) should be encouraged to take their medication at a time most convenient to their activities.

Evaluation

Daily nursing evaluation of diuretic effectiveness is accomplished by weighing the patient, monitoring the intake and output of fluid, and measuring blood pressures. In addition, nursing evaluation should focus on observing the patient for behavioral or physiological evidence of hypokalemia (muscle weakness, constipation or rectal impaction, postural hypotension, dyspnea, or cardiac arrhythmias), hyperglycemia (glycosuria), hyperuricemia (acute pain in a single joint — gout) and hyponatremia (muscle weakness, leg cramps, dry mouth, dizziness and gastric disturbances).

Teaching

Patients should be informed (and forewarned) of the effects of the drugs so that they can plan their days accordingly and not be alarmed by the diuresis. They should also be told of the danger of severe hypotension when alcohol is consumed concomitantly with a diuretic. Similarly, patients should be warned that ingesting licorice while on a thiazide, chlorthalidone or metolazone increases the risk of hypokalemia. Nurses should inform patients to increase fluid intake to two to three liters per day unless this is otherwise contraindicated.

Furosemide (Lasix)

Furosemide is a high-ceiling or loop diuretic, more potent than the thiazides, chlorthalidone or metolazone. However, in contradistinction to these drugs, furosemide does not dilate arterioles and therefore is not as effective as an antihypertensive. As a result, its routine use in the treatment of hypertension is not appropriate. The use of furosemide should be restricted to patients with renal damage who do not obtain adequate diuresis from hydrochlorothiazide or chlorthalidone.

In general, furosemide's contraindications and adverse effects are similar to those of the thiazides and chlorthalidone (Chapter 16). However, because of its potent diuretic effects, furosemide has a greater potential for producing serious electrolyte disturbances. Hyponatremia, hypokalemia and hypovolemia are among the adverse effects of the drug. Other adverse effects of furosemide are various forms of dermatitis, tinnitus and reversible deafness.

Nursing Process

The nursing process for furosemide is similar to those for the thiazides and chlorthalidone. Nurses should remember that furosemide is a more potent diuretic than the others and the likelihood of experiencing electrolyte disturbances is proportionately greater.

Vasodilators

Angiotensin-Converting Enzyme (ACE) Inhibitors

Mechanism of Action and Pharmacologic Effects

Captopril (Capoten), enalapril (Vasotec) and lisinopril (Prinivil, Zestril) are orally effective angiotensin-converting enzyme inhibitors. Renin, released from the kidney, is converted to angiotensin I, which in turn is changed to the vasoconstrictor angiotensin II. Captopril, enalapril and lisinopril inhibit the enzyme responsible for the conversion of angiotensin I to angiotensin II. Because they dilate arterioles but not veins, ACE inhibitors reduce peripheral resistance without producing postural hypotension. ACE inhibitors may also prevent the degradation of the vasodilator bradykinin and increase the production of vasodilator prostaglandins.

One additional effect of these drugs also deserves mention. Angiotensin II increases aldosterone secretion. By reducing the formation of angiotensin II, ACE inhibitors decrease aldsoterone secretion. As a result of a reduction in the secretion of the mineralocorticoid aldosterone, salt and water retention is reduced and blood pressure falls.

Captopril is effective without need for conversion to another form. Enalapril is a prodrug that is de-esterified in the liver to the active chemical enalaprilat. This fact has little clinical significance, except for the fact that the initial effect of enalapril may take longer to appear as the body converts the drug to its active metabolite. In addition, it is not clear what effect hepatic damage may have on the ability of the liver to convert enalapril to enalaprilat.

Lisinopril is the lysine derivative of enalaprilat. It is absorbed more slowly than enalapril after oral administration, but it does not require hydrolysis in the liver to form an active compound.

Enalapril and lisinopril have longer half-lives (eleven to twelve hours) than captopril (three hours) and may be administered once a day, compared to the twice-daily regimen currently recommended for captopril. This convenience factor must be counterbalanced with the knowledge that the initial hypotensive effect seen in approximately fifty per cent of patients taking an ACE inhibitor may be longer in duration if enalapril or lisinopril is used.

Therapeutic Uses

ACE inhibitors represent a major advance in the development of antihypertensive therapy. As effective alone as beta blockers or diuretics, these drugs often produce fewer adverse effects than other antihypertensives. The alterations in blood chemistry, bradycardia, intermittent claudication, fatigue, cold extremities, and decrease in libido produced by either diuretics and/or beta blockers are not experienced by patients on ACE inhibitors. As a result, many patients taking ACE inhibitors experience an increase in quality of life.

In addition to being effective alone, ACE inhibitors can be used to complement the antihypertensive effects of a diuretic or a beta blocker. ACE inhibitors also have an additive antihypertensive effect when combined with a calcium channel blocker.

Adverse Effects

Overall, the incidence of adverse effects is usually lower with ACE inhibitors than with other forms of antihypertensive therapy. Although initial clinical trials with relatively large doses of captopril found that one to two per cent of patients developed proteinuria and a smaller number demonstrated renal insufficiency, renal failure, polyuria, oliguria and urinary frequency, the cause-and-effect relationship with captopril is uncertain. Neutropenia and agranulocytosis that was probably drug-related occurred in about 0.3% of patients treated with captopril. Other adverse effects include skin rash, angioedema and dysgeusia. If the dose of captopril is restricted to a maximum of 150 mg per day, the incidence of adverse effects is reduced significantly. In addition to dose, the other factors that predispose patients to captopril-induced adverse effects are renal impairment and connective tissue disorders.

Severe symptomatic hypotension can occur after the first dose of captopril, particularly in diuretic-treated patients who are salt depleted. This effect can be reduced, or prevented, if the diuretic is stopped, or its dose reduced, in the three to four days prior to captopril treatment. Patients previously treated with diuretics should be started on low doses of captopril, in the range of 6.25 – 12.5 mg per day, before increasing the dose of captopril gradually over the next few days and reinstituting diuretic therapy slowly.

Enalapril may cause headache, dizziness, nausea, diarrhea and hyperkalemia. Similarly to captopril, severe symptomatic hypotension can occur after the first dose of enalapril. Again, the effect is more prevalent in salt-depleted patients. Because enalapril has a slower onset and longer duration of action than captopril, several hours may be required to produce the initial hypotensive effect, and this effect may last longer than that produced by captopril. Rash and taste disturbances may be less common with enalapril than captopril.

Lisinopril can also produce symptomatic hypotension, particularly in patients who are volume- or sodium-depleted as a result of diuretic therapy, salt restriction, diarrhea or vomiting. Similarly to enalapril, this effect may be delayed until four to six hours after taking lisinopril.

Nursing Process

Nurses must remain cognizant of the major adverse effects of captopril. If early signs of these appear, the physician should be contacted at once. Patients and their families should also be advised of the nature of the adverse effects of the drug and their symptoms.

Assessment

Prior to administering an ACE inhibitor, the nurse should review the patient's history for contraindications to their use. These include hypersensitivity, pregnancy, lactation and heart block. Blood studies for neutrophils, decreased platelets, renal and liver function, and electrolyte balance should be carried out prior to therapy.

Administration

ACE inhibitors should be stored in tight containers at 30°C or less. Oral preparations of captopril should be given one hour before meals. The absorption of enalapril is not affected by food. If intravenous therapy is ordered, ACE inhibitors must be administered slowly, using the diluent provided. Nurses must place the patient in the supine or Trendelenburg position for severe hypotension.

Evaluation

Observations for therapeutic response include a decrease in blood pressure in hypertensive patients and a reduction in edema and moist rales in patients with congestive heart failure. Daily evaluations should include fluid intake and output, body mass/weight and edema in feet and legs. Nurses should remain alert for possible allergic reactions, such as rash, fever, pruritis and urticaria.

Teaching

Patients should be instructed to take captopril one hour before meals, not to discontinue an ACE inhibitor abruptly, and not to use over-the-counter products unless directed by the physician. Nurses must stress the importance of compliance with the dosage schedule and instruct the patient to rise slowly from a sitting or lying position. Patients should be advised to avoid sunlight and told to report signs of allergic reaction (mouth sores, fever, swelling of hands or feet, irregular heart beat, chest pain) to the physician. Nurses must ensure that patients understand that dizziness and fainting may occur during first few days of therapy.

Calcium Channel Blockers

Mechanism of Action and Pharmacologic Effects

Diltiazem (Cardizem), nifedipine (Adalat, Procardia), nicardipine (Cardene) and verapamil (Isoptin) are calcium channel blockers. These drugs have previously been discussed as antianginal agents in Chapter 12. The material presented here will relate to their effects on the peripheral vasculature.

The antihypertensive effect of this group of drugs is believed to be related to their specific cellular action of selectively inhibiting transmembrane influx of calcium ions into vascular smooth muscle. The contractile process of vascular smooth muscle depends on the movements of extracellular calcium into the cells through specific ion channels. Diltiazem, nifedipine, nicardipine and verapamil block transmembrane influx of calcium through the slow channel without affecting to any significant degree the transmembrane influx of sodium through the fast channel. This reduces free calcium ions available within vascular smooth muscle cells, with the result that contractile processes are blocked, precapillary resistance vessels (arterioles) dilate and peripheral resistance falls.

Therapeutic Uses

Next to ACE inhibitors, the introduction of the calcium channel blockers for the treatment of hypertension represents the most significant advance in the treatment of this disease in the past twenty years. Similarly to ACE inhibitors, the calcium channel blockers are effective vasodilators and not encumbered by many of the adverse effects commonly associated with the older drugs, such as diuretics, beta blockers and central sympathetic inhibitors. Although official monographs state that calcium channel blockers should normally be used in patients in whom treatment with diuretics or beta blockers is contraindicated or have been associated with unacceptable adverse effects, physicians may soon begin to choose patients who would benefit from one of these drugs and start without trying first the diuretic or the beta blocker. If additional antihypertensive effects are required, a calcium channel blocker may be combined with a diuretic. In addition, nifedipine and nicardipine are often used with a beta blocker. However, verapamil and diltiazem have myocardial depressant effects and are not recommended in combination with beta blocker therapy.

Diltiazem, nifedipine and verapamil are prepared in a slow-release form for the treatment of hypertension, and prescriptions should indicate this form (see Table 15). The rapidly absorbed regular tablets or capsule forms of these drugs are intended primarily for the treatment of angina pectoris and not for hypertension.

Adverse Effects

Diltiazem can produce bradycardia, dizziness, weakness, headache, flushing, dryness of the mouth and pedal edema. In addition, gastrointestinal disturbances and dermatological reactions have occurred with the drug. Diltiazem is contraindicated in patients with: sick sinus syndrome, except in the presence of a functioning ventricular pacemaker; second- or third-degree A-V block; hypersensitivity to diltiazem; or severe hypotension (less than 90 mm Hg systolic pressure).

Nifedipine and nicardipine are the most potent peripheral vasodilators of the four calcium channel blockers. Their adverse effects include headache, dizziness, tachycardia and peripheral edema. These effects are minimized with the sustained-release product.

Constipation is very prevalent with verapamil. The drug also produces headache, vertigo, weakness, nervousness, pruritus, flushing, rash and gastric disturbances. Orthostatic hypotension and pedal edema are also encountered. As explained in Chapter 11, verapamil is a potent myocardial depressant with the ability to delay A-V conduction. As a result, it can produce bradycardia, A-V block, A-V dissociation, congestive heart failure and pulmonary edema. Usually verapamil should not be prescribed for patients with sick sinus syndrome, second- or third-degree A-V block, cardiogenic shock, or advanced congestive heart failure. Verapamil is also contraindicated in the presence of acute myocardial infarction; severe left ventricular dysfunction (unless secondary to a supraventricular tachycardia amenable to oral verapamil therapy); severe hypotension; and marked bradycardia.

Nursing Process

The nursing processes for calcum channel blockers found in Chapter 11 (verapamil) and in Chapter 12 (nifedipine, nicardipine and diltiazem) can be applied to use of these drugs to treat hypertension. The teaching points outlined in the other chapters are equally important with the hypertensive patient. It is advised that patients be taught to take their own blood pressure in order to monitor drug and therapy effects.

Hydralazine (Apresoline)

Mechanism of Action and Pharmacologic Effects

Hydralazine relaxes arteriolar smooth muscles by activating guanylate cyclase, resulting in the accumulation of cyclic guanosine monophosphate (cGMP). It has relatively little effect on veins. Thus, it decreases peripheral resistance and blood pressure without producing postural hypotension. Unfortunately, the fall in blood pressure triggers a reflex sympathetic response, resulting in an increase in heart rate and renin release and offsetting, in part, the primary hypotensive effects of the drug.

Hydralazine is metabolized in the liver. Acetylation is the major route of inactivation. The population in general may be divided into those in whom acetylation occurs quickly (rapid acetylators) and those in whom it occurs slowly (slow acetylators). During chronic therapy, hydralazine will accumulate in the slow acetylators unless lower doses are given.

Therapeutic Uses

The use of hydralazine alone to treat hypertension is limited because of reflex tachycardia. It is often used together with a beta blocker and a diuretic in what has been called **standard-triple therapy,** with hydralazine dilating arterioles, the beta blocker preventing hydralazine-induced reflex tachycardia and the diuretic increasing salt and water excretion. Hydralazine is contraindicated in patients with coronary artery disease, mitral valvular rheumatic heart disease, and acute dissecting aneurysm of the aorta.

Adverse Effects

Hydralazine's adverse effects include headache (due to vasodilatation), tachycardia, anorexia, nausea, dizziness and sweating. The most serious adverse effect of hydralazine is a lupus-like syndrome that has been reported in ten to twenty per cent of patients receiving doses in excess of 400 mg daily. This is seen most often in patients in whom the drug is slowly metabolized (slow acetylators). Unless these individuals receive lower doses, toxic levels of hydralazine may accumulate, giving rise to the lupus erythematosus-like syndrome.

Nursing Process

Assessment

Prior to administering the first dose of hydralazine, nurses should assess patients for contraindications to its use. The patient's history should be reviewed for indications of previous hypersensitivity to hydralazine, coronary disease, lupus erythematosus, current pregnancy and renal or hepatic disease. The patient's emotional status should be assessed and baseline blood pressure and body mass/weight measurements established.

Administration

Hydralazine is usually administered orally. One source suggests that taking hydralazine with food reduces first-pass metabolism by the liver. Therefore, in order to regulate the dosage, the drug must be taken consistently on either an empty or a full stomach.

Evaluation

Once therapy is started, nurses must assess the effect of the drug daily by monitoring blood pressure, body mass/weight and fluid intake and output. The patient should also be observed carefully for evidence of adverse effects, particularly hypersensitivities (rash, urticaria, itching, chills or elevated temperature), depression or lupus erythematosus (fever, arthralgia, malaise, enlarged spleen or lymphadenopathy).

Teaching

Because hydralazine can produce dizziness, nurses should advise patients to be extra careful in driving cars or using power tools. They should also be warned to stand up and lie down slowly. Patients and their families should be told that abrupt hydralazine withdrawal can cause a sudden rise in blood pressure. It is imperative, therefore, that sufficient supplies of the drug be available at all times. Patients and their families should be advised of the importance of routine blood monitoring. In addition, they should be supplied with a list of hydralazine's adverse effects and instructed to contact their physician if any of these occur. The patient should be warned to avoid over-the-counter preparations unless directed by the physician.

Prazosin (Minipress)

Prazosin decreases peripheral resistance by blocking alpha$_1$ receptors. Although the drug lowers blood pressure in both the upright and supine positions, its effect is greater when the patient stands. In contrast to hydralazine, prazosin produces only a small increase in heart rate, and little change in cardiac output and plasma renin levels. However, similarly to other vasodilators, fluid retention occurs during chronic therapy and this effect offsets, in part, the primary antihypertensive action of prazosin. Prazosin is usually given in combination with a diuretic and a beta blocker.

The adverse effects of prazosin include weakness, dizziness, headache, palpitations and lack of energy. The incidence of postural hypotension, indicating venodilatation, can be high if the starting dose is more than 1 mg per day.

Nursing Process

The nursing process related to prazosin use is discussed in detail in Chapter 8. It is summarized in Table 15 at the end of this chapter.

Terazosin (Hytrin)

Terazosin lowers blood pressure by dilating arterioles. This action appears to be produced by the selective blockade of alpha$_1$ receptors. Systolic and diastolic blood pressures are lowered in both the supine and standing positions. Terazosin is indicated for the treatment of mild to moderate hypertension. It is employed in a general treatment program in conjunction with a thiazide diuretic and/or other antihypertensive drugs as needed for proper patient response. Terazosin may be tried as a sole therapy in those patients in whom other agents caused adverse effects or are inappropriate.

Terazosin can cause marked hypotension, especially postural hypotension, and syncope in association with the first dose or first few doses of therapy. A similar effect can occur if therapy is reinstated following interruption for more than a few doses. Syncope has also occurred in association with rapid dosage increases or the introduction of another antihypertensive agent into the regimen of a patient taking high doses of terazosin. Patients should be advised to lie down when these symptoms occur and then wait for a few minutes before standing, to prevent their recurrence.

Syncope is the most severe adverse reaction to terazosin. The common reactions are dizziness, headache, asthenia, somnolence, nasal congestion and palpitations.

Nursing Process

The nursing process related to the use of terazosin is presented in Chapter 8 and summarized in Tables 8 and 15.

Labetalol (Normodyne, Trandate)

Labetalol blocks both alpha$_1$ and beta receptors. Although more potent as a beta blocker, labetalol's antihypertensive effects are due primarily to alpha$_1$ receptor antagonism, resulting in a decrease in peripheral resistance. The reflex tachycardia normally seen with arteriolar dilatation is prevented by the partial beta blockade. Bradycardia, usually seen with beta blocker therapy, does not occur with labetalol. Presumably the increase in sympathetic stimulation to the heart, secondary to vasodilatation, competes with the beta-blocking effects of the drug, the one offsetting the other.

Labetalol is usually added to other therapeutic regimens, notably diuretic therapy. The most serious adverse effects of labetalol reported are severe postural hypotension, jaundice and bronchospasm. Nausea and vomiting may also be experienced with the drug. Labetalol is contraindicated in uncontrolled congestive heart failure because sympathetic stimulation is a vital component supporting circulatory function in congestive heart failure, and inhibition with beta blockade carries the potential hazard of further depressing myocardial contractility and precipitating cardiac failure. Because of its ability to block both alpha$_1$ and beta receptors, the drug is also contraindicated in severe chronic obstructive lung disease, A-V block greater than first degree, cardiogenic shock and other conditions associated with severe and prolonged hypotension, and sinus bradycardia.

Nursing Process

Assessment
Nurses should review the patient's history for asthma, chronic obstructive pulmonary disease (COPD), cardiovascular or liver disease and diabetes mellitus. Nurses should also establish baseline measures of the patient's blood pressure and pulse in both lying and standing positions.

Administration
When administered orally, labetalol should either follow a meal or be accompanied by food. When given intravenously, the patient should be lying down during and for three hours after receiving the medication. The use of an infusion pump or other similar device for accurate measurement of intravenous administration is highly recommended.

Evaluation
Blood pressure measurements, both lying and standing, are compared to the baseline measures in order to determine the effectiveness of the drug.

Teaching
Patient teaching associated with labetalol revolves around its antihypertensive effect. Therefore, the nurse should implement the same teaching measures as those previously identified in relation to the use of hydralazine. Patients and their families should be counselled to consult their physician or pharmacist before taking over-the-counter medications.

Diazoxide (Hyperstat) and Sodium Nitroprusside (Nipride)

Diazoxide and sodium nitroprusside are given parenterally to treat hypertensive crises. Diazoxide dilates arterioles primarily, and sodium nitroprusside relaxes both arterioles and veins. Although many physicians and nurses may see little of these drugs, one or both are usually stocked in all hospitals. Given to the patient suffering through a hypertensive crisis, either drug may be life saving. Both drugs are contraindicated in compensatory hypertension, such as that associated with aortic coarctation or A-V shunt.

Drugs That Depress Venous Return

Guanethidine (Ismelin)

Mechanism of Action and Pharmacologic Effects

Guanethidine is an adrenergic neuron blocker that impairs sympathetic nervous system activity. Its mechanism of action, pharmacologic effects and adverse effects are explained in Chapter 8. Guanethidine dilates veins, reducing venous return and cardiac output, as well as arterioles, decreasing peripheral resistance. The drug produces both supine and postural hypotension in addition to causing a reduction in renal blood flow and glomerular filtration rate. The resulting increase in blood volume reduces the antihypertensive effect of guanethidine.

Therapeutic Uses

Although guanethidine is an effective antihypertensive drug, it is now used **only after standard therapy** (consisting of such drugs as hydrochlorothiazide, a beta blocker, an ACE inhibitor, a calcium channel blocker, hydralazine or methyldopa) has failed. When used, guanethidine is usually administered with a diuretic, such as hydrochlorothiazide. Guanethidine is contraindicated in proved or suspected pheochromocytoma or frank congestive heart failure not due to hypertension.

Adverse Effects

The adverse effects of guanethidine result from its ability to block sympathetic nerve endings. They include orthostatic (postural) hypotension, impaired erection/ejaculation, diarrhea and nasal stuffiness. Guanethidine does not cross the blood-brain barrier and sedation is not common.

Nursing Process

The nursing actions related to the use of guanethidine are presented in Chapter 8. They are briefly summarized in Table 15 at the end of this chapter.

Guanadrel (Hylorel)

The mechanism of action and hemodynamic effects of guanadrel are similar to those of guanethidine. It has a more rapid onset and shorter duration of action than guanethidine. Guanadrel is as effective an antihypertensive as guanethidine, but causes morning orthostatic hypotension and diarrhea less frequently. It has a reduced likelihood of causing impaired erection/ejaculation. In all other regards, including the nursing process related to its use, guanadrel seems similar to guanethidine.

Reserpine (Serpasil)

Reserpine is an adrenergic neuron blocker with mild antihypertensive activity. It crosses the blood-brain barrier and causes severe depression. Once depression is established, several drug-free weeks are required for the patient to recover. Few new patients should be started on reserpine. Reserpine is contraindicated in mental depression, active peptic ulcer, ulcerative colitis, digitalis intoxication and aortic insufficiency. Detailed discussion of the nursing actions related to reserpine are presented in Chapter 8 and summarized in Table 15 at the end of this chapter.

Drugs That Decrease Cardiac Output

Beta Blockers

Mechanism of Action and Pharmacologic Effects

Beta blockers are given to reduce beta$_1$ receptor mediated effects. By blocking beta$_1$ receptors, these drugs reduce cardiac output, thereby lowering blood pressure. Propranolol (Inderal), the prototype beta blocker, blocks both beta$_1$ and beta$_2$ receptors. By blocking beta$_2$ receptors on the bronchioles, it exposes the asthmatic or bronchitic patient to increased risk of bronchoconstriction. Blocking beta$_2$ receptors on blood vessels allows unopposed alpha$_1$ vasoconstriction, which may become clinically apparent especially in patients with Raynaud's phenomenon. Timolol (Blocadren) and nadolol (Corgard) are very similar to propranolol in their ability to block both beta$_1$ and beta$_2$ receptors.

The cardioselective beta blockers atenolol (Tenormin) and metoprolol (Betaloc, Lopresor, Lopressor) preferentially block beta$_1$ receptors, with less effect on beta$_2$ sites. As a result, atenolol and metoprolol have less effect on the bronchioles. However, this fact is largely of academic interest, because no beta blocker should be given to an asthmatic patient.

The cardioselective beta blockers are preferred in a diabetic patient. Normally, the hypoglycemic action of insulin is counterbalanced, in part, by the hyperglycemic effect of epinephrine — a beta$_2$ receptor mediated effect. Nonselective beta blockers prevent the epinephrine effect and accentuate the hypoglycemia produced by insulin. Atenolol and metoprolol, which do not affect the beta$_2$ effects of epinephrine, are preferred. Both cardioselective and nonselective beta blockers reduce the tachycardia and tremor that may be early signs of hypoglycemia.

Patients who experience cold extremities following administration of propranolol, timolol or nadolol may prefer a cardioselective beta blocker. By blocking beta$_2$ receptors in peripheral arterioles, nonselective beta blockers predispose patients to alpha$_1$ receptor mediated vasoconstriction. If atenolol or metoprolol are taken, vessel tone remains a balance between beta$_2$ receptor-induced vasodilatation and alpha$_1$ receptor mediated constriction.

Pindolol (Visken) and oxprenolol (Trasicor) are beta blockers with partial-agonist or intrinsic sympathetic activity (ISA). They are not true competitive inhibitors of beta receptors. Instead, the drugs are very weak beta stimulants that compete with the more potent chemicals epinephrine and norepinephrine at receptor sites, with the result that they reduce beta receptor mediated responses. Beta blockers with ISA may not reduce resting heart rate as much as other beta blockers. Acebutolol (Monitan, Sectral) is a cardioselective partial agonist, exerting its ISA only on beta$_1$ receptors.

It is also possible to classify beta blockers on the basis of their lipid solubility. Propranolol, timolol, metoprolol, pindolol and oxprenolol have significant lipid solubility and cross the blood-brain barrier readily. Nadolol, atenolol and acebutolol, on the other hand, have poor lipid solubility and are far less able to enter the brain. It has been argued that this gives the latter three a definite advantage because they may produce fewer central nervous system adverse effects.

The effects produced by a beta blocker are determined, to a major extent, by the degree of sympathetic stimulation normally present. Beta blockers lower maximal exercise heart rate and cardiac output in all patients. In the resting individual, when sympathetic tone is low, the consequences of their actions on heart rate are not so obvious. In the stressed or exercising human, who normally depends heavily on increased sympathetic stimulation, the effects of a beta blocker are very apparent when the cardiac rate and output fall well below the needs of the body.

Therapeutic Uses

Beta blockers can be used as initial drugs in the treatment of hypertension. If a beta blocker alone proves inadequate, a diuretic such as hydrochlorothiazide or chlorthalidone may be added. Alternatively, a diuretic can be used first, with the beta blocker added when required. When the combination of a beta blocker and a diuretic fails to suffice, a vasodilator is usually added as a third drug.

Adverse Effects

Bradycardia, fatigue, congestive heart failure and reduction in or loss of libido are the most obvious effects of a beta blocker. A block of beta$_2$ receptors in the bronchioles can produce bronchoconstriction in asthmatic patients. Beta blockers can precipitate cardiac failure in patients with congestive heart failure. The other adverse effects of beta blockers include nausea, vomiting, constipation, diarrhea, depression, disturbed sleep and nightmares. Allergic reactions such as rashes, fever and purpura may also be seen. Finally, peculiar inflammatory reactions with fibrosis have been reported.

Beta blockers are contraindicated in bronchospasm, including bronchial asthma. Other contraindications to the use of beta blockers include: allergic rhinitis during the pollen season, sinus bradycardia, A-V block greater than first degree, cardiogenic shock, right ventricular failure secondary to pulmonary hypertension, and congestive heart failure.

Nursing Process

The nursing process related to the administration of a beta blocker is presented in detail in Chapter 8. With respect to their use to treat hypertension, the evaluation and patient teaching aspects of the nursing process should receive major emphasis.

Evaluation

Evaluation of the patient's response should focus on assessing the efficacy of the beta blocker and early identification of adverse effects. Thus, extreme importance is attached to accurate measurement of apical/radial pulses, fluid intake and output, daily body mass/weight, blood pressure, respirations and circulation of the extremities (including color, warmth, blanching of the skin, and peripheral pulses).

Teaching

Patients and their families should be taught to observe for drug efficacy and adverse effects. The sudden withdrawal of beta blockers can result in a rapid increase in heart rate, myocardial infarction or arrhythmias. It is essential to have sufficient quantities of medication on hand at all times so that sudden accidental withdrawal of the drug will not occur.

When beta blockers are used to alter blood pressure, patients should be discouraged from smoking, drinking alcohol and using over-the-counter medications for colds, coughs or allergies. Safety precautions related to the potential drowsiness and dizziness often associated with these medications should be emphasized.

Central Sympathetic Inhibitors

Clonidine (Catapres)

Clonidine is believed to stimulate alpha$_2$ receptors in the brain, thereby reducing norepinephrine release from central nervous system sympathetic neurons. Inhibition of sympathetic tone decreases arterial pressure and heart rate. Postural hypotension is not common. Plasma renin activity is reduced because sympathetic stimulation to the kidney is decreased. Clonidine is a very potent antihypertensive. As little as 0.2 mg orally may be effective. Clonidine is usually added to diuretic therapy, if a beta blocker is contraindicated. Abrupt withdrawal of clonidine may lead to severe rebound hypertensive episodes; therefore, if clonidine therapy is discontinued for any reason, withdrawal should be done gradually over several days.

The adverse effects of clonidine include dry mouth, sedation or drowsiness. Impotence may occur rarely. Sodium, chloride and water retention often occur on clonidine treatment.

Nursing Process

Patients should be cautioned not to discontinue the drug abruptly, as severe rebound hypertension may occur. Other nursing processes related to the use of clonidine are the same as those for reserpine (Chapter 8), and are summarized in Table 15 at the end of this chapter.

Methyldopa (Aldomet)

Methyldopa reduces central sympathetic activity (see Chapter 8). The drug produces a significant reduction in blood pressure and total peripheral resistance, while cardiac output and renal blood flow are maintained. Because sympathetic reflexes are maintained fairly well when the patient stands, methyldopa does not produce the same degree of postural hypotension as guanethidine. Methyldopa has been used as a standard antihypertensive drug for more than twenty-five years. Clinically, its effects are similar to those of clonidine. Methyldopa is usually considered a second-line antihypertensive. It is employed when a diuretic alone is insufficient.

Methyldopa's adverse effects include sedation, edema, impotence and postural hypotension. Drug fever, hepatic dysfunction, hemolytic anemia and lactation are seen rarely. Up to twenty-five per cent of patients taking 1000 mg of methyldopa daily for six months or more develop a positive Coombs' test. This has little clinical significance. Methyldopa may decrease high-density lipoprotein (HDL) cholesterol levels. The drug is contraindicated in patients with active hepatic disease. It should also not be used in persons in whom previous methyldopa therapy has been associated with liver disorders or hemolytic anemia.

Nursing Process

The nursing process for methyldopa is presented in Chapter 8 and summarized in Table 15 at the end of this chapter.

Pharmacologic Approach to the Treatment of Hypertension

Drug therapy for mild to moderate hypertension should be attempted only after nonpharmacological measures (weight loss and reduction in dietary sodium intake) have failed. Weight loss by patients who are only slightly obese can reduce blood pressure significantly, independently of salt intake. With respect to salt, an intake in excess of approximately 10 g per day may aggravate hypertension, and dietary salt intake below normal intake levels may produce a small reduction in blood pressure. Furthermore, if drug therapy is required, reducing salt intake may increase the activity of antihypertensive drugs. Therefore, not only should excessive sodium intake be discouraged but in addition, mild sodium restriction (the "no added salt" diet or less than 5 g of sodium chloride daily) should be advised for hypertensive patients. As well, reducing dietary fat and increasing the ratio of polyunsaturated to saturated fat may also reduce blood pressure.

Mild hypertension may often be treated with one antihypertensive. More severe hypertension often may justify the use of two or more drugs. Two drugs, acting by different mechanisms, can often lower the blood pressure more than higher doses of each drug used alone. Drugs should be selected so that their mechanisms of action complement each other and reduce the consequences of the physiological response mechanisms evoked by each agent.

Hydrochlorothiazide or chlorthalidone may be adequate to treat patients with mild hypertension, with diastolic pressures between 90 – 100 mm Hg. However, because they increase both blood sugar and uric acid levels, diuretics should be avoided in patients with either diabetes or gout. Diuretics also increase renin release, and the resulting increase in angiotensin II and aldosterone levels may be sufficient to keep the patient hypertensive. If this happens, a beta blocker that will block beta$_1$ receptors in the kidney and the heart can be added to the therapeutic regimen. The beta blocker will reduce renin release and decrease cardiac output, resulting a further decrease in blood pressure. Alternatively, an ACE inhibitor can be combined with the diuretic.

Some physicians elect to treat essential hypertension with a beta blocker first. A beta blocker should be avoided in patients with congestive heart failure, diabetes, asthma or peripheral vascular disease. Beta blockers decrease renal perfusion and may increase blood volume. In this situation a diuretic, such as hydrochlorothiazide, can be added to the beta blocker therapy. Alternative combination therapy involves the use of a calcium channel blocker, such as nifedipine, with the beta blocker.

More physicians are turning to an ACE inhibitor as the first drug of choice in the treatment of essential hypertension. These agents are effective peripheral vasodilators and appear to improve the overall quality of life more than diuretics, beta blockers or methyldopa. Furthermore, they are not contraindicated in diabetes or gout (as are diuretics), heart failure, diabetes, asthma, peripheral vascular disease (as are beta blockers), or depression or liver disease (as is methyldopa). Obviously, if a second drug is required, a diuretic represents the logical choice for combination therapy with an ACE inhibitor.

The future may see increased use of calcium channel blockers for the treatment of hypertension. The availability of sustained-release tablets has greatly increased their usefulness as antihypertensives. Because experience with calcium channel blockers as antihypertensives is less than that with ACE inhibitors, they will probably be used as second- or third-line drugs in combination therapy until physicians gain more experience with their effects.

Other vasodilators, such as hydralazine, prazosin or terazosin, are usually reserved for patients with moderate hypertension (diastolic pressures between 100 – 110 mm Hg). They are often added to a regimen consisting of a diuretic and a beta blocker. The beta blocker will reduce the reflex tachycardia produced by the vasodilator, and the diuretic will ensure that an increase in blood volume does not occur.

Methyldopa or clonidine may be used in place of the vasodilator in the patient with moderate hypertension. These drugs are effective antihypertensives and are usually combined with hydrochlorothiazide or chlorthalidone. Their selection over a vasodilator is determined largely on the basis of the clinical response of the particular patient to one drug or the other, or the adverse effects that are best tolerated. Contraindications to the use of methyldopa have already been mentioned. Clonidine should be avoided in patients who suffer from depression.

Adrenergic neuron-blocking drugs, such as guanethidine, are usually reserved for the severely hypertensive patient, with a diastolic pressure in excess of 110 mm Hg, whose hypertension is not controlled on other drugs. These agents are often added to pre-existing treatment regimens consisting of a diuretic and a vasodilator. The adverse effects of blocking all peripheral sympathetic nerve endings are often so galvanizing that many physicians are reluctant to resort to guanethidine unless all other agents have been tried.

Further Reading

Ames, R. P. (1986). The effects of antihypertensive drugs on serum lipids and lipoproteins. I: Diuretics. *Drugs 32* :260-278.

Ames, R. P. (1986). The effects of antihypertensive drugs on serum lipids and lipoproteins. II: Non-diuretic drugs. *Drugs 32* :335-357.

Brodgen, R. N., Todd, P. A. and Sorkin, E. M. (1988). Captopril: An update of its pharmacodynamic and pharmacokinetic properties, and therapeutic use in hypertension and congestive heart failure. *Drugs 36* :540-600.

Buhler, F. R. (1988). Antihypertensive treatment according to age, plasma renin and race. *Drugs 35* :495-503.

Drugs for hypertension. (1989). *The Medical Letter 31* :25-30.

Drugs for hypertension. Drugs of choice. (1989). *The Medical Letter 31* :46-62.

Drugs for hypertensive emergencies. (1989). *The Medical Letter 31* :32-34.

Freis, E. D. (1986). The cardiovascular risk of diuretic-induced hypokalemia and elevated cholesterol. *Rational Drug Therapy 20* (3):1-6.

Ganten, D. and Reid, J. L. (1990). Cardiovascular considerations in hypertension: Effects of the angiotensin system. A seminar-in-print. *Drugs 39* (Suppl. 1):1-79.

Jessup, M. (1989). Angiotensin-converting enzyme inhibitors: Are there significant clinical differences? *J. Amer. Coll. Cardio. 13* :1248-1250.

Joseph, Jutta J. and Schuna, Arthur A. (1990). Management of hypertension in the diabetic patient. *Clinical Pharmacy 9* :864-872.

Less, K. R. (1988). Angiotensin-converting enzyme inhibitors. *Rational Drug Therapy 22* (9):1-5.

McLeod, A. A. and Jewet, D. E. (1986). Drug treatment of primary pulmonary hypertension. *Drugs 31* :177-184.

Moser, M. (1989). Relative efficacy of, and some adverse reactions to, different antihypertensive regimens. *Amer. J. Cardiol. 63* (4):2B-7B.

Moser, M., Black, H. and Stair, D. (1986). The dilemma of mid hypertension. *Drugs 31* :279-287.

Scriabine, A. (1987). Current and potential indication for Ca++ antagonists. *Rational Drug Therapy 21* (Nov.):1-7.

Spence, J. D. (1989). Stepped care for hypertension is dead but what will replace it? *Canad. Med. Assoc. J. 140* :1133-1136.

Todd, P. A. and Heel, R. C. (1986). Enalapril: A review of its pharmacodynamic and pharmacokinetic properties, and therapeutic use in hypertension and congestive heart failure. *Drugs 31* :198-248.

Table 15
Antihypertensive drugs.

Generic Name (Trade Name)	Use (Dose)	Action	Adverse Effects	Drug Interactions	Nursing Process
Pharmacologic Classification: Thiazide and Thiazide-like Diuretics					
Hydrochlorothiazide (Esidrex, Hydrodiuril)	Tx of edema and hypertens'n (**Oral:** Adults - 25-50 mg/day. Us. dose should be restricted to 25 mg; higher doses us. fail to produce addit'nal antihypertensive effects yet incr. adv. effects of hydrochlorothiazide. Children - 1-2 mg/kg/day in 2 divided doses)	Decr. peripheral resistance, incr. renal excret'n of NaCl and H₂O, resulting in decr. blood volume and BP.	Hypovolemia, hypokalemia, hyponatremia, renal colic, hematuria, crystalluria, hypersensitivity, pancreatitis, jaundice, hepatic coma, gout	**Angiotensin-converting enzyme (ACE) inhibitors:** Used tog. w. a diuretic, can produce a powerful hypotensive effect, poss. leading to postural hypotens'n. Avoid by stopping diuretic a few days before starting w. low doses of ACE inhibitor. Thereafter, it may be poss. to reintroduce the diuretic and incr. dose of ACE inhibitor slowly. **Antidiabetic drugs:** Their effects can be antagonized by thiazides and thiazide-like drugs, which can incr. blood glucose in diabetics and prediabetics and reduce or block effect of antidiabetic drugs.	**Assess:** Pt hx for contraindicat'ns to use (kidney or liver disease, low serum K or Na levels, chronic respiratory disease, pregnancy); establish baseline BP and weight; document extent of edema. **Administer:** In early a.m. **Evaluate:** Effectiveness of medicat'n (daily weight, fluid intake/output, BP); for evidence of adv. effects (hypokalemia, hyperglycemia, hyperuricemia, hyponatremia). **Teach:** Expected outcome of medicat'n (diuresis); not to consume licorice or alcohol while on thiazide diuretics.
Chlorthalidone (Hygroton)	Tx of edema and hypertens'n (**Oral:** Adults - 25-50 mg/day. Us. dose should be restricted to 25 mg; higher doses us. fail to produce addit'nal antihypertensive effects yet incr. adv. effects of chlorthalidone)	Thiazide-like diuretic; actions sim. to hydrochlorothiazide.	As for hydrochlorothiazide	**Colestipol:** May inhibit absorpt'n of a thiazide. **Corticosteroids:** Plus thiazides or thiazide-like drugs, may result in excess. loss of K. Also, a corticosteroid incr. hyperglycemic effect of the diuretic. **Digoxin:** May have incr. toxicity in presence of a thiazide or thiazide-like drug because of diuretic-induced deficiencies of K and Mg.	As for hydrochlorothiazide
Metolazone (Zaroxolyn)	Tx of edema and hypertens'n (**Oral:** Adults - 2.5-5 mg daily)	Thiazide-like diuretic; actions sim. to hydrochlorothiazide.	As for hydrochlorothiazide	**Ethanol:** May potentiate diuretic-induced orthostatic hypotens'n. **Lithium carbonate:** May undergo incr. renal reabsorpt'n in presence of a diuretic. **Narcotics:** May potentiate diuretic-induced orthostatic hypotens'n.	

Pharmacologic Classification: Loop Diuretic

Furosemide (Lasix)

Tx of edema and hypertens'n (Oral: Adults - 20-40 mg bid. Incr. gradually, if nec., to 200 mg/day in 2 doses)

Incr. renal excret'n of Na and Cl plus accompanying volume of H_2O, resulting in decr. blood volume.

Hypovolemia, electrolyte imbalance (see thiazide diuretics), gout, deafness, fluid deplet'n and dermatitis

ACE inhibitors: See thiazides, above. **Clofibrate:** And furosemide may compete for plasma albumin binding sites, resulting in incr. activities of both drugs. **Corticosteroids:** And furosemide may lead to excess. loss of K. Also, a corticosteroid incr. hyperglycemic effect of the diuretic. **Digoxin:** Can demonstrate incr. toxicities in presence of furosemide due to diuretic-induced loss of K and Mg. **Lithium carbonate:** May undergo incr. renal reabsorpt'n in presence of a diuretic.

Uricosurics: May have reduced effect in presence of a thiazide or thiazide-like drug because of diuretic-induced decr. in renal uric acid clearance.

As for hydrochlorothiazide

Pharmacologic Classification: Potassium-Sparing Diuretics

Spironolactone (Aldactone)

Tx of edema, hypertens'n and primary hyperaldosteronism (Oral: Adults - Initially, 50-100 mg daily in divided doses. Maint. dose, up to 200 mg/day)

Aldosterone antagonist; blocks Na-retent'n effects of aldosterone.

Amenorrhea, gynecomastia, hyperkalemia, hyponatremia, GI irritat'n, hypersensitivity

Lithium chloride: Spironolactone may incr. plasma Li and Li toxicity. **Potassium chloride:** Hyperkalemia may result if K supplements are also given. Pts treated w. K must be monitored very closely.

Assess: Pt hx for hypersensitivity to spironolactone, kidney disease, hyperkalemia, anuria; review other medicat'ns being taken for K supplements; establish baseline weight and BP. **Administer:** From light-resistant container; w. food to reduce gastric irritat'n and improve bioavailability of drug. **Evaluate:** Efficacy of tx (fluid intake/output, BP, daily weight); for adv. effects, esp. hypersensitivity, hyperkalemia. **Teach:** Expected outcome of medicat'n (diuresis); avoid overeating high-K foods; s/s of hyperkalemia should be reported to physician.

Generic Name (Trade Name)	Use (Dose)	Action	Adverse Effects	Drug Interactions	Nursing Process
Spironolactone 25 mg + hydrochlorothiazide 25 mg; spironolactone 50 mg + hydrochlorothiazide 50 mg (Aldactazide)	Tx of edema, hypertens'n, primary hyperaldosteronism (**Oral:** Initially, 1 lower-strength tablet daily. May incr. to 50 mg of ea. ingred. daily in a single dose or in divided doses. Adjust dose in accordance w. BP and serum K levels)	Aldosterone antagonist; blocks Na-retent'n effects of aldosterone and counteracts hypokalemic effects of hydrochlorothiazide.	As for spironolactone and hydrochlorothiazide	As for spironolactone and hydrochlorothiazide.	As for spironolactone and hydrochlorothiazide.
Triamterene 50 mg + hydrochlorothiazide 25 mg (Dyazide)	Tx of edema or hypertens'n (**Oral:** Initially, 1 tablet daily. Incr. or decr. dose prn)	Acts directly on tubular transport in distal convoluted tubules and collecting ducts to inhibit Na reabsorp'n and K secret'n.	Hyperkalemia, nausea, vomiting, leg cramps, dizziness	**Lithium:** Plasma levels and toxicities may incr. if amiloride or triamterene are used concomitantly w. Li. **Potassium chloride:** And either amiloride or triamterene administrat'n can lead to hyperkalemia.	**Administer:** Nurses are cautioned to be aware of the combinat'n of the 2 drugs in Dyazide and Moduret, and to assess and monitor for the actions and adv. effects of both drugs.
Amiloride 5 mg + hydrochlorothiazide 50 mg (Moduret)	Tx of edema or hypertens'n (**Oral:** Initially, 1 tablet daily. Adjust dose in accordance w. BP and serum K levels)	As for triamterene	Hyperkalemia, headache, dizziness, confusion, insomnia, depress'n, somnolence and decr. libido	See triamterene + hydrochlorothiazide.	See triamterene + hydrochlorothiazide.

Pharmacologic Classification: Vasodilator — Angiotensin-Converting Enzyme (ACE) Inhibitors

Generic Name (Trade Name)	Use (Dose)	Action	Adverse Effects	Drug Interactions	Nursing Process
Captopril (Capoten)	Tx of essential hypertens'n and CHF (**Oral:** Adults, *for mild to moderate hypertens'n* - initially, 12.5 mg bid or tid. *For severe hypertens'n,* initially 25 mg bid or tid. This can be incr. gradually over 1-2 weeks to 50 mg bid or tid. In volume-depleted or hyponatremic pts, initial dose should be 6.25-12.5 mg tid. Reduce dose in elderly pts or pts w. renal impairment)	Blocks convers'n of angiotensin I to angiotensin II, decr. peripheral resistance and aldosterone secret'n.	Low incidence of nephrotoxicity, neutropenia/agranulocytosis reported; skin rashes, angioedema, gastric irritat'n, nausea, vomiting, dysgeusia	**Diuretics:** Tog. w. an ACE inhibitor, can produce a powerful hypotensive effect, poss. leading to postural hypoten's'n. Avoid by stopping the diuretic a few days before starting w. low doses of the ACE inhibitor. Thereafter, it may be poss. to reintroduce the diuretic and incr. the dose of ACE inhibitor slowly. **Nonsteroidal anti-inflammatory drugs (NSAIDs):** Can reduce ability of ACE inhibitors to dilate blood vessels. **Potassium supplements and**	**Assess:** For hx of renal or hematologic abnormalities. **Administer:** 1 h ac. **Evaluate:** For efficacy of tx (decr. BP, edema, reduct'n of moist rales in CHF pts). For poss. allergic react'ns — rash, fever, pruritus and urticaria. Protein in urine, WC counts. **Teach:** Not to discontinue drug abruptly; not to use OTC drugs unless directed by physician. Stress importance of compliance to dose schedule. To rise slowly from sitting to standing. To avoid sunlight. S/s of impending neutropenia or agranulocytosis.

Drug	Use/Dosage	Action	Side Effects	Interactions	Nursing Process
Enalapril (Vasotec)	Tx of essential hypertens'n and CHF **(Oral: Adults** - initially, 2.5 mg for pts on a diuretic, or 5 mg for pts not on a diuretic. Maint. dose, 10-40 mg daily. In elderly pts the starting dose should be 2.5 mg)	As for captopril	Headache, dizziness, nausea, diarrhea, hyperkalemia. Severe symptomatic hypoten's'n can occur after first dose; this effect is more prevalent in salt-depleted pts. Rash and taste disturbance may be less common w. enalapril than captopril.	**potassium-sparing diuretics** (amiloride, spironolactone, triamterene): Should not be used w. ACE inhibitors. Because ACE inhibitors decr. aldosterone secret'n, they cause K to be retained. As a result, hyperkalemia can occur in pts receiving K supplements or K-sparing diuretics.	As for captopril
Lisinopril (Prinivil, Zestril)	Tx of essential hypertens'n **(Oral: Adults**, *normal renal function* - initially, 10 mg 1x/day; incr. gradually to 20-40 mg. *Impaired renal function* (serum creatinine ≥ 3 mg/mL or creatinine clearance < 3 mL/min) - init. dose should be 5 mg/day)	As for captopril	Symptomatic hypotens'n, particularly in pts who are volume- or salt-depleted as a result of diuretic tx, salt restrict'n, diarrhea or vomiting	As for captopril and enalapril	As for captopril and enalapril

Pharmacologic Classification: Vasodilator — Calcium Channel Blockers

Drug	Use/Dosage	Action	Side Effects	Interactions	Nursing Process
Diltiazem (Cardizem SR)	Tx of essential hypertens'n **(Oral: Adults** - 120-360 mg/day, administered in 2 equal doses. Av. dose in elderly pts may be somewhat lower)	Blocks entry of Ca into blood vessels, producing peripheral vasodilatat'n in arterioles and decr. peripheral resistance and BP.	Bradycardia, dizziness, weakness, headache, flushing, dryness of the mouth and pedal edema. In addit'n, GI disturbances and dermatological react'ns have occurred w. the drug.	**Beta blockers:** And diltiazem, can lead to severe sinus bradycardia, hypotens'n and heart failure. **Nitroglycerin** (time-release): And diltiazem, can produce exaggerated hypotens'n.	**Assess:** Baseline ECG, lab. tests for renal and hepatic funct'n; BP and pulse; current drug profile for use of digitalis, procainamide or quinidine; check hx for severe hypotens'n, cardiogenic shock, cardiomegaly, digitalis toxicity, AV block, severe CHF or pregnancy. **Administer:** Parenterally in coronary ICU only; orally, bid. **Evaluate:** BP and pulse. **Teach:** Indicators of efficacy and adv. effects; to avoid driving and using power equipment until effects are recognized; not to take OTC drugs without physician's advice; strict adherence to exercise regimen.

Generic Name (Trade Name)	Use (Dose)	Action	Adverse Effects	Drug Interactions	Nursing Process
Nifedipine (Adalat PA 20, Procardia PA)	Tx of essential hypertens'n (**Oral:** Adults - 1 [20 mg] tablet, swallowed whole, bid. Dose may be incr. prn to 2 [20 mg] tablets bid. Max. daily dose 80 mg; should not be exceeded)	As for diltiazem. Produces more profound peripheral vasodilatat'n than diltiazem. Also produces greater reflex tachycardia than diltiazem.	Dizziness, lightheadedness, peripheral edema, nausea, weakness, headache, flushing, transient hypotens'n, palpitat'ns, syncope	**Antihypertensives:** Nifedipine or nicardipine may potentiate effects of hypotensive agents. **Beta blockers:** Antihypertensive effect of beta blockers may be augmented by nifedipine's or nicardipine's reduct'n of peripheral vascular resistance. **Cimetidine:** May reduce clearance of nifedipine.	*As for diltiazem, plus:* **Administer:** From light-resistant containers stored at room temp.; protect from moisture.
Nicardipine (Cardene)	As for diltiazem (**Oral:** Adults - 20 mg tid initially; incr. after 3 days prn to 30 mg tid and then 40 mg tid. Pts w. impaired hepatic funct'n should start w. 20 mg bid)	As for diltiazem. Sim. to nifedipine. Produces more profound peripheral vasodilatat'n than diltiazem. Also sim. to nifedipine, nicardipine produces greater reflex tachycardia than diltiazem.	Headache, dizziness, lightheadedness, giddiness, flushing, heat sensat'n, peripheral edema and hypotens'n	As for nifedipine	*As for diltiazem, plus:* **Teach:** Pt to limit caffeine consumpt'n and avoid OTC drugs unless directed by physician. Notify physician of irreg. heart beat, SOB, swelling of hands/feet, dizziness, hypotens'n, nausea, constipat'n.
Verapamil sustained-release tablets (Isoptin SR)	As for diltiazem (**Oral:** Us. dose, 240 mg od, in a.m. w. food. Upward titrat'n should be based on tx efficacy and safety. If adequate response is not obtained, dose may be titrated upward in the following manner: 240 mg ea. a.m. w. food; 240 mg ea. a.m. plus 120 mg ea. p.m. w. food; 240 mg q12h w. food)	As for diltiazem; dilates arterioles and lowers BP. In addit'n, verapamil depresses myocardium and prolongs A-V conduct'n time.	Transient asystole, hypotens'n, development or worsening of heart failure, rhythm disturbances, stenocardia (angina), flushing, peripheral edema and pulmonary edema, dizziness, headache, fatigue, excitat'n, vertigo, syncope, tremor, constipat'n	**Antihypertensive drugs:** In pts using antihypertensive drugs the addit'nal hypotensive effect of verapamil should be considered. **Beta blockers:** Generally, verapamil should not be given to pts receiving beta blockers. If concomitant use is essential, such use should be started gradually in hospital under careful supervis'n. **Digoxin:** Plasma levels are incr. by chronic oral verapamil use. **Rifampin:** Reduces oral verapamil bioavailability.	As for diltiazem

Pharmacologic Classification: Vasodilator

Hydralazine (Apresoline)	Tx of essential hypertens'n (**Oral:** Adults - initially, 10-25 mg bid or tid. Incr. dosage by 10-25 mg prn. Children - initially, 0.75 mg/kg/day in 4 divided doses. **IV/IM:** See manufacturer's monograph)	Vasodilatat'n caused by direct relaxat'n of vascular smooth muscle, preferentially more effective on arterioles.	Tachycardia, angina, palpitat'ns, headache, anorexia, vomiting, nausea, dizziness, sweating, drug-induced lupus erythematosus, edema, hypersensitivity, blood dyscrasias, psychological react'ns	**Diazoxide:** And hydralazine may exhibit additive hypotensive effects. Concomitant use of diazoxide and hydralazine should be undertaken w. caution and adequate monitoring for excessive hypotens'n. **MAOIs:** Should be used w. caution in pts receiving hydralazine.	**Assess:** Pt hx for contraindicat'ns (hypersensitivity, coronary disease, lupus erythematosus, renal or hepatic disease, pregnancy); establish baseline weight and BP. **Administer:** Orally whenever possible. **Evaluate:** Response to tx (daily BP, weight, fluid intake/output); for evidence of side effects (hypersensitivity, lupus erythematosus). **Teach:** Safety precaut'ns for dizziness (see prazosin); need to keep enough drug on hand; need for gradual w'drawal of drug; s/s that should precipitate medical contact.

Pharmacologic Classification: Vasodilator — Alpha₁ Receptor Blockers

Prazosin (Minipress)	Tx of essential hypertens'n (**Oral:** Adults - initially, 1 mg given hs [w. instruct'ns that pt remain in bed for several hours], followed by 1 mg bid; incr. to tid prn. The dose may be incr. gradually to 20 mg/day prn. Children - 0.1 mg/kg/day)	Blocks alpha₁ receptors; stims. alpha₂ receptors, resulting in decr. peripheral resistance and less rebound tachycardia than w. hydralazine.	Reflex tachycardia, postural hypotens'n, nasal congest'n, GI hypermotility, inhibit'n of erect'n/ejaculat'n, fluid retent'n, weakness, dizziness, headache, palpitat'ns, lethargy	**Antihypertensive drugs:** Reduce dose of other antihypertensive agents and initiate prazosin at 0.5 mg bid or tid. When adding another antihypertensive agent to pre-existing prazosin tx, reduce prazosin dose to 1-2 mg bid or tid and retitrate. **Diuretics:** Incr. hypotensive effects of prazosin. Reduce dose of the diuretic to maint. level for that agent and initiate prazosin at 0.5 mg bid or tid. Gradually incr. prazosin dosage prn.	**Assess:** For pt hx of chronic renal failure; pregnancy; lactat'n; establish BP, weight. **Administer:** W. food and/or milk. **Evaluate:** Following initial dose, an incr. in dose or addit'n of other antihypertensives: watch for syncope w. sudden unconsciousness. 4-6 weeks may be required for full tx effects. Drug efficacy; adv. effects. **Teach:** To move from recumbent to standing posit'n slowly w. a stop in sitting posit'n before rising to feet; to lie down quickly if dizzy, faint or weak; not to drive a vehicle, operate power tools or work w. heavy machinery until dose is established and indiv. response indentified; to seek medical advice before taking OTC drugs for coughs, colds or allergies.
Terazosin (Hytrin)	Tx of essential hypertens'n (**Oral:** 1 mg hs initially. Slowly incr. dose to achieve desired effect. Us. dose range, 1-5 mg 1x/day. Some pts may benefit from doses up to 20 mg/day)	As for prazosin	Syncope, dizziness, headache, asthenia, somnolence, nasal congest'n, palpitat'n		

Generic Name (Trade Name)	Use (Dose)	Action	Adverse Effects	Drug Interactions	Nursing Process

Pharmacologic Classification: Vasodilator — Alpha and Beta Blockers

Generic Name (Trade Name)	Use (Dose)	Action	Adverse Effects	Drug Interactions	Nursing Process
Labetalol HCl (Normodyne Trandate)	Tx of hypertens'n (**Oral: Adults** - initially, 100 mg bid. Adjust dose thereafter semiweekly or weekly according to response. Us. maint. dose, 200-400 mg bid. **IV:** Initially, 20 mg given by slow inject'n over 2 min. Addit'nal inject'ns of 40-80 mg can be given at 10-min intervals until desired effect is attained or a total dose of 300 mg has been administered)	Blocks both alpha and beta receptors. Antihypertensive effects due primarily to alpha$_1$ receptor antagonism (decr. in peripheral resistance). Reflex tachycardia prevented by partial beta blockade.	Severe postural hypotens'n, jaundice, bronchospasm, fatigue/malaise, headache, nausea/vomiting, angina pectoris, dyspnea, drug rash, impotence, muscular aches and pains, blurred vision	**Antidiabetic agents:** May have more prolonged hypoglycemic effect when labetalol is used concomitantly. **Antihypertensive agents and diuretics:** Incr. hypotensive effects of labetalol. **Cimetidine:** Incr. bioavailability of labetalol. Use special care in establishing dose in these pts. **Halothane:** Incr. hypotensive effects of labetalol. High doses of halothane (3%) w. labetalol predispose pts to myocardial depressant effects of halothane and an undesirable reduct'n in myocardial performance. **Nitroglycerin:** Adds to hypotensive effects of labetalol.	**Assess:** Pt hx for asthma, COPD, CV or liver disease, diabetes mellitus; establish baseline BP and pulse lying and standing. **Administer, Evaluate, Teach:** As for hydralazine.

Pharmacologic Classification: Drugs That Depress Venous Return — Adrenergic Neuron Blockers

Generic Name (Trade Name)	Use (Dose)	Action	Adverse Effects	Drug Interactions	Nursing Process
Reserpine (Serpasil)	Tx of essential hypertens'n (**Oral: Adults, not receiving other antihypertensive agents,** initially, 0.5 mg daily for 1-2 weeks. Maint. dose, 0.1-0.25 mg od. Administer w. food, meals or milk)	Adrenergic neuron blocker; inhibits format'n, storage and release of norepinephrine from postganglionic sympathetic nerve endings; dilates arterioles and veins; decr. venous return, peripheral resistance, heart rate and BP. Crosses blood-brain barrier and causes depress'n.	Nasal congest'n, postural hypotens'n, incr. blood and extracellular fluid volume, diarrhea, male impotence, decr. libido, sedat'n, depress'n, suicide, extrapyramidal adv. effects	**Methotrimeprazine:** May have an additive hypotensive effect w. reserpine and produce orthostatic hypotens'n. **Monoamine oxidase inhibitors (MAOIs):** Plus reserpine, cause excitat'n and hypertens'n. Avoid MAOI use w. reserpine.	**Assess:** Family hx for breast cancer; pt hx of depress'n, peptic ulcer, ulcerative colitis, epilepsy, COPD, renal disease, cardiac arrhythmias; pregnancy or lactat'n; establish baseline levels of BP and pulse, sleep patterns, dietary habits, weight. **Administer:** From airtight, light-resistant container, w. meals or milk to minimize gastric irritat'n. If nausea accompanies administrat'n, give pc and NPO for 2-3 h. **Evaluate:** Supine and standing BP and pulse 2 h after oral dose; mental status, fluid intake/output, edema, daily weight. **Teach:** Family and pt to observe for s/s of adv. effects; that tx effect may take 3 weeks after starting drug and last for up to 4 weeks after stopping; precaut'ns related to postural hypotens'n.

Drug	Action	Side effects	Interactions	Nursing considerations
Guanethidine (Ismelin)	Tx of moderate to severe hypertens'n, except in presence of pheochromocytoma (**Oral:** Adults - initially, 10 mg/day. Maint. dose, us. 25-50 mg/day. Children - initially, 0.2 mg/kg/day; incr. by same am't q7-10 days prn)	Adrenergic neuron blocker resulting in reduced venous return, heart rate and cardiac output.	Reduced kidney perfus'n, salt and fluid retent'n; as for reserpine, except for CNS effects	**Amphetamines, tricyclic antidepressants, ephedrine, methylphenidate and phenothiazines:** Antagonize adrenergic blockade produced by guanethidine. **Antidiabetic agents:** Have incr. hypoglycemic effects in presence of guanethidine. **Ethanol:** Enhances orthostatic hypotensive effects of guanethidine. **Levarterenol** (norepinephrine): Has its pressor effects incr. by guanethidine. **Monoamine oxidase inhibitors (MAOIs):** Should not be used w. guanethidine because MAOIs may antagonize antihypertensive effects of guanethidine. **Phenylephrine:** May be a more potent pressor substance in presence of guanethidine.	As for reserpine, except for nsg activities rel. to CNS effects.

Pharmacologic Classification: Drugs That Decrease Cardiac Output — Beta Blockers

Drug	Action	Side effects	Interactions	Nursing considerations
Propranolol (Inderal)	Tx of hypertens'n (**Oral:** Initially, 40 mg bid, incr. prn to 80-160 mg bid)	Blocks both beta$_1$ and beta$_2$ receptors. Effects depend on level of sympathetic nervous activity. Decr. heart rate, ventr. systolic pressure, myocardial contractility and cardiac output; reduces coronary blood flow and O$_2$ consumpt'n; lowers BP; reduces sinus rate, slows AV conduct'n, decr. spontaneous rate of ectopic pacemakers.	Bronchoconstrict'n in asthmatics; potentiates effects of insulin; asystole, A-V block, bradycardia, heart failure, nausea, vomiting, constipat'n, diarrhea, depress'n, sleep disturbances, allergic react'ns	*Reference is made to propranolol, but drug interact'ns apply to all beta blockers unless otherwise indicated.* **Antiarrhythmic drugs** (disopyramide, lidocaine, tocainide, other Class 1 antiarrhythmics): Plus beta blocker, can result in exaggerated unwanted effects of antiarrhythmic agents – enhanced myocardial depress'n, hypotens'n, bradycardia, AV blockade, asystole. **Antiasthmatics** (beta$_2$ stimulants, e.g., albuterol/salbutamol, fenoterol, terbutaline): Are antagonized by nonselective beta blockers, incl. those w. partial-agonist activity. Cardioselective beta blockers are less likely to	**Assess:** Pt hx of CHF, bradycardia, heart block, asthma, hay fever, obstructive lung disease, liver or kidney disease, diabetes, myasthenia gravis; use of MAOIs within preceding 2 weeks; record apical/radial pulses (incl. rate, rhythm), BP, respirat'ns (incl. rate, rhythm), circulat'n to extremities (incl. color, warmth, blanching effect and peripheral pulses) as baseline for evalu-at'n of indiv. pt response. **Administer:** From airtight, light-resistant containers; ac and hs in order to facili-tate absorpt'n of medicat'n from stomach into circulatory system. **Evaluate:** Apical/radial pulses, fluid intake/output, daily weight, BP, respirat'ns, circulat'n to extremities for indicat'ns of adv. effects and to assist physician in establishing best indiv.
Nadolol (Corgard)	Tx of hypertens'n (**Oral:** Adults - initially, 80 mg 1x/daily; incr. at weekly intervals prn. Max. daily dose, 320 mg)			As for propranolol and nadolol	
Timolol (Blocadren)	Tx of hypertens'n (**Oral:** Adults - in pts already receiving another antihypertensive, initially 5-10 mg bid; incr. prn q2weeks by 5 mg bid. Max. daily dose, 60 mg. If used alone, initially 10 mg bid, incr. prn)				

Generic Name (Trade Name)	Use (Dose)	Action	Adverse Effects	Drug Interactions	Nursing Process
Atenolol (Tenormin)	Tx of hypertens'n (**Oral: Adults -** 50 mg 1x/daily; incr. within 1-2 weeks to 100 mg 1x/day prn)	Cardioselective beta blocker preferentially blocks beta$_1$ receptors in heart to decr. heart rate, ventr. systolic pressure, myocardial contractility and cardiac output; decr. BP; reduces coronary O$_2$ consumpt'n.	As for propranolol, nadolol and timolol, except has less effect on bronchioles, peripheral blood flow and insulin.	affect actions of beta$_2$ stimulants. **Antidiabetic agents:** Have their react'ns incr. by nonselective beta blockers, which reduce glycogen breakdown and delay rise in blood glucose level after insulin - or oral hypoglycemic-induced hypoglycemia. Furthermore, nonselective beta blockers modify normal physiologic react'ns to hypoglycemia. In presence of nonselective beta blocker, hypoglycemic react'n is accompanied by bradycardia rather than tachycardia and by a rise in diastolic BP as well as us. systolic pressor response.	dose; monitor diabetic pts for hypoglycemic and insulin shock; monitor ECG of pts receiving IV propranolol. **Teach:** Family and pt to observe responses to physical and psychological stress and to develop an indiv. appropriate level, pace and am't of activity; importance of avoiding abrupt w'drawal of drug because of danger of myocardial infarct or arrhythmias; to avoid alcohol, smoking and OTC medicat'ns for colds, coughs or allergies because of their potential effects on BP; caution to avoid driving vehicles, using power tools or working w. industrial machinery during regulat'n of dosage; instruct to move from recumbent to standing posit'n before rising to feet; teach family to seek medical attent'n if s/s of adv. effects occur.
Metoprolol (Betaloc, Lospresor, Lopressor)	Tx of hypertens'n (**Oral:** Initially, 50 mg bid; incr. to 100 mg bid prn. Us. maint. dose, 100-200 mg/daily)	As for atenolol	As for atenolol	Atropine (and other anticholinergics): May prevent bradycardia produced by beta blockers. **Clonidine:** Plus nonselective beta blocker, can potentiate hypertensive response during clonidine w'drawal.	
Oxprenolol (Trasicor)	Tx of hypertens'n (**Oral: Adults -** initially, 20 mg tid, followed w. incr. of 60 mg/day prn q2-3weeks until BP is controlled. Us. range, 120-320 mg/day. Max. dose, 480 mg/day)	Weak beta agonist that competes w. epinephrine and norepinephrine at receptor sites, resulting in reduction in beta-mediated effects.	As for propranolol, nadolol and timolol	**Digoxin:** May demonstrate reduced inotropic effects in presence of beta blocker. Beta blockers and digoxin are additive in depressing A-V conduct'n. Use beta blockers w. caution in pts taking digoxin who develop bradycardia.	As for propranolol
Pindolol (Visken)	Tx of hypertens'n (**Oral: Adults -** initially, 5 mg bid w. breakfast and evening meal, incr. after 1-2 weeks by a 10-mg increment in 2 equal doses. If nec., after an addit'nal 1-2 weeks, incr. to 15 mg bid. If total daily dose of 10-20 mg is adequate, pindolol may be given 1x/daily w. breakfast)	As for oxprenolol	As for propranolol, nadolol and timolol	**Epinephrine:** Can incr. BP in pts taking nonselective beta blockers. **Nifedipine, nicardipine:** Plus beta blocker, can occ. provoke severe hypotens'n and overt heart failure in susceptible pt w. poor myocardial reserve.	As for propranolol
Acebutolol (Monitan, Sectral)	Tx of hypertens'n (**Oral: Adults -** 100 mg bid. If nec., incr. after 1 week to 200 mg bid. In some cases, daily dose may need further increments of 100 mg	Cardioselective partial agonist. Competes w. epinephrine and norepinephrine at beta$_1$ receptor sites.	As for atenolol	**Prazosin:** And beta blocker, can result in incr. postural hypotens'n	

bid at intervals of not less than 2 weeks, to a max. of 400 mg bid. Maint. dose, 400-800 mg/daily. Pts w. satisfactory response to 400 mg or less per day can be given total dose 1x/daily in a.m.)

			after 1st dose of prazosin. **Sympathomimetics:** Plus nonselective beta blocker, can result in hypertens'n when large doses of sympathomimetic are used. **Verapamil:** Plus beta blocker, can result in enhanced myocardial depress'n, hypotens'n, bradycardia, A-V blockade and asystole.	As for reserpine

Pharmacologic Classification: Central Sympathetic Inhibitors

Drug	Indications / Dosage	Action	Adverse Effects	Interactions
Clonidine (Catapres)	Tx of hypertens'n, migraine headache, dysmenorrhea (**Oral:** Adults [hypertens'n] - initially, 50-100 µg qid. Incr. every few days according to response and tolerance. Give last dose hs to ensure BP control during sleep. Final dose range, 0.2-1.2 mg/day in divided doses. **Transdermal:** 1 Catapres-TTS patch applied weekly)	Alpha$_2$ stimulat'n, decr. central sympathetic secret'n, produces decr. BP.	Sedat'n, dry mouth, fluid retent'n, weight gain, dizziness, headache; dryness, itching or burning of eyes; corneal ulcerat'n (rare), nocturnal unrest, nausea, euphoria, constipat'n, impotence (rare), agitat'n upon w'drawal of tx	**Antidepressants, tricyclic:** May antagonize antihypertensive effects of clonidine. **Beta blockers, nonselective:** May exaggerate vasoconstrictor response when clonidine is w'drawn. W'draw beta blocker before stopping clonidine. **Levodopa:** May have its antiparkinsonian activity inhibited by clonidine.
Methyldopa (Aldomet)	Tx of hypertens'n (**Oral:** Adults - initially, 250 mg bid or tid for the first 48 h, then adjusted at intervals of not < 2 days until adequate response is achieved. Us. daily maint. dose, 500 mg in 2–4 doses. Incr. or decr. prn. Children - Initially, 10 mg/kg/day in 2–4 doses. Incr. or decr. prn. Max. daily dose 65 mg/kg or 3 g, whichever is less)	Converted to methyl-noradrenaline within brain. Methyl-noradrenaline stims. alpha$_2$ receptors to decr. central sympathetic secret'n, producing fall in BP.	Sedat'n, postural hypotens'n, edema, impotence, drug fever, hepatic dysfunct'n, hemolytic anemia, lactat'n; others as for reserpine	**Beta blockers:** May produce hypertensive react'ns w. methyldopa if pt experiences catecholamine release induced by physiologic stress, cholinesterase inhibit'n or administrat'n of indirect sympathomimetics.	As for reserpine

CHAPTER 15

Drugs for the Treatment of Hypotension and Shock

Teaching Objectives

Following completion of this chapter, the reader should be able to:

1. Briefly describe shock, listing the types of shock and the forms of therapy used in correcting each condition.
2. Discuss tissue perfusion during hypotension and shock, differentiating between the factors controlling blood flow to the heart, brain and kidneys.
3. Discuss the mechanisms of action, pharmacologic effects, therapeutic uses, adverse reactions and nursing processes for epinephrine, levarterenol, dobutamine, dopamine, sodium nitroprusside and nitroglycerin, when these drugs are used to treat shock.

Shock

Shock is a condition of acute peripheral circulatory failure. Broadly divided into anaphylactic shock, hypovolemic shock, cardiogenic shock, bacteremic shock, and neurogenic hypotension and shock, it can result from the loss of circulatory control or circulating fluid. Therapy is aimed at correcting the hypoperfusion of vital organs. Hypovolemic shock is treated by volume replacement; bacteremic shock by intensive antibiotic therapy, corticosteroids and volume replacement. In addition, sympathomimetic drugs or vasodilators (which either increase cardiac output or alter peripheral resistance, or both) may be appropriate. This chapter discusses the use of sympathomimetics or vasodilators in shock.

With regard to tissue perfusion during hypotension and shock, the heart, brain and kidneys deserve special comment. The major factor regulating blood flow through the coronary and cerebral vessels is the mean diastolic pressure. In the presence of hypotension, myocardial and cerebral perfusion are compromised. In this situation, sympathomimetics that increase blood pressure will improve the perfusion of both organs. Sympathomimetics can be used without concern that they might constrict the blood vessels in the heart and brain. The caliber of these vessels is determined by the metabolic needs of the tissue, not by stimulation of adrenergic receptors. The heart differs from the brain in one important aspect. Although the heart normally uses an aerobic metabolic pathway, it can operate for a short time anaerobically. The brain needs oxygen for its metabolism and is particularly susceptible to the consequence of acute hypotension and shock.

In contrast to the heart and brain, the kidney extracts only a relatively small amount of the oxygen provided to it under resting conditions, which means it can withstand, within limits, a reduction in blood flow by extracting a higher percentage of the oxygen supplied. However, sympathetic stimulation causes renal vasoconstriction. Adrenergic vasoconstrictors also reduce blood flow, possibly leading to renal ischemia.

Sympathomimetics are used to improve blood flow to vital organs. These drugs stimulate (1) alpha$_1$ receptors, increasing venous return and peripheral resistance, (2) beta$_1$ receptors, producing an increase in heart rate and cardiac output (if venous return is adequate), or (3) dopamine receptors, causing vasodilatation in the renal and splanchnic beds. The pharmacologic actions of these drugs are described in detail in Chapter 7. Readers are encouraged to refer to this chapter if additional information is required on any of the drugs presented below.

Sympathomimetics are used to improve tissue perfusion and not to maintain blood pressure at an arbitrary level. That fact notwithstanding, the infusion rate must be titrated to ensure that the desired level of blood pressure is not exceeded. Usually, systolic pressures between 90 – 100 mm Hg should be maintained. Somewhat higher levels may be established for hypertensive patients.

Vasodilators are also employed in selected patients with shock. These involve individuals with severe pump failure following acute myocardial infarction and patients with refractory chronic congestive heart failure. A vasodilator is used to increase cardiac output by reducing peripheral vascular resistance (afterload reduction), to relieve pulmonary congestion by increasing venous capacitance (preload reduction), and to limit the extent of ischemic damage by reducing myocardial oxygen demand and increasing myocardial oxygen supply. Drugs that dilate both veins and arteries are more useful than those with little effect on veins.

Sympathomimetics

Epinephrine, Adrenaline (Adrenalin)

Mechanism of Action and Pharmacologic Effects

Epinephrine stimulates beta$_1$ receptors in the heart and increases both heart rate and cardiac output. In small doses it dilates precapillary resistance vessels (arterioles) in skeletal muscles (beta$_2$ receptors) and constricts capacitance vessels (veins), an alpha$_1$ receptor mediated effect. The result is a decrease in peripheral resistance and an increase in venous return. Larger doses stimulate alpha$_1$ receptors on precapillary resistance vessels, producing a generalized vasoconstriction and an increase in peripheral resistance. Epinephrine also dilates the bronchioles.

Therapeutic Uses

Histamine, released from mast cells during anaphylactic shock, constricts bronchioles and dilates blood vessels. Epinephrine is a physiologic antagonist of histamine and is the drug of choice for the treatment of anaphylactic shock. By stimulating beta$_2$ receptors epinephrine prevents, or reverses, a histamine-induced bronchoconstriction. The ability of therapeutic doses of epinephrine to stimulate alpha$_1$ receptors enables this drug to reverse the histamine-induced vasodilatation. In an action unrelated to the treatment of anaphylactic shock, epinephrine's inotropic actions have led to its use in resuscitating the depressed heart.

Epinephrine should be given with caution to elderly patients and to those with cardiovascular disease, hypertension, diabetes or hyperthyroidism. It must be used with extreme caution in patients with long-standing bronchial asthma and emphysema who have developed degenerative heart disease. Epinephrine is contraindicated in patients with organic brain damage, cardiac dilatation or coronary insufficiency.

Adverse Effects

Anxiety, headaches, fear, palpitations, weakness and precordial pain are among the adverse effects of epinephrine. These are more prevalent in hyperthyroid patients.

Nursing Process

Assessment

In the treatment of anaphylactic shock there are virtually no contraindications to the use of epinephrine. Nursing assessment should establish baseline measurements of blood pressure, rate and rhythm of pulse, and color and temperature of the patient's extremities.

Administration

Epinephrine should be administered from light-proof containers using a tuberculin syringe. Always aspirate from the injection site to ensure that the needle has not entered a blood vessel because epinephrine is very toxic if inadvertently given intravenously. If repeated administration is required, rotate injection sites to prevent tissue necrosis.

Evaluation

Blood pressure should be taken and recorded at frequent intervals. If the decision is taken to inject epinephrine intravenously, the nurse should measure the blood pressure constantly until it stabilizes and at five-minute intervals thereafter. Accurate recording of urinary output will detect urinary retention. Nurses should also be aware that careful evaluation and monitoring after the crisis will be required in pregnant patients and those with a history of glaucoma, cardiovascular, circulatory or cerebrovascular disease, prostatic hypertrophy, diabetes mellitus or hyperthyroidism. Because of potential drug interactions, careful monitoring will also be required for patients who are simultaneously receiving tricyclic antidepressants, antidiabetic drugs, antihistamines, beta blockers or l-thyroxine.

The patient's posture, frequency of changes in position and respiratory rate will often provide early indications of anxiety. Feelings of anxiety and tension that are disproportionate to the situation may reflect excessive doses of epinephrine.

Levarterenol, Norepinephrine, Noradrenaline (Levophed)

Mechanism of Action and Pharmacologic Effects

Levarterenol stimulates alpha$_1$ receptors, constricting both capacitance and precapillary resistance vessels. The resulting increase in blood pressure activates the carotid sinus and aortic arch pressor receptors to stimulate reflexly the vagus nerve. The result is a fall in heart rate and cardiac output. Although levarterenol stimulates beta$_1$ receptors in the heart and might be thought to increase heart rate, this effect is not sufficient to override reflex stimulation of the vagus.

Therapeutic Uses

Levarterenol is indicated for the maintenance of blood pressure in acute hypotensive states, surgical and nonsurgical trauma, central vasomotor depression and hemorrhage. Its use in patients who are hypotensive from blood volume deficit is contraindicated, except as an emergency measure to maintain coronary and cerebral artery perfusion until blood volume replacement can be completed.

Adverse Effects

Because of its ability to produce marked vasoconstriction, levarterenol can cause tissue necrosis at the site of injection. This danger is minimized by administering the drug through a catheter into a deeply seated vein and changing the infusion site when prolonged treatment is required. Phentolamine (Regitine, Rogitine) can be injected to overcome the effects of extravasation.

Nursing Process

The nursing process related to the use of levarterenol is essentially the same as that identified above in association with the use of epinephrine.

Dobutamine (Dobutrex)

Mechanism of Action and Pharmacologic Effects

Dobutamine stimulates beta$_1$ receptors, with relatively less effect on beta$_2$ receptors and alpha receptors. Dobutamine does not stimulate dopaminergic receptors. Moderate doses of dobutamine increase myocardial contractility and cardiac output. The drug may also reduce peripheral resistance and ventricular filling pressure when administered in moderate doses. Large doses of dobutamine increase heart rate and blood pressure.

Therapeutic Uses

Dobutamine is used primarily to treat severe refractory chronic congestive heart failure. It is also employed as inotropic support after cardiac surgery. The drug may be valuable in acute circulatory failure secondary to depressed myocardial contractility. Generally, however, either dopamine or norepinephrine is preferred when marked hypotension is present.

Adverse Effects

The most common adverse effects of dobutamine are tachycardia and systolic hypertension. These effects can usually be controlled by reducing the dose of the drug. Dobutamine can occasionally cause ventricular arrhythmias. Because dobutamine increases A-V conduction, it can increase ventricular rate in patients with atrial fibrillation. The other adverse effects of dobutamine include nausea, headache, palpitations, anginal pain and shortness of breath.

Nursing Process

Detailed discussion of the nursing process related to the use of dobutamine is provided in Chapter 7. Readers are advised to review that material.

Dopamine (Dopastat, Intropin)

Mechanism of Action and Pharmacologic Effects

The effect of dopamine is dose dependent. In doses less than 5 µg/kg/min it stimulates dopaminergic receptors in the renal and mesenteric beds to produce vasodilatation and increase renal and mesenteric blood flow. Doses of 5 – 10 µg/kg/min also increase renal and mesenteric blood flow, while at the same time stimulating beta$_1$ receptors to increase myocardial contractility, heart rate and cardiac output. At doses above 10 µg/kg/min dopamine produces a generalized alpha$_1$ receptor mediated vasoconstriction and a reduction in renal blood flow.

Therapeutic Uses

Dopamine is preferred for the treatment of shock when the patient does not require the pronounced vasoconstrictor effects of norepinephrine. It is more potent than dobutamine as a pressor agent and is therefore preferred in patients with marked hypotension and shock. Because it can dilate renal vessels, dopamine is preferred over other sympathomimetics in patients with impaired renal function.

Adverse Effects

Dopamine can produce tachyarrhythmias, anginal pain, central nervous system stimulation, nausea, vomiting and headache. It may also increase myocardial oxygen consumption in patients with cardiogenic shock. However, it is less likely than norepinephrine to cause necrosis following extravasation. Phentolamine (Regitine, Rogitine; 5 – 10 mg in 10 mL) can be used to infiltrate the site if extravasation occurs.

Nursing Process

Detailed discussion of the nursing process related to the use of dopamine is provided in Chapter 7. Readers are advised to review that material.

Vasodilators

Sodium Nitroprusside (Nipride, Nitropress)

Mechanism of Action and Pharmacologic Effects

Nitroprusside dilates venous and arterial beds. Because it has a greater effect on afterload than nitroglycerin, nitroprusside is more likely to increase cardiac output. However, because its primary action on the coronary circulation is on the resistance rather than the conductance vessels, intravenous nitroprusside can cause coronary steal.

Therapeutic Uses

Nitroprusside can be used to treat severe persistent pump failure in patients with markedly reduced cardiac output and increased peripheral vascular resistance. The drug is particularly valuable in patients with severe acute decompensated chronic congestive heart failure, refractory to digoxin and diuretics. It should not be used in the treatment of compensatory hypertension, e.g., A-V shunt or coarctation of the aorta.

Adverse Effects

Nitroprusside may produce hypotension and tachycardia. Prolonged infusion of nitroprusside can lead to the accumulation of thiocyanate. Blood thiocyanate levels should be determined daily if nitroprusside is infused for more than seventy-two hours.

Nursing Process

Assessment
Before beginning drug treatment with nitroprusside, the patient should be assessed for baseline vital signs, blood pressure, body mass/weight and fluid intake and output. Blood studies for electrolytes and kidney and liver function should be done. In addition, a baseline electrocardiogram should be taken.

Administration
Administration should be by infusion pump with the solution wrapped in aluminum foil to protect it from light. Observe for color change in the solution and discard if discolored green, blue or dark red. Monitor blood pressure continuously.

Evaluation
The nurse should observe for the therapeutic effects of decreased peripheral resistance and increased cardiac output, absence of bleeding and progress of rales, dyspnea and edema of feet and legs. Assess the state of patient hydration (skin turgor and dryness of mucous membrane).

Nitroglycerin (Nitro-Bid IV, Nitrostat IV, Tridil)

Nitroglycerin is a vasodilator of both the venous and arterial circulation, with its effect being greater on the venous side. Intravenous nitroglycerin relieves pulmonary congestion, decreases myocardial oxygen consumption, and reduces ST-segment elevation. Intravenous nitroglycerin can be used to decrease myocardial ischemia and improve hemodynamics in severe left ventricular dysfunction complicating acute myocardial infarction. Its primary use is in patients with recurrent ischemic pain or marked elevation of left ventricular filling pressure and pulmonary edema. The major adverse effects of nitroglycerin stem from its vasodilating properties. These include headache, flushing, dizziness, hypotension and tachycardia. Nitroglycerin is contraindicated in hypotension or uncorrected hypovolemia.

Nursing Process

The nursing process for nytroglycerin is essentially the same as that outlined for nitrates in Chapter 12.

Further Reading

Chatterjee, K. and Parmley, W. W. (1977). Vasodilator treatment for acute and chronic heart failure. *Br. Heart J. 39* : 706-720.
Cohn, J. N. and Franciosa, J. A. (1977). Vasodilator therapy of cardiac failure. *New Engl. J. Med. 297* : 27-31, 254-258.
Johnson, S. A. and Gunnar, R. M. (1977). Treatment of shock in myocardial infarction. *J. Amer. Med. Assoc. 237* :2106-2108.

Table 16

Drugs for the treatment of hypotension and shock.

Pharmacologic Classification: Sympathomimetics

Generic Name (Trade Name)	Use (Dose)	Action	Adverse Effects	Drug Interactions	Nursing Process
Dobutamine (Dobutrex)	Tx of cardiac decompensat'n due to depressed contractility from organic heart disease or surgical procedures (**IV:** 8-24 μg/kg/min)	Stims. beta₁ receptors in heart; incr. cardiac output w. minimal effects on heart rate. Does not produce renal vasodilat'n, incr. GFR or Na excret'n.	Tachycardia, angina, cardiac arrhythmias, headache, hypertens'n, nausea, vomiting	*For drug interact'ns involving tricyclic antidepressants, diuretics, halogenated anesthetics, monoamine oxidase inhibitors and sympathomimetics, see dopamine in Table 5.*	**Assess:** Pt hx of tachycardia, ventr. fibrillat'n, pregnancy, diabetes, hypothermia; establish baseline BP, pulses, color and temp. of extremities. Check for potential drug interact'ns. **Administer:** Freshly mixed dilut'n, through patent IV, avoiding extravasat'n which can cause necrosis; provide constant nsg observat'n. **Evaluate:** BP, pulse (apical/peripheral), color and temp. of extremities, urinary output, mental'n.
Dopamine (Dopastat, Intropin)	To incr. cardiac output and improve renal blood flow in shock due to myocardial infarct, sepsis or trauma as well as in acute renal failure, open heart surgery or chronic CHF (**IV:** 2-5 μg/kg/min; incr. gradually to 20-30 μg/kg/min for seriously ill pts. Monitor urine output and ECG if doses larger than 20-30 μg/kg/min are used)	Stims. beta₁ receptors in heart to incr. both heart rate and stroke volume. Low to intermed. doses have no effect on peripheral resistance. Stims. specific dopamine receptors on renal blood vessels to incr. GFR, renal blood flow and Na excret'n.	Tachycardia, angina, cardiac arrhythmias, headache, hypertens'n, nausea, vomiting; high doses cause vasoconstrict'n of renal blood vessels.	*For drug interact'ns involving tricyclic antidepressants, diuretics, halogenated anesthetics and monoamine oxidase inhibitors, see Table 5.*	
Epinephrine, adrenaline (Adrenalin)	To relieve respiratory distress due to bronchospasm; provide rapid relief of hypersensitivity react'ns to drugs and other allergens; incr. BP in CPR (**IM/SC:** Adults - 0.2-1 mL epinephrine HCl 1/1000 solut'n. Start w. small doses and incr. prn. **IV or intracardiac:** *Cardiac resuscitation,* 0.5 mL diluted to 10 mL w. NaCl inject'n can be administered IV or intracardially to restore myocardial contractility. Children - **IM/SC:** Initially, 0.01	Bronchodilat'n due to beta₂ stimulat'n; incr. respiratory rate and tidal volume, reduced alveolar CO_2 concentrat'ns; reduced mucosal congest'n due to vasoconstrict'n of bronchiolar blood vessels.	Anxiety, headache, fear and palpitat'ns	**Antidepressants, tricyclic (TCA):** May incr. pressor response to epinephrine. Pts receiving TCA should be given epinephrine IV only w. great caution and beginning w. small doses. **Antidiabetic drugs:** Epinephrine incr. blood glucose and should be used cautiously in diabetic pts. **Beta blockers:** Blockade of beta receptors incr. alpha₁ (vasoconstrictor) effects of epinephrine. Give epinephrine cautiously to pts on propranolol and other nonse-	**Assess:** For pt hx of glaucoma; CV, circulatory or cerebrovascular disease; prostatic hypertrophy; diabetes mellitus; hyperthyroidism; pregnancy. Establish baseline BP, rate and rhythm of pulse, color and temp. of extremities. Check for potential drug interact'ns. **Administration:** Parenterally, from light-resistant vial using a tuberculin syringe; aspirate carefully; use SC route preferentially; rotate sites. **Evaluate:** BP and pulse carefully, esp. when IV route used; urine output, mental'n, color.

Drug	Indications/Dosage	Effects/Side Effects	Interactions	Nursing Considerations
	mL/kg [max. 0.3 mL]. If nec., 0.01 mL/kg is repeated q5-15 min prm)		lective beta blockers. Interact'n is less w. cardioselective beta blockers. **MAOIs:** And epinephrine use is contraindicated.	As for epinephrine
Levarterenol, noradrenaline, norepinephrine (Levophed)	To maintain BP in acute hypotensive states, surgical and nonsurgical trauma, cerebral vasomotor depress'n and hemorrhage (**IV: Adults** - 0.03 - 0.15 µg/kg/min)	Vasoconstrict'n due to stimulat'n of $alpha_1$ receptors. Headache, restlessness, anxiety, weakness, pallor, dizziness, tremor, precordial pain, palpitat'ns, respiratory distress, convuls'ns, cerebral hemorrhage and bradycardia	**Amphetamine:** May incr. pressor response to levarterenol. **Antidepressants, tricyclic:** May incr. several-fold pressor response to levarterenol. Give levarterenol only w. great caution. **Guanethidine:** Incr. response to levarterenol. Administer levarterenol very cautiously. **Methyldopa:** Can incr. and prolong pressor effect of levarterenol. Pts receiving methyldopa should be given levarterenol cautiously, beg. w. small doses.	

Pharmacologic Classification: Vasodilators

Drug	Indications/Dosage	Effects	Side Effects	Nursing Considerations
Sodium nitroprusside (Nipride, Nitropress)	Tx of severe persistent pump failure in pts w. markedly reduced cardiac output and incr. peripheral resistance (**IV: Adults** - initially, a dilute solut'n is infused at a rate of 16 µg/min. Subsequent infus'n rate should be determined by hemodynamic monitoring. *Infuse only w. sterile D5W. Not for direct inject'n.*)	Dilates venous and arterial beds. Because it has a greater effect on afterload than nitroglycerin, nitroprusside is more likely to incr. cardiac output. However, because its primary action is on resistance rather than conductance vessels, IV nitroprusside can cause coronary steal.	Hypotens'n, tachycardia. Prolonged infus'n can lead to accumulat'n of thiocyanate. Blood thiocyanate levels should be determined daily if nitroprusside is infused for more than 72 h.	**Assess:** Baseline reading for electrolytes: K^+, Na^+, Cl^-, CO_2. Renal funct'n; BP; weight; fluid intake/output. **Administer:** Acc. to BP readings q15min. By infus'n pump only, w. aluminum foil wrap to bottle to protect from light. Observe for color changes in infus'n solut'n. Discard if highly discolored (green, blue, dark red). **Evaluate:** For tx response of decr. BP and absence of bleeding. Monitor for adv. effects of nausea, vomiting, diarrhea, pedal edema. Skin turgor, dryness and hydrat'n. Check for rales, dyspnea and orthopnea.

Generic Name (Trade Name)	Use (Dose)	Action	Adverse Effects	Drug Interactions	Nursing Process
Nitroglycerin (Nitro-Bid IV, Nitrostat IV, Tridil)	To reduce myocardial ischemia and improve hemodynamics in pts w. severe left ventr. dysfunct'n complicating acute myocardial dysfunct'n (**IV:** Adults - initially, 5 μg/min infused in a dilute solut'n; incr. by 5 μg/min q3-5 min, prn. If no response is noted w. 20 μg/min, increments of 10 or even 20 μg/min may be employed)	Dilates both venous and arterial circulat'n, w. greater effect on venous side. Relieves pulmonary congest'n, decr. myocardial O_2 consumpt'n and reduces ST-segment elevat'n.	Headache, flushing, dizziness, hypotens'n, tachycardia	**Ethanol:** Plus nitrates may lead to more profound hypotens'n. **Nitrates, long-acting:** Administered chronically, can produce tolerance to nitroglycerin.	Follow nsg process for nitroglycerin preparat'n in Table 13, w. the added precaut'ns for IV administrat'n. Be sure to use special nonabsorbing tubing supplied by manufacturer as up to 80% of drug can be absorbed by regular plastic tubing. Be sure to prepare in a glass bottle or container and use infus'n pump. Monitor VS closely during administrat'n.

S E C T I O N   4

Renal Pharmacology

The kidney is an important organ in the body. In addition to eliminating sodium, chloride, water and body wastes, the kidney works in concert with the cardiovascular system to regulate blood pressure and cardiac function. Kidney failure leads to the accumulation of salt and water in the extracellular spaces of the body and this can precipitate hypertension and congestive heart failure. The kidney is also responsible for the secretion of renin which is subsequently converted into the vasopressor chemical angiotensin II. In view of the close working relationship between the cardiovascular and renal systems, the effects of drugs on the kidney are considered immediately after the section on cardiovascular pharmacology.

CHAPTER 16

Diuretics

Reabsorption of Sodium, Chloride and Water from the Nephron

Diuretics are drugs that increase the rate of urine formation. They are used primarily to decrease extracellular fluid volume. Diuretics work by reducing the ability of nephrons to reabsorb water. Before discussing the mechanisms of action of diuretics, it is essential to review the role of the nephron in the reabsorption of sodium, chloride and water. Particular attention is paid to sodium and chloride because they are the major electrolytes found in extracellular fluid. When they are reabsorbed from the nephron, water is also returned to the body. When they are lost in urine, they carry with them water molecules. All major diuretics decrease, in one way or another, the renal reabsorption of sodium and chloride, thereby promoting the excretion of water.

The following discussion of the physiology of the kidney is tortuous. For this we apologize. However, there is no simple way to lead someone through the nephron. That is just the way it is constructed. Our explanations will be facilitated by reference to Figure 17 and Table 17.

The functional unit of the kidney is the nephron. It is composed of the glomerulus, the proximal convoluted tubule, the loop of Henle, the distal convoluted tubule and the collecting duct. The initial process in urine formation is the filtration of plasma by renal glomeruli. The glomerular filtration rate (GFR) in normal humans is approximately 120 mL/min. Sodium and chloride are

Figure 17
Reabsorption of electrolytes and water from the nephron.

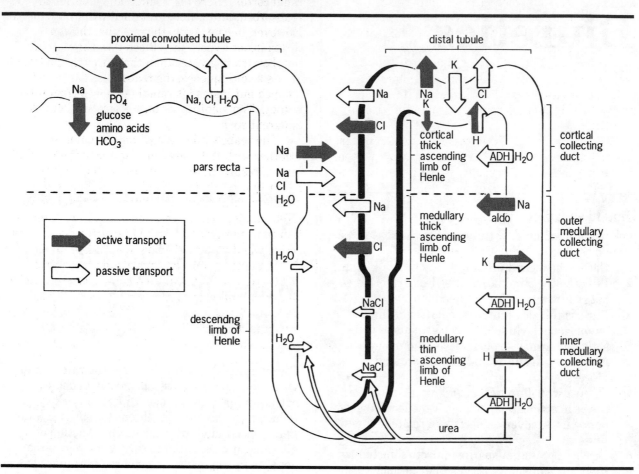

From: H. R. Jacobson and J. R. Kokko (1976), Diuretics: Sites and mechanisms of action. *Ann. Rev. Pharmacol. Toxicol.16* :201-214. Reproduced with permission.

Table 17
Percentage of water and sodium remaining at different points in the nephron.

	% H$_2$O Remaining	% Sodium Remaining
End of proximal tubule	20	20
End of loop of Henle	14	7
End of distal tubule	2 – 5	1 – 5
Excreted urine	0.1 – 1	0 – 1

filtered through the glomeruli and their concentrations in the glomerular filtrate reflect their plasma levels.

Following the filtration of plasma by renal glomeruli, most of the sodium, chloride and water is reabsorbed from subsequent sections of the nephron. Under normal conditions, approximately 99 – 99.5% of the sodium, chloride and water filtered through renal glomeruli is reabsorbed into the systemic circulation from subsequent sections of the nephron. Any decrease in the percentage of material reabsorbed, regardless of how small it may appear in relation to the quantities filtered, may increase significantly the amount of urine voided. For example, a decrease in the amount of sodium and chloride reabsorbed from 99.5% to 98.0% will cause a four-fold increase in urine production.

The mechanics of salt and water reabsorption differ depending on the section of the nephron involved. Approximately 80% of the glomerular filtrate is reabsorbed in the proximal convoluted tubule. This section of the nephron is permeable to water. As a result, when glucose, amino acids, phosphate and sodium are actively reabsorbed from the proximal convoluted tubule, water is drawn along with them to maintain the isotonicity of the fluid remaining in the lumen. Chloride is also reabsorbed passively in the proximal tubule. Chloride carries a negative charge and it accompanies positively charged sodium to maintain electrical neutrality.

The medulla of the kidney is hypertonic. Water descending down the loop of Henle is drawn into the hypertonic medulla in response to the higher osmotic pressure in this portion of the kidney. The descending loop of Henle is not permeable to sodium and chloride. These ions do not leave and, as a result, the liquid remaining in the tubule at the bend of the loop of Henle is hypertonic.

The ascending loop of Henle has characteristics opposite to those of the descending limb. It is permeable to sodium and chloride but impermeable to water. As fluid travels up the ascending loop, chloride is actively reabsorbed into the medulla of the kidney with sodium accompanying it to maintain electrical neutrality. Water is not reabsorbed because, as just stated, the ascending limb of Henle's loop is impermeable to it.

Before proceeding further on our safari through the nephron, let us pause for a moment to investigate the reasons for, and the consequences of, the aforementioned hypertonicity of the renal medulla. One reason is the previously described selective reabsorption of sodium and chloride from the ascending limb of the loop of Henle. The second reason is the reabsorption of urea from the collecting ducts into the medullary tissue. It may seem a little premature to digress and consider the collecting ducts at the end of our golden stream while we are still working our way up Henle's loop. However, if readers will cast their eyes to a point just before our river empties into the Bay of Bladder, they will see that urea is absorbed into the renal medulla at this point.

Now that we have established the reasons for the hypertonic medulla, what are its consequences? Stated simply, the hypertonic medulla provides the kidney with its final opportunity to concentrate urine. Under the influence of the antidiuretic hormone (ADH, vasopressin), water is drawn out of the collecting ducts into the hypertonic renal medulla and then reabsorbed into the blood. If anything, such as a loop diuretic, reduces the hypertonicity of the medulla, the ability of the nephron to concentrate urine is diminished and the kidney excretes increased quantities of this fluid.

Returning now to our story, we pick up our fluid

as it emerges from the renal medulla and travels up the ascending limb of the loop of Henle through the renal cortex. Here too, sodium and chloride are reabsorbed, and water is retained within the lumen. However, in contrast to the medulla, the renal cortex is not hypertonic. Blood flow through the renal cortex is greater than that through the medulla. As a consequence, the reabsorbed salt is not trapped but instead is rapidly removed from the kidney. The significance of this fact will become apparent soon.

The reabsorption of sodium and chloride, together with the retention of water in the tubular lumen, results in the dilution of water, with the result that a hypotonic fluid is presented to the distal convoluted tubule. Within the distal convoluted tubule, sodium, chloride and water reabsorption continues, with electrolyte transport occurring actively and water following in a passive manner.

In addition, an exchange of ions occurs in the last section of the distal tubule and collecting ducts. Under the influence of the mineralocorticoid aldosterone, sodium is reabsorbed in exchange for potassium and hydrogen, which are secreted into the lumen. This aspect of renal function has great clinical significance. All thiazide and loop diuretics reduce the reabsorption of sodium before it reaches the distal convoluted tubule. The higher levels of sodium in the fluid presented to the distal tubule cause an increase in sodium-potassium exchange. The increase in potassium secretion and excretion can produce hypokalemia. This will be discussed in more detail shortly.

The final process in the formation of urine has been referred to above. It occurs as fluid passes down the renal collecting ducts through the hypertonic medulla. The permeability of the collecting ducts to water is controlled by the secretion of the antidiuretic hormone (ADH, vasopressin) by the pituitary. When ADH is secreted, the collecting ducts are permeable to water, which is drawn from the lumen by the hypertonic medulla into medullary tissue and subsequently reabsorbed into the general circulation. In the absence of ADH, water cannot pass through the collecting ducts into the medulla. As a result, the concentration of urine does not occur. In this case an increased amount of urine is presented to the bladder.

Most nurses have experienced the full bladder that accompanies ingestion of ethanol. The explanation behind this phenomenon can be found in the fact that alcohol depresses the release of ADH by the pituitary, bringing with it diuresis. Another consequence is secondary dehydration. Think back and remember how much water you drank on the "day after".

Sites of Action of Diuretics within the Nephron

It is pertinent now to consider the possible sites where diuretics may act. Reference to Figure 18 will assist the reader. Because the majority of the glomerular filtrate is reabsorbed from the proximal convoluted tubule (site I), students cannot be faulted if they conclude that drugs which reduce the percentage of salt and water reabsorbed from the proximal convoluted tubule produce a marked diuresis. However, this is not the case, because salt and water retained in the proximal convoluted tubule are reabsorbed in the subsequent portions of the nephron.

Figure 18
Sites of sodium reabsorption and diuretic action in the nephron.

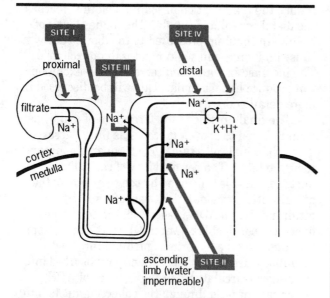

I = proximal tubule; II = ascending limb of Henle's loop;
III = cortical diluting site; IV = distal Na⁺/K⁺H⁺ exchange site.

From: A. F. Lant and G. M. Wilson (1974), Modern diuretic therapy. *Excerpta Medica*. Reproduced with permission.

On the other hand, drugs that inhibit the reabsorption of sodium and chloride from the medullary component of the ascending limb of the loop of Henle (site II) are most effective. Because they reduce the hypertonicity of the renal medulla, these drugs, called **loop diuretics** or high-ceiling diuretics, impair the ability of the nephron to concentrate urine in the collecting ducts.

Drugs that block the reabsorption of sodium and chloride in the cortical diluting segment (site III) will also produce marked diuresis. However, they are not as effective as the loop diuretics because they modify neither the hypertonicity of the renal medulla nor the concentrating ability of the collecting ducts.

By the time urine reaches the distal convoluted tubule (site IV), very little sodium and chloride remain to be reabsorbed. Therefore, drugs that block sodium and chloride reabsorption only in the distal convoluted tubule have limited effectiveness as diuretics. They are important, however, in reducing the renal secretion, and subsequent excretion, of potassium. Remember that potassium is normally exchanged for some of the sodium arriving in the distal convoluted tubules and collecting ducts. Potassium-sparing diuretics act in the distal convoluted tubules and collecting ducts to reduce this exchange. They are often used together with a loop diuretic or a drug that acts at site III to reduce the increased potassium-sodium exchange that would normally occur as a result of increased concentrations of sodium arriving in the distal segments of the nephron.

The reabsorption of water from the collecting ducts depends on the secretion of ADH. Patients with diabetes insipidus are deficient in this hormone and excrete large amounts of water. Few drugs depress ADH secretion. The effects of ethanol have already been mentioned. However, its other actions make it impractical to use on a long-term basis as a diuretic.

Groups of Diuretics

Thiazides, Chlorthalidone (Hygroton) and Metolazone (Zaroxolyn)

Mechanism of Action and Pharmacologic Effects

Thiazides were introduced in the mid-1950s. Chlorothiazide (Diuril) was the first drug on the market and it was rapidly followed by many others, such as hydrochlorothiazide (Hydrodiuril, Esidrix), hydroflumethiazide (Naturetin) and cyclothiazide (Anhydron). Qualitatively, all thiazides are identical. They differ only in the doses required to produce diuresis. Hydrochlorothiazide is currently the most popular member of the group.

Two additional drugs, chlorthalidone (Hygroton) and metolazone (Zaroxolyn), have actions very similar to those of the thiazides. They differ from thiazides only in the fact that they have longer durations of action and are therefore given less often.

Thiazides, chlorthalidone and metolazone block sodium and chloride reabsorption in the cortical diluting segment of the loop of Henle and in the proximal section of the distal convoluted tubule. As a result, water is also retained in the lumen of the nephron because of the osmotic drawing power of sodium and chloride. By blocking sodium reabsorption, thiazides, chlorthalidone and metolazone also increase potassium secretion. With more sodium arriving at the latter sections of the distal convoluted tubules and collecting ducts, increased quantities of potassium are secreted into the tubular lumen, in exchange for sodium, which is reabsorbed from the lumen into the systemic circulation. As a result of the increased excretion of potassium, serum potassium levels can fall and the patient may become hypokalemic.

The thiazides, chlorthalidone and metolazone decrease the renal excretion of uric acid, thereby increasing its concentration in plasma and predisposing patients to gout.

These diuretics may also induce hyperglycemia and aggravate pre-existing diabetes mellitus. The exact mechanism by which they produce this effect is still in doubt. It has been postulated that they inhibit the pancreatic release of insulin and block the peripheral utilization of glucose.

Therapeutic Uses

These drugs are used, together with salt restriction, to treat edema. Their efficacy depends on the condition being treated. Diuretics are used in the treatment of ascites, particularly when it is secondary to cirrhosis. They may eliminate the need for paracentesis or reduce the number of occasions this procedure is performed. Thiazides, chlorthalidone or metolazone may correct edema in chronic renal disease, if enough nephrons remain functional. However, if a significant number of nephrons have been destroyed, a loop diuretic may be required. Diuretic therapy has often been disappointing in the treatment of the nephrotic syndrome. Thiazides, chlorthalidone and metolazone are contraindicated in anuria. They should be discontinued if increasing azotemia and oliguria occur during treatment of severe progressive renal disease.

The treatment of hypertension with diuretics is discussed in Chapter 14. Thiazides or chlorthalidone are usually the drugs of choice because they decrease blood volume and dilate arterioles. Metolazone may have similar actions. Although loop diuretics are more effective diuretics, they do not dilate arterioles and usually are less effective in hypertension.

The use of diuretic therapy in the treatment of congestive heart failure is discussed in Chapter 10; diuretics are appropriate first-line agents for all grades of cardiac failure when sinus rhythm is present. They are usually sufficient alone in mild heart failure. When the patient is afflicted with more severe heart failure, diuretics are usually given with other drugs, such as a vasodilator or digoxin, or both.

Adverse Effects

Thiazides, chlorthalidone or metolazone can produce hypovolemia, hyponatremia and hypokalemia. In addition, they can precipitate attacks of gout because they reduce the elimination of uric acid by the kidney. These drugs also produce hyperglycemia and aggravation of pre-existing diabetes mellitus.

Other adverse reactions are anorexia, gastric irritation, nausea, vomiting, cramping, diarrhea, constipation, jaundice and pancreatitis. Patients may experience the central nervous system effects of dizziness, vertigo, paresthesias, headache and xanthopsia. Hypersensitivity reactions include purpura, photosensitivity, rash, urticaria, necrotizing angiitis, fever, respiratory distress including pneumonitis, and anaphylactic reactions.

Leukopenia, thrombocytopenia, agranulocytosis, aplastic anemia and hemolytic anemia have also been reported. In spite of this list, these drugs are generally considered to be quite safe when used in normal therapeutic doses.

Nursing Process

Assessment

Nursing assessment prior to the administration of a thiazide, chlorthalidone or metolazone should begin with a review of the patient's history for evidence of conditions that would contraindicate use of these drugs. These include kidney or liver disease, low serum potassium or sodium levels, or chronic respiratory disease. In the presence of any of these conditions, nurses should withhold the medication until its use is reconfirmed with the physician. Patient assessment includes baseline measurements of blood pressure, body mass/weight, as well as the site and extent of edema.

Administration

Diuretics should be administered in the morning to avoid interference with sleep. Potassium replacement should be given if serum potassium is less than 3.0 mEq/L. If nausea occurs, give the drug with food, although absorption may be decreased slightly.

Evaluation

Nursing evaluation of the patient following drug administration involves first observing the efficacy of the medication. This can be done by measuring the patient's daily body mass/weight, fluid intake and output and blood pressure. If the drug is effective, both the weight and the blood pressure (if previously elevated) should fall and the output of fluid should exceed the intake.

Patient evaluation should also emphasize the adverse effects of the drugs, such as hypokalemia (muscular weakness, constipation, postural hypotension, dyspnea, cardiac arrhythmias), glucosuria and hyperglycemia, hyperuricemia and gout (periodic monoarticular episodes of pain, swelling and inflammation), and hyponatremia (CNS disturbances — confusion, stupor, loss of sensorium, coma, poor skin turgor, postural hypotension).

Teaching

Patient teaching related to the use of the thiazides, chlorthalidone and metolazone should include alerting the patient to the expected effects of the drugs, particularly diuresis. Those patients whose lifestyles involve limited access to toilet facilities (e.g., crane operators, bus drivers) should be encour-

aged to take their medication at a time most convenient to their activities. Patients who experience dry mouth may be tempted to increase their fluid intake. They should be advised not to do so without consulting their physician. Patients should be advised to monitor their weight as a means of evaluating diuresis.

Patients should also be advised to seek instructions from their physician regarding dietary restriction of sodium and the need for increased dietary intake of potassium. Referral for consultation with a dietician might be considered. The patient should also be advised to refrain from consuming alcohol, which increases dehydration, or natural licorice, which increases the hypokalemic effects of these drugs.

The Loop Diuretics — Furosemide (Lasix), Ethacrynic Acid (Edecrin), and Bumetanide (Bumex)

Mechanism of Action and Pharmacologic Effects

Loop, or high-ceiling, diuretics inhibit the reabsorption of sodium and chloride in the ascending limb of the loop of Henle as it passes through the renal medulla. The resulting reduction in the hypertonicity of the renal medulla impairs the concentrating ability of the collecting ducts. As a consequence, loop diuretics are the most potent of the diuretics, surpassing the effects produced by thiazides, chlorthalidone and metolazone.

Because loop diuretics increase the concentration of sodium presented to the distal convoluted tubules and collecting ducts, they also promote greater sodium-potassium exchange. As a consequence, potassium excretion is increased and patients may experience hypokalemia.

Therapeutic Uses

The major therapeutic use of loop diuretics is to treat edema in patients with severe edema or renal impairment where the thiazides, chlorthalidone or metolazone may be ineffective. Furosemide is the most popular drug. Loop diuretics are sometimes used for the treatment of hypertension, in place of a thiazide, chlorthalidone or metolazone. Often this is not appropriate because loop diuretics do not dilate arterioles and are not as effective as the thiazides, chlorthalidone or metolazone in lowering blood pressure.

Loop diuretics are contraindicated in the

presence of complete renal shutdown. If increasing azotemia and oliguria occur during treatment of severe progressive renal disease, the loop diuretic should be discontinued. In hepatic coma and conditions producing electrolyte depletion, loop diuretic therapy should not be instituted until the underlying condition has been corrected or ameliorated. These drugs are also contraindicated in severe hypokalemia, hypovolemia or hypotension. Because furosemide has the potential to displace bilirubin from plasma albumin, it is contraindicated in newborns with jaundice or infants with conditions that might induce hyperbilirubinemia or kernicterus.

Adverse Effects

Electrolyte depletion is a major concern with the use of these drugs. This manifests as weakness, dizziness, lethargy, leg cramps, sweating, bladder spasms, anorexia, vomiting and/or mental confusion. Loop diuretics reduce uric acid secretion in the proximal convoluted tubules, predisposing patients to increased plasma uric acid levels and attacks of gout. Various forms of dermatitis and skin rashes have occurred with these drugs. Cases of vertigo, tinnitus and reversible deafness have also been reported.

Ethacrynic acid has also been reported to affect adversely the gastrointestinal tract, with symptoms of anorexia, malaise, abdominal discomfort or pain, dysphagia, nausea, vomiting and diarrhea.

Bumetanide produces similar electrolyte changes to those caused by furosemide or ethacrynic acid. It may also cause azotemia, hyperuricemia and rarely, impaired glucose tolerance. Large doses may cause myalgia in patients with renal failure. Nausea, vomiting, abdominal pain and rashes have also been reported with bumetanide.

Nursing Process

Assessment

The administration of furosemide, ethacrynic acid or bumetanide must be preceded by a nursing assessment to identify any contraindications to their use. Contraindications include previous hypersensitivity to the drug in question, diabetes mellitus, anuria and laboratory reports that indicate azotemia or electrolyte depletion. The diagnosis of diabetes mellitus in a patient receiving these drugs should alert the nurse to the need for particularly stringent nursing evaluation following administration of the medication. Baseline data including fluid intake and output, blood pressure and body mass/weight should also be collected at this time to allow for evaluation of drug effectiveness.

Administration

With any loop diuretic a single daily morning dose is preferred. If divided doses are necessary, they should be given in the early morning and early afternoon. This schedule is least likely to interfere with the normal sleeping pattern of the patient. The drugs should be stored in light-resistant containers and oral solutions should be refrigerated.

Intravenous administration of these medications should occur over a period of one to two minutes. Intramuscular injection is painful and should also be given slowly, preferably using a "Z-track" injection technique.

Evaluation

Nursing evaluation following administration of these drugs should aim at establishing the effectiveness of the medication. Weight loss, fluid intake versus fluid output, and reduced edema provide the best reflection of diuretic effectiveness. Nurses should also be alert for the adverse effects identified above in the preceding section. Urine should be tested for glucosuria, especially in the diabetic and prediabetic patient. It must also be remembered that these drugs are extremely effective diuretics and can produce severe dehydration resulting in circulatory collapse. Nurses should guard against this possibility by observing the skin turgor of the patient, as well as monitoring the aforementioned pulse, blood pressure, daily body mass/weight and fluid input/output ratio. Potassium blood levels should be evaluated and a potassium supplement considered if potassium levels fall below 3.0 mEq/L.

Teaching

Nurses should alert patients to the expected outcome of the drug (diuresis). Patients should also be instructed to move slowly from the supine to the standing position with a brief pause in the sitting position to reduce the possibility of postural hypotension. Because loop diuretics can produce gout, patients should be instructed to report monoarticular joint swelling, pain or inflammation.

Nurses should inform patients and their families to report weakness, dizziness, lethargy, leg cramps, perspiration, bladder spasms, anorexia, vomiting and mental confusion to their physicians because these symptoms can be due to electrolyte depletion. Similarly, the physician should be contacted immediately if patients experience ringing in the ears, severe abdominal pain, sore throat and fever or a skin rash.

Patients should also be advised to seek medical advice before taking aspirin or any other over-the-counter medicine that contains aspirin, because furosemide can reduce salicylate excretion and increase the possibility of aspirin poisoning.

Potassium-Sparing Diuretics — Spironolactone (Aldactone)

Mechanism of Action and Pharmacologic Effects

Spironolactone is similar in structure to aldosterone and acts as a competitive inhibitor of the mineralocorticoid in the distal convoluted tubules and collecting ducts. As a result, it prevents the aldosterone-induced loss of potassium.

Therapeutic Uses

Spironolactone may be given to treat conditions of excessive aldosterone levels, such as primary aldosteronism or cirrhosis accompanied by edema or ascites, or both. Spironolactone is used in the treatment of congestive heart failure in which edema and sodium retention are only partially responsive to, or intolerant of, other therapeutic measures. It does not affect the basic pathologic process of the nephrotic syndrome but may be used for inducing a diuresis in patients not responding to glucocorticoids or other diuretics.

The drug is most often combined with a thiazide, chlorthalidone, metolazone, furosemide or ethacrynic acid to prevent hypokalemia produced by these compounds. A popular product, marketed under the trade name of Aldactazide, contains a fixed ratio of either 25 mg of hydrochlorothiazide and 25 mg of spironolactone or 50 mg of hydrochlorothiazide plus 50 mg of spironolactone. The use of spironolactone in the treatment of hypertension is discussed in Chapter 14.

Spironolactone is contraindicated in anuria, acute renal insufficiency, significant impairment of renal function and hyperkalemia. It should not be used with potassium supplements.

Adverse Effects

In addition to hyperkalemia, the most common adverse effects for which nurses must evaluate patients using spironolactone include gynecomastia and gastrointestinal symptoms, such as nausea, cramping and diarrhea. Concern has surfaced over the use of spironolactone with the report of carcinoma of the breast in both men and women receiving the drug. At the present time no cause-and-effect relationship between the use of the drug and the appearance of the carcinoma has been established. Other adverse effects of spironolactone include drowsiness, dizziness, lethargy, headache, maculopapular or erythematous cutaneous eruptions, urticaria, mental confusion, drug fever, ataxia, mild androgenic effects including hirsutism, irregular menses, deepening of the voice, amenorrhea, postmenopausal bleeding, alterations in libido and sweating. These are usually reversible if the drug is discontinued.

Nursing Process

Assessment

Nursing assessment related to the prescription of spironolactone begins with a review of the patient's history for contraindications, such as hypersensitivity to the drug or renal disease. Use of this drug to treat elderly patients should alert the nurse to the need for particularly stringent evaluation following administration of the medication. Laboratory reports should be reviewed for evidence of electrolyte imbalance and records of fluid intake and output should be reviewed for indications of anuria. Baseline data, including the patient's body mass/weight, blood pressure and extent of edema, is gathered at this time to assist in evaluating the drug's effectiveness.

Administration

Spironolactone is stored in light-resistant containers and administered with meals to reduce gastrointestinal distress and enhance absorption. The drug is best given in the morning to avoid interference with sleep.

Evaluation

Nurses should observe the patient for evidence of the adverse effects mentioned before. Hypersensitivity reactions often manifest as sore throat, rash or jaundice. Progressive muscle flaccidity and paralysis, dyspnea, dysphasia and cardiac arrhythmias indicate hyperkalemia.

Teaching

Nurses should alert patients to the expected outcome of spironolactone treatment (diuresis). Patients should be instructed to use moderation in the consumption of foods high in potassium and to seek dietary counselling if necessary. A list of warning signs and adverse effects, including hypersensitivity reactions, hyperkalemia, hyponatremia, gastrointestinal irritation, amenorrhea and gynecomastia, should be given to patients. If any of these appear, patients should call their physician immediately.

Potassium-Sparing Diuretics — Triamterene (Dyrenium) and Amiloride (Midamor)

Mechanism of Action and Pharmacologic Effects

Triamterene and amiloride act directly on tubular transport in the distal convoluted tubules and collecting ducts to inhibit the reabsorption of sodium and the secretion of potassium. They work independently of aldosterone and are not competitive inhibitors of the mineralocorticoid.

Therapeutic Uses

Either drug may be used alone. Triamterene is indicated for the treatment of edema associated with congestive heart failure, hepatic cirrhosis, nephrotic syndrome, idiopathic edema, steroid-induced edema and edema due to secondary hyper-aldosteronism. The indications for the use of amiloride are much the same. However, their major clinical use is in combination with a thiazide, chlorthalidone, metolazone or a loop diuretic to reduce or prevent the hypokalemia produced by these agents. A most popular product, marketed under the trade name of Dyazide, contains a fixed ratio of 50 mg of triamterene and 25 mg of hydrochlorothiazide. The product Moduret contains 5 mg of amiloride and 50 mg of hydrochlorothiazide.

Triamterene and amiloride are contraindicated in the presence of elevated serum potassium levels, anuria, acute renal failure and severe or progressive renal disease. Triamterene should not be used in severe or progressive hepatic dysfunction. It should not be given to nursing mothers. Amiloride should not be given to patients with diabetic nephropathy. Neither drug should be used with potassium supplements.

Adverse Effects

Hyperkalemia is the major adverse effect of triamterene and amiloride. Relatively few other adverse effects are seen. The most common are nausea, vomiting, leg cramps and dizziness. Amiloride produces adverse central nervous system effects in about ten per cent of patients. These include headache, dizziness, confusion, insomnia, depression, somnolence and decreased libido.

Nursing Process

Nurses should guard against the possibility of hyperkalemia developing. The baseline measures previously mentioned should be taken to assist later in assessing drug effectiveness. As with all diuretics, patients should be informed of the expected effects of the drugs.

Osmotic Diuretics — Mannitol

Mechanism of Action and Pharmacologic Effects

Osmotic diuretics, such as mannitol, are pharmacologically inert nonelectrolytes that are freely filtered by the renal glomerulus and not reabsorbed from the nephron. When the diuretic is excreted in urine, it carries with it an amount of water equivalent to its osmotic drawing power.

Therapeutic Uses

Mannitol is the osmotic diuretic used most extensively. It must be injected and is available alone and in combination with sodium chloride. Mannitol is used to increase urine production when the renal filtration rate is acutely reduced. In this situation a higher percentage of sodium, chloride and water are reabsorbed. Loop diuretics and the thiazides may prove ineffective because they cannot reduce the reabsorbing capacity of the nephron for sodium and chloride sufficiently to increase urine flow. Osmotic diuretics may prove effective in this situation.

Mannitol is also employed for the reduction of cerebrospinal fluid pressure and volume. In this situation, the drug increases plasma osmolality, with the result that water diffuses from the cerebrospinal fluid into the plasma to be excreted by the kidneys.

Adverse Effects

A major adverse effect of mannitol is an increase in the extracellular fluid volume. By administering a large volume of hypertonic mannitol, which distributes throughout the extracellular space, fluid is drawn from the cells into the extracellular compartment. Hypersensitivity reactions, diverse in nature, have been reported with mannitol.

Nursing Process

Assessment
Prior to the administration of mannitol, nurses should attempt to identify any contraindications to its use. These include pregnancy, renal or cardiac disease, intracranial bleeding and dehydration.

Nursing assessment should also include baseline measurements, such as fluid intake and output, blood pressure, pulse, respirations, electrolyte levels and patient's body mass/weight, to determine potential risks and permit comparison with observations following administration in order to evaluate the effectiveness of the diuretic.

Evaluation

Following administration of mannitol, the nursing evaluation should have two major objectives. The first is to evaluate the effectiveness of the medication. This is accomplished by observing the patient's fluid intake and output and body mass/weight. The second objective is to identify early evidence of adverse effects, i.e., changes in: pulse rate, rhythm or quality; blood pressure; rate, rhythm or quality of respirations. Nurses should also observe patients for extravasation or phlebitis at the infusion site, patient-reported chest pain and signs of metabolic acidosis (drowsiness or restlessness).

Teaching

Patients should be told to increase fluids to two to three liters per day unless otherwise contraindicated. Warn patients to rise showly from sitting or lying position.

Further Reading

Birkenhagen, W. H. and Moser, M. (eds.) (1986). Symposium on diuretics in the 1980s. Issues and insights. *Drugs 31* :1-211.

DePew, C.L. et al. (1989) Furosemide: Update on a commonly used drug. *Critical Care Nurse 9* (2): 63-64.

Freis, E. D. and Papademetriou, V. (1985). How dangerous are diuretics? *Drugs 30* :469-474.

Lant, A. (1985). Diuretics, clinical pharmacology and therapeutic use, parts I and II. *Drugs 29* :162-188.

Szerlip, H. M. and Singer, I. (1989). The physiology of diuretics: Know what you're using. *Perspectives in Cardology 5* (5):43-54.

Table 18
Diuretics.

Pharmacologic Classification: Thiazide and Thiazide-like Diuretics

Generic Name (Trade Name)	Use (Dose)	Action	Adverse Effects	Drug Interactions	Nursing Process
Chlorothiazide (Diuril)	Tx of edema, hypertens'n (**Oral:** Adults - 500-1000 mg od or bid. Children - 22 mg/kg/day in 2 divided doses. Infants under 6 months - up to 33 mg/kg/day in 2 divided doses)	Incr. renal excret'n and Na, Cl and H_2O. Decr. blood volume. Reduces peripheral resistance.	Hypovolemia, hypokalemia, hyponatremia, hyperglycemia, hyperuricemia, renal colic, hematuria, crystalluria, hypersensitivity, pancreatitis, jaundice, hepatic coma, gout	**Angiotensin-converting enzyme (ACE) inhibitors** (enalapril, captopril, lisinopril): Tog. w. a diuretic, can produce powerful hypotensive effect, poss. leading to postural hypotens'n. Avoid by stopping diuretic a few days before starting w. low doses of ACE inhibitor. Thereafter it may be poss. to reintroduce the diuretic and incr. dose of ACE inhibitor slowly. **Corticosteroids:** Potentiate K-lowering effects of diuretics. **Digoxin:** Toxicity is incr. by diuretic-induced hypokalemia. Incr. sensitivity to digoxin appears rel. to rate of fall in plasma K and extracellular/intracellular concentra'n ratio. **Insulin, oral hypoglycemics:** May have reduced effects in presence of diuretics because diuretics can incr. blood sugar, thereby necessitating higher doses of insulin or oral hypoglycemics. **Lithium:** Diuretics can incr. levels of Li. **Nonsteroidal anti-inflammatory drugs (NSAIDs):** May inhibit natriuretic response to diuretics.	**Assess:** Pt hx for contraindicat'ns to use (incl. kidney or liver disease, low serum K or Na levels, chronic respiratory disease), establish baseline BP, weight, fluid intake/output to determine subsequent fluid loss and extent of edema. **Administer:** Pref. in early a.m. **Evaluate:** Efficacy of tx (daily weight, fluid intake/output, BP); for evidence of adv. effects. Evaluate rate, depth and rhythm of respira'ns and effect of exert'n. **Teach:** Expected outcome of medicat'n (diuresis). Not to consume licorice or alcohol while on diuretics. To eat foods rich in K. Advise pt to avoid sudden postural changes and to wear a sunscreen.
Hydrochlorothiazide (Esidrex, Hydrodiuril)	As for chlorothiazide (**Oral:** Adults - initially, 25-200 mg/day; maint. dose, 25-100 mg/day. Children - 2 mg/kg/day in 2 divided doses. Infants under 6 months - up to 3 mg/kg/day in 2 divided doses)	As for chlorothiazide	As for chlorothiazide		
Bendroflumethiazide (Naturetin)	As for chlorothiazide (**Oral:** Adults - initially, 5 mg daily, pref. in a.m.; may incr. to 20 mg as a single dose or 2 divided doses. Maint., 2.5-15 mg od or intermittently. Children - initially, up to 0.4 mg/kg/day in 2 divided doses. Maint., 0.05-0.1 mg/kg/day in a single dose)	As for chlorothiazide	As for chlorothiazide		As for chlorothiazide
Methyclothiazide (Aquatensen, Enduron)	As for chlorothiazide (**Oral:** Adults - initially, 2.5-10 mg od; same dose range is used for maint. Children - 0.05-0.2 mg/kg/day)	As for chlorothiazide	As for chlorothiazide	As for chlorothiazide	As for chlorothiazide

Generic Name (Trade Name)	Use (Dose)	Action	Adverse Effects	Drug Interactions	Nursing Process
Chlorthalidone (Hygroton)	As for chlorothiazide (**Oral:** 50-200 mg/day)	As for chlorothiazide	As for chlorothiazide	As for chlorothiazide	As for chlorothiazide
Metolazone (Zaroxolyn)	As for chlorothiazide (**Oral:** 5-20 mg/day)	As for chlorothiazide	As for chlorothiazide	As for chlorothiazide	As for chlorothiazide
Indapamide (Lozide)	As for chlorothiazide (**Oral:** Adults - initially, 2.5 mg/day; incr. prn to 5 mg/day)	As for chlorothiazide	As for chlorothiazide	As for chlorothiazide	As for chlorothiazide

Pharmacologic Classification: Loop Diuretics

Generic Name (Trade Name)	Use (Dose)	Action	Adverse Effects	Drug Interactions	Nursing Process
Furosemide (Lasix)	Tx of edema (**IV:** *For acute pulmonary edema,* adults - 40 mg repeated in 60-90 min prn. Infants and children - initially, 1 mg/kg; incr. prn by 1 mg/kg no earlier than 2 h after previous dose. *For acute renal failure,* adults - 40-80 mg. **Oral:** *For edema,* adults - initially, 20-80 mg. If adequate response is not obtained, incr. dose. Infants and children - initially, 2 mg/kg; incr. prn by 1-2 mg/kg 6-8 h after previous dose. Max. 6 mg/kg)	Inhibits reabsorpt'n of Na and Cl in ascending limb of loop of Henle, reducing hypertonicity of renal medulla and impairing concentrating ability of collecting ducts.	Hypovolemia, electrolyte imbalance (see thiazide diuretics), gout, deafness, fluid deplet'n, dermatitis	**ACE inhibitors:** As for thiazides, above. **Cephalosporins:** Furosemide may enhance nephrotoxicity of cephaloridine. **Clofibrate:** And furosemide may compete for albumin binding sites, increasing actions of both drugs. **Corticosteroids:** Furosemide may produce excessive K loss when given w. corticosteroids. Special attent'n should be given to K balance. **Digitalis products:** Furosemide can produce deficiency of K and/or Mg w. resultant predisposit'n to digitalis toxicity. Replacement tx should be undertaken prn. **Lithium carbonate:** Furosemide reduces Li excret'n. More frequent serum Li tests may be required. **Skeletal muscle relaxants:** Furosemide may incr. neuromuscular blockade produced by tubocurarine.	**Assess:** For pregnancy; pt hx of hypersensitivity, diabetes mellitus; lab. reports for evidence of azotemia, electrolyte deplet'n; establish baseline fluid intake/output, BP, weight. **Administer:** From light-resistant container (refrigerate oral solut'ns); single daily dose in a.m. or divided doses a.m. and early p.m., orally if possible. **Evaluate:** Weight loss, BP, fluid intake/output; for evidence of electrolyte deplet'n, hearing change, glucosuria, gout, severe dehydrat'n. **Teach:** Precaut'ns rel. to change from supine to standing posit'n; which foods are high in K; expected outcome (diuresis); s/s gout; to seek medical advice before taking OTC medicat'ns containing aspirin.

Drug	Action & Dosage	Adverse Effects	Interactions	Nursing Considerations
Ethacrynic acid (Edecrin)	Tx of edema (**IV:** *For acute pulmonary edema,* adults - 50 mg [0.5-1 mg/kg]. In critical situat'ns, 100 mg. **Oral:** Adults - initially, 50-100 mg daily. Incr. prn, us. in increments of 25-50 mg)	As for furosemide	As for furosemide, plus severe GI disturbances (anorexia, nausea, vomiting, severe watery diarrhea, GI bleeding)	**ACE inhibitors:** As for furosemide. **Aminoglycoside antibiotics:** Ethacrynic acid can produce ototoxicity that may potentiate ototoxicity of aminoglycosides. **Anticoagulants, oral:** Ethacrynic acid has been shown, in vitro, to displace warfarin from human albumin binding sites. It should be given w. caution to pts receiving oral anticoagulants, esp. in presence of hypoalbuminemia. **Corticosteroids:** As for furosemide. Ethacrynic acid may also incr. corticosteroid gastric hemorrhage. **Digitalis:** As for furosemide. **Lithium carbonate:** As for furosemide.	**Assess:** As for furosemide. **Administer:** Reconstitute IV solut'n according to manufacturer's instruct'ns; discard if not used within 24 h or if solut'n is hazy or opalescent. Avoid IV administrat'n concurrently w. blood or blood derivatives. Oral preparat'n w. meals. **Evaluate:** As for furosemide; for evidence of GI disturbance (see adv. effects) **Teach:** As for furosemide; reportable signs of GI adv. effects.
Bumetanide (Bumex)	Tx of edema (**IV:** *For pulmonary edema,* adults - initially, 0.5-1 mg. Repeat dose prn in 20 min. **Oral:** *For edema,* adults - initially, 1 mg daily in a.m. A second dose can be given prn, 6-8 h later. Incr. dose in refractory cases)	As for furosemide	Hypovolemia, hypokalemia, hypochloremia, hyponatremia, hyperuricemia, hyperglycemia, GI distress	As for furosemide and ethacrynic acid	As for furosemide and ethacrynic acid.

Pharmacologic Classification: Potassium-Sparing Diuretics

Drug	Action & Dosage	Adverse Effects	Interactions	Nursing Considerations
Spironolactone (Aldactone); spironolactone 25 mg + hydrochlorothiazide 25 mg (Aldactazide 25); spironolactone 50 mg + hydrochlorothiazide 50 mg (Aldactazide 50)	Tx of edema, hypertens'n, primary hyperaldosteronism (**Spironolactone oral:** *For edema,* adults - 50-100 mg daily in single or divided doses. Children - 1 mg/kg tid. **Aldactazide tablets:** Initially, 1 lower-strength tablet daily. May incr. to 50 mg of ea. ingred. daily in a single dose or in divided doses. Adjust dose in acc. w. BP and serum K levels)	Aldosterone antagonist; blocks Na retent'n and K secret'n.	Amenorrhea, gynecomastia, hyperkalemia, GI irritat'n, hypersensitivity	**Lithium chloride:** Spironolactone may incr. serum Li levels. **Potassium chloride:** Hyperkalemia may result if K supplements are also given. Pts so treated for severe K deficiency must be monitored very closely to detect hyperkalemia.	**Assess:** Pt hx for hypersensitivity to spironolactone, kidney disease, hyperkalemia, anuria; review other medicat'ns for K supplements; establish baseline weight, BP. **Administer:** From light-resistant container; w. food to reduce gastric irritation and improve drug bioavailability. **Evaluate:** Tx effectiveness (fluid intake/output, BP, daily weight); for adv. effects (esp. hypersensitivity, hyperkalemia). **Teach:** Expected effect (diuresis); to avoid overeating high-K food, taking OTC drugs; s/s that should be reported to physician.

Generic Name (Trade Name)	Use (Dose)	Action	Adverse Effects	Drug Interactions	Nursing Process
Triamterene (Dyrenium); triamterene 50 mg + hydrochlorothiazide 25 mg (Dyazide)	Tx of edema, hypertens'n [when combined w. a thiazide, chlorthalidone or metolazone] (**Triamterene oral:** *For edema*, adults - 100 mg bid pc. Children - 2-4 mg/kg/day in divided doses. **Dyazide tablets/capsules:** Initially, 1-2 tablets/capsules daily)	Inhibits secret'n of K and reabsorpt'n of Na in distal convoluted tubules.	Hyperkalemia, nausea, vomiting, leg cramps, dizziness, weakness, headache, dry mouth, anaphylaxis, blood dyscrasias, photosensitivity, rash	**Lithium:** Diuretics enhance cardiotoxicity and neurotoxicity of Li. **Potassium chloride:** Hyperkalemia can occur if used concurrently w. K supplements. If nec. to use both concomitantly, K balance should be monitored very closely.	**Assess:** Review other medicat'ns for K supplements, establish baseline weight, BP. **Evaluate:** Tx effectiveness. **Teach:** As for spironolactone.
Amiloride (Midamor); amiloride 5 mg + hydrochlorothiazide 50 mg (Moduret)	Tx of edema, hypertens'n [when combined w. a thiazide, chlorthalidone or metolazone] (**Amiloride oral:** Adults - 5-10 mg daily. **Moduret oral:** Initially, 1 tablet daily)	As for triamterene	Hyperkalemia, nausea, anorexia, diarrhea, vomiting, abdominal pain, appetite changes, jaundice, GI bleeding, GI disturbances, dizziness, encephalopathy, paresthesias, tremors, CNS disturbances, muscle cramps, weakness, somatic pain	As for triamterene	As for triamterene

CHAPTER 17

Drugs That Increase the Renal Conservation of Water

Teaching Objectives

Following completion of this chapter, the reader should be able to:

1. Discuss the action of vasopressin (the antidiuretic hormone) on the kidney.
2. Describe the pharmacologic effects of vasopressin on the other parts of the body.
3. List the dosage forms of vasopressin that are available for therapy and describe their differences.
4. Discuss the therapeutic uses and adverse effects of vasopressin therapy.
5. Describe the nursing process related to the use of vasopressin.
6. Discuss the use of thiazides in the treatment of diabetes insipidus and the nursing processes related to this use.

Vasopressin (Antidiuretic Hormone, ADH)

Mechanism of Action and Pharmacologic Effects

Vasopressin, also called the antidiuretic hormone (ADH), is secreted by the posterior pituitary gland in response to an increase in plasma osmolality or a decrease in extracellular volume. Its actions on the kidney have been described in Chapter 16. Briefly, vasopressin increases the permeability of the collecting ducts to water and thereby enables the kidney to conserve water in the face of dehydration.

When the tubular fluid reaches the collecting ducts it is hypotonic because of the reabsorption of sodium and chloride in the ascending limb of the loop of Henle. If an individual is well hydrated, vasopressin secretion is low, the collecting duct is impermeable to water and a large volume of hypotonic urine is voided. However, if the extracellular fluid volume is low, or the osmolality of the plasma is high, vasopressin is secreted and water reabsorption occurs from the collecting ducts.

In addition to its actions on water retention, vasopressin has a pronounced vasoconstrictor effect, affecting all parts of the vascular system. This effect is seen with doses of vasopressin greater than those necessary for maximal water conservation. The increase in blood pressure is not mediated through the autonomic nervous system. It cannot be blocked by adrenergic receptor blockers or sympathetic denervation.

Therapeutic Uses

A major therapeutic use of vasopressin is the treatment of diabetes insipidus, a condition caused by a deficiency of vasopressin and characterized by the excretion of large volumes of dilute urine and increased osmolality of the blood. In this condition, vasopressin therapy provides effective and immediate treatment and urine volume returns to normal.

Vasopressin is a polypeptide containing eight amino acids. If given orally, it is rapidly inactivated within the gastrointestinal tract. To be effective, vasopressin must be given parenterally or by insufflation. Vasopressin is available for intramuscular or subcutaneous administration in both aqueous solution or peanut oil suspension. The effects of the water-soluble form of vasopressin (Pitressin) last only a few hours. The repository form in oil (Pitressin Tannate) is effective for twenty-four to forty-eight hours. Desmopressin acetate (DDAVP) is a vasopressin analogue formulated in an isotonic aqueous solution for parenteral or intranasal administration.

Adverse Effects

The vasoconstrictor effects of vasopressin may reduce myocardial perfusion. Patients suffering from coronary artery disease should receive only small doses of vasopressin. Parenteral therapy is contraindicated in patients with cardiovascular and renal disease with hypertension, advanced arteriosclerosis, coronary thrombosis, angina pectoris, epilepsy and toxemia of pregnancy. The other adverse effects of vasopressin include facial pallor, headaches and increased uterine activity.

Several drugs have been shown to interact with vasopressin. Indomethacin, chlorpropamide and acetaminophen enhance the effects of the hormone. Lithium carbonate and methoxyflurane antagonize the effects of vasopressin on the kidney and can produce a vasopressin-resistant polyuria. The ability of demeclocycline to block the actions of vasopressin has led to its use in the treatment of patients with water intoxication due to high levels of vasopressin.

Nursing Process

Assessment

Nursing assessment should attempt to identify any contraindications to the use of vasopressin. Included in these is pregnancy, because one of vasopressin's adverse effects is uterine cramps or contractions. In addition, nursing assessment should establish baseline measurements of blood pressure, fluid intake and output, specific gravity of the urine (usually in the range of 1.001 – 1.006), skin turgor, frequency of urination and sleep patterns before the first administration of vasopressin. This information will provide the basis for later evaluation of the effectiveness or adverse effects of vasopressin therapy.

Administration

Various vasopressin preparations are available and it is important to differentiate between each. **Pitressin** is an injection solution of vasopressin, intended for intramuscular or subcutaneous injection. Its effects last only a few hours. **Vasopressin tannate** (Pitressin Tannate) is provided as a repository form, suspended in peanut oil for intramuscular use. As stated previously, the effects of vasopressin tannate may be seen for twenty-four to forty-eight hours. It must *never* be administered intravenously. Because of the potency of these preparations, care must also be taken to administer the correct dose. Vasopressin preparations should be stored in the refrigerator and parenteral solutions warmed slowly to room temperature prior to administration. Shaking the suspension thoroughly before loading the syringe will ensure that the drug is evenly dispersed in the suspension.

Lypressin (Diapid) is a solution designed for intranasal administration. To reiterate what has already been mentioned in Therapeutic Uses, **desmopressin acetate** (DDAVP) is a vasopressin analogue formulated in an isotonic solution for intravenous, intramuscular, subcutaneous or intranasal administration.

Evaluation

Nursing evaluation of the patient following the administration of vasopressin should focus on observing indicators of effectiveness, including an increased fluid intake/output ratio, improved skin turgor, reduced urinary frequency, urine specific gravity of more than 1.020 and a sleep pattern uninterrupted by waking to void. Nursing evaluation should also attempt to identify adverse effects of the medication, specifically, excessive fluid retention, increased intestinal peristalsis (abdominal cramps and diarrhea), uterine cramps and contractions, elevated blood pressure and hypersensitivity.

Teaching

Nurses should teach patients the correct techniques for self-administration at home. Patients and their families should be instructed to observe and report the effectiveness of the drug and the occurrence of adverse effects.

Thiazides

The pharmacology of the thiazides and their nursing processes are presented in Chapter 16. In view of their diuretic properties, it might seem unusual, to say the least, to include thiazides in a chapter dealing with drugs that increase the conservation of water. However, by producing mild volume depletion, thiazides enhance proximal tubular reabsorption of glomerular filtrate. This action reduces delivery of water to the distal parts of the nephron that are dependent on the secretion of vasopressin for water reabsorption. As a result, the consequences of a reduction in the secretion of vasopressin are not so readily apparent.

Chlorothiazide (Diuril) and hydrochlorothiazide (Esidrix, HydroDiuril) are the two drugs used most often. They are employed primarily in the treatment of nephrogenic diabetes insipidus. The usual doses of chlorothiazide or hydrochlorothiazide are 1 – 1.5 g or 50 – 150 mg, respectively, in daily divided doses. Thiazides are not effective unless dietary sodium is restricted.

Further Reading

Cobb, W. E., Spare, S. and Reichlin, S. (1978). Neurogenic diabetes insipidus: Management with DDAVP. *Ann. Intern. Med. 88* : 183-188.

Table 19
Drugs that increase the renal conservation of water.

Generic Name (Trade Name)	Use (Dose)	Action	Adverse Effects	Drug Interactions	Nursing Process
Pharmacologic Classification: Antidiuretic Hormone					
Vasopressin (Pitressin)	Symptomatic control of diabetes insipidus (**IM/SC**/*not IV*: Adults - 5-10 units [0.25-0.5 mL] tid or qid. Children - 2.5-10 units [0.125-0.5 mL] tid or qid)	Incr. permeability of collecting ducts to H₂O; permits water reabsorpt'n, retent'n.	Focal or systemic allergic react'ns, anaphylaxis, tremor, sweating, vertigo, circumoral pallor, "pounding" in head, abdominal cramps, flatulence, nausea, vomiting, urticaria, bronchiole constrict'n	**Corticosteroids:** Vasopressin incr. plasma cortisol levels. **Drugs affecting BP:** Vasopressin is a vasoconstrictor and will modify the actions of other drugs that influence BP.	**Assess:** Pregnancy; pt hx of CV disease, hypersensitivity. Establish baseline fluid intake/output levels, skin turgor, urinary frequency, BP, sleep patterns. **Administer:** Precise dose via proper route. Store in refrigerator. Slowly warm parenteral solut'ns to room temp. before injecting. Have pt clear nasal passages prior to intranasal administrat'n. **Evaluate:** Indicators of effectiveness; for adv. effects. **Teach:** Proper self-administrat'n; to observe and report adv. effects.
Vasopressin tannate (Pitressin Tannate)	As for vasopressin (**IM:** Adults - 1.25-5 units [0.25-1 mL suspension in peanut oil containing 5 pressor units/mL] prn, us. q1-3 days. Children - 1.25-2.5 units [0.25-0.5 mL] in peanut oil prn, us. q1-3 days)	As for vasopressin	As for vasopressin	As for vasopressin	As for vasopressin
Lypressin (Diapid)	As for vasopressin (**Intranasal:** One or more sprays of solut'n containing 50 pressor units [0.185 mg] per mL applied to one or both nostrils. Us. tid or qid, but dose and interval bet. applicat'ns must be determined individually)	As for vasopressin	As for vasopressin	As for vasopressin	As for vasopressin
Desmopressin acetate (DDAVP)	Antidiuretic hormone replacement tx for central diabetes insipidus, 1° and 2°. W'draw pt from previous medicat'n and establish baseline polyuria and	As for vasopressin	As for vasopressin	As for vasopressin	As for vasopressin

polydipsia. **(IV/IM/SC:** Adults -
0.25-1.0 mL [1-4 µg] od.
Children - 0.1 mL [0.4 µg] od.
Intranasal: Requires a higher
dose than IV administrat'n,
since only 10% of intranasal
desmopressin is absorbed.
Intranasal dosage is therefore
10x larger than IV dosage)

SECTION 5

Water, Electrolytes and Acid-Base Balance

It is unusual to consider water, sodium, potassium, calcium, magnesium and hydrogen as drugs. However, alterations in the amounts of any of these substances in the body can have profound effects on our ability to carry out normal biological functions. In the face of either an excess or a deficit in their levels, appropriate steps must be taken to restore normal concentrations. Nurses play a vital role in any corrective measures taken. Section 5 discusses the consequences of alterations in body water and electrolyte levels, the effects of metabolic and respiratory alkalosis and acidosis, the pharmacologic interventions available and the nursing process associated with these interventions.

C H A P T E R   1 8

Water, Electrolytes and Acid-Base Balance

General Considerations

Body water may be divided into intracellular and extracellular compartments. Extracellular water is composed of interstitial water and plasma. Electrolytes are dissolved in these water compartments and they contribute to the osmolality, pH and volume of liquid found at each site. Under normal conditions the kidneys and lungs combine to control electrolyte concentrations and water volume in the body. However, conditions may arise that alter either water volume or concentrations of electrolytes, or both. When this occurs, prompt attention may be required to prevent irreparable damage. This chapter will discuss the conditions that alter water and/or electrolyte balance in the body and the measures that can be taken to restore them to normal.

Total body water varies from 50% of body mass/weight in obese adults to 70% in lean adults. Major differences exist in both the volume and content of the intracellular and extracellular water compartments. Approximately 55% of the total body water is found intracellularly and 35% extracellularly. The remaining 10% can be divided between inaccessible bone water (7.5%) and transcellular water (2.5%) compartments. These latter compartments will not be discussed further, as they play little role in the maintenance of osmolality and pH.

The composition of electrolytes and protein in plasma water is given in Table 20. Sodium is the major cation found in plasma. Chloride and bicarbonate are the anions existing in highest concentrations. Potassium levels are low in plasma. The

Table 20
Comparison of electrolytes and protein in plasma (mEq/L).

	Cations			Anions
Sodium	135 – 145	Chloride		98 – 106
Potassium	3.5 – 5.0	Bicarbonate		24 – 28
Calcium	4.5 – 5.3	Phosphate and sulfate	2 – 5	
Magnesium	1.5 – 2.0	Organic anions		3 – 6
		Protein		15 – 20

plasma concentrations of these electrolytes differ only slightly from their levels interstitially.

Potassium and magnesium are the major cations in the intracellular water. The prominent anions are phosphate and protein. Little sodium chloride and bicarbonate are found intracellularly. Table 21 presents the concentrations of electrolytes in intracellular water of muscle tissue. They represent the approximate levels of electrolytes within other tissues.

The difference in the concentrations of sodium and potassium in the extracellular and intracellular water compartments is the result of the active transport of sodium out of, and potassium into, the cells. Osmotic pressure is the major factor responsible for the transport of water from one compartment to the other. An increase in sodium concentration in the body, together with its inability to enter body cells in high amounts, will draw water from the intracellular compartment into the extracellular space. By the same token, the accumulation of higher concentrations of potassium within cells causes water to diffuse from the extracellular compartment into the intracellular water space.

Table 21
Composition of electrolytes and protein in muscle intracellular water (mEq/L).

	Cations		Anions
Sodium	10	Bicarbonate	10
Potassium	150	Phosphate and sulfate	150
Magnesium	40	Protein	40

Dehydration and Water Intoxication

Dehydration

Dehydration is a water deficit that occurs either as a result of inadequate intake or increased loss of water. The former is most often encountered in unconscious patients or patients with esophageal or pyloric obstruction who are unable to ingest water. Increased water loss results from such situations as fever, a hot environment, low levels of antidiuretic hormone (ADH) secretion or insensitivity of the kidney to the actions of ADH (see Section 4). Other causes of increased water loss include renal disease, impaired capacity to reabsorb water (secondary to potassium depletion) and intensive diuretic treatment.

Water deficit is treated by administering water. It can be given alone or with electrolytes. If it is required alone, water can be given with 2.5 – 5% dextrose. The latter substance, a sugar, is oxidized in the body to produce water. Two to three liters of water can be given per day if renal function is normal. In the face of dehydration with increased serum sodium concentration, water can be given to restore the normal osmolality of the serum.

Nursing Process
Assessment
Nursing assessment of patients experiencing water deficit will reveal thirst, a dehydrated appearance, dry skin, dry mucous membranes, flushed skin, increased heart rate, oliguria, concentrated urine (specific gravity greater than 1.030) and hyperpnea. Additional observations will include weight loss, fever, lowered blood pressure and postural hypotension. Pushed to the extreme, hallucinations, delirium and coma occur.

Administration
Regardless of the pharmacologic intervention initiated by the physician to treat the dehydrated patient, the nursing responsibilities will emphasize safe intravenous and oral administration of the fluids and patient evaluation.

Evaluation

Nursing evaluation of patients being treated for dehydration should include careful monitoring of the patient's fluid intake and output and regular reassessment of the patient in order to evaluate the progress towards normal hydration, and to prevent excess hydration resulting in water intoxication.

Water Intoxication

Water intoxication is water excess that occurs if intake exceeds elimination. The most common causes are the parenteral administration of large volumes of water or reduced elimination of water due to renal insufficiency, congestive heart failure or liver disease accompanied by ascites.

Water excess is treated by restricting its intake. If severe water intoxication is present, the patient may be given a hypertonic solution of sodium chloride to increase water movement from the intracellular to the extracellular space and decrease intracellular water volume.

Nursing Process

Assessment

Nursing assessment of patients experiencing water intoxication will reveal polyuria, progressive deterioration in the level of consciousness (lethargy, confusion, stupor, coma), neuromuscular hyperexcitability (increased reflexes, muscular twitching, convulsions), headache, gastrointestinal disturbances (nausea, vomiting, gastrointestinal cramps), high skin turgor and edema.

Evaluation

Nursing actions at this stage are the same as for patients who are dehydrated. However, the purpose of the action is different. Monitoring of the fluid intake and output of the water-intoxicated patient is conducted for the purpose of maintaining fluid restriction; reassessment of the patient focuses on the return to normal hydration and prevention of dehydration.

Hyponatremia and Hypernatremia

Hyponatremia

Hyponatremia occurs when the plasma sodium concentration falls below 130 – 135 mEq/L. This can occur as a result of loss of sodium or retention of water. In either case, the concentration of sodium in the plasma falls. In the first situation a marked loss of sodium can result from the overenthusiastic application of diuretic therapy. Other causes of sodium loss include excessive sweating, a high level of gastrointestinal secretions and renal or adrenocortical insufficiency.

When hyponatremia is the result of water retention instead of sodium loss, it is called **dilutional hyponatremia.** Water may be retained in large quantities following the use of ADH. Chronic severe heart failure, cirrhosis of the liver with ascites and the nephrotic syndrome may also result in water retention.

The treatment of hyponatremia depends on its etiology. If hyponatremia is a result of a sodium deficit, it may be treated by the administration of sodium chloride, with or without sodium bicarbonate. Moderate deficits in adults are usually handled by administering 0.9% sodium chloride, which contains 155 mEq of sodium and chloride per liter. Ringer's solution may also be used, with or without lactate. More severe sodium deficits usually require 3% or 5% solutions of sodium chloride, which contain 513 and 855 mEq per liter, respectively. If water retention is the cause of the hyponatremia, water intake should be reduced. Sodium should not be administered in dilutional hyponatremia, as the total body sodium is normal or even elevated.

Nursing Process

Assessment

When a nursing assessment is conducted, patients with hyponatremia will demonstrate muscle weakness, leg cramps, dry mouth, dizziness and gastrointestinal disturbances (nausea, vomiting, cramps).

Evaluation

Nursing responsibilities related to the evaluation phase of the nursing process emphasize observing for positive responses to therapy, including changes in laboratory results, and being alert for excessive responses that might result in hypernatremia.

Hypernatremia

Hypernatremia is defined as serum or plasma sodium levels above the normal range. This usually means concentrations of sodium in excess of 150 mEq/L. The increased sodium levels may be a result of either an increased sodium intake without a commensurate increase in water, or a loss of water, without a corresponding increase in sodium elimination. On nursing assessment, evidence of hypernatremia will be displayed as central nervous system disturbances (confusion, stupor, coma), poor skin turgor and, possibly, postural hypotension (if the hypernatremia is due to water loss).

Hypernatremia resulting from an increase in sodium intake may be treated by reducing the amount of sodium provided to the patient. Diuretics may also be used to hasten sodium elimination. However, in this case, the water lost as a result of the diuretic must be replaced. If hypernatremia is due to a deficit of water, it is treated by administering water.

Nursing Process

Just as with the treatment of sodium depletion, nursing responsibilities related to the treatment of patients with hypernatremia should stress monitoring of the fluid intake and output, observing for evidence of alleviation of the negative findings of nursing assessment and prevention of hyponatremia.

Hypokalemia and Hyperkalemia

Hypokalemia

Hypokalemia occurs when serum potassium levels fall below 3.5 mEq/L. A fall in serum potassium usually indicates a decrease in total body potassium. However, this is not always the case. Acute alkalosis, treatment with insulin or stimulation of beta receptors may lower serum potassium values without decreasing the total body potassium content. By the same token, total body potassium may fall without producing a decrease in serum potassium concentrations. This can be explained by the fact that most body potassium is found intracellularly, not extracellularly.

It is not possible in this text to list and explain all the possible causes of a total body potassium deficit. In short, they include reduced potassium intake or increased potassium elimination. In the first instance, conditions such as starvation, upper gastrointestinal obstruction, steatorrhea and regional enteritis will decrease potassium intake. Increased potassium loss may occur through the gastrointestinal tract if emesis or diarrhea occurs, or via the kidneys, in conditions involving congenital tubule malfunction or diuresis from diabetes or diuretics. Metabolic alkalosis, burns and increased secretion of adrenocortical hormones may also increase potassium loss. The administration of large amounts of sodium chloride without potassium will increase potassium loss as it is exchanged for some of the increased sodium presented to the renal distal convoluted tubules.

Hypokalemia can be treated by administering potassium, either orally or parenterally. Potassium is toxic and care must be taken to prevent hyperkalemia. The kidneys are the main route for the elimination of potassium and their status must be assessed prior to beginning potassium therapy.

Hypokalemia is common when thiazide or loop diuretics are used (Chapter 16). Potassium-sparing diuretics are often combined with these drugs to minimize their hypokalemic effects. An alternate approach to prevent hypokalemia is the administration of sustained-release potassium chloride preparations. Slow-K and Micro-K Extencaps contain 600 mg (8 mEq K^+) per tablet or capsule, respectively. Klotrix and K-Tabs contain 750 mg of potassium chloride (equivalent to 10 mEq K^+). K-Lyte effervescent tablets contain 25 mEq or 50 mEq potassium as the bicarbonate and citrate salts.

The dosage of potassium must be individualized according to the patient's needs. Approximately 20 – 40 mEq of potassium is given to prevent hypokalemia. Potassium depletion is treated with approximately 40 mEq to a maximum of 100 mEq per day. In general, a daily dose exceeding 60 mEq of potassium should not be required. Potassium salts should be administered with milk or after meals in two or three divided doses per day to minimize gastric irritation and too-rapid absorption. Nausea, vomiting, diarrhea and abdominal cramps are the most frequent adverse effects.

Nursing Process

Assessment
Nursing assessment of patients with hypokalemia will display impaired neuromuscular function, including postural hypotension, weakness, flaccid paralysis and difficulty breathing; progressive disturbance of mental functioning (lethargy,

irritability, confusion); abnormal myocardial function (arrhythmias, congestive heart failure, heart block, cardiac arrest); and progressive gastrointestinal disorders (anorexia, intestinal distention, paralytic ileus).

Administration

Oral solutions of potassium should be diluted in strongly flavored drinks to disguise their taste and decrease gastric distress caused by the irritating ion. Whenever possible, dietary measures should be used to the greatest extent possible to treat hypokalemia.

Potassium chloride may be given parenterally, either in saline or glucose solution, in a dose of 1 – 3 mEq per kilogram of body mass every twenty-four hours. Intravenous solutions should never be administered undiluted; they should be highly diluted to provide a maximum of 20 mEq per hour. In addition, these solutions must be well mixed to prevent "crowning" in the intravenous bag. The rate of administration should be checked every fifteen minutes to assure that the patient's changing of position or some other factor does not alter the intravenous flow rate. The use of a perfusion pump is advised and highly desirable with children. Potentially fatal hyperkalemia, with the resultant cardiac arrhythmias, could result from too-rapid infusion. Patient reports of pain at the infusion site should be responded to by slowing the rate of infusion.

Evaluation

Nurses who are evaluating patients receiving oral potassium should observe for abdominal pain, distention, gastrointestinal bleeding or other evidence of stenosis or ulcers of the small intestine. All patients receiving potassium should have their fluid intake and output ratios monitored carefully. Any evidence of oliguria, anuria, or azotemia should result in withholding the medication. Nurses caring for these patients should observe carefully for clinical and laboratory evidence of hyperkalemia.

Hyperkalemia

Hyperkalemia denotes a serum potassium concentration above 5 mEq/L. It is caused by either increased potassium intake or decreased potassium elimination. Excessive potassium administration, either parenterally or orally, can cause hyperkalemia. Kidney failure reduces potassium elimination and can produce hyperkalemia. Other causes include the release of intracellular potassium in burns, severe infections and crush injuries. In these situations potassium moves from the intracellular to extracellular water compartments and serum potassium levels increase. Metabolic acidosis also causes potassium to move from the intracellular water to the extracellular compartment.

The major consequence of hyperkalemia is its deleterious effect on heart function. Depending on the degree of hyperkalemia, minor alterations in conduction may proceed through a lengthening of A-V conduction to a depression of impulse generation and conduction in all heart tissue. Asystole is the eventual outcome. This may be preceded by ventricular tachycardia and/or fibrillation. Plasma potassium levels of 5 – 7 mEq/L produce major depression in heart function.

Potassium is withheld from patients with hyperkalemia. A potassium exchange resin, sodium polysterene sulfonate (Kayexalate), may be given either orally or by enema. It is less effective when given rectally. This material retains potassium in the gastrointestinal tract and is eliminated in the feces.

If hyperkalemia is very severe and an emergency arises, insulin or calcium may be given intravenously. Insulin causes a deposition of potassium in the liver, thereby lowering plasma potassium levels. Calcium has the opposite actions to those of potassium on the heart and serves as an antagonist. Sodium bicarbonate, given intravenously, raises the pH of the extracellular fluid and, as a result, causes potassium to move from extracellular water into intracellular water. The resulting fall in serum potassium reduces its effect on the heart. Hemodialysis may be used in patients with renal insufficiency.

Nursing Process

Assessment

Nursing assessment of hyperkalemic patients prior to pharmacological intervention will reveal irritability (progressing from central nervous system irritability through muscular irritability to cardiac arrhythmias if untreated), gastrointestinal disturbances (nausea, intestinal colic, diarrhea), neuromuscular disruptions (weakness, flaccid paralysis, dysphasia), oliguria or anuria.

Administration

Orally administered Kayexalate should be mixed with a small amount of water or syrup to facilitate its administration. Although less effective, Kayexalate is infrequently administered rectally. In such cases it should be inserted deep (20 cm) into the sigmoid colon.

Evaluation

Nursing evaluation of patients receiving treatment for hyperkalemia should monitor carefully the patient's fluid intake/output ratios, because increased urinary output might indicate increased potassium excretion and potential hypokalemia if therapy is maintained. Nursing evaluation should also emphasize reassessment of the patient for positive evidence of response to therapy and for evidence of excessive elimination of potassium resulting in hypokalemia. Frequent monitoring of the patient is essential. Nurses should conduct a physical examination of the patient's signs and symptoms every two to four hours. Nurses caring for these patients should expect physicians to order daily laboratory testing of electrolytes. If cardiac irregularities have been evident, nurses should anticipate the physician ordering an electrocardiogram or even ECG monitoring.

Hypocalcemia and Hypercalcemia

Approximately 2% of the body's mass is calcium. Only 1% of this amount of calcium is in solution in body fluids. The normal total plasma or serum concentration of calcium ranges between 4.5 – 5.5 mEq/L. Levels above 5.8 mEq/L are classified as hypercalcemia, and concentrations below 4.5 mEq/L constitute hypocalcemia.

Hypocalcemia

The causes of hypocalcemia include hypoparathyroidism, chronic renal insufficiency and malabsorption syndromes. Hypocalcemia may produce rickets and osteomalacia. Calcium is an essential ion for many enzymes. It is important in membrane function and plays a vital role in neuromuscular function.

The treatment of hypocalcemia involves correcting the primary disease causing the low plasma levels. Thus, hypoparathyroidism is treated with vitamin D and calcium. This is discussed in more detail in Chapter 27. If tetany is present, calcium gluconate in a 10% solution can be given intravenously. A variety of different calcium salts are available for oral administration to treat less severe symptoms. These include calcium chloride, lactate, gluconate and carbonate.

Nursing Process

Assessment

Low plasma calcium concentrations will result in patients whose nursing assessment shows muscle hyperirritability (which can proceed to tetany and convulsions), alterations in the ECG, with the Q-T interval lengthening and the S-T segment being prolonged (owing to decreased myocardial contractility), stridor and dyspnea, abdominal cramps, urinary frequency and diplopia.

Administration

The major nursing responsibility is to administer oral doses of calcium salts approximately one hour after meals so that absorption will be least interfered with by alkalis and fats. Intravenous administration should be used only when oral administration is absolutely impossible, and then only at a very slow infusion rate accompanied by careful monitoring of vital signs for bradycardia and hypotension.

Evaluation

Patient response to therapy is evaluated by nursing assessment that reveals normal serum levels of calcium. Patients should also be carefully observed for evidence of hypercalcemia.

Hypercalcemia

Hypercalcemia also alters neuromuscular function. However, in contradistinction to hypocalcemia, which causes skeletal muscle hyperirritability, hypercalcemia produces muscle weakness as excitability is diminished.

If possible, the cause of hypercalcemia should be treated. Hypercalcemia is caused by hyperparathyroidism, bone neoplasms, sarcoidosis, multiple myeloma and vitamin D intoxication. Symptomatic hypercalcemia carries a high mortality rate and must be treated quickly. Calcium excretion can be increased by the use of diuretics. Obviously water, sodium, potassium and possibly also magnesium may need to be replaced when large diuretic doses are administered. Once the primary disease is treated, diuretic therapy may be discontinued. If hypercalcemia is a result of sarcoidosis or neoplasm activity, corticosteroid therapy, such as prednisone, may be used.

Nursing Process

Hypercalcemic patients undergoing nursing assessment show an increase in myocardial contractility and ventricular extra beats, possibly proceeding to idioventricular rhythm; polyuria, with accompanying thirst; anorexia and vomiting; occasionally, constipation; stupor and coma.

Nursing responsibilities are primarily related to the proper administration of the prescribed pharmacological agent such as calcitonin, EDTA, intravenous saline, sulfate and citrate salts, corticosteroids, or furosemide. The evaluation of the patient emphasizes positive response to the therapy or early detection of hypocalcemia. The reader should refer to appropriate sections of this book, or to package literature or specialty texts for further information about those pharmaceutical products used to treat hypercalcemia in specialized critical care settings.

Hypomagnesemia and Hypermagnesemia

Magnesium is an ion that receives relatively little attention when compared with sodium, potassium and calcium. However, aberrations in magnesium plasma concentrations can cause alterations in body function. Magnesium is essential to the action of many enzymes. Peripherally, it blocks the release of acetylcholine and decreases neuromuscular excitability. Normal plasma magnesium levels vary from 1.5 – 2.5 mEq/L.

Hypomagnesemia

Hypomagnesemia may be seen following starvation, diarrhea, malabsorption and primary aldosteronism. It may also be present in the alcoholic patient or following enthusiastic diuretic therapy. Hypoparathyroidism can produce hypomagnesemia. The ingestion of large doses of calcium and vitamin D will also lower plasma magnesium levels.

The treatment of hypomagnesemia involves administering magnesium chloride or sulfate parenterally in a dose of 10 – 40 mEq per day initially to overcome the severe deficiency. Thereafter, a maintenance dose of 10 mEq per day can be given.

Nursing Process

Low levels of magnesium result in patient assessment that reveals neuromuscular irritability and contractability (hyperactive reflexes, facial twitching, tetany, convulsions) and progressive psychological disorders (hallucinations, delusion, confusion). Nurses should evaluate the effectiveness of the magnesium supplement and observe any adverse effects.

Hypermagnesemia

Magnesium is eliminated from the body by the kidneys. Hypermagnesemia occurs when renal function is impaired and the body cannot eliminate the magnesium absorbed from food. Elevated plasma magnesium levels produce central and peripheral nervous system depression. Deep tendon reflexes are decreased if plasma magnesium levels exceed 4 mEq/L. In addition, changes in heart function may appear if the concentration of the ion reaches 10 – 15 mEq/L. These include an increase in the P-R interval, broadened QRS complexes, and elevated T-waves. However, death is usually not due to a depressed cardiac function. Rather, it results from respiratory muscle paralysis because of the decreased release of acetylcholine at the motor end-plates. Respiratory paralysis is a potential hazard as plasma magnesium levels reach 12 – 15 mEq/L.

Treatment involves the administration of calcium to antagonize the effects of magnesium on skeletal muscle, and extracorporeal or peritoneal dialysis to clear magnesium from the body. Nursing evaluation focuses on monitoring the effectiveness of the treatment in removing excess magnesium and on identification of early indications of hypomagnesemia.

Hydrogen Ion Concentration, Acidosis and Alkalosis

Food metabolism results in the production of the strongly acidic anions phosphate and sulfate. In addition, lactic acid and acetoacetic acid are formed as a result of the metabolism of fat and carbohydrates. Under normal circumstances these acids are buffered in the body and the hydrogen ion concentration, or pH, of the body fluids does not change. Both the kidneys and the lungs play a vital role in regulating body pH. The kidney eliminates both bicarbonate and hydrogen ions. The lungs expire carbon dioxide, thereby lowering the concentration of carbonic acid in the body.

Nursing assessment parameters related to acidosis and alkalosis are briefly summarized at the end of this chapter. Detailed information related to the relevant nursing actions and responsibilities is beyond the scope of this book. Readers seeking such information are advised to consult a medical-surgical nursing text.

Respiratory Acidosis

Respiratory acidosis results from the failure of the lungs to eliminate CO_2. As a result, pCO_2 rises in the alveoli and arterial blood. The usual causes include asthma, emphysema, suppression of the respiratory center by drugs or central nervous system disease, weakness of the respiratory muscles or inadequate ventilation during anesthesia.

Treatment involves improving ventilation. This can be done with bronchodilators (see Chapter 32) or mechanical aids. If drugs are responsible for the respiratory depression, steps should be taken to reverse their effects. In the case of anesthetics or most other central nervous system depressants, this may mean simply reducing the dose or stopping treatment. Narcotics may be reversed by the use of specific antagonists, such as naloxone (Narcan). If respiratory acidosis is severe, it may be necessary to infuse sodium bicarbonate to correct the pH quickly.

Respiratory Alkalosis

Respiratory alkalosis occurs when the pCO_2 falls due to hyperventilation. As a result, the pH of the extracellular fluid increases. The most common cause of hyperventilation is anxiety or fear. Although the body responds to the decrease in pCO_2 by excreting more bicarbonate base via the kidneys, this process occurs too slowly to attenuate the effects of hyperventilation. The increase in pH can produce increased neuromuscular irritability, asterixis and tetany. Treatment of spontaneous hyperventilation due to anxiety can involve the

administration of antianxiety drugs. The immediate problems of tetany can be handled by having the patient breathe into a bag. By inhaling the expired CO_2 the patient will increase the pCO_2 and terminate the respiratory alkalosis.

Metabolic Acidosis

Metabolic acidosis is caused by the overproduction of acid. This occurs in severe diabetes mellitus accompanied by ketosis. The excessive loss of base, such as is seen when bicarbonate is eliminated in large amounts in diarrhea, can also produce acidosis. Renal insufficiency reduces the capacity of the kidney to excrete hydrogen ions and this, too, may cause metabolic acidosis. In addition, kidney failure limits the ability of the body to excrete phosphate and sulfate. This, combined with the increased loss of sodium due to the failure of the kidney to exchange it for hydrogen ions, increases metabolic acidosis.

Treatment of metabolic acidosis involves correcting the specific condition causing the acidosis. Thus, diabetes is treated with insulin and electrolytes, such as sodium, potassium and bicarbonate, together with water replacement. In renal insufficiency, water and electrolyte deficits are corrected. If serum phosphate levels are high, aluminum-containing preparations can be given orally to reduce phosphate absorption from the gastrointestinal tract. Hyperkalemia, if present, can be treated as described earlier.

Metabolic Alkalosis

Metabolic alkalosis can result from the loss of gastric acid or the ingestion of large amounts of sodium bicarbonate. It can also occur as a result of potassium deficiency. As indicated in Chapter 16, potassium and hydrogen are secreted in the distal convoluted tubules and collecting ducts of the nephron in exchange for the reabsorption of sodium. In the face of low potassium levels, increased quantities of hydrogen are exchanged for sodium and metabolic alkalosis can ensue.

Metabolic alkalosis is treated by replacing either chloride, if its loss from the stomach is the cause of alkalosis, or potassium, if its deficiency precipitated the increased renal elimination of hydrogen ions. Obviously, water and other electrolytes should also be replaced if their levels are low.

Further Reading

Hamilton, Helen (1987). *Monitoring Fluid and Electrolytes Precisely.* Horsham, Pennsylvania: Intermed Communications.

Luckman, Joan and Sorenson (1980). "Fluid and Electrolytic Imbalances." In: *Medical-Surgical Nursing: A Psychophysiologic Approach,* pp. 171-228. Toronto: W. B. Saunders.

Steel, J. (1983). Too fast or too slow: The erratic IV. *Am. J. Nurs. 83* : 898-901.

White, S. (1979). IV fluids and electrolytes: How to head off the risks. *R.N. 42* (11):60-64.

Table 22
Water, electrolytes and acid-base balance.

Physiological State	Description	Cause	Pharmacologic Intervention	Findings of Nursing Assessment	Nursing Process
Dehydration	Water deficit	1. Inadequate fluid intake • unconsciousness • esophageal or pyloric obstruct'n 2. Incr. water loss • fever • heat • low ADH levels • renal disease • K deplet'n • diuretic overdose	2000-3000 mL H_2O w. 2.5% or 5% dextrose IV per day	• low fluid intake and/or high output • poor skin turgor • dry mucous membranes • thirst • flushed skin • incr. pulse rate • oliguria; conc. urine, specific gravity > 1.030 • hyperpnea • sudden excess. weight loss • elevated temp. • lowered BP, postural hypotens'n • eyeballs sunken, darkening of skin under eyes • prog. CNS disturbances: anxiety, apprehens'n, restlessness, hallucinat'ns, delirium, coma	1. **Monitor:** fluid intake carefully 2. **Observe** for: • return to normal findings in nsg assessment • water intoxication
Water intoxication	Water excess	1. Excess. intake; infus'n of large volumes of fluid 2. Reduced eliminat'n • renal insufficiency • CHF • liver disease w. ascites	• restrict'n of fluid intake • hypertonic NaCl solut'n • diuretics (see Chapter 16)	• polyuria • prog. deter. in LOC: lethargy, confus'n, stupor, coma • neuromuscular hyperexcitability: incr. reflexes, musc. twitching, convuls'ns • headache • nausea, vomiting, GI cramps • high skin turgor, edema	1. **Monitor:** fluid intake/output carefully 2. **Observe** for: • return to normal findings in nsg assessment • dehydrat'n
Hyponatremia	Serum Na < 130-135 mEq/L	1. Loss of Na • diuretic overdose • excess. sweating • high level of secret'ns • renal insufficiency • adrenocortical insufficiency	Determined by cause: 1. Administrat'n of • 0.9% NaCl solut'n containing 155 mEq NaCl/L • Ringer's solut'n • 3% or 5% NaCl solut'ns containing 513 and 855 mEq/L	• muscle weakness, leg cramps • dry mouth • dizziness • GI disturbances: nausea, vomiting, cramps	1. **Monitor:** fluid intake/output carefully 2. **Observe** for: • return to normal findings in nsg assessment • hypernatremia

Condition	Etiology	Treatment	Signs/Symptoms	Nursing Care
Hypernatremia Serum Na > 150 mEq/L	2. Water retent'n • use of ADH (vasopressin) • heart failure • cirrhosis • nephrotic syndrome 1. Incr. Na intake 2. Incr. fluid loss	2. Restrict fluid intake 1. Restrict Na intake; combine diuretics w. fluid replacement 2. Administer fluids	• CNS disturbances: confusion, stupor, coma • poor skin turgor • postural hypotens'n	1. **Monitor:** fluid intake/output carefully 2. **Observe for:** • return to normal findings in nsg assessment • hyponatremia
Hypokalemia Serum K < 3.5 mEq/L	1. Reduced K intake • starvat'n • upper GI obstruct'n • steatorrhea • regional enteritis 2. Incr. K loss • vomiting • diarrhea • diuresis • metabolic acidosis • burns • excess. adrenocortical hormones	1. KCl • oral: us. 40-100 mEq/day • parenteral: 1-3 mEq KCl/kg in glucose or saline solut'n q24h 2. Potassium gluconate • oral: 40-100 mEq/day	• impaired neuromuscular funct'n: postural hypotens'n, weakness, flaccid paralysis, dyspnea • prog. disturbance of mental funct'n: lethargy, irritability, confus'n • abnormal myocardial funct'n: arrhythmias, CHF, heart block, cardiac arrest • prog. GI disturbances: anorexia, intestinal distent'n, paralytic ileus	1. **Monitor:** urine output; discontinue IV K if output < 1 mL/h 2. **Observe for:** • indicat'ns of stenosis or ulcers of small intestine • oliguria • hyperkalemia 3. **Administer:** • IV — never give undiluted • rate should be adjusted to provide max. 20 mEq/h • if pain in vein, slow rate
Hyperkalemia Serum K > 5.5 mEq/L	1. Incr. K intake • parenteral • oral 2. Decr. K eliminat'n • kidney failure • burns • infect'ns • crush injuries • metabolic acidosis	1. Restrict K intake 2. Kayexalate • oral: 15-60 g/day, divided into 4 doses • rectal: 30 - 50 g/day 3. Insulin	• prog. deter. in cardiac funct'n: minor conduct'n changes, lengthened A-V conduct'n, depressed myocardial impulse generat'n, ventr. tachycardia, ventr. fibrillat'n, asystole • irritability • nausea, intestinal colic, diarrhea • weakness, flaccid paralysis, dysphasia • oliguria, anuria	1. **Monitor:** fluid intake/output carefully 2. **Administer:** mix Kayexalate w. small am't water or syrup to give orally 3. **Observe for:** • return to normal findings in nsg assessment • hypokalemia
Hypocalcemia Serum Ca < 4.5 mEq/L	• hypoparathyroidism • chronic renal insufficiency • malabsorpt'n syndromes	1. Correct'n of underlying condit'n 2. Calcium gluconate for tetany • oral: 1-2 g tid • IV: 0.5-2 g 3. Calcium acetate • oral: 0.325-1.3 g tid 4. $CaCO_3$ • oral: 1-2 g tid	• muscle hyperirritability, proceeding to tetany and convuls'ns • altered cardiac funct'n: decr. myocardial contractility, lengthened Q-T interval, prolonged S-T segment • stridor, dyspnea	1. **Administer:** • orally: Ca salts 1 h pc • IV: very slowly 2. **Observe for:** • return to normal findings in nsg assessment • hypercalcemia

Physiological State	Description	Cause	Pharmacologic Intervention	Findings of Nursing	Nursing Process
				• abdominal cramps • urinary frequency • diplopia • rickets • osteomalacia	
Hypercalcemia	Serum Ca > 5.8 mEq/L	• hyperparathyroidism • bone neoplasms • sarcoidosis • multiple myeloma • vitamin D intoxicat'n	• tx underlying cause • diuretics to incr. Ca excret'n • parenteral isotonic saline • steroids • isotonic disodium phosphate • monopotassium phosphate • isotonic sodium sulfate in water [2 L IV]	• dim. muscle excitability, muscle weakness • incr. myocadial contractility, extraventr. contract'ns, proceeding to idioventr. rhythm • polyuria w. accompanying thirst, proceeding to renal failure • anorexia, nausea, vomiting lethargy, exhaust'n, confus'n, irritability	**Observe** for: • return to normal findings in nsg assessment • hypocalcemia
Hypomagnesemia	Serum Mg < 1.5 mEq/L	• starvat'n • diarrhea • malabsorpt'n • chronic alcoholism • chronic nephritis • hypoparathyroidism	• tx underlying cause • magnesium chloride, 10-40 mEq/day to overcome deficiency; maint. dose, 10 mEq/day	• incr. neuromuscular irritabili- ty and contractility; hyperac- tive reflexes, facial twitching, tetany, convuls'ns • prog. psychological disorders: hallucinat'ns, delus'n, confus'n	**Observe** for: • return to normal findings in nsg assessment • hypermagnesemia
Hypermagnesemia	Serum Mg > 2.5 mEq/L	• impaired renal funct'n • excess. replacement follow- ing hypomagnesemia • excess. use of antacids containing Mg, e.g., Gelusil	• calcium gluconate 10%	• CNS and PNS depress'n: sedat'n, hypnosis, paralysis of skeletal and respiratory muscles • warm sensat'n throughout body • fall in BP • cardiac irregularities: incr. P-R inteval, broadened QRS complexes, elevated T-waves	**Observe** for: • return to normal findings in nsg assessment • hypomagnesemia
Respiratory acidosis	Elevated pCO_2 levels	Failure to eliminate CO_2 via lungs, owing to • asthma • emphysema	1. Bronchodilators (see Chapter 32) 2. W'drawal of drugs w. depres- sive effect on CNS	• dyspnea on exert'n, hyper- ventilat'n at rest, wheezing, cyanosis • tachycardia	**Observe** for: • depressed respirat'ns, tetany, GI disturbances • hyperkalemia, depressed

Condition	Defining values	Causes	Treatment	Signs and symptoms / Observe for

(continued)		• respiratory depress'n (drugs, CNS disease)
		• weakness of respiratory muscles
		• inadequate ventilat'n during anesthesia
			3. NaHCO₃
			  • oral: 5 g q30min
			  • IV: 0.25 g/kg
			4. THAM - IV, 300 mL/h
			5. Sodium lactate, 20 mg/kg IV, until urine is alkaline
				• respirat'n, apnea, hypoglycemia
				• metabolic acidosis
				• urine pH < 6.0

Respiratory alkalosis	Decreased pCO₂ levels	Hyperventilat'n owing to • anxiety • fear	Anxiolytics (see Chapter 46)	• neuromuscular irritability, asterixis, tetany • urine pH > 7.45

Metabolic acidosis	Blood pH < 7.35; plasma HCO₃ < 25 mEq/L	• diabetic coma
		• severe diarrhea
		• renal insufficiency
			Depends on cause:
			1. Diabetes
			  • insulin
			  • Na
			  • K
			  • HCO₃
			  • H₂O
			2. Renal insufficiency
			  • H₂O
			  • electrolytes
				• prog. deter. of LOC: apathy, disorientat'n, delirium, stupor, coma
				• nausea, vomiting, abdominal pain
				• headache
				• hyperpnea
				• s/s volume deplet'n: poor skin turgor, soft eyeballs, dry tongue, weakness
				• urine pH < 6.0

Metabolic alkalosis	Blood pH > 7.45; plasma HCO₃ > 29 mEq/L	• loss of gastric acid through vomiting, suct'n
		• excess. use of NaHCO₃
		• K deficiency
			Depends on cause:
			1. Loss of gastric acid
			  • Cl⁻ replacement
			  • Ringer's solut'n (10 mEq Cl/L)
			  • 0.9% NH₄Cl, IV
			  • water or other electrolytes prn
				• neuromuscular hyperexcitability: heightened reflexes, muscle twitching, tetany
				• prog. CNS excitat'n: belligerence, irritability, disorientat'n, convuls'ns
				• prog. respiratory deteriorat'n: shallow, slow respirat'ns, cyanosis, intermittent apnea
				• paralytic ileus
				• prog. cardiac arrhythmias
				Observe for:
				• rebound acidosis

SECTION 6

Drugs and the Blood

The importance of the blood for the transport of
drugs to body tissues has been mentioned.
However, blood is more than just a vehicle in which
drugs are dissolved, or a highway on which they are
carried throughout the body. Blood is also a tissue
and like all other tissues it, too, is subject to human
frailty. Section 6 discusses the use of drugs to treat
disorders of the blood. Blood physiology includes
the role of blood in transport of lipoproteins and
oxygen and the means by which blood coagulates.
Accordingly, we have chosen to discuss the use of
antihyperlipidemic drugs in Chapter 19. Chapter
20 deals with the use of iron, folic acid and vitamin
B_{12} in the treatment of anemias. Finally, Chapter
21 discusses the use of anticoagulant and
antiplatelet drugs, as well as fibrinolytic agents and
vitamin K.

CHAPTER 19

Antihyperlipidemic Drugs

Teaching Objectives

Following completion of this chapter, the reader should be able to:

1. List three factors contributing to the development of atherosclerosis.
2. Name the plasma lipids implicated in the development of atherosclerosis.
3. Describe the forms in which triglycerides and cholesterol are carried in the plasma.
4. List the four kinds of lipoproteins found in the plasma as determined by ultracentrifugation, and describe their composition of triglycerides and cholesterol.
5. List the four kinds of lipoproteins found in the plasma as determined by electrophoresis, and describe their composition of triglycerides and cholesterol.
6. Discuss the formation of the chylomicrons, very low-density lipoproteins (VLDL) and low-density lipoproteins (LDL) in the body.
7. Discuss briefly the origin of exogenous and endogenous hyperlipidemias.
8. Discuss the mechanism of action, clinical uses, adverse effects and related nursing process for clofibrate, gemfibrozil, cholestyramine, colestipol, lovastatin, simvastatin, pravastatin, niacin and probucol.

Atherosclerosis

Myocardial infarction, caused by atherosclerosis, is the most common cause of death in the Western world. At least three factors have been implicated in the development of atherosclerosis. These are hypertension, smoking and high plasma lipid levels. Individuals with high plasma lipid levels are more likely to suffer a myocardial infarct. A reduction in elevated plasma lipids decreases the risk of an infarct. Drugs are used to lower plasma lipids with the intent of preventing myocardial infarcts.

Classification of Plasma Lipoproteins

The plasma lipids implicated in the development of atherosclerosis are cholesterol and the triglycerides. Insoluble in the plasma, they form complexes with proteins and phospholipids and are carried in the plasma as lipoproteins. Two techniques have been used to classify plasma lipoproteins. Nurses should understand the value of these tests in diagnosing plasma lipoprotein abnormalities.

Ultracentrifugation

One method of classifying lipoproteins involves drawing a plasma sample and subjecting it to ultracentrifugation. The more dense lipoproteins are found at the bottom of the centrifuge tube and the lighter ones near the top. The **lipoprotein fractions** are constituted as follows:

1. **Chylomicrons**, which consist of eighty to ninety per cent triglycerides and remain at the top of the centrifuge tube. Chylomicrons are formed in the intestine from food containing fatty acids that have more than twelve carbons.
2. **Very low-density lipoproteins** (VLDL, prebeta lipoproteins), which consist of fifty to seventy per cent triglycerides. VLDL are formed in the liver from free fatty acids, cholesterol and carbohydrate.
3. **Intermediate-density lipoproteins** (IDL, broad-beta lipoproteins) are formed by the catabolism of VLDL and are intermediate products in the formation of low-density lipoproteins (LDL). As intermediates between VLDL and LDL they contain, percentage-wise, lesser amounts of triglycerides and more cholesterol than VLDL, but greater amounts of triglycerides and less cholesterol than LDL. IDL are not found in high concentrations in plasma, unless their subsequent catabolism is delayed.
4. **Low-density lipoproteins** (LDL, beta lipoproteins), which contain mainly cholesterol, are formed by the removal of triglycerides from VLDL.
5. **High-density lipids** (HDL, alpha lipoproteins) contain twenty per cent cholesterol, eight per cent triglycerides and seventy-two per cent phospholipids and proteins. An inverse relationship exists between plasma HDL levels and the incidence of coronary heart disease in subjects over age fifty.

Electrophoresis

A second method of differentiating between the various plasma lipoprotein complexes utilizes electrophoresis. If a plasma sample is placed on an electrophoresis plate and subjected to an electrical charge, the different lipoproteins can be separated on the basis of their ability to move in an electrical field into the following fractions:

1. The fastest-moving fraction can be found the farthest distance down the plate. This is called the **alpha lipoprotein fraction** and is composed of HDL.
2. The next fraction, called the **beta lipoprotein fraction,** moves more slowly than the alpha fraction. The beta lipoprotein band on the electrophoresis plate contains LDL.

3. Moving more slowly than the beta fraction are the **prebeta lipoproteins.** They are found between the beta band and the origin where the plasma sample was applied to the plate. The prebeta band is composed of VLDL.
4. Finally, one lipoprotein band does not migrate in an electrical field. This band is found at the origin. It is composed of **chylomicrons.**

Table 23 summarizes the comparative classification of lipoproteins.

Table 23
Comparative classification of lipoproteins.

Ultracentrifugation		Electrophoresis
1. Chylomicrons, found near the top of the tube. Contain 80-90% triglycerides (TG).	=	Band that remains at the origin of the electrophoresis plate.
2. VLDL, containing 50-70% TG and cholesterol.	=	Prebeta band; moves slowly down the electrophoresis plate.
3. LDL, responsible for 75% of cholesterol found in plasma.	=	Beta band; moves farther down the electrophoresis plate than the prebeta band.
4. HDL, containing about 20% cholesterol and 8% TG. An inverse relationship exists between HDL levels and incidence of coronary heart disease in subjects over 50.	=	Alpha lipoproteins; move farthest down the electrophoresis plate.

Origins of the Various Lipoproteins

The formation of the various lipoprotein complexes is shown in Figure 19. Chylomicrons are formed in the intestine from food and contain mainly triglycerides. They are synthesized from fatty acids having more than twelve carbons, and smaller amounts of cholesterol. Once absorbed into the lymph and transported into the plasma, chylomicrons are acted upon by the enzyme lipoprotein lipase to release their triglycerides, which are subsequently stored as fat or converted to fatty acids.

Figure 19
Diagrammatic description of the physiology of lipid transport in humans.

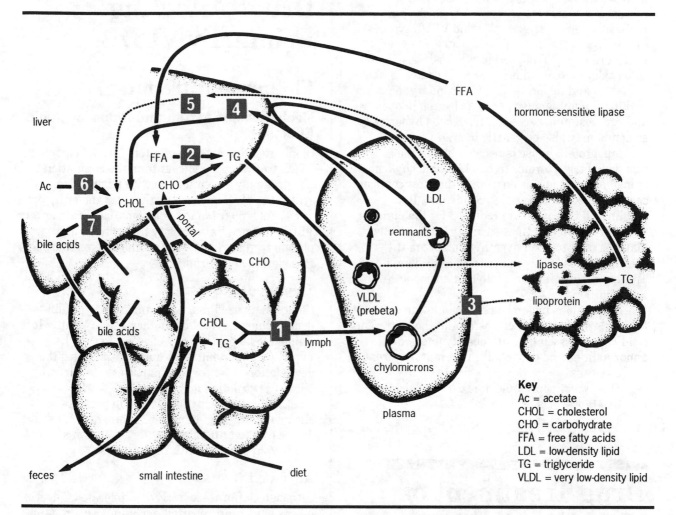

Key
Ac = acetate
CHOL = cholesterol
CHO = carbohydrate
FFA = free fatty acids
LDL = low-density lipid
TG = triglyceride
VLDL = very low-density lipid

From: W. R. Hazzard (1976), A pathophysiologic approach to managing hyperlipemia. *Am. Fam. Phys. 14* (2):78-87. Reproduced with permission.

VLDL are formed in the liver from free fatty acids, cholesterol and carbohydrate. The VLDL are subsequently stripped of some of their triglycerides and converted to intermediate-density lipoproteins or remnants. As the intermediate-density proteins lose more triglycerides they are converted to LDL, which contain mainly cholesterol.

Causes of Hyperlipidemias

Hyperlipidemias may be of exogenous or endogenous origin. Exogenous hyperlipidemia results from the ingestion of a meal high in content of fatty acids having twelve or more carbons. The chylomicrons formed are released into the circulation by the intestinal lymphatics. Exogenous hyperlipidemia can be reduced by eating food containing fatty acids having fewer than twelve carbons, because these are absorbed directly into the portal circulation and carried to the liver.

Endogenous hyperlipidemia results from an increase in the synthesis of lipoproteins or a decrease in their rate of removal from the plasma. Excessive hepatic triglyceride and VLDL synthesis in the liver is the most common cause of hypertriglyceridemia. Triglyceride synthesis is stimulated by caloric excess, dietary carbohydrates, ethanol, estrogens and hyperinsulinism secondary to peripheral insulin antagonism, such as is seen in obesity and corticosteroid excess. Endogenous hypertriglyceridemia may also be genetic in origin.

Lipoprotein lipase is responsible for the removal of triglycerides from VLDL and chylomicrons. A defect in this enzyme is the most common cause of massive hypertriglyceridemia. Both insulin and thyroxine are required for the maintenance of lipoprotein lipase activity. Uncontrolled diabetes mellitus and hypothyroidism are the leading causes of severe hypertriglyceridemia. Treatment with insulin or thyroid hormone reverses the condition.

Endogenous hypercholesterolemia can result from overproduction of cholesterol in the liver. This condition is associated with obesity and genetic abnormalities and can result in premature coronary heart disease.

The hyperlipoproteinemias can be classified into five types, as shown in Table 24.

Drug Treatment of Hyperlipidemias

Initial treatment for hyperlipidemia should include a specific diet, weight reduction and an exercise program. For patients with diabetes mellitus good diabetic control must be maintained. Drug therapy is often not recommended until diet and exercise have been tried for two to three months. The institution of drug therapy should not mean that nondrug therapy can be discontinued. Nonpharmacologic means of controlling hyperlipidemias must remain an integral part of the treatment regimen.

Drugs Affecting Primarily VLDL

Clofibrate (Atromid-S)

Mechanism of Action and Pharmacologic Effects

Clofibrate stimulates lipoprotein lipase to increase VLDL triglyceride removal from the circulation. The drug may also interfere with triglyceride synthesis, VLDL release by the liver and/or lipolysis in fat. As a result of these actions, clofibrate lowers VLDL, intermediate-density lipoproteins and plasma triglycerides. Its hypocholesterolemic effect is moderate and variable.

Therapeutic Uses

Clofibrate is used in the treatment of hyperlipidemias characterized by an increase in VLDL. It is claimed to be particularly effective in type III hyperlipoproteinemias because it stimulates the degradation of beta VLDL particles. Its clinical efficacy is still disputed.

Clofibrate is contraindicated in pregnancy. It should not be given to nursing mothers because it can be excreted in milk. Clofibrate should also not be given to patients with renal disease.

Adverse Effects

Although clofibrate is fairly well tolerated, adverse effects have been reported, including weight gain, alopecia, leukopenia, nausea, dysphagia and allergic reactions.

Nursing Process

Assessment
The nursing assessment of the patient prior to the administration of clofibrate should focus on review of the patient's history for contraindications to its use. These include evidence of past history of peptic ulcer or gout. Nurses should also review the patient's history for evidence of diabetes mellitus treated with oral hypoglycemics. Renal and hepatic functions should also be checked. Nurses should enquire whether the patient is pregnant or likely to become pregnant, because birth control should be practised during drug therapy. Bowel pattern requires daily assessment for increase in bulk. Water should be added to the diet if constipation develops.

Table 24
Types of hyperlipoproteinemia.

	Lipoprotein Characteristics of Plasma	Metabolic Defect	Appearance of Fasting Plasma After Standing Overnight at 4°C	Cholesterol/ Triglyceride Ratio
Type I Exogenous hyperlipidemia (hyperchylomicronemia)	Major incr. in chylomicrons. Us. decr. LDL, VLDL, HDL.	Decr. chylomicron clearance due to deficiency of lipoprotein lipase or abnormality of apo-CII.	Creamy supernatant w. clear infranate	< 0.2/1
Type IIa Hyperbetalipoproteinemia (hypercholesterolemia)	Incr. LDL; normal VLDL; absence of chylomicrons.	Incr. LDL synthesis, decr. clearance due to deficiency of or defect in LDL receptors.	Clear	> 1.5/1
Type IIb Combined hyperlipidemia (mixed hyperlipidemia)	Incr. LDL; incr. VLDL; absence of chylomicrons.	Same defect as Type IIa but also incr. VLDL.	No creamy layer on top but infranate may range from clear to turbid.	Variable
Type III Broad-beta (dysbetalipoproteinemia)	Incr. IDL; poss. presence of chylomicrons.	Incr. IDL product'n or decr. clearance. Incr. total plasma apo-E plus deficiency of apo-E-III. Poss. deficiency of hepatic lipase.	Faint creamy supernatant w. turbid infranate	Range 0.3/1 - 2.0/1, with 1/1 often found
Type IV Endogenous hyperlipidemia (hypertriglyceridemia)	Incr. VLDL; normal or decr. LDL; absence of chylomicrons.	Incr. VLDL product'n or decr. clearance or both. Poss. abnormal apo-I/C-III complex.	No creamy supernate, clear to turbid infranate	Variable
Type V Mixed hyperlipidemia	Incr. VLDL; incr. chylomicrons; normal or decr. LDL.	Incr. product'n or decr. clearance of chylomicrons and VLDL. Poss. imbalance bet. apo-CII and CIII, as well as poss. abnormal apo-E.	Clear supernate and turbid infranate	0.15/1 - 0.6/1

Administration
Clofibrate should be administered from a light-resistant container. Administer with meals to reduce gastric distress.

Evaluation
First, nurses should evaluate the effectiveness of clofibrate therapy. This is demonstrated by a decrease in plasma triglycerides. Second, the safety of clofibrate must be established. Recent reports have questioned its safety. Nurses should remain alert for all reported adverse effects of the drug. Nursing evaluation of the patient following administration of the medication should emphasize observation for evidence of adverse effects: flu-like musculoskeletal symptoms (aching joints, general weakness and fatigue), increased bleeding tendencies in people who are also taking oral anticoagulants, and increased effectiveness of oral hypoglycemic agents in diabetics.

Teaching
The importance of patient teaching related to dietary knowledge and habits, and daily exercise patterns as a means of treating hyperlipidemias, cannot be overemphasized. Compliance with drug therapy is important to prevent drug toxicity. As an in-depth discussion of patient teaching is beyond the scope of this text, readers are advised to consult a medical-surgical nursing text for nursing interventions related to patient teaching in these areas.

Gemfibrozil (Lopid)

Mechanism of Action and Pharmacologic Effects

Gemfibrozil lowers elevated serum lipids primarily by decreasing serum triglycerides with a variable reduction in total serum cholesterol level. These decreases occur in the VLDL and LDL fractions. In addition, gemfibrozil may increase the HDL cholesterol fraction. Gemfibrozil appears to have a greater depressant effect on the VLDL, which are rich in triglycerides, than on the LDL, which are rich in cholesterol.

Gemfibrozil's mechanism of action has not been definitely established. In humans, it has been shown to inhibit peripheral lipolysis and to decrease the hepatic extraction of free fatty acids, thus reducing hepatic triglyceride production. The drug also inhibits synthesis of VLDL-carrier apoprotein, leading to a decrease in VLDL.

Therapeutic Uses

Gemfibrozil is indicated as an adjunct to diet and other therapeutic measures in the management of patients with type IV hyperlipidemia who are at high risk of sequelae and complications from their hyperlipidemia. If a significant serum lipid response is not obtained in three months, gemfibrozil should be discontinued. Gemfibrozil is contraindicated in the presence of hepatic or renal dysfunction, including primary biliary cirrhosis. It is also contraindicated in patients with pre-existing gall bladder disease. *Strict birth control procedures must be exercised by women of childbearing potential.* If pregnancy occurs, gemfibrozil must be discontinued. Women who are planning pregnancy should discontinue gemfibrozil several months prior to conception.

Adverse Effects

The incidence of adverse effects with gemfibrozil is low. Nausea, vomiting, abdominal and epigastric pain appear to be the most common effects, with approximately five per cent of patients encountering these problems.

Nursing Process

Assessment

The patient's history should be reviewed for documentation of possible contraindications. In the event of evidence of liver, kidney or gall bladder disease, the nurse should withhold gemfibrozil pending consultation with the attending physician. Nurses should anticipate that the physician will order blood studies prior to administering the first dose of gemfibrozil. The patient's chart should be checked to ensure that blood has been drawn for serum LDL and VLDL, triglycerides, total cholesterol, complete blood count, blood glucose and liver function tests. These tests assist the physician in detecting contraindications to gemfibrozil use and in establishing baseline levels for determining drug efficacy.

Administration

Ordinarily, gemfibrozil is stored at room temperature. It is taken in two divided doses one-half hour before breakfast and before dinner.

Evaluation

Drug efficacy is determined by means of blood tests of serum LDL and VLDL, triglycerides, total cholesterol, complete blood counts, blood glucose and liver function tests. Patients should be carefully monitored for evidence of cholelithiasis or cholecystitis, which often occurs during the night or early morning. Such evidence includes some or all of the following: right upper quadrant pain, epigastric pain radiating to the right shoulder blade, nausea, vomiting, flatulence, jaundice.

Teaching

Patients should be alerted that gemfibrozil may cause blurred vision and vertigo; therefore, they should avoid driving and the use of power tools until their individual response to this medication is determined. Compliance with drug therapy is important to prevent drug toxicity.

In collaboration with the physician and dietician, nurses should work with the patient to facilitate nonpharmacologic interventions known to contribute to successful treatment of lipid disorders. Detailed discussion of these measures is beyond the scope of this book. Readers should refer to a medical-surgical nursing text for further information on dietary, lifestyle, and behavioral interventions related to nursing care of patients with lipid disorders.

Drugs Affecting Primarily LDL

Cholestyramine (Questran) and Colestipol Hydrochloride (Colestid)

Mechanism of Action and Pharmacologic Effects

Cholestyramine and colestipol hydrochloride are nonabsorbed resins that sequester bile acids in the intestine, preventing their absorption. The reduced levels of bile acids increase the rate of conversion of cholesterol to bile acids in the liver, thereby increasing LDL receptor activity and apoprotein B catabolism. Unfortunately, the decrease in LDL is offset, at least in part, by a compensatory increase in cholesterol synthesis in the liver and intestine.

Therapeutic Uses

Cholestyramine and colestipol are used to treat hyperlipidemias characterized by an increase in beta lipoproteins or LDL. They are used in conditions where the increase is seen only in LDL or in situations where the increase in LDL is also accompanied by a rise in prebeta lipoproteins or VLDL. Cholestyramine is a drug of choice for type IIa (hyperbetalipoproteinemia). When used with dietary control, cholestyramine reduces LDL an additional twenty to forty per cent.

Adverse Effects

The adverse effects of cholestyramine and colestipol hydrochloride include abdominal discomfort, bloating, nausea, dyspepsia, steatorrhea, and possibly either constipation or diarrhea.

Nursing Process

Assessment

Before the initial administration of either of these drugs, the patient's history should undergo nursing review aimed at identifying conditions that might contraindicate use of these medications (i.e., renal disease, peptic ulcer or gout). Since cholestyramine and colestipol are not absorbed systemically, they are not expected to cause fetal harm when administered in recommended doses during pregnancy. There are, however, no adequate and well-controlled studies in pregnant women, and the known interference with the absorption of fat-soluble vitamins may be detrimental even in the presence of supplementation. The patient's drug regimen should be examined, in consultation with the pharmacist, for drugs listed above and any others that might interact with cholestyramine and colestipol. Prior to administering the first dose of these medications, nurses should ensure that blood has been drawn for laboratory tests to establish baseline levels of blood lipids.

Administration

Administration of cholestyramine or colestipol hydrochloride must be timed so that it either precedes by at least one hour the administration of the aforementioned drugs, or follows them by at least four hours.

Oral doses of this medication are prepared by adding the prescribed amount to 200 mL (approximately 6 oz) of liquid of the patient's preference and allowing it to stand for two to three minutes to absorb the fluid. Thereafter, stir the mixture vigorously to distribute the medication uniformly. Have the patient drink quickly and immediately. Follow with 100 – 150 mL of additional fluid from the same glass to ensure that no medication remains in the glass.

Evaluation

Nursing evaluation should focus on identifying adverse effects. In addition, any evidence of bleeding should be reported to the physician at once. Patients should be monitored for signs of deficiency in vitamins A, D and K.

Teaching

Patient teaching related to the use of either of these drugs should emphasize the necessity for continuation of the prescribed diet and exercise programs. Patients should also be advised of dietary interventions that might assist in reducing or relieving constipation, such as prunes, rhubarb and other high-bulk foods, accompanied by increased fluid intake. Patients should be alerted to the danger of increased bleeding tendencies and urged to contact their physician immediately if these appear.

Lovastatin (Mevacor), Simvastatin (Zocor) and Pravastatin (Pravachol)

Mechanism of Action and Pharmacologic Effects

Lovastatin, simvastatin and pravastatin are cholesterol-lowering agents. After oral ingestion these drugs, or their active metabolites, inhibit specifically 3-hydroxy-3-methylglutaryl-coenzyme A (HMG-CoA) reductase. This enzyme catalyzes the conversion of HMG-CoA to mevalonate, which is an early and rate-limiting step in the biosynthesis of cholesterol.

Lovastatin, simvastatin and pravastatin reduce cholesterol production by the liver and induce some changes in cholesterol transport and disposition in the blood and tissues. The mechanism of this effect is believed to involve both reduction of the synthesis of LDL and an increase in LDL catabolism as a result of the induction of LDL receptors. In addition, these drugs may increase HDL levels.

Therapeutic Uses

Lovastatin, simvastatin and pravastatin are indicated as adjuncts to diet for the reduction of elevated total and low-density lipoprotein cholesterol (LDL-C) levels in patients with primary hypercholesterolemia (types IIa and IIb), when the response to diet and other measures alone has been inadequate. Types IIa and IIb hyperlipoproteinemias are characterized by elevated serum cholesterol levels, in association with normal triglyceride levels (type IIa) or elevated serum cholesterol levels plus increased triglyceride levels (type IIb).

Lovastatin is contraindicated in patients with active liver disease with unexplained persistent elevations of serum transaminase levels. It is recommended that liver function tests be performed at baseline and every four to six weeks during the first fifteen months of therapy with lovastatin, and periodically thereafter. If the transaminase levels show evidence of progression, particularly if they rise to three times the upper limit of normal and are persistent, the drug should be discontinued.

The contraindications to the use of simvastatin and pravastatin include acute liver disease or unexplained persistent elevations of serum transaminases.

Adverse Effects

In spite of the preceding comments, lovastatin is generally well tolerated, and adverse reactions are usually mild and transient. The most frequently encountered adverse reactions involve the gastrointestinal tract (constipation, diarrhea, dyspepsia, flatus, abdominal pain or cramps, heartburn and nausea). Muscle cramps and myalgia are sometimes observed. Headache has been reported in nine to ten per cent of patients taking the drug. Transient elevations of creatinine phosphokinase (CK) are commonly seen in lovastatin-treated patients but have usually been of no clinical significance. Rhabdomyolysis has occurred rarely. Lovastatin therapy should be discontinued if marked elevation of CK levels occurs, and appropriate therapy should be instituted.

Simvastatin's adverse effects include constipation, flatulence, nausea, headache, and abdominal pain. Elevations of creatinine phosphokinase levels three or more times the normal values on one or more occasions have been reported in approximately five per cent of patients taking simvastatin. This is attributable to the noncardiac fraction of CK. Myopathy has been reported rarely. In clinical trials, marked persistent increases (to more than three times the upper limit of normal) in serum transaminases have occurred in one per cent of adult patients who received simvastatin. It is recommended that liver function tests be performed at baseline, and periodically thereafter, in all patients taking pravastatin. If the transaminase levels show evidence of progression, particularly if they rise to three times the upper limit of normal and are persistent, simvastatin should be discontinued. Simvastatin should be used with caution in patients who consume substantial quantities of alcohol and/or have a past history of liver disease.

Similar to the other HMG-CoA reductase inhibitors, liver function tests should be performed at baseline and periodically thereafter in all patients. Special attention should be given to patients who develop increased transaminase levels. Liver function tests should be repeated to confirm an elevation and subsequently monitored at more frequent intervals. If increases in alanine aminotransferase (ALAT) and aspartate aminotransferase (ASAT) equal or exceed three times the upper limit of normal and persist, therapy should be discontinued. In view of these concerns, it is not surprising that caution should be exercised when pravastatin is administered to patients with a history of liver disease or heavy alcohol ingestion. As previously explained, HMG-CoA reductase inhibitors, including pravastatin, have been associated with elevations of CK. Myalgia has been associated with pravastatin therapy. Interruption of therapy with pravastatin should be considered in any patient with an acute, serious condition, suggestive of a myopathy or having a risk factor predisposing to the development of renal failure or rhabdinomyolysis, such as severe acute infection, hypotension, major surgery, trauma, severe metabolic, endocrine or electrolyte disorders and uncontrolled seizures.

Nursing Process

Assessment
During drug administration, cholesterol levels should be periodically checked, liver function studies monitored and renal function tests performed in patients with compromised renal systems. Eyes should be tested with a slit lamp one month after treatment begins and annually, as lens opacities may occur.

Administration
Administration of the drug is advised with the evening meal. If the dose is increased, it can be taken with breakfast and supper. These drugs should be stored in a tight light-protected container in a cool environment.

Evaluation
Cholesterol levels are monitored after eight weeks for attainment of desired levels.

Teaching
Patient teaching includes stressing the importance of reporting blurred vision and the necessity of eye examinations. Treatment may continue for several years, as the necessities of a low-cholesterol diet and an exercise program need constant emphasis.

Niacin

Niacin reduces the rate of synthesis of LDL and apoprotein B by depressing the synthesis of VLDL. As a result, VLDL and LDL cholesterol levels decrease and HDL cholesterol increases. Niacin may be effective in all types of hyperlipoproteinemia except type I. Niacin may produce a greater fall in triglycerides in patients with type V hyperlipoproteinemia than other drugs.

Flushing occurs in almost all patients when niacin is started. Although it often subsides, about ten to fifteen per cent of patients experience this effect throughout the duration of therapy. Other adverse effects of niacin include pruritus, dry skin with scaling, and acanthosis nigrans. Gastrointestinal effects attributed to niacin include nausea, vomiting, flatulence and diarrhea. Reactivation of peptic ulcer is a more serious gastrointestinal effect. Other serious reactions to niacin include impaired glucose tolerance, hyperuricemia and liver dysfunction, including cholestatic jaundice. Liver tests should be performed periodically.

Nursing Process

Assessment
It is imprtant to carry out liver function studies (AST, ALT, bilirubin, alkaline phosphatase) and blood glucose levels before and during therapy. Assess niacin levels during drug administration to monitor therapeutic response.

Administration
Niacin should be taken with meals to reduce gastrointestinal upset.

Evaluation
Nurses should monitor the effects of decreased lipids. These include warm extremities and the absence of numbness in the extremities. Observe for signs of liver dysfunction, such as clay-colored stools, itching, dark urine or jaundice. Finally, patients should be evaluated for central nervous system adverse effects — headache, paresthesias and blurred vision.

Teaching
Nurses should prepare the patient for the flushing and increased feeling of warmth that occur several hours after oral intake or immediately after intramuscular, intravenous or subcutaneous administration. Patients should be told to remain recumbent if postural hypotension occurs. They should also be cautioned to refrain from taking alcohol and told to avoid sunlight if skin lesions are present.

Probucol (Lorelco)

Probucol reduces elevated cholesterol levels. It is used in the treatment of patients with elevated LDL and combined hyperlipidemias. Probucol's adverse effects are diarrhea, flatulence, abdominal pain and nausea.

Nursing Process

Assessment
Nurses should anticipate that the physician will

order blood studies prior to administration of the first dose of this medication. The patient's chart should be checked to ensure that blood has been drawn for serum LDL and VLDL, triglycerides and total cholesterol. Birth control should be practised while on the drug.

Administration
Gastrointestinal discomfort is minimized if the drug is taken with breakfast and dinner.

Evaluation
The patient's pulse should be carefully monitored during the initial period of therapy because of the risk of idiosyncratic effects of the drug on the cardiovascular system. The extent of gastrointestinal effects of this drug must be determined in order to permit early detection of fluid and electrolyte imbalances that might accompany prolonged nausea, vomiting and diarrhea. Any unexplained bleeding or increased bruising tendencies may indicate adverse hematologic effects.

Teaching
Patients and their families should be aware of the importance of proper self-administration of this drug (see section above on Administration). In addition, they should be taught the indicators of adverse effects, with emphasis on reporting the presence of any of these to the physician immediately. Also, they should be alerted to the importance of laboratory tests in determining drug efficacy.

Patients being treated with probucol should be advised to abstain from alcohol. Taken together, alcohol and probucol produce gastric irritation, with a high risk of gastrointestinal bleeding.

In collaboration with the physician and dietician, nurses should work with the patient to facilitate nonpharmacological interventions known to contribute to successful treatment of lipid disorders. Detailed discussion of these measures is beyond the scope of this book. Readers should refer to a medical-surgical nursing text for further information on dietary, lifestyle and behavioral interventions related to nursing care of patients with lipid disorders.

Further Reading

Baron, R. B. (1989). Management of hypercholesterolemia. A primary care perspective. *West. J. Med. 150* :562-568.

Berglund, G., Lithell, H., Olsson, A. G. and Vessby, B. (1988). Symposium on prevention of atherosclerosis. Strategies for the 90s. *Drugs 36* (Suppl. 3):1-122.

Blum, C. B. and Levy, R. I. (1986). Rational drug therapy of hyperlipoproteinemias. Part I. *Rational Drug Therapy 20* (9):1-7. Part II. *Rational Drug Therapy 20* (10):1-4.

Choice of cholesterol-lowering drugs (1988). *The Medical Letter 30* :85-88.

Choice of cholesterol-lowering drugs (1989). *The Medical Letter 31* :26-31.

Choice of cholesterol-lowering drugs (1991). *The Medical Letter 33* :1-4.

Dart, A. M. (1990). Managing elevated blood lipid concentrations: Who, when and how? *Drugs 39* :374-387.

Fidge, N. H. (1990). Lipid-lowering drugs — Mechanisms of action. *Australian Prescriber 13* :73-77.

Frishman, S. H., Zimetbaum, P. and Nadelmann, J. (1989). Lovastatin and other HMG CoA reductase inhibitors. *J. Clin. Pharmacol. 29* :975-982.

Henwood, J. M. and Heel, R. C. (1988). Lovastatin. A preliminary review of its pharacodynamic properties and therapeutic uses in hyperlipidemia. *Drugs 36* :429-454.

Illingworth, D. R. (1987). Lipid-lowering drugs. An overview of indications and optimum therapeutic use. *Drugs 33* :259-276.

Krukemeyer, J. J. and Talbert, R. L. (1987). Lovastatin. A new cholesterol-lowering agent. *Pharmacotherapy 7* :198-210.

O'Conner, P., Feely, J. and Shepherd, J. (1990). Lipid-lowering drugs. *Brit. Med. J. 300* :667-672.

Roberts, W. C. (1989). Lipid-lowering therapy after an atherosclerotic event. *Amer. J. Cariol. 64* :693-695.

Simons, L. A. (1990). Lipid-lowering drugs — Clinical applications. *Australian Prescriber 13* :77-80.

Stoy, D.B. (1989). Helping patients take cholesterol-lowering drugs. *Amer. J. Nursing 89* (12) :1631-1633

Todd, P. A. and Ward, A. (1988). Gemfibrozil. A review of its pharmacodynamic and pharmacokinetic properties, and therapeutic uses in dyslipidemia. *Drugs 36* :314-339.

Table 25
Antihyperlipidemic drugs.

Generic Name (Trade Name)	Use (Dose)	Action	Adverse Effects	Drug Interactions	Nursing Process
Pharmacologic Classification: Drugs Affecting Primarily VLDL					
Clofibrate (Atromid-S)	As an adjunct to diet and other measures for reduct'n of severely elevated plasma lipids in pts at high risk of sequelae due to hyperlipidemia who do not respond adequately to diet, exercise, weight loss and other tx. Used to treat hyperlipidemia characterized by an incr. in VLDL. **(Oral:** *For adults only -* 500 mg bid or qid)	Lowers VLDL, IDL and plasma TG, exact mechanism unknown; thought to stim. **lipoprotein lipase** to incr. VLDL TG removal from circulat'n. May also interfere w. TG synthesis, VLDL release by liver and/or lipolysis in fat.	Nausea, diarrhea, GI upset, fatigue, weakness, drowsiness, dizziness, headache, myalgia, arthralgia, skin react'ns, leukopenia, anemia, eosinophilia, cardiac arrhythmias, swelling and phlebitis at site of xanthomata, cholelithiasis and cholecystitis, impotence, decr. libido, weight gain, polyphagia	**Anticoagulants, oral:** May demonstrate incr. effect in presence of clofibrate. Dosage of oral anticoagulant should be reduced by 50% to maintain prothrombin time. **Antidiabetic drugs, oral:** May demonstrate incr. effect in presence of clofibrate. **Furosemide:** And clofibrate may compete for plasma albumin, resulting in painful or stiff muscles and marked diuresis.	**Assess:** Pt hx for renal disease, peptic ulcer, gout; pt drug regimen for oral hypoglycemics or oral anticoagulants. **Administer:** From light-resistant container. **Evaluate:** Diabetics on oral hypoglycemics; for adv. effects (bleeding, flu-like symptoms). **Teach:** Tx interact'n w. diet, exercise regimen, nonsmoking and medicat'n. *Birth control should be practised.*
Gemfibrozil (Lopid)	As an adjunct to diet and other measures in management of pts w. type IV hyperlipidemia at high risk of sequelae and complicat'ns **(Oral:** Adults - 1200 mg in 2 divided doses 30 min before a.m and p.m. meal. Max. recom. daily dose, 1500 mg)	Lowers elevated serum lipids; decr. primarily serum TG. Variable reduct'n in total serum cholesterol. Decr. VLDL and LDL fract'ns. May incr. HDL cholesterol. Mechanism of action not established. Inhibits peripheral lipolysis and decr. hepatic extract'n of free fatty acids, thus reducing hepatic TG product'n. Also inhibits synthesia of VLDL carrier apoprotein.	GI disturbances (abdominal pain, diarrhea, nausea, epigastric pain, vomiting) and rash	**Anticoagulants, oral:** Must be administered w. caution to pts taking gemfibrozil. Dosage of anticoagulant should be reduced to maintain prothrombin time in desired range to prevent bleeding complicat'ns. Frequent prothrombin determinat'ns are advisable until it has been definitely established that prothrombin level has stabilized. **Lovastatin:** And gemfibrozil used tog. have been reported to produce severe myositis w. markedly elevated serum creatinine phosphokinase (CK) and myoglobinuria rhabdomyolysis. When myoglobinuria is severe, acute renal failure may ensue. *Therefore, lovastatin should not be used concomitantly w. gemfibrozil.*	**Assess:** Hx for contraindicat'ns (liver, kidney or gall bladder disease); ensure blood drawn for serum LDL and VLDL, TG, total cholesterol, CBC, blood glucose and liver funct'n tests. **Administer:** At room temp. in 2 divided doses 1 h before breakfast and dinner. **Evaluate:** Drug efficacy using blood tests; monitor cholelithiasis or cholecystitis. **Teach:** Not to drive or use power tools until effect on vision determined; nonpharmaceutical control of lipid diseases. Importance of compliance w. drug tx to prevent drug toxicity.

Generic Name (Trade Name)	Use (Dose)	Action	Adverse Effects	Drug Interactions	Nursing Process
Pharmacologic Classification: Drugs Affecting Primarily LDL					
Cholestyramine (Questran)	To reduce serum cholesterol concentrat'ns, particularly type II hyperlipidemia (**Oral:** Mix w. fruit juice, water, milk, apple sauce or pureed fruit just before administrat'n and take ac. Adults - initially, 4 g bid for 1st week; incr. to 8 g bid on 2nd week and 12 g bid thereafter. Take other drugs at least 1 h before or 4-6 h after cholestyramine to avoid impeding their absorpt'n)	Lowers plasma beta lipoprotein levels by preventing reabsorpt'n of bile acids in intestine, causing incr. cholesterol to be converted to bile acids.	Nausea, vomiting, constipat'n, diarrhea, abdominal pain and distent'n, pyrosis; rash and irritat'n of skin, tongue, perianal area; impaired vitamin K and Ca absorpt'n	**Acidic compounds** (incl. warfarin, phenylbutazone, digoxin, thiazides, phenobarbital and thyroid hormones): Bind to cholestyramine and colestipol in GI tract. As a result, cholestyramine and colestipol can block their absorpt'n. **Tetracyclines and fat-soluble vitamins:** Have their absorpt'n blocked by cholestyramine and colestipol.	**Assess:** For pregnancy; bowel habits, drug regimen. **Administer:** Thoroughly dissolved in strong-flavored liquid at least 1 h before or 4 h after other prescribed medicat'ns. **Evaluate:** For constipat'n, bleeding tendencies, s/s of deficiencies in vitamins A, D or K. **Teach:** Necessity for concurrent diet and exercise tx, proper self-administrat'n, dietary intervent'ns for relief of constipat'n; to observe and report bleeding tendencies.
Colestipol hydrochloride (Colestid)	As for cholestyramine (**Oral:** Adults - 15-30 g daily, taken bid-qid w. meals. Take other drugs at least 1 h before or 4-6 h after colestipol to avoid impeding their absorpt'n)	As for cholestyramine	As for cholestyramine	As for cholestyramine	As for cholestyramine
Lovastatin (Mevacor)	As an adjunct to diet for reduct'n of elevated total and LDL cholesterol levels in pts w. primary hypercholesterolemia (types IIa and IIb), when response to diet and other measures has been inadequate (**Oral:** Adults - us. starting dose, 20 mg per day, given as single dose w. evening meal. Adjustments in dosage should be made prn at intervals of not < 4 weeks, to a max. of 80 mg/day given in a single dose or divided doses w. morning and evening meals. Measure cholesterol levels periodically and consider reducing lovastatin dose if cholesterol levels fall below targeted range)	Principal metabolite of lovastatin is a specific inhibitor of enzyme that catalyzes conversion of 3-hydroxy-3-methylglutaryl-coenzyme A (HMG-CoA) to mevalonate, which is an early and rate-limiting step in biosynthesis of cholesterol. Lovastatin reduces cholesterol product'n by liver. May also incr. LDL catabolism as a result of induct'n of LDL receptors. Lovastatin may incr. HDL levels.	*Contraindicated in pts w. active liver disease w. unexplained persistent elevat'ns of serum transaminase levels.* Most frequent adv. effects are constipat'n, diarrhea, dyspepsia, flatus, abdominal pain or cramps, heartburn and nausea. Other effects include muscle cramps and myalgia. Rhabdomyolysis has occurred rarely. Lovastatin should be stopped if marked elevat'n of CK levels	**Anticoagulants, oral:** May interact w. lovastatin. Careful monitoring of prothrombin time is recommended. **Cholestyramine and colestipol:** May produce additive effects w. lovastatin. **Gemfibrozil and niacin:** May incr. incidence of myopathy associated w. lovastatin. Risks and benefits of using lovastatin w. fibrates or lipid-lowering doses of niacin should be carefully considered. **Immunosuppressants:** Incr. incidence of myopathy w. lovastatin. Benefits and risks of using lovastatin concomitantly w. immunosuppressive drugs should be considered carefully.	**Assess:** Throughout tx, cholesterol levels for drug efficacy, liver funct'n studies, renal funct'n test. Eyes should be tested for lens opacities. **Administer:** Give w. evening meal. If dose incr., take w. breakfast and supper. Store in tight light-resistant container in cool room. **Evaluate:** Cholesterol levels for tx effect. **Teach:** Stress importance of reporting blurred vision and having eyes examined. Continue low-cholesterol diet and exercise program.

occurs. Headache is seen in 9-10% of pts taking lovastatin. *Lovastatin is contraindicated in pregnancy. Women taking lovastatin should not breast-feed.*

Drug	Dose	Action	Adverse effects	Drug interactions	Nursing considerations
Pravastatin (Pravachol)	As for lovastatin (**Oral:** Initially, 10-20 mg od hs. If serum cholesterol is markedly elevated, dose may be initiated at 40 mg/day. Drug can be taken without regard to meals)	Pravastatin inhibits HMG-CoA reductase. This enzyme catalyzes the convers'n of HMG-CoA to mevalonate, which is an early and rate-limiting step in biosynthesis of cholesterol.	Elevated transaminase, ALAT, ASAT or CK levels may be seen. Myalgia can occur. *Pravastatin is contraindicated during pregnancy. Women taking pravastatin should not breast-feed.*	**Antacids:** Reduce bioavailability of pravastatin. **Cholestyramine and colestipol:** May reduce absorpt'n of pravastatin. Give pravastatin either 1 h or more before or at least 4 h after either drug. **Cimetidine:** Incr. bioavailability of pravastatin. **Coumarin anticoagulants:** Used w. pravastatin, requires careful monitoring of prothrombin times. **Immunosuppressive drugs, fibrates, erythromycin, niacin:** Administered concomitantly w. lovastatin, incr. risk of myopathy or rhabdomyolysis associated w. lovastatin. Because of similarities bet. pravastatin and lovastatin, concomitant use of these drugs w. pravastatin should be considered carefully.	As for lovastatin
Simvastatin (Zocor)	As for lovastatin (**Oral:** Initially, 10 mg/day, given as a single dose hs. Adjustments of dose should be made prn at intervals of not < 4 weeks, to a max. of 40 mg daily, given as a single dose hs)	As for lovastatin	Constipat'n, flatulence, nausea, headache, abdominal pain. Elevat'ns of CK and serum transaminase have been seen. *Simvastatin is contraindicated in pregnancy. Women taking simvastatin should not breast-feed.*	**Cholestyramine:** Appears to have additive cholesterol-lowering effects w. simvastatin. **Immunosuppressive drugs, fibrates, niacin:** Administered concomitantly w. lovastatin, incr. risk of myopathy or rhabdomyolosis w. lovastatin. Because of similarities bet. simvastatin and lovastatin, concomitant use of these w. simvastatin should be considered carefully.	As for lovastatin

Generic Name (Trade Name)	Use (Dose)	Action	Adverse Effects	Drug Interactions	Nursing Process
Niacin	Used as adjunctive tx in all types of hyperlipoproteinemias except type I (Oral: Adults - initially, 100 mg tid; incr. to 3-9 g/day, given in 3-4 divided doses, with or without meals)	Reduces rate of synthesis of LDL and apoprotein B by depressing synthesis of VLDL. As a result, VLDL and LDL cholesterol decr. and HDL cholesterol incr.	Flushing, pruritus, dry skin, nausea, vomiting, flatulence, diarrhea, reactivat'n of peptic ulcer, impaired glucose tolerance, hyperuricemia, liver dysfunct'n (including cholestatic jaundice)		**Assess:** Liver funct'n and blood glucose levels. Niacin levels during tx. **Administer:** W. meals to reduce GI upset. **Evaluate:** Effects of decr. lipids, such as warm extremities and absence of numbness in extremities. Observe for s/s of liver dysfunct'n, CNS disturbances. **Teach:** Prepare pt for flushing and feelings of incr. warmth following drug administrat'n. Pt to remain recumbent if postural hypotens'n occurs. Caution pt to refrain from alcohol and to avoid sunlight if skin lesions are present.
Probucol (Lorelco)	Tx of type II hyperlipidemias and combined hyperlipidemias (Oral: Adults - 500 mg bid with a.m. and p.m. meals)	Reduces elevated plasma cholesterol; exact mechanism unknown.	Mild to moderate adv. effects of short durat'n, incl. diarrhea, GI react'ns (flatulence, abdominal pain, nausea, vomiting), hyperhidrosis, fetid sweat, angioneurotic edema	**Clofibrate:** And probucol are not recommended concomitantly because an incr. in serum TG can occur.	**Administer:** W. meals a.m. and p.m.; from light-resistant container stored in cool dark place. **Teach:** To consult physician if side effects are persistent and severe; benefits of concurrent diet and exercise tx. Caution pt that *birth control must be practised while taking this drug.*

CHAPTER 20

Antianemic Drugs

Teaching Objectives
Following completion of this chapter, the reader should be able to:

Teaching Objectives
Following completion of this chapter, the reader should be able to:

1. Describe the difference between iron-deficiency anemia and anemia due to folic acid or vitamin B_{12} deficiency.
2. Discuss the absorption, distribution and storage of iron.
3. Describe the iron requirements of infants, children, adolescents, adult men and nonmenstruating women, menstruating women and pregnant women.
4. Discuss the causes and characteristics of iron-deficiency anemia.
5. List the various types of iron preparations that may be taken orally or parenterally; discuss their relative therapeutic merits and identify the nursing process related to their use.
6. Describe the characteristics of iron toxicity, its treatment and the nursing process related to the use of deferoxamine.
7. Discuss the actions of folic acid and vitamin B_{12} on DNA synthesis and the consequences of a deficiency in either chemical.
8. State the daily folic acid requirements for an adult and describe the availability of folic acid in food.
9. Discuss the absorption, distribution, elimination and actions of folic acid.
10. Discuss the therapeutic uses of folic acid supplements and identify the nursing process related to their use.
11. Describe the dietary requirements for vitamin B_{12} and its availability in food.
12. Discuss the absorption, distribution, elimination and actions of vitamin B_{12}.
13. Discuss the therapeutic uses of vitamin B_{12} and identify the nursing process related to its use.

Body Iron Requirements

Iron Metabolism

Although iron absorption may occur throughout the gastrointestinal tract, most takes place from the duodenum. Usually the amount of iron absorbed equals the quantity eliminated by the kidneys. Iron absorption increases in response to iron-deficiency anemia or pyridoxine deficiency. It is also increased during the latter months of pregnancy. Normally, between five to ten per cent of the iron ingested in food is absorbed. This increases to approximately twenty per cent in iron-deficient subjects given normal amounts of iron in the diet.

Once absorbed, iron is usually carried in the blood bound to the transport alpha$_1$ globulin protein transferrin. This protein is usually about one-third saturated with iron and, as a result, if more iron is absorbed it, too, can be carried on the transferrin. A decrease in plasma iron level, together with an increase in the iron binding capacity, is encountered in iron deficiency. Hemosiderosis and hemochromatosis, on the other hand, present pictures of high levels of plasma iron, with transferrin being almost completely saturated.

The quantity of iron in the body varies according to the age of the individual. At birth it ranges from 200 – 300 mg, depending on the weight of the child. Thereafter, it builds slowly to 2 – 6 g in adults.

Iron is present in many forms in the body. Hemoglobin accounts for approximately seventy per cent of the total body iron. Myoglobin, the heme protein of skeletal and cardiac muscle, amounts to about three per cent of total body iron.

Table 26
Daily iron requirements.*

	Iron Need for Erythropoiesis (mg/day)	Food Iron Requirement (mg/day)
Infants	0.5 – 1.5	1.5 mg/kg**
Children	0.4 – 1	4 – 10
Adolescents	1 – 2	10 – 20
Menstruating women	1 – 2	7 – 20
Pregnant women	2 – 5	20 – 50†
Normal men and nonmenstruating women	0.5 – 1	5 – 10

* Modified slightly from report of the ad hoc Committee of the Council on Foods and Nutrition of the American Medical Association.
** To a maximum of 1.5 mg daily.
† This amount of iron cannot be provided in the diet and requires supplementation with medicinal iron.

From: V. F. Fairbanks, J. L. Fahey and E. Beutler, *Clinical Disorders of Iron Metabolism*. Grune and Stratton, 1971. Reproduced with permission.

Approximately twenty-five per cent of body iron is found in the storage forms of ferritin and hemosiderin. Although transferrin is important in the transport of iron in plasma, it accounts for only 0.1% of the body iron content. In addition to its role in the transport of oxygen in the blood, iron is important in many enzyme functions, such as those mediated by cytochrome *c* catalase. The amounts of iron needed for these functions are very small, and parenchymal iron accounts for only 0.2% of the total body content.

Iron is transferred from transferrin to specific receptor sites on the membrane of erythrocyte precursors, after which it is incorporated into the protoporphyrin molecule to form heme. Heme is subsequently coupled with globin to form the oxygen carrying material hemoglobin. The normal erythrocyte has a life span of approximately 120 days. About 21.5 mg of iron, or 6.25 g of hemoglobin, turn over each day.

The capacity of the body to eliminate iron is limited. Only 0.5 – 1 mg of iron is lost each day by adult males and nonmenstruating females from the 21.5 mg liberated from erythrocytes. The remainder is reutilized. Menstruating females may lose an additional 0.5 – 0.6 mg of iron daily.

Dietary iron requirements vary throughout life.

In the adult, they approximate the daily loss. During periods of growth, menstruation or pregnancy, the requirements for iron are greater. Table 26 presents the estimated dietary iron requirements for men and women at different ages.

Although dietary iron should provide most men and postmenopausal women in North America with sufficient iron, adolescent girls and, to a lesser degree, mature premenopausal women may require iron supplementation. Infants between six and twenty-four months of age and pregnant women also require additional iron.

Iron-Deficiency Anemia

The expression iron-deficiency anemia is almost as much a part of North Americana as hot dogs, beer and baseball. The intellect of the public is constantly insulted with ads for one or another "iron tonic". It is apparent from the preceding discussion that most people obtain sufficient iron from their diet. Furthermore, iron deficiency does not always produce anemia. Small decreases in total body iron may have no effect on hemoglobin.

Progressing in severity, iron deficiency may (a) decrease only the iron stores without lowering serum iron concentration, (b) deplete the iron stores and produce a fall in serum iron levels insufficient to cause anemia, or (c) deplete the iron stores and produce a fall in serum iron concentration of sufficient magnitude to produce anemia. The red cells in iron deficiency are usually hypochromic and microcytic.

Iron deficiency is a symptom rather than a disease. It is caused by either the inadequate absorption or increased elimination of iron. The presence of iron-deficiency anemia in adult males or postmenopausal women indicates significant blood loss, and these patients should be investigated to determine the cause of the blood loss. Excessive menstrual flow or multiple pregnancies are the most common causes of iron-deficiency anemia in women of childbearing age. Iron provided by the diet may be inadequate to meet the growth needs of infants and children. Other causes of inadequate iron absorption include diseases or surgical alterations of the gastrointestinal tract.

Oral Iron Preparations

Therapeutic Uses and Adverse Effects

Many iron-containing products are available. There is little to choose between them. The correct product for a particular patient is the one that he or she can tolerate best. Iron may cause nausea, abdominal cramps and either diarrhea or constipation. Patients may be obliged to try several different salts of iron before they find the one they tolerate best. Generally speaking, the gastric intolerance is closely related to the iron content of each salt. Products that produce a reduced incidence of gastrointestinal distress usually contain less iron.

Several sustained-release formulations of iron are available that are designed to release iron slowly as the tablet progresses down the gastrointestinal tract. This type of formulation should produce less gastrointestinal irritation. Unfortunately, many sustained-release tablets may not allow for optimal absorption because iron is best absorbed from the duodenum. These products are best reserved for patients who have demonstrated intolerance to standard iron-containing tablets.

After selecting the iron salt most compatible with the continued gastrointestinal peace of the patient, the next question is how much and for how long. At maximum rates of red cell formation during the treatment of iron-deficiency anemia, about 40 – 60 mg of iron are necessary for optimum hemoglobin production in adults. Allowing for twenty per cent absorbtion in iron-deficient patients, approximately 200 – 300 mg of iron should be required on a daily basis for maximum hemoglobin production. However, hemoglobin production seldom continues at maximum rates for long periods of time. As a result, 180 – 240 mg of iron daily should suffice to produce an optimal response of a one per cent increase in hemoglobin concentration per day.

Ferrous sulfate is the standard iron salt against which all other preparations should be compared. It is usually prepared in 300-mg tablets. Many physicians and nurses feel that ferrous sulfate is the most irritating of all iron salts. This may be due to the fact that it contains more iron per milligram of salt than most of its competitors.

Ferrous gluconate is a popular iron salt because it produces less gastric irritation than ferrous sulfate. However, 300 mg of ferrous gluconate contains only 35 mg of iron compared to the 60 mg in ferrous sulfate. This can explain its reduced incidence of gastric intolerance.

Ferrous fumarate contains 33% iron, with a 200-mg tablet providing 65 mg of the element. Although it is popular with some people, there seems to be little reason for selecting it over the cheaper ferrous sulfate.

Ferrous succinate contains 35% iron and is usually provided in 100-mg tablets. It is usually more expensive than ferrous sulfate and there is little evidence to suggest that it is superior, either in efficacy or in reduced gastrointestinal adverse effects.

Nursing Process

Assessment
Prior to the administration of iron, nursing assessment should emphasize a review of the patient's history for evidence of peptic ulcer, regional enteritis, ulcerative colitis or cirrhosis. In the presence of any of these conditions, the medication should be withheld pending consultation with the attending physician. Baseline blood studies of hematocrit (HCT), hemoglobin (HGB), reticulocytes and bilirubin should be done before and during treatment.

Administration
Oral iron preparations should be administered with meals to prevent gastric irritation. Administration with a glass of citrus juice may also be advisable since ascorbic acid has been reported to facilitate iron absorption. Simultaneous administration of antacids or milk with iron inhibits its absorption. Patients, or parents, should be advised that liquid iron preparations stain the teeth black. Therefore, preparations should be well diluted and administered through a straw. Rinsing the mouth with water will ensure that none of the medication is left on the teeth.

Evaluation
Nursing evaluation of the patient following the initiation of iron therapy focuses on identifying a positive response to the medication. In addition to laboratory tests to measure therapeutic response, the efficacy of the drug can be evaluated by patient reports of increased energy, reduced lethargy and fatigue, and improved appetite. Nurses should monitor the bowel habits of patients, as well as the feces for changes in color, diarrhea or constipation.

Teaching
Patients should be alerted to expect black tarry stools and to report gastrointestinal disturbances. Dietary sources of iron should be reviewed with patients and their families. Referral for dietary counselling should be considered. Finally, patients should be instructed to keep iron tablets out of the reach of children because of the severe and often fatal effects of iron toxicity.

Parenteral Iron Preparations

Therapeutic Uses and Adverse Effects

Parenteral iron is required for patients who are unable to tolerate oral iron or absorb it from the gastrointestinal tract. Patients with chronic inflammatory bowel disease or colostomies may be unable or unwilling to ingest iron. Idiopathic or postresection malabsorption syndromes may be another indication for parenteral iron because patients with these problems may be unable to absorb iron. Very occasionally, some patients with severe iron deficiency discovered late in a pregnancy may qualify for parenteral iron treatment. Patients suffering from severe uncontrollable gastrointestinal bleeding may also receive parenteral iron.

Parenteral iron has advantages and drawbacks. Although one can correct iron deficiency quickly with parenteral iron therapy, the ability of the body to eliminate iron is limited. Care must be taken to calculate the dose accurately to avoid iron overload with hepatic damage.

Iron dextran (Imferon) is a parenterally formulated complex of ferric hydroxide and low molecular weight dextran that can be given either intramuscularly or intravenously. Iron sorbitol (iron sorbitex) injection (Jectofer) must be administered intramuscularly only.

Nursing Process

Assessment
The parenteral administration of iron dextran is contraindicated in patients whose nursing assessment reveals a current pregnancy, previous hypersensitivity or a history of arthritis, ankylosing spondylitis, liver disease or leukemia. A small initial test dose of iron dextran (25 mg in adults) should always be given prior to administration of the prescribed therapeutic amount. This will permit assessment of the patient for potential anaphylactic responses.

Administration
Iron dextran should be administered by deep intramuscular injection in the upper outer quadrant of the gluteus maximus using a two-inch needle that has been changed following withdrawal of the solution from the vial. The needle should be inserted into the muscle using the Z-track method, as shown in Figure 20, which involves displacing the skin and subcutaneous tissue laterally over the muscle, inserting the needle, and then releasing the skin and subcutaneous tissue. This method

produces a needle track which is Z-shaped and thus prevents leakage of the medication up the needle track into the subcutaneous tissue and skin where it can cause staining lasting up to two years. Nurses should also aspirate carefully to avoid inadvertent intravenous injection. Individuals who have small muscle mass should have this medication injected intravenously by a physician.

Figure 20
Illustration of Z-track injection method.

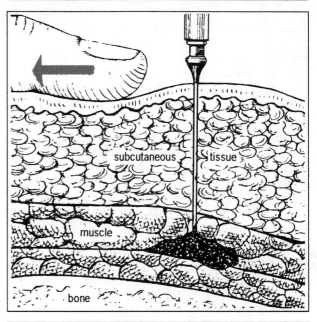

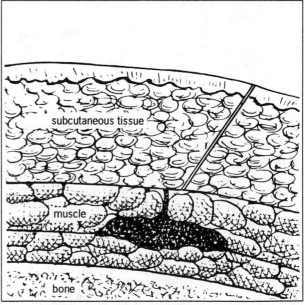

Evaluation

Nursing evaluation of patients should focus on identifying the adverse effects of iron dextran, including anaphylactic reactions. Severe febrile reactions, as well as arthralgia and myalgia, have also been observed, as have variable degrees of soreness and inflammation at the injection site following intramuscular injection. Other observations during nursing evaluation might include peripheral vascular flushing with overly rapid intravenous administration; hypotensive reactions; and possible arthritic reactivation in patients with quiescent rheumatoid arthritis. Observation of the patient's vital signs at fifteen-minute intervals for two hours following the first administration of parenteral iron will permit early identification of these adverse reactions. Thereafter, the patient should be observed at half-hour intervals for two hours following each parenteral administration of iron. Nurses should also evaluate patients for minor adverse reactions to iron dextran, including headache, transitory paresthesias, nausea, shivering, itching and rash. Brown skin discoloration may occur at the injection site. Local phlebitis has been reported after intravenous administration.

The adverse effects of iron sorbitol include headache, dizziness, flushing, nausea and vomiting, as well as more severe systemic reactions consisting of generalized pain, precordial pressure sensations, palpitations and a fall in blood pressure in some patients.

Nursing evaluation of the effectiveness of these medications is the same as that outlined for oral iron products. Specifically, it includes laboratory tests to measure therapeutic response, and subjective reports by the patient of increased energy, reduced lethargy and tiredness, and improved appetite.

Teaching

Patient teaching should assist the individual and family in identifying dietary sources of iron. Collaboration with, or referral to, a dietician may be beneficial. Patients should be instructed to report unusual symptoms occurring within twenty-four hours following injection of iron.

Acute Iron Toxicity

Nurses may encounter children who have accidentally swallowed large numbers of iron tablets. This is a relatively common occurrence because iron is prescribed often for mothers and also may be obtained without prescription in a variety of over-the-counter products. Depending on the size of the child, as few as ten to thirty tablets have been reported to produce death.

The irritant effects of iron on the gastrointestinal tract have already been mentioned. When large amounts are consumed, iron can produce a necrotizing gastroenteritis. Bleeding and transudation into the lumen can occur. Shock may ensue as a result of fluid loss or vasodilatation. The latter effect has been attributed either to the actions of large amounts of ferritin on the blood vessels or the consequences of bacterial toxins crossing the damaged intestine.

Initially, the patient may experience acute enteritis and shock. This is evidenced by vomiting and diarrhea together with dyspnea and lethargy. After this initial period, which may last from one to six hours, the patient may recover. However, some subjects proceed to metabolic acidosis and coma. First-aid treatment should include attempts to have the subject vomit. Gastric lavage may be attempted in a hospital setting. Gavage with 5% sodium bicarbonate to form an insoluble nonabsorbable complex.

Deferoxamine (Desferal)

Deferoxamine (Desferal) is a material that chelates with iron to make a nontoxic complex. It can be given intramuscularly or intravenously to reverse the effects of systemic iron toxicity. However, deferoxamine can be toxic in its own right (see Table 27) and should be used only if symptoms of systemic iron poisoning appear. In the presence of a nursing assessment that reveals a current pregnancy, anuria or history of pyelonephritis or other kidney disease, the danger of using this medication must be weighed against the risk of fatality due to iron toxicity. Only fully dissolved medication should be administered and at the specific infusion rate specified by the physician.

Nursing evaluation should monitor vital signs and fluid intake and output for evidence of adverse reactions (fever, hypotension, shock). Reddish-colored urine following administration of deferoxamine indicates high serum iron levels and the necessity for continuing therapy. Long-term therapy necessitates careful monitoring of ophthalmic function, since deferoxamine has been shown to cause blurred vision and cataracts.

Folic Acid and Vitamin B_{12} Deficiency

Discussion of the actions of folic acid and vitamin B_{12} follows logically that of iron. A deficiency in any of the three can cause anemia. However, in the case of iron deficiency, the anemia is usually hypochromic and microcytic, whereas folic acid or vitamin B_{12} deficiency produce hyperchromic megaloblastic anemia. Both folic acid and vitamin B_{12} are essential for the synthesis of deoxyribonucleic acid (DNA) in the nucleus of cells. In their absence cell mitosis stops. The consequences of vitamin B_{12} deficiency exceed those of a lack of folic acid. Although both conditions produce similar changes in bone marrow, a lack of vitamin B_{12} produces pernicious anemia, a condition marked by megaloblastic anemia, gastrointestinal symptoms (including glossitis and dyspepsia) and neurological abnormalities.

Folic Acid

Metabolism

Folic acid is widely distributed in animal and vegetable foods. Although the conjugated form of the vitamin found in food is less readily absorbed than folic acid in tablets, humans can usually absorb sufficient amounts in their diet to meet the needs of the body. The chemical is absorbed in the first third of the small intestine. Its absorption may be inadequate in patients with diseases of the small intestine. Once absorbed, folic acid is distributed throughout the body and eliminated by the kidneys. When normal amounts are ingested, only small amounts of folic acid are lost in the urine. As the dose is increased, more of it may find its way through the nephrons.

The healthy adult requires about 50 µg of folic acid daily, which is usually supplied by the diet. During pregnancy the requirements for folic acid increase to 100 – 200 µg per day and may exceed the dietary supply. Supplemental folic acid is usually given at this time.

As mentioned earlier, folic acid is essential for the synthesis of DNA by the nucleus of cells. In its absence the DNA content of cell nuclei falls and the ability of cells to divide by mitosis is reduced. This is seen first in rapidly dividing cells, such as those responsible for the formation of new erythrocytes.

Therapeutic Uses

Supplemental folic acid is administered when inadequate amounts of the vitamin are absorbed, as a result of either a dietary deficiency or a malabsorption syndrome. The former situation is not common because of widespread distribution of the vitamin in food. It is seen more often in chronic alcoholics and the elderly who may fail to eat a balanced diet. The latter condition occurs following partial gastrectomy or diseases of the small intestine, such as tropical sprue, steatorrhea or celiac disease. Regional ileitis, irradiation damage and intestinal tuberculosis are other causes of folic acid malabsorption.

The replacement of folic acid in the diet of patients who fail to eat adequate amounts of food requires only 100 – 200 µg daily. Larger quantities, in the range of 0.5 – 1 mg (500 – 1000 µg) daily, are warranted for patients with malabsorption problems.

Increased requirement for folic acid during pregnancy has already been mentioned. Failure to provide patients with adequate amounts of folic acid during pregnancy may result in megaloblastic anemia. Not surprisingly, this condition is more prevalent in less developed countries and poorer areas of North America. Occurring during the third trimester, and more often during twin pregnancies, folic acid deficiency results from the increased fetal requirements placed on the mother. The dose of folic acid required during pregnancy is similar to that recommended for malabsorption syndromes — 0.5 – 1 mg daily.

The age of polypharmacy is upon us and with it the opportunity for drug interactions. Several drugs have been shown to inhibit folic acid absorption. These include phenytoin, primidone, carbamazepine and mephobarbital, all antiepileptics. Oral contraceptives may also, on rare occasions, reduce folic acid absorption. If supplemental folic acid is not provided, megaloblastic anemia may occur.

Nursing Process

Assessment

If the nursing assessment of the patient prior to the administration of folic acid supplements reveals gastrointestinal disturbances (glossitis, dyspepsia), degenerative changes of the spinal cord and peripheral nerves including disturbances of the vibratory sense, proprioception and pyramidal tract function, and psychological disturbances (irritability, overactivity, excitement, depression, disorientation, poor decision making), the medication should be withheld pending consultation with the physician because these symptoms indicate vitamin B_{12} deficiency rather than lack of folic acid.

Evaluation

Nursing evaluation should emphasize determining folic acid's effectiveness. This is inferred from patient reports of an increased sense of well-being. Patients may also report the alleviation of such symptoms as glossitis, weight loss, irritability, fatigue, insomnia, forgetfulness and pallor. Following administration of folic acid, a patient evaluation that reveals continued gastrointestinal disturbances, degenerative neurological changes or psychological disturbances should be reported to the physician because these indicate vitamin B_{12} deficiency.

Teaching

Patient teaching should stress counselling regarding dietary sources of folic acid, such as yeast, liver, fresh raw green vegetables and fresh fruits. Referral to, or collaboration with, a dietitian may be appropriate. Patients and their families should also be instructed in the desired therapeutic effects of folic acid to enable them to judge the effectiveness of the medication.

Vitamin B_{12}

Metabolism

Vitamin B_{12}, or cyanocobalamin, is found only in food of animal origin. Its absorption in the lower part of the ileum depends upon the secretion of a glycoprotein, called the intrinsic factor, by the parietal cells of the fundus and body of the stomach. In the absence of the intrinsic factor, very little vitamin B_{12} is absorbed and pernicious anemia occurs. Once absorbed, vitamin B_{12} is stored in the liver and eliminated in the bile.

Daily requirements for vitamin B_{12} are minute. The normal diet provides from $1 - 85$ µg daily, with the amount lost in the bile being only 1 µg every twenty-four hours. The amount stored in the body is about 5 mg. It follows from these figures that several years free of vitamin B_{12} are required before a patient develops a deficiency of clinical significance.

In some ways the actions of vitamin B_{12} and folic acid overlap. Both chemicals are required for the synthesis of DNA. As a result, patients with pernicious anemia demonstrate a megaloblastic anemia similar to that described previously for folic acid deficiency. However, the consequences of pernicious anemia involve also the neurological and gastrointestinal systems.

The neurological signs of vitamin B_{12} deficiency include degenerative changes of the dorsal and lateral columns of the spinal cord and peripheral nerves. As a result, patients experience disturbances of vibratory sense, proprioception and pyramidal tract function. In addition, mental disturbances, ranging from mood swings to psychosis, may appear. Optic atrophy can also occur.

The consequences of vitamin B_{12} deficiency on the gastrointestinal system include glossitis and dyspepsia. They reflect gastric mucosal atrophy and result from the inability of normally rapidly developing cells to form sufficient DNA for mitosis.

Vitamin B_{12} injection reverses these effects. Folic acid will treat the megaloblastic anemia but has no effect on the other consequences of vitamin B_{12} deficiency. For this reason, it should not be used to treat megaloblastic anemia until it is clear that a vitamin B_{12} deficiency is not the cause of the anemia. If folic acid is used inappropriately to treat a megaloblastic anemia due to vitamin B_{12} deficiency, the physician and nurse may be lulled into a false sense of security by the improvement in the blood picture while the gastrointestinal and neurological systems continue to deteriorate.

Therapeutic Uses

Vitamin B_{12} is used to treat pernicious anemia and other vitamin B_{12} deficiency states. The effects of vitamin B_{12} are often rapid. Mental symptoms often improve within hours and the megaloblastic anemia disappears in a few weeks. The neurologic effects respond more slowly. Peripheral neuropathy usually disappears and subacute degeneration of the spinal cord stops, but improvement is slow.

Vitamin B_{12} can be given orally to the very unusual patients (generally vegans — strict vegetarians) in whom symptoms are due to dietary deficiency, not an absence of the intrinsic factor. The dosage range for oral therapy is $1 - 25$ µg/day, accompanying meals. If patients are unwilling to take oral vitamin B_{12} daily to replace the quantity normally consumed in the diet, monthly injections can be given.

Nursing Process

Administration

The administration of vitamin B_{12} is preceded by a nursing assessment that establishes pretherapeutic levels of neurological and psychological integrity. As mentioned above, oral administration usually accompanies meals in order to benefit from stimulation of intrinsic factor production, essential to the absorption of vitamin B_{12}. Nursing evaluation of the effectiveness of the medication is based on amelioration of the symptoms of deficiency. Refer to Table 27 for administrative details.

Teaching

Patients with pernicious anemia must be treated parenterally. They should be informed that they will require vitamin B_{12} treatment for the duration of their lives and should also be taught the consequences of failure to comply with the therapeutic regimen. In addition, nurses should alert the patient and the family to the need to inform the physician of other diseases or infections that occur, since the dosage of vitamin B_{12} might require adjustment.

Further Reading

Arthur, C. K. and Isbister, J. P. (1987). Iron deficiency: Misunderstood, misdiagnosed and mistreated. *Drugs 33* :171-182.

Finch, C. A. and Huebers, H. (1982). Perspectives in iron metabolism. *New Engl. J. Med. 306* :1520-1528.

Table 27
Antianemic drugs.

Pharmacologic Classification: Oral Iron-Containing Preparations

Generic Name (Trade Name)	Use (Dose)	Action	Adverse Effects	Drug Interactions	Nursing Process
Ferrous sulfate (Feosol, Fer-In-Sol, Fer-Grad, Ferro-Gradumet, Fesofor, Mol-Iron)	Tx of uncomplicated Fe-deficiency anemia (**Oral:** Adults - initially, 30-60 mg elemental Fe; incr. prn in 30-mg increments to max. 180 mg/day in 3-4 doses. Children *6-12 yrs* - 24-120 mg [3 mg/kg] elemental Fe/day in 3-4 divided doses; *2-5 yrs* - 15-45 mg [3 mg/kg] of elemental Fe/day in 3-4 divided doses; *6 mos-2 yrs* - up to 6 mg/kg/day of elemental Fe in 3-4 divided doses; *infants* - 10-25 mg of elemental Fe/day, given in 3-4 divided doses. Consult product monographs for indiv. product)	Replenishes depleted Fe stores produced by inadequate diet, inadequate absorpt'n or incr. eliminat'n.	GI upset, nausea, abdominal cramps, diarrhea, constipat'n	**Antacids:** Given concomitantly w. Fe compounds, decr. Fe absorpt'n. Administrat'n of antacids and Fe preparat'ns should be spaced as far apart as possible. **Tetracyclines:** Can suffer from reduced absorpt'n if ingested within a few hours of Fe.	**Assess:** HCT, HGB, reticulocytes and bilirubin before and during drug tx. For tx of peptic ulcer, regional enteritis, ulcerative colitis, cirrhosis. **Administer:** Liquid Fe well diluted via a straw, w. meals or citrus juice. **Evaluate:** For positive responses to tx (incr. energy, appetite; less fatigue). Monitor eliminat'n patterns for changes. **Teach:** To expect black tarry stools; to report GI disturbances; to eat foods high in Fe; to store this medicat'n out of reach of children.
Ferrous gluconate (Fergon)	As for ferrous sulfate (**Oral:** Adults - 300-600 mg [35-70 mg elemental Fe] tid. Children *6-12 yrs* - 300-900 mg [35-105 mg elemental Fe] od or bid; *infants and children under 6 yrs* - 100-300 mg [12-35 mg elemental Fe] daily)	As for ferrous sulfate	As for ferrous sulfate	As for ferrous sulfate	As for ferrous sulfate
Ferrous fumarate (Feostat, Feroton, Ferrofume, Fersamel, Hematon, Toleron)	As for ferrous sulfate (**Oral:** Adults - 100-400 mg [approx. 33-133 mg elemental Fe] daily in 1-4 doses. Children *6-12 yrs* - 100-300 mg [33-100 mg elemental Fe] daily in 1-4 doses; *1-5 yrs* - initially, 15 mg elemental Fe/day; incr. prn gradually to max 45 mg elemental Fe/day in 3-4 divided doses; *infants* - 10-20 mg elemental Fe/day, divided into 2-4 doses)	As for ferrous sulfate	As for ferrous sulfate	As for ferrous sulfate	As for ferrous sulfate

Generic Name (Trade Name)	Use (Dose)	Action	Adverse Effects	Drug Interactions	Nursing Process
Ferrous succinate (Cerevon)	As for ferrous sulfate **(Oral:** Adults and children over 12 - 100-300 mg [35-105 mg elemental Fe] daily)	As for ferrous sulfate	As for ferrous sulfate	As for ferrous sulfate	As for ferrous sulfate

Pharmacologic Classification: Parenteral Iron-Containing Preparations

Generic Name (Trade Name)	Use (Dose)	Action	Adverse Effects	Drug Interactions	Nursing Process
Iron dextran (Imferon)	Severe Fe-deficiency anemias when oral tx is contraindicated or ineffective **(IV** by physician or **IM:** Highly individual; consult manufacturer's inform'n for details on dosage)	As for ferrous sulfate	Anaphylactic react'ns, severe febrile react'ns, arthralgia and myalgia, soreness, inflammat'n and brown skin discolorat'n at inject'n site, hypotensive react'n, arthritic reactivat'n in pts w. quiescent rheumatoid arthritis. **Tx:** Prompt IV epinephrine and suitable antihistamine. If BP still remains low, use IV levarerenol.		**Assess:** For pregnancy; hx of hypersensitivity, arthritis, ankylosing spondylitis, liver disease or impaired funct'n, leukemia. **Administer:** 25-mg test dose initially; change needle after w'drawing solut'n from container; administer IM deep into outer quadrant of gluteus maximus using Z-track method and 2" needle; aspirate on barrel of syringe to prevent accidental IV infus'n. **Evaluate:** BP and pulse for 2 h; drug efficacy as for oral Fe preparat'ns. **Teach:** Foods high in Fe; to report unusual s/s occurring within 24 h.
Iron sorbitol, iron sorbitex (Jectofer)	Tx of Fe-deficiency anemia whenever parenteral administrat'n of Fe is preferred (determine dose from manufacturer's product monograph)	As for ferrous sulfate	Flushing, nausea and vomiting, dysgeusia; more severe systemic react'ns incl. gen. pain, precordial pressure sensat'ns, palpitat'ns, fall in BP.		

Pharmacologic Classification: Iron Antidote

Generic Name (Trade Name)	Use (Dose)	Action	Adverse Effects	Drug Interactions	Nursing Process
Deferoxamine (Desferal)	Tx of [a] acute Fe intoxicat'n, as adjunct to standard tx measures; [b] chronic Fe overload due to transfus'n	Chelates w. Fe to make a nontoxic complex.	Allergic skin react'n (urticaria, gen. erythema), hypotens'n, tachycardia, shock,	**Ascorbic acid:** Administered orally for 3 or more days before deferoxamine, doubles urinary Fe excret'n.	**Assess:** For pregnancy, anuria, hx of pyelonephritis or renal disease. **Administer:** Only fully dissolved drug at specifically prescribed flow rate.

	dependent anemias (**IM:** *For acute Fe intoxicat'n* - initially, 90 mg/Kg. This may be followed by 45 mg/Kg q4-12h prn. Max. single dose should not exceed 1 g. In general, not more than 6 g should be given in 24 h. Adults and children - **IV:** For pts in shock and those beginning to show signs of CV collapse. Infus'n rates should be adapted to severity of poisoning. Rate of infus'n should not exceed 15 mg/Kg/h)	dizziness, convuls'ns, abdominal discomfort, diarrhea, thrombocytopenia, blurred vision, impaired hepatic/renal funct'n, dysuria, pyrexia		**Evaluate:** For adverse react'ns, vital signs (fever, hypotens'n, shock), fluid intake/output, color of urine, ophthalmic funct'n.

Pharmacologic Classification: Parenteral Iron-Containing Preparations

Folic acid (Folvite)	Tx of folate deficiency (**Oral/IM/SC:** Adults and children - up to 1 mg/day. When clinical symptoms have subsided and blood tests have become normal, a maint. dose of 0.1-0.25 mg/day should be given orally)	Required for DNA synthesis for bone marrow mature'n and cell mitosis.	Allergic responses	**Antiepileptic drugs:** May inhibit folic acid absorpt'n. **Contraceptives, oral:** May rarely reduce folic acid absorpt'n.	**Assess:** For GI disturbances, degenerative neurological changes, psychological abnormalities. **Evaluate:** Tx effectiveness, psychological status, neurological integrity. **Teach:** Dietary sources of folic acid.
Vitamin B$_{12}$ cyanocobalamin (Betalin 12 Crystalline, Redisol, Rubramin PC, Ruvite, Sytobex)	Pernicious anemia with or without neurologic complicat'ns; anemias due to malabsorpt'n of vitamin B$_{12}$ (**IM/SC:** Adults - 30 µg/day for 5-10 days, followed by 100-200 µg monthly until remiss'n is complete; thereafter, 100 µg q4weeks. Children - 1000-5000 µg total, given in divided doses of 30-50 µg/day over 2 or more weeks. Thereafter, give folic acid early in tx w. vitamin B$_{12}$ unless folic acid levels are adequate)	Required for DNA synthesis for bone marrow mature'n and cell mitosis.	Mild transient diarrhea, polycythemia vera, peripheral vascular thrombosis, itching, transitory exanthema		**Assess:** Establish baseline indicators of psychological status and neurological integrity. **Administer:** Parenteral route essential for tx of pernicious anemia. Oral route may be used in pts who do not lack intrinsic factor but fail to ingest sufficient quantities of vitamin B$_{12}$ in food; orally, mixed with juice and accompanying meals. **Evaluate:** VS for pulmonary edema; neurological and psychological status. **Teach:** Necessity in pernicious anemia for lifetime parenteral tx; consequences of failure to comply w. regimen; need to inform physician of other diseases or infect'ns that occur and might require vitamin B$_{12}$ dosage adjustment.

CHAPTER 21

Anticoagulant and Antiplatelet Drugs, Fibrinolytic Agents and Vitamin K

Teaching Objectives

Following completion of this chapter, the reader should be able to:

1. Describe the etiologies of arterial and venous thromboses.
2. Describe the mechanism of action, pharmacologic effects, therapeutic uses and adverse effects of heparin and the nursing process related to its use.
3. Describe the mechanism of action, pharmacologic effects, therapeutic uses and adverse effects of oral anticoagulants and the nursing process related to their use.
4. Discuss the means by which aspirin reduces platelet adhesion and/or aggregation, its efficacy in the treatment of cerebrovascular or coronary artery disease and the nursing process related to its use.
5. Discuss the means by which sulfinpyrazone reduces platelet adhesion and/or aggregation, its efficacy in the treatment of cerebrovascular or coronary artery disease and the nursing process relating to its use.
6. Describe briefly the use of dipyridamole as an antiplatelet drug and the nursing process related to its use.
7. Explain the mechanism of action, pharmacologic effects, therapeutic uses and adverse effects of fibrinolytic drugs and the nursing process related to their use.
8. Discuss vitamin K, describing its occurrence in nature, absorption from the gastrointestinal tract, action in the body, therapeutic uses, adverse effects and the nursing process related to its use.

Thromboses and Emboli

Three groups of drugs can be used in the management of thromboses and emboli. These are (1) anticoagulants, which inhibit the formation of fibrin, (2) antiplatelet drugs, which reduce platelet adhesion and/or aggregation and (3) fibrinolytic and thrombolytic agents, which digest fibrin. This chapter discusses all three groups. In addition, the use of vitamin K is discussed because of its importance in the process of coagulation.

Formation of Arterial and Venous Thromboses

Venous and arterial thromboses have different causes. Venous thrombi usually form in regions of slow or disturbed flow. They begin as small deposits in either the venous sinuses of the deep veins of the legs or of the valve cusp pockets. Coagulation of the blood plays a major role in the formation and extension of venous thrombi.

Arterial thromboses are formed after damage to the endothelium of the artery allows platelets to adhere to the vessel wall, serving as the focus for thrombus formation. The adhesion of a few platelets to the vessel wall is followed by the aggregation of increased numbers of thrombocytes. Fibrin, formed by coagulation, subsequently encases the platelets, giving rise to a platelet-fibrin plug. Because blood flow in the arteries is rapid, arterial thrombi stay close to vessel walls and have been termed **mural thrombi.**

A mural thrombus may either remain at its original site or be sheared away by the rapid blood flow to locate in other parts of the body. If it remains at its site of origin, the mural thrombus can serve as a focus for further platelet aggregation. In that case, a platelet-fibrin plug may be formed, which becomes incorporated into the vessel wall to produce atherosclerosis-like lesions.

From the preceding discussion it is apparent that these vascular problems are treatable by different types of drugs. Anticoagulants are employed to prevent thrombus formation in the veins, where blood coagulation plays an important role. Antiplatelet drugs are used to stop microemboli forming in the arteries and arterioles, where platelet adhesion is involved.

Anticoagulant Drugs

Blood coagulation is a complex process. Its intricacies are illustrated in Figure 21. Clotting can be precipitated either by contact activation through the intrinsic system or by the traumatic release of tissue thromboplastin via the extrinsic system. The importance of vitamin K is evident from the fact that clotting factors II, VII, IX and X depend upon it for their synthesis.

Table 28
Antithrombotic drugs.

Anticoagulants

1. Coumarin and indanedione anticoagulants — reduce the activity of vitamin K-dependent clotting factors II, VII, IX and X.
2. Heparin — increases the activity of antithrombin III and so potentiates the naturally occuring plasma inhibitor of activated factors IX, X, XI and of thrombin.
3. Ancrod — converts fibrinogen to an unstable form of fibrin, the plasma fibrinogen level being markedly reduced.

Antiplatelet agents

4. Drugs that inhibit some platelet functions (e.g., aspirin, indomethacin, sulfinpyrazone, dipyridamole, possibly dextran).

Thrombolytic agents

5. Streptokinase — activates plasminogen to form plasmin indirectly (via the formation of an activator complex with plasminogen or plasmin).
6. Urokinase — activates plasminogen to form plasmin directly.

Fibrinolytic stimulants

7. Ethyloestrenol + phenformin; stanozolol alone — enhance plasma fibrinolytic activity (possibly by increasing activator content of the walls of superficial veins).

Antifibrinolytic agents

8. Aminocaproic acid, tranexamic acid, aprotinin — competitively inhibit plasminogen activation and noncompetitively inhibit plasmin; aprotinin also has vasoactive properties.

Heparin

Mechanism of Action and Pharmacologic Effects

Heparin is a very potent anticoagulant. Heparin works by means of a plasma cofactor, the heparin cofactor or antithrombin III, which neutralizes several activated clotting factors: XIIa, kallikrein, XIa, IXa, Xa, IIa and XIIIa. Heparin must be injected to be effective. Once it is injected its effects are immediate but fleeting, with fifty per cent being dissipated within the first hour.

Heparin also decreases plasma turbidity normally seen after the ingestion of a fat-containing meal. This effect is attributed to a release of a lipase from capillary walls that breaks down chylomicrons and free fatty acids in plasma. At the present time it is not clear whether this action of heparin has any therapeutic significance.

Figure 21

Diagrammatic representation (simplified) of the human blood coagulation and fibrinolytic enzyme system.

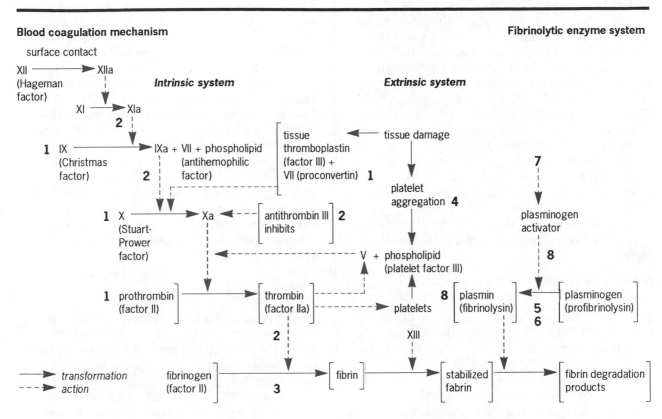

Blood coagulation mechanism

Fibrinolytic enzyme system

For clarity, the role of calcium in the activation reactions of coagulation factors is not included in this diagram. Calcium is not required for the activation of factor XII or for action of factor XI.

From: A.S. Gallus and J. Hirsh (1976), Antithrombotic drugs: Part 1. *Drugs 12* :41-68. Reproduced with permission.

Therapeutic Uses

The clinical uses of heparin are based on its ability to prevent new clot formation and limit the propagation of existing thrombi. Lower doses of heparin are used to prevent a thrombosis and higher doses to treat an established thrombosis. The doses and routes of administration used are summarized in Table 30 at the end of this chapter. They are, however, only estimates and should be altered in accordance with the results of coagulation tests, such as whole blood clotting time, thrombin time, or activated partial thromboplastin time (PTT). If an oral anticoagulant is also used, a prothrombin test also should be performed. When heparin is given continuously intravenously, the coagulation test should be performed about every four hours in the early stages of treatment. If heparin is given intermittently, a coagulation test is performed before each injection. Once the dosage range has been stabilized, daily coagulation tests are generally satisfactory.

Heparin is contraindicated in the presence of hemophilia, severe clotting disorders and uncontrollable bleeding. It is also contraindicated in patients with severe liver damage, individuals in shock and those who are hypersensitive to the drug. The administration of large doses of heparin should be delayed four hours postoperatively.

Adverse Effects

Bleeding is the major complication of heparin therapy. In addition, patients receiving more than 15 000 USP units per day on a long-term basis may develop osteoporosis. A small number of patients on heparin develop a thrombocytopenia of unknown origin, and platelet counts should be done during heparin therapy. In many cases the adverse effects can be terminated simply by stopping the drug. If it is necessary to inhibit heparin's effects immediately, protamine sulfate can be administered. Protamine sulfate binds to heparin to form an inactive complex. Because protamine is itself an anticoagulant, it must not be administered in excess of the amount required to neutralize heparin. Each milligram of protamine neutralizes approximately 90 USP units of heparin activity derived from lung tissue or about 115 USP units of heparin activity derived from intestinal mucosa. Protamine should be given by very slow intravenous infusion in doses not to exceed 50 mg of protamine in any ten-minute period. Too-rapid administration of protamine can cause severe hypotensive anaphylactoid-like reactions. Facilities to treat shock should be available. Because of the anticoagulant effect of protamine it is unwise to give more than 100 mg over a short period unless a larger requirement is certain.

Nursing Process

Assessment

Before administering heparin, nurses should review the patient's history to verify that there are no contraindications to its use, e.g., active bleeding or conditions associated with bleeding tendencies: leukemia, thrombocytopenic purpura, hemophilia; hepatic disease; alcoholism; neurological, ophthalmic or spinal surgery; menstruation, pregnancy, postpartum; ulcerative conditions of the gastrointestinal tract; open wounds; or uncontrolled hypertension. In addition, the patient's chart should be checked to ensure that blood for baseline laboratory studies has been drawn.

Administration

The procedure of administering heparin begins with a thorough examination of the label because of the wide variety of strengths and preparations available. The intravenous or subcutaneous routes are preferred. Withdrawal of heparin from the vial should be followed by changing the needle so that no medication will be left along the needle track. Use of a tuberculin syringe will ensure greater accuracy in measuring the amount of the medication. The ideal site is the abdominal fat pad; not in arms and not intramuscular. An injection site that is at least two inches away from the umbilicus and from any scar tissue should be chosen. Use of a 25-gauge half-inch needle and the Z-track method of injection (see Figure 20, Chapter 20) will prevent leakage of heparin back up the needle track. The injection site should not be massaged following withdrawal of the needle; this can cause local bleeding and bruising.

Evaluation

The primary purpose of the nursing evaluation of the patient during heparin therapy is early identification of any adverse effects of the medication. Foremost among these is bleeding, which occurs most frequently with high doses of the drug. It is a nursing responsibility to coordinate laboratory phlebotomy appropriately with injection time, to monitor partial thromboplastin times (PTTs) and to draw the physician's attention to abnormal values. Nurses should be alert for occult blood in the urine and stools; fever, increased pulse rate, a drop in blood pressure or other changes in the vital signs, which might indicate undetected bleeding; unexplained, persistent low back pain, which could indicate abdominal bleeding; petechiae, purpura, excessive bruising or bleeding gums, which can indicate heparin overdose; and excessive menstrual flow.

Teaching

Patients receiving heparin should be told of its diuretic effect and informed that an increase in menstrual flow can ensue. They should also be aware that the drug can produce a transient alopecia. Patients should be instructed to report bleeding immediately. They should also be informed that cigaret and alcohol use can alter heparin's effects. Similarly, they should be advised not to use over-the-counter medications without consulting the pharmacist or physician regarding the possibility of drug interactions. Patients should carry a Medic-Alert ID identifying the drug taken.

Oral Anticoagulants

Mechanism of Action and Pharmacologic Effects

Oral anticoagulants are similar in structure to vitamin K. They competitively inhibit the action of this vitamin and thereby reduce the synthesis of factors II, VII, IX, and X in the liver. In contrast to the immediate onset of action of heparin, the effects of oral anticoagulants are delayed until the coagulation factors formed prior to treatment disappear. This usually requires thirty-six to forty-eight hours. The dosages and plasma half-lives of several oral anticoagulants are summarized in Table 29.

Oral anticoagulant dosage should be controlled by periodic determination of the prothrombin time. A prothrombin test should be ordered forty-eight hours after starting treatment and every one to two days thereafter until the patient's prothrombin time is stable at 1.5 – 2.5 times the control value (e.g., 21 – 35 s with a control of 14 s). Heparin can prolong the one-stage prothrombin time. Four to five hours should elapse between the last intravenous dose and twelve to twenty-four hours after the last subcutaneous dose of heparin before a sample is drawn for a prothrombin test.

Therapeutic Uses

Oral anticoagulants are used to prevent the formation of new fibrin thrombi and reduce the extension of already formed clots. In the treatment of an acute deep venous thrombosis, heparin is used first, followed by three to six months of therapy with an oral anticoagulant. Low-dose heparin has been shown to be effective in preventing thrombosis before and after surgery in certain high-risk patients. Patients with rheumatic valve disease experience a lower incidence of pulmonary or systemic emboli if treated with an oral anticoagulant. Oral anticoagulants have also been used in patients recovering from myocardial infarcts, but evidence for their efficacy is not conclusive. They are also given to patients suffering from cerebrovascular disease to reduce the incidence of transient cerebral ischemic attacks.

At the earliest signs of bleeding, the oral anticoagulant should be withdrawn. Conditions associated with increased risk include severe to moderate hepatic or renal insufficiency, infectious diseases or disturbances of intestinal flora, moderate to severe hypertension, and surgery or trauma resulting in large exposed raw surfaces. Congestive heart failure may increase sensitivity to oral anticoagulants.

Adverse Effects

Hemorrhage is the major adverse effect of oral anticoagulants. Although bleeding may occur anywhere in the body, the gastrointestinal tract is the most common site. Patients with undiagnosed peptic ulcers or gastrointestinal neoplasms are at greater risk. Intracerebral hemorrhage is another major cause of death. Sudden neurologic or psychiatric problems are of concern and should be reported to the physician because of the risk of a subdural hematoma. Hemorrhages are treated by stopping the drug and administering vitamin K_1. In emergencies, plasma derivatives containing vitamin K-dependent clotting factors can be given.

Allergic reactions may occur with oral anticoagulants, particularly with phenindione. Other adverse effects of oral anticoagulant drugs include rashes, diarrhea, pyrexia, neutropenia, thrombocytopenia, agranulocytosis, hepatitis and nephritis.

Drug Interactions with Oral Anticoagulants

Many drugs interact with oral anticoagulants. Some influence the ability of anticoagulants to antagonize vitamin K in the body. Others alter the absorption, distribution or elimination of the anticoagulants. It is beyond the scope of this text to discuss all drugs that have been shown to interact with oral anticoagulants. Nurses are encouraged to refer to Table 31 at the end of this chapter for a list of interacting drugs. Collaboration and consultation with a pharmacist will ensure nurses access to the most current information on drug interactions.

Table 29
Characteristics of some oral anticoagulant drugs.

Drug	Plasma Half-life (h)	Initial Dose	Day 2 Dose	Maintenance Dose		Time for PT to Reach 2x Control Value (h)	Length of Action
				Average	Range		
Warfarin	42	20 – 40 or 10 – 15†	– 10 – 15†	8 8	3 – 20 3 – 20	36 – 48 96 – 120†	Intermediate
Dicoumarol	24	300	200	75	25 – 120	36 – 48	Intermediate
Phenprocoumon	160	24	–	4	0.75 – 6	36 – 48	Long
Ethylbiscoumacetate	2.5	900 – 1200	900 – 1200	450	300 – 600	18 – 30	Short
Phenindione	5	200	100	100	25 – 200	36 – 48	Intermediate

†   Warfarin regimen when loading dose is not used. Doses are expressed in milligrams.
From: A. S. Gallus and J. Hirsh (1976), Antithrombotic drugs: Part 1. *Drugs 12* :41-68. Reproduced with permission.

Nursing Process

Assessment

Nursing assessment of patients for whom oral anticoagulants have been prescribed is similar to that previously discussed for heparin. In addition, nurses should try to estimate the probability of patient compliance with the prescribed regimen following discharge from hospital. Patients with a history of alcoholism, senility or mental illness are less likely to be dependable, both with respect to taking the drug regularly and appearing for routine laboratory evaluation. Nurses should identify a reliable family member who will assist in monitoring patient compliance and observing for adverse effects of the drug in the home. In addition, nursing assessment should include a review of the medication history to identify potential drug interactions with the oral anticoagulants.

Administration

Oral anticoagulants should be administered from light-proof and moisture-proof containers. They should be given at the same time each day in acute care settings and in response to the daily prothrombin times.

Evaluation

Nurses are expected to recognize prothrombin times that are beyond the desired range and communicate them to the attending physician. Nurses should also monitor blood pressure for changes.

Nursing responsibilities related to the evaluation of treatment involve the aforementioned determination of patient compliance, assisting with measurement of drug effectiveness, maintaining an up-to-date medication history and the identification of adverse reactions. Patients should be observed for bleeding gums, nose bleeds, excessive bruising or petechiae, hematuria, tarry stools, hematemesis and the sudden appearance of lumbar or abdominal pain. The appearance of any of these effects should be reported to the physician immediately. They indicate impending spontaneous hemorrhage, which is a medical emergency requiring urgent intervention.

Teaching

The importance of patient compliance was mentioned earlier. Nurses must teach patients and their families the importance of compliance with the prescribed therapeutic regimen, including the accompanying laboratory tests. Patients and their families should also be instructed to watch for evidence of spontaneous bleeding. A check list can be given as a memory aid. The importance of contacting the physician immediately, should any of the effects on the list be noted, must be impressed on patients and their families.

Patient teaching should also emphasize the fact that response to anticoagulants can be altered by many factors, including nonprescription and prescription drugs, illness, diet, exposure to insecticides or even prolonged periods of hot weather. Any of these circumstances should be promptly brought to the attention of the attending physician. The ability of common household remedies, particularly those containing aspirin, to alter dramatically the effect of oral anticoagulants should be stressed. Patients should also be instructed to exert extra caution when working in the kitchen with knives or when shaving. It may be most difficult to stop a cut from bleeding.

Patients should be instructed to tell their dentist that they are receiving anticoagulants before dental work is initiated. They should also be strongly urged to wear a medical alert bracelet.

Antiplatelet Drugs

The pathogenesis of arterial thrombi was presented in the initial paragraphs of this chapter. To review briefly, a few platelets adhere to the damaged section of a blood vessel and secrete chemicals that allow other platelets to aggregate around the original thrombocytes. This triggers blood coagulation and soon the platelets are encased in fibrin. The fast flow of blood in the arteries may shear some of the platelet-fibrin mass free of the vessel wall to be carried away in the circulation. At this time the platelet-fibrin mass may completely disintegrate, with the individual platelets returning to their original form. It is also possible, however, that the small platelet-fibrin mass may not disintegrate. Instead, it may be carried to a very small blood vessel, where it can lodge and block the microcirculation to a small area of the body. This process is depicted in Figure 22.

Figure 22
Microcirculation obstruction.

The microcirculation of an organ can be obstructed by emboli arising from mural thrombi composed of platelets and fibrin. Intravascular platelet aggregates may have a similar effect. Obstruction of the microcirculation is known to occur in transient attacks of monocular blindness and cerebral ischemia, and may also be responsible for kidney damage associated with atherosclerotic lesion of the aorta above the renal arteries, and some cases of myocardial infarction.

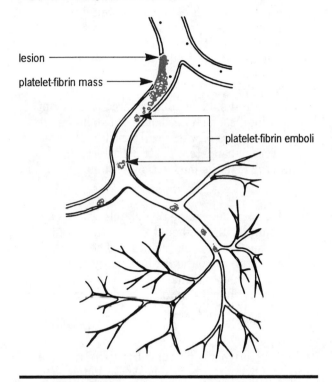

From: J.F. Mustard and M.A.Packham (1975), Platelets, thrombosis and drugs. *Drugs 9* :19-76. Reproduced with permission.

Microemboli blocking the blood flow to small areas of the heart have been blamed for starting cardiac arrhythmias. In the brain they have been accused of producing transient ischemic attacks, uniocular visual loss and cerebrovascular accidents. For these reasons, it is in the patient's best interest to deter platelets from adhering to damaged walls or arteries. It should also be noted that if a platelet-fibrin plug is not sheared from the wall by the force of the circulation it will enlarge until it occludes blood flow at its original site or provides a focus for subsequent atherosclerosis formation.

At the present time three drugs are being studied actively for their effects on platelet adhesion and/or aggregation. They are aspirin (acetylsalicylic acid, ASA), sulfinpyrazone and dipyridamole. All three have been on the market for other clinical indications for several years. Aspirin is a tried-and-true analgesic/anti-inflammatory agent, used to relieve mild to moderate pain, inflammation or both. Sulfinpyrazone (Anturan, Anturane) was introduced as a uricosuric drug to treat gout. Dipyridamole (Persantine) was originally used to prevent angina pectoris attacks.

Aspirin

Mechanism of Action and Pharmacologic Effects

Aspirin inhibits platelet aggregation by inactivating cyclo-oxygenase, the enzyme responsible for synthesizing the prostaglandin-like substance thromboxane A_2 in platelets. Thromboxane A_2 promotes platelet aggregation. Aspirin's effects are irreversible, lasting for the lifetime of the platelet (seven to ten days).

Therapeutic Uses

Aspirin has been used to prevent cardiovascular disease. For primary prevention, benefit has been demonstrated conclusively in men for myocardial infarction, but evidence concerning stroke and vascular death remains inconclusive because of inadequate numbers of endpoints in the trials conducted to date. For secondary prevention, the evidence concludes that aspirin is beneficial for men in myocardial infarction, stroke and vascular death. Dosages for women have not yet been determined.

Adverse Effects

The pharmacology of aspirin is detailed in Chapter 54. Readers are encouraged to refer to this chapter for the adverse effects of aspirin, before participating in the management of patients receiving the drug for its antiplatelet effects.

Nursing Process

The nursing process related to the use of aspirin is also presented in Chapter 54. Nursing responsibilities related to patient assessment, drug administration, patient evaluation and patient teaching are summarized in Table 30 at the end of this chapter.

Sulfinpyrazone (Anturan, Anturane)

Sulfinpyrazone prevents platelet adhesion and aggregation by inhibiting thromboxane A_2 synthesis in platelets. It differs from aspirin in that its effects are brief. Once the concentration of sulfinpyrazone in the blood falls, platelets are able to synthesize thromboxane A_2 again. It is essential, therefore, that sulfinpyrazone be given continually if it is to have an effect on platelet function. Sulfinpyrazone has been reported to have a beneficial effect in transient cerebral ischemia and to improve survival in patients who have experienced a myocardial infarct. However, much work must be done before its efficacy in the treatment of arterial thrombi is established.

Sulfinpyrazone is discussed in Chapter 58, dealing with drugs for the treatment of gout. Its adverse effects are presented there and need not be detailed again. They are briefly summarized in Table 30 at the end of this chapter.

Nursing Process

Detailed discussion of the nursing actions initiated by the prescription of sulfinpyrazone can also be found in Chapter 58. The nursing process related to its use as an antiplatelet drug is summarized in Table 30 at the end of this chapter.

Dipyridamole (Persantine)

Dipyridamole appears to block platelet aggregation, but its mechanism of action is still not clear. When tested in patients with cerebral vascular disease, dipyridamole had no effect. Similar results were obtained when the drug was given to patients with coronary artery disease. In one study, patients given dipyridamole plus aspirin had significantly fewer fatal and nonfatal myocardial infarcts than placebo-treated patients. Dipyridamole, together with warfarin, has been shown to reduce platelet adhesion or aggregation in patients with mitral valve replacement.

Oral dipyridamole may cause headache or gastric irritation at high dosage levels. An intravenous bolus of dipyridamole may be associated with chest pain/angina, headache and/or dizziness.

Nursing Process

Assessment
Nursing assessment should begin with a review of the patient's history for evidence of contraindications, specifically, acute myocardial infarct, current pregnancy or lactation, and hypotension. Consultation with the pharmacist in reviewing the patient's current drug therapy will reveal drug incompatabilities. A past history of aspirin sensitivity should alert the nurse to the need for particularly stringent evaluation of the patient during the initial phases of therapy with this medication. Baseline measurement of blood pressure should be performed because dipyridamole is a vasodilator.

Administration
Dipyridamole should be administered on an empty stomach, that is, one hour before or two hours after meals. A full glass of water will assist in absorption. In the event of persistent gastric distress, the patient may take the medication with meals.

Evaluation
Drug efficacy is determined by platelet counts and clotting times. Nurses should know the desired range for these laboratory values and be prepared to communicate the patient's laboratory results to the physician. As explained above, the vasodilator effects of dipyridamole require the nurse to monitor the patient's blood pressure.

Teaching
Patients experiencing postural hypotension should be advised to change positions slowly. Patients should be taught to notify their physician of adverse effects as identified above.

Fibrinolytic Drugs

Three fibrinolytic, or thrombolytic, drugs have been studied during the past few years. They are urokinase, found in human urine; streptokinase (Kabikinase, Streptase), produced by beta-hemolytic streptococci; and tissue plasminogen activator [TPA] (Activase). The actions of streptokinase and TPA are discussed here.

Streptokinase (Streptase)

Mechanism of Action and Pharmacologic Effects

Blood contains plasminogen. When plasminogen is activated it releases plasmin, which lyses fibrin clots. Streptokinase activates the plasminogen-plasmin system, giving rise to increased amounts of plasmin. Streptokinase is administered to remove formed thrombi or emboli.

Therapeutic Uses

The indications for the use of streptokinase include pulmonary embolism, deep vein thrombosis, arterial thrombosis and embolism, arteriovenous cannula occlusion and coronary artery thrombosis. Streptokinase treatment of coronary thrombosis should be instituted as soon as possible after the onset of symptoms of acute myocardial infarction, preferably within six hours. Streptokinase is contraindicated in patients with a predisposition to bleeding. Because thrombolytic therapy increases the risk of bleeding, streptokinase is contraindicated in active internal bleeding, recent cerebrovascular accident (within two months), intracranial or intraspinal surgery and intracranial neoplasm.

Adverse Effects

Hemorrhage is a danger when streptokinase is used. Aminocaproic acid (Amicar) is an antidote for overdose of a fibrinolytic agent. It should be given in a loading dose of 5 g, either orally or intravenously by slow infusion, followed by 1 – 1.25 g/h until the bleeding is controlled. Streptokinase also depletes the blood of its normal pool of plasminogen. As a result, spontaneous thrombosis can occur after the effects of streptokinase disappear. To prevent secondary clot formation, heparin should be given immediately after the effects of the fibrinolytic agent cease, followed by oral anticoagulants for seven days, during which time the blood plasminogen levels return to normal.

Because streptokinase is a bacterial protein elaborated by group C beta-hemolytic streptococci, it can produce allergic reactions. Reactions attributed to possible anaphylaxis have been observed rarely in patients treated with streptokinase. These range in severity from minor breathing difficulty to bronchospasm, periorbital swelling, or angioneurotic edema. Other, milder allergic effects such as urticaria, itching, flushing, nausea, headache and musculoskeletal pain have been observed. Approximately thirty-three per cent of patients treated with streptokinase have shown

increases in body temperature of greater than 0.83°C. Symptomatic treatment is usually sufficient to alleviate discomfort. The use of acetaminophen rather than aspirin is recommended.

Nursing Process

Assessment

Prior to the administration of a fibrinolytic drug, nursing assessment of the patient should be conducted with the aim of estimating the risk of, and potential sites for, hemorrhage. A patient whose history reveals recent surgery, parturition within the preceding ten days, gastric or intestinal ulcers, liver disease, active tuberculosis or other hemorrhagic conditions is at great risk of hemorrhage following the administration of fibrinolytic drugs. Patients whose drug histories indicate extensive use of aspirin, use of anticoagulants, indomethacin or phenylbutazone should also be considered at increased risk of hemorrhage if given a fibrinolytic drug.

Administration

Streptokinase that has been reconstituted within the preceding twenty-four hours using isotonic saline as a diluent can be used. This enzyme is destroyed by vigorous shaking of the vial. When reconstituting streptokinase, swirl the vial gently after adding the diluent rather than agitating energetically. Administration of an intravenous bolus of this medication should be followed by application of manual pressure and a pressure dressing for fifteen minutes. The pressure dressing should be maintained for another hour and checked for hemorrhage every ten minutes. Bed rest is necessary during the entire course of treatment.

Evaluation

Nursing evaluation of patients receiving fibrinolytic medications should include observation for drug effectiveness (relief of symptoms, decreased thrombin time) and for adverse effects (hemorrhage, allergic responses or fever). Allergic responses are of particular concern when streptokinase is administered to hypersensitive individuals. Patients should be observed closely for signs of bleeding, including hematuria, hematemesis and epistaxis, especially during the first hour of treatment.

Tissue Plasminogen Activator (Activase)

Mechanism of Action and Pharmacologic Effects

Recombinant tissue plasminogen activator (TPA) is a synthetic fibrinolytic protein that activates plasminogen or converts plasminogen to plasmin specifically in the presence of fibrin. The **clot selectivity** of TPA enables it to lyse clots without having a significant effect on circulating plasminogen. TPA has a half-life of about five minutes, compared to about twenty-three minutes for streptokinase.

Therapeutic Uses

TPA's current indications are for the lysis of suspected occlusive coronary artery thrombi associated with evolving transmural myocardial infarction, and the improvement of ventricular function and reduction in the incidence of congestive heart failure associated with acute myocardial infarction. Clinical trials have demonstrated that TPA is effective in patients in whom therapy is initiated within six hours of onset of symptoms.

The immediate benefits of TPA treatment include a prompt reperfusion and restoration of coronary artery patency in patients with total coronary artery occlusion. Electrocardiographic changes in cardiac enzymes and alterations in the pattern of chest pain indicate that rapid perfusion afforded by TPA may limit the size of the infarct.

Adverse Effects

Bleeding is the most significant adverse effect with TPA. In most cases, bleeding has been minor. Contraindications include active internal bleeding, history of cerebrovascular accident, recent intracranial or intraspinal surgery or trauma (within two months), intracranial neoplasm, arteriovenous malformation or aneurysm, known bleeding diathesis, or severe uncontrolled hypertension.

Nursing Process

Assessment

During administration of tissue plasminogen activator nurses must monitor vital signs, blood pressure and neurologic signs. Body temperature should be monitored every four hours because a temperature greater than 40°C (104°F) may indicate internal bleeding. Observe patients for signs of bleeding during the first hour of treatment. These include hematuria, hematemesis, bleeding from the mucous membranes and epistaxis.

Administration

Tissue plasminogen activator is reconstituted using the provided diluent, adding appropriate amounts of sterile water for injection (no preservatives) to 1 mg/mL. Mix by slow inversion. Intravenous solution should be reconstituted after eight hours. For best results, the drug should be administered within six hours of coronary occlusion. Pressure should be applied for thirty seconds to minor bleeding sites. The physician should be informed if this does not control bleeding. Apply pressure dressing to such sites. Tissue plasminogen activator powder is stored at room temperature and protected from excessive light.

Evaluation

Nurses must monitor patients for changes in blood studies and for desired prothrombin and bleeding times. Patients must be observed for allergy, fever, rash, itching, chills and mild reactions.

Teaching

Prepare the patient for the procedure by explaining its process and possible reactions throughout treatment.

Vitamin K₁, Vitamin K₂, and Menadione

Mechanism of Action and Pharmacologic Effects

Although vitamin K is not a single chemical, it is often convenient to refer to it as such, as in vitamin K deficiency. This is acceptable so long as we recognize the fact that there are two naturally occurring substances, vitamin K_1 (phytonadione) and vitamin K_2, which stimulate the hepatic synthesis of vitamin K-dependent clotting factors. Both vitamin K_1 and vitamin K_2 are found in plant leaves and vegetable oils and synthesized in large quantities by bacteria in the intestinal tract. In addition to these naturally occurring substances, the synthetic chemical menadione, or vitamin K_3, is included in the general term "vitamin K".

Vitamins K_1 and K_2 are well absorbed from the gastrointestinal tract if bile salts are present. Vitamin K_1 is also formulated for subcutaneous, intramuscular or intravenous administration. Menadione does not require bile for absorption. It is also available as a water-soluble salt, menadione sodium bisulfite, for parental administration. Menadiol tetrasodium diphosphate (Kappadione, Synka-Vite) is another water-soluble salt of menadione, intended for oral or parenteral administration.

Therapeutic Uses

Vitamin K is given to treat a deficiency resulting from its inadequate intake, absorption or utilization. It is also given to antagonize the actions of oral anticoagulants.

Vitamin K is also sometimes given during the first days of life to newborn infants, who have only twenty to forty per cent of the adult levels of prothrombin. For prophylaxis and treatment of hemorrhagic diseases of the newborn, the water-soluble vitamin K analogues are not as safe as phytonadione. Doses of menadiol sodium diphosphate in excess of 10 mg have been associated with hyperbilirubinemia in infants.

Patients with intrahepatic or extrahepatic biliary obstruction may not absorb naturally occurring forms of vitamin K. Treatment with oral vitamin K_1 plus bile salts will usually correct the problem. Vitamin K_3 does not require bile for absorption. Broad-spectrum antibacterials can kill vitamin K-producing bacteria in the colon, leading to hypoprothrombinemia and hemorrhage. Treatment with vitamin K can reverse the hypoprothrombinemia. Hepatocellular disease may produce hypoprothrombinemia. Vitamin K is of no value in this condition because the problem lies in the inability of the liver to synthesize clotting factors, even in the presence of adequate amounts of the vitamin.

Menadiol sodium diphosphate should not be administered to the mother during the last few weeks of pregnancy. Menadiol should not be administered to infants.

Adverse Effects

As might be expected, the administration of a vitamin K product may cause temporary refractoriness to anticoagulant therapy. An overdose of vitamin K in an infant can produce hemolytic anemia or kernicterus.

Nursing Process

Assessment
Prior to administration of any vitamin K preparation, nurses must identify previous hypersensitivity to the medication or severe liver disease. Either of these situations warrants withholding the drug until the physician verifies its administration. Evidence of hypersensitivity or allergic tendencies should alert nurses administering the medication to intensify their observations and evaluations of the patient's response to the drug.

Administration
Nurses should administer only those vitamin K preparations which have been stored in a cool, dark place. Intravenous solutions should be diluted with only 0.9% normal saline, 5% dextrose in 0.9% normal saline, or 5% dextrose in water. Unused solutions should be discarded immediately. Intravenous solutions of vitamin K_1 can be protected from light during infusion by wrapping the container in tinfoil or by poking a hole in the bottom of a paper bag and inverting it over the hanger suspending the intravenous solution.

Intramuscular injections of vitamin K_1 can be administered to preteens, teenagers and adults in the gluteus maximus; intramuscular injections of vitamin K_1 in infants and small children are best administered in the quadratus lateralus (anterior lateral thigh) or deltoid. Insertion of the needle into the muscle must be followed by aspiration in order to prevent inadvertant intravenous injection.

Oral preparations of vitamins K_1 and K_2 should be administered with bile salts in order to facilitate their absorption.

Evaluation
During and immediately following intravenous administration of vitamin K_1, patients should be evaluated constantly for acute anaphylactic reactions. Their vital signs should be monitored at frequent intervals for such preliminary indications of shock as peripheral vasodilatation (including flushing of the face, feelings of constriction in the chest, weakness, tachycardia and hypotension). These may be followed by anaphylactic shock, including respiratory and cardiac arrest. Patients receiving vitamin K_3 should be observed for evidence of nausea, vomiting, headache or allergic skin reactions. Drug effectiveness of all vitamin K preparations is evaluated using laboratory reports of prothrombin times.

Further Reading

Aspirin for prevention of myocardial infarction and stroke (1989). *The Medical Letter 31* :77-79.

Collen, D., Lijnen, H.R., Todd, P.A. and Goa, K.L. (1989). Tissue-type plasminogen activator: A review of its pharmacology and therapeutic use as a thrombolytic agent. *Drugs 38* :346-388.

Coller, B.S.C. (1990). Platelets and thrombolytic therapy. *New Engl. J. Med. 322* :33-42.

Ginsberg, J.S. and Hirsh, J. (1988). Optimum use of anticoagulants in pregnancy. *Drugs 36* :505-512.

Hennekens, C.H. and Buring, J.E. (1988). Aspirin and risk of cardiovascular disease. *Rational Drug Therapy 22* (11):1-6.

Loscalzo, J. (1989). Thrombolysis in the management of acute myocardial infarction and unstable angina pectoris. *Drugs 37* :191-204.

Reilly, I.A.G. and FitzGerald, G.A. (1988). Aspirin in cardiovascular disease. *Drugs 35* :154-176.

Roger, S.D., Reimersma, L.B. and Clements, S.D. (1987). Tissue plasminogen activator: An evaluation of clinical efficacy in acute myocardial infarction. *Pharmacotherapy 7* :111-121.

Sherry, S. (1987). Thrombolytic agents for acute evolving myocardial infarction: Comparative effects. *Rational Drug Therapy 21* (1):1-9.

Steering Committee of the Physicians' Health Study Research Group (1988). Preliminary report: Findings from the aspirin component of the ongoing Physicians' Health Study. *New Engl. J. Med. 318* :262-264.

Tissue-type plasminogen activator for acute coronary thrombosis (1987). *The Medical Letter 29* :107-109.

Turpie, A.G.G. (1989). Examining the role of anticoagulants in post-AMI. *Perspectives in Cardiology 5* (5):31-41.

Table 30
Anticoagulant and antiplatelet drugs, fibrinolytic agents and vitamin K.

Generic Name (Trade Name)	Use (Dose)	Action	Adverse Effects	Drug Interactions	Nursing Process
Pharmacologic Classification: Anticoagulant					
Heparin	Tx of thrombophlebitis, phlebothrombosis and cerebral, coronary and retinal vessel thrombosis. To prevent extens'n of clots and thromboemboli. To prevent occurrence of thromboembolism, clotting during dialysis and other surgical procedures **(IV:** Adults - 5000 USP units initially, followed by individualized doses of 5000-10 000 USP units q4-6h. *For disseminated intravascular coagulat'n,* adults - 50 USP units/kg q6h. Children - 25 USP units/kg q6h. **IV infus'n:** Adults - loading dose of 5000 USP units into tubing, then 20 000-30 000 units at an initial rate of 0.5 units/kg/min in D5W or isotonic NaCl inject'n. Adjust rate subsequently according to clotting time results. Children - 50 USP units/kg initially, followed by 100 USP units/kg q4h. **SC:** Adults - 10 000-12 000 USP units q8h or 14 000-20 000 units q12h. *For low-dose prophylaxis,* 5000 units 2 h before surgery and q12h thereafter until pt is discharged or is fully ambulatory)	Works by means of a plasma cofactor, the heparin cofactor or antithrombin III, which neutralizes several activated clotting factors: XIIa, kallikrein, XIIa, XIa, Xa, IXa and IIa. Its effects are immediate but fleeting: 50% dissipated in 1st hour.	Hemorrhage; local irritat'n, mild pain or hematoma at inject'n site; hypersensitivity; osteoporosis; alopecia; thrombocytopenia; aldosterone suppress'n.	**Anticoagulants, oral:** Interact w. heparin. Heparin administrat'n may prolong prothrombin time in pts receiving oral anticoagulants. Blood for prothrombin time should not be drawn within about 4-5 h of IV heparin and 12-24 h after last SC dose of heparin. **Antihistamines:** May partially counteract effects of heparin. **Ethacrynic acid:** Incr. incidence of heparin-induced GI bleeding. **Dextran:** And heparin, may act synergistically when administered concurrently. **Digoxin:** May partially counteract anticoagulant effects of heparin. **Salicylates and other NSAIDs:** May induce bleeding; should be used w. caution in pts on heparin. **Tetracycline antibiotics:** May partially counteract anticoagulant effects of heparin.	**Assess:** For active bleeding or condit'ns associated w. bleeding tendencies; hepatic disease, alcoholism; neurological, ophthalmic or spinal surgery; menstruat'n, pregnancy, postpartum; ulcerative condit'ns of GI tract; open wounds. Check to ensure that blood for baseline lab. studies has been drawn. **Administer:** Examine label carefully; IV or SC routes preferred; change needles after w'drawing medicat'n from vial; use tuberculin syringe; inject'n site should not be within 2" of umbilicus or scar tissue; use Z-track inject'n procedure w. 25-gauge 1/2" needle; do not massage inject'n site. **Evaluate:** Urine and stools for occult blood. **Teach:** Pts should report bleeding immediately, avoid OTC drugs and wear Medic-Alert ID.

Generic Name (Trade Name)	Use (Dose)	Action	Adverse Effects	Drug Interactions	Nursing Process
Pharmacologic Classification: Oral Anticoagulants					
Warfarin (Athrombin-K Potassium, Coumadin Sodium, Warfilone Sodium, Warnerin Sodium)	To induce hypoprothrombinemia in prophylaxis and tx of venous thrombosis and its extens'n; tx of embolizat'n. In AMI for pts at high risk for thromboembolic complicat'ns. Adjunct in TIA, cerebral embolism and coronary occlus'n **(Oral/IV:** Adults - 15 mg, 10 mg and 10 mg on first 3 days. Us. maint. dose, 5-7.5 mg/day thereafter. Use prothrombin time determinat'ns as guide)	Competitively inhibits action of vitamin K and thus blocks synthesis in liver of clotting factors II, VII, IX and X.	Minor or major hemorrhage from any tissue or organ; alopecia, urticaria, dermatitis, fever, nausea, diarrhea, abdominal cramping, hypersensitivity react'ns; hemorrhagic infarct'n and necrosis of skin	See Table 31	**Assess:** As for heparin; est. probability of pt compliance w. prescribed regimen; identify family member(s) to assist in monitoring pt compliance; medicat'n hx to identify potential drug interact'ns. **Administer:** Only preparat'ns that have been stored in tightly closed, light-resistant containers that have been protected from moisture and humidity. **Evaluate:** BP changes; pt compliance; for evidence of spontaneous bleeding; drug efficacy; drug hx for interact'ns that might alter drug efficacy. **Teach:** Pt and family the importance of compliance w. prescribed regimen, incl. lab. tests; to report immediately any signs of bleeding; that many nonprescript'n and prescript'n drugs, illness, diet, exposure to insecticides or prolonged hot weather can cause altered response to this medicat'n, in which case physician should be contacted; to shave w. an electric razor.
Bishydroxycoumarin (Dicoumarol)	As for warfarin **(Oral:** Adults - 200-300 mg 1st day, followed by 25-200 mg daily. Use prothrombin time determinat'ns as guide. Maint. dose, 25-150 mg od)	As for warfarin	As for warfarin	See Table 31	
Phenprocoumon (Marcumar, Liquamar)	As for warfarin **(Oral:** Adults - 24 mg on lst day. Maint. dose varies bet. 0.75-6 mg, as determined by prothrombin time)	As for warfarin	As for warfarin	See Table 31	
Pharmacologic Classification: Antiplatelet Drugs					
Aspirin, acetylsalicylic acid, ASA	Tx of coronary artery disease, transient cerebral ischemia, cerebral vascular accident, myocardial infarct'n **(Oral:** *Platelet antiaggregant, cerebral and retinal ischemic attacks -* Men, 650 mg bid. *Prophylaxis of venous thromboembolism after total hip replacement -* Men, 650 bid started 1 day before surgery and continued for 14 days. *Adjunctive tx (w.*	Interferes w. enzyme responsible for synthesis of thromboxane A$_2$, thereby inhibiting platelet adhes'n and aggregat'n.	GI irritation, allergy, salicylism, tinnitus, vision disturbances, confus'n, sweating, thirst, nausea, vomiting, diarrhea	**Anticoagulants, oral:** Interact w. salicylates. Large doses of salicylates reduce plasma prothrombin and displace oral anticoagulants from plasma proteins. Salicylates can produce GI bleeding. Avoid concomitant use of salicylates and oral anticoagulants. For drug interact'ns involving antidiabetic agents, methotrexate, spironolactone and uricosurics, see Table 77.	**Assess:** Hx of allergy or sensitivity, peptic ulcers, anticoagulant tx, bleeding tendencies, salicylism. **Administer:** With meals. **Evaluate:** Drug effectiveness; adv. effects. **Teach:** Self-evaluat'n for adv. effects; need for compliance.

Drug	Use and dosage	Action	Side effects	Interactions	Nursing considerations
(continued)	*dipyridamole) to incr. platelet survival in pts w. prosthetic heart valves -* 975 mg daily w. 100 mg dipyridamole daily, in divided doses. *For prophylaxis after myocardial infarct -* Men, 325 mg tid. **May be supplemented w. dipyridamole 75 mg tid)**				
Sulfinpyrazone (Anturan, Anturane)	Tx of clinical states in which abnormal platelet behavior is a causative or associated factor (**Oral:** *For amaurosis fugax [TIA] -* 600-800 mg/day in 3-4 divided doses w. meals. Do not exceed 1000 mg [20 mg/kg for a 50-kg man] daily)	Inhibits prostaglandin synthesis, thus blocks thromboxane A_2 format'n, inhibiting platelet adhes'n and aggregat'n.	Gastric disturbances; may aggravate or reactivate peptic ulcer; impairment of renal funct'n; skin rashes	**Salicylates:** May cause unpredictable and at times serious prolongat'n of bleeding time; in combinat'n w. sulfinpyrazone, may cause bleeding episodes. **Sulfonamides:** May have their actions potentiated by sulfinpyrazone.	**Assess:** For pt hx of renal calculi, hypersensitivity, kidney disease, use of oral hypoglycemics, peptic ulcers, liver disease. **Administer:** With meals. **Evaluate:** For adv. effects (GI disturbances or hypersensitivity), retroperitoneal pain in light of renal colic, incidence of hypoglycemia in diabetics using oral hypoglycemics. **Teach:** To drink large volumes of fluids, at least 3 L (12 8-oz. glasses)/day; to continue medicat'n unless otherwise instructed by physician; s/s hypersensitivity; not to take aspirin or other OTC medicat'ns without consulting physician.
Dipyridamole (Persantine)	Prevent'n of postoperative thromboembolic complicat'ns associated w. prosthetic heart valves (**Oral:** *Thromboembolic disease -* 100 mg qid, 1 h ac; or 100 mg/day + 1 g aspirin/day. *Coronary artery disease -* 75 mg dipyridamole + 325 mg aspirin tid in pts who have suffered a previous myocardial infarct. *Coronary artery bypass graft surgery -* For 2 days preop, dipyridamole 100 mg qid. Day of surgery: morning of operat'n, dipyridamole100 mg. 1 h postop: dipyridamole 100 mg [via NG tube]. 7 h postop: 75 mg dipyridamole + 330 mg ASA. Daily maint. dose for next 12 mos: dipyridamole 75 mg + ASA 330 mg tid)	Appears to block platelet aggregat'n but mechanism of action is not clear.	Headache, dizziness, nausea, flushing, syncope or weakness, skin rash, gastric irritat'n, emesis, abdominal cramping		**Assess:** Review pt hx for evidence of contraindicat'ns, myocardial infarct, pregnancy/lactat'n, hypotens'n, ASA sensitivity. Baseline measurements of BP and VS. **Administer:** 1 h ac. **Evaluate:** Evidence of effectiveness; adv. effects. **Teach:** Need for compliance; s/s hypotens'n.

Generic Name (Trade Name)	Use (Dose)	Action	Adverse Effects	Drug Interactions	Nursing Process
Pharmacologic Classification: Fibrinolytic Drug					
Streptokinase (Kabikinase, Streptase)	Lysis of acute massive pulmonary emboli, extensive thrombi of deep veins, acute arterial thrombi obstructing coronary arteries associated w. evolving myocardial infarct. For clearing of occluded arteriovenous cannulas as an alternative to surgery when absolutely necessary. (For dosage inform at'n, consult manufacturer's monograph.)	Activates plasminogen-plasmin system to cause breakdown of thrombi or emboli.	Severe internal bleeding. Tx may include stopping drug, administering packed RBC and cryoprecipitate or fresh frozen plasma plus aminocaproic acid. Anaphylaxis has been observed rarely.		**Assess:** For hemorrhage risk (recent surgery, postpartum, gastric ulcers, liver disease, active TB, etc.); drug hx for use of aspirin, anticoagulants, indomethacin, phenylbutazone, baseline thrombin time. **Administer:** Only freshly reconstituted, using isotonic saline. Do not shake. Bed rest throughout tx. **Evaluate:** For drug effectiveness (thrombin time); for hemorrhage, allergic react'ns, fever.
Tissue plasminogen activator (TPA, Alteplase, Activase)	Indicated for thrombolysis in evolving myocardial infarct (**IV:** Total dose, 100 mg over 3 h; 60 mg in 1st hour, w. 6-10 mg as an initial bolus [over 1-2 min] and the rest infused slowly over remaining hour; 20 mg should be infused in the 2nd hour, and 20 mg more in the 3rd hour)	Converts plasminogen to plasmin specifically in presence of fibrin. Plasmin subsequently lyses the fibrin clot.	Bleeding is most significant adv. effect.		**Assess:** BP, VS and neurologic signs throughout tx. Observe for signs of bleeding, esp. in 1st hour of tx. **Administer:** Reconstitute by aseptically adding to vial the appropriate volume (50 mL) of accompanying vial of sterile water for injection. Mix by slow invers'n. **Evaluate:** For bleeding sites, apply pressure for 30 s; notify physician if bleeding continues. Use pressure dressing. Monitor changes in blood status for prothrombin, bleeding and clotting times. Observe for allergic react'ns. **Teach:** Prepare pt for procedure; explain possible react'ns.
Pharmacologic Classification: Vitamin K					
Phytonadione, vitamin K₁ (Aqua Mephton, Konakion, Mephyton)	Management of coagulat'n disorders due to faulty format'n of factors II, VII, IX and X when caused by vitamin K deficiency or interference w. vitamin K activity (For hypoprothrombinemic states, adults and children - **Oral:** 2.5-25 mg. For prophy-	Essential for synthesis of factors required for clotting; overcomes actions of oral anticoagulants.	Flushing sensat'ns, rapid and weak pulse, sweating, hypotens'n, dyspnea, pain, swelling, tenderness at inject'n site, allergy, hyperbilirubinemia in newborn	**Anticoagulants, oral:** See Table 31.	**Assess:** Hx of hypersensitivity to drug; severe liver disease. **Administer:** Only solut'ns stored in cool, dark place; IM to preteens, adolescents and adults in gluteus maximus; IM to infants and young children in quadratus lateralus or deltoid muscles; aspirate carefully; apply gentle pressure only to

Drug	Dosage			Nursing implications
(phytonadione, continued)	laxis of hemorrhagic disease in newborn - **IV/IM/SC:** 0.5-1 mg immediately after birth; although less desirable, 1-5 mg may be given to mother 12-24 h before delivery. For tx of hemorrhagic disease in newborn - **IM/SC:** 1 mg. Overdosage w. oral anticoagulants - **IV** (slow): 0.5 -5 mg for mild overdose; up to 10 mg for moderate overdose; 25 mg for severe overdose. Adjust frequency and addit'nal doses in accordance w. prothrombin times or pt's condit'n. If Prothrombin time is not satisfactory after 6-8 h, repeat dose)			inject'n site; IV solut'ns diluted w. 0.9% saline or D5W; discard unused preparat'ns, protect IV solut'ns from light during infus'n. **Evaluate:** Constantly during and immediately following IV administrat'n; VS for indicat'ns of shock; for adv. react'ns. Monitor drug effectiveness using lab. reports of prothrombin times.
Menadione (Vitamin K₃)	As for phytonadione (**Oral:** 2-10 mg daily)	As for phytonadione	As for phytonadione. Menadione hemolyzes RBC in pts who are deficient in glucose-6-phosphate dehydrogenase as well as in newborn (esp. premature) infants.	**Assess:** As for phytonadione. **Administer:** With bile salts to pts w. bile deficiency. **Evaluate:** For adv. effects; monitor drug effectiveness.
Menadione sodium bisulfite (Hykinone)	As for phytonadione (**SC/IM/IV:** 2.5-10 mg daily)	As for phytonadione	As for phytonadione	As for phytonadione.
Menadiol sodium diphosphate (Synkavite)	As for phytonadione (**Oral; SC/IM/IV:** For management of hypoprothrombinemic hemorrhagic states, adults - 5-15 mg od or bid. Children - 5-10 mg od or bid)	As for phytonadione	As for phytonadione	As for phytonadione.

Table 31
Oral anticoagulant drug interactions.

Allopurinol may inhibit the metabolism and prolong the action of oral anticoagulants.

Aminoglycoside antibiotics may reduce vitamin K production by gut bacteria, thus enhancing the effects of oral anticoagulants.

Anabolic steroids increase patient sensitivity to oral anticoagulants.

Antidiabetic drugs may interact in different ways with oral anticoagulants. Dicumarol may inhibit the metabolism of tolbutamide and increase serum chlorpropramide levels. Tolbutamide may displace dicumarol from its binding sites in plasma proteins, increasing its effects.

Barbiturates may increase the metabolism of coumarin anticoagulants and decrease gastrointestinal absorption of dicumarol. Starting or stopping barbiturates may require readjustment of oral anticoagulant dosage.

Carbamazepine may increase warfarin metabolism.

Chloral hydrate has trichloroacetic acid as a major metabolite, which may displace warfarin from plasma protein binding sites.

Cholestyramine may impair both anticoagulant and vitamin K absorption. Giving warfarin at least six hours after cholestyramine avoids the impaired absorption. If concurrent use is necessary, patients should be monitored more frequently.

Clofibrate may enhance the effect of warfarin on vitamin K-dependent clotting factor synthesis or turnover of vitamin K.

Contraceptives (oral) may increase the activity of certain clotting factors in the blood and increase dosage requirements for oral anticoagulants.

Corticosteroids produce hypercoagulability of the blood and may antagonize the actions of oral anticoagulants.

Dextrothyroxine enhances the rate of factor II degradation. Avoid concomitant use, if possible.

Ethacrynic acid displaces warfarin from plasma albumin binding sites, thereby increasing its effect.

Ethanol may increase the activity of oral anticoagulants, but heavy drinkers metabolize warfarin faster than normal persons. Patients taking oral anticoagulants should avoid consuming large amounts of ethanol.

Glucagon may increase the hypoprothrombinemic response to warfarin.

Glutethimide increases the metabolism of oral anticoagulants.

Griseofulvin may inhibit the effect of warfarin.

Heparin may prolong further the prothrombin time in patients receiving oral anticoagulants.

Indomethacin can produce ulcers and inhibit platelet function. Obtain prothrombin times more frequently.

Metronidazole may inhibit the metabolism of warfarin and increase its pharmacologic activity. Avoid concomitant use, if possible.

Nonsteroidal anti-inflammatory drugs (NSAIDS) may displace warfarin from plasma albumin binding sites, thereby increasing its activity.

Phenylbutazone and oxyphenbutazone may inhibit warfarin metabolism, produce gastrointestinal ulceration, and impair platelet function. Avoid their use together.

Phenytoin can have its metabolism inhibited and its duration of action increased by dicumarol and possibly also by phenprocoumon. Phenytoin may stimulate dicumarol metabolism and displace dicumarol from its plasma protein binding sites. In addition, phenytoin may prolong prothrombin times in some patients. Avoid concomitant use of phenytoin and dicumarol or phenytoin and phenprocoumon. Warfarin is the oral anticoagulant of choice in patients taking phenytoin.

Quinidine may produce additive effects with oral anticoagulants.

Salicylates in large doses may reduce plasma prothrombin levels and displace oral anticoagulants from plasma protein binding sites. Salicylates are usually not recommended for patients receiving oral anticoagulants.

Rifampin increases warfarin metabolism.

Thyroid preparations increase the catabolism of vitamin K-dependent clotting factors.

Vitamin K antagonizes the effects of oral anticoagulants. A sudden increase in the intake of leafy vegetables or other foods high in vitamin K content will modify the hypoprothrombinemic response to oral anticoagulants.

SECTION 7

Drugs and the Gastrointestinal Tract

Stretching approximately 11 m (36 ft) in the adult, the gastrointestinal tract plays an important role in our general well-being. Like other organ systems, the gastrointestinal tract is subject to disease. The importance of placating it cannot be overstressed. Failure to restore peace and harmony within our entrails can divert attention from almost all other activities and make a normal life virtually impossible. This section pays heed to the problems of the gastrointestinal tract and discusses antiulcer therapy, drugs for the treatment of chronic inflammatory bowel disease, agents for the treatment of diarrhea and constipation, as well as antiemetic and antinauseant drugs.

CHAPTER 22

Antiulcer Drugs

Teaching Objectives

Following completion of this chapter, the reader should be able to:

1. Define the expression peptic ulcer.
2. List some of the causes of peptic ulcers.
3. Discuss the mechanism of action, pharmacologic effects, therapeutic uses and adverse effects of cimetidine, ranitidine, famotidine and nizatidine, and the related nursing process.
4. Discuss the mechanism of action of anticholinergic drugs, their use and adverse effects in the treatment of peptic ulcers, and the related nursing process.
5. Describe the rationale behind the use of misoprostol in the treatment of peptic ulcers, as well as its mechanism of action and pharmacologic effects, therapeutic uses, adverse effects and nursing process.
6. Discuss the mechanism of action of omeprazole, its pharmacologic effects, therapeutic uses, adverse effects and nursing process.
7. Discuss the mechanism of action, therapeutic uses and adverse effects of antacids, and the related nursing process.
8. Discuss the mechanism of action, therapeutic uses and adverse effects of sucralfate, and the related nursing process.

Ulcers

An ulcer is a hole in the tissue covering one of the surfaces of the body. Ulcers may be found in the skin, the cornea of the eye, and the lining of the gastrointestinal tract. Peptic ulcers appear in those parts of the gastrointestinal tract that are exposed to gastric juice containing acid and pepsin and extend at least through the entire thickness of the esophageal, gastric or duodenal mucosa. Duodenal ulcers are most common.

The consequences of an ulcer vary depending on its site and extent. For example, if an ulcer occurs close to a large artery it may erode the wall of the vessel and cause a severe hemorrhage. Although most ulcers do not penetrate deeper than the esophageal, gastric or duodenal muscle layers, a few, called penetrating ulcers, may perforate through the entire wall, allowing fluid to flow from the gastrointestinal tract into the peritoneal cavity. This can be a life-threatening situation. If the site of the penetrating ulcer occurs adjacent to another organ, such as the liver or pancreas, the escape of gastric secretions may damage these tissues.

The cause of an ulcer may not always be known. It is recognized that smoking predisposes a person to peptic ulcer formation. The ingestion of a nonsteroidal anti-inflammatory drug, such as aspirin, phenylbutazone or indomethacin may also cause an ulcer. It was believed for years that corticosteroid consumption could produce an ulcer. Recently, this view has been challenged. Caffeine stimulates gastric acid secretion, and it has been speculated that the heavy use of coffee can produce ulcers; however, no evidence can be found to implicate coffee consumption in the development of peptic ulcers. For those of us who also revel in chili or pepperoni, we are happy to report that no diet or food item has been shown to produce ulcers or cause sleeping ulcers to erupt. Alcohol has been implicated in the development of ulcers, and many people have indeed endured a bout or two of alcoholic gastritis. Although it is possible that just such an event can cause an exacerbation of ulcer symptoms, moderate and heavy ethanol use does not, in itself, increase the incidence of peptic ulcers.

Folklore has it that you can "worry yourself into an ulcer". This is not the case. There is no evidence that stressful occupations cause ulcers. This should be of no small satisfaction to the student preparing for an exam or the nurse gearing up for rounds with the chief of surgery.

The medical management of peptic ulcers has included the recommendation of "ulcer diets" consisting of soft, bland foods. There is little evidence that these diets, or the practice of eating frequently, does anything but complicate the patient's life. Drug therapy is aimed primarily at altering the pH of the gastric fluids. The edict "no acid, no ulcer" is still valid. The use of drugs that either reduce the secretion of acid or diminish the effects of the secreted acid will help the patient who suffers from the consequences of gastric acid or pepsin secretion. In all cases, regardless of the type of drug chosen, proper diagnosis is important because response to therapy does not rule out the presence of a gastric malignancy.

Drugs That Block the Secretion of Gastric Acid

The fasting stomach secretes acid continously, following a circadian rhythm. Peak amounts are released near midnight and lowest quantities shortly before awakening. The parietal cell is stimulated to secrete acid by activation of receptors in the basolateral membrane. At least three different receptor types have been identified on the parietal cell, which are activated by histamine, acetylcholine, or gastrin. After these three types of receptors have been stimulated, the actual secretion of gastric acid is driven by an enzyme in the secretory membrane of the parietal cell. This enzyme is an H^+, K^+-ATPase. Because this enzyme is actually responsible for the secretion of H^+ ions, and H^+ ions are protons, the H^+, K^+-ATPase enzyme is also called the **proton pump.**

This chapter discusses the pharmacology of drugs that inhibit the actions of histamine or acetylcholine or the activity of the proton pump. In addition, the effects of the prostaglandin E_1 (PGE_1) derivative misoprostol, which has antisecretory and cytoprotective effects, are presented.

Histamine$_2$ (H$_2$) Blockers

Cimetidine (Tagamet)

Mechanism of Action and Pharmacologic Effects

Histamine receptors in the stomach differ from those in other parts of the body. They are called H_2 receptors to separate them from the H_1 receptors found elsewhere. Drugs used to treat allergies block H_1 receptors and thereby reduce or prevent the effects of histamine on blood vessels, bronchioles, skin, nasal mucosa and conjunctiva. These drugs are called **antihistamines.** They have no effect on the actions of histamine in the stomach because the receptors in that organ are of the H_2 type. Cimetidine is a reversible, competitive antagonist of the actions of histamine on H_2 receptors. It inhibits, in a dose-dependent manner, histamine-evoked gastric acid secretion. It also inhibits secretion induced by gastrin and partially blocks that stimulated by acetylcholine. Cimetidine reduces both the volume of gastric juice secreted and its hydrogen ion concentration. The output of pepsin generally falls in parallel with the diminished volume of gastric secretion.

Therapeutic Uses

Cimetidine is indicated for the treatment of gastric and duodenal ulcers. A full course of therapy is normally six weeks. Patients who had suffered for years from gastric or duodenal ulcers were afforded relief when cimetidine appeared on the market. Cimetidine promotes both duodenal and gastric healing. Its major advantage over antacid therapy lies in taste and patient acceptance. Many patients relapse when cimetidine is stopped. If this occurs, long-term maintenance therapy, 300 mg once or twice daily, may be required. Cimetidine is also indicated as an adjunctive agent in the management of cystic fibrosis in children.

Adverse Effects

Cimetidine's adverse effects include diarrhea, muscular pain, skin rash, dizziness and mental confusion. It also blocks androgen receptors and can cause gynecomastia and breast tenderness. Rarely, cimetidine can cause hepatitis, bone marrow depression and elevation of serum creatinine levels.

Cimetidine reduces the microsomal metabolism of several drugs, thereby delaying their elimination and possibly increasing their effects. These include warfarin-type anticoagulants, phenytoin, propranolol, metoprolol, chlordiazepoxide, imipramine and theophylline.

Nursing Process

Assessment
Prior to the initial administration of cimetidine, women of childbearing age should undergo nursing assessment for the purpose of detecting a current pregnancy. Although there is no evidence to indicate that the drug is teratogenic, it should be used in pregnant or lactating patients or women of childbearing potential only when the anticipated benefits outweigh the risks.

Administration
Frequently, this drug is self-administered because the patient is not hospitalized for treatment of the ulcer. Oral administration should be separated by one hour from the administration of antacids because of possible drug interaction. In hospital medical and geriatric units, it is frequently given parenterally as well as orally.

Teaching
Because the patient is usually treated on an outpatient basis, the nursing responsibilities are primarily related to patient teaching regarding the importance of compliance with prescribed regimen. Patients are sometimes inclined to discontinue the medication as soon as they are asymptomatic. This must be discouraged because of the likelihood of relapse and its potentially dangerous consequences. Patients should be informed of the possible adverse effects of cimetidine and instructed to contact their physicians should any of these appear.

Ranitidine (Zantac)

Ranitidine is four to nine times more potent than cimetidine. Like cimetidine, ranitidine is very effective but there is no evidence that it is more effective than cimetidine. Ranitidine's major advantage over cimetidine is its failure to interfere with drug metabolism and its lack of antiandrogenic effects. Because ranitidine does not block androgen receptors, it does not produce the gynecomastia occasionally seen with cimetidine. In addition, rantidine does not produce drowsiness and confusion.

The nursing process associated with the prescription of ranitidine is essentially the same as that identified for cimetidine. The occurence of jaundice indicates hepatotoxicity and should be reported at once.

Famotidine (Pepcid)

Famotidine is a competitive inhibitor of H_2 receptors and its effects are very similar to those of ranitidine. It is indicated in the treatment of acute duodenal ulcer, acute benign gastric ulcer, and the Zollinger-Ellison syndrome. Famotidine also is used prophylactically in duodenal ulcer patients. Famotidine is usually well tolerated; most adverse reactions have been mild and transient. These include headache, dizziness, constipation and diarrhea.

The nursing process for famotidine is similar to that for cimetidine and ranitidine, with the added caution to assess blood count during therapy and to be on the alert for possible blood dyscrasias (thrombocytopenia — fatigue, bruising, bleeding and poor healing).

Nizatidine (Axid)

Nizatidine is another agent that has competitive, reversible inhibition action on the H_2 receptors of gastric acid-secreting cells. Its properties are similar to those of ranitidine and famotidine. Nizatidine is indicated in the treatment of acute duodenal ulcer and acute benign gastric ulcer and for the prevention of duodenal ulcer.

The nursing process for nizatidine is essentially the same as that for ranitidine.

Anticholinergic Drugs

Mechanism of Action and Pharmacologic Effects

The pharmacology of anticholinergics and their implications for nursing care have been detailed in Chapter 6. Anticholinergics block muscarinic receptors in the stomach, thereby preventing acetylcholine, released by the vagus, from stimulating gastric acid secretion. Unfortunately, high doses of most anticholinergics are usually required, with the result that a general parasympathetic block is often produced throughout the body.

Therapeutic Uses

The value of most anticholinergics is limited by relatively poor efficacy and unacceptable adverse effects. Pirenzepine (Gastrozepin) is an interesting anticholinergic. More effective than its predecessors, it has little CNS toxicity and minimal peripheral adverse effects. The appearance of the H_2 blockers has reduced greatly the use of anticholinergics. With the possible exception of pirenzepine, anticholinergics are less effective and more toxic than either cimetidine or ranitidine.

Combination products are available containing both an anticholinergic and a CNS depressant. Donnatal (hyoscyamine, atropine, scopolamine and phenobarbital) and Librax (clidinium and chlordiazepoxide) are two examples. These products are used as adjunctive therapy in the treatment of peptic ulcers, irritable bowel syndrome and acute enterocolitis. The therapeutic rationale for combining a CNS depressant with an anticholinergic must be questioned.

Anticholinergic drugs, including pirenzepine, are contraindicated in glaucoma, obstructive uropathy due to prostatism, and obstructive diseases of the gastrointestinal tract.

Adverse Effects

A major drawback to the use of anticholinergics for the treatment of peptic ulcers is the variety of adverse effects seen. With the exception of pirenzepine, anticholinergic treatment often blocks all cholinergic innervation, and the patient experiences a dry mouth, mydriasis, cycloplegia, anhidrosis, tachycardia, urinary retention and decreased intestinal motility.

Nursing Process

The nursing process associated with the prescription of anticholinergic drugs is discussed in Chapter 6. Readers are advised to refer to that chapter.

Prostaglandin Analogues

Misoprostol (Cytotec)

Mechanism of Action and Pharmacologic Effects

Misoprostol is a synthetic analogue of PGE_1. The drug has both gastric antisecretory and cytoprotective effects. The antisecretory effect occurs through a direct action on the parietal cells. Misoprostol exerts its cytoprotective effect by enhancing natural mucosal defense mechanisms. Misoprostol can protect the gastric mucosa against various irritants such as alcohol, acetylsalicylic acid and some nonsteroidal anti-inflammatory drugs (NSAIDs).

Therapeutic Uses

Misoprostol is indicated for the treatment of duodenal ulcer and also for the treatment and prevention of NSAID-induced gastric ulcers (≥ 0.3 cm in diameter). Misoprostol is contraindicated in pregnancy. Women should be advised to use strict contraceptive measures while taking misoprostol. If pregnancy is suspected, the use of misoprostol should be discontinued and the pregnancy followed very closely (weekly) for the next four weeks.

Adverse Effects

Diarrhea and abdominal pain are the most common adverse effects of misoprostol. Other adverse effects of the drug are nausea, headache and dizziness.

Nursing Process

Nursing assessment should involve monitoring gastric pH during treatment to ensure that the pH is maintained at a level greater than 5. It is also recommended that fluid intake and output be assessed. In addition, blood studies for BUN and creatinine are recommended. Misoprostol can be stored at room temperature prior to drug administration. Patient evaluation by the nurse involves monitoring for therapeutic response to misoprostol (absence of pain or gastrointestinal symptoms). Patient teaching includes cautioning the patient to avoid over-the-counter preparations, alcohol, coffee and harsh spices. Patients should be told to take misoprostol only as directed and not to share the drug with anyone else. Finally, nurses must emphasize that patients must not take misoprostol if they are pregnant.

H⁺, K⁺ – ATPase (Proton Pump) Inhibitors

Omeprazole (Losec, Prilosec)

Mechanism of Action and Pharmacologic Effects

Omeprazole inhibits the gastric enzyme H^+, K^+-ATPase (the proton pump) which is responsible for secretion of H^+ by the parietal cells of the stomach. It produces a dose-dependent inhibition of both basal acid secretion and stimulated acid secretion. Daily oral doses of 20 mg of omeprazole reduce twenty-four-hour intragastric acidity by approximately eighty per cent. Neither food nor antacids have any effect on the bioavailability of omeprazole.

Therapeutic Uses

Omeprazole is indicated in the treatment of conditions for which a reduction of gastric acid secretion is required, such as duodenal ulcer, gastric ulcer, reflux esophagitis and Zollinger-Ellison syndrome. Experience with long-term administration of omeprazole to patients with duodenal and gastric ulcers and reflux esophagitis is limited, and its used in maintenance therapy cannot be recommended until further data become available.

Adverse Effects

Omeprazole is well tolerated. The incidence of adverse reactions is low. When they have occurred, most adverse reactions have been mild and transient, and there has been no consistent relationship with treatment. The adverse reactions experienced with omeprazole include nausea, headache, diarrhea, constipation, abdominal pain, dyspepsia, flatulence and vomiting. Omeprazole is metabolized in the liver via the cytochrome P_{450} system. It can interact with other drugs that are also metabolized by cytochrome P_{450} (see Drug Interactions under Table 33).

Nursing Process

Nurses should begin their assessment by checking the patient's history for previous hypersensitivity to this drug, and for hepatic and renal insufficiency. Drug therapy is not advised during pregnancy. Prior to administration, omeprazole capsules should be stored in tightly capped containers in a dry place and swallowed whole with sufficient water. The assessment process involves monitoring the therapeutic effects of omeprazole throughout therapy. Elderly patients should receive particularly close attention because they may show increased sensitivity to omeprazole and require alterations in drug dosage. Nurses should teach patients about possible drug interactions with tranquillizers. Patients should also be advised to avoid over-the-counter drugs and alcohol.

Drugs That Reduce the Effects of Secreted Gastric Acid and Pepsin

Antacids

Mechanism of Action and Pharmacologic Effects

Prior to the introduction of cimetidine, antacids were the standard treatment of peptic ulcers because they relieved pain and promoted healing. As the pH of the stomach increases, the action of pepsin decreases. At pH values between 4 and 5 the proteolytic action of pepsin is completely inhibited.

Therapeutic Uses

Although antacids are still widely used in the treatment of gastric and duodenal ulcers, the popularity of H_2 blockers has decreased their use. However, for patients who can tolerate their taste and consume adequate amounts on a regular basis, antacids provide an effective form of treatment. A full course of therapy is six weeks, unless radiology or endoscopy demonstrates healing.

In choosing the appropriate antacid for a patient, five factors should be considered. The first involves the **selection of a nonsystemic over a systemic antacid.** Sodium bicarbonate is rapidly absorbed. Although it will increase the pH of the stomach, it will also change the systemic pH of the body and as a result is not recommended. Calcium carbonate is partially absorbed and for this reason its use, on a chronic basis, is not recommended. The nonsystemic antacids are salts of aluminum and magnesium. They are not absorbed and are preferred for chronic therapy.

The second consideration in selecting an antacid is the **dosage form** used. Although most antacids are available in both liquids and tablets, a better response is obtained with the liquid formulations. This must be counterbalanced with the knowledge that most liquids have an insipid, nauseating taste. For this reason, patients often find tablets more acceptable.

The **acid-neutralizing capacity** of the various products is the third consideration. Not all products neutralize acid equally. The acid-neutralizing capabilities of several popular products are given in Table 32.

Cost is a fourth consideration. Most patients must consume large quantities of antacids on a regular basis for many months, or even years. This can place a heavy burden on their pocketbook and may be a major reason for stopping treatment.

The fifth consideration is **taste.** No antacid has a pleasant flavor. Consideration should be directed to just how bad each tastes. Choosing a product a patient prefers improves compliance.

Table 32
Approximate amounts of several antacid products required to neutralize 150 mmoles of hydrochloric acid.

Antacid Product	mL Required to Neutralize HCl
Amphogel	100
Gelusil	60
Maalox	50
Mylanta II	30
Riopan	60

Adverse Effects
Systemic antacids are absorbed. If used chronically they can change the systemic pH of the patient. Nonsystemic antacids are salts of aluminum and magnesium. Both affect the bowel, but in different ways. Aluminum produces constipation; magnesium causes diarrhea. In an attempt to counterbalance the constipating effects of one with the laxative properties of the other, many antacid products contain both aluminum and magnesium salts.

Nursing Process
Sodium bicarbonate is an effective antacid but can produce metabolic alkalosis. In addition, it tends to cause rebound gastric acidosis. The primary nursing responsibility is patient teaching to caution patients not to use this home remedy.

Because antacids are usually self-administered on an outpatient basis, nurses should ensure that the patient is taking the medication properly. If tablets are the dosage form required, proper administration means chewing the tablets and washing them down with at least 250 mL (8 oz.) of water. Refrigerating antacid suspensions often makes them more palatable. Suspensions should be well shaken before measuring to ensure proper distribution. Nurses should evaluate the relief of symptoms produced by the use of the medication. In addition, any adverse effects should be identified and patients instructed regarding the circumstances in which medical advice should be sought. Nurses should identify any adverse effects produced by calcium carbonate-containing products.

Sucralfate (Carafate, Sulcrate)

Mechanism of Action and Pharmacologic Effects
Sucralfate is not absorbed from the gastrointestinal tract. The drug is claimed to coat the ulcer crater and protect it from the corrosive actions of acid and pepsin. Sucralfate can also protect the gastric mucosa against various irritants, such as alcohol and acetylsalicylic acid (aspirin) Further claims for the product include its ability to inactivate pepsin.

Therapeutic Uses
Sulcralfate is indicated for the treatment of duodenal and nonmalignant gastric ulcer and to prevent recurrence of duodenal ulcer. At present, the place of sulcrafate in the treatment of peptic ulcer appears to be as an alternative for the patient who either cannot tolerate the adverse effects of cimetidine, or the cost of ranitidine, famotidine, nizatidine, misoprostol or omeprazole.

Adverse Effects
Sulcralfate's adverse effects are mild and rarely lead to discontinuing the drug. Constipation, seen in about two per cent of patients, is the main complaint. Other adverse effects reported include diarrhea, nausea, gastric discomfort, indigestion, dry mouth, skin rash, pruritus, back pain, dizziness, sleepiness and vertigo.

Nursing Process

Evaluation
Establish baseline description of patient's subjective perceptions of symptoms as a means of later evaluating drug efficacy.

Administration
Administer from an airtight container that has been stored at room temperature. Ensure two hours between administration of sucralfate and medications with which it chemically binds. When this medication is to be administered via nasogastric tube, the pharmacist should be requested to dissolve it in an appropriate solution. Otherwise, an improperly crushed and dissolved tablet may form an ineffective and nontherapeutic mass in the patient's stomach or intestines.

Evaluation
Note patient's subjective reports related to the relief of symptoms as a means of evaluating drug efficacy.

Teaching
Emphasize to the patient the importance of continuing the prescribed dosage regimen. Omission of a dose, alteration of dosage or changing of administration times may decrease the effectiveness of this medication.

Further Reading

Bianchi, P.G. and Parente, F. (1991). Long-term treatment of duodenal ulcer. A review of management options. *Drugs 41* :38-51.

Clissold, S.P. (1986). Famotidine. Pharmacodynamic and pharmacokinetic properties and a preliminary review of its therapeutic use in peptic ulcer disease and Zollinger-Ellison syndrome. *Drugs 32* :197-221.

Clissold, S.P. and Campoli-Richards, D.M. (1986). Omeprazole. A preliminary review of its pharmacodynamic and pharmacokinetic properties, and therapeutic potential in peptic ulcer disease and Zollinger-Ellison syndrome. *Drugs 32* :15-47.

Flier, J.S. and Underhill, L.H. (1990). Pathogenesis of peptic ulcers and implications for therapy. *New Engl. J. Med. 322* :909-916.

Monk, J.P. and Clissold, S.P. (1987). Misoprostol. A preliminary review of its pharmacodynamic and pharmacokinetic properties, and therapeutic efficacy in the treatment of peptic ulcer disease. *Drugs 33* :1-30.

Omeprazole (1990). *The Medical Letter 32* :19-21.

Price, A.H. and Brogden, R.N. (1988). Nizatidine. A preliminary review of its pharmacodynamic and pharmacokinetic properties, and its therapeutic use in peptic ulcer disease. *Drugs 36* :521-539.

Sontag, S.J. (1986). Prostaglandins in peptic ulcer disease. An overview of current status and future directions. *Drugs 32* :445-457.

Wardell, T. (1991). Assessing and managing a gastric ulcer. *Nursing 21* (3): 34-41

Table 33
Antiulcer drugs.

Generic Name (Trade Name)	Use (Dose)	Action	Adverse Effects	Drug Interactions	Nursing Process
Pharmacologic Classification: Histamine2 (H2) Antagonists					
Cimetidine (Tagamet)	Tx of duodenal ulcer, benign gastric ulcer and reflux esophagitis (*For duodenal ulcer, nonmalignant gastric ulcer* - **Oral:** Adults - 800 mg hs, or 600 mg bid at breakfast and hs, or 300 mg qid w. meals and hs. *Prophylaxis of recurrent ulcer* - **Oral:** Adults - 400 mg hs, or 300 mg bid at breakfast and hs. *Gastroesophageal reflux disease* - **Oral:** Adults - 800 mg hs, or 600 mg bid at breakfast and hs, or 300 mg qid w. meals and hs for 8-12 weeks. *Upper GI tract hemorrhage* - **IV or intermittent infus'n:** Adults - 300 mg q6h until 48 h after active bleeding has stopped; thereafter, 600 mg PO bid at breakfast and hs, or 300 mg q6h)	Blocks histamine receptors (H$_2$) in stomach, thereby preventing histamine secreted by stomach from increasing gastric acid secret'n.	Mild and transient diarrhea, fatigue, dizziness and rash; mild, reversible, nonprogressive gynecomastia during prolonged tx. Confus'n in elderly.	**Anticoagulants, oral; chlordiazepoxide; diazepam; lidocaine; phenytoin; propranolol; theophyline:** May have their hepatic metabolism reduced by cimetidine. As a result, their eliminat'n is reduced and blood levels increased. Dosages of these drugs may require adjustment when starting or stopping concomitantly administered cimetidine, to maintain safe optimum blood levels.	**Assess:** For pregnancy, lactat'n. **Administer:** With food; separate from antacids by 1 h. **Teach:** Importance of taking drug for prescribed period; smoking decr. efficiency.
Ranitidine (Zantac)	As for cimetidine (*For duodenal ulcer and benign gastric ulcer* - **Oral:** 300 mg od hs. In most pts healing occurs in 4 weeks, although a few may require further course of tx. Pts w. hx of recurrent ulcer - **Oral:** 150 mg od hs. *Reflux esophagitis* - **Oral:** 150 mg bid or 300 mg hs for up to 8 weeks)	As for cimetidine	None serious. May include fatigue, headache, dizziness, diarrhea and skin rashes.		As for cimetidine
Famotidine (Pepcid)	As for cimetidine (*For tx of duodenal ulcer* - **Oral:** Initially, 40 mg od hs for 4-8 weeks.	As for cimetidine	Headache, dizziness, constipat'n, diarrhea		As for cimetidine, w. added caution that nurses be alert for blood dyscrasias and thrombocytopenia.

Drug	Uses / Dosage	Side Effects	Action	Nursing Considerations
	Maint. tx for duodenal ulcer - **Oral:** 20 mg od hs for up to 6-12 months. *Tx of benign gastric ulcer -* **Oral:** 40 mg od hs. Tx should be given for 4-8 weeks, but durat'n of tx may be shortened if healing can be documented. *Pathologic hypersecretory condit'ns (e.g., Zollinger-Ellison syndrome) -* **Oral:** Initially, 20 mg q6h; incr. prn. Doses up to 160 mg q6h have been administered. *In some hospitalized pts w. pathological hypersecretory condit'ns or intractable ulcers, or in pts unable to take oral medicat'n -* **IV:** 20 mg q12h. Change to oral tx as soon as acute situat'n is under control)	As for cimetidine		
Nizatidine (Axid)	As for cimetidine (*For duodenal or benign gastric ulcer -* **Oral:** 300 mg od hs. *Maint. tx in duodenal ulcer -* **Oral:** 150 mg od hs for up to 6-12 months)	Low incidence	As for cimetidine	

Pharmacologic Classification: Anticholinergic Drugs

Drug	Uses / Dosage	Side Effects	Action	Nursing Considerations
Prenzepine (Gastrozepin)	Tx of duodenal and nonmalignant gastric ulcer (**Oral:** 50 mg bid, a.m. and p.m. In pts w. more pronounced symptoms, 50 mg tid can be given. In pts requiring long-term tx, pirenzepine can be given continuously for up to 3 months)	Dryness of mouth, visual disturbances, fatigue, heartburn or digestive complaints, dizziness, constipat'n, diarrhea, nausea, vomiting	Competitive antagonist of acetylcholine at muscarinic receptors in stomach. Blocking muscarinic receptors prevents normal acetylcholine-induced stimulat'n of gastric acid secret'n.	**Assess:** Hx glaucoma, hypertens'n, coronary artery disease, chronic GI condit'n, asthma or pulmonary disease, urinary retent'n. **Administer:** With meals; w. liquid diet initially for pts w. edematous duodenal ulcer, after pt has voided. **Evaluate:** Effectiveness, toxicity, fluid balance and electrolyte status prn for pts on long-term tx. **Teach:** Initially, to avoid driving or using heavy machinery; proper mouth care.

Generic Name (Trade Name)	Use (Dose)	Action	Adverse Effects	Drug Interactions	Nursing Process

Pharmacologic Classification: Prostaglandin Analogue

Misoprostol (Cytotec)	Indicated for duodenal ulcer; tx and prevent'n of NSAID-induced gastric ulcers (*For duodenal ulcer* - **Oral**: Adults, 200 µg qid [pc, hs] for 4 weeks. In pts who are not healed after 4 weeks, tx may be continued for another 4 weeks. *Tx and prevent'n of NSAID-induced gastric ulcers* - **Oral**: 400-800 µg/day in divided doses. When appropriate, misoprostol and NSAIDs are to be taken simultaneously. Misoprostol should be taken after food)	Synthetic analogue of PGE₁. It has both antisecretory and cytoprotective effects. Antisecretory effect occurs through direct action on parietal cells. Misoprostol exerts its cytoprotective effect by enhancing natural mucosal defense mechanisms.	Diarrhea and abdominal pain are most common. Others incl. nausea, headache, dizziness. *Misoprostol is contraindicated in pregnancy.*		**Assess:** Monitor gastric pH (> 5), fluid intake/output, blood studies for BUN and creatinine. **Administer:** Store drug at room temperature. **Evaluate:** Monitor for tx effect and absence of pain and GI symptoms. **Teach:** Caution pt to avoid OTC preparat'ns, alcohol, coffee and harsh spices. Drug should be taken as directed and *never* shared. Do not take if pregnant.

Pharmacologic Classification: H⁺, K⁺-ATPase (Proton Pump) Inhibitor

Omeprazole (Losec, Prilosec)	Condit'ns for which a reduct'n of gastric acid secret'n is required (*Duodenal ulcer, acute tx* - **Oral**: Adults - 20 mg od. For pts whose ulcers are not healed after 2 weeks, an add'l 2 weeks of tx is recommended. *Duodenal ulcer, refractory cases* - **Oral**: Adults - 40 mg 1x/daily. *Gastric ulcer, acute tx* - **Oral**: Adults - 20 mg od. Healing us. occurs within 4 weeks. For pts whose ulcers have not healed after this initial course of tx, an add'l 4 weeks of tx is recommended. *Gastric ulcer, refractory cases* - **Oral**: Adults - 40 mg od. Healing is us. achieved within 8 weeks. *Reflux esophagitis, acute tx* - **Oral**: Adults - 20 mg od. *Reflux esophagitis, refractory tx* - **Oral**: 40 mg od for 8 weeks.	Inhibits enzyme responsible for final step in secret'n of acid by parietal cells of stomach. Can block stimulus to acid secret'n produced by acetylcholine, gastrin or histamine.	Incidence low. May include nausea, headache, diarrhea, constipat'n, abdominal pain, dyspepsia, flatulence, vomiting. Can interact w. other drugs that are also metabolized by cytochrome P₄₅₀ (see Drug Interactions).	**Diazepam:** Can experience incr. half-life after repeated dosing w. 40 mg/kg of omeprazole. **Phenytoin:** Has shown incr. half-life after repeated dosing w. 40 mg/day of omeprazole.	**Assess:** Pt hx for hypersensitivity to drug; for hepatic/renal insufficiency. This drug not advised during pregnancy. **Administer:** Swallow capsule w. full glass water. Store in tightly capped container in dry place. **Evaluate:** For tx effects. Pay close attention to elderly pts for reduced levels of tolerance. **Teach:** Caution pts about interact'n w. tranquilizers; to avoid OTC drugs and alcohol.

Zollinger-Ellison syndrome - **Oral:** Adults - initially, 60 mg od; incr. prn. With doses > 80 mg, dose should be divided and given bid. Doses up to 120 mg tid have been administered)

Pharmacologic Classification: Gastroduodenal Cytoprotective Agent

Drug	Use / Dosage	Action	Side Effects	Interactions	Nursing Process
Sucralfate (Carafate, Sulcrate)	Tx of duodenal and nonmalignant gastric ulcer (**Oral:** 1 g qid, 1 h ac and hs. *Prophylaxis of duodenal ulcer recurrence - 1 g bid on empty stomach)*	Inhibitory action on proteolytic activity of pepsin. An adherent and cytoprotective barrier at ulcer site.	Constipat'n, diarrhea, nausea, gastric discomfort, indigest'n, dry mouth, skin rash, pruritus, back pain, dizziness, sleepiness, vertigo	**Antacids:** Should not be taken within 0.5 h before or after sucralfate because binding of sucralfate within ulcer crater may decr. as a consequence of a change in intragastric pH. **Digoxin:** Absorpt'n may be reduced by concomitant administrat'n of sucralfate.	**Evaluate:** Relief of symptoms. **Teach:** Importance of compliance to dosage regimen.

Pharmacologic Classification: Antacids

Drug	Use / Dosage	Action	Side Effects	Interactions	Nursing Process
Aluminum hydroxide (Amphogel)	Adjunct in tx of gastric and duodenal peptic ulcers to relieve pain (**Oral:** *Liquid containing 320 mg/5mL* - 10 mL 5-6x/day bet. meals and hs. *Tablets containing 600 mg* - 1 tablet 5-6x/day)	Neutralizes gastric acid and raises pH to a level where pepsin activity is reduced.	Constipat'n, dysgeusia, fatigue	**Iron preparat'ns:** May have decr. absorpt'n when taken shortly before, with or within a few hours after Al-containing antacids. **Isoniazid:** May not be absorbed if taken before, with or a few hours after $Al(OH)_3$ and magaldrate (Riopan). **Phenothiazines:** May not be absorbed if taken shortly before, with or within a few hours of an antacid. **Tetracyclines:** Have reduced absorpt'n if taken shortly before, with or within a few hours of an antacid.	**Administer:** Cold. **Evaluate:** Relief of symptoms; for adv. effects; amount consumed.
Magnesium hydroxide (Milk of Magnesia)	As for $Al(OH)_3$ (**Oral:** 5-10 mL qid)	As for $Al(OH)_3$	Diarrhea, nausea, vomiting, abdominal pain		As for $Al(OH)_3$
Aluminum and magnesium hydroxide (Maalox, Mylanta, Gelusil, Riopan)	As for $Al(OH)_3$ (**Oral:** 10-20 mL ac and hs, or more often prn)	As for $Al(OH)_3$	As for $Al(OH)_3$ and $Mg(OH)_2$		As for $Al(OH)_3$ and $Mg(OH)_2$

CHAPTER 23

Drugs for the Treatment of Chronic Inflammatory Bowel Disease

Teaching Objectives:

Following completion of this chapter, the reader should be able to:

1. Divide chronic inflammatory bowel disease into ulcerative colitis and Crohn's disease and compare the two with respect to etiology, location within the gastrointestinal tract and presentation of colonic and extracolonic symptoms.
2. Discuss the mechanisms of action, therapeutic uses and adverse effects of sulfasalazine and mesalamine (5-aminosalicylic acid), as well as the related nursing processes.
3. Discuss the mechanism of action, therapeutic uses, routes of administration and adverse effects of corticosteroids in the treatment of chronic inflammatory bowel disease, as well as the related nursing processes.
4. Discuss the mechanism of action, therapeutic uses, adverse effects and nursing process associated with use of azathioprine and mercaptopurine in the treatment of chronic inflammatory bowel disease.
5. Describe the rationale for the use of antibiotics and antibacterials in the treatment of chronic inflammatory bowel disease and the evidence for their efficacy.
6. Describe the mechanism of action, therapeutic use, adverse effects and nursing process associated with the use of cromolyn in the treatment of chronic inflammatory bowel disease.
7. List the groups of drugs used to assist in the normalization of bowel habit and discuss their mechanisms of action, therapeutic uses, adverse effects and related nursing process.

Chronic Inflammatory Bowel Disease

Chronic inflammatory bowel disease may be divided into ulcerative colitis and Crohn's disease. With an annual incidence in North America and Europe between five and ten new cases per 100 000 population for ulcerative colitis and three to five new cases per 100 000 for Crohn's disease, these conditions are not among the most common medical disorders. However, for those patients afflicted, chronic inflammatory bowel disease can be devastating, not only altering lifestyle but also presenting the prospect of death. Nursing these individuals presents special problems. It is important that nurses understand the nature of the two diseases and the drugs used to treat them if they are to provide appropriate nursing care.

Ulcerative colitis and Crohn's disease have many similarities. They are both ulcerating inflammatory diseases of the intestine of unknown etiology that often present with diarrhea, rectal bleeding, abdominal pain, fever or weight loss. Ulcerative colitis and Crohn's disease have identical extracolonic manifestations that include arthritis, ankylosing spondylitis, eye damage, venous thromboses, skin problems and kidney, liver and pancreas deterioration. Ulcerative colitis differs from Crohn's disease in that it involves only the mucosa of the large intestine. In contrast, Crohn's disease is not restricted to only the mucosa. It affects the entire gastrointestinal wall. Furthermore, although the ileum and colon are its most common sites, Crohn's disease can also be found in the stomach, duodenum, jejunum and rectum.

The cause or causes of ulcerative colitis and Crohn's disease are unknown. Speculation involves genetic factors, infectious agents or immunological disturbances. It is possible that hereditary factors play a role because there is a familial incidence in the disease. This is not to say that parents with chronic inflammatory bowel disease always give birth to children who later develop the condition. The probability is less than ten per cent that a patient afflicted will have a child similarly bothered. However, it is not uncommon for families to have more than one member with inflammatory bowel disease, some with ulcerative colitis and others with Crohn's disease.

The argument in favor of the role of an infectious agent is supported by an increased incidence of lymphocytotoxic antibodies in patients with ulcerative colitis. In addition, there appears to be an increased incidence of these antibodies in blood relatives and spouses of patients, suggesting that they may have contracted an infectious agent from the patients. Further support for this hypothesis can be obtained from the observation that antibacterial therapy can provide at least partial symptomatic relief. At the present time, however, no micro-organism has been found in abnormal amounts in patients with ulcerative colitis.

The immunological hypothesis is perhaps the most exciting. It is based on the fact that patients with ulcerative colitis and Crohn's disease demonstrate a number of immunological abnormalities. It has already been mentioned that the extracolonic manifestations of ulcerative colitis resemble those seen in the autoimmune group of diseases, such as rheumatoid arthritis. This fact, plus the knowledge that immunosuppressive drugs are effective in treating inflammatory bowel disease, gives credence to the view that ulcerative colitis and Crohn's disease are due to immunological defects in the patient.

Drug Treatment of Chronic Inflammatory Bowel Disease

Drug therapy of ulcerative colitis or Crohn's disease involves the use of anti-inflammatory agents, immunosuppressants and antibiotics or antibacterials. No drug is curative and there is some doubt whether treatment even alters the course of these diseases, especially Crohn's disease. The use of these drugs, alone or in combination, is based on the previously stated assumption that ulcerative colitis and Crohn's disease are inflammatory disorders that may have an immunological or infectious basis, or both. Other forms of drug treatment include the use of cromolyn to reduce the release of histamine from mast cells in the gastrointestinal tract and narcotics to treat diarrhea symptomatically.

It is not the place of this book to discuss other forms of therapy. Readers should refer to a medical-surgical nursing text to familiarize themselves with the use of elemental diets and parenteral hyperalimentation, since they may form an important component of complete therapeutic regimen for patients with chronic inflammatory bowel disease.

Anti-Inflammatory Agents

Sulfasalazine (Azulfidine, Salazopyrin, SAS-500)

Mechanism of Action and Pharmacologic Effects

Sulfasalazine is split by bacteria in the lower colon into sulfapyridine, a sulfonamide antibacterial, and mesalamine (5-aminosalicylic acid), an anti-inflammatory chemical. It is believed that sulfasalazine owes its therapeutic value to the actions of the mesalamine component.

Therapeutic Uses

The primary established value of sulfasalazine in ulcerative colitis is the prevention of relapse once remission is attained. In Crohn's disease, sulfasalazine appears to be of more use when the colon is involved. It is of debatable value when Crohn's disease is limited to the small intestine. Sulfasalazine is contraindicated in patients who are hypersensitive to sulfonamides or salicylates. It should also not be used in infants under two.

Adverse Effects

The common adverse effects of sulfasalazine are nausea and vomiting. Other effects include arthralgia, skin rash, fever, headache and renal impairment. Sulfasalazine may also cause blood dyscrasias, the most common being hemolytic anemia.

Nursing Process

Assessment

Before administering sulfasalazine, nurses should assess the patient's history for evidence of previous hypersensitivity to sulfonamides, allergies or asthma, and for liver or kidney disease. These conditions provide sufficient justification to seek verification of the order from the physician. If the drug order is confirmed, the patient should be evaluated very carefully for adverse effects. The benefit/risk ratio must be carefully evaluated when the drug is given during pregnancy, especially at term or to a woman who is breastfeeding, because kernicterus may be produced in the newborn.

Administration

Administration of sulfasalazine following meals or a snack will prevent some of the mild, but unpleasant, gastric effects. In order to maintain sufficient therapeutic levels of the medication in the gastrointestinal tract at all times, sulfasalazine should be administered at equal intervals twenty-four hours a day. Sulfasalazine should be given with a full glass of water to maintain adequate hydration.

Evaluation

Fever, headache and skin rash occurring together could indicate Stevens-Johnson syndrome, which is fatal in about 25% of cases. A nurse who observes any of the preceding adverse effects should withhold any further doses of sulfasalazine and contact the physician immediately. Additional nursing evaluation of patients taking this medication should emphasize urinary output of at least 1500 mL/24-h period because of the danger of crystalluria.

Teaching

Patients should be alerted to the possibility that sulfasalazine will turn their urine an orange color. They should also be taught the importance of maintaining adequate fluid intake to ensure a urinary output of more than 1500 mL per day. Patient teaching should alert the patient and family to the indicators of drug effectiveness and to the adverse effects produced by sulfasalazine. The likelihood of photosensitivity should be emphasized and patients encouraged to avoid sunlight or to use a sunscreen.

Mesalamine, 5-Aminosalicylic Acid (Asacol, Salofalk)

Mechanism of Action and Pharmacologic Effects

As noted earlier, sulfasalazine is a combination of sulfapyridine linked to mesalamine (5-aminosalicylic acid). Intestinal bacteria in the ileum and colon break sulfasalazine down to these two components. Sulfapyridine is absorbed and metabolized in the liver, whereas mesalamine is excreted in the feces. As mentioned above, mesalamine is responsible for the anti-inflammatory effects and sulfapyridine for many of the adverse effects of sulfasalazine. It is therefore reasonable to expect that 5-aminosalicylic acid should be as effective as sulfasalazine, but with a reduced incidence of adverse effects.

Therapeutic Uses

In North America 400-mg enteric-coated tablets of mesalamine are available and are indicated as adjunctive therapy in the treatment of ulcerative colitis. Rectal suppositories and a rectal suspension are also available. The suppositories are indicated in the management of ulcerative proctitis and as adjunctive therapy in more extensive distal ulcerative colitis. The rectal suspension is used in the management of distal ulcerative colitis extending to the splenic flexure including refractory distal ulcerative colitis. In addition, the rectal suspension is approved as adjunctive therapy in more extensive disease as well as for the prevention of relapse in distal ulcerative colitis. Long-term mesalamine therapy may be necessary to prevent recurrent relapses of active colitis. These products are contraindicated in patients with a history of sensitivity to salicylates and in patients under the age of two years.

Adverse Effects

Because mesalamine does not contain the sulfonamide sulfapyridine, its side effects are much less frequent and less severe than those of sulfasalazine. Occasionally patients may have mild nausea, colic or headache.

Nursing Process

Assessment

Assess patients for adverse gastrointestinal effects, rectal pain, cramps, gas, nausea or diarrhea. If these occur, the drug may have to be discontinued.

Administration

Suppositories should be stored at room temperature and administered two or three times daily. If the rectal suspension is ordered, it should be give at bedtime and retained by the patient until morning.

Evaluation

Nurses should monitor patients for the therapeutic effects of mesalamine. These include absence of pain and bleeding from the gastrointestinal tract, as well as decreased number of diarrhea stools.

Teaching

If rectal preparations are ordered, the nurse should instruct the patient or family member in the method of administration. Patients should also be told to notify the physician of any adverse gastrointestinal symptoms.

Corticosteroids

Mechanism of Action and Pharmacologic Effects

The pharmacology of corticosteroids and the nursing actions related to their use are presented in Chapter 29. Table 34 at the end of this chapter contains a brief synopsis of this information. The anti-inflammatory effects of glucocorticoids account, at least in part, for their effectiveness in chronic inflammatory bowel disease. Their immunosuppressive actions may also play a role in their ability to placate the irritated intestine.

Therapeutic Uses

Corticosteroids are indicated in ulcerative colitis to reduce acute inflammation. Their value in preventing recurrence is still debatable. Once a decision is made to use corticosteroid treatment, the initial dose should be sufficient to produce remission and therapy should be maintained for a period of time to ensure success. Thereafter, an attempt should be made to withdraw the drug.

Corticosteroid enemas may be effective if the condition is restricted to the left side of the colon. Their use reduces greatly the risk of systemic adverse effects. Hydrocortisone (Cortenema), methylprednisolone (Medrol Enpak) and betamethasone (Betnesol) are available in enema form. The enema can be attempted once nightly for two to four weeks. If nightly treatment for two to four weeks does not prove successful, oral steroid therapy should be introduced. On the other hand, success within this time may be followed by enema treatment every other night for seven days and then every third night for an additional week. The intermittent use of corticosteroid enemas may be successful in the management of many patients with mild chronic ulcerative colitis.

Moderate inflammatory bowel disease may need oral corticosteroid treatment. Although many steroids could be used, prednisone is most often prescribed because it is effective and usually cheap. Triamcinolone is not recommended because effective doses produce profound nitrogen loss.

If the patient presents for the first time in acute distress and requires hospitalization, intravenous corticosteroid treatment, such as hydrocortisone sodium succinate, may be required.

Adverse Effects

Caution should be exercised in the use of corticosteroids. These drugs are double-edged swords. Although they can provide dramatic relief for patients, corticosteroids also produce many adverse effects. These include pituitary-adrenal suppression, increased susceptibility to infection, osteoporosis, hyperglycemia, "buffalo hump", "moon face" and the possibility of psychotic disturbances. Their systemic use is justified only after other methods of treatment have failed. The adverse effects and drug interactions of corticosteroids are presented in greater detail in Chapter 29.

Nursing Process

Nurses charged with the responsibility of administering corticosteroid therapy to patients should read Chapter 29 dealing specifically with the actions of these drugs.

Immunosuppressants

Azathioprine (Imuran) and Mercaptopurine (Purinethol)

Azathioprine and mercaptopurine are immunosuppressants and reduce the proliferation of B-lymphocytes, T-lymphocytes and macrophages. Their use is based on the belief that chronic inflammatory bowel disease may be the result, at least in part, of an immunological disorder. Azathioprine and mercaptopurine are used most often with corticosteroids in Crohn's disease because they reduce the dose of steroid required.

The adverse effects of azathioprine and mercaptopurine are attributable to their ability to impair cell multiplication. In addition to their immunosuppressant effects, azathioprine and mercaptopurine can depress bone marrow and produce pancreatitis, alopecia and rashes. These effects are rarely seen with the low dosages of the drugs used to treat Crohn's disease.

Nursing Process

Assessment
Prior to administering the initial dose, nurses should establish baseline measures of vital signs, particularly the range of normal temperatures for the individual patient. They should also review the patient's history for evidence of contraindications, specifically, current pregnancy, previous hypersensitivity or pancreatitis. The presence of kidney or liver disease in the patient's history should alert the nurse to the need for particularly attentive evaluation for adverse effects. Regular nursing assessment before the administration of any dose of these medications should emphasize continuous clinical observation for evidence of infection, such as elevated temperature, changes in other vital signs, nasal or sinus congestion, sore throat, fever, chills, malaise and wounds that produce discharge and do not heal.

Administration
These drugs should be administered from airtight, light-resistant containers that have been stored at room temperature. Administration of these medications with or immediately after meals will reduce gastric irritation. If gastric upset persists, request the physician to change the order so that the daily dose is divided into two smaller doses given at different times.

Evaluation
Obviously, nursing evaluation of patients receiving either azathioprine or mercaptopurine must be concerned with their possible adverse effects. Any drug that diminishes the ability of rapidly dividing cells to multiply will affect not only the immune system but any other area of the body with cells that multiply rapidly. Thus, in addition to an increased susceptibility to infections, as a result of their immunosuppressant effects, azathioprine and mercaptopurine can produce bone marrow depression. Although this is not usually seen in the doses of azathioprine used to treat ulcerative colitis, it should always be borne in mind. Nurses caring for patients receiving these drugs may expect the physician to order complete blood counts and kidney and liver function tests routinely as a means of detecting these adverse effects. Nurses must be alert constantly for clinical manifestations of thrombocytopenia, specifically, increased tendency to bruising, bleeding gums, petechiae, purpura, melena, epistaxis, hemoptysis and hematemesis. In addition, the importance of observing for clinical indications of infection cannot be overemphasized.

Monitoring of fluid intake and output as well as color and specific gravity of urine is important, because toxicity is increased in patients with reduced urinary output. Adverse effects on the liver may be indicated by clinical observations of pruritus, abdominal pain, distention, clay-colored stools, tea-colored urine and jaundice. Other adverse effects for which nurses should evaluate users of the drug include pancreatitis, alopecia and rashes.

Teaching
The importance of strict adherence to the prescribed drug regimen and evaluative laboratory testing must be impressed on the patient. Patients and their families should be advised of the importance of avoiding crowds and individuals with colds, flu or other infectious conditions. In addition, they should be instructed in the early detection of infection as identified in the preceding section on assessment. The importance of personal hygiene in preventing infection should also be emphasized. Patients should be taught self-evaluation for evidence of kidney or liver effects. Finally, patients of child-bearing age should be advised to practise birth control scrupulously during and for four to six months following a course of treatment with these medications because of their teratogenic potential.

Antibiotics

The use of antibiotics or antibacterials in the treatment of chronic inflammatory bowel disease is based on the premise that an infectious agent may be the cause of the disorder. The evidence to support this view is, at best, tenuous. Ampicillin, the tetracyclines, trimethoprim plus sulfamethoxazole (Bactrim, Septra) and chloramphenicol have been tried, with questionable success. Metronidazole (Flagyl) is indicated in the treatment of Crohn's disease not responsive to sulfasalazine.

Nurses should identify and be familiar with the specific drugs used in their particular area. Attention should be paid to the adverse effects of each. The pharmacology and the related nursing responsibilities of each drug are presented in Section 14.

Histamine-Release Inhibitor

Cromolyn/Sodium Cromoglycate (Nalcrom)

Cromolyn, or sodium cromoglycate, reduces the release of histamine from mast cells. It is marketed in an oral dosage form (Nalcrom) for the treatment of food allergies and chronic inflammatory bowel disease. The initial dose for adults is 200 mg four times daily before meals.

Cromolyn produces few adverse effects. Unfortunately, it is also often ineffective. Comparative studies have shown cromolyn to be less effective than sulfasalazine. Some patients respond to cromolyn, but more improve on sulfasalazine. Cromolyn must be used more extensively before we can establish its place in the treatment of chronic inflammatory bowel disease. It now appears justified only in those patients who either have not responded to, or are allergic to, sulfasalazine.

Drugs to Assist in the Normalization of Bowel Habit

Drugs can be used to treat the diarrhea of chronic inflammatory bowel disease. However, this form of treatment is secondary to the more specific therapy outlined earlier. In addition, antidiarrheal drugs should not be used in acute colitis because they can precipitate toxic dilatation of the colon under these circumstances.

Narcotics

Mechanism of Action and Pharmacologic Effects

As anyone can attest who has taken codeine tablets as an analgesic for more than a day, narcotics have a constipating action. Narcotics decrease the propulsive motility of the colon. Although most narcotics could be used for this purpose, diphenoxylate (Lomotil) and loperamide (Imodium) are preferred because they are poorly absorbed from the gastrointestinal tract.

Therapeutic Uses

Diphenoxylate has been on the market for many years. It is the favorite of many physicians. Loperamine was introduced later. It is at least as effective as diphenoxylate. These drugs should be used as adjuncts to rehydration therapy, for the symptomatic control of chronic diarrhea associated with inflammatory bowel disease. They are contraindicated in the treatment of diarrhea associated with pseudomembranous entercolitis. Diphenoxylate must be kept out of the reach of children because accidental overdosage may cause severe or even fatal respiratory depression. The use of diphenoxylate or loperamide is not recommended in children under two years of age.

Adverse Effects

The systemic adverse effects of diphenoxylate include nausea, drowsiness, lethargy, sedation, respiratory depression, dizziness, vomiting, anorexia, pruritus and skin eruptions. These reactions are characteristic of most narcotics. They are less likely to occur when a poorly absorbed drug like diphenoxylate is administered. However, abdominal bloating and cramps, paralytic ileus and toxic megacolon can also occur if care is not taken to monitor the patient. The most frequent effect of loperamide is constipation, a sign of overdosage. Loperamide can also produce toxic megacolon.

Nursing Process

Assessment
Nursing assessment of patients prior to the administration of diphenoxylate or loperamide should include reviewing the patient's history for evidence of contraindications including liver disease or a current pregnancy. Baseline measures of fluid and electrolyte status must be established.

Evaluation
Following administration of these drugs, the nurse assigned to care for the patient should evaluate the individual for central nervous system depression. Although neither diphenoxylate nor loperamide are significantly absorbed under normal conditions, the possibility that they may undergo appreciable absorption in the presence of inflammatory bowel disease should not be overlooked. If this occurs, central nervous system depression may occur. This is particularly important in those patients who are also receiving other narcotics or central nervous system depressants.

Following administration of either of these medications, patients with a history of liver disease should be carefully evaluated for evidence of threatening hepatic coma (minor psychomotor disturbances; disorientation to time, place and person; coarse hand tremor; inattentiveness or lack of ability to concentrate). Abdominal distention in patients receiving either of these medications suggests toxic megacolon. Any of the preceding observations should cause the nurse to withhold further medication and contact the physician immediately.

Teaching
Patient teaching should emphasize the importance of taking only the prescribed amount when self-administering the drug at home. Nurses should also stress the importance of storing the drugs out of the reach of children. Fatalities have resulted from accidental overdose in children. As with other drugs that are self-administered, the patient and family should be instructed regarding evaluation of the drug's effectiveness and identification of adverse effects. Nurses should caution patients to avoid over-the-counter drugs, especially those containing alcohol.

Anticholinergics

Anticholinergic drugs can also be used to reduce diarrhea. Their pharmacology and the nursing process related to their use are discussed in detail in Chapter 6. Propantheline, marketed as Pro-Banthine, is an example of an anticholinergic. A dose of 15 mg or more of this drug has been used to decrease the incidence and degree of diarrhea. However, all anticholinergics produce a variety of adverse effects that include dry mouth, absence of saliva, lack of sweat, mydriasis, cycloplegia and tachycardia. Under these circumstances, it might be hard for patients to remember why they took the drug in the first place.

Cholestyramine (Questran)

Cholestyramine is a nonabsorbed resin that sequesters bile acids and may be of considerable assistance to the patient following ileal resection. The pharmacology of this drug, together with its drug interactions and doses, is discussed in Chapter 19.

Further Reading

Drug treatment of Crohn's disease (1986). *Drugs &Therapeutics Bulletin 24* (4):13-15.

Jarnerto , G. (1989). Newer 5-aminosalicylic acid-based drugs in chronic inflammatory bowel disease. *Drugs 37* :73-86.

Peppercorn, M.A. (985). Inflammatory bowel disease, role of sulfasalazine and 5-aminosalicylic acid. *Drug Therapy* :62-70.

Riis, P. (1983). Treating ulcerative colitis: What to choose from the therapeutic supermarket. *Acta Med. Scand. 213* :161-163.

Sack, D.M. and Peppercorn, M.A. (1983). Drug therapy of inflammatory bowel disease. *Pharmacotherapy 3* :158-176.

Table 34
Drugs for the treatment of chronic inflammatory bowel disease.

Generic Name (Trade Name)	Use (Dose)	Action	Adverse Effects	Drug Interactions	Nursing Process
Pharmacologic Classification: Anti-Inflammatory Drugs					
Sulfasalazine (Azasulfidine, Salazopyrin, SAS-500)	Tx of severe ulcerative colitis, proctitis or distal ulcerative colitis (**Oral: Adults** - Severe, acute attacks - 1-2 g tid-qid. *Moderate and mild attacks* - 1 g tid-qid. *Prophylaxis* - 1 g bid-tid. **Children**, 25-35 kg - 500 mg tid; 35-50 kg - 1 g bid-tid. *Prophylaxis* - 25-35 kg - 500 mg bid; 35-50 kg - 500 mg bid-tid. For proctitis and distal ulcerative colitis, **Adults** - **Rectal:** 1 enema daily, pref. hs)	Split by bacteria in colon to release anti-inflammatory chemical 5-aminosalicylic acid, which provides relief.	Anorexia, nausea, vomiting, gastric distress, blood dyscrasias, skin erupt'ns, headache, vertigo, tinnitus, peripheral neuropathy	**Digoxin:** Oral absorpt'n may be decr. by sulfasalazine. Pts receiving both drugs should be observed closely for evidence of reduced digoxin effect.	**Assess:** For hx hypersensitivity to sulfonamides, allergies, asthma, liver/kidney disease, 3rd trimester pregnancy, lactat'n. **Administer:** With food or pc, w. full glass water, at equal intervals during day. **Evaluate:** For drug effectiveness, adv. effects, adequate urinary output (>1500 mL), renal funct'n. **Teach:** Importance of adequate fluid intake; indicators of adv. effects and drug effectiveness; that urine may turn orange color.
Mesalamine, 5-aminosalicylic acid (Asacol, Salofalk)	Adjunct. tx in ulcerative colitis (**Oral: Adults** - 1200-2400 mg daily in divided doses. Max. dose, 4000 mg/day. **Rectal suspens'n:** 4 g hs, retained during entire rest period. **Rectal suppositories:** 2 [250-mg] or 1 [500-mg] suppositories bid-tid. Us. adult dose, 1-1.5 g/day)	5-aminosalicylic acid is major active component of sulfasalazine and has topical anti-inflammatory effect on colon.	Mild nausea, colic, headache		**Assess:** For adv. GI effects, rectal pain, cramps, gas, nausea, diarrhea. If these occur, drug may have to be stopped. **Administer:** Rectal suspens'n hs only. Store at room temp. **Evaluate:** Monitor for tx effect, absence of pain, bleeding from GI tract and decr. no. of diarrhea stools. **Teach:** If rectal preparat'n is ordered, instruct pt or family in method of administr'n. Advise pt to notify physician if adv. GI symptoms occur.
Pharmacologic Classification: Corticosteroids					
Prednisone	To assist during critical period in ulcerative colitis or Crohn's disease (**Oral: Adults** - initially, 40 mg/day in 4 equal doses for 4-6 days. Reduce by 5 mg/week to 20 mg/day. Maintain for 1 month, then w'draw at rate of 5 mg/week)	Anti-inflammatory effects	Acute adrenal insufficiency from rapid w'drawal, fluid/electrolyte imbalance, hyperglycemia, glycosuria, incr. susceptibility to infect'ns, peptic ulcer, Cushing's syndrome, growth arrest	**Anticoagulants, oral:** Interact w. corticosteroids because corticosteroids incr. blood coagulability and antagonize action of anticoagulant. Conversely, corticosteroids can incr. danger of hemorrhage because of their effects on vascular integrity. Monitor pts closely. **Antidiabetic agents:** May have	**Assess:** For pregnancy; evidence of infect'n; pt hx diabetes mellitus, hypertens'n, CHF, nephritis, thrombophlebitis, peptic ulcer, psychosis, Cushing's syndrome, active TB, herpes simplex; establish baseline weight, BP, sleep pattern. **Administer:** Prednisone w. meals during initial doses; give maint. dose in early a.m. (06:30-07:00) w. food;

Drug	Use	Action	Adverse Effects	Drug Interactions	Nursing Process
Hydrocortisone enema (Cortenema)	Adjunct in tx of nonspecific inflammatory disease involving rectum, sigmoid and left colon, such as idiopathic ulcerative colitis, ulcerative proctitis, regional enteritis (granulomatous colitis) w. left-side involvement, proctitis, proctocolitis and radiat'n proctitis (**Rectal:** 1 retent'n enema, containing 100 mg hydrocortisone in 60 mL, od hs for 2-3 weeks, and qod thereafter)	As for prednisone	As for prednisone	reduced effects in presence of corticosteroids because corticosteroids incr. blood sugar levels. Monitor pts carefully for decr. control. **Diuretics:** May cause excessive K loss in pts also receiving corticosteroids. Watch K balance in these pts. **Indomethacin:** Is ulcerogenic. Combined effects of this drug w. corticosteroids may incr. incidence or severity of GI ulcerat'n. *For drug interact'ns involving amphotericin B, barbiturates, oral contraceptives, phenytoin, salicylates and rifampin, see Table 46.*	regularly — never w'draw medicat'n abruptly; store in light-proof container. **Evaluate:** Response; weight, daily muscle strength and mass in limbs; for hyperglycemia; BP bid until dosage is stabilized; for s/s infectious diseases or inflammat'n; wound healing; diet for K, protein and NaCl intake; refer to dietician prn; emotional status and sleep pattern; for GI irritat'n; for evidence of adv. effects. **Teach:** Nec. of medical supervis'n and importance of personal hygiene in preventing infect'ns; need for caution to prevent fractures resulting from osteoporosis; danger of/precaut'ns against abrupt w'drawl of medicat'n; indicators of adv. effects.
Methylprednisolone acetate retent'n enema (Medrol Enpak)	As for hydrocortisone enema (**Rectal:** 1 retent'n enema, containing 40 mg methylprednisolone acetate, od or bid)	As for prednisone	As for prednisone		As for prednisone
Betamethasone disodium phosphate (Betnesol)	As for hydrocortisone enema (**Rectal:** 1 retent'n enema, containing 5 mg betamethasone/100 mL, nightly for 2-4 weeks)	As for prednisone	As for prednisone		As for prednisone

Pharmacologic Classification: Immunosuppressant Drug

Drug	Use	Action	Adverse Effects	Drug Interactions	Nursing Process
Azathioprine (Imuran)	Restricted to pts w. inflammatory bowel disease for whom convent'nal drug tx is inadequate or for whom continuous systemic corticosteroid tx is required and surgery inappropriate (**Oral/parenteral: Adults -** 2 mg/kg/day or 100-200 mg/day)	Reduces proliferat'n of B- and T-lymphocytes and macrophages.	*High doses:* Leukopenia, anemia, thrombocytopenia, bleeding, oral lesions, rashes, drug fever, alopecia, pancreatitis, arthralgia, steatorrhea, nausea, vomiting, diarrhea, anorexia, jaundice	**Allopurinol:** Interacts w. azathioprine. Azathioprine is metabolized first to 6-MP, which is then converted to inactive products. Allopurinol increases 6-MP blood levels by reducing its metabolism. Reduce dose of azathioprine to approx. 25-33% usual am't administered if allopurinol is also given.	**Assess:** Establish baseline VS; check for hx pancreatitis, kidney/liver disease, hypersensitivity; for clinical evidence of infect'n. **Administer:** From airtight, light-resistant container stored at room temp.; with or immediately following meals. **Evaluate:** For evidence of infect'n, unusual bleeding tendencies (incr. tendency to bruising, bleeding gums, petechiae, purpura, melena, epistaxis, hemoptysis, hematemesis), liver effects (pruritus, abdominal pain, distent'n, clay-colored stools, tea-colored urine, jaundice, pancreatitis), alopecia, rashes. **Teach:** Strict adherence to drug regimen and scheduled lab. testing; to avoid crowds and people w. colds, flu or other infectious condit'ns; early detect'n of infect'n; importance of personal

Generic Name (Trade Name)	Use (Dose)	Action	Adverse Effects	Drug Interactions	Nursing Process
					hygiene in preventing infect'n; self-evalu-at'n for s/s kidney/liver effects; to practise birth control scrupulously during and for 4-6 months after course of tx.

Pharmacologic Classification: Narcotic Antidiarrheal Drugs

Generic Name (Trade Name)	Use (Dose)	Action	Adverse Effects	Drug Interactions	Nursing Process
Diphenoxylate (Lomotil)	Adjunct in management of diarrhea (**Oral:** Adults - initially, 5 mg tid or qid. Max. dose, 20 mg/24 h in divided doses. Lower dosage as soon as initial control of symptoms is achieved. Maint. dose may be as low as 25% of dose required for initial control. Children - 300-400 µg/kg daily in divided doses)	Narcotics decr. propulsive motility of colon.	Nausea, drowsiness, coma, lethargy, sedat'n, respiratory depress'n, dizziness, vomiting, anorexia, pruritus, skin erupt'ns, giant urticaria, angioneurotic edema, restlessness, insomnia, abdominal bloating and cramps, paralytic ileus, toxic megacolon, numbness of extremities, headache, blurring of vision, gum swelling, euphoria, depress'n, general malaise	**Barbiturates, benzodiazepines and other CNS depressants:** May have their actions potentiated by diphenoxylate. **MAOIs:** May precipitate hypertensive crisis in pts receiving diphenoxylate.	**Assess:** Pt hx for liver disease. **Evaluate:** For abdominal distent'n; CNS depress'n; concurrent barbiturate tx; for impending coma in pts w. liver disease. **Teach:** Nec. to take precise recommended dosage; evaluat'n of drug effectiveness; adv. effects. *Keep out of reach of children.*
Loperamide (Imodium)	Symptomatic control of acute and chronic diarrhea and of intestinal transit time in pts w. ileostomies, colostomies and other intestinal resect'ns (**Oral:** Adults - 4 mg initially, followed by 2 mg after each unformed stool. Max. dose, 16 mg/day. Children - 1st-day dosage, 2-5 years [10-20 kg] - 1 mg tid [3 mg/day]; 5-8 years [20-30 kg] - 2 mg bid [4 mg/day]; 8-12 years [> 30 kg] - 2 mg tid [6 mg/day]. Following 1st-day tx - 1 mg/10 kg, administered only after a loose stool)	As for diphenoxylate	Constipat'n		**Assess:** For current pregnancy; as for diphenoxylate. **Evaluate:** As for diphenoxylate. **Teach:** As for diphenoxylate. Caution pt to avoid OTC drugs, esp. those containing alcohol.

CHAPTER 24

Laxatives and Antidiarrheal Drugs

CHAPTER 24

Laxatives and Antidiarrheal Drugs

Teaching Objectives

Following completion of this chapter, the reader should be able to:

1. Describe the frequency of bowel movements in healthy individuals.
2. List the causes of functional diarrhea.
3. List the mechanisms of action for antidiarrheal drugs.
4. List the antidiarrheal drugs that work within the intestinal lumen; explain their mechanisms of action and the nursing process related to the use of each drug.
5. Discuss the cause, prevention and treatment of travelers' diarrhea.
6. List the antidiarrheal drugs that work on the gut wall; explain their effects, contraindications and the nursing process related to their use.
7. Define the terms cathartic and laxative.
8. Discuss the appropriate and inappropriate use of laxatives and cathartics.
9. List the means by which carthartics and laxatives may work.
10. List the bulk laxatives; describe their effects and the nursing process related to their use.
11. List the stool softeners; describe their effects and the nursing process related to their use.
12. List the chemical stimulants; describe their effects and the nursing process related to their use.
13. List the osmotic laxatives and cathartics; describe their effects and the nursing process related to their use.

The Bowels

The actions of the bowels have weighed heavily on the collective mind of humankind since the beginning of time. No organ system has been so much subjected to human idiosyncrasy as the lower regions of the intestines. They have been coddled and cursed, irrigated and irritated, placated and purged — all in the interest of ensuring the daily bowel movement.

Our fascination with colonic function is understandable. Despite their distance from the brain, the bowels can be real attention-getters. Everyone has had the experience of enduring several feces-free days. The profound sense of relief that follows that first bowel movement is an experience to be treasured for many a moon. Today's frenetic lifestyle presents the colon with ever greater challenges. People travel more now than ever before and travel often upsets the colonic humors, presenting problems of economic and social significance. Many an executive has flown half-way around the world to chair a meeting, only to be rendered nonoperational by a seemingly continuous flow of stools. Others have experienced just the opposite effect: in these individuals, travel pulls tight the strings of the anal sphincter. Still others suffer alternately the bullet of constipation and the torrent of diarrhea. There is nothing quite like flying from Los Angeles to New York on a Monday, only to have one's bowels arrive with a clap of thunder on Friday evening, just in time for your after-dinner speech at the windup banquet. Experienced travelers cannot be blamed if they are unsure whether to buy a bit of internal dynamite to break the logjam on days three to four, or a medicated cork to stem the tide on day five.

The frequency of bowel movements and the consistency of stools have been discussed for centuries. Folklore holds that one, and only one, bowel movement per day is essential for good health. Fortunately, this is not true, or many of us would be quite ill. In one study of 1100 post office employees, it was found that only 53 had regular daily bowel movements. Obviously, other explanations must be sought for the failure of the mail to arrive on time! Lest we snicker unfairly at the posties, a survey of 440 nurses yielded essentially the same results. Other studies have shown that 99% of people have between three movements per week and three per day. It is the nurse's responsibility to explain this fact to patients. If this is understood, much of the perceived need for laxatives or antidiarrheal preparations will disappear.

It is easier to count stools than to measure their consistency. Yet it is just as important to know something of their nature. Forcing a cardiac patient to strain in producing a hard torpedo can be just as dangerous as neglecting the patient with liquid diarrhea as he quickly dehydrates. Although it may be convenient simply to ask the patient about the physical nature of his stools, it may also be unreliable. Most patients are not experienced stool gazers and may have little to compare against their own efforts. Thus an individual may claim, incorrectly, that his movements are not hard if he has been used to clearing cannon balls. Nurses should be well experienced stool watchers and, unpleasant as this may be, are often in the best position to study their consistency.

It must be apparent to even the casual observer that laxatives and antidiarrheal preparations are overused. Patients must be advised that the daily bowel movement is not sacred. Deviations from this pattern may be quite normal. There are, however, indications for the use of drugs that modify the bowels. The means by which these agents produce their effects, and their appropriate uses, will form the basis for the rest of this chapter.

Functional Diarrhea

It is important to differentiate between functional and organic diarrhea. The former condition requires minimal investigation; the latter an extensive workup. The use of an antidiarrheal preparation to treat organic disease may initially alleviate the patient's symptoms, but delay more appropriate treatment.

The causes of diarrhea may vary from patient to patient. They include: (1) increased water arriving at the colon, (2) decreased colonic water reabsorption, (3) increased pressure gradient from cecum to anus, or (4) decreased sigmoid segmentation. The last-named cause is best understood when it is recognized that the sigmoid section of the colon acts like a sphincter or valve, regulating the passage of material to the rectum. Decreased sigmoid segmentation reduces the valve effect and increases the volume of material presented to rectum. Drugs given to treat diarrhea act to reduce either the volume of material arriving at the rectum or the peristaltic activity of the intestine. In either case, the urge to defecate is reduced.

Drugs That Act within the Intestinal Lumen

Psyllium (Hydrocil, Metamucil)

Psyllium is capable of treating constipation or diarrhea. In the latter situation it absorbs water from the developing feces in the intestine to form a gel, thereby reducing the possibility of a watery diarrhea. Psyllium also absorbs bile acids. This may be important for its antidiarrheal action because bile acids can stimulate the colon. Nursing evaluation of patients following the administration of psyllium must document the number of stools per day and describe the characteristics of the fecal material. This information is essential in order to establish the effectiveness of the drug.

Pectin

Pectin is a dietary fiber obtained from citrus rind. The mechanism by which it reduces diarrhea is not clear, as it is destroyed within the intestine. Pectin is usually used in conjunction with kaolin in products such as Kaopectate.

Kaolin

Kaolin is hydrated aluminum citrate. Combined with pectin, it has formed a time-honored treatment for diarrhea. Although its mechanism of action is not clear, explanations for its effects include an ability to bind bacteria, toxins, bile acids and other material in the gut. It has also been claimed that the astringent effect of aluminum contributes to the action of kaolin. An **astringent** is an agent that contracts body tissue and blood vessels. A styptic pencil, used to stem the flow of blood after shaving, is an astringent. In that sense one could think of kaolin ingestion as swallowing a styptic pencil. That should be enough to pucker anyone's intestines and reduce diarrhea!

Bismuth Subsalicylate

Pepto Bismol, containing bismuth subsalicylate, has been used for years to treat diarrhea. It has found favor with North Americans visiting Mexico. Pepto Bismol has reduced complaints of diarrhea, nausea and abdominal cramping caused by toxigenic *Escherichia coli* and shigella. At the present time it is not clear if the beneficial results are due to the bismuth or the subsalicylate — undoubtedly a purely academic point to the unfortunate soul who is watching his intestines being washed away by Mexico's finest water. Obviously, much work remains to be done before the actions of this old remedy are completely understood.

A note of caution about Pepto Bismol: the use of 240 mL daily has been suggested for prevention of travelers' diarrhea. This contains the equivalent salicylate content to 2.6 g of aspirin (ASA) or, put another way, eight 325-mg (5-grain) tablets. If this dose of Pepto Bismol is given to patients taking large doses of aspirin for arthritis, toxic concentrations of salicylate can accumulate in the body. In addition, patients taking oral anticoagulants, uricosuric drugs or methotrexate may experience adverse drug interactions if they consume the recommended dose of Pepto Bismol.

Cholestyramine (Questran)

Cholestyramine binds bile salts. Its use in the treatment of hyperlipidemia and the nursing processes related to its use are discussed in Chapter 19. The drug has been reported to be effective in the treatment of patients with irritable bowel problems secondary to bile salt malabsorption. Although cholestyramine has varyingly been described as tasting like plastic or dehydrated horse manure, relatively small amounts are used to treat diarrhea, thereby reducing the taste problem. Four to six grams per day of the drug have been recommended in this situation. A brief synopsis of information related to the use of this drug is presented in Table 35 at the end of this chapter.

Antibiotics/Antibacterials

Travelers' diarrhea is caused by an infection and, as a result, would not normally be discussed in a section dealing with chronic functional diarrhea. However, this is the most appropriate location in the book for this topic. Bacterial infection from enterotoxigenic *Escherichia coli* is the most common cause of travelers' diarrhea. Other pathogens include shigella, salmonella and viruses. Any tourist who has undergone the three-dimensional experience (nausea, vomiting and diarrhea) of travelers' diarrhea must have wondered if there was not something that he or she could have taken to prevent such a plague.

Some studies have suggested that the tetracycline antibiotic doxycycline (Vibramycin) is effective as a prophylactic. Although a definite dose has not been established, it would appear that 100 – 200 mg daily of doxycycline will suffice for most individuals. To the purist, this use of a "therapeutic umbrella" might not seem justified. It is often pointed out by such individuals that travelers' diarrhea is a self-limited illness of several days' duration. Presumably, all one has to do is to wait out the storm. However, after passing more than ten loose stools per day the patient may become self-limited! Sulfonamides and trimethoprim-sulfamethoxazole (Bactrim, Septra) have also been reported to prevent travelers' diarrhea.

It is one thing to try to protect a patient from the scourge of the "Aztec Two-Step" and quite another to cure the problem once it has settled in. Antimicrobial treatment begun after the symptoms have started probably does not reduce the number of days the patient is incapacitated if the diarrhea is due to enterotoxigenic *E. coli*. Obviously, stool cultures should be taken from patients experiencing severe diarrhea (more than ten loose stools per day) with blood and mucus in the stools. Between the time of taking the cultures and obtaining the results, co-trimoxazole (Bactrim or Septra, one tablet every twelve hours) or ampicillin (500 mg four times daily) could be given. These medications will be discussed in detail in Section 14.

Nursing Process

Assessment

Nurses working in physicians' offices will most frequently come in contact with those patients for whom doxycycline is prescribed as prophylaxis for travelers' diarrhea. Nursing assessment should attempt to determine previous tetracycline hypersensitivity. Tetracycline antibiotics combine with calcium to discolor developing teeth and should not be given to pregnant or lactating women or to children younger than ten to twelve years of age.

Administration

Doxycycline that has passed the manufacturer's expiry date must *never* be administered to patients. Severe renal problems have been associated with the administration of outdated tetracycline and its derivatives.

Evaluation

Nursing evaluation of patients who have been taking doxycycline should emphasize identification of overgrowth of nonsensitive micro-organisms. Characteristic observations related to microbial overgrowth include: lingua nigra, pruritus vulva, proctitis and gingivitis. The number and characteristics of the patient's daily stools are important means of differentiating between the early irritant effect of the medication and a bowel infection caused by nonsensitive micro-organisms. The patient's fluid intake and output should be monitored for evidence of oliguria, which indicates adverse renal effects and requires immediate discontinuation of the drug.

Teaching

Patient teaching related to the prescription of doxycycline should emphasize avoiding ultraviolet light, either natural or artificial, because phototoxicity can result. This fact in itself might discourage vacationers from using the drug. No one wants to pay enormous sums for a tropical vacation only to discover that because of doxycycline-induced photosensitivity he or she must either wrap up like a mummy or risk being fried like a lobster and spend-

ing the rest of the vacation indoors in the dark recovering! Those travelers who persist in taking the medication should be instructed to store it in airtight, light-resistant, moisture-proof containers in a cool, dry place. Individuals should also be warned to discard all unused doxycycline because of outdated doxycycline's deleterious effects on the kidneys.

Drugs That Act on the Gut Wall

Narcotics

Narcotics decrease the propulsive action of the colon and increase distal segmentation, improving the valve action of the sigmoid section of the colon. Although they are undoubtedly effective, caution should be exercised in their use to treat diarrhea. In particular, narcotics should not be used in any bacterial infection causing diarrhea, including travelers' diarrhea, because they can worsen the condition by reducing or preventing the clearance of pathogens from the intestines. Narcotics can worsen antibiotic-induced colitis or precipitate toxic megacolon in severe ulcerative colitis.

Although most narcotics could be selected for their actions on the bowels, a few have been chosen for the treatment of diarrhea. Tincture of opium or camphorated tincture of opium (paregoric) in the past were the favorites of many physicians.

Codeine has also been used on many occasions for the treatment of functional diarrhea. It is effective and considerably cheaper than diphenoxylate or loperamide. The constipating action of codeine is obvious to anyone who has taken the drug for the relief of pain. Thirty milligrams of codeine three times daily will cement the bowels of most mortals.

Diphenoxylate (Lomotil) is a popularly prescribed narcotic for the treatment of diarrhea. It is less well absorbed than codeine but is still capable of producing systemic effects. Many nurses and mothers have come to depend on this drug for the treatment of diarrhea and colic in children. Lomotil is formulated in a palatable cherry-flavored liquid containing 2.5 mg of diphenoxylate per 5 mL.

Loperamide (Imodium) is a very popular antidiarrheal narcotic. It is very poorly absorbed and has few systemic effects. Loperamide is more potent and longer-acting than diphenoxylate.

Nurses should caution parents to keep narcotics away from children because accidental poisoning has often occurred. With the exception of loperamide, narcotics can produce nausea, sedation and dizziness. The nursing process for these drugs is discussed in detail in Chapter 23.

Drug Treatment of Constipation

A **cathartic** is an agent that causes the evacuation of the bowels. A **laxative** can also be defined this way, but is usually considered to be milder in action than a cathartic. In this book, the terms laxative and cathartic will be used interchangeably. Regardless of the name used, these drugs are often abused. Many in our society equate purging with purifying. In the U.S. alone, over $100 million per year is spent on laxatives, and much of this money is wasted. At least one study has shown that most patients, previously taking laxatives daily, continued to be "regular fellows" when switched to identical-looking placebos.

The above statements notwithstanding, laxatives do have a small place in health care. First, however, it must be emphasized that all laxatives are contraindicated in patients with cramps, colic, nausea, vomiting, fever or undiagnosed abdominal pain. Also, since some laxatives can be shared by a nursing mother with her infant, nurses should teach lactating mothers to use diet and exercise as well as other nondrug remedies to prevent constipation or to treat it. The role of laxatives in the treatment of functional constipation is always secondary to a fiber-rich diet and other nondrug procedures. Laxatives may be indicated for the maintenance of soft feces, to prevent straining, especially in patients with cardiovascular problems or anorectal disorders. They can also be used to evacuate the bowels prior to diagnostic procedures or surgery.

Laxatives act by (1) retaining water in the intestine, thereby liquefying the feces (bulk laxatives and osmotic laxatives), (2) softening the stools to facilitate their evacuation (stool softeners) or (3) irritating the colon to increase peristalsis (chemical stimulants). Although we may not agree with much of the use of laxatives, it is essential to review how they produce their effects.

Bulk Laxatives

Bran

Bran has been known as a laxative for at least 2500 years. Found in cereals such as All-Bran and Fine Bran, bran mixes with food where its hydrophilic action enables it to retain water in the intestine and increase stool volume. A major disadvantage to the use of bran is its taste. Many users claim that it tastes like a mixture of sawdust and cardboard. This can make it difficult for the constipated patient to ingest sufficient quantities of bran for it to work. About 20 g of bran daily are required; this can be obtained from two to three heaping tablespoonsful of Fine Bran or All-Bran, respectively. If the patient prefers, bran alone may be purchased and incorporated into other foods.

Psyllium

Psyllium is obtained from the seed coat of an Indian plant. It is found in several products including Metamucil, Hydrocil, Effersyllium and Serutan. Psyllium has the capacity to hold water in the intestinal lumen and swell to many times its original volume. Given in a dose of 2 – 6 g three times daily, psyllium may soften hard stools. The drug is best taken in juice at mealtimes and accompanied by an additional 200 mL (8 oz.) of water.

Agar and Karaya

The gums agar and karaya attract water. They are incorporated in several laxative products. Many patients feel that they have derived benefit from products containing these substances. Nurses should evaluate patients receiving karaya for allergic reactions such as urticaria, rhinitis, dermatitis and asthma.

Osmotic Laxatives

Osmotic laxatives are not well absorbed from the intestinal tract. As a result of the osmotic pressure created by the nonabsorbed solute, water is also retained in the intestinal lumen. The increased volume of water liquefies developing feces and promotes easy defecation.

Magnesium Sulfate and Magnesium Hydroxide

The expression "a dose of salts" was common many years ago. The introduction and extensive marketing of newer laxatives has reduced both the use of this expression and the drugs to which it referred. Saline laxatives are poorly absorbed from the gastrointestinal tract and retain water in the intestine by their osmotic action.

Magnesium sulfate (Epsom salts) is commonly used, in spite of the fact that it has a bitter, unpleasant taste. When taken in 5 – 15 g quantities it produces a semifluid cartharsis within three hours. Low doses of magnesium hydroxide (Milk of Magnesia) neutralize stomach acid. Larger amounts produce catharsis. It is important for the user to understand this dose-dependent response. Otherwise, the overzealous use of magnesium hydroxide by the patient seeking antacid relief may yield an entirely unexpected effect with a well-defined endpoint. If absorbed, magnesium is eliminated from the body by renal excretion. Although the absorption of magnesium from these salts is not more than 25% of the dose, they should not be administered to patients with renal impairment because the concentration of magnesium can climb into the toxic range (see Chapter 18).

Lactulose (Cephalac, Chronulac)

Lactulose is a disaccharide, composed of galactose and fructose. It is not hydrolyzed in the small intestine and therefore not absorbed. The osmotic pressure caused by the retention of lactulose in the intestinal lumen results in the retention of water and electrolytes.

Prior to administration, nursing assessment of the patient should be undertaken to establish any previous history of diabetes or the presence of an existing pregnancy. In both cases, lactulose administration is contraindicated.

Although lactulose may be effective in relieving constipation, quantities up to 8 g daily may be required. Some patients find these quantities difficult to take because the drug has a sweet, syrupy taste. For this reason administration often includes diluting the drug in water or other juices, given with the patient's dessert at meal time.

Lactulose is also marketed under the trade name of Cephalac. This product provides symptomatic improvement and some normalization of the electroencephalogram in about three-fourths of patients with portal systemic encephalopathy associated with chronic liver disease. Concentrations of ammonia in the blood are reduced by 25 – 50 % because of the ability of lactulose to reduce the absorption of ammonia and possibly other toxic amines from the intestinal tract.

Stool Softeners

Mineral Oil

The very name stool softeners conjures up an image of their mechanism of action. Obviously soft stools are easier for those tender tissues down below to clear than hard stools. The oldest stool softener in use is mineral oil. This substance is also marketed as liquid petrolateum or liquid paraffin. It is used to lubricate stools, for stools, like pistons, run easier and faster when they are oiled.

In spite of its place in history, mineral oil is not a good laxative. It may slither into the lungs and produce acute pneumonitis, chronic diffuse pneumonitis or localized granulomas. This is more prevalent in the young and elderly who take the product chronically. Mineral oil will also block absorption of the fat-soluble vitamins A, D, E and K. Finally, oil may leak through the anal sphincter. In addition to being unpleasant itself, the leakage of oil can cause pruritus. The primary nursing responsibility related to the use of mineral oil is patient teaching to inform the patient of these adverse effects.

Dioctyl Sodium Sulfosuccinate, Docusate Sodium (Colace)

Docusate is a detergent and although it is tempting to state that it cleans patients out, we will not yield to the impulse. It is incorporated into too many products for all to be listed here. Probably the most commonly used is Colace; the one with the most intriguing name is Afko-Lube. Other common trade names include Comofax and Modane Soft. Docusate is claimed to soften the stool by the accumulation of water in the intestine. It can disrupt the gastric mucosal barrier and is best reserved for situations in which a stool softener is required for a short period. Implications for nursing actions are summarized in Table 35 at the end of this chapter.

Chemical Stimulants

Chemical stimulants are taken for the purpose of irritating the intestine and thereby increasing its motility. Once irritated, the intestine can be a difficult beast to tame. Many a sorry soul has taken a drug in this category only to wish later that he could restrain the tiger in his tank. After all, enough is enough. All chemical stimulants produce griping, increased mucus secretion, and in some people, excessive evacuation of fluid.

Phenolphthalein

Phenolphthalein is the active ingredient in many products, including such household remedies as Ex-Lax, Feen-A-Mint and Phenolax. The drug produces its irritant effect on the colon. As a result, a period of several hours is required before the effects of phenolphthalein are seen. For this reason, it is best taken at night before retiring.

Bisacodyl (Dulcolax, Theralax)

Bisacodyl is similar to phenolphthalein in its effects on the colon. It is given orally or rectally. In the colon it initiates repetitive peristalsis. A soft, formed stool is usually produced six to ten hours after oral administration and fifteen to sixty minutes after insertion in the rectum. The usual oral dose should be administered from an airtight container that has been stored in a cool place (at temperatures below 30°C or 86°F). Patient teaching should include instructions to swallow the tablets whole. Chewing destroys the enteric coating and results in gastric irritation. Taking the tablets within one hour of ingesting either milk or an antacid may also destroy the enteric coating and produce gastric irritation.

Castor Oil

Castor oil — the very name used to strike fear in the hearts of many youngsters. Untold numbers of children grew to adulthood in spite of a weekly purgation with castor oil. Derived from the naturally occurring *Ricinus communis* seed and containing the active ingredient ricinoleic acid, castor oil acts on the small intestine. It is usually prescribed only when prompt, thorough evacuation of the bowel is desired. Castor oil will produce abdominal cramps and loose bowel movements within two hours. It is usually administered on an empty stomach. Castor oil is not given during pregnancy because it has been associated with the onset of labor. Possessing an unpleasant taste, castor oil can be made more palatable if it is offered in a large glass to which is added 125 mL (4 - 5 oz.) of citrus juice and 2 mL (1/2 teaspoon) of baking soda. This mixture is stirred rapidly and consumed quickly.

Nursing Process

The nursing process in relation to the use of laxatives by patients must consider the action of the specific laxative prescribed in order to administer it at the least disruptive time for the patient. For example, magnesium sulfate, which acts in two to three hours, would not be administered at bedtime; however, bisacodyl (Dulcolax, Theralax), which requires six to eight hours to work, is best administered at bedtime so that it will have its effect early in the morning and not disrupt daily activities. Nursing evaluation of patients taking laxatives should always include the frequency of bowel movements and characteristics of the fecal material. Nurses are advised to follow the norms for individual bowel patterns as described in this chapter and medicate for constipation *only* as necessary, not by institutional routine.

Nurses deal with constipation frequently in their clinical practice. There are many causes of constipation. Constipation is a common adverse effect of narcotic and nonsterioidal anti-inflammatory drugs. The following nursing process is suggested for the nursing diagnosis.

Nursing Process Related to Drug Effects on Bowel Function

Assessment
Nursing assessment should include an investigation to obtain baseline data for normal bowel, dietary and fluid patterns before initiation of therapy. Chronic use of medications, laxatives and enemas

needs investigation. Include an assessment of what dietary measures have been successful to relieve constipation in the past. Changes in meal routines, immobility, emotional disturbances and lack of privacy should also be investigated. Assess changes in physical activity and exercise routines before and during drug therapy.

Administration

Establish a regular bowel evacuation program with the patient, based on his or her individual patterns and needs. Administer appropriate laxative, stool softener or bowel evacuation procedure as necessary, following consultation with patient, pharmacist and physician.

Evauation

Evaluate frequency of bowel elimination, characteristics of stools, blood in stools, presence of straining, pain, abdominal distention, palpable mass, rectal pressure and appetite impairment. Monitor effects of medications and/or evacuation treatment to reach the established goal of a regular bowel program.

Teaching

Provide instruction for appropriate use of bulk in the diet, adequate daily fluid intake and appropriate level of exercise for age and physical condition. Emphasize the need to recognize stimulus behaviors such as warm fluids and the importance of immediate response to the urge to defecate. For the hospitalized patient, provide privacy and effective positioning with adequate support (elevation of feet on footstool as necessary). Long-term instruction should include exercises to strengthen abdominal muscles, plans for carrying out dietary regimen, exercise and other lifestyle changes to establish a continuing evacuation plan.

Further Reading

Curry, Clarence E., Jr. (1982). "Laxative Products." *Handbook of Nonprescription Drugs, 7th ed.*, pp. 69-72. Washington: American Pharmaceutical Association.

Longe, R. Leon (1982). "Antidiarrheal and Other Gastrointestinal Products." *Handbook of Nonprescription Drugs, 7th ed.*, pp. 53-67. Washington: American Pharmaceutical Association.

Kronborg, I.J. and Howard, A. (1981). Diarrhea: Causes and specific treatment. *Drugs 21* :62-68.

Thompson, W.G. (1979). *The Irritable Gut: Functional Disorders of the Alimentary Canal.* University Park Press.

Thompson, W.G. (1980). Laxatives: Clinical pharmacology and rational use. *Drugs 19* :49-58.

Travelers' diarrhea (1979). *Medical Letter 21* :41-43.

Table 35
Laxatives and antidiarrheal drugs.

Generic Name (Trade Name)	Use (Dose)	Action	Adverse Effects	Drug Interactions	Nursing Process
Pharmacologic Classification: Antidiarrheal Drugs					
Psyllium (Hydrocil, Metamucil)	Relief of chronic, atonic, spastic and rectal constipat'n. May also be used to treat diarrhea (**Oral:** 7 g mixed with glass of water or other suitable fluid 1-3x/day. Second glass of water enhances drug's effects)	Absorbs water from developing feces in intestine to form gel, thereby reducing possibility of watery diarrhea. Also absorbs bile salts. This may be important for its antidiarrheal action.			**Assess:** For severe abdominal pain, intestinal obstruct'n, no. and characteristics of stools. **Administer:** Mixed w. 200 mL (8 oz.) fluid. **Teach:** Record no. and characteristics of stools.
Kaolin-pectin mixture (Kaopectate)	Simple diarrhea (**Oral:** *After each movement* - Adults - 60-120 mL. Children - over 12 years - 60 mL; 6-12 years - 30-60 mL; 3-6 years -15-30 mL; under 3 years - 5 mL or more prn)	Uncertain; poss. due to its ability to bind intestinal contents; might possess an astringent quality.		**Digitalis glycosides:** Undergo reduced absorp't'n in presence of kaolin-pectin preparat'ns.	
Bismuth subsalicylate (Pepto-Bismol)	Tx of diarrhea (**Oral:** *Suspension* - Adults - 30 mL; children -10-14 years - 20 mL; 6-10 years - 10 mL; 3-6 years -5 mL; repeat every half-hour to one hour prn to 7-8 doses. *Tablets* - Adults - 2 tablets; children -10-14 years - 1 tablet; 6-10 years - 2/3 tablet; 3-6 years - 1/3 tablet; repeat q30 min, not to exceed 8 doses)	Mechanism of action poorly understood.	High doses may produce salicylate toxicity.	**Anticoagulants, oral; ASA and other salicylates; hypoglycemics, oral:** Activities may incr. in presence of bismuth subsalicylate because latter can displace them from plasma proteins. **Uricosurics:** May have reduced activity in presence of bismuth subsalicylate because latter can decr. tubular secret'n of uricosurics.	**Assess:** For hx of arthritis treated w. aspirin or other NSAIDs; use of oral anticoagulants, uricosurics.
Diphenoxylate (Lomotil)	As an adjunct in management of diarrhea (**Oral:** Adults - initially, 5 mg tid or qid. Max. dose, 20 mg/24 h in divided doses. Lower dosage as soon as initial	Narcotics decr. propulsive motility of colon.	Nausea, drowsiness, coma, lethargy, sedat'n, respiratory depress'n, dizziness, vomiting, anorexia,	**Barbiturates, benzodiazepines, ethanol and other CNS depressants:** May have their actions potentiated by diphenoxylate.	**Assess:** For bacterial bowel infect'ns, antibiotic-induced colitis, hx of liver disease. **Evaluate:** For abdominal distent'n; for CNS depress'n in pts also receiving

Generic Name (Trade Name)	Use (Dose)	Action	Adverse Effects	Drug Interactions	Nursing Process
	control of symptoms is achieved. Maint. dose may be as low as 25% of dose required for initial control. Children - 300-400 μg/kg/day in divided doses)		pruritus, skin erupt'ns, giant urticaria, angioneurotic edema, restlessness, insomnia, abdominal bloating and cramps, paralytic ileus, toxic megacolon, numbness of extremities, headache, blurring of vision, gum swelling, euphoria, depress'n, general malaise	**MAOIs:** Tog. w. diphenoxylate, may precipitate hypertensive crisis.	barbiturates; for impending coma in pts w. liver disease; no. and characteristics of stools. **Teach:** Nec. for recommended dosage; evaluat'n of drug effectiveness; adv. effects; keep out of reach of children.
Loperamide (Imodium)	For symptomatic control of acute and chronic diarrhea and intestinal transit time in pts w. ileostomies, colostomies and other intestinal resect'ns **(Oral:** Adults - initially, 4 mg followed by 2 mg after each unformed stool. Max. dose, 16 mg/day for 10 days)	As for diphenoxylate	Constipat'n		As for diphenoxylate

Pharmacologic Classification: Laxative

Generic Name (Trade Name)	Use (Dose)	Action	Adverse Effects	Drug Interactions	Nursing Process
Magnesium sulfate (Epsom salts)	Constipat'n **(Oral:** Adults - 5-15 g prn)	Poorly absorbed in intestine; incr. water level because of osmotic gradient. Stim. peristalsis by incr. bulk.	Dehydrat'n; Mg toxicity. See Chapter 18, Table 22.		**Administer:** Dissolved in ice water or juice.
Magnesium hydroxide (Milk of Magnesia)	Constipat'n **(Oral:** Adults - 15-30 mL prn)	As for magnesium sulfate	As for magnesium sulfate		
Mineral oil	Constipat'n **(Oral:** Adults - 15-45 mL daily)	Penetrates and softens fecal material.	Aspirat'n may produce acute pneumonitis, chronic diffuse pneumonitis, localized granulomas; blocks absorpt'n of vitamins; pruritus.		**Evaluate:** For adv. effects; frequency and characteristics of stools.

Drug	Uses/Dosage	Action	Side effects	Interactions	Nursing considerations
Lactulose (Chronuluc)	Constipat'n (**Oral:** Adults - 10-40 g daily prn)	Nonabsorbed disaccharide; results in retent'n of water and electrolytes in intestine.			**Assess:** Hx for evidence of diabetes or pregnancy. **Evaluate:** Diluted w. water or other fluids, or w. dessert.
Docusate sodium; dioctyl sodium sulfosuccinate (Colace)	Management of constipat'n due to hard stools (**Oral:** Adults and children over 12 years - 100-200 mg; children - 6-12 years - 40-120 mg; 36 years - 20-60 mg; 0-3 years - 10-40 mg. **Retent'n enema:** 5 mL of drops and 90 mL of edema fluid. **Flushing enema:** 1 mL of drops and 100 mL enema fluid)	Softens stools by accumulat'n of water in intestine.	Rarely, can enhance absorpt'n of orally administered drugs.	**Mineral oil:** Absorpt'n and hepatotoxicity may incr. w. concomitant administrat'n of docusate.	**Administer:** Oral solut'ns mixed w. milk or juice. **Evaluate:** Frequency and characteristics of stools.
Phenolphthalein (Ex-Lax, Feen-A-Mint, Phenolax)	Constipat'n (**Oral:** Adults - 60 mg; children - 15-30 mg)	Local irritat'n of intestines and incr. intestinal motility.	Gripping; incr. mucus secret'n; excess. evacuat'n of fluids resulting in electrolyte deficiency; allergic react'ns		**Evaluate:** Frequency and characteristics of stools. **Teach:** Might cause alkaline urine or stools to turn red; oral dose might produce effects over several days.
Bisacodyl (Dulcolax, Theralax)	Acute or chronic constipat'n (**Oral:** Adults - 10-15 mg hs or before breakfast. *Protoscopic, radiographic or preoperative preparat'n* - 10-15 mg evening before and 10-mg suppository, or 1 μenema, 1-2h before procedure. Children - > 6 years - 10-mg suppository or 1 μenema, or 5-10 mg orally. Infants and children under 6 years - 5-mg suppository or 1/2 μenema)	As for phenolphthalein	Mild cramping; mild irritat'n of rectum after using suppository for several weeks.		**Administer:** From airtight container, stored in cool place. **Teach:** To swallow tablets without chewing; that taking w. milk or antacid might cause gastric irritat'n.

CHAPTER 25

Antinauseant and Antiemetic Drugs

Teaching Objectives

Following completion of this chapter, the reader should be able to:

1. List the types of drugs used to reduce nausea and vomiting.
2. Discuss the mechanism of action, pharmacologic effects, therapeutic uses and adverse effects of scopolamine in the treatment of nausea and vomiting and the nursing process related to its use.
3. Describe the pharmacologic effects, therapeutic uses and adverse effects of antihistamines used in the treatment of nausea and vomiting and the nursing process related to their use.
4. Discuss the mechanism of action, pharmacologic effects, therapeutic uses and adverse effects of phenothiazines and haloperidol in the treatment of nausea and vomiting and describe the nursing process related to their use.
5. Describe the mechanism of action, pharmacologic effects, therapeutic uses and adverse effects of metoclopramide and domperidone in the treatment of nausea and vomiting and describe the nursing process related to their use.
6. Discuss the mechanism of action, pharmacologic effects, therapeutic uses, adverse effects and nursing process for cisapride.
7. Describe the mechanism of action, pharmacologic effects, therapeutic uses and adverse effects of trimethobenzamide and the nursing process related to its use.

Nausea, Vomiting and Motion Sickness

This chapter reviews the treatment of nausea, vomiting and motion sickness. Drugs used to treat these conditions may be classified as (1) anticholinergics, (2) antihistamines, (3) antidopaminergics and (4) miscellaneous drugs. For the first three groups, only their use to reduce nausea, vomiting or motion sickness will be discussed. The detailed pharmacology of these agents can be found in Chapters 6, 35 and 44, respectively.

Anticholinergic Drugs

Mechanism of Action and Pharmacologic Effects

Anticholinergic drugs block competitively muscarinic receptors throughout the body (Chapter 6). They also reduce the excitability of the labyrinth receptors, depressing conduction in vestibular pathways or preventing recruitment of impulses at the chemoreceptor trigger zone. Stimulation of the chemoreceptor trigger zone in the brain activates the vomiting center. Drugs, such as anticholinergics, that reduce the sensitivity of the chemoreceptor trigger zone are often effective in the treatment of nausea and vomiting.

Therapeutic Uses

Scopolamine (hyoscine) is the anticholinergic used most frequently. Its value as an antinauseant is counterbalanced by its adverse effects resulting from a generalized cholinergic block. The introduction of the transdermal therapeutic system (Transderm-SCOP, Transderm-V) has been a significant advance. These flat circular units continuously release scopolamine over thirty-six to forty-eight hours. Applying one disc behind the ear often provides effective protection of nausea and vomiting associated with motion sickness, without undue systemic adverse effects. An anticholinergic should not be used by persons suffering from glaucoma or when it causes pressure pain behind the eye.

Adverse Effects

Dryness of the mouth, cycloplegia and drowsiness are the most common adverse effects of scopolamine. They are experienced less frequently if the transdermal delivery system is used. Infrequently, patients may experience disorientation, memory disturbances, restlessness, giddiness, hallucinations and confusion when scopolamine is administered systemically. Because of the central nervous sytem depression that scopolamine can produce, patients should be cautioned about engaging in activities that require mental alertness, such as driving a car or operating dangerous machinery.

Nursing Process

The nursing process related to the use of anticholinergic medications is discussed in detail in Chapter 6. Readers are advised to review that content.

Antihistamines

Mechanism of Action and Pharmacologic Effects

Several antihistamines are used to prevent vertigo, motion sickness and the nausea of pregnancy. These include cyclizine (Marezine, Marzine), dimenhydrinate (Dramamine, Gravol), hydroxyzine (Atarax, Orgatrax, Vistaril), meclizine (Antivert, Bonamine, Bonine) and promethazine (Phenergan, Remsed). Their mechanism of action is not completely understood. They may affect neural pathways originating in the labyrinth.

Therapeutic Uses

The therapeutic indications differ slightly from product to product, but all are indicated for the prevention and relief of the nausea or vomiting of motion sickness. The drugs are also recommended for the treatment of vertigo. With the exception of hydroxyzine, all antihistamines are effective in treating the nausea of pregnancy. However, antiemetics are generally not recommended during pregnancy. Hydroxyzine and promethazine are indicated for the treatment of postoperative emesis. Finally, dimenhydrinate, meclizine and promethazine may be used in the treatment or prophylaxis of the nausea and vomiting of radiation sickness.

Adverse Effects

Drowsiness is the most common adverse effect of antihistamines. Dizziness may also occur. All antihistamines possess appreciable anticholinergic activity. Patients may experience dry mouth, nose and throat; blurred vision; difficult or painful urination; thickening of bronchial secretion; and tachycardia. Depending on the drug used, patients may also complain of headache, loss of appetite, nervousness, restlessness, skin rash, upset stomach or stomach pain, excitement and nausea.

Nursing Process

Antihistamines are discussed in Chapter 35. Readers are advised to refer to that chapter for details related to the nursing process associated with their use.

Antidopaminergic Drugs

Antipsychotic Drugs

Mechanism of Action and Pharmacologic Effects

Dopamine is the neurotransmitter in the chemoreceptor trigger zone. By blocking dopamine receptors, phenothiazines and haloperidol (Haldol) reduce nausea or vomiting, or both. Only thioridazine (Mellaril), of the commonly used phenothiazines, appears devoid of antinauseant activity. These drugs also block dopaminergic and alpha$_1$ receptors throughout the body, accounting for many of the peripheral effects (see Chapters 4 and 44).

Therapeutic Uses

Dopaminergic blocking drugs reduce the sensitivity of the chemoreceptor trigger zone to numerous emetic stimuli, such as antineoplastics, radiation, uremia, estrogens, tetracyclines and narcotics. They do not appear to be effective in controlling motion sickness or treating vertigo. The contraindications to their use are described in Chapter 44.

Adverse Effects

The adverse effects of phenothiazines and haloperidol are discussed in detail in Chapter 44. Drowsiness is the most common adverse reaction when these drugs are used as antinauseants. Other commonly encountered effects are orthostatic hypotension, dryness of the mouth and nasal congestion. Extrapyramidal reactions resulting from inhibition of dopaminergic receptors in the basal ganglia are well-recognized adverse effects of phenothiazines and haloperidol. The drugs are also capable of producing cholestatic jaundice, granulocytopenia, urticaria, dermatitis, thrombocytopenia, leukopenia, agranulocytosis, purpura, pancytopenia, gastroenteritis, photosensitivity, galactorrhea and edema of the extremities.

Patients with a hypersensitivity to one phenothiazine should not be treated with any of these drugs. They are contraindicated in patients with bone marrow depression and in pregnant women with a history of pre-eclampsia. Care should be taken if the patient is already receiving another central nervous system depressant or antihypertensive agents.

Nursing Process

Antipsychotic drugs are discussed in Chapter 44. Readers are advised to consult that chapter for details related to the nursing process associated with their use.

Metoclopramide (Maxeran, Reglan) and Domperidone (Motilium)

Mechanism of Action and Pharmacologic Effects

Metoclopramide also has an antidopaminergic effect at the chemoreceptor trigger zone, but it also increases gastrointestinal motility. Metoclopramide increases the strength of contractions of the gastric antrum and speeds gastric emptying. It appears to relax the duodenal bulb and accelerate upper gastrointestinal tract transit, thereby alleviating gastric stasis. These actions explain the use of metoclopramide in the treatment of delayed gastric emptying and may also play a role in its antinauseant properties.

Domperidone is a peripheral dopamine antagonist. It has antiemetic activity similar to that of metoclopramide, although the incidence of extrapyramidal side effects is lower because domperidone does not readily cross the blood-brain barrier. The administration of domperidone increases lower esophageal sphincter pressure, the duration of antral and duodenal contractions, and the gastric emptying of liquids and semisolids.

Therapeutic Uses

Injectable metoclopramide may be used for the prevention of nausea and vomiting associated with the chemotherapy of malignancies. Domperidone is indicated in the symptomatic management of upper gastrointestinal motility disorders associated with chronic and subacute gastritis and diabetic gastroparesis. Domperidone may also be used to prevent gastrointestinal symptoms associated with the use of dopamine-agonist antiparkinsonian agents (see Chapter 52). Neither metoclopramide nor domperidone should be used whenever stimulation of gastrointestinal motility might be dangerous, e.g., in the presence of gastrointestinal hemorrhage, mechanical obstruction or perforation.

Adverse Effects

Drowsiness, fatigue and lassitude occur in about ten per cent of patients receiving metoclopramide. Less frequent adverse reactions are insomnia, headache, dizziness and bowel disturbances. Parkinsonism or extrapyramidal symptoms, or both, have been reported in about one per cent of patients.

The overall incidence of side effects with domperidone was less than seven per cent. The more serious or troublesome side effects (galactorrhea, gynecomastia, menstrual irregularities) are dose-related and gradually resolve after lowering the dose or discontinuing therapy.

Nursing Process

Assessment
Nursing assessment related to the use of either metoclopramide or domperidone should begin with a review of the patient's history for documentation of seizure disorders or a current pregnancy. In the presence of such documentation, these medications should be withheld pending consultation with the physician. In consultation with the pharmacist, the

current drug regimen should be reviewed for concurrent use of drugs causing extrapyramidal symptoms. A patient history of congestive heart failure, hypokalemia, kidney disease or gastrointestinal hemorrhage should signal particularly attentive monitoring following administration of either drug. Because domperidone is a newer agent, nurses are advised to check with the pharmacist when giving this drug for current drug information and for the manufacturer's literature enclosed with the product.

Administration

Administer these drugs one-half hour before meals and at bedtime from a light-resistant container that has been stored at room temperature. Consult with the pharmacist before mixing other injectable solutions in the same syringe. Solutions added to intravenous infusions should be protected from light by wrapping the solution bag in aluminum foil or enclosing in a brown paper bag. Unused portions of ampules should be discarded immediately.

Evaluation

Patients should be evaluated for extrapyramidal symptoms such as restlessness, involuntary movements, facial grimacing, rigidity or tremors. Drug effectiveness is determined by absence of vomiting and by patients' subjective reports of relief of anorexia or nausea. Monitor patients carefully for evidence of sodium retention and hypokalemia.

Teaching

Patients should be cautioned to avoid driving and the use of power tools because of the possiblity of extrapyramidal effects. Recommend the use of gum, hard candy or frequent rinsing of mouth to relieve dryness.

Miscellaneous Drugs

Cisapride (Prepulsid)

Mechanism of Action and Pharmacologic Effects

The inclusion of cisapride in this chapter is open to criticism because cisapride is not indicated in the treatment of nausea. However, the similarity of cisapride to metoclopromide and domperidone dictates that here is the most appropriate place to present this interesting compound.

Cisapride is a gastrokinetic drug whose activity is considered to be due to enhancement of the physiological release of acetylcholine at the myenteric plexus. The drug increases esophageal peristaltic activity and lowers esophageal sphincter tone, thereby decreasing reflux of gastric contents into the esophagus and improving esophageal clearance. Gastric and duodenal emptying are also enhanced by cisapride as a consequence of increased gastric and duodenal contractility and antroduodenal coordination. Cisapride decreases duodenogastric reflux. The drug also enhances intestinal propulsive activity and improves both small and large bowel transit. Cisapride is free of dopamine receptor blocking activity. Because it is not a cholinomimetic, cisapride does not increase basal or pentagastrin induced gastric acid secretion.

Therapeutic Uses

Cisapride is indicated in the symptomatic management of gastrointestinal motility disorders, including gastroesophageal reflux disease; gastroparesis, idiopathic or associated with diabetic neuropathy; and intestinal pseudo-obstruction. Like metoclopramide and domperidone, cisapride is contraindicated whenever gastrointestinal stimulation might be dangerous.

Adverse Effects

The most frequent adverse effects of cisapride involve the gastrointestinal tract — diarrhea and abdominal discomfort. Most adverse effects are transient and rarely necessitate discontinuation of therapy.

Nursing Process

Assessment

Before administering this drug, review the patient history for gastrointestinal bleeding, hepatic or renal insufficiency or a current drug regimen of anticoagulants. Drug therapy is not advised with pregnancy and lactation.

Administration

Cisapride should be stored at room temperature and protected from moisture and light.

Evaluation

Following administration of cisapride, nurses should monitor blood levels of the drug, particularl in elderly patients because levels tend to be higher than in younger persons.

Teaching

Caution the patient about the increased sedative effect of medication when cisapride is taken with tranquillizers or alcohol.

Trimethobenzamide HCl (Tigan)

Trimethobenzamide depresses the chemoreceptor trigger zone. It has been promoted for alleviating nausea and reducing the frequency of vomiting in the immediate postoperative period, in radiation sickness and in gastroenteritis. It is not as effective as phenothiazines postoperatively. Trimethobenzamide has little or no value in the prevention or treatment of vertigo, motion sickness or nausea and vomiting due to cancer chemotherapy.

Trimethobenzamide's adverse effects are infrequent and seldom require stopping the drug. They include hypersensitivity, drowsiness, blurring of vision, depression, headache, dizziness and jaundice.

Nursing Process

Assessment

Establish baseline measures of vital signs, particularly blood pressure. Check for evidence of existing viral condition, particularly in children and adolescents.

Administration

Administer with water or fluid. The capsule may be emptied and mixed with food or fluid if necessary. Intramuscular injections should be given deep in the upper outer quadrant of the buttock or in the ventrolateral gluteal site.

Evaluation

Monitor surgical patients carefully for hypotension when they are receiving this medication parenterally. Be alert for rash or other evidence of allergic hypersensitivity. There is a suspicion that the use of this medication in children with viral diseases is associated with Reyes' syndrome. Discontinue trimethobenzamide immediately and summon the physician at once if the early signs of Reyes' syndrome develop in children — specifically, persistent vomiting, hyperpnea, lethargy, confusion, disorientation or irrational behaviour, convulsions, unconsciouness.

Teaching

Patient teaching should emphasize the avoidance of driving or operating power tools because of the risk of dizziness or drowsiness. Patients should be advised to contact the physician immediately if adverse effects occur, especially those associated with hypersensitivity or Reyes' syndrome. Patients should be told that this medication is incompatible with alcohol.

Further Reading

Barbezat, G.O. (1981). The vomiting patient: A rational approach. *Drugs 22* :246-253.

Chemotherapy-induced emesis. Focus on metoclopramide (1983). *Drugs 25* (Suppl. 1):1-88.

"Drugs Used in Vertigo, Motion Sickness and Vomiting." (1986). *AMA Drug Evaluations*, 6th ed.

Table 36
Antinauseant and antiemetic drugs.

Generic Name (Trade Name)	Use (Dose)	Action	Adverse Effects	Drug Interactions	Nursing Process
Pharmacologic Classification: Anticholinergic Drug					
Scopolamine, hyoscine	Prevent'n and tx of motion sickness (**SC:** Adults - 0.6 mg initially, followed by 0.3 mg q6h. Children - 0.006 mg/kg)	Reduces excitability of labyrinth receptors, depressing conduct'n in vestibular pathways or preventing recruitment of impulses at chemoreceptor trigger zone.	Xerostomia, flushing, bradycardia, mydriasis, blurred vision, urinary retent'n, tachypnea, scarlatinoform rash, delirium, fever, stupor, coma, respiratory failure, death	**Methotrimeprazine:** Plus scopolamine, has been reported to produce extrapyramidal symptoms. Anticholinergics should be administered w. caution in pts receiving methotrimeprazine.	**Assess:** Hx glaucoma, hypertens'n, coronary artery disease, chronic GI condit'ns, asthma, pulmonary disease. **Administer:** From light-resistant container. **Evaluate:** Drug efficacy by absence of vomiting.
Transdermal scopolamine (Transderm-SCOP, Transderm-V)	As for scopolamine (**Transdermal patches containing 1.5 mg scopolamine:** Adults - Apply 1 disc to postauricular skin approx. 12 h before antiemetic effect is required)	As for scopolamine	As for scopolamine		As for scopolamine
Pharmacologic Classification: Antihistamines					
Cyclizine (Marezine, Marzine)	Prophylaxis and tx of motion sickness, radiat'n sickness, vertigo; nausea and vomiting assoc. w. childhood diseases; drug-induced vomiting (**IM:** *Postoperative vomiting* - Adults - 50 mg 15-30 min before end of operat'n; repeat tid prn. Children - *up to 6 years* - 25% adult dose; *6-10 years* - 50% adult dose. **Oral:** *Motion sickness* - Adults - 50 mg 30 min before departure, then q4-6h prn [max. 200 mg daily]. Children - *6-10 years* - 3 mg/kg divided into 3 doses throughout 24-h period)	May affect neural pathways originating in labyrinth.	Large doses may cause drowsiness and dryness of mouth.	**CNS depressants:** Have additive depressant effects w. antihistamines. Pts should be cautioned against taking ethanol, hypnotics, sedatives, psychotherapeutic agents or other drugs w. CNS-depressant effects during antihistamine tx)	**Assess:** For current pregnancy; hx hypersensitivity; establish baseline BP. **Administer:** Orally w. food or milk; from light-resistant container stored at room temp.; aspirate IM inject'ns carefully. **Evaluate:** Postop. pts carefully for hypotens'n; drug efficacy by absence of vomiting. **Teach:** To avoid driving or using power tools; to beware of combining w. alcohol, barbiturates, narcotics or other CNS depressants.

Drug	Action/Indication/Dosage		Side Effects	Interactions	
Dimenhydrinate (Dramamine, Gravol)	Prevent'n and relief of motion sickness, nausea and vomiting of radiat'n sickness, postoperative vomiting, drug-induced nausea and vomiting; also for symptomatic tx of nausea, vomiting and vertigo of Meniere's disease and other labyrinth disturbances. (*Motion sickness* - **Oral:** Adults - 50-100 mg 30 min before departure, repeated q4h prn. **IM:** 50 mg q3-4h prn. **IV:** 50 mg in 10 mL NaCl inject'n over 2 min. Children - **Oral/IM:** 1-1.5 mg/kg q6h. Max. 300 mg/day)	As for cyclizine	Drowsiness; dizziness; dry mouth, nose, throat; blurred vision; dysuria; headache; nervousness, restlessness; skin rash; thickening of bronchial secret'ns; tachycardia; upset stomach	*As for cyclizine, plus:* **MAOIs:** May prolong and intensify antimuscarinic effects of dimenhydrinate.	As for cyclizine
Meclizine (Antivert, Bonamine, Bonine)	Control of nausea, vomiting and vertigo due to motion sickness, pregnancy, radiat'n, Meniere's syndrome, labyrinthitis **(Oral:** *Motion sickness* - 25-50 mg od, 1 h prior to departure. *Labyrinth and vestibular disturbances* - 25-100 mg daily in divided doses, depending on clinical response. *Radiat'n sickness* - 50 mg 2-12 h prior to radiat'n tx)	As for cyclizine	As for dimenhydrinate	As for dimenhydrinate	As for cyclizine
Promethazine (Phenergan, Remsed)	Antiemetic in control of nausea and vomiting of varied etiology (*Motion sickness* - Adults - **Oral/rectal:** 25 mg bid, 30 min - 1 h before departure. Children - **Oral/rectal:** 12.5-25 mg bid. *Nausea and vomiting* - Adults - **IM/rectal:** Initially, 25 mg, then 12.5-25 mg prn q4-6h. Children under 12 years - **IM/rectal:** Adjust dose on basis of age, weight of pt and severity of condit'n. Administer no more than 50% adult dose)	As for cyclizine	As for dimenhydrinate and cyclizine	As for cyclizine	As for cyclizine

Pharmacologic Classification: Antidopaminergic Drugs — Antipsychotic Drugs

Generic Name (Trade Name)	Use (Dose)	Action	Adverse Effects	Drug Interactions	Nursing Process
Perphenazine (Trilafon)	Effective in nausea and vomiting caused by surgery, cytotoxic drugs, radiat'n and toxins (**Oral:** Adults - 2-4 mg q4-6h. **IM:** Adults - 5 mg; rarely, 10 mg)	Dopamine is a neurotransmitter in the chemoreceptor trigger zone of the brain. By blocking dopamine receptors, perphenazine reduces nausea and vomiting. Also blocks dopaminergic and alpha receptors throughout body, accounting for many of the peripheral effects.	When used as antinauseant, most common adv. effect is drowsiness. For others commonly encountered, see Table ??	*See Table 65, plus:* **Antacids:** May inhibit absorpt'n of antidopaminergics. **Anticholinergics:** May decr. absorpt'n of antidopaminergics. **Antihypertensives:** May produce a greater fall in BP if given concomitantly w. an antipsychotic drug. **CNS depressants:** Such as general anesthetics, opiates, barbiturates, alcohol and benzodiazepines, will have additive brain depressant effects if combined w. an antipsychotic. **Levodopa:** Will have its effects reduced by concomitant use of an antipsychotic because latter blocks dopamine receptors in brain.	**Assess:** Pt hx and drug regimen for contraindicat'ns. **Administer:** *Oral* - 1 h before or after antacids or antidiarrheals; extended-release tablets should be swallowed whole; dilute oral concentrate in water, orange juice, milk or carbonated soft drinks. *IM* - Deep in gluteal muscle. Keep pt supine for 1 h. **Evaluate:** BP for hypotens'n; for extrapyramidal effects (restlessness, weakness of extremities, involuntary movements, facial grimacing, muscle rigidity or tremors), tardive dyskinesia in elderly females, jaundice, sudden rise in temp. **Teach:** To avoid sunlight, OTC drugs, driving or use of power tools; to take only prescribed am't; that urine may turn reddish-brown.
Prochlorperazine (Compazine, Stemetil)	As for perphenazine (**Oral:** Adults - 5-10 mg tid or qid. Children - 9-14 kg - 2.5 mg q12-24h; 14-18 kg - 2.5 mg q8-12h; 18-39 kg - 2.5 mg q8h or 5 mg q12h. **IM:** Adults - 5-10 mg q3-4h. Max. 40 mg/day. Children - over 10 kg - 0.13 mg/kg once. **Rectal:** Adults - 25 mg bid. Children - 9-14 kg - 2.5 mg q12-24h; 14-18 kg - 2.5 mg q8-12h; 18-39 kg - 2.5 mg q8h)	As for perphenazine	As for perphenazine	As for perphenazine	
Thiethylperazine (Torecan)	As for perphenazine (**Oral/Rectal/IM:** 10 mg od-tid)	As for perphenazine	As for perphenazine	As for perphenazine	As above
Haloperidol (Haldol)	As for perphenazine (**Oral/IM:** Adults - 1, 2 or 5 mg q12h prn)	As for perphenazine	As for perphenazine	As for perphenazine	As above

Pharmacologic Classification: Antidopaminergic Drugs — Metoclopramide, Domperidone

Metoclopramide (Maxeran, Reglan)	Prevent'n of nausea and vomiting assoc. w. chemotherapy of malignancies (*Alleviat'n of nausea and vomiting induced by moderately emetic cancer chemotherapeutic agents* - Adults - **IV:** 0.5-0.75 mg/kg diluted in 50 mL of a large-volume parenteral solut'n and infused slowly over a 15-min period 30 min prior to chemotherapy and at intervals of 2, 5 and 8 h after 1st dose. *For highly emetic regimens containing cisplatin* - Adults - **IV:** 2-3 mg/kg 30 min before chemotherapy, and then at 2- and 4-h intervals. *Delayed-onset nausea and vomiting caused by cisplatin* - Adults - **Oral:** 0.5 mg/kg qid for 6 days beginning 24 h after chemotherapy. *Delayed gastric emptying* - Adults - **Oral:** 5-10 mg tid or qid ac. **IM/IV** (slowly): 10 mg, repeated bid or tid prn. Children -5-14 years - **Oral:** 2.5-5 mg tid ac)	Claimed to depress chemoreceptor trigger zone, nuclei of vagal nerve, or reticular format'n in brain. These actions may account for antinauseant effects.	Drowsiness, fatigue and lassitude; occas'nally, agitat'n, irritability, constipat'n or diarrhea, urticarial maculopapular rash, dry mouth.	**Anticholinergics:** Antagonize metoclopramide's GI effects. **Cholinergics:** May incr. metoclopramide's effects. **CNS depressants:** May produce additive sedative effects w. metoclopramide. **Digoxin:** May have decr. absorpt'n in presence of metoclopramide. **Neuroleptics:** Have potentiated effects in presence of metoclopramide.	**Assess:** Hx for seizures, current pregnancy, CHF, kidney disease, GI bleeding, hypokalemia. **Administer:** 30 min ac and hs, from light-resistant container; store at room temp.; protect solut'ns diluted for IV infus'n from light w. aluminum foil or paper bag; discard unused port'ns of ampules. **Evaluate:** For extrapyramidal symptoms (see perphenazine, above); monitor for Na retent'n and hypokalemia. **Teach:** To avoid driving and use of power tools.
Domperidone (Motilium)	Symptomatic management of upper GI motility disorders assoc. w. chronic and subacute gastritis and diabetic gastroparesis (*Upper GI motility disorders* - Adults - **Oral:** 10 mg tid or qid, 15-30 min ac and hs prn. Up to 20 mg tid or qid for severe or resistant cases. *Nausea and vomiting assoc. w. dopamine agonists and antiparkinsonian agents* - Adults - **Oral:** Usually, 20 mg tid or qid)	Dopamine antagonist. Has antiemetic effects sim. to metoclopramide, w. lower incidence of extrapyramidal side effects because domperidone does not cross blood-brain barrier.	Overall incidence low. Most serious are galactorrhea, gynecomastia and menstrual irregularities.	**Antacids and H₂ blockers:** Should be avoided because absorpt'n of domperidone requires gastric acidity. **Anticholinergic drugs:** May compromise beneficial effects of domperidone. **MAOIs:** Should be administered w. care in pts taking domperidone.	**Administer:** When administering domperidone, nurses are advised to check w. pharmacist to obtain current informat'n from enclosed manufacturer's literature.

Generic Name (Trade Name)	Use (Dose)	Action	Adverse Effects	Drug Interactions	Nursing Process
Pharmacologic Classification: Miscellaneous Drugs					
Cisapride (Prepulsid)	Symptomatic management of GI motility disorders, including gastroesophageal reflux disease, gastroparesis and intestinal pseudo-obstruct'n (Gastroesophageal reflux disease - Adults - **Oral:** 5-10 mg tid or qid, 15 min ac and hs w. beverage. Gastroparesis/pseudo-obstruct'n - **Oral:** 10 mg tid-qid, 15 min ac and hs w. beverage)	Enhances physiologic release of acetylcholine at myenteric plexus. Incr. esophageal peristaltic activity and lowers sphincter tone, thereby decr. gastric reflux into esophagus and improving esophageal clearance. Also enhances gastric and duodenal emptying as a consequence of incr. gastric and duodenal contractility and antroduodenal coordinat'n. Decr. duodenal gastric reflux. Enhances intestinal propulsive activity and improves both small- and large-bowel transit.	Diarrhea and abdominal discomfort	Drug absorpt'n from the intestine may be accelerated by cisapride. **Anticholinergics:** Antagonize effects of cisapride on GI motility. Incr. esophageal peristaltic activity. **Anticoagulants:** May have incr. effects in presence of cisapride. **Anticonvulsants:** Blood levels should be monitored carefully when cisapride is given concomitantly. **CNS depressants:** May show incr. activity in presence of cisapride. **H₂ blockers:** Such as cimetidine or ranitidine, can incr. slightly the oral bioavailability of cisapride.	**Assess:** Pt hx for GI bleeding, hepatic and renal insufficiency; check if pt is receiving anticoagulants. Drug should not be given to pregnant or lactating pt. **Administer:** Store at room temp.; protect from moisture and light. **Evaluate:** Monitor blood levels of drug, esp. in elderly pts. **Teach:** Caution about incr. sedative effect when taking tranquilizers or alcohol.
Trimethobenzamide (Tigan)	Prevent'n and tx of nausea and vomiting due to infect'ns, toxicoses, underlying disease processes, drug administrat'n, radiat'n tx, travel sickness, postop. stage in labyrinthitis, Meniere's syndrome or psychic disturbances (**Oral:** Adults - 250 mg tid or qid. Children - 4-5 mg/Kg q6-8h. **IM:** Adults - 200 mg tid or qid. To prevent postop. vomiting - A single dose of 200 mg may be given before or during surgery. Repeat prn 3 h after stopping	Depresses chemoreceptor trigger zone in brain.	Hypersensitivity react'ns, drowsiness, blurred vision, depress'n, headache, dizziness, jaundice, hypotens'n, disorientat'n, muscle cramps, convuls'ns, opisthotonus and coma		**Assess:** Baseline VS; check for pre-existing viral condit'n, esp. in children and adolescents. **Administer:** With water or fluid; IM deep in gluteal muscle. **Evaluate:** BP for hypotens'n; for hypersensitivity; for indicat'ns of Reyes' syndrome in children (persistent vomiting, hyperpnea, lethargy, confus'n, disorientat'n, irrat'nal behavior, convuls'ns, unconsciousness).

surgery. Do not give IM to children. **Rectal:** Adults - 200 mg tid or qid. Children - 4-5 mg/kg q6-8h. Do not administer rectally to premature or newborn infants)

SECTION 8

Endocrine Pharmacology

By definition, an endocrine gland produces one or more internal secretions that are introduced directly into the blood stream and carried to other parts of the body whose functions they regulate or control. The endocrine glands are the thyroid, parathyroid, pancreas, adrenal cortex and gonads. This section discusses the use of drugs as replacement therapy in cases of endocrine deficiency. It also considers their use to reduce endocrine function in situations of hypersecretion. In the case of the adrenal cortex, we also discuss in detail the anti-inflammatory actions of the glucocorticoids and their importance in health care.

CHAPTER 26

Drugs and the Thyroid

Teaching Objectives

Following completion of this chapter, the reader should be able to:

1. Describe the function of the thyroid gland.
2. Discuss the synthesis, storage, secretion, transport and actions of the thyroid hormones.
3. List the symptoms of hypothyroidism.
4. Compare the various pharmaceutical preparations available for the treatment of hypothyroidism.
5. Identify the nursing process associated with drugs used in the treatment of hypothyroidism.
6. Discuss special problems in the treatment of hypothyroidism.
7. Describe the symptoms and causes of hyperthyroidism.
8. Discuss the mechanism of action, therapeutic uses and adverse effects of propylthiouracil and methimazole, as well as the nursing process related to their use.
9. Discuss special problems in the treatment of hyperthyroidism.
10. Explain the use of adjunctive drugs in the treatment of hyperthyroidism and identify the nursing process related to their use.

The Thyroid Gland

The thyroid is the largest endocrine gland. Normally weighing about 20 g, it can increase its size twenty- to thirty-fold if a goiter develops. The major function of the thyroid gland is the synthesis, storage and secretion of the iodinated chemicals l-tri-iodothyronine (T_3) and l-thyroxine (T_4). To accomplish this task, the thyroid actively extracts iodide from the plasma, oxidizes it to iodine before coupling the iodine to the amino acid tyrosine, forming either monoiodotyrosine or di-iodotyrosine. T_3 is formed from one molecule each of monoiodotyrosine and di-iodotyrosine. T_4 is produced from two molecules of di-iodotyrosine. Once synthesized, both T_3 and T_4 are stored within the thyroid as thyroglobulin and released into the circulation following stimulation of the gland by the thyroid-stimulating hormone (TSH). Some of the T_4 released is subsequently converted to T_3.

Thyroid activity is controlled by TSH, released from the pituitary. For its part, TSH release is triggered by the secretion of the thyrotrophic-releasing hormone from the hypothalamus. TSH increases both the synthesis and secretion of T_3 and T_4. Removal of the anterior pituitary leads to a diminished thyroid mass as well as decreased production and secretion of thyroid hormones. The administration of pituitary extracts to hypophysectomized patients restores normal TSH levels and returns thyroid structure and function to normal.

A balance exists between the secretion of TSH and the thyroid hormones. An increase in circulating levels of T_3 and T_4 decreases TSH secretion. The reverse is also true: a decrease in circulating T_3 and T_4 increases TSH secretion.

Once secreted, T_3 and T_4 are highly bound to specific plasma proteins called thyroid-binding globulin and thyroid-binding prealbumin. T_3 and T_4 are also bound nonspecifically to albumin. A smaller percentage of T_3 is bound, and as a result more of this hormone is found free in blood. Only T_3 and T_4 molecules free in plasma water can enter body cells and exert an effect. Thus, T_3 produces a more rapid effect than T_4.

Hospital laboratories routinely determine total plasma T_3 and T_4 levels. These measurements may be meaningless if they reflect only changes in amounts of T_3 and/or T_4 bound to plasma proteins. For example, the thyroid-binding globulin is increased by the consumption of estrogens and during pregnancy, and reduced by the administration of androgens. As a result, the total T_3 and T_4 levels in plasma are increased or decreased, respectively, but the free levels are not altered. The patients are neither hyperthyroid nor hypothyroid.

T_3 and T_4 increase tissue metabolic rate. In addition to activating mitochondrial protein synthesis, they stimulate the cell membrane sodium pump, causing an expenditure of energy. Thyroid hormones are also necessary for general growth and for maturation and development of the central nervous and skeletal systems. Thyroid deficiency in childhood results in cretinism, a condition characterized by growth failure and mental retardation.

Diseases of the thyroid can be divided into those that involve only a change in gland size (adenamatous goiter, thyroid cancer or nontoxic diffuse goiter) and those that involve an alteration in its secretion (hypothyroidism or hyperthyroidism). In hypothyroidism or hyperthyroidism, drug therapy plays an important role in restoring health.

Drug Treatment of Hypothyroidism

Nursing assessment of patients with hypothyroidism reveals fatigue, swelling of the hands and the area around the eyes, constipation, dry skin and menstrual irregularities. These symptoms can range from mild to severe. If mild, they may be inapparent to the patient and detectable only by laboratory examination. When severe, they can extend to a characteristic gutteral voice, thickened boggy skin (myxedema), slow mental processes, loss of body hair, intolerance to cold, ascites, pericardial effusion, frank myxedema, coma and death.

Hypothyroidism can be primary or secondary. If primary, the disorder lies within the gland itself. This may occur as a result of radioiodine therapy, partial or total surgical removal of the gland, or treatment with antithyroid drugs. Primary hypothyroidism is also caused by the autoimmune destruction of the gland (Hashimoto's thyroiditis). Secondary hypothyroidism results from the failure of the pituitary to secrete adequate amounts of TSH.

Regardless of the cause, thyroid hormone therapy is essential to reverse the clinical abnormalities and restore euthyroidism. Several products are available that provide T_3 or T_4, or both. Their pharmacologic actions, therapeutic uses and adverse effects are identical. They differ only in their actual content of T_3 and T_4, the speed with which they produce their effects, the absolute doses used and their cost.

Desiccated Thyroid Tablets (Thyrar)

Desiccated thyroid tablets are prepared by removing fat and water from hog or beef thyroids. They are the cheapest form of therapy but have several drawbacks. The tablets are standardized on the basis of their iodine content rather than on the amounts of T_3 and T_4 present. Because the major portion of iodine in the gland is in the form of inert iodotyrosines, the iodine assay does not reflect the biologic potency of the tablets. In addition, the ratio of T_4 to T_3 can vary from 2:1 to 3:1, depending on the particular batch of tablets. The iodine assay will not measure the actual levels of each hormone or the relative ratios of one to the other.

L-Thyroxine, Levothyroxine (Eltroxin, Levothyroid, Synthroid)

Oral and injectable forms of l-thyroxine (T_4) are the preferred treatment. The advantages of these preparations over desiccated thyroid include reliable potency and the absence of wide swings in serum T_3 and T_4 levels. Converted in part to T_3 in the body, T_4 provides a reliable source of both thyroid hormones. 0.1 mg of T_4 is usually considered equivalent to 60 mg of desiccated thyroid or 25 µg of liothyronine sodium (T_3).

Liothyronine — L-Tri-iodothyronine (Cytomel)

Liothyronine (T_3) is 2.5 to 3.3 times more potent than l-thyroxine (T_4). Its effects are seen sooner, and at first glance liothyronine may seem more attractive than T_4. However, stabilization of a patient on T_3 may be more difficult because it is cleared from the body faster than T_4. Furthermore, treatment with T_4 provides a reliable source of both T_3 and T_4. Finally, although most clinical laboratories can measure T_4 in serum, many cannot measure T_3.

Combinations of Liothyronine and L-Thyroxine, Liotrix (Euthroid, Thyrolar)

These preparations contain the sodium salts of T_4 and T_3 in a 4:1 ratio and are designed to mimic normal thyroid secretion. However, the patient-to-patient variations in normal serum T_3 levels make it difficult to achieve this goal. It is difficult to see how these products provide any advantage over the cheaper T_4-containing tablets which are converted, at least in part, to T_3 in the body.

Thyroglobulin (Proloid)

Obtained from frozen hog thyroid, thyroglobulin meets USP standards for iodine, as assayed biologically. Its indications, adverse effects, precautions and doses are the same as those for thyroid tablets, with which it is equipotent.

Special Treatment Problems

The treatment of the hypothyroid neonate or child presents a special problem. Children, particularly neonates, are at risk if thyroid activity is low. If hypothyroidism is suspected in the neonate or child, serum should be drawn for thyroid function tests and therapy begun immediately without waiting for the results. The risk of giving thyroid hormone to a neonate who does not require it is minimal compared to the danger of withholding the drug if the baby is hypothyroid. One protocol calls for 10–12 µg of T_4 to be given for every kilogram of body weight, initially. This can be reduced to 8–10 µg/kg after three months. Thereafter, the dose may be reduced according to the manufacturer's directions.

Although myxedema coma is rare, it can have a fifty per cent mortality rate. To handle this situation, an initial intravenous dose of 300–500 µg of T_4 can be given, followed by 50–100 µg intravenously daily.

Nursing Process

Regardless of the thyroid preparation used, the nursing process is the same.

Assessment

Nursing activities are initiated with a review of the patient's history for evidence of angina pectoris, hypertension, kidney disease or current pregnancy. If any of these conditions are documented, the prescription must be verified with the attending physician and the nursing evaluation of the patient intensified following administration of the medication. Similarly, if nursing review of the patient's current drug regimen reveals concurrent use of catecholamines, the prescription of a thyroid substitute or supplement must be verified with the physician and evaluation of the patient's response to the medication intensified. Finally, nursing assessment should establish baseline measures against which the patient's response to the drug can be measured. These include blood levels, body mass/weight, vital signs, and height and growth rate in children as well as fluid intake and output.

Administration

Thyroid medication should be administered from an airtight and light-resistant container to protect it from exposure to light or moisture. Because of the severe consequence of accidental overdosage, it is imperative that precisely the prescribed amount be administered. Administration before breakfast will enhance absorption from the intestinal lumen.

Evaluation

The patient's response to the thyroid substitute should be evaluated by monitoring fluid intake and output for evidence of diuresis, daily body mass/weight for weight loss, and vital signs for increased pulse, respirations and blood pressure. Observation of the patient should reveal increased levels of physical activity and mental alertness following administration of thyroid substitutes. Nursing evaluation should also emphasize identification of evidence of overdose. The assessment parameters for overdose are the same as those for thyrotoxicosis, i.e., nervousness, agitation, irritability and elevated metabolic rate (as indicated by weight loss in spite of large food intake), frequent loose bowel movements, fever, heat intolerance, diaphoresis, elevated blood pressure, tachycardia and palpitations, irregular rapid pulse, tremor and insomnia.

Teaching

Nurses should teach patients and their families to take precisely the prescribed amount of thyroid substitute. This is essential if the medication is to produce the desired effect. If larger quantities are taken, patients may experience adverse effects due to chronic or acute overdose. Patients and families should be instructed how to take and record the patient's pulse so that it can be reported to the physician during regular checkups to assist in monitoring the patient's progress. They should also be taught to note the adverse effects of the drug and the importance of contacting the physician immediately if these appear. Nursing instruction of patients should emphasize the life-long need for thyroid replacement. The drug should neither be discontinued nor its dosage altered without medical advice. Any illness that results in prolonged diarrhea may interfere with drug absorption and should be reported to the physician. Patients should also be taught to avoid over-the-counter preparations with iodine, as well as iodine-rich foods.

Drug Treatment of Hyperthyroidism

The major signs and symptoms of hyperthyroidism are well known. They include heat intolerance, loss of weight, bruit over the thyroid, a hyperkinetic circulatory state and dyspnea. Unusual muscle fatigue, irritability and the presence of eye signs, such as lid lag, weakness of the extraocular muscles and proptosis may also be seen. The great majority of North American patients with hyperthyroidism suffer from either Graves' disease or toxic adenoma of the thyroid. The distinction between the two is important. Graves' disease is an autoimmune disorder caused by the existence in the blood of thyroid-stimulating antibody (TSAb). It may be treated surgically, with iodine-131 (^{131}I), or with antithyroid drugs. A toxic adenoma of the thyroid is a benign neoplasm that requires ablation to produce a cure.

Propylthiouracil (Propacil, Propyl-Thyracil) and Methimazole (Tapazole)

Mechanism of Action and Pharmacologic Effects

Propylthiouracil and methimazole block the oxidative iodination of tyrosine, thereby preventing the formation of T_3 and T_4. Propylthiouracil also impairs the peripheral conversion of T_4 to T_3. Methimazole does not affect the conversion of T_4 to T_3.

Therapeutic Uses

Propylthiouracil and methimazole are used to prepare patients for surgery, to assist in the management of patients in thyrotoxic crisis and to treat hyperthyroidism chronically. Relatively high doses are required to return chronically hyperthyroid patients to the euthyroid state. Thereafter, the dosage may be reduced. Some physicians prefer to give enough propylthiouracil or methimazole to block thyroid function completely and then administer sufficient T_4 to maintain a euthyroid state. TSAbs persist in the blood of most patients treated with either drug; a clinical relapse may occur if treatment is stopped.

Both propylthiouracil and methimazole are

contraindicated in nursing mothers. Concerns over the use of either drug in pregnancy are expressed later in this chapter under the heading Special Treatment Problems. It goes without saying that in the treatment of thyrotoxicosis during pregnancy, propylthiouracil or methimazole should be used in the smallest possible doses. Rare cases of aplasia cutis, as manifested by scalp defects, have occurred in infants born to mothers who have used methimazole during pregnancy. Because scalp defects have not been reported in offspring of patients treated with propylthiouracil, this drug may be preferable to methimazole in pregnant women requiring treatment with antithyroid drugs.

Adverse Effects

Propylthiouracil produces numerous adverse effects, including skin rash, urticaria, fever, granulocytopenia, agranulocytosis, pancytopenia, hepatitis, myalgia and headache. Methimazole's adverse effects include nausea, vomiting, epigastric distress, headache, fever, arthralgia, pruritus, edema and pancytopenia. Overtreatment with either propylthiouracil or methimazole can result in goiter. The decrease in serum T_3 and T_4 increases TSH secretion, producing hyperplasia of the thyroid.

Nursing Process

Assessment

Prior to the administration of propylthiouracil or methimazole, nursing assessment should aim at identifying patients who are pregnant or breastfeeding. The difficulty of treating pregnant women is described below. Patients who are breastfeeding should be advised to wean their babies, because both propylthiouracil and methimazole will cross into breast milk and impair thyroid hormone production in nursing infants.

Nursing assessment should seek to identify those patients whose drug regimen also includes the use of anticoagulants. Propylthiouracil can cause hypoprothrombinemia and result in bleeding tendencies in patients taking anticoagulants. In addition, nursing assessment should include establishing baseline measurements of vital signs and body mass/weight for later use in determining the drug's effectiveness or in identifying its adverse effects.

Administration

If patients are bothered by drug-induced gastric distress, propylthiouracil and methimazole can be taken with meals. Store these drugs in light-resistant containers. Recommend to patients a fluid intake of three to four liters daily unless otherwise contraindicated.

Evaluation

Following the administration of either drug, weight gain and a decrease in pulse rate, accompanied by a calmer manner, usually indicate drug effectiveness. Drug overdose is suggested by nursing evaluations that demonstrate a sudden weight gain, peripheral and periorbital edema, depression and intolerance to cold. Other adverse effects that might appear during nursing evaluation include sore throat, fever, rash, nose bleed, excessive bruising, and unexplained or prolonged bleeding. These can reflect agranulocytosis, pancytopenia and lowered prothrombin levels.

Teaching

Patient teaching related to the use of propylthiouracil and methimazole should stress the importance of keeping regularly scheduled appointments with the physician for evaluation and laboratory studies. Nurses should also emphasize the importance of taking these drugs at the times and in the amounts specified to maintain proper blood T_3 and T_4 levels. Patients and their families should be instructed in the proper method of measuring pulse rate and taught to record the pulse rate at regular intervals. These findings, together with the patient's weight, should be reported to the physician at scheduled visits. The adverse effects of the drugs should be explained to both patients and families and emphasis given to the importance of reporting any that appear immediately to the physician. Patients should be instructed to avoid over-the-counter products containing iodine and iodine-rich foods.

Potassium Iodide, Sodium Iodide, Strong Iodine Solutions

Mechanism of Action and Pharmacologic Effects

Large doses of iodide or iodine inhibit, at least temporarily, organic iodine formation and thyroid hormone release. High doses may also prevent the effects of TSH on the thyroid gland.

Therapeutic Uses

Iodine or iodide is given after treatment with an antithyroid drug such as propylthiouracil, to prepare hyperthyroid patients for thyroidectomy. Iodide is also given intravenously approximately two to three hours after an antithyroid drug to treat thyrotoxic crisis or neonatal thyrotoxicosis.

Adverse Effects

These drugs produce an unpleasant taste of iodine and a burning in the mouth. Patients may experience a sore mouth and throat, as well as hypersalivation, painful sialadenitis, acne and other rashes. Diarrhea and a productive cough may also be seen. Sensitive individuals may experience angioedema with swelling of the larynx and dyspnea.

Nursing Process

Assessment

When the patient's history indicates evidence of hypersensitivity or idiosyncrasy to iodine, hyperkalemia, acute bronchitis or pregnancy, nurses should verify the order with the physician before administering the first dose of these medications. Evidence in the patient's history of renal impairment, cardiac disease, tuberculosis or Addison's disease should alert the nurse to the need for particularly close monitoring and evaluation following administration of these medications. Nurses should expect the physician to order baseline serum potassium levels and therefore should ensure that blood has been drawn prior to the administration of the first dose of these drugs.

Administration

Use only solutions stored in airtight and light-resistant containers. Discard brownish-yellow solutions because they have been exposed to light and contain free iodine. When these medications are being administered preoperatively in preparation for thyroid surgery, nurses should comply strictly with the schedule of administration.

These medications should be administered following meals and diluted in 250 mL (8 oz.) of fluid in order to minimize gastric distress. Enteric-coated tablets are infrequently used because of their tendency to cause small bowel lesions. If this form is used patients should take at least 250 mL (8 oz.) of fluid with the medication. Administer liquid preparations through a straw to prevent tooth discoloration.

Teaching

Instruct patients to contact the physician immediately if evidence of gastrointestinal bleeding, abdominal pain, distention, nausea or vomiting appears. Advise the patient to report adverse effects (see above) to the physician quickly. Instruct patients to consult the pharmacist or physician before using over-the-counter drugs, because many of these preparations contain iodine which could increase the total amount ingested beyond acceptable levels. Similarly, patients using these medications over extended periods of time should avoid foods that are high in iodine (for example, shellfish) and iodized salt. Such patients should also avoid sudden withdrawal from the medication because of the risk of thyroid storm.

Special Treatment Problems

Hyperthyroidism in pregnancy is a special treatment problem. In the nongravid state, hyperthyroidism may be treated by ablation of the gland either surgically or with ^{131}I or by treating the patient with propylthiouracil or methimazole. In pregnancy, however, most physicians prefer not to subject the patient to the stress of surgery. Radioactive iodine is also not appropriate because it crosses the placenta and can damage the fetal thyroid. Therefore, the only treatment remaining is propylthiouracil or methimazole. As stated earlier, because methimazole administration during pregnancy has been associated with rare cases of aplasia cutis, many physicians prefer to use propylthiouracil. In using either of these drugs, however, it is important to titrate the dose carefully to guard against producing a hypothyroid goiter in the fetus. Reducing the dose of the antithyroid drug by one-half during the second month of treatment has been recommended to keep the free serum thyroxine concentration in the upper range of normal.

Severe hyperthyroidism, often called **thyroid storm,** must be treated quickly as it represents a danger to life. Propylthiouracil may be preferred to methimazole because of its ability to reduce the peripheral conversion of T_4 to T_3. A dose of 200 mg every six hours has been suggested. Iodide can be administered one hour after the first dose of propylthiouracil. The addition of iodide reduces the production and secretion of T_3 and T_4 faster than can be achieved solely by propylthiouracil. The mechanism by which high doses of iodide produce this effect is still not clear. Beta-blocker therapy may also be used to remove many of the sympathetically mediated consequences of the thyroid storm.

Adjunctive Drugs

Many of the effects of hyperthyroidism resemble excessive sympathetic nervous system stimulation. These include tachycardia, palpitations, sweating, tremor and nervousness. The use of beta blockers has been mentioned in the treatment of thyroid storm. Their administration should not be restricted to the acute needs of patients with severe hyperthyroidism. Drugs such as propranolol (Inderal) can benefit many hyperthyroid patients by reducing or abolishing some or all of the effects mentioned earlier. It should be recognized, however, that a beta blocker provides only symptomatic treatment. The activity of the thyroid gland and the concentrations of serum T_3 and T_4 still remain elevated. More specific treatment, such as surgery, ^{131}I or antithyroid drugs, is still required to reduce thyroid function.

The nursing process related to the use of beta blockers is detailed in Chapter 8. A synopsis of their nursing implications is contained in Table 6 at the end of that chapter.

Benzodiazepines may also play a role in the treatment of hyperthyroidism to reduce the anxiety of patients. The drug of choice is probably one with a relatively long half-life, such as diazepam. Nursing responsibilities related to benzodiazepine use are discussed in Chapter 46.

Further Reading

Campbell, A.J. (1986). Thyroid disorders in the elderly. Difficulties in diagnosis and treatment. *Drugs 31* :455-461.

Potency of oral thyroxine preparations (1984). *The Medical Letter 26* :41.

Rakel, R.W. (1984). *Conn's Current Therapy.* Philadelphia: W.B. Saunders.

Zaritsky, A. (1989). Hyperthyroidism: Current therapy. *Drugs 37* :375-381.

Table 37
Drugs and the thyroid.

Pharmacologic Classification: Thyroid Preparations

Generic Name (Trade Name)	Use (Dose)	Action	Adverse Effects	Drug Interactions	Nursing Process
Thyroid USP (Thyrar)	Replacement tx for decr. or absent thyroid funct'n (**Oral:** *For myxedema* - Initially, 30-180 mg daily. *Other hypothyroid states* - 60-300 mg daily. Us. maint. dose, 30-125 mg/day. Desiccated thyroid 60 mg is equivalent to 60 mg thyroglobulin, 0.1 mg [100 µg] levothyroxine sodium, or 25 µg liothyronine sodium)	Replaces or substitutes for reduced or absent thyroid hormone product'n due to malfunct'ning thyroid gland	*Overdose:* Same s/s as thyrotoxicosis, e.g., nervousness, tremors, headache, insomnia, palpitat'ns, tachycardia, cardiac arrhythmias, angina pectoris, diarrhea and abdominal cramps, sweating, heat intolerance, fever, weight loss	**Anticoagulants, oral:** May have their effects incr. by all forms of thyroid replacement. Reduce anticoagulant dose by one-third when thyroid replacement is started. Subsequently, anticoagulant dosage should be adjusted on the basis of frequent prothrombin determinat'ns. **Antidiabetic agents:** May have their effects reduced by thyroid replacement tx. May be nec. to incr. dose of the antidiabetic if thyroid tx is started. Conversely, decreasing dose of the thyroid preparat'n may cause hypoglycemic react'ns if the dosage of the oral hypoglycemic is not adjusted. **Cholestyramine and colestipol:** Bind thyroxine and liothyronine in intestine, thus impairing their absorpt'n. 4-5 h should elapse bet. administrat'n of cholestyramine or colestipol and thyroid hormones. **Estrogens and progestins:** May incr. serum thyroxine-binding globulin, poss. increasing required dose of thyroxine replacement tx. **Insulin:** May require an incr. in dosage if thyroid replacement tx is used. **Phenytoin:** May displace thyroxine from plasma protein binding sites, thereby temporarily	**Assess:** For angina pectoris, hypertens'n, kidney disease, pregnancy; drug hx for concurrent use of sympathomimetics; establish baseline measures for clinical symptoms of hypothyroidism (or myxedema). Also: baseline body weight, VS, fluid intake/output. **Administer:** From light-resistant container w. tight-fitting lid; precisely the prescribed dosage, before breakfast. **Evaluate:** For drug effectiveness as indicated by diuresis, weight loss, moderat'n of emot'nal state, incr. pulse rate, incr. physical/mental activity, absence of constipat'n and relief of other clinical symptoms; for evidence of overdose (see Adverse Effects). **Teach:** To take precisely the prescribed amount; to record and report pulse rate; to note and report adv. effects; that replacement tx is life-long and should not be discontinued; that dosage should not be altered without medical supervision; to contact physician if prolonged diarrhea is experienced.
L-Thyroxine, levothyroxine (Eltroxin, Levothyroid, Synthroid)	As for thyroid USP (*For mild hypothyroidism* - Young and middle-aged adults - **Oral:** Initially, 50-100 µg/day; incr. by 50 µg or less at 3-4 week intervals to 100 µg/day. Av. maint. dose, 125-150 µg/day. For *severe hypothyroidism* - Initially, 25 µg/day; incr. by 25 µg at 2-week intervals to 100 µg/day. Further increases by increments of 50-100 µg may be made at 2-week intervals prn. Us. maint. dose, 100-200 µg/day. Older adults - Initially, 12.5-50 µg/day for 3-6 weeks; incr. by 12.5-25 µg q3-8weeks prn. *For congenital hypothyroidism* - **Oral:** Children - 0-6 months - 8-10 µg/kg/day; 6-12 months - 6-8 µg/kg/day; 1-5 years - 5-6 µg/kg/day; 6-12 years - 4-5 µg/kg/day. In cretinism, not below 100 µg/day. *In myxede-*	As for thyroid USP	As for thyroid USP		

Drug	Dosage	Action/Use	Side/Adverse Effects	Interactions	Nursing Considerations
(continued)	ma, coma or stupor - Adults - **IV:** 200-500 µg. An addit'nal 100-300 µg or more may be given on 2nd day prn)	As for thyroid USP	As for thyroid USP	As for thyroid USP. increasing free or active levels of thyroxine. As a result, phenytoin may incr. activity of thyroxine.	As for thyroid USP
Liothyronine, l-tri-iodothyronine (Cytomel, Tertroxin)	As for thyroid USP (*For mild hypothyroidism* - **Oral:** Initially, 25 µg/day; incr. by 12.5-25 µg q1-2weeks prn. Us. maint. dose, 25-75 µg/day. *For myxedema* - **Oral:** Initially, 5 µg/day; may incr. by 5-10 µg/day q1-2weeks. When 25 µg/day is reached, dosage may often be incr. by 12.5-25 µg q1-2weeks. Us. maint. dose, 50-100 µg/day. *For cretinism* - **Oral:** Initiate tx as early as poss. to avoid permanent physical/mental changes. Initially, 5 µg/day, w. a 5-µg increment q3-4days prn. Infants may require only 20 µg/day for maint. At 1 year, 50 µg/day may be required. Above 3 years, full adult dosage may be required)	As for thyroid USP	As for thyroid USP	As for thyroid USP	As for thyroid USP

Pharmacologic Classification: Antithyroid Drugs

Drug	Dosage/Use	Action	Side/Adverse Effects	Interactions	Nursing Considerations
Propylthiouracil (Propacil, Propyl-Thyracil)	Medical tx of hyperthyroidism and in preparat'n for subtotal thyroidectomy or radioactive iodine tx (**Oral:** *For hyperthyroidism* - Adults - Initially, 300-600 mg/day in divided doses q6-8h to a max. of 1.2 g/day. After pt is euthyroid, 100-300 mg/day is given in 3 divided doses. Children - *10 years and over* - intially, 150-300 mg/day in divided doses q6-8h until pt is euthyroid, followed by 100-300 mg/day in 2 doses for maint. *6-10 years* - Initially, 50-150 mg/day in divided doses q6-8h. *Under 6 years* - Initially, 120-	Prevents format'n of tri-iodothyronine (T_3) and thyroxine (T_4) by blocking oxidative iodinat'n of tyrosine in thyroid gland. Also blocks peripheral convers'n of thyroxine to tri-iodothyronine.	Skin rash, urticaria, fever, granulocytopenia, jaundice, hepatitis, headache, pruritus, drowsiness, neuritis, edema, vertigo, alopecia, pigmentat'n, periarteritis, hypoprothrombinemia, nausea, vomiting, epigastric distress, arthralgia, paresthesias and loss of taste	**Sulfonamides:** Should not be administered w. propylthiouracil antithyroid drugs because both may cause agranulocytosis.	**Assess:** For current pregnancy; concurrent use of anticoagulants; establish baseline measures of VS and weight. **Administer:** With meals. Store in light-resistant containers. **Evaluate:** For drug efficacy as indicated by slow, steady, regular weight gain, peripheral and periorbital edema, depress'n, cold intolerance; for indicat'ns of adv. effects, esp. sore throat, fever, rash, nose bleeds, excess. bruising, unexplained or prolonged bleeding. **Teach:** Importance of keeping regular appointments w. physician for blood studies; to note evidence of adv. effects (see Evaluate, above) and report these

Generic Name (Trade Name)	Use (Dose)	Action	Adverse Effects	Drug Interactions	Nursing Process
	175 mg/m²/day in divided doses q8h. *For neonatal thyrotoxicosis - 10 mg/kg/day in divided doses. For thyrotoxic crisis -* Adults - 600 mg - 1.2 g/day in divided doses.				to physician immediately. To measure, record and report pulse rate and weight; importance of taking drug at correct time and in amount specified. Avoid OTC products that contain iodine or iodine-rich foods.
Methimazole (Tapazole)	Medical tx of hyperthyroidism and to ameliorate hyperthyroidism in preparat'n for subtotal thyroidectomy or radioactive iodine tx (**Oral:** Adults - Initially, 15-60 mg/day in divided doses q6-8h until pt is euthyroid. Maint. dose, 10-30 mg/day in 1-3 doses. Children - *6-10 years - Initially, 0.4 mg/kg/day in divided doses q6-8h. Under 6 years - 12-17.5 mg/m²/day in divided doses q8h. For thyrotoxic crisis - 60-120 mg/day in divided doses)*	Prevents format'n of tri-iodothyronine (T₃) and thyroxine (T₄) by blocking oxidative iodinat'n of tyrosine in thyroid gland.	Skin rash, urticaria, nausea, vomiting, epigastric distress, arthralgia, paresthesias, loss of taste, abnormal loss of hair, myalgia, headache, pruritus, drowsiness, neuritis, edema, vertigo, skin pigmentat'n, jaundice, sialadenopathy, lymphadenopathy, drug fever, lupus-like syndrome, hepatitis, periarteritis and hypoprothrombinemia		As for propylthiouracil
Potassium iodide, sodium iodide, strong iodine solution	Orally, after an antithyroid drug, to prepare hyperthyroid pts for thyroidectomy, and IV to treat thyrotoxic crisis or neonatal thyrotoxicosis. These drugs should not be used alone (**Oral:** *To prepare hyperthyroid pts for thyroidectomy -* Strong iodine solut'n USP [2-6 drops tid] or KI solut'n USP [5 drops tid] can be given to adults and children for 10 days before surgery. **IV:** *For thyrotoxic crisis -* 250-500 mg/day of NaI USP, beginning 1 h after initial dose of propylthiouracil and propranolol has been given)	Large doses of iodide or iodine inhibit, at least temporarily, organic iodine format'n and thyroid hormone release. High doses may also prevent effects of TSH on thyroid gland.	Risk of thyrotoxicosis, respiratory obstruct'n of infant by enlarged thyroid (if mother treated w. iodide during pregnancy), iodide myxedema, hypothyroidism	**Lithium carbonate:** May have synergistic antithyroid activity when used w. iodide preparat'ns. If it is nec. to administer both drugs concomitantly, nurses should be alert for s/s hypothyroidism.	**Assess:** For hx hypersensitivity to iodine, hyperkalemia, acute bronchitis or pregnancy. Also check for renal impairment, cardiac disease, TB, Addison's disease. Take baseline serum K levels. **Administer:** On strict schedule, following meals, through straw. Store in airtight, light-resistant container. Discard discolored solut'n. Give w. 250 mL (8 oz) of fluid. **Teach:** To report immediately evidence of GI bleeding, abdominal pain, nausea/vomiting. To avoid OTC preparat'ns w. iodine and iodine-rich foods.

Pharmacologic Classification: Adjunctive Therapy

For a discussion of the use of propranolol in the treatment of hyperthyroidism, refer to Chapter 26. Details on the dosage, adverse effects, drug interactions and nursing process for propranolol can be obtained from Table 8 at the end of Chapter 8. For a discussion on the use of benzodiazepines in the treatment of hyperthyroidism, refer to Chapter 26. Details on the dosage, adverse effects, drug interactions and nursing process of these drugs can be obtained from Table 69 at the end of Chapter 46.

CHAPTER 27

Drugs and the Parathyroid Gland

Plasma Calcium

The parathyroid hormone (PTH), vitamin D and calcitonin regulate calcium and phosphate metabolism. Calcium serves both mechanical and metabolic functions in the body. Mechanically, it is the main constituent in bone, where the great majority of body calcium is found. Metabolically, calcium is essential for nerve and muscle function, cardiac activity, the actions of cell membranes and the clotting of blood.

It is with respect to the metabolic functions of calcium that attention is focused on its plasma concentration. The plasma levels of calcium depend on its absorption from the intestine, the quantity stored in bone, and the amount eliminated by the kidneys. Forty per cent of plasma calcium is bound to albumin and not able to diffuse into tissues. Another ten per cent is present as citrate or phosphate salts. The remainder of plasma calcium is present in its ionic form and it is this fraction that leaves the vascular bed to influence metabolic functions.

Normal plasma calcium levels range from approximately 9 – 10.5 mg/100 mL (2.2 – 2.65 mmol/L). PTH is secreted in response to a fall in the levels of ionized plasma calcium. It increases the intestinal absorption of calcium, mediates the transfer of calcium from bone to blood, and decreases the renal excretion of calcium. If it can be stated that a fall in ionized calcium concentration in plasma triggers the release of PTH, the converse is also true: high levels of ionized calcium in plasma decrease PTH secretion.

For its part, vitamin D stimulates the absorption of calcium and phosphate. Vitamin D is not active itself. Rather, it is a prohormone, converted to 25-hydroxy vitamin D in the liver. Its subsequent metabolism in the kidney to the active 1,25-dihydroxy vitamin D (calcitriol) stimulates calcium absorption.

Calcitonin is a hormone secreted by the thyroid gland. Released in response to an increase in plasma-ionized calcium, it decreases bone resorption and increases calcium excretion.

Hypoparathyroidism

In the past this condition often resulted from total, or partial, surgical thyroidectomy. Located behind both the upper and lower poles of the thyroid gland, the parathyroids are "sitting ducks" to be removed inadvertently during thyroidectomy. The use of radioactive iodine, propylthiouracil or methimazole to reduce thyroid function has decreased the incidence of hypoparathyroidism. In idiopathic hypoparathyroidism, the gland ceases to function for unknown reason(s).

Vitamin D and Calcium Supplements

Mechanism of Action and Pharmacologic Effects

Hypoparathyroidism is characterized by hypocalcemia and hyperphosphatemia with a history of tetany. Preparations of PTH are not available for therapeutic use. Patients may be treated by giving vitamin D_2 or vitamin D_3 plus elemental calcium. The goal of therapy is to stabilize plasma calcium levels at no higher than 9 mg/100 mL (2.2 mmol/L) to prevent hypercalciuria.

Adverse Effects

The primary adverse effects resulting from the use of vitamin D or calcium, or both, is hypercalcemia manifesting as muscle weakness, increased myocardial irritability, polyuria with accompanying thirst, anorexia, nausea, vomiting, bone pain, either constipation or diarrhea, lethargy, exhaustion, mental confusion and irritability.

Nursing Process

Assessment

For patients whose hypoparathyroidism is to be treated using vitamin D, calcium and dietary therapy, nurses must first nutritionally assess the patient. Particular emphasis must be paid to dietary calcium and vitamin D intake. Referral to a nutritionist for assessment and counselling is usually the most appropriate procedure. Prior to treatment, nurses should also document the patient's vital signs and fluid intake/output ratio as indicators of the extent of the hypoparathyroidism.

Before administering calcium supplements, nurses should review the patient's current drug profile, in consultation with the pharmacist, for concurrent use of digoxin (Lanoxin) or other digitalis glycosides. Calcium potentiates the effects of these drugs. The use of a tetracycline should also be noted because calcium inhibits tetracycline absorption. The patient's history should be examined for previous incidents of renal calculi.

Evaluation

Nursing evaluation is the same, regardless of whether calcium supplements and/or vitamin D and diet therapy are used. The effectiveness of treatment is indicated by a nursing assessment that reveals less muscular irritability; stabilization of cardiac function; relief of stridor, dyspnea, abdominal cramps, urinary frequency and diplopia. If constipation occurs, increase bulk and fluids in diet.

Teaching

Patients should be advised that the benefits of treatment do not accrue for approximately one week. Nurses should emphasize the life-long necessity for therapy and the importance of compliance with the prescribed regimen in order to prevent relapse. Patients and their families should be carefully instructed regarding the indicators of drug efficacy and of drug overdose. They should also be taught the importance of regular monitoring of blood calcium levels to permit accurate dosage regulation.

Hyperparathyroidism

More than eighty-five per cent of cases of primary hyperparathyroidism are due to a chief cell adenoma of the parathyroid gland. Patients often present with symptoms of hypercalcemia, bone disease and renal calculi. The diagnosis of hyperparathyroidism is usually made in the clinical laboratory. Serum calcium levels are usually in the range of 11 – 14 mg/100 mL. In some cases, they may be higher.

Pharmacologic Treatment

Hyperparathyroidism is usually treated by surgical removal of the hyperfunctioning tissue. If this is not possible, medical treatment may ameliorate the symptoms caused by the hypercalcemia. An attempt is often made to restore body fluids, electrolytes and renal function to normal. This involves the administration of fluids, with or without saline, and large doses of loop diuretics, such as furosemide or ethacrynic acid, to increase calcium excretion. Nursing responsibilities related to the use of these medications were discussed in depth in Chapter 16. Readers are advised to refer to that material. A synopsis of that information is contained in Table 18 at the end of that chapter. Neutral phosphate solutions, given either orally or intravenously, will also lower plasma calcium levels as the element moves into bone.

Corticosteroids, such as prednisone, which decrease calcium absorption, and calcitonin may be tried in the treatment of hyperparathyroidism. The nursing activities initiated as the result of the prescription of corticosteroids are presented in detail in Chapter 29 and Table 46.

Mithramycin is a cytotoxic anticancer drug that also has a potent hypocalcemic effect because it reduces bone resorption. Although the effects of mithramycin are seen within a few hours, the maximum fall in plasma calcium levels does not occur for several days. As with all anticancer drugs, mithramycin has pronounced toxicities. When used for the treatment of hypercalcemia, however, it has few adverse effects. Used on a long-term basis, it can cause nausea, vomiting and platelet depression, leading to hemorrhage. Nursing assessment should include review of the patient's chart for documentation of blood clotting disorders, electrolyte imbalance or an existing pregnancy. The drug order should be verified with the physician if these conditions are present. When the patient's chart contains evidence of liver or kidney disease or prior abdominal or mediastinal radiation treatment, the patient should be evaluated with particular vigilance for adverse effects. This drug is administered via an intravenous infusion that has been established by a physician. Nurses should evaluate the infusion site and terminate the infusion immediately if extravasation occurs. Patients should be carefully evaluated for evidence of electrolyte imbalance (refer to Chapter 18 and Table 22 for nursing assessment of hyperkalemia and hypokalemia), thrombocytopenia (epistaxis, hematemesis, hemoptysis, purpura, petechiae), bowel function and dehydration.

Further Reading

Rakel, R.E. (1985). *Conn's Current Therapy*. Philadelphia: W.B. Saunders.

Ryan, W.G. (1975). *Endocrine Disorders*. Year Book Publishers.

Table 38
Drugs and the parathyroid.

Pharmacologic Classification: Vitamin D and Vitamin D-like Preparations

Generic Name (Trade Name)	Use (Dose)	Action	Adverse Effects	Drug Interactions	Nursing Process
Vitamin D_2, ergocalciferol, calciferol (Deltalin, Drisdol)	Tx of hypoparathyroidism and vitamin D deficiency; adjunct in osteomalacia assoc. w. hypophosphatemia and renal tubular disease (**Oral:** For hypoparathyroidism - Adults - Initially, 50 000 - 200 000 IU daily after acute tetany is controlled w. IV Ca. Maint. dose, 25 000 - 100 000 IU/day. Children - 10 000 - 25 000 IU daily)	Facilitates absorpt'n of Ca and PO_4 from small intestine.	GI and CNS disturbances and soft tissue calcificat'n, poss. widespread; renal complicat'ns, anorexia, nausea, weakness, weight loss, stiffness, convuls'ns, mental retardat'n, anemias, mild acidosis, impairment of renal funct'n, decline in av. rate of linear growth, incr. mineralizat'n of bones in infants and children (dwarfism).		**Assess:** Diet for Ca intake; establish extent of hypocalcemia, incl. VS and fluid intake/output. **Evaluate:** For ameliorat'n of hypocalcemia; for early evidence of hypercalcemia. **Teach:** To observe for adv. effects; that tx effects occur in approx. 1 week; nec. for life-long tx and regular medical monitoring. Incr. bulk and fluids if constipat'n occurs.
Vitamin D_3, cholecalciferol, dihydrotachysterol (Hytakerol)	As for vitamin D_2 (**Oral:** For hypoparathyroidism - Adults - Initially, 0.75 - 2.5 mg/day. Maint. dose, from 0.25 - 1.75 mg/week. Larger doses in some pts)	As for vitamin D_2	As for vitamin D_2		As for vitamin D_2
Calcitriol (Rocaltrol)	Management of hypocalcemia and osteodystrophy in pts w. chronic renal failure undergoing dialysis; vitamin D-resistant rickets (**Oral:** Initially, 0.25 µg/day. Measure serum Ca levels 2x/week during titrat'n period. W'draw drug if pt is hypercalcemic)	Vitamin D_3 must be metabolized in the liver and kidneys before it is fully active on its target tissue. Calcitrol is the major active metabolite. It is indicated in the management of hypocalcemia and osteodystrophy in pts w. chronic renal failure who cannot convert vitamin D_3 to calcitriol.	As for vitamin D_2		As for vitamin D_2

Pharmacologic Classification: Mineral

Drug	Action	Use/Dosage	Side Effects	Interactions	Nursing Implications
Calcium (available in various salt forms)	Incr. plasma Ca concentrat'n.	Tx of Ca deficiency, incl. hypoparathyroidism (**Oral:** Adults - approx. 2 g elemental Ca/day in divided doses. **IV:** Adults - Initially 20 mL of 10% solut'n of calcium gluconate, injected slowly, followed by a slow infus'n of a 0.3-0.8% solut'n [30-40 mL of a 10% solut'n in 500-1000 mL of isotonic NaCl or D5W inject'n] over 3-12 h. Infants - 2 mL/kg of a 10% solut'n)	Anorexia, nausea, weakness, weight loss, vague aches and stiffness, constipat'n, diarrhea, convuls'ns, mental retardat'n, anemia, mild acidosis	**Corticosteroid:** Administrat'n may interfere w. Ca absorpt'n. **Digitalis:** And Ca^{+2} ions have sim. effects on myocardium. Inject'n of Ca preparat'ns is strictly contraindicated in digitalized pts. **Tetracyclines:** Absorpt'n is reduced by oral Ca preparat'ns.	**Assess:** Establish extent of hypocalcemia; establish baseline VS and fluid intake/output ratio; for hx renal calculi; diet for Ca intake; for concurrent use of tetracyclines or digitalis preparat'n. **Administer:** With meals to avoid gastric irritat'n. **Evaluate:** For relief of s/s hypocalcemia; for evidence of hypercalcemia. **Teach:** As for vitamin D (see above).

Pharmacologic Classification: Hormonal Therapy

Drug	Action	Use/Dosage	Side Effects	Interactions	Nursing Implications
Calcitonin (Calcimar)	Calcitonin is a hormone secreted by the thyroid gland, released in response to an incr. in ionized plasma Ca. It decr. bone resorpt'n and incr. Ca excret'n.	Tx of symptomatic Paget's disease of bone; rapid tx of hypercalcemic emergencies [along w. other appropriate agents] (**SC/IM:** For hypercalcemia - 4 IU/kg q12h; incr. to 8 IU/kg q12h if response is not satisfactory within 1-2 days. If response is still unsatisfactory after 2 more days, a max. of 8 IU/kg may be given q6h)	Nausea w. or without vomiting. Local inflammatory react'ns at inject'n site, facial flushing, metallic taste, tingling of hands	See Table 46	**Assess:** For hx allergy to fish, esp. salmon; administer skin test for allergic response. **Administer:** Solut'n reconstituted w. diluent provided by manufacturer; store reconstituted solut'n in refrigerator; discard any unused solut'n after 2 weeks; warm refrigerated solut'n before preparing inject'n. **Evaluate:** Drug effectiveness as indicated by ameliorat'n of s/s hypercalcemia; for evidence of adv. effects, esp. systemic hypersensitivity react'ns and early evidence of hypocalcemia. **Teach:** That nausea and vomiting in initial period of tx will resolve as tx progresses; proper sterile inject'n technique for self-administrat'n at home; indicators of adv. effects.
Prednisone	Decr. Ca absorpt'n.	Hyperparathyroidism (**Oral:** Initially, 5-60 mg/day, divided into 4 equal doses. Maint. dose, 5-10 mg/day)	See Table 46	See Table 46	See Table 46

CHAPTER 28

Insulin and Oral Hypoglycemics

Teaching Objectives

Following completion of this chapter, the reader should be able to:

1. Define diabetes mellitus.
2. Discuss the effects of insulin on intermediary metabolism.
3. Describe the consequences of insulin deficiency in diabetes mellitus.
4. Explain the diagnostic criteria for diabetes mellitus.
5. List the subclasses of diabetes mellitus and describe the symptoms of each.
6. Explain the therapeutic objectives in the treatment of diabetes mellitus.
7. Describe the different preparations of insulin and explain the use of each.
8. Discuss the nursing process associated with the use of insulin.
9. Discuss insulin resistance and its treatment.
10. Describe the adverse effects of insulin and their treatment.
11. List the two groups of oral hypoglycemic drugs and describe their mechanisms of action, therapeutic uses and adverse effects.
12. Discuss the nursing process related to the use of oral hypoglycemics.
13. Compare glucagon with insulin and describe its therapeutic use.

Diabetes mellitus, or diabetes as it is often called, is being diagnosed with increasing frequency. Although it is not completely understood, it has been established that diabetes mellitus is a genetically and clinically heterogeneous group of disorders characterized by high blood sugar concentrations.

The actions of insulin and the metabolism of glucose are interwoven. A 70-kg human has only 350 – 400 g of glucose and glycogen. In spite of this, glucose plays a vital role in body metabolism. It is the major source of energy for all cells and the only source for brain and nerve tissue. Glucose is also readily converted to fats and may supply carbon atoms for the synthesis of some amino acids.

Under normal conditions glucose absorption from the gastrointestinal tract stimulates insulin release. However, the blood level of glucose is not the only factor determining the extent of insulin release. Insulin release is greater if glucose is absorbed through the gastrointestinal tract, when compared to an equivalent rise in plasma glucose following intravenous infusion. It is likely that intestinal factors involved in the absorption of glucose also play a role in the release of insulin. In addition to glucose and intestinal factors, amino acids increase insulin secretion.

Insulin is synthesized in islets of the pancreas and stored in two compartments in beta cells. The smaller compartment, containing approximately 2% of the insulin, releases the hormone quickly in response to stimulation. The larger compartment, containing 98% of the insulin, serves as a store for the hormone, replenishing the smaller compartment as it secretes its supply. Insulin-dependent diabetics have little or no insulin in either compartment. Noninsulin-dependent diabetics are not insulin deficient but may have a reduced capacity to secrete the hormone in response to metabolic stimulation. In these individuals the problem may lie in

Table 39
Diagnostic criteria for diabetes mellitus.

Diabetes Mellitus in Nonpregnant Adults

Any of the following are considered diagnostic of diabetes:

A. Presence of classic symptoms of diabetes, such as polyuria, polydipsia, ketonuria and rapid weight loss, together with gross and unequivocal elevation of plasma glucose.

B. Elevated fasting glucose concentration on more than one occasion:
venous plasma   ≥ 140 mg/dL (7.8 mmol/L)
venous whole blood   ≥ 120 mg/dL (6.7 mmol/L)
capillary whole blood   ≥ 120 mg/dL (6.7 mmol/L)

If the fasting glucose concentration meets these criteria, the oral glucose tolerance test (OGTT) is *not required.* Indeed, virtually all persons with fasting plasma glucose (FPG) > 140 mg/dL will exhibit an OGTT that meets or exceeds the criteria in C, below.

C. Fasting glucose concentration less than that which is diagnostic of diabetes (B, above) but sustained elevated glucose concentration during the OGTT on more than one occasion. *Both* the 120-min sample *and* some other sample taken between administration of the 75-g glucose dose and 120 min later must meet the following criteria:
venous plasma   ≥ 200 mg/dL (11.1 mmol/L)
venous whole blood   ≥ 180 mg/dL (10.0 mmol/L)
capillary whole blood   ≥ 200 mg/dL (11.1 mmol/L)

Impaired Glucose Tolerance (IGT) in Nonpregnant Adults

Three criteria must be met: the fasting glucose concentration must be below the value that is diagnostic for diabetes; the glucose concentration 120 min after a 75-g oral glucose challenge must be between normal and diabetic values; and a value between 30-min, 60-min or 90-min OGTT value later must be unequivocally elevated.

Fasting value:
venous plasma   < 140 mg/dL (7.8 mmol/L)
venous whole blood   < 120 mg/dL (6.7 mmol/L)
capillary whole blood   < 120 mg/dL (6.7 mmol/L)

30-min, 60-min or 90-min OGTT value:
venous plasma   ≥ 200 mg/dL (11.1 mmol/L)
venous whole blood   ≥ 180 mg/dL (10.0 mmol/L)
capillary whole blood   ≥ 200 mg/dL (11.1 mmol/L)

120-min OGTT value:
venous plasma of between   140 – 200 mg/dL
(7.8 – 11.1 mmol/L)
venous whole blood of between   120 – 180 mg/dL
(6.7 – 10.0 mmol/L)
capillary whole blood of between   140 – 200 mg/dL
(7.8 – 11.1 mmol/L)

Normal Glucose Levels in Nonpregnant Adults

Fasting value:
venous plasma   < 115 mg/dL (6.4 mmol/L)
venous whole blood   < 100 mg/dL (5.6 mmol/L)
capillary whole blood   < 100 mg/dL (5.6 mmol/L)

120-min OGTT value:
venous plasma   < 140 mg/dL (7.8 mmol/L)
venous whole blood   < 120 mg/dL (6.7 mmol/L)
capillary whole blood   < 140 mg/dL (7.8 mmol/L)

OGTT values between 30-min, 60-min or 90-min OGTT value later:
venous plasma   < 200 mg/dL (11.1 mmol/L)
venous whole blood   < 180 mg/dL (10.0 mmol/L)
capillary whole blood   < 200 mg/dL (11.1 mmol/L)

Glucose values above these concentrations but below the criteria for diabetes or IGT should be considered nondiagnostic for these conditions.

Diabetes Mellitus in Children

Either of the following are considered diagnostic of diabetes:

A. Presence of classic symptoms of diabetes, such as polyuria, polydipsia, ketonuria and rapid weight loss, together with a random plasma glucose greater than 200 mg/dL.

B. In asymptomatic individuals, *both* an elevated fasting glucose concentration *and* a sustained elevated glucose concentration during the OGTT on more than one occasion. Both the 120-min sample *and* some other sample taken between administration of the glucose dose (1.75 g/kg ideal body weight, up to a maximum of 75 g) and 120 min later must meet the criteria below:

Fasting value:
venous plasma   ≥ 140 mg/dL (7.8 mmol/L)
venous whole blood   ≥ 120 mg/dL (6.7 mmol/L)
capillary whole blood   ≥ 120 mg/dL (6.7 mmol/L)

120-min OGTT value and an intervening value:
venous plasma   ≥ 200 mg/dL (11.1 mmol/L)
venous whole blood   ≥ 180 mg/dL (10.0 mmol/L)
capillary whole blood   ≥ 200 mg/dL (11.1 mmol/L)

Impaired Glucose Tolerance (IGT) in Children

Two criteria must be met: the fasting glucose concentration must be below the value that is diagnostic of diabetes, and the glucose concentration 120 min after an oral glucose challenge must be elevated.

Fasting value:
venous plasma   < 140 mg/dL (7.8 mmol/L)
venous whole blood   < 120 mg/dL (6.7 mmol/L)
capillary whole blood   < 120 mg/dL (6.7 mmol/L)

120-min OGTT value:
venous plasma   > 140 mg/dL (7.8 mmol/L)
venous whole blood   > 120 mg/dL (6.7 mmol/L)
capillary whole blood   > 120 mg/dL (6.7 mmol/L)

Normal Glucose Levels in Children

Fasting value:
venous plasma   < 130 mg/dL (7.2 mmol/L)
venous whole blood   < 115 mg/dL (6.4 mmol/L)
capillary whole blood   < 115 mg/dL (6.4 mmol/L)

120-min OGTT value:
venous plasma   < 140 mg/dL (7.8 mmol/L)
venous whole blood   < 120 mg/dL (6.7 mmol/L)
capillary whole blood   < 140 mg/dL (7.8 mmol/L)

the inability of the pancreas to store or release insulin from the smaller compartment.

Insulin regulates the entry of glucose into many tissues. Under its influence, glucose enters skeletal and cardiac muscle and fat to act as a source of energy. In the absence of insulin, glucose cannot enter these tissues. Not all tissues depend on insulin for the entry of glucose. Glucose can enter nerve tissue, kidney tubules, liver and intestinal mucosa cells, even in the absence of insulin.

Insulin can also influence glucose metabolism. In its presence, glucose is converted in the liver to its storage form, glycogen. The absence of insulin, and the consequent inability of the body to use glucose as an energy source, forces the body to move to other food stores. Triglycerides are broken down to fatty acids which are then metabolized in the liver and elsewhere to provide energy. The increased utilization of fat results in the accumulation of its metabolic byproducts, ketone bodies. Betahydroxybutyric acid and acetoacetate are the two main ketone bodies to accumulate. Insulin deficiency causes muscles to waste because protein is converted to amino acids which are then metabolized to provide energy.

Diagnosis of Diabetes Mellitus

The medical diagnosis of diabetes mellitus can be based on the unequivocal elevation of plasma glucose concentration, together with the classic symptoms of polyuria, ketonuria, polydipsia and weight loss. Patients whose nursing assessment reveals these symptoms should be immediately referred to a physician for further assessment and diagnosis. The physician may also diagnose diabetes mellitus on the basis of elevated fasting plasma glucose concentrations on more than one occasion or elevated plasma glucose concentrations after an oral glucose challenge on more than one occasion. Table 39 sets out the diagnostic criteria for diabetes mellitus in nonpregnant adults and children; it also establishes the criteria for impaired glucose tolerance in nonpregnant adults and children. These patients are in a gray area between normals and diabetics. They should be monitored by the physician to determine whether diabetes mellitus will ensue.

Classes of Diabetes Mellitus

Patients suffering from diabetes mellitus may be placed in one of two subclasses. The first, referred to as **type I** or **insulin-dependent** diabetes mellitus, includes patients who usually experience an abrupt onset of symptoms, insulin deficiency and dependency on injected insulin to sustain life. They are prone to ketosis. In the past this condition was usually called juvenile or growth-onset diabetes because it occurred most often in juveniles; however, it can occur at any age. Thus, it is inappropriate to classify it by age.

In **type II, maturity-onset** or **noninsulin-dependent** diabetes mellitus, patients are not prone to ketosis. Ketosis may occur during stress brought on by infections or trauma. If diet or oral hypoglycemic drugs are not sufficient to correct symptomatic, or persistent, fasting hyperglycemia, these patients will require insulin. Noninsulin-dependent diabetics may show a range of insulin responses to glucose, ranging from low to above-normal secretion of the hormone. They may be asymptomatic for years with only a slow progression of the disease. In spite of this, noninsulin-dependent diabetics demonstrate the typical chronic associations and complications of diabetes. These are atherosclerosis, microangiopathy, neuropathy and cataracts. Formerly called adult-onset diabetes mellitus because it most often occurs after the age of forty, it is now recognized to occur as well in young persons.

Gestational diabetes (see Table 40) refers to the onset of glucose intolerance in women during pregnancy. By definition it excludes women who were diabetic before pregnancy. If patients remain diabetic after pregnancy, they must be reclassified as type I (insulin-dependent) or type II (noninsulin-dependent) diabetics.

Table 40
Gestational diabetes.

Two or more of the following values after a 100-g oral glucose challenge must be met or exceeded:

	Venous Plasma	Venous Whole Blood	Capillary Whole Blood
Fasting	105 mg/dL (5.8 mmol/L)	90 mg/dL (5.0 mmol/L)	90 mg/dL (5.0 mmol/L)
1 h	190 mg/dL (10.6 mmol/L)	170 mg/dL (9.5 mmol/L)	170 mg/dL (9.5 mmol/L)
2 h	165 mg/dL (9.2 mmol/L)	145 mg/dL (8.1 mmol/L)	145 mg/dL (8.1 mmol/L)
3 h	145 mg/dL (8.1 mmol/L)	125 mg/dL (7.0 mmol/L)	125 mg/dL (7.0 mmol/L)

Pharmacologic Treatment of Patients with Diabetes Mellitus

The treatment of patients with diabetes mellitus has two goals. The initial or short-term objective of treatment is to relieve the symptoms of the disease, to overcome ketoacidosis, and to restore normal growth, weight gain and resistance to infections by achieving normal blood sugar levels. This goal has been achieved with more success than the long-term objective, which is to avoid the complications of diabetes mellitus, particularly those affecting the vascular and nervous system that often appear after fifteen to twenty years of the disease. Insulin-dependent diabetics obviously require treatment with the hormone. Noninsulin-dependent patients may respond to changes in the diet or to oral hypoglycemic drugs.

Insulin

Pharmacokinetics of Insulin Preparations

Most commercial preparations of insulin are made from a combination of beef and pork zinc insulin crystals and are formulated to provide effects that are rapid, intermediate or prolonged. The pharma-cokinetic characteristics of these insulins are summarized in Table 41. These values should not be taken to indicate specific times in hours for the onset and duration of action of the various insulins because of the great intra- and interpatient variability observed. They do, however, provide an approximate comparison of the pharmacokinetics of the various insulin preparations.

Regular crystalline insulin is clear in appearance. Its peak activity can be seen in two to four hours and its duration of action is six to eight hours. Longer-acting insulins are complexed with protamine (NPH, PZI) or formulated as large crystals (Lente series) to reduce their rates of absorption. Semilente insulin is turbid and has a rapid onset of action. However, its actions are more prolonged than regular crystalline insulin.

NPH and Lente insulins are intermediate-acting products. Peak activity occurs six to twelve hours after injection. Durations of action last from twenty-four to twenty-eight hours. Protamine zinc insulin and Ultra Lente insulin are prolonged-acting products. Peak activity is seen fourteen to twenty-four hours after injection. Durations of action extend to thirty-six hours or more.

The Iletin II insulins are highly purified insulins. Iletin II insulins are particularly suitable for patients now taking beef-pork insulin who have persistent local or systemic allergy, or those currently taking beef-pork insulin or beef insulin who have developed insulin lipodystrophy.

Human biosynthetic insulin (Humulin) is a highly purified insulin formed by recombinant DNA. Identical to human insulin and free of animal pancreatic impurities, it is less likely to induce immunoglobulin E and G (IgE and IgG) production. Its use should result in a reduced incidence of allergies and resistance. Humulin is recommended by its manufacturer for (1) newly diagnosed insulin-

Table 41
Characteristics of available insulins.

Type of Insulin	Source	Action (Hours)		
		Onset	Peak Effect	Duration
Regular Iletin I (IV, SC)	Beef/Pork	0.5	2 - 4	5 - 7
Regular Ietin II (IV, SC)	Pork	0.5	2 - 4	5 - 7
Semi Lente II (SC)	Pork	1 - 2	2 - 4	12 - 16
NPH Iletin I (SC)	Beef/Pork	1 - 2	6 - 12	24 - 28
NPH Iletin II (SC)	Pork	1 - 2	6 - 12	24 - 28
Lente Iletin I (SC)	Beef/Pork	1 - 3	6 - 12	24 - 28
Lente Iletin II (SC)	Pork	1 - 3	6 - 12	24 - 28
Ultralente Iletin I (SC)	Beef/Pork	4 - 6	18 - 24	36 or more
Protamine Zinc Iletin I (SC)	Beef/Pork	4 - 6	14 - 24	36 or more
Portamine Zinc Iletin II (SC)	Pork	4 - 6	14 - 24	36 or more
Human Insulins				
Humulin R (IV, SC)	Recombinant DNA	0.5	2 - 4	5 - 7
Humulin N (SC, IM)	Recombinant DNA	1 - 2	6 - 12	18 - 24
Humulin 30/70 (SC, IM)	Recombinant DNA 30% Regular insulin 70% NPH insulin			up to 24
Humulin L (SC, IM)	Recombinant DNA	4 - 6	14 - 24	up to 24
Humulin U (SC, IM)	Recombinant DNA			24 or more

Iletin II = Highly purified insulins containing < 1/1 000 000 parts proinsulin, compared with < 20 parts proinsulin in normal insulin. Human insulin formed by recombinant DNA is less likely to induce IgE and IgG.

IV = intravenous; SC = subcutaneous; IM = intramuscular

Prepared from information provided in *Yesterday, Tomorrow — Total Commitment to Total Diabetes Care*. Indianapolis: Eli Lilly. Reproduced with permission.

dependent patients, (2) newly diagnosed insulin-requiring patients with maturity-onset diabetes and (3) patients with existing maturity-onset diabetes who are new to insulin therapy.

Humulin is formulated as a rapidly acting preparation with a short duration (five to seven hours) of action (Humulin-R). It is also produced in the form of two intermediate-acting products. Humulin-N is an NPH insulin and Humulin-L is a Lente insulin. Both products have durations of action of up to twenty-four hours. Humulin-U is an Ultralente insulin with a slower onset of action than regular insulin and a longer duration of action (at least twenty-four hours or more.)

Therapeutic Uses of Insulin Preparations

Insulin must be used in patients with insulin-dependent diabetes and should be considered for individuals afflicted with diabetes mellitus before thirty years of age. Any patient with ketosis, persistent ketonuria, or ketoacidosis should be treated with insulin. Insulin should be administered to diabetics with severe infections and gangrene. It is also indicated in noninsulin-dependent diabetics in whom diet or oral hypoglycemics, or both, have failed. Insulin should also be used in noninsulin-dependent diabetics who are taking corticosteroids or suffering from reduced kidney or liver function.

Gestational diabetes should be treated with insulin if diet alone is unsuccessful. Oral hypoglycemics are not indicated because they will cross the placenta and stimulate fetal insulin production abnormally.

The choice of the appropriate insulin preparation(s) depends on the unique needs of each patient. Rapidly acting insulin is the preparation of choice when an immediate effect is required, such as in the treatment of ketoacidosis and coma, following surgery, or in the treatment of acute infections with fever. Several doses of insulin per day could also be used as maintenance therapy. However, many patients find several daily injections unacceptable. In these situations, the intermediate- or prolonged-acting formulations may be selected to meet the requirements of each patient.

Insulin Resistance

Insulin resistance is caused by the presence of large amounts of IgG insulin-binding antibodies. Most patients require less than 50 – 60 units of insulin per day. This is slightly more than the 30 – 40 units of insulin a normal human secretes per day. Doses in excess of 100 units daily are uncommon. If the dosage requirements reach 200 units per day, insulin resistance is said to have occurred.

Insulin resistance usually is self-limiting, lasting from less than a month to a year or more. It is usually treated by increasing the daily dose of insulin. Another approach involves switching the source of insulin from beef or beef-pork to purified pork. Human insulin may be used extensively in the future. If these steps fail, corticosteroid therapy, usually 40 – 80 mg of prednisone daily, may be given for a maximum of one month to reduce antibody formation. Corticosteroids have an intrinsic hyperglycemic effect. As a result, insulin requirements may rise initially and then fall as IgG levels are reduced. Corticosteroid therapy should be started in a hospital or conducted carefully on an outpatient basis.

Obesity reduces target organ sensitivity and can induce chronic insulin resistance. A reduction in weight or food intake will usually restore normal insulin sensitivity. Cushing's disease and hyperthyroidism will increase the dosage of insulin required.

Acute insulin resistance can occur during stress. Surgery, trauma, emotional upheaval or infections are common causes of acute insulin resistance. Large doses of insulin, water and electrolytes may be required while attention is directed to treating the precipitating cause.

Adverse Effects

Hypoglycemic reactions are of the greatest concern. The signs of hypoglycemic reactions depend, at least in part, on the speed at which plasma glucose levels fall. A rapid drop in plasma glucose concentration releases epinephrine from the adrenal medulla, resulting in pallor, sweating, trembling, tachycardia, weakness and hunger. A more gradual fall in plasma glucose levels does not trigger the same release of epinephrine. In this case the signs of hypoglycemia are headache, blurred vision, diplopia, incoherent speech, mental confusion, coma and convulsions. These effects are due to a lack of substrate for the brain. As mentioned before, the brain depends entirely on glucose for its source of energy. Severe insulin-induced hypoglycemia can decrease brain oxygen consumption by almost fifty per cent.

Allergic reactions, both local and systemic, are also of great concern. Drug sensitivity, usually beginning several weeks after starting therapy and characterized by an erythematous, indurated area around the injection site, is the most common reaction. Generalized reactions usually start with urticaria and may rarely proceed through angioedema and anaphylaxis. Patients who are allergic to standard insulin preparations may be tried on either the "highly purified" insulins (Iletin II) or human insulin (Humulin).

Lipodystrophies, involving either atrophy or hypertrophy of fat, can occur at sites in which insulin is injected repeatedly.

Nursing Process

Assessment

Nursing assessment of patients prior to the administration of insulin should seek evidence of hypersensitivity to the insulin being used. Patients who have developed systemic allergic reactions to insulin from one source (e.g., beef insulin) will usually benefit from being changed to insulin from another source (e.g., pork). Human insulin will be used extensively in the future, particularly for individuals who are allergic to beef and pork insulin. The patient's dietary intake should be assessed, in consultation with a dietician, in order to identify any changes that might influence the amount of insulin required. Similarly, periods of emotional stress or a change in the patient's activity or exercise level might require an alteration in the dose of insulin required.

The patient's drug regimen should be reviewed, in consultation with the pharmacist, as part of the nursing assessment for the addition or deletion of drugs that modify the hypoglycemic effect of insulin. Steroids (corticosteroids or anabolic steroids), diuretics (furosemide, ethacrynic acid, thiazides), hormones (thyroid, estrogen, oral contraceptives), monoamine oxidase inhibitors (pargyline, tranylcypromine) and beta blockers (propranolol) all alter the effect of insulin.

Nurses should also test the patient's urine for sugar and acetone to detect early indications of hyperglycemia or ketosis, e.g., dry flushed skin, dry mouth and excessive thirst, anorexia, shortness of breath, acetone breath odor, low blood pressure, weak and rapid pulse, and dimness of vision. In addition, if a review of the patient's history reveals a gradual progression of symptoms over a period of several days, excessive food intake, insufficient insulin intake (perhaps due to omission of a dose), infection, fever, or vomiting, withhold the prescribed dose of insulin until the physician is contacted.

Administration

The procedure for the administration of insulin is initiated by examining the contents of the vial. Any medication that is outdated, discolored, clumped, cloudy, unused after being opened for several weeks, or has been exposed to extremes of temperature (either heat or cold) or strong sunlight should be discarded. Vials containing insulin precipitates should be rolled between the palms and gently turned end for end in order to assure that the precipitate is evenly dispersed. Vigorous agitation of these vials is to be avoided since it will result in the formation of froth on the surface and the uneven suspension of the precipitate. After the suspension has been prepared in the preceding fashion, select an insulin syringe calibrated in units corresponding to the strength of the insulin (e.g., a 40-unit syringe to administer 40 IU insulin). Usually the barrels of disposable syringes are color coded. This color matches the color on the label of the corresponding insulin strength. In order to prevent lipoatrophy, injection sites should be carefully rotated according to a prearranged and documented plan.

Insulin should be administered 15 – 60 min before a meal, depending on the type of insulin being used. The actual injection procedure is the same as for any sterile subcutaneous injection. A half-inch needle is used and inserted at a 45° angle to the surface of the bunched skin. Some authorities advise stretching the surface of the skin when injecting over adipose tissue such as on the abdomen. Subcutaneous injection is essential in order to ensure that the insulin is absorbed at the appropriate rate. If insulin is injected intramuscularly or intravascularly it is absorbed too rapidly and hypoglycemia can occur. Always aspirate carefully on the barrel of the syringe in order to ensure that accidental intravascular injection is prevented.

Evaluation

When patient evaluation reveals evidence of hypoglycemia, nurses may administer 10 g of fast-acting carbohydrate immediately, e.g., a small box of raisins, 125 mL (4 oz.) fruit juice, four or five dried fruit pieces. Slowly digested carbohydrates (e.g., three saltines, 33 g (0.5 oz.) cheese, 250 mL (8 oz.) nonfat yogurt may be needed after 10 g of fast-acting source. The frequency and intensity of hypoglycemic incidents should be noted along with relevant information about dietary intake, level of activity or psychological stressors associated with the events. This information is essential in determining whether or not a dosage adjustment is required. Nurses should also investigate for hyperglycemia because its presence indicates the need for adjustment of the therapeutic regimen.

The nurse who discovers an unconscious diabetic should immediately summon a physician. Unconsciousness in a diabetic can be due to hypoglycemia, hyperglycemia, ketosis or unrelated causes. In view of the fact that intravenous glucose will rapidly reverse the effects of hypoglycemia and not harm patients with other causes of coma, nurses can anticipate that the physician will administer this first without waiting for the results of blood sugar levels. Sometimes 0.5 – 1 mg of glucagon can be prescribed intravenously in place of glucose.

Teaching

Patient teaching related to the pharmacological aspects of the treatment of diabetes mellitus is very important. The reader is referred to a medical-surgical nursing textbook for detailed information regarding the total teaching needs of patients with diabetes mellitus. The first priority for patient education related to insulin-dependent diabetes must be teaching proper sterile injection procedures. Nurses should emphasize the importance of maintaining adequate supplies of insulin and syringes on hand, especially when traveling or over long weekends when pharmacies may be closed. Patient teaching will include instruction in the use of capillary blood glucose equipment, the need to monitor blood glucose versus urine glucose, reading and recording blood glucose levels, and the increased need for testing if the patient is sick or meals are missed.

Patients and their families should be instructed in the early identification of insulin's adverse effects. Patients who are taking insulin should be advised to wear a medical identification bracelet or carry a card that contains pertinent medical information. Patients should be instructed to carry raisins or dried fruit as first aid treatment for hypoglycemic incidents. They should also be instructed to seek medical advice for any change in health status. In the event of illness, bed rest and high fluid intake are indicated until a physician is available.

During the initial period of insulin therapy, visual disturbances may occur. These are a result of fluctuations in blood glucose levels which cause osmotic changes in the lens and the vitreous and aqueous humors. Patients should be counselled to expect this and to persevere for approximately two months until the condition stabilizes, rather than seek an immediate change of glasses.

Patients should be referred for dietary counselling with particular emphasis on the interaction between insulin and diet. A referral to a home health or public health agency for evaluation and followup after discharge from hospital will identify those areas of patient teaching which require further emphasis or clarification.

Oral Hypoglycemic Drugs

Oral hypoglycemic drugs can be divided into sulfonylureas and biguanides. Table 42 lists some of the oral hypoglycemics available in North America.

Mechanism of Action and Pharmacologic Effects

Sulfonylureas require the presence of insulin to be effective. These drugs (1) stimulate the release of insulin from the pancreas; (2) increase the action of insulin on the liver to decrease hepatic glucogenesis; and (3) increase the action of insulin on muscle to increase glucose utilization.

Sulfonylureas are well absorbed when taken orally. They differ mainly in their respective durations of action. With the exception of chlorpropamide, all sulfonylureas are extensively metabolized in the body. Chlorpropamide is not significantly metabolized. It is cleared largely unchanged by the kidneys. This drug has the longest half-life of the sulfonylureas and can be given on a once-daily basis.

Metformin also requires the presence of insulin to lower blood sugar. Its mechanism of action is not clear. Metformin may decrease the absorption of glucose from the intestinal tract or increase its utilization in the body by stimulating anaerobic glycolysis, or both.

Table 42
Some oral hypoglycemic drugs used in North America.

Drug and Class	Duration of Action (h)
Sulfonylureas	
Acetohexamide (Dimelor)	10 – 16
Chlorpropamide (Chloronase, Diabinese)	20 – 60
Glyburide (Diabeta, Euglucon)	10 – 15
Tolazamide (Diabewas, Tolinase)	10 – 16
Tolbutamide (Mobenol, Orinase)	6 – 10
Biguanide	
Metformin (Glucophage)	5 – 6

Therapeutic Uses

Oral hypoglycemics are used only in patients with noninsulin-dependent diabetes mellitus. Many authorities believe further that these drugs should be restricted to those who are not treated effectively by diet alone and who are unwilling to take insulin. Contraindications to the use of oral hypoglycemics include ketoacidosis; coma; stress conditions such as severe infection, trauma or surgery; or the presence of frank jaundice, liver disease, or renal disease or impairment. Oral hypoglycemics should not be administered during pregnancy or lactation. No evidence exists that they are more effective than diet control. Oral hypoglycemics do not prevent the cardiovascular complications of diabetes mellitus.

Adverse Effects

The adverse effects of the sulfonylureas appear to be minor and involve between one to five per cent of patients. Only one to two per cent of patients are required to discontinue therapy. The adverse effects mentioned most frequently involve hypoglycemia, allergic skin reactions, gastrointestinal problems, blood dyscrasias and liver dysfunction. Sulfonylureas may also produce disulfiram (Antabuse)-type reactions when taken with alcohol.

The adverse effects of metformin involve primarily the gastrointestinal tract. These include a metallic taste, anorexia, nausea and vomiting, as well as diarrhea.

Nursing Process

Assessment

Prior to the administration of a sulfonylurea, nurses should review the patient's history for evidence of recent or impending stressful life events, either physical (surgery, infection, trauma, fever) or psychosocial (death of a close friend or relative, examinations, business reverses, divorce, marriage). Any of these situations may require a short-term alteration in the therapeutic regimen. These patients should be subjected to particularly cautious and careful nursing evaluation following the initiation of therapy.

The nursing assessment should also include a review of the patient's total drug regimen, in consultation with the pharmacist, for recent additions, deletions or dosage changes that alter the efficacy of the oral hypoglycemic. The simultaneous use of diuretics, corticosteriods, oral contraceptives (estrogen/progestin combinations) or nicotinic acid reduces the hypoglycemic effect of sulfonylureas. The concurrent use of long-acting sulfonamides, tuberculostatics, phenylbutazone, clofibrate,

monoamine oxidase inhibitors, coumarin derivatives, salicylates, probenecid or propranolol potentiates the hypoglycemic effect of sulfonylureas.

A nursing assessment that reveals a history of ketosis, type I diabetes mellitus, malnutrition, liver or kidney disease, pregnancy, cardiovascular disease, retinopathy or neuropathy necessitates withholding the drug until the attending physician verifies the prescription.

Nursing assessment of patients prior to the administration of metformin resembles that described for sulfonylureas. Specifically, a patient history of ketosis, type I diabetes mellitus, malnutrition, liver or kidney disease, diabetic complications (e.g., retinopathy, neuropathy), cardiovascular or respiratory disease, pregnancy, alcohol abuse, lactic acidosis, or the imminent occurrence of diagnostic procedures leading to temporary oliguria should result in withholding the drug pending clarification with the attending physician. The patient's drug use profile should be reviewed for anticoagulants (which are potentiated by their use with metformin) and for diuretics, corticosteroids, oral contraceptives (estrogen/progestin) and nicotinic acid, which potentiate the hypoglycemic effect of metformin.

Administration

All sulfonylureas should be given in the morning in order to prevent nocturnal hypoglycemic reactions. They should be administered with breakfast to diminish the gastric disturbances that frequently accompany their use.

As with the sulfonylureas, metformin should be administered with food and at times that will reduce the occurrence of nocturnal hypoglycemia.

Evaluation

Nursing evaluation of the patient receiving one of these drugs is essentially the same as that identified for patients treated with insulin. Additional factors to be considered include observation of the patient for evidence of severe gastric distress (nausea, vomiting, pain, diarrhea); allergic reactions (itching, photophobia, rash); blood dyscrasias (fever, sore throat); liver dysfunction (tea-colored urine, light-colored stools). Any of these situations may require alteration in the dosage, selection of a different sulfonylurea preparation, or replacing the medication with insulin. The fact that these adverse effects are claimed to occur in only one to five per cent of patients should not reduce nursing vigilance in the evaluation of a patient following drug administration. As suggested earlier, nurses should monitor the patient for stressful life events that might alter the efficacy of the therapeutic regimen.

Nurses should evaluate patients receiving metformin for gastrointestinal distress. Patient evaluation should also include observation for early signs of hypoglycemia (note the frequency and severity of such occurrences), hyperglycemia, recent or impending stressful events, bleeding tendencies in the presence of the simultaneous use of anticoagulants, alcohol abuse or lactic acidosis, when the patient has a history of alcohol abuse.

Teaching

Patient teaching in relation to the use of sulfonylureas is similar to that identified for patients who are receiving insulin therapy. In addition, patients should be advised that concurrent use of alcohol and a sulfonylurea may result in a reaction similar to that seen with the combination of alcohol and disulfiram (Antabuse). Therefore, the use of alcohol should be discouraged.

Patient education in relation to the use of metformin is the same as that identified in relation to the use of insulin. In addition, nurses should warn patients of the danger of lactic acidosis when alcohol is consumed during metformin therapy.

Glucagon

Mechanism of Action and Pharmacologic Effects

Glucagon is a hormone synthesized and stored in the alpha cells of the pancreatic islets. The contrasts between it and insulin are striking, in spite of the fact that the two are stored in adjacent pancreatic cells. Insulin secretion is increased when glucose is absorbed from the gastrointestinal tract. The release of glucagon is depressed by glucose absorption. Once released, insulin facilitates the storage of food energy. Glucagon, released when blood sugar levels fall, acts to mobilize glucose to provide energy. Accordingly, insulin secretion is increased and glucagon release decreased following a meal. During a fast, the reverse is true: glucagon secretion is increased and insulin decreased.

Therapeutic Uses

Glucagon is useful in counteracting severe hypoglycemic reactions in diabetic patients, but only if liver glycogen is available. Glucagon is of little or no value in states of starvation, adrenal insufficiency or chronic hypoglycemia. The patient with insulin-dependent diabetes may not have as

great a response in blood glucose levels as the noninsulin-dependent stable diabetic. Both should be given supplementary carbohydrate as soon as possible.

A dose of 0.5 – 1 mg of glucagon given subcutaneously, intramuscularly or intravenously usually awakens the unconscious hypoglycemic patient in five to twenty minutes. If the response is delayed, there is no contraindication to the administration of one or two additional doses of glucagon; however, the use of parenteral glucose must be considered. Intravenous glucose should be given if the patient fails to respond to glucagon.

Adverse Effects

Glucagon is largely free of untoward effects. Nausea and vomiting may occur with large doses. Since glucagon is a protein, the possibility of hypersensitivity reactions remains.

Nursing Process

Assessment

When glucagon is prescribed for a patient, it is often ordered as a p.r.n. medication to be administered at the discretion of the nurse. Glucagon is also ordered in emergency situations. In either case, the nurse should be familiar with any patient history of allergies, kidney or liver disease, or current use of oral anticoagulants. Any of these conditions, or the presence of emaciation or malnutrition, prohibits the administration of glucagon by a nurse.

Administration

Freeze-dried glucagon is reconstituted using the solvent provided by the manufacturer. If refrigerated, the reconstituted solution is stable for three months. The date of reconstitution must be placed on the label. Glucagon should never be administered in a syringe containing any other medication. Immediately following the patient's return to consciousness, oral carbohydrates should be given to prevent rebound hypoglycemia.

Evaluation

Patient evaluation by nursing personnel should emphasize monitoring the level of consciousness, observing for early evidence of hypersensitivity reactions, nausea, vomiting or aspiration. Frequent use of glucagon by patients who are also receiving oral anticoagulants might result in hypoprothrombinemia; therefore, such patients should be observed carefully for increased bleeding tendencies.

Teaching

When glucagon is prescribed as emergency treatment in the home, a responsible member of the patient's family must be taught the signs of hypoglycemia which require the use of the medication. They should also be taught the technique of preparing and administering the medication. The importance of seeking immediate medical assistance following such hypoglycemic episodes must be stressed, so that any necessary adjustments to the therapeutic regimen can be made.

Further Reading

Asmal, A.C. and Marbles, A. (1984). Oral hypoglycemic agents: An update. *Drugs 28* :62-78.

Benon, J.E. (1989). Oral hypoglycemic agents. *New Engl. J. Med. 321* :1231-1245.

Brogden, R.N. and Heel, R.C. (1987). Human insulin. Review of its biologic activity, pharmacokinetics and therapeutic use. *Drugs 34* :350-371.

Diabetes Mellitus, 8th ed. (1980). Indianapolis: Eli Lilly.

Galloway, J. (1980). Insulin treatment of the early '80s. *Diabetes Care 3* :615-622.

Melander, A., Bitzen, P.-O., Faber, O. and Groop, L. (1989). Sulphonylurea antidiabetic drugs: An update of their clinical pharmacology and rational therapeutic use. *Drugs 37* :58-72.

National Diabetes Data Group (1979). Classification and diagnosis of diabetes mellitus and other categories of glucose intolerance. *J. Diabetes 28* :1039-1057.

Robertson, C. (1989). The new challenges on insulin therapy. *R.N. 52* (2):34-38.

Ward, G.M. (1987). The insulin receptor concept and its relation to the treatment of diabetes. *Drugs 33* :156-170.

Zimmerman, B.R. (1989). Influence of the degree of control of diabetes on the prevention, postponement and amelioration of late complications. *Drugs 38* :941-956.

Table 43
Insulin and oral hypoglycemics.

Generic Name (Trade Name)	Use (Dose)	Action	Adverse Effects	Drug Interactions	Nursing Process
Pharmacological Classification: Hormone					
Rapid-acting insulins: Regular insulin (Insulin-Toronto, Insulin-Toronto [Beef], Insulin-Toronto [Pork], Iletin I)	*Rapid-acting insulin:* Onset of action, 30 min - 1 h after inject'n. Approx. peak effect bet. 2-4 h. Durat'n of action, approx. 5-7 h (**SC:** Individualized according to blood or urine glucose. **IV:** *For ketoacidosis* - Adults - 6-10 U/h, infused. Children - 0.1 U/kg/h [w. limitat'n being up to adult dose], given by continuous infus'n. **IM:** *For ketoacidosis when facilities for continuous IV infus'n are limited* - Initially, 10-20 U administered IV, followed by 5-10 U hourly, IM)	Insulin regulates entry of glucose into many tissues. Under its influence, glucose enters skeletal and cardiac muscle and fat, to act as a source of energy. In its absence, glucose cannot enter these tissues. Insulin also influences metabolism of glucose. In its presence, glucose is converted in the liver to its storage form, glycogen. The absence of insulin, and the consequent inability of the body to use glucose as an energy source, forces the body to move to other food stores. Triglycerides are broken down to fatty acids, which are then metabolized in the liver and elsewhere to provide energy. The incr. utilizat'n of fat results in the accumulat'n of its metabolic byproducts, ketone bodies. Beta-hydroxy-butyric acid and acetoacetate are the	Hypoglycemia (manifested by hunger, nervousness, warmth, sweating and palpitat'ns); headache, confus'n, drowsiness, fatigue, anxiety, blurred vision, diplopia; numbness of lips, nose or fingers; local and systemic allergic reactions; fat dystrophies.	**Beta blockers (nonselective):** Enhance the hypoglycemia produced by insulin by interfering w. catecholamine-induced glycogenolysis. Also, the warning sign of tachycardia that may accompany hypoglycemia is us. not seen in beta blocker-treated pts. Concomitant use of a beta blocker and insulin should be avoided if possible. Otherwise, pts should be monitored carefully. **Contraceptives, oral:** Used concomitantly w. oral contraceptives, insulin can cause a decr. in glucose tolerance in diabetic women, poss. resulting in incr. daily insulin requirements. **Diuretics:** May incr., decr. or not change daily insulin requirements. **Epinephrine:** Incr. blood sugar levels and reduces effects of insulin. **Ethanol:** Can incr. insulin's hypoglycemic actions. **Guanethidine:** Can incr. insulin's hypoglycemic actions. **Hormones** (incl. growth hormone, corticotrophin, glucocorticoids, thyroid hormone and glucagon): Reduce hypoglycemic effects of insulin. **MAOIs:** Can incr. hypoglycemic actions of insulin. **Phenytoin:** May antagonize hypoglycemic effects of insulin.	**Assess:** For evidence of hypersensitivity to insulin; urine for sugar and acetone; for alterat'n in dietary intake; for change in activity or exercise level; for incr. stress; for concurrent use of drugs that enhance insulin's hypoglycemic effect; for evidence of hyperglycemia (impending diabetic coma). **Administer:** Solut'n that is *not* outdated, discolored, clumped, cloudy, partially used after being open for several weeks; solut'n that *has* been stored in a cool place and *not* exposed to extremes of temp. (either heat or cold) or to strong sunlight. Disperse suspens'n evenly by rolling vial bet. palms and gently turning end for end; avoid shaking; use an insulin syringe calibrated in units corresponding to strength of insulin; rotate inject'n sites to reduce lipoatrophy; administer 15-60 min before a meal depending on type of insulin; use half-inch needle inserted at a 45° angle to skin surface; avoid IM inject'n; aspirate on barrel of syringe to prevent accidental IV inject'n resulting in immediate, severe hypoglycemia. **Evaluate:** For hypoglycemia (note frequency and severity of occurrences), hyperglycemia, lipoatrophy, local or systemic allergic responses; for recent or impending stressful life events. **Teach:** Proper sterile technique for administrat'n (as above); instruct in technique and interpretat'n of blood glucose readings; importance of keeping adequate supplies on hand,
Highly purified insulin (Velosulin, Regular Iletin II Pork)					
Human biosynthetic insulin (Humulin R)					
Semilente insulin (Semilente Insulin, Semilente Iletin I)	Onset of action, approx. 1-2 h. Peak effect bet. 2-4 h. Durat'n of action 12-16 h (**SC:** *For newly diagnosed mild diabetics* - Initially, 10-20 U 30 min before breakfast. At least 2 daily doses may be nec. No standard dose can be cited for this drug)				
Intermediate-acting insulins: NPH insulin, isophane insulin (NPH Insulin, NPH Iletin, NPH Insulin [Beef], NPH Insulin [Pork], NPH Insulin [Isophane])	*Intermediate-acting insulin:* NPH has onset of action within 1-2 h and lente within 1-3 h. Approx. peak effects, bet. 6-12 h after administrat'n. Durat'n of NPH and lente insulins is us. 24-28 h (**SC:** Individualize dosage. Initially, 10-20 U 30-60 min before breakfast, often combined w. regular insulin. If needed, NPH and regular insulin				

Highly purified insulin (Insulatard NPH, Iletin II Pork)

Human biosynthetic insulin (Humulin N)

Lente insulin (Lente Insulin, Lente Iletin I, Lente Insulin Pork), lente insulin highly purified (Lente Iletin II Pork)

Long-acting insulins: Protamine zinc insulin (Protamine Zinc Insulin, Protamine Zinc Iletin, Protamine Zinc [Beef], Proamine Zinc [Pork])

Ultra lente insulin (Ultra Lente Insulin, Ultra Lente Iletin)

Human biosynthetic insulin (Human L Lente)

may be given in divided doses to provide approx. one-third of daily requirement 30 min before evening meal or hs)

PZI and ultra lente insulins have onset of action 4-6 h following injectn. Approx. peak effects, bet. 14-24 h [PZI] and 18-24 h [ultra lente] following tx. Durat'n of action, 36 h or longer (**SC:** As for NPH [isophane] suspens'n)

main 2 ketone bodies to accumulate. Insulin deficiency causes muscles to waste because protein is converted to amino acids that are metabolized to provide energy.

esp. when traveling or at times when pharmacies may be closed; self-evaluat'n for adv. effects; to wear medical ID bracelet; to carry dried fruit or raisins as first aid tx for hypoglycemia; to seek medical advice for any change in health status; in case of illness, bed rest and high fluid intake should be 1st actions until physician examines pt; no OTC drugs or other medicat'ns without consulting physician; during initial period of insulin tx, vision disturbances may occur. Advise newly diagnosed diabetics to expect this and to persevere until condit'n stabilizes, rather than seek immed. change of spectacle lenses; refer to nutritionist for dietary counseling; refer to home health or public health agency for evaluat'n after discharge from hospital.

Salicylates: In daily doses of 1.5-6 g, can incr. insulin's hypoglycemic effects in some pts.

Steroids, anabolic: Can incr. insulin's hypoglycemic effects in some pts.

Pharmacologic Classification: Oral Hypoglycemics — Sulfonylureas

Acetohexamide (Dimelor, Dymelor)

To control hyperglycemia in responsive diabetes mellitus of the stable, mild, nonketosis-prone, noninsulin-dependent type that cannot be controlled by proper dietary management and exercise, and when insulin tx is not appropriate (**Oral:** 500 mg - 1.5 g daily)

Incr. secret'n of insulin from pancreas, acts w. insulin to decr. hepatic gluco-genesis and incr. glucose utilizat'n in skeletal muscle.

Hypoglycemia, nausea, epigastric fullness and heart-burn, jaundice of both cholestatic and mixed types, allergic skin react'ns, leukopenia, agranulocytosis, thrombocytopenia, hemolytic and aplastic anemia, headache

Anticoagulants, oral: May interact in diff. ways w. oral hypoglycemics. Dicumarol may inhibit metabolism of tolbutamide and incr. serum chlorpropamide levels. Tolbutamide may displace dicumarol from plasma protein binding sites and thus incr. its effects.

Beta blockers: Enhance hypoglycemia produced by oral hypoglycemics, by interfering w. catecholamine-induced

Assess: For recent or impending stress-ful life events, both physical and psychological; hx of ketosis, type I diabetes, malnutrit'n, liver or kidney disease, pregnancy or cardiac disease; review current drug regimen w. pharmacist for recent addit'ns or delet'ns that might alter drug efficacy.

Administer: In a.m. with breakfast.

Evaluate: For hypoglycemia (note frequency and severity of occurrences); for hyperglycemia, GI distress; for itching, photophobia, rash, fever, sore

Generic Name (Trade Name)	Use (Dose)	Action	Adverse Effects	Drug Interactions	Nursing Process
Chlorpropamide (Chloronase, Diabinese)	As for acetohexamide (Oral: Once daily w. breakfast. Middle-aged pts us. begin w. 250 mg/day; older pts begin w. 100-125 mg/day. Dosages may incr. or decr. by 50-125 mg at 3-5 day intervals. Us. range, 100-500 mg daily)	As for acetohexamide	As for acetohexamide	glycogenolysis. Also, warning sign of tachycardia which may accompany hypoglycemia is us. not seen in beta blocker-treated pts. Concomitant use of a beta blocker and an oral hypoglycemic should be avoided. When this is not poss., pts should be monitored carefully. **Chloramphenicol:** Reduces tolbutamide metabolism and incr. half-life of chlorpropamide. **Clofibrate:** Incr. hypoglycemic effects of sulfonylureas.	throat, tea-colored urine, light-colored stools, diarrhea, vomiting; for recent or impending stressful life events. **Teach:** As for insulin; that alcohol consumpt'n concurrently w. sulfonylurea tx may result in a react'n similar to that seen w. disulfiram (Antabuse).
Gliclazide (Diamicron)	As for acetohexamide (Oral: 80–320 mg/day. Dosage of 160 mg and above should be divided int 2 equal pts for bid treatment	As for acetohexamide	As for acetohexamide	**Contraceptives, oral:** Impair glucose tolerance. **Corticosteroids:** Incr. blood sugar levels and may decr. diabetic control.	
Glyburide (Diabeta, Euglucon)	As for acetohexamide (Oral: Us. starting dose in newly diagnosed diabetics is 5 mg/day [2.5 mg in pts over 60 years] for 5-7 days; incr. or decr. in increments of 2.5 mg. Max. dose, 20 mg/day. Maint. dose, us. 5-10 mg/day, given as single dose during or immed. after breakfast or, in the event of light breakfast, at lunch. If dosage > 10 mg is required, take excess w. evening meal)	As for acetohexamide	As for acetohexamide	**Dextrothyroxine:** May incr. blood glucose levels in diabetic pts. **Epinephrine:** Incr. blood glucose levels. Use cautiously. **Guanethidine:** Can incr. oral hypoglycemic's hypoglycemic actions. Pts receiving guanethidine plus an antidiabetic drug should be watched closely for incr. antidiabetic effect. **Halofenate:** May displace sulfonylureas from plasma protein binding sites, thereby incr. their pharmacologic effects.	
Tolazamide (Diabewas, Ronase, Tolinase)	As for acetohexamide (Oral: Initially, 100-250 mg daily w. breakfast, adjusted q4-6 days prn. Administer am'ts > 500 mg/day in 2 doses)	As for acetohexamide	As for acetohexamide	**MAOIs:** Plus oral hypoglycemics, may produce excess. hypoglycemia.	
Tolbutamide (Mobenol, Orinase)	As for acetohexamide (Oral: Initially, 500 mg bid. Adjust dose gradually until minimal effective am't is determined. Maint. dose, 250 mg - 3 g/day. Total daily dose should be given in divided am't throughout day)	As for acetohexamide	As for acetohexamide	**NSAIDs:** Can protentiate actions of oral hypoglycemics. **Phenothiazines:** Can produce hyperglycemia and lead to loss of diabetic control.	

Phenylbutazone: Incr. half-life of acetohexamide's active metabolite; decr. tolbutamide metabolism and displaces tolbutamide from plasma protein binding, increasing its pharmacologic activity.

Rifampin: Stimulates tolbutamide metabolism.

Salicylates: Decr. hyperglycemia of diabetics and displace tolbutamide and chlorpropamide from plasma proteins. Give cautiously.

Steroids, anabolic: Decr. blood sugar levels in diabetic pts. May also inhibit metabolism of oral hypoglycemics.

Sulfonamides: May inhibit metabolism of tolbutamide and displace it from plasma protein binding sites.

Sympathomimetics: May produce hyperglycemia and result in loss of diabetic control.

Thiazides: May inhibit insulin secret'n and produce hyperglycemia.

Thyroid hormones: Incr. dosage requirements for insulin or oral hypoglycemics.

CHAPTER 29

Adrenal Corticosteroids

Teaching Objectives

Following completion of this chapter, the reader should be able to:

1. List the three types of steroids secreted by the adrenal cortex.
2. Discuss the factors controlling the release of cortisol and aldosterone.
3. Describe the actions of glucocorticoids and mineralocorticoids.
4. Explain the basis for the anti-inflammatory effects of glucocorticoids.
5. Explain the rationale for the synthesis of newer glucocorticoids.
6. Describe the use of corticosteroids in replacement therapy.
7. Identify the nursing process associated with corticosteroid replacement therapy.
8. Differentiate between the use of high-dose, short-term; low-dose, long-term; and high-dose, long-term glucocorticoid suppressive therapy.
9. Explain the rationale for alternate-day glucocorticoid therapy.
10. Identify the nursing process related to the use of glucocorticoids for immunosuppressive or anti-inflammatory therapy.
11. Discuss glucocorticoid use in the treatment of rheumatoid arthritis, osteoarthritis, allergic diseases and bronchial asthma.

Physiological Control of Adrenal Cortical Hormone Release

The adrenal cortex secretes glucocorticoids, mineralocorticoids and sex hormones. Glucocorticoids are so named because they have important actions on glucose metabolism. However, their effects are not limited to glucose. These hormones exert major actions on all aspects of carbohydrate, fat and protein metabolism. They also modify cardiovascular function and reduce the response to inflammatory stimuli. Mineralocorticoids increase the renal reabsorption of sodium, chloride and water, while promoting the excretion of potassium. Although the expression corticosteroid can be taken to mean any chemical, natural or synthetic, that possesses glucocorticoid and/or mineralocorticoid properties, it is usually used to refer to drugs with predominantly glucocorticoid effects. In this chapter the words glucocorticoid and corticosteroid are used interchangeably.

Many drugs have been synthesized to mimic, in part or in whole, the effects of the glucocorticoids. These drugs are used to treat many diseases. Their use in the treatment of bronchial asthma, rheumatoid arthritis, chronic inflammatory bowel disease and skin disorders, to mention but four areas, is discussed in separate chapters. Glucocorticoids owe their therapeutic usefulness to their marked metabolic, anti-inflammatory and immunosuppressive actions. This chapter discusses the pharmacologic properties of glucocorticoids and the general principles and nursing process underlying their systemic use.

Regulation of Glucocorticoid Release

Cortisol, also called hydrocortisone, is synthesized in the adrenal cortex and released in response to stimulation from the hypothalamus and pituitary. The hypothalamus releases a chemical called the corticotrophin-releasing factor (CRF), which stimulates secretion of the adrenocorticotrophic hormone (ACTH) from the pituitary. ACTH, in turn, stimulates the adrenal cortex to synthesize and release cortisol. A major factor controlling the release of CRF and ACTH is the circulating level of glucocorticoids. In the face of low plasma cortisol concentrations, CRF and ACTH secretion increase. By way of contrast, high levels of cortisol or synthetic glucocorticoids depress CRF and ACTH release.

Stress increases the release of corticosteroids. In response to stress, blood levels of ACTH increase rapidly. Shortly thereafter cortisol secretion is increased.

Cortisol secretion is subject to diurnal variation. High blood levels of cortisol are found in the early morning hours around 06:00 (a stressful time for most of us), and low levels in the late evening. Individuals who work from midnight to 08:00 and sleep throughout the day show peak plasma cortisol levels just after arising, around 16:00, and low levels just prior to retiring.

Regulation of Mineralocorticoid Release

Aldosterone increases the reabsorption of sodium, chloride and water and the elimination of potassium and hydrogen ions by the kidney. Its actions and the pharmacology of aldosterone antagonists are discussed in Chapter 16. If plasma sodium falls or plasma potassium increases, or blood pressure drops, the adrenal cortex releases aldosterone. This results in an increase in sodium, chloride and water reabsorption and potassium elimination.

Actions of Glucocorticoids

Metabolic Effects

Glucocorticoids produce a variety of effects. They influence the intermediary metabolism of carbohydrates, fats and proteins and modify salt and water balance. In supraphysiological doses, glucocorticoids have marked anti-inflammatory and immunosuppressive effects.

The metabolic actions of glucocorticoids are complex and involve both anabolic and catabolic effects. They increase glucose synthesis and impair its utilization. As a result, blood sugar levels rise. Glucocorticoids have a catabolic action on fat and muscle, releasing free fatty acids, glycerol and amino acids from these tissues and increasing their levels in the blood. Gluconeogenesis – the formation of glucose from fatty acids and amino acids – increases. In addition to their catabolic actions on muscle, glucocorticoids reduce amino acid uptake into this tissue, resulting in muscle wasting. In response to the increase in blood amino acids, glucagon is secreted, further accelerating hepatic glucose output.

The effects of glucocorticoid therapy on fat tissue are apparent to any nurse who has participated in the clinical management of patients receiving these drugs. As mentioned before, the direct effects of glucocorticoids on fat tissue are antianabolic (a decrease in glucose uptake into fat) and catabolic (a breakdown of fat already formed, with an increase in free fatty acid production). These actions are counterbalanced, at least in part, by insulin released in response to the increase in blood glucose levels. Insulin has opposite effects to glucocorticoids. It stimulates lipogenesis and inhibits lipolysis. The consequence of the antagonism between a glucocorticoid and insulin is a redistribution of fat in the body. At sites in which the actions of the corticosteroid predominate, fat is lost; in areas in which insulin dominates, fat accumulates. Nurses will notice a characteristic "moon face" and "buffalo hump" in patients on high-dose glucocorticoid therapy as fat accumulates around the face and in the supraclavicular area following prolonged treatment.

Glucocorticoids interfere with the metabolic actions of vitamin D, causing a reduction in calcium absorption and an increase in its renal clearance. These actions account for the osteroporosis induced by glucocorticoids.

Anti-inflammatory and Immunosuppressive Effects

Glucocorticoids owe much of their therapeutic usefulness to their marked anti-inflammatory effects. These actions are nonspecific and can be directed against inflammatory responses to immunologically mediated disorders as well as to mechanical or chemical injury, or infection. The anti-inflammatory and immunosuppressive responses to corticosteroids correlate with their glucocorticoid potency. In developing new corticosteroids for the treatment of inflammatory disorders, efforts are made to design drugs with marked glucocorticoid and minimal mineralocorticoid effects.

Inflammation was described nearly 1900 years ago as *rubor et tumor cum calore et dolore* (redness and swelling with heat and pain). Glucocorticoids treat each symptom. First, they potentiate the vasoconstrictor effects of circulating epinephrine and norepinephrine, thereby reducing blood flow and redness. The reduced blood flow to the inflamed area also diminishes heat at the affected site. Swelling is a result of increased capillary permeability and the leakage of fluid from blood vessels. Glucocorticoids decrease capillary permeability and reduce the loss of plasma into inflamed tissues. Finally, much of the pain is due to the release of two endogenous mediators of inflammation — histamine and bradykinin. Mast cells synthesize, store and release histamine. Glucocorticoids reduce histamine release by diminishing the accumulation of mast cells at the site of inflammation. The chemical prostaglandin E_2 is synthesized within neutrophils. It serves to increase the pain-producing activities of both histamine and bradykinin. Glucocorticoids reduce neutrophil migration to the site(s) of inflammation and decrease prostaglandin E_2 synthesis and release. Glucocorticoids also diminish T-lymphocyte levels in blood, thereby reducing the cell-mediated immunity response to an inflammatory stimulus.

To the description of inflammation as redness, swelling, heat and pain, may be added one more facet — disturbed function. As a result of fibrin deposition, capillary and fibroblast proliferation and the deposition of collagen and cicatrization, the ability of a joint to move normally is disturbed. Glucocorticoids reduce fibrin deposition and minimize both capillary and fibroblast proliferation. They also decrease the deposition of collagen and cicatrization. It is apparent from the preceding that no one action of glucocorticoids accounts for their anti-inflammatory effects. Rather, this action depends on a large number of glucocorticoid-induced effects.

The use of glucocorticoids to treat inflammatory conditions is a double-edged sword. Although the suppression of inflammation may afford considerable relief or even prove life saving, glucocorticoids can also suppress signs of an infection. Furthermore, patients on long-term, high-dose corticosteroid treatment regimens have a reduced immunologic capability and are at greater risk of infections.

Synthetic Corticosteroids

The introduction of cortisol (hydrocortisone) as a drug provided a major therapeutic advance. However, because cortisol possesses both significant glucocorticoid and mineralocorticoid actions, new steroids have been synthesized with the aim of accentuating glucocorticoid activity and reducing or abolishing mineralocorticoid properties. Table 44 lists the more commonly used glucocorticoids and compares them to cortisol with respect to their anti-inflammatory (glucocorticoid) and sodium-retaining (mineralocorticoid) potencies.

From Table 44 it is apparent that prednisone, for example, is 3.5 times more potent as a glucocorticoid than cortisol, but has only half the mineralocorticoid potency of cortisol. As useful as the data in Table 44 are, they must be reviewed carefully. Glancing along the line for cortisol, for example, might lead the nurse to conclude that this corticosteroid's mineralocorticoid potency is twice its glucocorticoid activity. This is not true. Although cortisol has mineralocorticoid actions, they are considerably less than its glucocorticoid effects. The purpose of providing the values in Table 44 is solely to enable the nurse to compare within the glucocorticoid and mineralocorticoid columns the relative potencies of the various corticosteroids.

Newer steroids have longer half-lives than cortisol. Their biological half-lives are considerably longer than their chemical half-lives because the consequences of steroid action outlast by many hours the presence of the drug in the tissues. Glucocortiods are classified as short-acting (cortisol and cortisone), intermediate-acting (prednisone, prednisolone, methylprednisolone and triamci-

Table 44
Adrenal corticosteroid preparations.

Drug	Anti-inflammatory Potency[1]	Equivalent Potency[1] (mg)	Sodium-retaining Potency	Daily Dose (mg) Above Which HPA Suppression Is Possible[2]		Plasma Half-life (min)	Biological Half-life (h)
				Males	Females		
Cortisol (hydrocortisone)	1	20	2+	20 – 30	15 – 25	90	8 - 12
Cortisone	0.8	25	2+	25 – 35	20 – 30	90	8 - 12
Prednisone	3.5	5	1+	7.5 – 10	7.5	200 or >	18 - 36
Prednisolone	4	5	1+	7.5 – 10	7.5	200 or >	18 - 36
Methylprednisolone	5	4	0	7.5 – 10	7.5	200 or >	18 - 36
Triamcinolone	5	4	0	7.5 – 10	7.5	200 or >	18 - 36
Paramethasone	10	2	0	2.5 – 5	2.5 – 5	300 or >	36 - 54
Betamethasone	25	0.6	0	1 – 1.5	1 – 1.5	300 or >	36 - 54
Dexamethasone	30	0.75	0	1 – 1.5	1 – 1.5	300 or >	36 - 54

[1]Potency is defined as milligram-for-milligram equivalence with cortisol.
[2]HPA means hypothalmic-pituitary-adrenal. Dosage intended as a guide only. The dose in an individual depends on the total body surface area. The figures quoted are those which apply in general.

Modified from: Swartz, S.L., Dluhy, R.G. (1978). Corticosteroids: Clinical pharmacology and therapeutic use. *Drugs 16* :238-255. Reproduced with permission.

nolone) and long-acting (betamethasone and dexamethasone) on the basis of their biological half-lives. Cortisone and prednisone are inactive. They are converted to cortisol and prednisolone, respectively, in the liver. The latter chemicals are responsible for the pharmacological effects of cortisone and prednisone.

Systemic Glucocorticoid Therapy

Replacement Therapy

Corticosteroids may be administered as replacement therapy in primary or secondary adrenal insufficiency. Primary adrenal insufficiency is characterized by inadequate cortisol production, despite the presence of large quantities of ACTH.

The most frequent cause of primary adrenal insufficiency, or Addison's disease, is idiopathic atrophy of the adrenal glands, which results in a deficiency of both cortisol and aldosterone. Treatment for this condition involves the use of both a glucocorticoid and a mineralocorticoid. An appropriate dosage regimen for the treatment of Addison's disease is 20 mg/day of cortisol and 0.1 mg/day of the mineralocorticoid fludrocortisone (Florinef).

Adrenal insufficiency secondary to pituitary insufficiency is characterized by low levels of both ACTH and cortisol and normal levels of aldosterone. Treatment involves replacement of the missing cortisol. Thirty-five to 40 mg of cortisone or 20 – 25 mg of cortisol can be given daily. The normal diurnal secretion of cortisol will be simulated if approximately two-thirds of the daily dose is given on arising in the morning and the remaining one-third around 16:00.

Congenital adrenal hyperplasia (adrenogenital syndrome) results from enzyme deficiencies in the synthesis of cortisol. As a result of low cortisol levels, ACTH secretion is increased, elevating the synthesis and secretion of adrenal androgens. Evidence of the condition in the female is often seen at birth as masculinization of the external genitalia. Diagnosis of the adrenal genital syndrome in males may not be made until later in infancy or in childhood. Treatment involves the administration of a glucocorticoid to suppress ACTH secretion. It may also be necessary to administer a mineralocorticoid if a reduction in both glucocorticoid and mineralocorticoid synthesis occurs.

Suppressive Therapy

General Considerations

Corticosteroids may be given either on a short-term, high-dose; long-term, low-dose; or long-term, high-dose basis for their anti-inflammatory or immunosuppressive effects. The short-term, high-dose regimen, as used for the treatment of emergencies such as status asthmaticus and anaphylactic shock, does not produce pituitary-adrenal suppression. Long-term, low-dose corticosteroid therapy is used in the treatment of chronic conditions, such as rheumatoid arthritis. Serious adverse effects can occur, but they are not as severe as when long-term, high-dose therapy is employed for conditions such as autoimmune hemolytic anemia and temporal arteritis, which require this regimen.

Alternate-day steroid therapy is intended to minimize the consequences of chronic high-dose glucocorticoid treatment. Patients are usually started on a daily corticosteroid regimen until relief is obtained. Thereafter, it may be possibe to convert them gradually to alternate-day treatment by doubling the daily glucocorticoid dose and administering it as a single dose on alternate mornings. Intermediate-acting steroids, such as prednisone (with a biologic half-life of 1.5 days), are most appropriate for alternate-day treatment. They provide protection for most of each forty-eight hour period but still allow enough drug-free time for pituitary-adrenal responsiveness to return before the next dose. Unfortunately, conditions requiring high-dose, long-term treatment often require daily therapy to respond. Short-acting steroids such as cortisol are inadequate for most patients, because the length of time between the cessation of their action and the next dose is usually too long to provide significant protection. On the other hand, long-acting steroids are also inappropriate when used on an alternate-day basis. Because their durations of action exceed forty-eight hours, the patient's pituitary-adrenal function cannot recover before the next dose is given.

The use of supraphysiological doses of a glucocorticoid (75 mg of cortisol or equivalent doses of a synthetic steroid) for longer than two weeks results in suppression of the pituitary-adrenal axis, which

may persist for as long as nine to twelve months following withdrawal of treatment. As a result, to avoid an acute adrenal crisis, glucocorticoid therapy should not be withdrawn abruptly. The first step is to administer the total daily dose on a once-daily basis. Thereafter, the dose can be decreased gradually to physiological levels.

Therapeutic Uses

Glucocorticoids are used nonspecifically in the treatment of inflammatory diseases of the intestine, bronchioles, nose, eyes, ears, skin and joints, as discussed in Chapters 23, 32, 33, 38, 39 and 57, respectively. Their use in these conditions is detailed in the relevant chapters and need not be repeated here. However, it bears pointing out that fear of their adverse effects has relegated glucocorticoids to a position behind other less effective, but also less toxic, drugs.

Corticosteroids are used to treat allergic diseases. However, they are indicated only in situations not controlled adequately by less dangerous agents, such as antihistamines. Since glucocorticoids do not act immediately, life-threatening situations, such as anaphylaxis and angioneurotic edema of the glottis, should be treated with subcutaneous epinephrine. Glucocorticoids are then used in short-term high doses as second-line treatment.

Corticosteroids may be used in the treatment of rheumatic carditis, collagen vascular diseases, renal diseases, cerebral edema, malignant hematological diseases, liver diseases and shock. None of these will be presented in detail in this book. Readers are encouraged to seek out relevant reference texts if they wish to understand the therapeutic value of steroids in the above conditions.

Adverse Effects

Table 45 lists some of the more important complications of long-term, suppressive corticosteroid therapy. The adverse effects are, in most cases, a direct consequence of the major pharmacologic properties of corticosteroids and more often seen when higher doses are used. Following chronic steroid therapy, myopathy presents as a proximal muscle weakness; marked wasting of the musculature is seen in the extremities.

Peptic ulceration is a commonly accepted adverse effect of glucocorticoid therapy. Some authorities dispute the view that glucocorticoids predispose patients to ulcers.

The central nervous system disturbances produced by corticosteroids vary from insomnia, nervousness and slight mood changes, to schizophrenia and suicide attempts. Reactions of

Table 45
Complications of corticosteroid therapy.

Musculoskeletal
    Myopathy
    Osteoporosis/vertebral compression
    Fractures
    Aseptic necrosis of bone

Gastrointestinal
    Peptic ulceration (often gastric)
    Gastric hemorrhage
    Intestinal perforation
    Pancreatitis

Ophthalmologic
    Glaucoma
    Posterior subcapsular cataracts

Cardiovascular and renal
    Hypertension
    Sodium and water retention, edema
    Hypokalemic alkalosis

Metabolic
    Precipitation of clinical manifestations of genetic diabetes
        mellitus, including ketoacidosis
    Hyperosmolar nonketotic coma
    Hyperlipidemia
    Induction of centripetal obesity

Endocrine
    Growth failure
    Secondary amenorrhea
    Suppression of hypothalamic-pituitary-adrenal system

Central nervous system
    Psychiatric disorders
    Pseudocerebral tumor

Inhibition of fibroblasts
    Impaired wound healing
    Subcutaneous tissue atrophy

Suppression of the immune response
    Superimposition of a variety of bacterial, fungal, viral and
        parasitic infections in steroid-treated patients

From: Melby, J.C. (1977). Clinical pharmacology of systemic steroids. *Ann. Rev. Pharmacol. Toxicol. 17*:511-527. Reproduced with permission.

this nature are generally more frequent and more severe in patients with known psychological difficulties.

As a result of their mineralocorticoid activity, many steroids can create problems in patients with pre-existing hypertension or cardiovascular disease. In these individuals, dexamethasone or triamci-nolone (corticosteroids with minimal mineralocorticoid activity) may be preferred, together with a restriction of dietary salt and/or the use of diuretics with supplementary potassium.

The ability of glucocorticoids to induce osteoporosis has already been explained. Patients who are more likely to develop osteoporosis, such as postmenopausal women, elderly, immobilized and diabetic patients, suffer a greater risk of compression fracture of the vertebral column. For these individuals, supplementary therapy with vitamin D and calcium is recommended.

Glucocorticoids stimulate the formation and diminish the utilization of glucose. Thus, latent diabetes mellitus may be unmasked by prolonged steroid therapy and pre-existing disease is often aggravated. Secondary to an alteration in adipose tissue metabolism, patients may accumulate fat in the supraclavicular area ("buffalo hump") and acquire a "moon face".

Corticosteroids can reduce significantly the host defense mechanism. Attention should be given to the possibility of a pre-existing infection before starting steroid therapy, not only for the systemic administration of drugs, but also for their topical use.

Nursing Process

The nursing process is much the same, regardless of whether glucocorticoids are used for replacement purposes or for their anti-inflammatory effects. The only major difference is that adverse effects are more likely to occur in the latter situation because considerably higher doses are needed to reduce inflammation.

Assessment
Prior to administering the first dose of a glucocorticoid, the nurse should review the patient's history for documentation of conditions that increase the risk of using this medication, such as diabetes mellitus, hypertension, congestive heart failure, nephritis, thrombophlebitis, peptic ulcer, psychosis and Cushing's syndrome. Patients' histories should also be reviewed for evidence of pre-existing infections (for example, active tuberculosis, herpes eruptions or fungal infections), pregnancy or lactation. If any of these conditions are found, the initial dose should be withheld, pending confirmation of the order by the physician. If they develop, or are discovered subsequent to the initiation of corticosteroid therapy, the medication should be administered but the physician informed immediately.

As suggested in Chapter 3, in order for nurses to contribute to the evaluation of the effectiveness of the drug, they must be familiar with the goal of therapy. Nowhere is this more important than with the use of glucocorticoids. These drugs are used to treat a wide variety of conditions; therefore, the goal of therapy will determine the baseline assessment data and descriptions to be gathered by nurses as a basis for comparison later during the evaluation phase of the nursing process in order to determine the effectiveness of treatment.

Nursing assessment should emphasize the establishment of baseline measurements of body mass/weight, blood pressure, serum potassium, blood sugar and urine glucose, as well as descriptions of the patient's emotional state and usual sleep pattern. This will allow later evaluation of any adverse effects of the drug.

The nurse should assess the patient already on chronic therapy for recent or impending stressful life events (either physical or psychosocial). Physical stress such as infections, herpes eruptions or pregnancy should be reported immediately to the attending physician. Psychological stresses, including the death of a relative or close friend, marital disruption or occupational pressures, should also be brought to the physician's attention. The doctor will usually order supplementary dosages of the corticosteroid if the crisis is severe.

Administration
Regardless of whether they are given daily or on alternate days, corticosteroids should be administered in the early morning to approximate the peak levels achieved normally. Depending on the needs of the patient and the duration of action of the steroid selected, additional doses may be required during the day. Ideally, the last dose of the day should be given by 16:00, again in order to approximate the natural cyclic levels. These drugs are usually administered with food, to minimize gastric irritation. Corticosteroids should be stored in light-proof containers to prevent deterioration. Intra-articular injections of corticosteroids are used infrequently for the treatment of the acute inflammatory phases of osteoarthritis. These are always administered by a physician. Intramuscular injection is given deeply into a large muscle mass, using a 19-gauge needle. Nurses should rotate the sites of intramuscular injection, avoiding the deltoid muscle.

Evaluation
Nursing evaluation of patients receiving glucocorticoids should consider first the therapeutic effectiveness of the medication. Relief of the symptoms of adrenal insufficiency, in the case of replacement therapy, or inflammation, in the case of anti-inflammatory treatment, are the primary indicators of drug effectiveness.

The importance of monitoring the patient for adverse effects cannot be overstated. The patient's body mass/weight, blood pressure, emotional state, sleep pattern, as well as muscle strength and limb mass should be noted daily. In addition, the patient should be observed for evidence of gastric irritation, infections, inflammation or delayed wound healing. Serious infections or illness often go unnoticed in patients on glucocorticoids because of the absence of inflammatory indicators. Nursing evaluation should also include routine glucose and acetone tests of urine samples for diabetics or those patients with a family history of diabetes. Other patients should have periodic, if less frequent, urine glucose and acetone tests performed to permit early detection of latent tendencies to diabetes, which may be aggravated by the use of glucocorticoids. Patients with congestive heart failure who are receiving these drugs should be observed for sudden weight gain and foot and ankle edema. The patient's diet should be evaluated for potassium, protein, salt and vitamin D intake. If necessary, the patient and family should be referred to a nutritionist for dietary counseling.

As mentioned before, nursing evaluation of the patient receiving corticosteroid therapy should also attempt to identify recent or impending stressful life events (psychological or physiological) which might reduce the response to therapy. Even with the benefit of increased dosage during periods of acute stress, patients on long-term therapy risk acute adrenal insufficiency. Nursing evaluation of patients experiencing this condition will reveal anorexia, nausea, vomiting, dehydration, weakness, lethargy, tachycardia, syncope and hypotension. This situation constitutes a medical emergency and requires the immediate attention of a physician.

It is extemely important that patients be rigorously evaluated for recurrence of the condition for which the drugs were originally prescribed when glucocorticoid therapy is withdrawn, dosage is reduced or frequency of administration is decreased (e.g., from daily to alternate-day administration).

Teaching
Nurses must emphasize to patients on long-term therapy the danger of abrupt drug withdrawal. Patients must be taught to take precautions against accidental abrupt withdrawal. Specifically, they should always wear, or carry, medical-alert jewellery or identification, and maintain adequate supplies of the drug at all times. Nurses should

also teach patients and their families the importance of regular medical supervision and the necessity for making and keeping appointments with the physician. Personal hygiene should be stressed as a means of preventing infection, as should the need to wear shoes at all times. Patients should also be counseled to take precautions against insect bites. They should be cautioned about the risk of osteoporosis and the need to take extra precautions against falling, especially during the winter in regions prone to heavy deposits of ice and snow. Finally, patients and their families should be instructed carefully in the identification of early signs of the adverse effects of corticosteroids.

Further Reading

Adrenal corticosteroids in nonendocrine diseases (1986). In: *AMA Drug Evaluations*, 6th ed., pp. 1089-1104.

Agents used to treat adrenal dysfunction (1986). In: *AMA Drug Evaluations,* 6th ed., pp. 661-687.

Fauci, A.S. (1983). Corticosteroids in autoimmune disease. *Hosp. Pract. 18* :99-114.

Giannotti, B. and Stuttgen, G., eds. (1988). Symposium on topical corticosteroids, today and tomorrow. *Drugs 36* (Suppl. 5):1-61.

Table 46
Adrenal corticosteroids.

Generic Name (Trade Name)	Use (Dose)	Action	Adverse Effects	Drug Interactions	Nursing Process
Pharmacologic Classification: Short-Acting Glucocorticoids					
Cortisol, hydrocortisone (Cortef, Hydrocortone, Solu-Cortef)	Replacement tx in acute or chronic adrenocortical insufficiency or salt-losing forms of congenital adrenal hyperplasia, or as anti-inflammatory agent in a variety of inflammatory disorders *(For chronic adrenocortical insufficiency -* **Oral:** 12-15 mg/m²/day, $2/3$ in a.m. on rising, $1/3$ in afternoon. *For congenital adrenal hyperplasia -* **Oral:** 25 mg/m²/24 h [$1/3$ q8h], or $1/3$ in a.m. and $2/3$ in evening. *For emergencies -* **IV:** Initially, 100 mg. Large doses [50 mg/kg] have been proposed for shock. *For salt-losing crisis in congenital adrenal hyperplasia -* **IV:** 50-100 mg w. IV fluids for 1-2 days until crisis is controlled. *For emergencies when IV route is not possible -* **IM:** 100-250 mg, repeated prn)*	Impairs glucose utilizat'n while incr. its synthesis. Incr. blood sugar. Catabolic actions on fat and muscle release fatty acids, glycerol and amino acids from these tissues and incr. their blood levels. Incr. gluconeogenesis. Reduces amino acid uptake into muscle; results in wasting. Causes redistribut'n of fat in body. Reduces Ca absorpt'n and incr. its renal clearance, causing osteoporosis. Possesses nonspecific anti-inflammatory effects that can be directed against immunologically mediated disorders, mechanical or chemical injury or infect'ns. W. infect'ns, tx must also include appropriate antibacterial, antifungal or antiviral medicat'n.	Na and H_2O retent'n, hypokalemic alkalosis, hyperlipidemia, redistribut'n of fat, myopathy, osteoporosis, growth failure, psychiatric disorders, impaired wound healing, pituitary-adrenal suppress'n, incr. susceptibility to infect'ns. For addit'nal adverse effects, see Table 45.	*The following apply to glucocorticoids in general, unless otherwise stated:* **Amphotericin B:** May have its K-depleting effects incr. by glucocorticoids. **Anticoagulants, oral:** Can have their effects antagonized by corticosteroids, which incr. blood coagulability. Conversely, corticosteroids can incr. danger of hemorrhage because of their effects on vascular integrity. Because of risk of GI tract ulcerat'n and poss. of hemorrhage, pts who receive both corticosteroids and oral anticoagulants should be monitored carefully. **Antidiabetic agents:** May have their effects reduced by glucocorticoids, which incr. blood sugar levels. Monitor pts taking both drugs carefully. **Barbiturates:** Particularly phenobarbital, may incr. metabolism of corticosteroids, necessitating an incr. in steroid dosage. **Diuretics** (thiazides, chlorthalidone, ethacrynic acid, furosemide): May cause an excess. loss of K in pts also receiving a glucocorticoid. **Estrogen-containing products** (such as oral contraceptives): Can incr. serum cortisol-binding globulin. **Indomethacin:** Is ulcerogenic.	**Assess:** For recent or impending stressful life events, either physical or psychological; check BP, sleep pattern, emot'nal status, weight. **Administer:** With food; $2/3$ daily dose in a.m. and remainder about 16:00. **Evaluate:** Proximal muscle strength, sleep pattern, emot'nal status and stability, BP, urine sugar and acetone; diet for K, Ca, protein, vitamin D; refer for dietary counseling prn; for inflammat'n, infectious diseases; herpes erupt'ns, nausea, vomiting, dehydrat'n, weakness, lethargy, tachycardia, hypotens'n. **Teach:** Nec. of medical supervis'n; importance of personal hygiene, esp. foot care, as means of preventing infect'ns; need for caution to prevent fractures resulting from osteoporosis; danger of and precautions against abrupt drug w'drawal; s/s side effects.
Cortisone (Cortone Acetate)	Various, as follows *(For chronic adrenal insufficiency -* **Oral:** 12-15 mg/m²/day, $2/3$ in a.m., $1/3$ in afternoon. *For congenital adrenal hyperplasia -* **Oral:** 20-30 mg/m²/day)*				

Pharmacologic Classification: Intermediate-Acting Glucocorticoids

Generic Name (Trade Name)	Use (Dose)	Action	Adverse Effects	Drug Interactions	Nursing Process
				Combined effects of this drug and corticosteroids may result in incr. incidence or severity of GI tract ulcerat'n. If poss., avoid concomitant use.	
Prednisolone (Delta-Cortef, Dua-Pred, Hydeltra-TBA, Hydeltrasol, Predaline RP, Meticortolone, Saracort, Sterane)	Various, as follows (*For replacement tx* - **Oral:** 4 mg/m²/day, ²/₃ in a.m. and ¹/₃ in afternoon. *For anti-inflammatory effects* - **Oral:** 5-60 mg/day. *For emergencies* - **IV:** 25-50 mg prednisolone sodium phosphate. *For arthritis or bursitis* - **Intra-articular/intrabursal inject'n:** 25 mg for larger joints; 10-15 mg for smaller joints)	As for short-acting glucocorticoids	As for short-acting glucocorticoids	**Phenytoin:** May incr. rate of corticosteroid metabolism. **Rifampin:** May incr. rate of metabolism of corticosteroids, thereby decr. their pharmacologic effects. **Salicylates:** May have their serum concentrat'ns reduced by corticosteroids. Although concomitant use of both drugs is not contraindicated, salicylism may occur if dose of corticosteroid is reduced.	**Assess:** For pregnancy or lactat'n; for hx diabetes mellitus, hypertens'n, hypokalemia, CHF, nephritis, thrombophlebitis, peptic ulcer, psychoses, Cushing's syndrome, active TB, herpes simplex; establish baseline BP, sleep pattern. **Administer:** With meals during initial doses; give maint. doses in early a.m. with food; regularly — never w'draw drug abruptly; store in light-proof container; IM inject'n given deep (not in deltoid); rotate sites; use 19-gauge needle. **Evaluate:** Tx effectiveness; daily weight, muscle strength, limb mass; for hyperglycemia; BP bid until dose is regulated; for infectious diseases, inflammat'n, wound healing; diet for K, protein and NaCl intake; refer to dietician prn; for recent or impending stressful life events; emot'nal status and stability; sleep pattern; for GI irritat'n; for adv. effects. **Teach:** As for cortisol.
Prednisone (Deltasone, Meticorten, Orasone)	Various, as follows (*Replacement tx* - **Oral:** 4 mg/m²/day, ²/₃ in a.m., ¹/₃ in afternoon. *Inflammatory condit'ns* - **Oral:** 5-60 mg/day)	As for short-acting glucocorticoids	As for short-acting glucocorticoids	As above	
Methylprednisolone (Medrol, Depo-Medrol, Solu-Medrol)	Various, as follows (**Oral:** Initially, 4-60 mg/day. *For severe shock* - **Oral:** Initially, 100 mg, repeated q2-6h. Alternatively, 200 mg initially, followed by 100 mg q4-6h. *For prolonged effects (allergic, dermatologic, collagen diseases)* - **IM:** 40-120 mg methylprednisolone acetate q1-4weeks. **Intra-articular:** 40-80 mg. **Intrales'nal:** 20-60 mg. **Soft tissue:** 4-30 mg)	As for short-acting glucocorticoids	As for short-acting glucocorticoids	As above	
Triamcinolone (Aristocort, Aristospan, Kenacort, Kenalog)	Various, as follows (**Oral:** Adults - 4-48 mg/day. After satisfactory response, reduce dose by 2 mg q2-3days, to opt.	As for short-acting glucocorticoids	As for short-acting glucocorticoids	As above	As for cortisol and prednisolone.

maint. level. **Oral: Children** - under 27 kg - 4-12 mg/day; over 27 kg - adult dose. Maint. level in children is regulated by clinical respose. **IM:** Adults - 40-80 mg triamcinolone acetonide. Children - 6-12 years - 40 mg initially. As durat'n is variable, subsequent doses for adults and children should be given when s/s recur. **Intra-articular/intrabursal:** Adults - up to 10 mg triamcinolone acetonide for smaller areas; up to 40 mg for larger areas. Tx should be repeated on recurrence of symptoms. **Intrales'nal:** Max., 1 mg/injectn site of triamcinolone acetonide)

Pharmacologic Classification: Long-Acting Glucocorticoids

Drug	Dosage				
Betamethasone (Celestone, Celestone Phosphate, Celestone Soluspan)	Various, as follows (**Oral:** 0.25-1 mg tid or qid. **IM/IV:** Initially, up to 9 mg betamethasone sodium phosphate/day. Parenteral dose is us. one-third to one-half the 12-h oral dose. **IM suspens'n:** 6-12 mg betamethasone acetate-betamethasone sodium phosphate. **Intra-articular:** 1.5-12 mg betamethasone acetate-betamethasone sodium phosphate. **Intrales'nal:** 0.2 mL/cm² betamethasone acetate-betamethasone sodium phosphate suspens'n, containing 3 mg betamethasone acetate and 3 mg betamethasone sodium phosphate per mL. Max. dose, 1 mL. **Soft tissue inject'n:** 1.5-6 mg betamethasone acetate-betamethasone sodium phosphate suspens'n)	As for short-acting glucocorticoids	As for short-acting glucocorticoids	As for short-acting glucocorticoids	As for cortisol and prednisolone

Generic Name (Trade Name)	Use (Dose)	Action	Adverse Effects	Drug Interactions	Nursing Process
Dexamethasone (Decadron, Delalone, Dexone, Hexadrole)	Various, as follows (**Oral:** 0.75-9 mg/day initially, divided into 2-4 doses. **IV/IM:** 4-20 dexamethasone sodium phosphate initially for emergencies)	As for short-acting glucocorticoids	As for short-acting glucocorticoids	As for short-acting glucocorticoids	As for cortisol and prednisolone
Paramethasone (Haldrone)	(*For antiinflammatory effects -* **Oral:** 2-24 mg/day)	As for short-acting glucocorticoids	As for short-acting glucocorticoids	As for short-acting glucocorticoids	As for cortisol and prednisolone
Pharmacologic Classification: Mineralocorticoids					
Desoxycorticosterone acetate (Doca Acetate) Desoxycorticosterone pivalate (Percorten Pivalate)	Addison's disease; congenital adrenal hyperplasia (**IM:** *For chronic primary adrenal cortical insufficiency* - 1-2 mg desoxycorticosterone acetate. For salt-losing congenital adrenal hyperplasia - 1-2 mg/day for first 3-4 days, adjusted thereafter prn; 25 mg desoxycorticosterone pivalate equals 1 mg desoxycorticosterone acetate solut'n in oil. Av. dose for desoxycorticosterone pivalate is 25-100 mg q4weeks)	Has almost no glucocorticoid activity. Decr. excret'n of Na; incr. excret'n of K; incr. blood volume and extracellular fluid; decr. hematocrit.	Hypertens'n, edema, hypokalemia, cardiac enlargement, CHF. All result from Na and H_2O retent'n and K loss.	As for glucocorticoids	As for cortisol and prednisolone
Fludrocortisone acetate (Florinef Acetate)	(*Chronic primary adrenal cortical insufficiency* - **Oral:** 0.05-0.1 mg fludrocortisone acetate/day. Salt-losing forms of congenital adrenal hyperplasia - Initially, doses up to 0.2 mg/day, reduced gradually over several months to 0.05-0.1 mg/day)	Very potent mineralocorticoid, w. moderate glucocorticoid effects. Only mineralocorticoid available for oral administrat'n)	As for desoxycorticosterone.	As for glucocorticoids	As for cortisol and prednisolone

CHAPTER 30

The Sex Hormones

The Physiological Secretion and Action of the Sex Hormones

No organs are the subject of so much social comment as the ovaries and testes. Never content to carry on their work quietly, these organs occupy center stage as they promote both the reproductive and recreational activities of men and women. Students of gonadal function readily recognize the exocrine and endocrine importance of the ovaries and testes. The exocrine activities are manifest in the synthesis and release of ova or sperm and their endocrine prowess is demonstrated by the formation and secretion of estrogens, progesterone and androgens.

Role of the Pituitary

Behind every successful gonad stands a good pituitary. **Follicle stimulating hormone (FSH)** and **luteinizing hormone (LH),** secreted by the anterior pituitary, control both the exocrine and endocrine functions of the ovaries and testes. In females, FSH stimulates the ovaries to produce ova and estrogens. LH acts first in concert with FSH in females to promote ovulation and later alone to stimulate progesterone and estrogen synthesis by the corpus luteum. In males, FSH increases growth of the seminiferous tubules and LH stimulates production of testosterone by Leydig's cells in the testes. FSH, LH and testosterone act together to stimulate spermatogenesis. In the absence of FSH and LH, humans would find this world much less crowded and a lot less interesting.

Estrogens and Progesterone

The word estrogen is used to describe a chemical that possesses female sex hormone properties. The human ovary secretes two estrogens, **estradiol,** sometimes called estradiol-17-beta, and **estrone.** A third estrogen, **estriol,** is a metabolic product of both estradiol and estrone. Estradiol is the estrogen of greatest biological significance in humans.

Once secreted, estrogens have pronounced effects on the body. Among other things, their presence or absence determines an individual's sex. Few tissues in the body are not affected by estrogens. In the female, estrogens are responsible for the physiologic changes that occur at puberty and are essential for the development of the reproductive organs. They increase the mitotic activity and stratification of the cells of the vaginal epithelium and cause a proliferation of the uterine cervical mucosa. Estrogens produce endometrial mitoses, increase the height of the epithelium, and improve the blood supply and capillary permeability of uterine vessels. In response to estrogen stimulation, uterine water and electrolyte content increase. In contrast, ovariectomy produces atrophic changes in all uterine tissues. Estrogens also stimulate stromal development and ductal growth in the breasts.

Estrogens are responsible for the accelerated growth phase in maturing females and for closing the epiphyses of the long bones at puberty. The other metabolic actions of the estrogens include at least a partial responsibility for the maintenance of normal skin and blood vessel structure in females. Although estrogens do not stimulate bone formation, they decrease the rate of bone resorption in ovariectomized women.

Progesterone is also secreted by females. It is synthesized and secreted by the corpus luteum and placenta. Progesterone's effects are usually seen only when tissues have been stimulated previously by estrogens. Both hormones are important in establishing the proper uterine environment for the fertilized egg. Whereas estrogens act to stimulate the growth of sensitive tissues, progesterone, released later in the menstrual cycle, converts the newly formed cells into secretory tissue. For example, estrogens increase stromal and ductal development in the breasts and progesterone subsequently prepares the mammary glands for lactation. Progesterone reduces uterine motility and prepares the estrogen-stimulated endometrium for egg implantation and gestation.

In view of their importance to ovulation, fertilization and implantation, it is not surprising that FSH, LH, estrogens and progesterone show cyclic surges in secretion. FSH and LH secretions peak shortly before ovulation occurs (Figure 23). Plasma estradiol levels (E_2) rise quickly before FSH and LH release occurs. Thereafter, plasma estradiol falls, only to rise again six to eight days after ovulation, before decreasing once more prior to menstruation. In contrast to the biphasic pattern of estrogen release, progesterone secretion remains low during the first half of the cycle and increases markedly after ovulation and corpus luteum formation. **17-hydroxyprogesterone (17-OHP)** is a progesterone metabolite. Its levels reflect progesterone release. This secretory pattern (Figure 23) is understood when it is remembered that a function of progesterone is to prepare the estrogen-stimulated endo-metrium for the implantation of the fertilized egg and gestation. If fertilization does not occur, progesterone secretion falls and menstruation ensues.

Figure 23

Schematic representation of the plasma levels of gonadotropins and gonadal steroids during the human menstrual cycle.

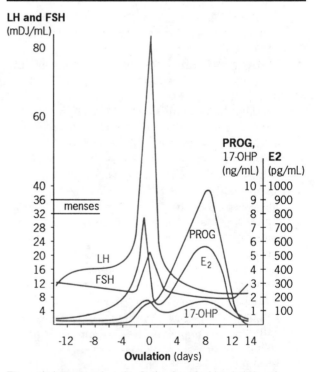

The cycle is centered on day 0, the day of midcycle LH peak. LH = leuteinizing hormone; FSH = follicle-stimulating hormone; PROG = progesterone; E_2 = plasma estradiol; 17-OHP = 17-hydroxyprogesterone.

From: L. Speroff and R.L. Vande Wiele (1971), Regulation of the human menstrual cycle. *Amer. J. Obstet. Gynec. 109* : 234-247. Reproduced with permission.

Androgens

Male sex hormones are collectively called androgens. **Testosterone** is the major androgen secreted
by males. The secretion of androgens begins in
earnest at the time of puberty and is responsible for
the conversion of the boy to the man. The testes are
the main source of androgens in males and they
secrete large amounts of testosterone. Many other
organs, such as the skin, salivary and adrenal
glands, can also secrete androgens. Under normal
conditions, however, their contribution to the total
androgen pool in the male is small.
Androstenedione is secreted by female adrenals
and accounts for most of the androgens found in
women. Under normal conditions, androgen secretion in women is much lower than the quantities of
estrogens released.

Testosterone is responsible for the full morpho-
logical and functional development of the male
reproductive tract, including the accessory glands
and external genitalia. Castration removes the
major source of androgens from the body and it is
impossible for the skin, salivary glands or adrenals
to pick up the slack. In the face of such a calamity
the seminal vesicles and prostate suffer a marked
reduction in size and secretory capacity.

Androgens are also responsible for many of the
other characteristics that distinguish males from
females. They initiate recession of the male
hairline (setting up the rumor that bald men are
more virile) and determine distribution and growth
of hair on the face, body and pubes. Androgens can
also take credit for the bass section in the church
choir because they enlarge the larynx and thicken
the vocal chords.

The effects of androgens on sexual development
in the male are more obvious than their actions on
body metabolism, but these should not be forgotten.
The secretion of testosterone increases protein
anabolism and decreases protein catabolism.
Androgens increase the ability of muscles to work
by stimulating the number, thickness and tensile
strength of muscle fibers. Following the separation
of a male from his testicles, most skeletal muscles
either stop accumulating protein or accumulate it at
a reduced rate.

Pharmacologic Preparations of the Sex Hormones

Estrogens

Pharmacokinetics

The naturally occurring estrogens are estradiol,
estrone and estriol. Only estradiol is used as a drug
and its action is greatly reduced by significant
metabolism as it passes through the liver in the
portal circulation (the first-pass effect). Several
approaches may be used to overcome this problem.
It may be injected as estradiol benzoate, estradiol
cypionate (Depo-Estradiol, E-Ionate PA) and estradiol valerate (Delestrogen). In these forms estradiol
is absorbed slowly, misses the portal circulation and
has a long duration of action.

Another approach that facilitates oral administration and still circumvents first-pass metabolism
is to administer synthetic estrogenic drugs that are
not rapidly inactivated by the liver. These include
ethinyl estradiol (Estinyl, Feminone), diethylstilbe-
strol (Honvol, Stibilium, Stiphosterol) and quine-
strol (Estrovis). A popular oral product, Premarin,
is obtained from pregnant mares' urine. Premarin
contains the sodium salts of conjugated estrogen
sulfates.

The most recent development in estrogen therapy is the development of a transdermal therapeutic
system (Estraderm). The 17-ß-estradiol is held in a
reservoir between an occlusive backing and micro-
porous membrane that controls the rate of release
of the drug. A contact adhesive holds the system to
the skin through which the estradiol then passes,
entering the blood of the dermis. In appropriately
selected postmenopausal women Estraderm is both
effective and well tolerated.

Therapeutic Uses

Estrogens are used for several therapeutic indications. The most common use of estrogens is in oral
contraceptives. As this involves the concomitant
administration of a progestin, the subject of oral
contraceptives is discussed later in this chapter.
Estrogen use is contraindicated in patients with
active hepatic dysfunction or disease, especially of
the obstructive type. They are also contraindicated
in patients with a personal history of breast or
endometrial cancer. Endometrial hyperplasia also

contraindicates estrogen therapy without accompanying progestagen. Other contraindications for estrogen use include undiagnosed vaginal bleeding, a history of cerebrovascular accident, coronary thrombosis, the presence of classical migraine, a history of thrombophlebitis or thromboembolic disease, partial or complete loss of vision or diplopia arising from ophthalmic vascular disease, and suspected pregnancy.

Estrogens can be used as replacement therapy. This is most commonly seen in treating the symptoms of menopause. The decline in ovarian function often produces characteristic hot flashes that may alternate with chills. Inappropriate sweating and paresthesias can also occur. Other symptoms of menopause are muscle cramps, myalgias, arthralgias, overbreathing, palpitation, anxiety, faintness and syncope. Estrogen treatment relieves the hot flashes and other vasomotor effects as well as atrophic vaginitis. Postmenopausal osteoporosis may also be offset for at least one year by estrogen administration. Therapy usually involves estrogen administration for three to four weeks followed by a week without treatment. This procedure is often repeated for six to nine months.

Replacement estrogen therapy is indicated when the ovaries fail to develop. In Turner's syndrome ovarian dysgenesis with dwarfism occurs. Treatment with an estrogen produces breast enlargement and menses but does not cause the normal growth spurt or ovarian maturation. Hypopituitarism causes ovarian, thyroidal and adrenal cortical failure. Replacement therapy in girls involves treatment with thyroxine, adrenal cortical hormones and an estrogen.

Estrogens can provide relief from dysmenorrhea by inhibiting ovulation. Cyclic therapy with oral contraceptives is often successful. However, the current trend is to treat primary dysmenorrhea with inhibitors of prostaglandin E_2alpha synthesis. Prostaglandin E_2alpha accumulates in the uterus immediately before menstruation and provokes uterine contractions. Drugs such as aspirin, ibuprofen (Motrin, Rufen), naproxen (Naprosyn), naproxen sodium (Anaprox) and mefenamic acid (Ponstan, Ponstel) block prostaglandin synthesis. They are given for three to four days each month, just before and during the first one or two days of menstruation.

Estrogens are often used to suppress postpartum lactation because they inhibit prolactin secretion. However, bromocriptine (Parlodel) is gaining popularity because of its lack of estrogenic adverse effects. This drug has dopaminergic properties and mimics the action of the prolactin-inhibiting factor (PIF) secreted by the hypothalamus. As a result, the release of prolactin by the pituitary is reduced and galactorrhea stopped. However, some experts maintain that, because of fear of adverse effects, neither sex hormones nor bromocriptine should be used routinely for lactation suppression.

An estrogen, often combined with a progestin in an oral contraceptive tablet, can be used to treat endometriosis by reducing FSH secretion. Although some patients can be withdrawn from this treatment after four to six months and remain symptom free, most relapse and require additional estrogen therapy or surgery. The drug danazol (Cyclomen, Danocrine) also prevents FSH secretion. It appears more effective in endometriosis treatment with a lower rate of relapse once withdrawn. Danazol is also used in the treatment of benign fibrocystic breast disease.

Adverse Effects

Nausea is the most frequent adverse effect of estrogen treatment. This can be compared with the morning sickness experienced during the early months of pregnancy. If large doses of an estrogen are used, patients may suffer anorexia, mild diarrhea and/or vomiting. The effects of estrogens on blood coagulation are discussed later in this chapter under the topic oral contraceptives.

Nursing Process

Assessment

Prior to administration of estrogen replacement therapy, the nurse should review the patient's history for any evidence of an undisclosed malignant breast lesion, cardiovascular disease, calcium or potassium imbalance, and family history of malignancies of the breast or reproductive organs. Physical assessment should emphasize detection of blood dyscrasias, hepatic disease, thyroid disease, pregnancy or lactation. A nursing assessment that reveals any of these justifies withholding the medication pending verification by the physician. Nursing assessment prior to estrogen administration should also establish the patient's age, weight and sleep patterns.

Administration

Estrogen replacement therapy is usually self-administered by the patient on a cyclic schedule depending on the preparation prescribed by the physician. Readers are advised to consult the particular product monograph for detailed information. Titration of the estrogen dose is recommended, with the patient using the lowest effective dose. Estrogen preparations should be given with food or milk to decrease gastrointestinal symptoms.

Evaluation

Evaluation

During and following a course of estrogen therapy patients should be evaluated for possible adverse effects. Early identification of unilateral leg pain, swelling, redness or Homans' sign is important because these observations suggest thrombophlebitis. Other effects of estrogens on blood coagulation are discussed later in this chapter under oral contraceptives. Changes in emotional status or sleep patterns indicate psychological effects of the medication. Evidence of abdominal pain, cramps or discomfort should be documented and reported to the attending physican. Nurses should also evaluate changes in the amount and duration of vaginal bleeding, as these indicate therapeutic effectiveness.

Teaching

Patient teaching related to use of estrogen replacement therapy should emphasize the necessity of regular medical supervision during prolonged therapy, proper administration of the drug according to the prescribed cyclic schedule, and self-evaluation for therapeutic effectiveness and adverse effects. Nurses should advise the patient to measure her body mass/weight weekly and report gains greater than 2 kg (approximately 5 lb.).

Antiestrogens — Clomiphene (Clomid, Serophene)

Mechanism of Action and Pharmacologic Effects

Stimulation of the estrogenic receptors by estradiol, estrone and estriol reduces FSH and LH secretion. Clomiphene competes with estrogens for their receptor sites in the body. By blocking the actions of endogenous estrogens, clomiphene prevents the normal "feedback inhibition" of FSH and LH secretion. Increased quantities of the gonadotropins are secreted, leading to ovarian stimulation, ovulation and sustained corpus luteum formation.

Therapeutic Uses

Clomiphene is effective in the treatment of infertility due to anovulation. It is used in cases of female infertility when anatomical causes have been ruled out. Clomiphene is ineffective in women who have ovarian or pituitary failure or who suffer from undeveloped ovaries. Animal studies have demonstrated teratogenicity at doses twenty to thirty times the dose recommended for humans. As a result, clomiphene should not be administered during pregnancy. In addition, clomiphene is contraindicated in patients with liver disease or a history of liver dysfunction and in patients with bleeding of undetermined origin.

Adverse Effects

The adverse effect of clomiphene results from hyperstimulation of the ovaries. Multiple cysts are formed, resulting in a higher incidence of multiple births. However, the 6 – 8% incidence of multiple births produced by clomiphene is not as high as the 15 – 25% seen after Pergonal (FSH, LH) gonadotrophin administration. Approximately three-quarters of the multiple births resulting from clomiphene treatment are twins.

Nursing Process

Assessment

Prior to administration of clomiphene, nursing assessment should include a review of the patient's history for evidence of hepatic disease, bleeding tendencies, ovarian cysts, neoplastic disease or retinal disorders. The presence of any of these conditions is sufficient reason to reconsider the decision to use the drug. Patients should also be assessed for an existing pregnancy.

Administration

Clomiphene is usually self-administered in the home. The drug is to be taken at the same time every day to maintain drug levels.

Teaching

Patient teaching is of the utmost importance. Patients should be taught to identify an ovulatory response using a basal temperature chart. They should also be alerted to the importance of reporting pelvic pain, abdominal pain or visual disturbances to the physician immediately. Patients should be told that if pregnancy is suspected, they must notify the physician immediately.

Progestins

Pharmacokinetics

Progesterone is rapidly inactivated by the liver and has little activity if given orally. The hormone may be administered intramuscularly to circumvent first-pass liver metabolism. A progestin is a drug that mimics some properties of progesterone. Although some progestins have properties that resemble progesterone very closely, others have inherent estrogenic and androgenic effects. It is beyond the scope of this text to detail the properties of each progestin. Instead, we will describe the therapeutic uses of some of the more commonly used chemicals (see Table 48).

Medroxyprogesterone acetate (Depo-Provera) and hydroxyprogesterone caproate (Delalutin) are two progestins designed for intramuscular injection. Several progestins are available for oral administration. These drugs are not rapidly inactivated when they pass through the liver in the portal circulation. They include megestrol acetate (Megace, Pallace), norethindrone (Micronor, Norlutin), norethindrone acetate (Norlutate) and norethynodrel.

Therapeutic Uses

The major therapeutic use of progestins is in oral contraceptive tablets. This application is discussed later in this chapter.

Dysfunctional uterine bleeding often results from the continuous action of estradiol, causing endometrial hyperplasia, with insufficient progesterone secreted to maintain the endometrium. Progestin therapy often assists the patient. It can be given orally or intramuscularly in the last half of the cycle for six months. After discontinuation, regular spontaneous menstruation may return.

The concomitant use of progestin and estrogen therapy for the treatment of dysmenorrhea, endometriosis and postpartum lactation has been discussed previously. Other indications for progestin therapy are endometrial carcinoma and early pregnancy (threatened abortion and habitual abortion). The use of a progestin for the prevention of abortion must be weighed against the fact that the drug may cause virilization and genital deformities in the fetus.

Progestin therapy is contraindicated in the presence of thrombophlebitis, thromboembolic disorders and cerebral apoplexy. These drugs are also contraindicated in patients with a past history of undiagnosed vaginal bleeding, breast pathology and urinary tract bleeding.

Adverse Effects

Inferential evidence suggests an association between progestin administration early in pregnancy and the occurrence of congenital malformations. Other adverse effects in women taking progestins include breakthrough bleeding, intercyclic spotting, changes in menstrual flow, amenorrhea, changes in cervical erosion and cervical secretion, and breast tenderness. Patients may experience edema and weight gain. Skin sensitivity reactions consisting of urticaria, pruritus, edema and generalized rash have occasionally occurred.

Nursing Process

Assessment

Nursing assessment of the patient receiving progestin therapy for dysfunctional uterine bleeding should establish the extent of the bleeding, including both the amount and duration of the bleeding. Progestins should not be administered to women who have a history of malignancy in the breasts or reproductive organs. Patients for whom this medication is prescribed should be thoroughly assessed to make sure that they are not pregnant because the administration of progestins during pregnancy may cause fetal virilization and genital deformities.

Administration

Progestins are usually self-administered in the home. It is recommended that the dose be titrated to the lowest effective amount. Progestins should be taken with food or milk to prevent gastrointestinal upsets.

Evaluation

Nursing evaluation of the progestin-treated patient should attempt to determine the therapeutic effectiveness of the medication. Evidence of a reduced volume of bleeding, shorter duration of bleeding, greater number of days without bleeding, and re-establishment of a regular menstrual cycle reflects treatment success.

Patient evaluation by nurses should also emphasize early detection of adverse effects. Leg pain, Homans' sign, swelling of one leg, or a red streak on one leg all suggest thrombophlebitis. Similarly, chest pain, an unexplained cough or difficulty in breathing suggest pulmonary embolism. Sudden excruciating headache, alteration in emotional status or an increase in the frequency and severity of headaches should also be noted, especially if accompanied by dizziness or blurred vision, because these symptoms could herald the development of cerebrovascular complications. Edema indicates fluid retention and potential electrolyte imbalance. The drug should be withdrawn immediately if the skin or sclera become jaundiced. Similarly, the discovery that the patient is pregnant should result in the immediate discontinuation of the drug.

Teaching

Patient teaching by nurses should emphasize proper self-administration of this medication. Patients should be taught to evaluate themselves for adverse effects, advised to avoid sunlight, and told to report suspected pregnancy immediately.

Oral Contraceptives

Oral contraceptive tablets became widely available in the early 1960s. Their use expanded rapidly: by 1965 approximately 15% of all married women 15 – 44 years of age in the United States were taking them. In 1973 this had increased to 25%, or about 6.6 million women. In 1977 it was estimated that 54 million women in the world were consuming oral contraceptive tablets. These figures should not come as a surprise. For centuries, humankind has sought a truly efficient method of birth control. Oral contraceptives meet that need, providing efficacy so near to 100% that closer estimates are not possible.

Types of Products and Patterns of Administration

Oral contraceptives contain either a combination of an estrogen plus a progestin, or a progestin alone. Table 47 presents a list of oral contraceptives currently on the market. Combination estrogen-progestin tablets are most popular. They prevent ovulation if taken the same time each day from the fifth to the twenty-sixth day of the cycle. Day one is the first day of menstruation. Bleeding occurs three or four days after stopping the tablets and the cycle is repeated, beginning on day five. Concern over the possible toxicity of estrogens has led to the introduction of products containing as little as 20 μg of estrogen.

Most recently, oral contraceptive tablets have been placed on the market containing variable amounts of estrogen and progestin (Ortho 7/7/7, Synphasic, Triphasil, Triquilar) in an attempt to mimic the normal patterns of estradiol and progesterone secretion. These products are very effective and have a reduced incidence of breakthrough bleeding.

Progestin-only tablets are available as oral contraceptives. Containing either 0.35 mg of norethindrone (Micronor, Nor QD) or 0.075 mg of norgestrel (Ovrette), these products must be taken every day of the cycle at the same time each day. They inhibit the secretion of pituitary gonadotropins, thereby preventing follicular maturation and ovulation, as well as causing changes in the cervical mucus and endometrium. The contraceptive efficacy of progestin tablets is ninety-seven to ninety-eight per cent, somewhat lower than conventional estrogen-progestin tablets. Progestin tablets may cause troublesome irregular bleeding. Contraindications to the use of oral contraceptives have been described earlier under the headings Estrogens and Progestins.

Table 47
Oral contraceptive products.

< 50 μg ethinyl estradiol plus a progestin

Brevicon
Demulen 30
Loestrin 1.5/30
Minestrin 1/20
Mini-Ovral
Ortho 0.5/35
Ortho 10/11
Ortho-Novum 1/35

50 μg ethinyl estradiol plus a progestin

Demulen 50
Norlestin 1/50
Norlestin 2.5/50
Ovral

50 μg mestranol plus a progestin

Norinyl 1/50
Ortho-Novum 1/50

> 50 μg mestranol plus a progestin

Norinyl 1/80
Norinyl 2

Only 0.35 mg norethindrone

Micronor

Variable amounts estrogen and progestin

Ortho 7/7/7
Synphasic
Triphasic
Triquilar

Adverse Effects

Concern has been expressed about the safety of oral contraceptives. This concern has centered in the past on the effects of the estrogen component in the tablets. The greatest attention has been given to the cardiovascular complications of oral contraceptive use. In particular, concern has been expressed that these drugs increase the likelihood of venous thromboembolic disorders, myocardial infarction and stroke. Oral contraceptives do increase the incidence of venous thromboembolism, with the risk of this increasing about three-fold during the first month of treatment. Thereafter the risk remains constant, falling to control levels within a month of stopping treatment. Obesity or moderate cigaret smoking increases the risk of oral contraceptive-induced venous thromboembolism in women over age thirty-five.

Other risk factors must also be considered. It is unlikely that obesity or moderate cigaret smoking (fifteen cigarets or less per day) increases the risk of venous thromboembolic disorders occurring in women under age thirty-five on oral contraceptives. On the other hand, venous thromboembolism may be more prevalent in women with blood groups of types A, B or AB.

The risk of thromboembolism may be reduced significantly by using low-dose estrogen preparations. Tablets containing $50 - 80$ µg of either ethinyl estradiol or mestranol are only one-third to one-half as likely to produce venous thromboses as preparations with $100 - 150$ µg of these estrogens.

The increased risk of myocardial infarction appears to be due to an estrogen-induced rise in platelet aggregation and platelet prothrombin-converting activity. These effects, combined with an increased formation of fibrin around the platelet aggregate, increase the risk of coronary thrombosis. Among current users of the pill between the ages of $30 - 39$ and $40 - 44$, the risks of myocardial infarction are increased approximately three-fold and four-fold, respectively. Decreasing the estrogen component from $100 - 150$ µg of ethinyl estradiol or mestranol per pill to 30 µg diminishes the risk of a myocardial infarct by as much as eighty per cent. In contradistinction to venous thromboembolism, in which the risk increases only during the time the pill is taken, the dangers of myocardial infarction remain higher for up to ten years after cessation of the medication.

Age and smoking increase the risk of a myocardial infarct and death. In women under age thirty-five the risk of death from oral contraceptive use is one-fourth the risk of death from pregnancy and similar to the risk of death associated with other means of contraception. As women age past thirty-five, the risk of death in nonsmokers increases to approach the risk of death associated with complications of pregnancy and exceed the risk of death associated with other means of contraception. In women over thirty-five, the risk of death among smokers on the pill exceeds the risk of death associated with the complications of pregnancy.

The risk of myocardial infarction in users of oral contraceptives is increased in patients with a history of pre-eclamptic toxemia, hypertension, type II hyperlipoproteinemia or diabetes. Hypertension increases the likelihood of oral contraceptive users experiencing a thrombotic stroke. Both cigaret smoking and hypertension increase the risk of a hemorrhagic stroke in women taking the pill.

Concern has also been raised of the possible increase in cancer in women taking oral contraceptives. Studies conducted by the World Health Organization (WHO) have found that oral contraceptives appear to have a protective effect against cancers of the endometrium and ovary. Furthermore, oral contraceptives, as they have been used in the past, appear to have produced little or no net increase in breast cancer in developed countries. The possibility that oral contraceptive use may increase the risk slightly in developing countries should be investigated further.

Oral contraceptives may increase cervical cancer risk, particularly the risk of invasive disease. Alternatively, the observed increase in risk in users may be due to behavioral characteristics of users or their sexual partners that increase the likelihood of exposure to sexually transmitted diseases. Any enhanced risk of cervical cancer due to oral contraceptive use is no greater in developing than in developed countries. Oral contraceptive use probably does not alter the risk of gall bladder cancer.

Nursing Process

Nursing responsibilities to patients for whom oral contraceptives have been prescribed begin in the physician's office. The patient must be fully informed by the nurse about birth control methods and the risks of oral contraceptives. This is essential if the patient is to make a fully informed and rational decision.

Assessment

Nursing assessment should determine whether the patient is intellectually capable of understanding and complying with the instructions for self-administration. The nurse should establish the patient's age, body mass/weight, smoking habits, blood pressure and emotional stability. The physician requires this information to determine the risk factors involved in prescribing oral contraceptives and to establish baseline measures for later comparison. Discovery during nursing assessment of a previously undisclosed history of cardiovascular disease or malignancy of the breast or reproductive organs should be immediately reported to the physician.

Administration

Generally, oral contraceptives are self-administered on an outpatient basis. Patients should be advised to take the drug at the same time every day.

Evaluation

Patients taking oral contraceptives should be examined by nurses for leg pain, Homans' sign, chest pain, difficulty breathing, unexplained cough, severe prolonged headache, increase in frequency and/or severity of headaches, dizziness, visual disturbances, nausea, vomiting, diarrhea, constipation, weight gain, edema, change in emotional status (especially the development of depression), excessive menstrual flow or breakthrough bleeding, vaginal discharge, pruritis vulvae and/or burning on urination. These observations suggest the various adverse effects of oral contraceptives. Other adverse effects are cardiovascular complications, including thrombophlebitis, pulmonary embolus, cerebrovascular disease; gastrointestinal disturbances; emotional instability; menstrual alterations; enlargement of existing fibroids; vaginal infections and fluid/electrolyte imbalances.

Teaching

The goals of patient teaching related to oral contraceptives are to ensure that the patient understands the proper method of self-administration, the criteria for self-evaluation for adverse effects and the importance of reporting the occurrence of adverse effects to the physician. Patients should be told to report suspected pregnancy to the physician immediately.

Androgens

Pharmacokinetics

Testosterone is the major androgen secreted by the testes. Similar to estradiol and progesterone, testosterone cannot be given orally because it is rapidly inactivated during its first pass through the liver in the portal circulation. To circumvent first-pass metabolism, testosterone may be injected intramuscularly as the propionate, enanthate or cypionate ester. Methyltestosterone (Metandren) can be taken either orally or sublingually. Other orally effective androgens are fluoxymesterone (Halotestin), oxandrolone (Anavar) and stanozolol (Winstrol).

Therapeutic Uses

Androgens are used for replacement therapy. Patients suffering from hypogonadism, associated with testicular failure, respond well to long-acting androgens, such as testosterone cypionate (Andro-Cyp, Depo-Testosterone, T-Ionate-PA) or testosterone enanthate (Delatestryl), with the development of secondary sex characteristics and increased potency. Androgens are also given at the age of puberty to males with hypopituitarism.

In view of the widespread use of estrogen therapy in postmenopausal women, it seems fair and reasonable to offer equal opportunity to men in the form of androgen treatment. It is well known that testicular function decreases gradually with advancing years. Signs of this include decreased libido, decreased sexual activity and reduced muscle mass and strength. Plasma testosterone levels decrease around the age of fifty. In cases where plasma testosterone levels are well below those expected, androgen replacement therapy may increase libido, keep the peace at home, and maintain secondary sex characteristics.

Androgens are known to stimulate erythropoiesis. Use has been made of this effect to treat patients with hypoplastic anemia, the anemia of cancer, aplastic anemia, red cell aplasia, hemolytic anemias and those related to renal failure, lymphomas, leukemias and myeloid metaplasias.

Androgens are used for the treatment of recurrent and metastatic carcinoma of the breast; the response is much better in tumors containing estrogen or progesterone receptors, or both.

Several androgens — ethylestrenol (Maxibolin), methylandrostenolone (Dianobol) and stanozolol (Winstrol) — are used for their anabolic effects. They are employed to help postoperative recovery and to treat chronic debilitating diseases. Although possibly beneficial on a short-term basis, they do not alter the outcome of the underlying disease. Their use to accelerate growth is the subject of great controversy. Some children undergo a growth spurt when treated with an anabolic androgen, but the epiphyses may close, compromising future growth.

Athletes may use anabolic androgens in an attempt to gain weight quickly. Although this may take place, much of the initial increase in weight results from the retention of sodium, chloride and water by the kidney. Androgens may increase muscle mass, weight and strength and can appeal to individuals with strong backs and weak brains. However, one cannot condone hormonal therapy in otherwise healthy young men and women. Long-term androgen therapy decreases FSH and LH secretion, leading to testicular atrophy. From the coach's point of view, this might not be a bad idea. It certainly will tend to reduce the desire for extracurricular activity and keep the athlete's mind only on sports.

Androgens are contraindicated in carcinoma of the male breast; known or suspected carcinoma of the prostate; and cardiac, hepatic or renal decompensation. Other contraindications to their use include hypercalcemia; impaired liver function; prepubertal males; patients easily stimulated sexually; pregnancy and lactation.

Adverse Effects

Women taking androgens experience menstrual irregularities. Masculinization can also occur. This is seen first as acne, growth of facial hair and deepening of the voice. Later, male-pattern baldness and excessive body hair may become evident. Marked development of the skeletal muscles and veins, together with hypertrophy of the clitoris, may subsequently ensue.

Androgens are sometimes given to children for their anabolic effects. Whereas the anabolic use of androgens in children may be justified in individual cases, nurses should be aware that serious disturbance of growth, and of sexual and bone development, can occur during chronic therapy. Androgens enhance closure of the epiphyses.

Androgens increase salt and water reabsorption by the kidneys. Edema can be a problem for patients receiving large doses for cancer. It is also undesirable in patients with congestive heart failure, kidney disease or hypoproteinemia.

The other adverse effects of androgens include biliary stasis, leading to jaundice, and hepatic adenocarcinoma. Impotence and azoospermia are also adverse effects of chronic androgen treatment. This may seem strange, given the fact that testosterone is required, together with FSH and LH, for spermatogenesis. However, the daily use of androgens leads to a decrease in FSH and LH secretion, leading to impotence and azoospermia.

Nursing Process

Assessment

Regardless of the purpose for which androgen therapy is initiated, nursing responsibilities begin with assessment of the patient. The goals of nursing assessment are to identify contraindications to androgen use and establish baseline measures for future evaluation of beneficial or adverse effects. Baseline measures include body mass/weight, blood pressure, fluid intake/output ratios and emotional status. The patient's history should be reviewed for previously undisclosed indications of epilepsy, migraine, cardiovascular disease or kidney pathology. Identification of any of these conditions should be reported to the physician immediately. In addition, females for whom this drug is prescribed should be examined for pregnancy or lactation.

Administration

A titrated dose is recommended to identify the lowest effective dose.

Evaluation

Nursing evaluation of patients during androgen therapy will be guided by the purpose for which the drug was prescribed and the sex of the patient. Thus, virilization in male patients is probably a desired therapeutic effect, or at least not an unpleasant one. Mild reversible virilization (mild hirsutism, reduced breast size, acne) in female patients might be tolerated. However, major irreversible virilization (deepened voice, clitoral hypertrophy, male-pattern baldness) in women would be acceptable only in the presence of severe, probably terminal, illness such as metastatic breast cancer. When anabolic androgens are given to children, nurses must remember that serious disturbances of growth and of sexual and bone development can occur during chronic therapy. Remember that androgens accelerate closure of the epiphyses. Edema is usually not a problem when androgens are used as replacement therapy in hypogonadism or hypopituitarism. However, because androgens increase salt and water reabsorption by the kidneys, patient evaluation by nurses should stress early identification of edema in patients receiving large doses for the treatment of malignancies. Obviously, salt and water retention must be detected early in patients who are suffering from congestive heart failure, kidney disease or hypoproteinemia. Other adverse effects requiring nursing evaluation were discussed earlier in this chapter.

Teaching

Patient teaching related to the use of androgens should stress that therapeutic effectiveness requires prolonged therapy. The nature of the desired therapeutic effect should also be described to patients and their families. Patients should be instructed in the importance of a diet high in protein, calories, vitamins and minerals, and if necessary, be referred for dietary counseling by a nutritionist. Female patients can be reassured that mild virilization will reverse when the drug is withdrawn. However, they should be instructed to report pronounced virilization promptly to the physician. Nurses should teach patients and their families to evaluate themselves for adverse effects, along with the importance of quickly reporting any of these observations to the physician.

Further Reading

American College of Sport Medicine (1984). Position stand on use of anabolic-androgenic steroids in sport. *Am. J. Sports Med. 12* :13-18.

Androgens and anabolic steroids (1986). *Drug Evaluations*, 6th ed., pp. 687. American Medical Association.

Choice of contraceptives (1988). *The Medical Letter 30* :105-108.

Choice of contraceptives (1989). Drugs of choice. *The Medical Letter 31* :63-69.

Dyment, P.G. (1984). Drugs and the adolescent athlete. *Ped. Ann. 13* :602-604.

Johnson, M.D., Jay, S. and Rickert, V.I. (1989). Anabolic steroid use by male adolescents. *Pediatrics 83* :921-924.

Medical factors in contraceptive choice (1986). *Drugs and Therapeutics Bulletin 24* (19):73-76.

Mellion, M.B. (1984). Anabolic steroids in athletics. *Am. Fam. Physician 30* (July):113-119.

Thomas, D.B. (1989). OCs and cancer risk: Comparing results from developing and developed countries. *Outlook 7* (4):2-6.

Utian, W.R. (1988). Transderm estradiol. A recent advance in oestrogen therapy. *Drugs 36* :383-386.

Wilson, J.D. and Griffin, J.E. (1980). The use and misuse of androgens. *Metabolism 29* :1278-1295.

Young, R.L. and Golzieher, J.W. (1987). Current status of postmenopausal oestrogen therapy. *Drugs 33* :95-106.

Table 48
Sex hormones.

Generic Name (Trade Name)	Use (Dose)	Action	Adverse Effects	Drug Interactions	Nursing Process
Pharmacologic Classification: Estrogens					
Estradiol (Estrace)	Tx of menopause or failure of ovarian development; also amenorrhea, dysmenorrhea, endometriosis, breast cancer. Prevent'n or cessat'n of postpartum lactat'n (**Oral:** *For menopausal symptoms -* Initially, 1-2 mg/day. Maint. dose, 0.5-2 mg/day, us. for 21 days, followed by 7-day rest. **Estraderm patches:** Apply to skin 2x weekly)	Estrogens are essential for development of reproductive changes that occur at puberty in the female. They incr. mitotic activity and stratificat'n of vaginal epithelial cells, cause proliferat'n of uterine cervical mucosa, produce endometrial mitoses (hyperplasia), incr. height of epithelium (hypertrophy) and improve blood supply and capillary permeability of uterine vessels. Estrogens incr. uterine water and electrolyte content. They stimulate stromal development and ductal growth in the breasts. Estrogens are responsible for accelerated	Nausea, anorexia, vomiting, cholestatic jaundice; Na and H_2O retent'n; breakthrough bleeding; incr. cervical mucus; endometrial hyperplasia; breast swelling and tenderness; incr. blood sugar levels and decr. glucose tolerance; headache, mental depress'n, altered libido, nervousness, dizziness, fatigue, irritability; incr. in BP, aggravat'n of migraine headache; thrombophlebitis, pulmonary embolism, cerebral thrombosis	*The following apply to all estrogenic products:* **Anticoagulants (oral):** Can interact w. estrogens. Estrogens may incr. activity of certain clotting factors in blood, thereby requiring incr. in oral anticoagulant dosage. For pts requiring oral anticoagulant tx, it is advisable to use another contraceptive method. **Corticosteroids:** May demonstrate incr. plasma binding if estrogens are administered. Estrogens can incr. cortisone-binding globulin in serum. They may also slow normal metabolism of hydrocortisdone. As a result, estrogens can produce excess. corticosteroid response. **Rifampin:** May incr. rate of metabolism of estrogens, thereby reducing their effectiveness. If pt is taking estrogen product for contracept'n, it is probably best to use another method.	**Assess:** Hx for evidence of malignant breast lesions, CV disease, Ca or K imbalance, family hx of breast or reproductive malignancy, blood dyscrasias, hepatic or thyroid disease, pregnancy or lactat'n; establish age, baseline weight, sleep pattern. **Administer:** Titrat'n of dose is advised to determine lowest effective dose. **Evaluate:** For weight gain, peripheral edema, thrombophlebitis (Homans' sign); change in mood or sleep pattern; am't, durat'n, discomfort of vaginal bleeding. **Teach:** Nec. for regular medical supervis'n during prolonged use; proper self-administrat'n; self-evaluat'n for adv. effects.
Estradiol cypionate (Depo-Estradiol, E-lonate PA)	As for estradiol (**IM:** *For replacement tx* - 1-5 mg weekly for 2 or 3 weeks)				
Estradiol valerate (Delestrogen)	As for estradiol (**Oral:** 10-40 mg every 1-4 weeks, depending on clinical indicat'n. *For cyclic tx* - 20 mg on day 1 of ea. cycle; 2 weeks after day 1, administer 250 mg hydroxyprogesterone caproate and 5 mg estradiol valerate; 4 weeks after day 1 is day 1 of next cycle)	growth phase in maturing females and for closing of epiphyses of long bones at puberty. They are partially responsible for maint. of normal skin and blood vessel structure in females. Estrogens decr. rate			
Estrone piperazine sulfate (Ogen)	As for estradiol (**Oral:** *Cyclically for replacement tx* - 0.35-1.5 mg/day. A progestin may be added on the last 10 days. **Vaginal:** *For atrophic vaginitis or kraurosis vulvae* - 2-4 g/day, cyclically)		As for estradiol	As for estradiol	As for estradiol
Conjugated estrogens (Premarin)	As for estradiol (**Oral:** *Menopausal symptoms* - 0.625-		As for estradiol	As for estradiol	As for estradiol

Drug	Dose			
(Estradiol, cont'd)	1.25 mg/day, cyclically; a progestin may be added during last 10 days. *Replacement tx in hypogonadism* - 0.625-1.25 mg/day cyclically for 25 days ea. month, w. a progestin added during last 10 days. *Dysfunct'nal uterine bleeding due to atrophic endometrium* - 2.5-5 mg/day in divided doses for 1 week. Regimen should also include a progestin. *Breast carcinoma in women > 5 years postmenopause* - 10 mg tid for at least 3 months. *Prostatic carcinoma* - 1.25-2.5 mg tid. **IV:** *For emergency tx of dysfunct'nal uterine bleeding in presence of denuded endometrium* - 25 mg q4h for 3 doses, followed by an estrogen-progestin preparat'n orally. **Vaginal:** *For atropic vaginitis, kraurosis vulvae* - 2-4 g/day)	of bone resorpt'n in overiectomized women. They are employed in tx of prostatic cancer and in managagement of 5-year postmenopausal breast tumors, in the belief that some cancers are hormone dependent. For example, if a prostatic cancer is androgen dependent, tx w. estrogens (tog. w. castrat'n) is reasonable.		
Ethinyl estradiol (Estinyl, Feminone)	As for estradiol (**Oral:** *Menopausal symptoms* - 0.02-0.5 mg/day for 21 days. A progestin may be added for last 10 days. This is followed by 7-day period without medicat'n. *Funct'nal uterine bleeding* - 0.5 mg od or bid until hemostasis is secured; then cyclic administrat'n of 0.05 mg od-tid during 1st 2 weeks of menstrual cycle; followed by progesterone for 5 days. 3 cycles may be given. *Carcinoma of breast in postmenopausal women* - 0.10 mg tid. *Prostatic carcinoma* - 0.15-3 mg/day hs)	As for estradiol	As for estradiol	As for estradiol
Diethylstilbestrol diphosphate (Honvol, Stilphosterol)	As for estradiol (**Oral:** *Hypogonadism or replacement tx* - 0.2-0.5 mg diethylstilbestrol/day and cyclically. A	As for estradiol	As for estradiol	As for estradiol

Generic Name (Trade Name)	Use (Dose)	Action	Adverse Effects	Drug Interactions	Nursing Process
	progestin may be added during last 10 days. *Breast cancer* - Initially, 15 mg/day; incr. according to tolerance of pt. *Prostatic carcinoma* - Initially, 1-3 mg diethylstilbestrol daily; incr. in advanced cases. **Vaginal suppositories:** *Replacement tx* - up to 7 mg/week.				

Pharmacologic Classification: Progestins

Generic Name (Trade Name)	Use (Dose)	Action	Adverse Effects	Drug Interactions	Nursing Process
Progesterone	*(Depending on the progestin)* Tx of funct'nal menstrual disorders; endometriosis; uterine cancer in nonpregnant women; metastatic cancer of the breast **(IM:** *Diagnostic use in amenorrhea* - 100-200 mg in oil. *Dysfunct'nal uterine bleeding* - 50-100 mg in oil)	*Although comments below refer to progesterone, they can also be taken to reflect actions of all progestins.* Progesterone is synthesized and secreted by corpus luteum and placenta. A progestin is a drug synthesized to mimic some of the actions of naturally occurring progesterone. Progesterone works in associat'n w. estrogens. Its effects are us. seen only when tissues have been stimulated by estrogens. Both hormones are important in establishing proper uterine environment for fertilized egg. Whereas estrogens stimulate growth of sensitive tissues, proges-	Breakthrough bleeding, spotting, change in menstrual flow, amenorrhea; edema, changes in weight; changes in cervical erosion and cervical secret'ns; cholestatic jaundice; rash with or without pruritus; melasma or chloasma; mental depress'n; pain at inject'n site		**Assess:** For pregnancy; review hx for evidence of malignancy of reproductive organs; establish am't and durat'n of uterine bleeding. **Administer:** Titrat'n advised to determine lowest effective dose. Often self-administered daily for 20 days, beg. on day 5 of menstrual cycle. **Evaluate:** For vascular disorders (thrombophlebitis, pulmonary embolism, cerebrovascular disease), edema, alter-at'n in emot'nal status, jaundice, pregnancy. **Teach:** Proper self-evaluat'n for tx efficacy and adv. effects. Advise pt to avoid sunlight; to report suspected pregnancy immediately.
Hydroxyprogesterone caproate (Delalutin)	**(IM:** *For menstrual disorders* - 125-250 mg/cycle)		As for progesterone		
Medroxyprogesterone acetate (Oral - Provera; IM - Depo-Provera)	Various, as follows **(Oral:** *For amenorrhea and dysfunct'nal uterine bleeding* - 5-10 mg/day for 10 days. *Endometriosis* - 30 mg/day. *Menopausal replacement tx* - 10 mg for last 10 days of estrogen adminis-trat'n. **IM:** *Endometriosis* - 150 mg q3months. *Endometrial carcinoma* - 400 mg - 1 g weekly during initial tx)				
Norethindrone (Norlutin)	Various, as follows **(Oral:** *Amenorrhea and dysfunct'nal uterine bleeding* - 5-20		As for progesterone		As for progesterone

	mg/day, starting on day 5 of cycle and ending on day 25. *Endometriosis* - Initially, 10 mg/day for 2 weeks; incr. by 5 mg/day q2weeks until dose of 30 mg/day is reached. Tx may be held at this level for 6-9 months or until breakthrough bleeding demands temporary terminat'n)	terone, released later in menstrual cycle, converts newly formed cells into secretory tissue. For example, estrogens incr. stromal and ductal development in breasts; progesterone subsequently prepares mammary glands for lactat'n. Progesterone reduces uterine motility and prepares estrogen-stimulated endometrium for egg implantat'n and maint. of gestat'n. Progestins can be used to treat kidney and endometrial cancer, on the belief that these cancers are hormone dependent.	As for progesterone	As for progesterone	
Norethindrone acetate (Norlutate)	Various, as follows (**Oral**): *Amenorrhea and dysfunct'nal uterine bleeding* - 2.5-100 mg/day, starting on day 5 of cycle and ending on day 25. *Endometriosis* - Initially, 5 mg/day for 2 weeks; incr. by 2.5 mg/day q2weeks until 15 mg/day is reached. Tx may be held at this level for 6-9 months or until breakthrough bleeding demands temporary terminat'n)				

Pharmacologic Classification: Androgens

Fluoxymesterone (Halotestin)	Androgens are administered to males as replacement tx in primary hypogonadism or testicular hypofunct'n 2° to hypopituitarism. Also used in palliative tx of postmenopausal women w. advanced, inoperable, androgenic-responsive, metastatic mammary carcinoma. Androgens may also be used as anabolic agents in condit'ns in which tissue-building action is desired (**Oral**: *Androgen deficiency* - 10-20 mg/day. *Malignant breast carcinoma in women* - 10-30 mg/day in divided doses. *Erythropoiesis stimulat'n* - 20-50 mg/day)	Testosterone is main androgen secreted by males. Synthetic androgens are designed to mimic some of the actions of testosterone. Testosterone is responsible for full morphological and funct'nal development of male reproductive tract, incl. accessory glands and external genitalia. Androgens are also responsible for initiating recess'n of male hairline and determining distribut'n	*In males:* Virilizat'n, phallic enlargement in prepubertal males. Inhibit'n of testicular funct'n; testicular atrophy in postpubertal males. *In females:* Hirsutism, deepening of voice, clitoral hypertrophy. *In both sexes:* Nausea, vomiting, diarrhea, jaundice, altered libido, leukopenia, acne, edema, premature closure of epiphyses	**Anticoagulants, oral:** Should be avoided, if poss., in pts taking anabolic steroids, because latter may decr. clotting-factor format'n, incr. clotting-factor degradat'n, and incr. affinity of receptor sites for anticoagulant. If essential to use both drugs, pts should be monitored more carefully for excess. anticoagulant response. **Antidiabetic drugs:** Interact w. anabolic steroids, which may decr. blood sugar levels in some diabetic pts. Also, they may reduce rate of metabolism of oral hypoglycemic drugs. Thus pts should be monitored closely for s/s of hypoglycemia if anabolic	**Assess:** Hx for epilepsy, migraine, CV or kidney disease; establish baseline BP, weight, fluid intake/output ratio, emot'nal status; for current pregnancy or lactat'n when used in females for anabolic purposes. **Administer:** Titrat'n is recommended to identify lowest effective dose. **Evaluate:** For peripheral edema, weight gain, alterat'n in fluid intake/output ratio; for virilizat'n; for tx effectiveness, diet; for incr. libido; emot'nal status. **Teach:** Expected outcome of tx; need for prolonged tx; need for diet high in calories, protein, vitamins and minerals; refer for diet counseling prn; that mild virilizat'n will reverse when drug is w'drawn; to report virilizat'n effects and change in emot'nal status.

Generic Name (Trade Name)	Use (Dose)	Action	Adverse Effects	Drug Interactions	Nursing Process
Methyltestosterone (Metandren, Testred)	Various, as follows (**Oral:** *Male hypogonadism* - 5-20 mg/day [linguets] or 10-40 mg/day [tablets]. *Eunuchoidism* - 5-20 mg/day [linguets] or 10-40 mg/day [tablets]. *Female carcinoma of breast* - 50 mg [linguets] or 100 mg [tablets] bid for 2-4 weeks; then halved, if response is evident)	and growth of hair on face, body and pubes. Androgens enlarge larynx and thicken vocal cords. Secret'n of testosterone incr. protein anabolism and decr. protein catabolism. Androgens incr. ability of muscles to work, by stimulating number, thickness, and tensile strength of muscle fibers. Androgens can be given to premenopausal women w. mammary cancer in the belief that this cancer is hormone dependent.	As for fluoxymesterone	steroids are added to an antidiabetic drug regimen. Consider poss. alterat'ns in antidiabetic dosage requirements.	As for fluoxymesterone
Testosterone enanthate (Delatestryl)	Various, as follows (**IM:** *In women, to enhance libido* - 100 mg q4weeks; use only if uterus is normal size. *For mammary cancer (in premenopausal women)* - 200-400 mg q2weeks or more; dosage to be adjusted depending on clinical response. *For hypogonadism in men* - 200-400 mg q4weeks. *For cryptorchidism* - 100-200 mg q4weeks. Chorionic gonadotropin us. should be tried first. Use only when no obstructive anatomic lesion exists. If descent has not occurred after 3-4 months of tx, surgical transplantat'n should be considered. *For oligospermia* - 100-200 mg q4-6weeks for development and maint. of testicular tubular funct'n; 200 mg every week for 6-12 weeks for suppress'n of spermatogenesis and rebound stimulat'n)		As for fluoxymesterone	As for fluoxymesterone	As for fluoxymesterone
Oxandrolone (Anavar)	Various, as follows (**Oral:** *Growth stimulat'n in children* - 0.1-0.25 mg/kg/day. *Anabolic effect in adults* - 5-10 mg/day)	As for fluoxymesterone	As for fluoxymesterone	As for fluoxymesterone	

Pharmacologic Classification: Dopamine Agonist

| Bromocriptine mesylate (Parlodel) | Galactorrhea w. or without amenorrhea due to hyperprolactinemia. Prolactin-dependent menstrual disorders and infertility. Prevent'n of postpartum and postabort'n lactat'n and suppress'n of established lactat'n. Tx of prolactin-secreting inoperable adenomas or prior to surgery. Prolactin-dependent male hypogonadism. Adjunctive tx in acromegaly (**Oral:** *Prevent'n or suppress'n of postpartum lactat'n* - 2.5 mg bid with a.m. and p.m. meals for 14 days. *Galactorrhea w. or without amenorrhea due to hyperprolactinemia* - 1.25-2.5 mg hs to establish tolerance; grad. incr. after 2-3 days to 2.5 mg bid w. meals. Dose may be incr. prn to 2.5 mg tid. Continue drug until milk secret'n disappears completely or, in the case of menstrual dysfunction, until menstrual cycle has returned to normal. *Prolactin-dependent menstrual disorders and infertility* - 1.25-2.5 mg hs to establish tolerance. Grad. incr. after 2-3 days to 2.5 mg bid w. meals. Dose may be incr. prn to 2.5 mg tid) | Stim. dopamine receptors in brain. Major effect is to inhibit prolactin synthesis and secret'n, either by direct action on pituitary or indirect action on hypothalamus. | Nausea, vomiting, vertigo and/or headache, drowsiness, nervousness, blurred vision, fatigue, listlessness, hot flashes, tinnitus, nasal congest'n, breast tenderness, abdominal cramps, constipat'n or diarrhea | **Ergot-containing products:** Are not recommended concomitantly w. bromocriptine. **Ethanol:** Should be avoided during tx w. bromocriptine because in some pts concomitant use has given rise to alcohol intolerance and incr. severity/incidence of bromocriptine's adv. effects. **Phenothiazines and haloperidol:** May decr. efficacy of bromocriptine. | **Assess:** Establish baseline BP and monitor closely, as this drug decr. BP. **Administer:** With meals; store at room temp. in tight containers. Safe use in pregnancy *not* established. **Evaluate:** For tx effect in Parkinson's disease (decr. in drooling, slow movements, dyskinesia). **Teach:** To change posit'n slowly; to avoid hazardous activity; that tx effect may take 2 months. |

Pharmacologic Classification: Inhibitor of FSH Secretion

| Danazol (Cyclomen, Danocrine) | Tx of endometriosis char. by dysmenorrhea, pelvic pain, infertility, indurat'n of cul de sac, or dyspareunia. For symptomatic relief of pain and tenderness assoc. w. fibrocystic breast disease. Only those | Suppresses pituitary-ovarian axis by inhibiting output of gonadotropins from pituitary gland and by interfering w. hormone target-tissue | Acne, edema, flushing, incr. growth of hair on face and extremities, changes in breast size, weight gain, sweating, voice change, oiliness of | **Anticoagulants, oral:** May have their effects potentiated by danazol. When such drugs are given concurrently w. danazol, careful attent'n to dosage is recommended, as is readjustment of dosage prn. | As for *androgens* |

Generic Name (Trade Name)	Use (Dose)	Action	Adverse Effects	Drug Interactions	Nursing Process
	pts should be selected who are unresponsive to, or intolerant of, other tx measures, or in whom such measures are otherwise inadvisable (**Oral:** *Endometriosis* - 200-800 mg/day in 2-4 divided doses, administered without interrupt'n for 3-6 months. *Fibrocystic breast disease* - 100-400 mg/day in 2 divided doses. Tx should continue uninterrupted until complete disappearance of symptoms or for 6 months, whichever occurs first)	interact'n. Both FSH and LH outputs are depressed, and preovulatory surge of these hormones is blocked.	skin and hair; rarely, clitoral hypertrophy		

Pharmacologic Classification: Ovulatory Drug

Generic Name (Trade Name)	Use (Dose)	Action	Adverse Effects	Drug Interactions	Nursing Process
Clomiphene citrate (Clomid, Serophene)	Induct'n of ovulat'n in pts w. persistent ovulatory dysfunct'n who desire pregnancy (**Oral:** 50 mg daily for 5 days, started at any time in pt who has had no recent uterine bleeding. If progestin-induced bleeding is planned or if spontaneous uterine bleeding occurs before tx, start 5-day regimen on or about 5th day of cycle. In absence of ovulat'n, give 100 mg/day for 5 days as early as 30 days after previous tx. Never give more than 100 mg for 5 days. If ovulatory menses have not occurred after 3 courses of tx, diagnosis should be re-evaluated)	Stim. release of pituitary gonadotropins (FSH and LH), resulting in maturat'n of ovarian follicle, ovulat'n, development of corpus luteum.	Multiple pregnancy, birth defects, ovarian hypertrophy, effects on liver funct'n, BSP retent'n in > 5% of pts. Common symptomatic adv. effects: hot flashes, abdominal discomfort, visual blurring, spots or flashes; nausea or vomiting; dizziness, lightheadedness; incr. nervous tens'n; depress'n, fatigue, headache, insomnia; urticaria or allergic dermatitis; breast soreness, heavier menses; incr. urinary frequency or volume; reversible hair loss and weight gain		**Assess:** For existing pregnancy; review hx for hepatic disease, bleeding tendencies, ovarian cysts, neoplastic disease, retinal disease. **Administer:** Self-administered. Take drug at same time every day. **Evaluate:** For ovulatory response using basal body temp. chart; for pelvic or abdominal pain, visual disturbances, pregnancy. **Teach:** Methods for and importance of self-evaluat'n for drug efficacy and adv. effects.

Drugs That Stimulate or Relax the Uterus

Teaching Objectives

Following completion of this chapter, the reader should be able to:

1. Discuss the actions, therapeutic uses and adverse effects of the uterine stimulants oxytocin, ergonovine maleate, methylergonovine maleate, dinoprostone, dinoprost tromethamine and carboprost tromethamine, and the nursing process related to their use.

2. Discuss the mechanism of action, pharmacologic properties, therapeutic uses and adverse effects of the uterine relaxants ritodrine and isoxsuprine, and the nursing process related to their use.

Uterine Stimulants

Although many drugs can stimulate the uterus, only oxytocin, the ergot alkaloids ergonovine and methylergonovine, and some prostaglandins have the selectivity and predictability of action required for this purpose.

Oxytocin (Pitocin, Syntocinon)

Mechanism of Action and Pharmacologic Effects

Specific oxytocin receptors are present in the uterus during pregnancy, particularly during the latter phases. At this time the uterus is highly responsive to oxytocin, which stimulates both the frequency and force of uterine contractions. These effects of oxytocin are estrogen dependent.

Specific receptor sites for oxytocin are also present in the mammary gland during lactation. At this time oxytocin stimulates myoepithelial cell contractions, forcing milk from the alveoli of the breast.

Oxytocin relaxes vascular smooth muscle, decreasing both systolic and diastolic blood pressure, as well as producing flushing and an increase in peripheral circulation.

Therapeutic Uses

Intravenous oxytocin is used to induce and augment labor. Oxytocin may be used in inevitable or incomplete abortion. Intramuscular oxytocin is used after delivery to prevent or control hemorrhage, restoring normal tone to the hypotonic uterus. Used as an intravenous bolus, it may cause transient hypotension. Intranasal oxytocin is used to stimulate milk letdown.

Adverse Effects

Oxytocin, given in labor, can cause uterine rupture. It rarely causes anaphylactoid or allergic reactions. Some studies indicate that neonates delivered from oxytocin-treated mothers have shown an increased incidence of jaundice. Prolonged use of high-dose oxytocin combined with dextrose and water can cause water intoxication.

Nursing Process

Assessment

Prior to administering oxytocin, the nurse should review the patient's history for contraindications to its use. These include previous cesarean section or uterine surgery, tendency to allergic drug responses, the presence of toxemia, or cardiovascular or renal disease. Women with any of these conditions are at increased risk, and oxytocin should be withheld pending clarification of the order with the attending physician.

Complications of delivery such as cephalopelvic disproportion, malpresentation, undilated cervix, abruptio placenta or fetal death also increase risk to the mother and provide sufficient rationale for withholding the medication.

Nursing assessment should establish baseline measures of maternal vital signs, body mass/weight, and quality of contractions, including frequency, duration and strength. Electronic monitoring should be established on women for whom oxytocin is ordered. In addition, baseline measures of fetal heart tone and rate should be established.

Administration

Oxytocin should be stored in a refrigerator and administered by nurses only when a physician is immediately available. The preferred method of administration during labor is intravenously via an infusion set using a Y-connector to join the solution containing the oxytocin to an unmedicated intravenous solution. In this way, the unmedicated solution can be used to maintain the patency of the vein when oxytocin is administered intermittently over an extended period of time.

The best means of precisely regulating the oxytocin dosage is through the use of an infusion pump. In preparing an oxytocin infusion, the intravenous bottle or bag should be rotated and tilted in order to ensure that the medication is distributed evenly through the solution. The infusion rate must be monitored continuously.

Intramuscular injection is not recommended; however, should it be necessary during delivery, it is best accomplished using a ventrolateral gluteal or deltoid site. Following intramuscular administra-tion, the nurse should massage the injection site to assist in drug absorption.

Prior to intranasal administration, the patient should be asked to blow her nose. She should then sit upright with her head in a vertical position, hold the container upright, insert it into her nostril and squeeze during the inspiratory phase of respiration, i.e., ventilation.

A crash cart should be available on the unit and magnesium sulfate available at the bedside.

Evaluation

Patients receiving oxytocin require continuous and rigorous evaluation of its efficacy. Contractions, maternal vital signs and fluid intake/output must be monitored. If these measurements deviate from the previously established baseline values, the nurse must immediately request the presence of the physician. If contractions last over one minute or disappear, turn the patient on her side and notify the physician. Continuous electronic fetal monitoring should be maintained, and the physician notified immediately of deviations. Evidence of fetal distress, prolonged (longer than 90 s) or excessively strong contractions (above 50 mm of mercury on an electronic monitor), fluid retention or other manifestations of impending water intoxication, allergic or anaphylactic reactions, or cardiovascular irregularities should be reported to the physician at once for immediate remedial action.

Teaching

When oxytocin is administered intranasally to stimulate lactation, patients should be taught the proper means of administration. They should also be carefully instructed concerning the drug's adverse effects and advised to seek assistance immediately should any of these appear.

Ergonovine Maleate (Ergotrate Maleate) and Methylergonovine Maleate (Methergine)

Mechanism of Action and Pharmacologic Effects

Ergonovine and methylergonovine are potent uterine stimulants. Although uterine sensitivity increases as pregnancy proceeds, even the immature uterus responds to these drugs. Within a few minutes of oral administration, firm tetanic contractions begin in the postpartum uterus which, in the course of about ninety minutes, gradually change to a series of clonic contractions that persist for another ninety minutes or more. Uterine contractions begin within one minute after intravenous or two to three minutes following intramuscular administration.

Ergot alkaloids can constrict blood vessels and should not be given to patients with chronic or pregnancy-induced hypertension.

Therapeutic Uses

Available orally and parenterally, erogonovine and methylergonovine are used for the prevention or treatment of postpartum or postabortal hemorrhage.

Adverse Effects

Both drugs can cause vasoconstriction, resulting in hypertension and headaches. Other cardiovascular effects include palpitations, dyspnea and transient chest pains. Gangrene can develop in patients with Buerger's or Raynaud's diseases. Patients may also experience vertigo, nausea, vomiting and diarrhea when ergonovine or methylergonovine are administered.

Nursing Process

Assessment
Vascular, hepatic or renal disease contraindicate the use of ergonovine and methylergonovine. The patient's history should be reviewed for evidence of these conditions. The patient should also be assessed for evidence of hypocalcemia, because this condition may antagonize the response to these drugs. In addition, baseline measurements of the height, consistency and location of the patient's fundus should be established prior to administering the medication. Baseline measurements of blood pressure and pulse, as well as character and amount of vaginal bleeding, must be established to assess changes indicating hemorrhage.

Administration
Ergonovine maleate should be administered from a refrigerated container. If no refrigeration is available, discard supplies of the drugs stored in the delivery room for more than sixty days because of decreased potency.

Evaluation
Evidence of drug efficacy will be provided by reduced fundus height, solid fundus consistency and the patient's subjective reports of abdominal cramping. Severe abdominal cramping indicates that drug dosage should be reduced.

The patient's vital signs and peripheral circulation should be monitored for evidence of adverse effects. Hypertension, palpitations, dyspnea, or patient reports of coldness, numbness or tingling of extremities, headache, vertigo or chest pains should all be reported immediately to the attending physician. Gastric distress manifested as nausea, vomiting or diarrhea should also be reported to the physician, and palliative nursing measures initiated.

Teaching
Patient teaching should emphasize the desired effect of the drug and the expectation of abdominal cramping. Patients should be instructed to inform the nurse if they feel cold, numb or tingling extremities, headache or dizziness, chest pain or nausea.

Dinoprostone (Prostin E$_2$)

Mechanism of Action and Pharmacologic Effects

Dinoprostone is a synthetic prostaglandin that stimulates the myometrium of the gravid uterus to contract in a similar manner to the spontaneous contractions seen during labor in the term uterus. Stimulation of the smooth muscles of the gastrointestinal tract can cause nausea, vomiting and diarrhea.

Therapeutic Uses

Dinoprostone is indicated as a uterine stimulant for induction of labor at or near term in (1) elective induction or (2) indicated induction, such as postmaturity, hypertension, toxemia of pregnancy, premature rupture of amniotic membranes, Rh incompatibility, diabetes mellitus, intrauterine death or fetal growth retardation.

Adverse Effects

Vomiting, with or without nausea and diarrhea, is the most common adverse effect of dinoprostone. Fetal heart rate changes have been reported in approximately six per cent of patients. Other adverse effects occur very rarely and include headache, hypertension, hypotension, hyperthermia, dizziness, chills, hiccough, flushing, tachycardia, dyspnea, bronchospasm and rash.

Nursing Process

Assessment
Nursing assessment of patients for whom dinoprostone has been prescribed should emphasize review of the patient's history for evidence of glaucoma, epilepsy, allergies or asthma, previous cesarean section or uterine surgery. The patient should undergo nursing physical assessment to determine

the presence of possible cephalopelvic disproportion, fetal malpresentation, fetal distress, multiple pregnancy, polyhydramnios or uterine hypertonus. Baseline measurements of blood pressure and pulse must be taken to monitor for subsequent changes and possible hemorrhage. At the same time, the patient's current drug regimen should be reviewed for possible concurrent use of other oxytocics. The occurrence of any of the preceding situations or conditions precludes nursing administration of this medication.

Administration
Vaginal suppositories should be be stored in a refrigerator. Prior to administration, they should be gradually warmed to room temperature. Nurses should have the patient empty her bladder before administration of this drug. After inserting the suppository high into the vagina, nurses should ensure that the patient remains supine for ten minutes.

Evaluation
Nursing evaluation following administration of this medication should emphasize drug efficacy, as evidenced by onset of labor. All usual nursing evaluations during labor should be conducted. Particular emphasis should be paid to the maternal vital signs for adverse effects such as hypertension or hypotension, fever, tachycardia, dyspnea or bronchial spasm. Fetal heart rate should also be monitored, and any changes reported immediately. Nurses caring for patients receiving this medication should also be alert for other adverse effects such as hiccoughs, nausea, vomiting or diarrhea; fever or chills; flushing or rash; or postpartum hemorrhage.

Dinoprost Tromethamine (Prostin F$_{2alpha}$) and Carboprost Tromethamine (Prostin/15M)

Mechanism of Action and Pharmacologic Effects

Dinoprost tromethamine and carboprost tromethamine are also prostaglandins. Dinoprost tromethamine stimulates uterine contractility. Carboprost is a synthetic analogue of prostaglandin F$_{2alpha}$ (PGF$_{2alpha}$) with a longer duration of action than the parent compound. Both drugs induce uterine contractions similar to those seen during term labor.

Therapeutic Uses

Dinoprost tromethamine is usually given intra-amniotically to induce midtrimester abortion. Carboprost tromethamine offers the advantage of intramuscular administration, circumventing the difficulties of intra-amniotic or extraovular injections with dinoprost. Concomitant administration of dinoprost and intravenous oxytocin has caused uterine hypertonus and cervical perforation in the presence of an undilated or poorly dilated cervix. Their concomitant use must be approached with caution in the absence of adequate cervical dilatation.

Adverse Effects

The adverse effects of these drugs are usually not severe. Cervical-vaginal fistulae, lower-segment uterine rupture, and retention of the placenta, with hemorrhage, are the most dangerous effects. These drugs should not be used in women who have had a cesarean section or hysterotomy, or who have a history of uterine fibroids or cervical stenosis. Nausea and vomiting occur in most patients. Other adverse effects include fever, hypotension and syncope, hypertension and headache.

Nursing Process

Assessment
Assessment prior to administration of dinoprost tromethamine or carboprost tromethamine should begin with a review of the patient's history for evidence of previous cesarean section or uterine surgery, uterine fibroids, cervical stenosis, pelvic inflammatory disease, asthma, allergies, respiratory disease, glaucoma, hypertension, diabetes, epilepsy, vascular, renal or hepatic disease. Physical assessment of the patient should attempt to identify any evidence of anemia or jaundice and should establish baseline vital signs that can be used subsequently in observing the patient for indications of hemorrhage.

Administration
These medications should be administered only by a physician from ampules that have been refrigerated at 2 – 8° Celsius for less than two years. Any supplies of these medications that have not been refrigerated, or which are more than two years old, should be discarded. Intramuscular injections should be given deep into muscle mass. Rotate injection sites.

Evaluation

As with other medications, patients who have received dinoprost tromethamine or carboprost tromethamine should be evaluated for both drug efficacy and adverse effects. Vaginal examination will ensure that the administration catheter has remained in position and has not prolapsed into the vagina. In addition, vaginal examination will permit determination of cervical dilatation as an indicator of drug efficacy and may provide early evidence of adverse effects such as cervical or lower uterine lacerations or rupture.

The patient's vital signs should be monitored every fifteen minutes for evidence of such adverse effects as fever, hypotension and syncope, hypertension and headache. The quality, frequency and duration of uterine contractions indicate drug efficacy. Immediate medical assistance should be sought if contractions become sustained or excessively strong.

Gastrointestinal disturbances such as nausea, vomiting and diarrhea are relatively common with these medications. They should be reported to the physician and palliative nursing measures initiated.

The abortion products should be evaluated to ensure that a complete abortion has occurred. Because these drugs do not interfere with the integrity of the fetal-placental unit, a live fetus may be born. Therefore, in collaboration with the physician, nurses must evaluate the vitality of the fetus, particularly when these drugs are administered late in the second trimester.

Teaching

Prior to treatment, patients must be advised of the benefits and risks of these drugs. They should be particularly alerted to their adverse effects. Patients should also be informed that if the abortion is unsuccessful, another means must be sought to terminate the pregnancy, because of the possible teratogenic effects of these medications.

Uterine Relaxants

Ritodrine HCl (Yutopar)

Mechanism of Action and Pharmacologic Effects

Ritodrine stimulates $beta_2$ receptors and decreases both the frequency and intensity of uterine contractions. To a lesser degree, ritodrine stimulates $beta_1$ receptors, resulting in a dose-related tachycardia.

Therapeutic Uses

Ritodrine inhibits uterine contractions associated with premature labor. It is titrated intravenously to control contractions. Thereafter, the patient may be placed on oral maintenance therapy. The use of ritodrine to reduce fetal asphyxia in the active stage of labor has also been advocated.

Adverse Effects

Ritodrine's adverse effects result mainly from its beta-adrenergic properties. These include (1) tachycardia, (2) an increase in systolic and a decrease in diastolic pressure, (3) a rise in blood glucose, insulin and free fatty acids, and (4) a decrease in serum potassium. Ritodrine also causes palpitations, tremor, nausea, vomiting, hyperglycemia, headaches, nervousness, anxiety, malaise, chest pains and tightness, and erythema.

Fetal tachycardia, neonatal hypoglycemia and hypocalcemia have been reported. In addition, the fetus can be affected by maternal ketoacidosis. These effects are more prevalent following parenteral treatment with ritodrine.

Nursing Process

Assessment

Women for whom ritodrine hydrochloride has been prescribed should be evaluated for the stage of their pregnancy. Ritodrine should be withheld from women found to be less than twenty weeks pregnant until the physician is consulted. The patient's drug regimen should be reviewed for concurrent use of corticosteroids, beta blockers and sympathomimetics because of undesirable drug interactions. Nurses should also review the maternal history for evidence of cardiovascular disease, pulmonary hypertension, hyperthyroidism, diabetes mellitus, asthma or allergic tendencies. The use of ritodrine hydrochloride in patients with these conditions is contraindicated.

Nursing assessment must establish baseline

measures of pulse, respiration and blood pressure as indicators of cardiovascular and respiratory status. In addition, nurses should ensure that baseline measures of blood glucose and electrolytes are determined.

Administration
Parenteral ritodrine is administered with the assistance of an infusion pump.

Evaluation
Nursing evaluation of patients receiving intravenous ritodrine should emphasize monitoring the frequency, duration and intensity of contractions every fifteen minutes as an indication of drug efficacy. At the same time, cardiovascular and respiratory status should also be established every fifteen minutes. This should include measurements of pulse, respirations and blood pressure. Patients should also be evaluated regularly for evidence of hypocalcemia and hypoglycemia.

Patients receiving oral maintenance doses of ritodrine should experience regular monitoring of blood glucose and electrolyte levels.

Because ritodrine crosses the placenta and enters the fetal circulation, fetal heart rate should be monitored at the same time as maternal heart rate. Neonates delivered to women who have received ritodrine should be evaluated for hypoglycemia and hypocalcemia.

Isoxsuprine HCl (Vasodilan)

Isoxsuprine is available for both oral and intravenous administration. The drug stimulates beta adrenergic receptors, inhibiting uterine contractility. It is used in the management of premature labor in suitable patients with intact membranes, cervix less than 4 cm and less than 80% effaced.

Maternal pulmonary edema has been reported in patients treated with isoxsuprine. A persistent tachycardia of 140 beats per minute or more, and a blood pressure below 90/50 mm Hg may be early signs of impending pulmonary edema. The adverse effects of isoxsuprine include tachycardia, nausea and vomiting, hypotension, cardiac arrhythmias, palpitations, dizziness, hyperglycemia and hypocalcemia.

Nursing Process

Assessment
The nursing process for patients receiving isoxsuprine to prevent spontaneous abortion are the same as those identified earlier for ritodrine.

Further Reading

Caritis, S.N., Edelstone, D.I. and Mueller-Heuback, E. (1979). Pharmacologic inhibition of preterm labor. *Am. J. Obstet. Gynecol. 133* :557-578

Davey, D.A. (1980). Induction of labor. *Clin. Obstet. Gynecol. 7* :481-509.

Nevin, M.M.D. (1988). Dangers of DES. *Canadian Nurse 84* (3):17-19.

Petrie, R.H. (1981). Pharmacology and use of oxytocin. *Clin. Perinatol. 8* :35-47.

Table 49
Drugs that stimulate or relax the uterus.

Pharmacologic Classification: Uterine Stimulants (Oxytocics)

Generic Name (Trade Name)	Use (Dose)	Action	Adverse Effects	Drug Interactions	Nursing Process
Oxytocin (Pitocin, Syntocinon)	Various, as follows (IV Infus'n: Use solut'n containing 10 mU/mL of normal saline or Ringer's solut'n. Induct'n of labor - Begin at rate of 1-2 mU/min; may incr. by 1-2 mU/min q15-30min to obtain opt. response. Av. dose to induce labor at term, 8-10 mU/min. Oxytocin challenge test - A dilute solut'n is infused IV starting at lowest pump setting, 0.5 mU/min; dose is doubled q20-30min until 3 contract'ns are observed q10min [max. rate, 20 mU/min] unless repetitive late deceler-at'n or fetal bradycardia occurs earlier. If either occurs, oxytocin should be discontinued stat. Prevent'n of postpartum uterine atony and hemorrhage - 20-40 mU/mL in an electrolyte solut'n given at a rate of 40 mU/min or sufficient to control uterine atony. Avoid bolus inject'n because of untoward CV effects, even in young healthy pts. IM: To control postpartum bleeding - 3-10 U. Nasal: For milk letdown - 1 spray in 1 or both nostrils 2-3 min before nursing)	Oxytocin exerts selec-tive action on smooth musculature of uterus, particularly toward end of pregnancy, during labor and immed. following delivery. Oxytocin stims. rhyth-mic contract'ns of uterus, incr. frequen-cy of existing contract'ns and raises tone of uterine muscu-lature. Oxytocin also stims. milk letdown process of postpar-tum pts.	Uterine rupture, aller-gic react'ns, sinus bradycardia, PVCs and other arrythmias in fetus; water intoxi-cat'n		**Assess:** Review hx for contraindicat'ns (previous cesarian births, tendency to allergic response, toxemia, CV or renal disease, complicat'ns of delivery); estab-lish baseline VS, weight, quality of contract'ns (incl. frequency, durat'n and strength); if contract'ns last > 1 min or disappear, turn pt on her side and notify physician at once; establish electronic monitoring; establish baseline fetal heart rate and tone. **Administer:** From vial stored in refriger-ator; only w. physician immed. available; IV via infus'n set using Y-connector, pref. using an infus'n pump; distribute drug evenly in IV solut'n by tilting and rotating bag; IM during labor should be given in ventrolateral gluteal site and massage to assist absorpt'n; intranasal administrat'n should be preceded by pt blowing nose; pt should sit up w. head in vertical posit'n, hold container upright, insert into nostril and squeeze during inspirato-ry phase of respirat'n. Crash cart should be available at unit and MgSO₄ available at bedside. **Teach:** Expected tx outcome; when given intranasally to stim. lactat'n, proper administrat'n/self-evaluat'n for adv. effects.

Generic Name (Trade Name)	Use (Dose)	Action	Adverse Effects	Drug Interactions	Nursing Process
Ergonovine maleate (Ergotrate Maleate); methylergonovine maleate (Methergine); methylergometrine maleate (Methylergobasine)	For prevent'n o tx of postabortal hemorrhage due to uterine atony (IV: *In emergencies when excess. uterine bleeding has occurred* - 0.2 mg. **IM:** *To control uterine hemorrhage* - 0.2 mg, repeated in 2-4 h if bleeding is severe. **Oral:** *To minimize late postpartum bleeding* - 0.2-0.4 mg ergonovine maleate bid-qid, us. for 2 days)	Produces rhythmic uterine contract'ns within 6-15 min. Oral ergonovine produces firm tetanic contract'n of postpartum uterus which, over about 90 min, grad. changes to series of clonic contract'ns that persist for another 90 min or more. Parenteral administrat'n causes uterine contract'ns to begin more rapidly in 2-3 min if given IM or 1 min if given IV)	Headache, vertigo, hypertens'n, palpitat'ns, dyspnea, transient chest pains, nausea, vomiting, diarrhea	**Vasopressors** (e.g. dopamine, epinephrine, metaraminol, methoxamine, norepinephrine, phenylephrine): May interact w. ergonovine, methylergonovine or methylergometrine to produce incr. vasoconstrict'n.	**Assess:** Review hx for vascular or hepatic disease; check for hypocalcemia; establish baseline for height, consistency and locat'n of fundus. Establish baseline BP, pulse and character/am't of vaginal bleeding; assess changes that indicate hemorrhage. **Administer:** From refrigerated container. **Evaluate:** Height, consistency and locat'n of fundus; pt percept'n of abdominal cramping; VS, peripheral circulat'n, sensat'n; for GI distress. **Teach:** Expected tx outcome; to report adv. effects.

Pharmacologic Classification: Uterine Stimulants (Prostaglandins)

Generic Name (Trade Name)	Use (Dose)	Action	Adverse Effects	Drug Interactions	Nursing Process
Dinoprostone (Prostin E$_2$)	Induct'n of labor at or near term; in elective induct'n or indicated induct'n (**Oral:** 0.5 mg followed in 1 h by 2nd dose of 0.5 mg; thereafter, hourly. *A single dose should never exceed 1.5 mg. Total tx period w. dinoprostone should not, in any instance, exceed 18 h.* **Vaginal:** One 20-mg suppository. Subsequently, at intervals of 3-5 h until abort'n occurs)	Stims. myometrium of gravid uterus to contract in a manner sim. to contract'ns observed in term uterus during spontaneous labor. Also stims. GI smooth muscle.	Vomiting w. or without nausea and diarrhea, fetal heart changes, headache, hypertens'n, hypotens'n, postpartum hemorrhage, fever, dizziness, chills, tachycardia, dyspnea, bronchospasm	**Oxytocin:** Should not be started until at least 1 h has elapsed following last oral dose of dinoprostone because prostaglandins may potentiate oxytocin's effect.	**Assess:** Review hx for glaucoma, epilepsy, allergies, asthma, previous cesarian birth or uterine surgery; physical assessment for complicat'ns of delivery; check for concurrent use of other oxytocics. Baseline BP, pulse to monitor for changes and possible hemorrhage. **Administer:** Have pt empty bladder *before* administrat'n. Suppositories stored in refrigerator, then warmed to room temp.; insert suppositories high into vagina; keep pt supine for 10 min. **Evaluate:** For onset of labor; monitor VS, fetus for adv. effects.
Dinoprost tromethamine (Prostin F$_{2alpha}$)	Given intra-amniotically to induce abort'n when size of uterus and am't of amniotic fluid is adequate, us. after 15 weeks of gestat'n (**Intra-amniotic:** 40 mg w. 1st mL containing 5 mg,	Induces uterine contract'ns sim. to those seen during term labor.	Cervical or lower uterine lacerat'n or rupture, retent'n of placenta, hemorrhage, nausea or vomiting, breast enlargement		

Drug	Dosage/Indications	Action	Adverse Effects	Interactions	Nursing Considerations
	injected over 1-2 min to determine sensitivity to drug and confirm that needle is placed correctly. If nec., a 2nd 10-20 mg dose is given after 6 h)		and lactat'n, fever, syncope, hypertens'n and hypotens'n and headache, pain at site of inject'n, bronchospasm, arrhythmias, hyperventilat'n, paresthesias and hyperesthesias		**Administer:** Give IM deep into muscle mass; rotate inject'n sites.
Carboprost Tromethamine (Prostin/15 M)	To stim. uterine contract'ns; to induce abort'n bet. weeks 12 and 20 (**IM:** Initially, 250 µg repeated prn at 1.5-3.5 h intervals. If several doses of 250µg fail, incr. to 500 µg. Total dose, not > 12 mg)	Carboprost is a synthetic analogue of dinoprostone, w. longer durat'n of action. Carboprost offers advantage of IM administrat'n.	Vomiting, diarrhea and fever		

Pharmacologic Classification: Adrenergic Uterine Relaxants

Drug	Dosage/Indications	Action	Adverse Effects	Interactions	Nursing Considerations
Ritodrine hydrochloride (Yutopar)	Management of preterm labor in suitable pts (**IV:** Initially, 100 µg/min; grad. incr. by 50 µg/min q10min until desired result. Max. dose, 350 µg/min. Continue infusing for 12 h after uterine contract'ns cease. **Oral:** 10 mg approx 30 min before terminat'n of IV tx. Us. dose for 1st 24 h is 10 mg q2h; thereafter, 10-20 mg q4-6h. Max. total daily dose, 120 mg)	Beta-receptor stimulant that exerts preferential effect on adrenergic receptors, influencing uterine contractility. Stimulat'n of receptors inhibits contractility of uterine smooth muscle. Beta-adrenergic stimulat'n in other body systems may lead to some CV or metabolic effects.	*Maternal effects:* Beta-adrenergic stimulat'ns incl. palpitat'ns, tremor, nausea, vomiting, headache, erythema, nervousness, jitteriness, restlessness, emot'nal upset or anxiety, chest pain or tightness, cardiac arrythmias. *Neonatal effects:* Hypoglycemia, ileus, hypocalcemia and hypotens'n. **Warning for use of ritodrine:** Closely monitor maternal pulse rate/BP and fetal heart rate. Monitor am't of IV fluids administered and rate of administrat'n to avoid circulatory fluid overload.	**Adrenergics:** May have additive effects w. ritodrine. **Anesthetics:** May have their hypotensive effects potentiated by ritodrine. **Antihypertensives:** May have their effects incr. by ritodrine. **Beta blockers:** Inhibit action of ritodrine; coadministrat'n of these drugs should be avoided. **Beta$_2$ bronchodilators:** May have additive effects w. ritodrine. **Corticosteroids:** Used concomitantly, may lead to pulmonary edema. **Diazoxide:** Potentiates ritodrine's hypotensive and arrhythmic effects. **Dobutamine and dopamine:** May have additive effects w. ritodrine. **Indapamide:** Potentiates ritodrine's hypotensive and arrhythmic effects.	**Assess:** Stage of pregnancy (should be ≥20 weeks); current drug regimen for corticosteroids, beta blockers, sympathomimetics; review hx for CV disease, pulmonary hypertens'n, hyperthyroidism, diabetes mellitus, asthma, allergies; ensure that blood has been drawn for baseline measures of blood glucose and electrolytes. **Administer:** With infus'n pump. **Evaluate:** Frequency, durat'n and intensity of contract'ns q15min; CV and respiratory status q15min; for hypocalcemia and hypoglycemia; neonate blood glucose and electrolytes.

Generic Name (Trade Name)	Use (Dose)	Action	Adverse Effects	Drug Interactions	Nursing Process
Isoxsuprine hydrochloride (Vasodilan)	Management of preterm labor in suitable pts w. > 20 weeks of gestat'n, who have intact amniotic membranes w. cervical dilatat'n ≤ 4 cm and < 80% cervical effacement (**IV:** Initial dose, 80 mg in 250 mL D5W, to run at 0.2 mg/min. After 15-20 min, if contract'ns have not been satisfactorily controlled, incr. isoxsuprine q15min by 0.1-0.2 mg/min, until no contract'ns or a max of 1 mg/min is reached. Following uterine relaxat'n, continue for 3 h, then decr. by 30% and continue as maintenance for 24 h, minimum. If no further contract'ns are present, decr. slowly and overlap w. 20 mg isoxsuprine IM q3h for 24 h and/or w. 1-2 10-mg tablets q6h. If uterine activity increases, return to IV tx)	As for ritodrine HCl. Isoxsuprine stims. beta receptors, inhibiting uterine contractility. Because of its ability to stim. beta receptors in blood vessels, isoxsuprine can cause vasodilatat'n. This effect has led to its use to provide symptomatic relief in peripheral and cerebral vascular disorders.	*Maternal adv. effects following parenteral tx:* Pulmonary edema, tachycardia, nausea and vomiting, hypotens'n, cardiac arrythmias, palpitat'ns, dizziness, hyperglycemia. *Maternal adv. effects following oral tx:* Mild tachycardia, palpitat'n or tremor; nausea. *Fetal adv. effects:* Tachycardia, hypotens'n at delivery, hypocalcemia, hypoglycemia (15-20%) and ileus (40%). **Warning:** Maternal pulmonary edema may occur in pts treated w. isoxuprine. Incidence incr. w. concomitant use of corticosteroids. Monitor pts closely. See ritodrine for warning relating to fluid overload. This warning also applies to isoxsuprine.	As for ritodrine HCl.	As for ritodrine HCl.

SECTION 9

Pharmacology of the Respiratory System

Nurses need not be reminded of the importance of the respiratory system. Charged with the responsibility for the exchange of oxygen and carbon dioxide between blood and the environment, its normal function is essential for a healthy body. Conditions such as bronchial asthma or the common cold reduce the capacity of the respiratory system to carry out its physiological function. When this happens, drug therapy may be required. Section 9 discusses the use of drugs to treat these conditions. In addition, it describes the actions of antihistamines. Although the use of these drugs is not restricted to respiratory medicine, a major use for antihistamines is in the treatment of coughs and colds. For this reason, antihistamines have been included in this section of the book.

CHAPTER 32

Antiasthmatic Drugs

Asthma

Asthma is a disease characterized by increased responsiveness of the trachea and bronchi to various stimuli and manifested by a widespread narrowing of the airways that changes in severity either spontaneously or as a result of therapy. The duration and severity of an asthmatic attack varies from patient to patient, from occasional wheezing to sustained airway occlusion, or cardiac arrest. Three factors account for the airway obstruction: (1) bronchiolar smooth muscle constriction, (2) edema of the bronchial mucosa, and (3) mucus plugging.

The etiology of asthma is not completely understood. Some patients suffer from **extrinsic,** or allergic asthma, having formed IgE antibodies in response to exposure to an allergen. Common allergens are pollen, animal dander, house dust, specific foods (e.g., shellfish) or medications (penicillin is notorious). When exposed to an allergen, the sensitized patient rapidly experiences an asthmatic attack. Allergic asthma is common in children. It is less prevalent in adults.

Other patients are not demonstrably allergic. The etiology of their disease, often called **intrinsic** asthma, is more difficult to explain. Intrinsic asthma often occurs later in life. It has been postulated that increased cholinergic stimulation may be a factor in intrinsic asthma. Certainly, the bronchioles are richly innervated with parasympathetic nerve fibers, and acetylcholine causes bronchiolar constriction. Increased secretion of this neurotransmitter or heightened sensitivity to its effects could explain asthma. However, much work remains to be done before cholinergic stimulation can be established as a cause of asthma.

Asthmatic attacks may be precipitated in

susceptible individuals by a variety of conditions. These include exposure to allergens, viral respiratory infections and emotional upset. With respect to the last factor, an improvement in asthma can often be correlated with emotional stability. Some types of exercise can precipitate an attack in some asthmatic patients. Other exercises, such as swimming, are used in its treatment. Nurses who practise in the northern United States or Canada will recognize the effects of cold on an asthmatic patient. There is nothing like -35° temperatures to tickle the airways into closing.

Drug therapy is designed to treat the factors responsible for airway obstruction. Treatment will be discussed under the categories of (1) bronchodilators, (2) anti-inflammatories, and (3) inhibitors of inflammatory-response mediators.

Bronchodilators

Beta-Adrenergic Drugs

Mechanism of Action and Pharmacologic Effects

Beta$_1$ receptors are found in the heart, and beta$_2$ receptors in the bronchioles and blood vessels. The pharmacology of these drugs is presented in detail in Chapter 7. Drugs that stimulate beta$_1$ receptors increase heart rate and force of contraction. Beta$_2$ stimulants dilate bronchioles and decrease peripheral resistance.

Examples of beta$_2$ stimulants used to treat asthma are orciprenaline/metaproterenol (Alupent, Metaprel), albuterol/salbutamol (Proventil, Ventolin), terbutaline (Brethine, Bricanyl), fenoterol (Berotec) and procaterol (Pro-Air). These drugs produce less tachycardia than isoproterenol, which was used extensively before their introduction. They may be taken orally or by inhalation.

Therapeutic Uses

Beta$_2$ stimulants are the most effective bronchodilators and are commonly used for the treatment of asthma. Administered by inhalation, they may be used regularly to prevent attacks or periodically to stop a developing attack. Although they are also available in oral dosage forms, they are more effective and more specific for beta$_2$ receptors when inhaled. Unfortunately, the effects of beta-adrenergic drugs often decrease when they are used chroni-

cally. Beta$_2$ stimulants are contraindicated in patients with tachyarrhythmias.

Albuterol or salbutamol (Proventil, Ventolin) is a very popular and effective bronchodilator. Usual doses produce little tachycardia or tremor. As with all beta$_2$ stimulants, it causes tachycardia in higher doses. Fenoterol (Berotec) usually has a slower onset and longer duration of action than most beta$_2$ stimulants. In all other respects it is similar to these drugs. Metaproterenol or orciprenaline (Metaprel, Alupent) is an effective bronchodilator but produces a relatively high incidence of tremors. Terbutaline (Brethine, Bricanyl) is an effective drug with properties similar to those of the other beta$_2$ stimulants. Procaterol HCl (Pro-Air) is the most recently introduced beta$_2$ agonist for the treatment of bronchial asthma. Administered orally, it is rapidly absorbed and shows bronchodilating activity for up to eight hours. When inhaled, procaterol has a rapid bronchodilating activity, commencing within five minutes and extending for up to eight hours.

Epinephrine (Adrenalin) stimulates alpha$_1$, beta$_1$ and beta$_2$ receptors. Bronchodilatation is complemented by alpha$_1$-mediated vasoconstriction, which reduces edema and mucus production. For usual control of asthma it has largely been replaced by the more selective beta$_2$ stimulants. However, epinephrine is still used for the treatment of acute exacerbations of asthma when inhaled beta$_2$ stimulants cannot be used.

Ephedrine also stimulates alpha$_1$, beta$_1$ and beta$_2$ receptors. Ephedrine has little place in modern medicine. Although it dilates bronchioles, the drug also increases heart rate, raises peripheral resistance and stimulates the central nervous system. Products such as Marax and Tedral contain fixed ratios of ephedrine, theophylline and a central nervous system depressant. There is no evidence that they are more effective than theophylline alone. Furthermore, the use of a central nervous system depressant is strongly discouraged.

Adverse Effects

Tachycardia is the major adverse effect of beta-adrenergic drugs. Although it is more common after use of drugs that stimulate both beta$_1$ and beta$_2$ receptors, it can also be seen with selective beta$_2$ agonists when large doses are used. Other adverse effects include headaches, dizziness, nausea and tremors.

Nursing Process

The role of the nurse is to counsel the patient regarding proper administration of the medication and the nature of its adverse effects. As mentioned in Chapter 7, nurses should advise patients to seek immediate medical attention if the beta$_2$ stimulant does not terminate an attack. The reader can refer to Chapter 7 or Table 50 for the complete list of nursing actions.

Theophylline, Aminophylline and Oxtriphylline (Choledyl)

Mechanism of Action and Pharmacologic Effects

Theophylline is a less effective bronchodilator than inhaled beta$_2$ stimulants. Theophylline was previously believed to increase levels of the bronchodilator chemical cyclic adenosine monophosphate (cyclic AMP) by inhibiting phosphodiesterase, the enzyme responsible for its inactivation. However, the concentration of theophylline required to inhibit phosphodiesterase is many times the levels attained in vivo. It is currently believed that the drug dilates bronchioles by acting as an adenosine antagonist. Theophylline also increases heart rate and stimulates the central nervous system.

Theophylline is sparingly soluble in water and as a result it is usually marketed in the form of water-soluble salts. These compounds dissolve more readily in the gastrointestinal tract and are better absorbed. Two popular salts are aminophylline (theophylline ethylenediamine) and oxtriphylline (choline theophyllinate). The latter compound is sold under the trade name Choledyl. Regardless of the salt used, theophylline is the active drug in the body.

Therapeutic Uses

Theophylline, aminophylline or oxtriphylline can be used alone for the treatment of mild asthma, or combined with a beta$_2$ stimulant, ipratropium bromide, cromolyn and/or a corticosteroid in patients requiring more than one drug. At the present time, theophylline, aminophylline or oxtriphylline are usually recommended for use in patients who have failed to respond adequately to an inhalable steroid plus an inhalable beta$_2$ agonist. The ability to measure plasma theophylline levels has assisted in its safe and effective use. Therapeutic serum concentrations of theophylline are accepted as 10 – 20 μg/mL (55 – 110 μmol/L). Levels above 20 μg/mL (110 μmol/L) are associated with toxic effects.

Theophylline is given parenterally, orally and rectally. Intravenous aminophylline is used in emergency situations. Careful individual dosing is required to prevent toxic effects. Oral preparations of theophylline, aminophylline or oxtriphylline are often given every six to eight hours. Several sustained-release formulations of theophylline (including Choledyl-SA, Phyllocontin, Quibron-T, Respid, Slo-Phyllin, Somophyllin-12, and Theo-Dur) are also available for use. These products offer the convenience of twice-daily dosing with a possible reduction in adverse effects. Rectal absorption is erratic and because the margin of safety with theophylline is narrow, this route is not recommended.

Theophylline-containing products are contraindicated in peptic ulcer and coronary artery disease. They should also not be used when myocardial stimulation could prove harmful.

Adverse Effects

The principle adverse effects of theophylline are dose dependent and include gastric irritation, nausea, tachycardia, cardiac arrhythmias, central nervous system excitation, insomnia, nightmares and convulsions. Nausea is due to both gastric irritation and stimulation of the chemoreceptor trigger zone in the brain. Adverse effects occur less frequently if either oxtriphylline or aminophylline are used. However, this can be explained on the basis that these salts contain only sixty-five or eighty-five per cent theophylline, respectively.

Nursing Process

Assessment
Prior to the initial administration of theophylline, nurses should review the patient's history for documentation of pre-existing conditions that are not compatible with the drug. The physician should be contacted for confirmation of the prescription if the patient is pregnant, suffers from hypotension, hypertension, coronary artery disease, angina pectoris, peptic ulcers, renal or hepatic disease, hyperthyroidism or glaucoma. The patient's vital signs, particularly respiratory rate, rhythm, depth and chest expansion should be assessed prior to the intial dose of theophylline. Theophylline blood levels should be monitored to ensure that they remain in the therapeutic range of 10 – 20 μg/mL (55 – 110 μmol/L). Nurses must be aware that toxicity may occur with small increases above 20 μg/mL (110 μmol/L).

Administration
Theophylline should always be administered following meals to reduce gastric irritation. It should also be accompanied by at least 250 mL (8 oz.) of water to help dissolve the drug.

Evaluation

Following theophylline administration, nurses should evaluate the patient's respiratory response and compare the rate, rhythm, depth of respiration and chest expansion with the observations made before treatment. The continuing evaluation of patients receiving theophylline should include monitoring of vital signs, intake and output of fluids, and behavior. These patients should also be observed for early indications of adverse effects including an accelerated pulse rate, sudden changes in blood pressure, fluid retention, anorexia, nausea, vomiting, dizziness, insomnia and irritability.

Teaching

Patient education should focus on safety precautions. The drug can produce slight transient dizziness and patients should be advised to avoid driving or using heavy motorized equipment, industrial machinery or power tools until the effects of theophylline are fully recognized. The use of aminophylline suppositories can produce rectal irritation. If this occurs, it should be brought to the attention of the physician. Nurses must emphasize the need for a patient to seek medical advice before taking over-the-counter remedies, especially those for the treatment of colds or nasal congestion. Patients who smoke should be advised to stop and be given general teaching related to the respiratory problems caused by smoking.

Anticholinergic Drugs

Ipratropium Bromide (Atrovent Inhaler)

Mechanism of Action and Pharmacologic Effects

Ipratropium is an anticholinergic drug (see Chapter 6) that is administered by inhalation or nasal aerosol. It competitively blocks the action of acetylcholine at parasympathetic (cholinergic) receptors. Ipratropium is poorly absorbed and has few systemic effects.

Therapeutic Uses

Ipratroprium may be given by inhalation for the treatment of bronchoconstriction associated with asthma or chronic obstructive pulmonary disease (COPD — chronic bronchitis or emphysema). For the treatment of asthma, it is a less effective bronchodilator than inhaled beta$_2$ stimulants, but has additive effects when used in conjunction with a beta$_2$ agonist. Ipratropium is an equally or more effective bronchodilator than a beta$_2$ agonist in the treatment of COPD.

It has a slower onset of action than beta$_2$ agonists, with its maximum effects appearing about two hours after inhalation. Its relatively long duration of action (approximately six hours) makes the drug suitable for maintenance therapy.

Tolerance does not appear to develop to ipratropium. Because of minimal effects on the cardiovascular system, it may be used as the initial bronchodilator in patients with heart disease, hypertension, cerebrovascular disease or thyrotoxicosis. An inhaled beta$_2$ stimulant, theophylline, cromolyn or corticosteroids may be added to ipratropium in patients requiring multiple-drug therapy.

Adverse Effects

Ipratropium bromide is well tolerated. Its most common adverse effects are dry mouth or throat or both, headache, bad taste and/or blurred vision.

Nursing Process

Ipratropium bromide is a relatively new drug and nursing experience with it is limited. Nurses are advised to consult the manufacturer's package insert material for latest information and clinical practice advice.

Assessment

Assess the patient for palpitations. If they occur, it may be necessary to stop ipratropium and begin alternative therapy.

Administration

Ipratropium should be stored at room temperature. Give frequent drinks and hard candy to relieve dry mouth.

Evaluation

Nurses should evaluate the breathing patterns of patients for therapeutic effects. Although tolerance is usually not a problem, nurses should monitor patients for possible drug tolerance and the need to alter dosage.

Teaching

Patients must be taught the importance of complying with the number of prescribed inhalations per twenty-four hour period to remove the possibility of drug overdose.

Anti-Inflammatory Drugs

Corticosteroids

Mechanism of Action and Pharmacologic Effects

The pharmacology of these drugs is presented in detail in Chapter 29. Corticosteroids are very effective anti-inflammatory drugs. In discussing the effects of chronic corticosteroid therapy in asthma it is important to differentiate between inhalable steroids, which provide effective relief of inflammation for many patients, with minimal or no systemic adverse effects, and the ingestion of drugs such as prednisone, which although effective as anti-inflammatories can produce severe systemic adverse effects.

Therapeutic Uses

The introduction of **inhaled** beclomethasone dipropionate (Beclovent, Vanceril) has provided many patients with the benefits of local corticosteroid therapy without systemic toxicities. Beclomethasone dipropionate owes its therapeutic value to two properties. First, it is a very effective anti-inflammatory drug. Second, in normal doses, the quantity of drug swallowed is extensively inactivated during its first pass through the liver. The success of this form of therapy cannot be questioned. Most patients who might otherwise have received systemic corticosteroid therapy can now be treated satisfactorily with beclomethasone dipropionate. Like beta$_2$ stimulants, inhalable corticosteroids work better if an "add-on" device is inserted between the mouthpiece of the meter dose inhaler and the patient. Many physicians believe that inhalable corticosteroid should be started if a patient requires beta-stimulant bronchodilator treatment more frequently than twice daily.

Budesonide (Pulmicort) is a second inhalable glucocorticoid used for asthma. Like beclomethasone dipropionate, budesonide has high topical anti-inflammatory potency with minimal systemic effects. This favorable separation between topical anti-inflammatory activity and systemic effect is due to strong glucocorticoid receptor affinity and an effective first-pass metabolism with a short half-life for the quantity of the drug that is inadvertently swallowed.

Systemic corticosteroids are usually reserved for patients who have not responded to other forms of treatment. Concern over adverse effects usually relegates their systemic use to patients in whom beta$_2$ stimulants, ipratropium bromide and/or theophylline are not capable of providing relief. Prednisone is usually the corticosteroid chosen when systemic steroid therapy is indicated. Its duration of action is approximately thirty-six hours. Given orally, it is metabolized in the liver to its active metabolite, prednisolone. If alternate-day therapy is effective, adrenal atrophy is reduced and the adverse effects of prednisone are minimized.

Soluble corticosteroids such as methyl prednisolone sodium succinate (Solu-Medrol) are administered intravenously, along with intravenous aminophylline and an inhaled beta$_2$ stimulant in the treatment of status asthmaticus.

Adverse Effects

The adverse effects of systemic corticosteroid therapy are described in Chapter 29. They include redistribution of body fat, leading to a "moon face" and a "buffalo hump", increased susceptibility to infection, and reduced growth rate in children. Osteoporosis can also occur and patients may show psychotic changes. The local effects of beclomethasone dipropionate include laryngeal myopathy and *Candida albicans* infections in the mouth and throat.

Nursing Process

This information is presented in Chapter 29 and Table 46. With respect to the use of inhalable beclomethasone dipropionate, continued use predisposes patients to fungal infections of the mouth. Nurses should recommend that patients rinse their mouths with an antiseptic mouthwash immediately following each inhalation to reduce this likelihood.

Inhibitors of Inflammatory-Response Mediators

Cromolyn/Sodium Cromoglycate (Intal)

Mechanism of Action and Pharmacologic Effects

Histamine, released from mast cells during an antigen-antibody reaction, constricts bronchioles and produces mucus. Cromolyn, or sodium cromoglycate, decreases histamine release from mast cells. It is inhaled in a microcrystalline powder or solution (Intal) or from a pressurized aerosol (Fivent). Cromolyn is not a bronchodilator.

Therapeutic Uses

Cromolyn is used chronically to prevent asthmatic attacks. In mild exercise-induced asthma, it can be used when needed before exercise. Cromolyn is not a bronchodilator and has no value in terminating an attack. Although cromolyn affords protection to some patients, particularly those with mild allergic asthma, many patients fail to respond to the drug. In general, younger patients fare better on the medication.

Adverse Effects

Cromolyn has few adverse effects. When given as a powder, it may cause irritation.

Nursing Process

Assessment
Nursing actions related to the prescription of cromolyn begin with a review of the patient's history for evidence of previous kidney or liver disease. Eosinophil counts should be monitored during therapy. The rate and rhythm of the respiratory status of patients should also be noted before and during therapy, as well as coughing, wheezing and dyspnea.

Administration
The powder medication is inhaled using a special "Spinhaler". Nurses are advised to consult the manufacturer's insert for detailed instruction on the administration of cromolyn. The capsules and their contents should be protected from heat and moisture during storage. These capsules should not be swallowed. Nurses should ensure that patients clear mucus before using cromolyn.

Teaching
Patient teaching should involve instruction on the use of the "Spinhaler". Nurses must stress to patients that the cromolyn capsules are not effective when taken orally. Similarly, nurses must emphasize the need for patients to take the medication every day, even if an attack has not occurred for some period of time. Failure to heed this advice may result in a recurrence of the asthmatic attacks.

Nedocromil Sodium (Tilade)

Mechanism of Action and Pharmacologic Effects

Nedocromil sodium inhibits the release of inflammatory mediators from a variety of cell types occurring in the lumen and in the mucosa of the bronchial tree. When it is administered topically to the bronchi, it displays specific anti-inflammatory properties. Nedocromil prevents the release of mediators, such as histamine, leukotriene C_4 (LTC_4) and prostaglandin D_2 from the cellular population of the chronically inflamed bronchus, especially from mast cells of the mucosal type.

Therapeutic Uses

When administered by inhalation, nedocromil is indicated as an adjunctive in the treatment of mild to moderate reversible obstructive airway disease, including bronchial asthma and bronchitis, particularly where allergic factors may be present. Nedocromil can also be used on a maintenance or occasional basis in the prevention of bronchospasm provoked by stimulants such as inhaled allergens, cold air, exercise and atmospheric pollutants.

Adverse Effects

Few adverse effects of nedocromil sodium have been reported. Patients may complain of an unpleasant taste, headache and nausea. However, in nearly all cases these have been mild and transient and insufficient to require discontinuation of treatment.

Ketotifen (Zaditen)

Mechanism of Action and Pharmacologic Effects

Ketotifen has a complex pharmacologic action. Its effects include blocking histamine$_1$ (H$_1$) receptors, stabilizing mast cells and thereby reducing histamine release, and inhibiting the effects of the platelet-activating factor. In addition, ketotifen may also antagonize calcium flux in smooth muscle, and enhance beta-adrenergic mediated effects in the bronchioles. The result of these actions is that the drug may reduce the severity and duration of asthma attacks.

Therapeutic Uses

Ketotifen is used as an adjunct to other drugs in the chronic prophylaxis of mild atopic (allergic) asthma in children. The efficacy of ketotifen in asthma prophylaxis in children is controversial. It does not appear to be more effective than cromolyn (Intal) and in some trials it appears to have been no more effective than placebo therapy. However, other studies claim significant effects for the drug. Six to twelve weeks of chronic treatment with ketotifen may reduce a patient's daily requirements for theophylline, a beta$_2$ agonist or corticosteroids.

Adverse Effects

Ketotifen produces few adverse effects. The most common are temporary sedation, weight gain, rash, dry mouth, dizziness, nausea and headache.

Drug Treatment of Status Asthmaticus

An acute attack of asthma, unresponsive to the patient's usual medications, is a serious medical emergency. Patients should be hospitalized and treated intensively. They should not receive any central nervous system depressants, such as a benzodiazepine or barbiturate, because these drugs have been associated with incidents of sudden death. A bronchodilator should be given parenterally. Either epinephrine, subcutaneously, or aminophylline, intravenously, are the drugs of choice. A soluble corticosteroid, such as methyl prednisolone sodium succinate (Solu-Medrol), should be given intravenously. Patients may also be treated regularly with an inhalation dose of a beta$_2$ stimulant, such as salbutamol. Detailed nursing interventions that are not pharmacologically based will be found in medical-surgical nursing texts.

Further Reading

Barnes, P.J. (1989). A new approach to the treatment of asthma. *New Engl. J. Med. 321* :1517-1527.

Dolovich, M.B. and Newhouse, M.T. (1988). Aerosols, generation, methods of administration and therapeutic applications in asthma. In: E. Middleton et al. (eds.), *Allergy, Principles and Practice,* 3rd ed., pp. 568-578. C.V. Mosby.

Drugs for asthma. Drugs of choice (1989). *The Medical Letter 31* :70-78.

Glynn-Barnhart, A., Hill, M. and Szefler, S.J. (1988). Sustained-release theophylline preparations: Practical recommendations for prescribing and therapeutic drug monitoring. *Drugs 35* :711-726.

Gregg, I. (1989). What has been the effect of modern therapy upon morbidity of asthma? *Eur. Resp. J. 2* :674-677.

Guyatt, G.H., Townsend, M., Norgradi, S., Pugsley, S.T., Keller, J.L. and Newhouse, M.T. (1988). Acute response to a bronchodilator. An imperfect guide for bronchodilator therapy in chronic airflow limitation. *Arch. Intern. Med. 148* :1949-1952.

Inhaled corticosteroids: Are higher doses better? (1986). *Drugs and Therapeutics Bulletin 24* (Jan. 13):1-2.

Knight, A. (1989). Preventing asthma deaths. *Modern Med. of Canada 44* :526-534.

Mawhinney, H. and Spector, S.L. (1986). Optimum management of asthma in pregnancy. *Drugs 32* :178-187.

Meltzer, E.O. (1990). To use or not to use antihistamines in patients with asthma. *Annals of Allergy 64* :183-186.

Newhouse, M.T. and Dolovich, M. (1987). Aerosol therapy of reversible airflow obstruction. Concepts and clinical applications. *Chest 91* (5)(Suppl.):58S-64S.

Sears, M.R., Taylor, D.R., Print, C.G., Lake, D.C., Quingquing, Li, Flannery, E.M., Yates, D.M., Lucas, M.K. and Herbison, G.P. (1990). Regular inhaled beta-agonist treatment in bronchial asthma. *The Lancet 336* :1391-1396.

Table 50
Antiasthmatic drugs.

Generic Name (Trade Name)	Use (Dose)	Action	Adverse Effects	Drug Interactions	Nursing Process
Pharmacologic Classification: Adrenergic Drugs					
Epinephrine, adrenaline (Adrenalin, Medihaler-Epi, Primatene Mist, Vaponephrin)	Parenteral tx for emergencies [status asthmaticus]. Inhalat'n tx for symptomatic relief of bronchospasm and mucus secret'ns (**SC:** Adults - 0.2-0.5 mL $1/1000$ solut'n q20min prn up to 3 doses. Children - 0.01 mg/kg. May be repeated q20min for 3 doses max. **Inhalat'n:** Us. 2 inhalat'ns; if no relief, repeat in 5 min)	Bronchodilatat'n due to stimulat'n of beta$_2$ receptors, incr. respiratory rate and tidal volume, reduced alveolar CO_2 concentrat'ns; reduced mucosal congest'n due to vasoconstrict'n of bronchiolar blood vessels assoc. w. alpha$_1$ stimulat'n	Fear, anxiety, tension, restlessness, headache, tremor, pallor, incr. intraocular pressure, respiratory difficulties, palpitat'ns, tachycardia, incr. cardiac output, hyperten's'n	**Antidepressants, tricyclic:** May incr. several-fold the pressor responses to epinephrine. **Antidiabetic drugs:** Will have reduced effects because epinephrine incr. glucose levels. **Antihistamines:** May potentiate actions of epinephrine. **Beta blockers:** May result in exaggerated alpha (vasoconstrictor) response to epinephrine. This can produce hypertension and reflex vagal-induced bradycardia. **L-thyroxine:** Can potentiate effects of epinephrine.	**Assess:** For pt hx of glaucoma; for CV, circulatory or cerebrovascular disease; prostatic hypertrophy, diabetes mellitus, hyperthyroidism or pregnancy. Establish baseline BP, rate and rhythm of pulse, color and temp. of extremities. **Administer:** From a light-resistant container, us. self-administered prn for asthmatic attacks. **Evaluate:** Respiratory effect; BP and pulse carefully; color; urine output; mental'n and orientat'n. **Teaching:** Use only no. of doses nec. to achieve relief; wait 2 min bet. doses; s/s adv. effects; sit or lie down after use; discard discolored solut'ns; count pulse rate.
Ephedrine	Administered chronically to prevent asthmatic attacks (**Oral:** Adults - 25-50 mg q6h. Children - 3 mg/kg q24h in 4 divided doses)	As for epinephrine	As for epinephrine	**Guanethidine:** May have its actions antagonized by ephedrine. **MAOIs:** And epinephrine can produce severe hypertensive react'n.	As for epinephrine
Isoproterenol (Isuprel, Vapo-Iso, Medihaler-Iso)	Symptomatic relief of bronchospasm in asthma and other chronic bronchopulmonary disorders in which bronchospasm is complicating factor (**Inhalat'n:** 1-2 puffs from preset nebulizer; max. 8x/day for adults)	Stimulat'n of beta$_2$ receptors in bronchioles causes incr. format'n of cAMP and produces bronchodilatat'n. Simultaneous stimulat'n of beta$_1$ receptors produces tachycardia.	Refractory bronchial obstruct'n, tachycardia, incr. cardiac output, cardiac arrhythmias, cardiac arrest, decr. BP, headache, nausea, palpitat'ns, tremor, insomnia	**Antidepressants, tricyclic:** And isoproterenol produce cumulative effects. **Beta blockers:** Can inhibit actions of isoproterenol.	**Assess:** As for epinephrine. **Administer:** From metered nebulizer by instructing pt to insert mouthpiece bet. teeth, close lips around mouthpiece, exhale through nose, inhale through mouth and simultaneously release dose from nebulizer, hold breath for as long as possible, then exhale slowly.

Drug	Action/Use	Side Effects	Dosage	Drug Interactions	Nursing Considerations
Albuterol, salbutamol (Proventil, Ventolin), fenoterol (Berotec), metaproterenol orciprenaline (Metaprel, Alupent) terbutaline (Brethine, Bricanyl), procaterol (Pro-Air)	Selective beta₂ stimulants w. same uses as isoproterenol. Selective beta₂ stimulant produces incr. cAMP format'n and resultant bronchodilat'n.	Palpitat'ns, tachycardia, nervousness, tremor, nausea, vomiting, headache, dizziness	**(Inhalat'n:** 1-2 puffs up to qid. More than 8 puffs/day not recommended. **Oral:** *Albuterol/salbutamol* - Adults - 2-4 mg tid or qid. Children [6-12 years] - 2 mg tid-qid. *Controlled release, 4- or 8-mg salbutamol tablets (Volmax)* - Adults and children [12 and over] - 8 mg q12h. *Fenoterol* - Adults - 2.5-5 mg bid-tid. *Orciprenaline* - Adults and children [over 12 years] - Initially, 20 mg tid-qid. Children 4-12 years - 10 mg tid. *Terbutaline* - Adults - 5 mg tid. Reduce to 2.5 mg tid in the event of adv. effects. *Procaterol* - Adults and children over 12 years - initially, 50 µg bid. For some pts, may incr. dose to 50 µg tid or 100 µg bid. Not to exceed 200 µg/day)	**Antidepressants, tricyclic:** Potentiate effects of beta agonists on vascular system. **Beta blockers:** Block effects of beta stimulants. **MAOIs:** Potentiate effects of beta agonists on vascular system.	As for isoproterenol

Pharmacologic Classification: Theophylline Products

Drug	Action/Use	Side Effects	Dosage	Drug Interactions	Nursing Considerations
Theophylline (Elixophylline, Bronkodyl, Theolar, etc.), aminophylline (Aminophyl, Aminophylline Suppositories), oxtriphylline (Choledyl)	Symptomatic tx of reversible bronchoconstrict'n, bronchial asthma, COPD and related bronchospastic disorders	Blockade of adenosine receptors, resulting in bronchodilatat'n. Other effects of theophylline include CNS excitat'n, incr. in heart rate and systemic vasodilatat'n.	Gastric irritat'n, nausea, vomiting, anorexia, diarrhea, CNS excitat'n, irritability, insomnia, nightmares, convuls'ns, palpitat'ns, tachycardia, cardiac arrhythmias, diuresis, respiratory distress	**(Oral:** Adults - 100-300 mg q6h. **Rectal:** Adults - 250-500 mg aminophylline suppositories tid. **IV:** *Aminophylline* - If no theophylline preparat'n taken for previous 24 h, loading dose is 6 mg/kg over 20-30 min. Maint. dose for nonsmoking adults, 0.5±0.2 mg/kg/h. For addit'nal dosage informat'n, consult manufacturer's monograph and adjust according to serum levels)	**Allopurinol:** Can elevate serum theophylline levels. **Beta stimulants:** May incr. bronchodilatat'n produced by theophylline and its salts but may also produce toxic synergism. **Epinephrine:** May produce toxic synergism w. theophylline and its salt. **Erythromycin:** Can elevate theophylline serum levels. **Estrogens:** Can elevate theophylline serum levels. **Phenobarbital:** Can incr. theophylline clearance. **Phenytoin:** Can incr. theophylline clearance. **Progestins:** Can elevate theophylline serum levels.	**Assess:** For pregnancy; review hx for hypotens'n, coronary artery disease, angina, peptic ulcer, renal or hepatic disease, hypertens'n, hyperthyroidism, glaucoma. Establish baseline VS, theophylline blood levels for efficacy and toxicity. **Administer:** With 250 mL (8 oz.) water, pc; w. antacid if GI irritat'n is pronounced. **Evaluate:** Respirat'ns (rate, rhythm, depth, chest expans'n); plasma theophylline levels; pulse, BP; fluid intake/output; for early signs of adv. effects (anorexia, nausea, vomiting, dizziness, irritability). **Teach:** Safety precaut'ns related to transient dizziness; report rectal irritat'n when drug given rectally; seek medical

Generic Name (Trade Name)	Use (Dose)	Action	Adverse Effects	Drug Interactions	Nursing Process
					advice prior to taking OTC drugs; importance of not smoking; us. general instruct'ns to pts w. respiratory problems.

Pharmacologic Classification: Anticholinergic

Generic Name (Trade Name)	Use (Dose)	Action	Adverse Effects	Drug Interactions	Nursing Process
Ipratropium bromide (Atrovent Inhaler)	Maint. tx of chronic reversible airway obstruct'n (**Inhalat'n:** 2 puffs [40 µg] tid-qid. Some may need up to 4 puffs [80 µg] at a time for max. benefit. Max. daily dose not to exceed 8 puffs [160 µg]. Min. interval bet. doses not less than 4 h)	By blocking action of vagus competitively, ipratropium dilates bronchioles, reduces mucus secret'n and decr. edema. Ipratropium is poorly absorbed and us. has few systemic effects. It is a less effective bronchodilator than inhaled beta₂ stimulants.	Dry mouth, headache, blurred vision, tremor, palpitat'ns, urinary retent'n		**Assess:** For palpitat'ns, as drug may have to be changed. **Administer:** Store at room temp. Give frequent drinks and hard candy to relieve dry mouth. **Evaluate:** Breathing patterns for tx effects. Monitor for poss. drug tolerance, indicating need for dose change. **Teach:** Importance of compliance to no. of inhalat'ns/24 h, as overdose may occur.

Pharmacologic Classification: Corticosteroids

Generic Name (Trade Name)	Use (Dose)	Action	Adverse Effects	Drug Interactions	Nursing Process
Prednisone (Deltasone, Meticorten, Orasone)	For bronchospasm not treated adequately by other medicat'ns (**Oral:** Adults - Initial daily dose, 5-60 mg)	Reduces inflammat'n and edema, potentiates bronchodilating effects of adrenergic drugs. For addit'nal actions, refer to Chapter 29 and Table 46.	Redistribut'n of body fat and fluid; hirsuitism; muscle wasting; K deplet'n; emot'nal disturbances; hypertens'n. For addit'nal adv. effects, refer to Table 45.	For drug interact'ns involving amphotericin B, oral anticoagulants, antidiabetic agents, barbiturates, oral contraceptives, diuretics, indomethacin, phenytoin, rifampin and salicylates, see Table 46.	**Assess:** For pregnancy or lactat'n; for hx diabetes mellitus, hypertens'n, CHF, nephritis, thrombophlebitis, peptic ulcer, psychoses, Cushing's syndrome, active TB, herpes simplex; establish baseline weight, BP, sleep pattern. **Administer:** Prednisone with meals during initial doses; give maint. doses in early a.m. w. food; regularly—never w'draw drug abruptly. **Evaluate:** Tx effectiveness; daily; muscle strength and mass in limbs; for hyperglycemia; BP bid until dosage regulated; for infectious diseases, inflammat'n, wound healing; diet for K, protein, salt intake; refer to dietician
Beclomethasome dipropionate (Beclovent, Vanceril)	Tx of steroid-responsive asthma (**Inhalat'n:** Adults - 2 puffs [100 µg] tid-qid. If this dose not sufficient, it can be doubled initially. Not to exceed 1 mg/day [20 puffs]. Children 6-14 years - 1 puff bid-qid. 3-5 years - 1 puff bid-tid)	As for prednisone. Beclomethasone dipropionate aerosol us. provides satisfactory antiasthmatic action without systemic adv. effects.	Above 1 mg daily, systemic adrenal suppress'n. Appearance of C. albicans in mouth and throat. Laryngeal myopathy.	As for prednisone	

Drug	Use / Dosage	Action	Adverse Effects	Nursing Implications	
Budesonide (Pulmicort Inhaler, Pulmicort SPACER)	**As for beclomethasone dipropionate (Inhalat'n: Adults and children over 12 years - 400-1600 µg/day, divided into 2-4 doses. Maint. dose is us. 200-400 µg bid, but higher may be nec. for longer or shorter periods in some pts. Children 6-12 years - Initially, 200-400 µg/day, in divided doses bid. Maint. tx is individualized at lowest effective dose)**	As for prednisone	Few adv. effects if used for a limited time.	As for prednisone	prn; for recent or impending stressful life events, emot'nal status and stability; sleep pattern; for GI irritat'n; for adv. effects. **Teach:** Nec. of medical supervis'n; importance of personal hygiene as means of preventing infect'ns; danger of and precaut'ns against abrupt w'drawl of medicat'n; s/s adv. effects.
Methyprednisolone sodium succinate (Solu-Medrol)	Emergency tx of steroid-responsive asthma (**IV:** Initially, 20-100 mg over a period of at least 10 min. Subsequent doses can be given q6h afterward)	As for prednisone	Few adv. effects.	As for prednisone	As for prednisone

Pharmacologic Classification: Inhibitors of Inflammatory Response Mediators

Drug	Use / Dosage	Action	Adverse Effects	Nursing Implications
Cromolyn, sodium cromoglycate (Intal)	As adjunct in management of intrinsic and extrinsic asthma, including exercise-induced asthma, cold air-induced asthma and occupat'nal asthma. Use continuously to prevent s/s these condit'ns (**Inhalat'n:** For adults and children - For Intal, 1 Spincap cartridge qid at 4-6 h intervals)	Reduces release of histamine from mast cells in response to an antigen-antibody react'n.	Inhalat'n of Intal powder may cause transient bronchospasm or irritat'n of throat or trachea.	**Assess:** For previous hypersensitivity, kidney or liver disease. Monitor eosinophil count during tx. Monitor respiratory status before and during tx for rate, rhythm and for coughing, wheezing and dyspnea. **Administer:** Follow manufacturer's direct'ns using special inhaler; protect from moisture and heat. Capsules *not* to be swallowed. Have pt clear mucus before administrat'n. **Teach:** Proper method of self-administrat'n; that capsules are *not* effective when taken orally; that up to 4 weeks may be required before tx benefits are seen; to consult w. physician before discontinuing.
Nedocromil sodium (Tilade)	Adjunct in tx of mild to moderate reversible obstructive airway disease, particularly where allergic factors may be present. Prevent'n of bronchospasm provoked by stimulants such as inhaled allergens, cold air, exercise and atmospheric pollutants (**Inhalat'n:** Adults and children over 12 - Two actuat'ns [4 mg] qid. Some pts can be maintained on 2 actuat'ns bid)	Inhibits release of inflammatory mediators from a variety of cell types in the lumen and mucosa of bronchial tree. Prevents release of histamine, LTC_4, and PGD_2.	Few adv. react'ns have been reported. Pts may complain of unpleasant taste, headache and nausea.	

Generic Name (Trade Name)	Use (Dose)	Action	Adverse Effects	Drug Interactions	Nursing Process
Ketotifen (Zaditen)	Adjunct to other drugs in chronic prophylaxis of mild atopic [allergic] asthma in children (**Oral:** Children 3 years and older - Initially, 0.5 mg bid or 1 mg hs. Incr. after approx. 5 days to 1 mg bid with a.m. and p.m. meals)	Blocks histamine₁ receptors. Stabilizes mast cells and reduces histamine release. May also antagonize Ca flux in smooth muscle and enhance beta-adrenergic effects.	Low incidence adv. effects. Temporary sedat'n, weight gain, rash, dry mouth, dizziness, nausea, headache	**Alcohol or sedatives:** Should be avoided w. ketotifen because of risk of additive CNS depress'n. **Antidiabetic agents, oral:** Plus ketotifen, may produce thrombocytopenia.	

CHAPTER 33

Nasal Decongestants

Teaching Objectives

Following completion of this chapter, the reader should be able to:

1. List the types of drugs used to treat nasal congestion.
2. Discuss the mechanism of action, pharmacologic effects, therapeutic uses and adverse effects of adrenergic vasoconstrictors, as well as the nursing process related to their use.
3. Describe the mechanism of action, pharmacologic effects, therapeutic uses and adverse effects of antihistamines in the treatment of nasal congestion, as well as the nursing process related to their use.
4. Discuss the mechanism of action, pharmacologic effects, therapeutic uses and adverse effects of corticosteroids in the treatment of nasal congestion, as well as the nursing process related to their use.
5. Explain the mechanism of action, therapeutic use and adverse effects of cromolyn in the treatment of nasal congestion, as well as the nursing process precipitated by its use.

An increase in nasal vascular congestion, resulting from such conditions as the common cold and inflammation of the nose and sinuses, reduces airflow. This chapter discusses the use of adrenergic vasoconstrictors, antihistamines, corticosteroids and histamine-release inhibitors in the treatment of nasal congestion.

Adrenergic Vasoconstrictors

Mechanism of Action and Pharmacologic Effects

Adrenergic vasoconstrictors stimulate alpha$_1$ receptors on blood vessels. When they are applied topically, their actions are restricted largely to the nasal mucosa. Administered orally, they may constrict vessels throughout the body, increasing peripheral resistance and blood pressure. Included in the adrenergic vasoconstrictors currently available are ephedrine sulfate, naphazoline HCl (Privine), phenylephrine HCl (Neo-Synephrine), pseudoephedrine HCl (Sudafed), tetrahydrozolone HCl (Tyzine) and xylometazoline HCl (Neo-Synephrine II, Otrivin).

Therapeutic Uses

Adrenergic vasoconstrictors offer the patient temporary, symptomatic relief of the acute rhinitis that accompanies the common cold, hay fever, nonseasonal allergic rhinitis and sinusitis. When used topically in the form of drops or spray, they have a rapid onset of action. However, not all areas of the mucosa may be exposed to the drug. Furthermore, the topical route is more likely to produce rebound congestion, especially with chronic use. Propylhexedrine vaporizer (Benzedrex) provides the patient with a volatile vasoconstrictor that can reach the desired area of the nasal mucosa and provide rapid decongestion.

Oral treatment may enable the vasoconstrictor to reach nasal areas not accessible if the drug is applied topically. Although the onset of action is slower following ingestion, the drug's duration of action is also longer. As mentioned before, oral therapy may result in a generalized vasoconstriction and an increase in blood pressure.

Adverse Effects

Applied topically, adrenergic vasoconstrictors can produce stinging, burning or dryness of the mucosa, and rebound hyperemia. Chronic abuse results in red, edematous mucosa. Systemic hypertension is usually not seen when the drugs are applied topically. However, systemic reactions can be seen, particularly in infants and children, if large doses are used. These drugs should be used with great care in the young.

The adverse effects of oral administration include hypertension, palpitations, dizziness, nervousness and central nervous system stimulation. Constriction of the coronary vessels can lead to cardiac arrhythmias. Young patients and individuals suffering from cardiovascular disease are at greater risk.

Nursing Process

The role of the nurse regarding the use of adrenergic vasoconstrictors is detailed in Chapter 7. Readers are advised to refer to that material.

Administration
Ordinarily these medications are self-administered, once in the morning and once at night. Patients should blow their nose before using the medication. For the administration of nose drops, the patient should lie down with the head turned to the side in order to prevent the nose drops from entering the throat. After every use and before returning the dropper to the container, the dropper should be thoroughly rinsed to prevent contamination of the solution with nasal secretions.

For the administration of nasal spray the patient should sit up and lean slightly forward. The nozzle should be placed in the nostril but not occluded. Patients should sniff vigorously during administration of the spray.

Teaching
Patients should be cautioned that swallowing medication that enters the throat may cause systemic effects. Patient teaching should alert the patient to the possibility that intranasal application of these medications may cause a stinging sensation in the nose. In addition, nurses should emphasize to patients the risk of rebound congestion that is associated with prolonged use of these medications.

Antihistamines

Mechanism of Action and Pharmacologic Effects

Antihistamines competitively block histamine$_1$ (H$_1$) receptors in the body, thereby preventing histamine from producing vasodilatation, increased capillary permeability and tissue edema. These drugs, which include diphenhydramine HCl (Benadryl), clemastine fumarate (Tavist), chlorpheniramine maleate (Chlor-Trimeton, Chlor-Tripolon), brompheniramine maleate (Dimetane), dexchlorpheniramine maleate (Polaramine), astemizole (Hismanal), terfenadine (Seldane) and loratadine (Claritin) can be used for a variety of conditions in which the release and action of histamine play an important role. The general pharmacology of antihistamines is presented in Chapter 35. This chapter deals with their use only in the treatment of nasal congestion.

Therapeutic Uses

Antihistamines reduce the symptoms of sneezing, rhinorrhea and pruritus of the eyes, nose, and throat in patients with allergic rhinitis. Their efficacy is better when the symptoms are of recent onset. Antihistamines are most effective when rhinorrhea is associated with nasal congestion. They may aggravate a dry stuffy nose, in which case patients are better treated with normal saline or a polyethylene glycol-propylene glycol solution, used alone or in combination with antihistamines.

The drugs are more effective in the treatment of seasonal allergic rhinitis than in nonseasonal, perennial allergic rhinitis. They are found in all cold preparations, but evidence for their effectiveness in this condition is not overwhelming. Antihistamines are often combined with adrenergic vasoconstrictors in products such as Actifed, Dimetapp, Drixoral and Ornade.

Adverse Effects

Sedation is the most common adverse effect of antihistamines. Astemizole, terfenadine and loratadine have minimal sedative effects. Except for individuals taking these three drugs, all patients should be warned of the dangers of driving a car or operating machinery and informed about the additive effects of alcohol and antihistamines. Other manifestations of central nervous system depression are dizziness, lassitude, incoordination, fatigue, tinnitus and diplopia. Some patients, particularly children, may experience euphoria, nervousness, irritability, insomnia, tremors and an increased tendency towards convulsions.

The gastrointestinal adverse effects of antihistamines include nausea, vomiting, abdominal discomfort, constipation and diarrhea. Loss of appetite may also occur. Most antihistamines have anticholinergic properties and can cause dryness of the mouth, throat and nasal airway; tightness of the chest; palpitations; headache; and urinary retention.

Nursing Process

The nursing process associated with the use of antihistamines is discussed in detail in Chapter 35. Readers are advised to refer to that material.

Corticosteroids

Mechanism of Action and Pharmacologic Effects

The general pharmacology of corticosteroids is presented in Chapter 29. They are potent anti-inflammatory drugs. Applied topically, they reduce erythema and edema in nasal passages.

Therapeutic Uses

Beclomethasone dipropionate (Beconase, Vancenase) and flunisolide (Nasalide, Rhinalar) are formulated for topical nasal use. Although they are offically indicated for the treatment of perennial and seasonal allergic rhinitis unresponsive to conventional therapy, many physicians use them as first-line drugs in allergic rhinitis because they have fewer side effects and are more effective than antihistamines.

Both products may also be helpful in the management of rhinitis of physical or chemical origin. The drugs have also been suggested for the treatment of rhinitis medicamentosa resulting from the overzealous use of topical vasoconstrictors. Polyposis originating in the nasal cavity may be controllable with topical steroids, but surgical excision is often still required. Both beclomethasone dipropionate and flunisolide may prevent or delay recurrent polyposis following polypectomy.

Adverse Effects

Local reactions include a burning sensation in the nose, sneezing attacks and, on occasion, a bloody nasal discharge. Patients may develop localized candidal infections. If high doses of these drugs are applied to the nose, sufficient quantities may be absorbed to depress the hypothalamic-pituitary-adrenal axis and produce generalized systemic effects. Long-term use may lead to atrophic rhinitis.

Nursing Process

Corticosteroids are very powerful medications. Their use should not be treated lightly. Readers are advised to consult Chapter 29, where detailed discussion of the nursing process related to the prescription and use of corticosteroids is presented.

Histamine-Release Inhibitors

Cromolyn/Sodium Cromoglycate (Rynacrom)

The pharmacology of cromolyn, or sodium cromoglycate, is discussed in greater detail in Chapter 32. The drug reduces the release of histamine following an antigen-antibody reaction. This property accounts for its prophylactic use in the treatment of seasonal rhinitis. Insufflated as either a powder or a two per cent solution, cromolyn affords relief to many patients afflicted with seasonal rhinitis. Other than slight irritation, cromolyn causes few adverse effects. The nursing process associated with the use of cromolyn is also presented in detail in Chapter 32.

Further Reading

Bryant, B.G. and Cormier, J. F. (1982). Cold and allergy products. In: *Handbook of Nonprescription Drugs,* 7th ed., pp. 123-169. Washington: American Pharmaceutical Association.

Decongestant, cough and cold preparations (1986). *AMA Drug Evaluations,* 6th ed., pp. 369-391.

First report of the expert advisory committee on nonprescription cough and cold remedies on antihistamines, nasal decongestants and anticholinergics (1989). *Information Letter No.764* (August 10). Ottawa: Health Protection Branch.

Hendeles, L., Weinberger, M. and Wong, L. (1980). Medical management of noninfectious rhinitis. *Amer. J. Hosp. Pharm. 37* :1496-1504.

Table 51
Nasal decongestants.

Pharmacologic Classification: Adrenergic Vasoconstrictors

Generic Name (Trade Name)	Use (Dose)	Action	Adverse Effects	Drug Interactions	Nursing Process
Oxymetazoline HCl (Afin, Duration, Neo-Synephrine 12 Hour)	Symptomatic relief of nasal congest'n due to sinusitis, rhinitis and the common cold (**Topical** [solut'n or spray]: Adults and children over 6 years - 2-4 drops or 2-3 squeezes 0.05% solut'n in each nostril, a.m. and hs. Children 2-5 years - 2-3 drops 0.025% solut'n in each nostril)	Stims. alpha₁ receptors on blood vessels. When applied locally, their actions are largely restricted to nasal mucosa. Administered orally, adrenergic vasoconstrictors may constrict blood vessels throughout body, incr. peripheral resistance and BP.	Burning, stinging, mucosal dryness, sneezing, palpitat'ns, tachycardia, hypertens'n, headache, nervousness, insomnia, blurred vision, drowsiness, CNS depress'n, rebound congest'n	The following interact'ns apply generally to all vasoconstrictors: **Antidepressants, tricyclic:** Can incr. activity of adrenergic vasoconstrictors. Because of poss. generalized vasoconstrict'n and tachycardia, vasoconstrictors should be used very cautiously in pts receiving TCAs. **MAOIs:** Are contraindicated in pts receiving adrenergic vasoconstrictors.	See Table 5. **Administer:** Self-administered a.m. and hs. Nose drops: Pt should blow nose before use; lie down w. head turned to side; rinse dropper thoroughly after each use. Spray: Pt should sit up, lean slightly forward, insert nozzle into nostril but not occlude it; sniff vigorously during administrat'n. **Teach:** Medicat'n that enters throat may cause systemic effects; that intranasal applicat'n may cause stinging sensat'n; risk of rebound congest'n w. prolonged use.
Phenylephrine HCl (Coricidin Nasal Mist, Neo-Synephrine HCl)	As for oxymetazoline (**Intranasal:** Adults - Several drops 0.25-1% solut'n or jelly q3-4h prn. Infants - Use 0.125% solut'n)	As for oxymetazoline	As for oxymetazoline	As for oxymetazoline	As for oxymetazoline
Phenylpropanolamine HCl (Propadrine, Propagest)	As for oxymetazoline (**Oral:** Adults - 25 mg q4h. Children - 12.5 mg q4h)	As for oxymetazoline	As for oxymetazoline	As for oxymetazoline	As for oxymetazoline
Pseudoephedrine HCl (Eltor, Neo-Synephrinol, Novafed, Sudafed)	As for oxymetazoline (**Oral:** Adults - 60 mg tid-qid. Children - 4 mg/kg/day in 4 divided doses)	As for oxymetazoline	As for oxymetazoline	As for oxymetazoline	As for oxymetazoline
Xylometazoline HCl (Neo-Synephrine II, Otravin, Sinutab Long-Lasting Nasal Spray)	As for oxymetazoline (**Intranasal:** Use q8-10h. Adults - 1-2 sprays [0.1%] or 2-3 drops [0.1%] into each nostril. Children over 6 years - 1-2 sprays [0.05%] or 2-3 drops [0.05%] in each nostril. Children under 6 years -1 spray [0.05%] or 1 drop [0.05%])	As for oxymetazoline	As for oxymetazoline	As for oxymetazoline	As for oxymetazoline

Generic Name (Trade Name)	Use (Dose)	Action	Adverse Effects	Drug Interactions	Nursing Process
Pharmacologic Classification: Antihistamines	*For all informat'n on antihistamines, refer to Table 53.*				
Pharmacologic Classification: Corticosteroids					
Beclomethasone dipropionate (Beconase, Vancenase)	Corticosteroid tx of perennial/seasonal allergic rhinitis unresponsive to convent'nal tx (**Intranasal:** 1 applicat'n [50 µg beclomethasone dipropionate] into each nostril tid-qid. Max. adult dose, 20 applicat'ns/day. Max. children's dose, 10 applicat'ns/day)	Nonspecific anti-inflammatory actions. For addit'nal actions, refer to glucocorticoids, Chapter 29, Table 46.	Nasal/throat irritat'n. For addit'nal adv. effects, refer to glucocorticoids, Table 45.	For drug interact'ns involving amphotericin B, oral anticoagulants, antidiabetic agents, barbiturates, oral contraceptives, diuretics, indomethacin, phenytoin, rifampin and salicylates, refer to Table 46.	See Table 46
Flunisolide (Nasalide, Rhinalar)	As for beclomethasone dipropionate (**Intranasal:** Adults - 2 sprays [50 µg flunisolide] in each nostril bid. Incr. to max. tid prn. Children 6-14 years - Max. dose, 1 spray to each nostril tid. For maint., use lowest effective dose.	As for beclomethasone dipropionate	As for beclomethasone dipropionate	As for beclomethasone dipropionate	See Table 46
Pharmacologic Classification: Histamine-Release Inhibitor					
Cromolyn, sodium cromoglycate (Rynacrom)	Prophylaxis of seasonal rhinitis (**Intranasal:** Initially, insufflate 1 cartridge in ea. nostril qid, or 1 squeeze nasal solut'n in ea. nostril 6x/day)	Reduces release of histamine from mast cells in response to antigen-antibody react'n	Occas'nally, slight irritat'n of nasal mucosa. Occas'nal headache, sneezing, cough, unpleasant taste in mouth. Cases of erythema, urticaria or maculopapular rash have been reported. These have cleared within a few days of w'drawing drug.		

CHAPTER 34

Antitussives

Nonproductive versus Productive Coughs

Many "cough medicines" are available; however, confusion exists as to the best product for the particular patient. This is not surprising, because most cough medicines are sold on the basis of their own "unique" ingredients, rather than on an analysis of the type of cough experienced. Nurses are well aware that patients can suffer from two types of coughs. The first, a dry hacking, nonproductive cough, torments the patient with its incessant tickling. Yielding to the temptation for just one more cough results in more irritation and distress before the tickle and urge return again. Productive coughs, by contrast, present the picture of a congested patient woofing up copious amounts of phlegm from a seemingly bottomless well. It is obvious that these two disparate, but equally pathetic, problems warrant different treatments.

Nonproductive, hyperactive coughs should be treated with a drug to stop the patient from coughing. In addition, the irritation of a nonproductive cough may be relieved by the demulcent action of an expectorant that increases respiratory secretions. Patients with congested, productive coughs should not receive a cough suppressant. It is bad enough to be drowning in your own secretions without being given a drug that removes the urge to cough them up. Such patients should be assisted in their attempts to clear phlegm. Often all that is required is adequate fluids and humid air. An expectorant may also help to remove phlegm.

The multitude of cough preparations on the market makes it impossible to discuss each separately. Instead, attention will be directed to the types of drugs often used to treat coughs.

Cough Suppressants

Mechanism of Action and Pharmacologic Effects

Cough suppressants depress the cough center in the medulla oblongata area of the brain. As a result, the urge to cough is significantly reduced: the tormenting tickle is, at least for the moment, set to rest. Narcotics are the most effective cough suppressants. Codeine and hydrocodone (Dicodid, Hycodan) are often used for this purpose. Dextromethorphan is an effective non-narcotic cough suppressant found in both prescription and over-the-counter products.

Therapeutic Uses

Cough suppressants should be used to treat nonproductive, dry, hacking coughs. Codeine syrup is excellent for this purpose. Hydrocodone is also very effective but it is more potent than codeine and has a greater abuse liability. Over the past decade hydrocodone has become a very popular street drug.

Dextromethorphan is popular as a cough suppressant in most over-the-counter products. It is effective and appears to have little dependence liability.

Adverse Effects

The adverse effects of narcotics are discussed in Chapter 53. Normal antitussive doses of codeine and hydrocodone are generally well tolerated. The most frequently encountered adverse reactions include nausea, vomiting, constipation and dizziness. Central nervous system depression is particularly likely to occur if the patient is also taking an antihistamine. Patients should be warned about the dangers of operating moving machinery or driving a car. Respiratory depression occurs when large doses are taken and is more prevalent in children under the age of five. Continuous use can lead to drug dependency, particularly with hydrocodone.

The adverse effects of dextromethorphan are usually mild. They include drowsiness, nausea and dizziness.

Nursing Process

Codeine is discussed in Chapter 53 with other narcotics. Readers should refer to that chapter for details of the nursing process related to its use.

The nursing process for patients using products containing dextromethorphan must emphasize patient teaching, especially patient safety. Patients should be cautioned to avoid exceeding the recommended dosage. They should also be instructed that products containing dextromethorphan often cause drowsiness; therefore, they should avoid driving or using power tools while taking them. Patients should be reminded not to take these or any drugs in the dark. Because cough preparations are often pleasantly flavored, nurses should remind patients to keep them out of the reach of children. Patient teaching should also include nonpharmaceutical nursing measures for the relief of nonproductive cough: limit talking, no smoking, high fluid intake, use of a vaporizer, sucking on hard candy.

Expectorants

Mechanism of Action and Pharmacologic Effects

An expectorant is a drug that increases the output of respiratory tract fluid. Guaifenesin (glyceryl guaiacolate) and potassium iodide are two of the most commonly used expectorants. However, little objective evidence can be found to support their effectiveness. Both drugs irritate the gastric mucosa. This action may reflexly stimulate the parasympathetic nervous system to increase respiratory secretions.

Therapeutic Uses

Expectorants are given to increase the flow of respiratory secretions, thereby decreasing the viscosity of phlegm and enabling the patient to clear congestion. It is also contended that the increased secretions will soothe the irritated membranes and reduce the stimulus to cough.

Adverse Effects

Guaifenesin can cause drowsiness and nausea. The adverse effects of potassium iodide are more numerous and include gastric irritation, rhinorrhea, or nasal stuffiness and lacrimation. Potassium iodide stimulates salivary gland secretion and can produce swollen glands. The drug may exacerbate acne and acneform eruptions. Erythema around the face, chest, mouth and throat may also be seen. Other adverse effects of potassium iodide are hemorrhage, bullous rashes with fever, adenopathy, suppression of thyroid function and, on rare occasions, hyperthyroidism. In addition, mental depression, nervousness, insomnia, parkinsonism, headache and impotence have been reported after potassium iodide.

Nursing Process

The nursing process related to the use of expectorants should emphasize patient safety and is essentially the same as that identified for cough suppressants. Patients should also be instructed in nonpharmaceutical nursing measures for relief from a productive cough: limit talking, no smoking, high fluid intake, use of a vaporizer.

Antihistamines

Mechanism of Action and Pharmacologic Effects

Antihistamines competitively block histamine$_1$ (H$_1$) receptors. The drugs used most often in cough preparations include chlorpheniramine, phenindamine, pyrilamine, doxylamine, methapyrilene, phenyltoloxamine and diphenhydramine. Diphenhydramine is particularly noteworthy because it is also an effective cough suppressant.

Therapeutic Uses

Antihistamines are incorporated into most cough preparations. Some of the more popular products are Actifed C Expectorant, Naldecon, Phenergan Expectorant with Codeine, Phenergan VC Expectorant with Codeine, and Tussionex. Coughs caused by allergies respond better to products containing antihistamines. Most antihistamines also have anticholinergic effects and these account for some of their drying effects. Diphenhydramine is often used to suppress the cough reflex.

Adverse Effects

Antihistamines depress the central nervous system. Patients should be advised of the additive depressant effects of ethanol and antihistamines. Not all antihistamines are equally depressant and patients who experience profound depression on one product should be given another.

The anticholinergic effects of antihistamines can cause urinary retention, constipation and dry mouth. Paradoxically, many patients experience diarrhea.

Nursing Process

The nursing process associated with the use of antihistamines is discussed in Chapter 35. Readers should refer to that chapter for detailed information.

Adrenergic Vasoconstrictors

Adrenergic vasoconstrictors are often combined with cough suppressants, expectorants and antihistamines in "shotgun" formulations. By stimulating alpha$_1$ receptors on blood vessels they reduce congestion and promote easier breathing. Three of the more popular drugs are phenylephrine, phenylpropanolamine and pseudoephedrine.

Applied topically, adrenergic vasoconstrictors can produce stinging, burning or dryness of the mucosa and rebound hyperemia. Chronic abuse results in red, edematous mucosa. Systemic hypertension is usually not seen when the drugs are applied topically. However, systemic reactions can be noted, particularly in infants and children, if large doses are used. These drugs should be used with great care in the young.

The nursing process associated with the use of adrenergic vasoconstrictors is discussed in detail in Chapter 7. Specific application to the respiratory tract is contained in Chapter 32. Readers should refer to those chapters for comprehensive information.

Further Reading

Bryant, B.G. and Cormier, J. F. (1982). Cold and allergy products. *Handbook of Nonprescription Drugs,* 7th ed., pp. 123-169. Washington: American Pharmaceutical Association.

Decongestant, cough and cold preparations (1986). *AMA Drug Evaluations,* 6th ed., pp. 369-391.

First report of the expert advisory committee on nonprescription cough and cold remedies on antihistamines, nasal decongestants and anticholinergics (1989). *Information Letter No.764* (August 10). Ottawa: Health Protection Branch.

Table 52
Antitussives.

Generic Name (Trade Name)	Use (Dose)	Action	Adverse Effects	Drug Interactions	Nursing Process
Pharmacologic Classification: Cough Suppressants					
Codeine	Control of exhausting, nonproductive cough (**Oral:** Adults - 5-10 mg q3-4h prn. Children - 1-1.5 mg/kg/day, divided into 6 doses)	Codeine and hydrocodone are narcotics. By depressing the cough center in the medulla oblongata of the brain, codeine and hydrocodone suppress the urge to cough. They are most effective in treating nonproductive dry, hacking coughs. For other effects of these narcotics, refer to Table 76.	*Codeine and hydrocodone:* Nausea, vomiting, constipat'n, dizziness, palpitat'ns, drowsiness, pruritus, hyperhidrosis, agitat'n, respiratory depress'n, dependence	**Antidepressants, tricyclic and phenothiazines:** May demonstrate incr. CNS depress'n in presence of codeine or hydrocodone. **Ethanol:** As for TCAs. **MAOIs:** May require lower dosage in presence of codeine or hydrocodone.	See Chapter 53 and Table 76
Hydrocodone bitartrate	As for codeine (**Oral:** Doses to be taken no less than 4 h apart, pc and hs, w. food or milk. Adults - 5 mg, not to exceed 30 mg in a 24-h period. Max. single dose, 15 mg. Children -> age 12 - 5 mg, not to exceed 30 mg/24 h. Max. single dose, 10 mg; *aged 2-12* - 2.5 mg, not to exceed 15 mg/24 h. Max. single dose, 5 mg; < *age 2* - 1.25 mg, not to exceed 7.5 mg/24 h. Max. single dose, 1.25 mg)				See codeine in Chapter 53 and Table 76
Dextromethorphan HBr (Benylin DM, DM Syrup and others)	As for codeine (**Oral:** Adults - 10-20 mg q4h. Children - 1 mg/kg/day in 3-4 divided doses)	Effective non-narcotic cough suppressant that depresses cough center in medulla oblongata.	Slight drowsiness, nausea and dizziness (infrequently)		**Teach:** Pt safety; to avoid exceeding recommended dosage; to avoid driving or using power tools; not to take this or any medicat'n in dark; remind pts to keep medicat'ns out of reach of children; nonpharmaceutical nursing measures.
Diphenhydramine hydrochloride (Benylin)	Used to suppress cough center in brain (**Oral:** Adults - 25 mg q4h. Max. dose, 150 mg/24 h. Children aged 6-11 - 12.5 mg q4h or 5 mg/kg/day in 4 divided doses. Max. dose, 75 mg/day)	Antihistamine that also depresses cough center in medulla oblongata. For its other actions, refer to Chapter 35, Table 53.	Drowsiness, dizziness, dryness of mouth, nausea, nervousness, vertigo, palpitat'n, blurring of vision, headache, restlessness, insomnia, thickening of bronchial secret'ns, diarrhea, vomiting and excitat'n	**CNS depressants** (e.g., ethanol, hypnotics, sedatives): Have additive CNS-depressant effects w. antihistamines. **Para-aminosalicylic acid:** Absorpt'n is impaired by diphenhydramine.	As for dextromethorphan

Pharmacologic Classification: Expectorants

Guaifenesin, glyceryl guaiacolate (Breonesin, Glycotuss, Robitussin and others)	Guaifenesin is an expectorant used in symptomatic relief of respiratory condit'ns assoc. w. dry nonproductive cough and in presence of mucus in respiratory tract (**Oral:** Adults - 200-400 mg q4h. Max. dose, 2.4 g/day. Children aged 6-12 - 50-100 mg q4-6h. Max. dose, 600 mg/day)	Incr. output of lower respiratory tract fluid. Enhanced flow of less viscid secret'ns promotes ciliary action and facilitates removal of mucus. Unfortunately, evidence for efficacy is often lacking.	Nausea, GI upset, drowsiness

Teach: Pt safety; as above for cough suppressants

CHAPTER 35

Antihistamines

Antihistamines, regardless of their chemical structures, have the same basic mechanism of action and
the same major adverse effects.

Mechanism of Action and Pharmacologic Effects

Antihistamines reversibly block histamine$_1$ (H_1)
receptors. They prevent histamine from contracting
smooth muscle, dilating blood vessels, increasing
capillary permeability, inducing tissue edema and
stimulating mucus secretion. Not all histamine-
mediated effects are blocked by these drugs.
Antihistamines do not inhibit histamine-induced
bronchiolar constriction. In addition, they do not
prevent histamine from stimulating gastric acid
secretion, an H_2 receptor-mediated effect.

Therapeutic Uses

Antihistamines are used to treat a variety of allergic disorders. However, because histamine is only
one mediator of allergic reactions, antihistamines
may provide only partial relief of many of the
symptoms. Patients with mild symptoms of recent
onset are generally more responsive to antihistamines. Patients with chronic illness derive less
benefit. Antihistamines are least effective in
controlling the symptoms of severe allergic or
immunologic disease, including anaphylaxis.

Foremost among the conditions for which
antihistamines are used are upper respiratory allergies, characterized by sneezing, rhinorrhea and
pruritus of the nose, eyes and throat.
Antihistamines usually relieve these symptoms,
particularly if they are of recent onset. Hay fever
(seasonal allergic rhinitis) responds better to
antihistaminic therapy than nonseasonal, perennial
allergic rhinitis. Patients with vasomotor rhinitis
experience variable relief from antihistamines.
Lower respiratory disorders with bronchospasm do
not respond well to antihistamines.

Although most cough and cold preparations contain antihistamines, their value is still the subject of considerable controversy. Any effect antihistamines may have in drying the nose likely results from their anticholinergic properties.

Antihistamines often relieve the pruritic component of acute urticaria. Although angioedema will respond, at least partly, to antihistamines, epinephrine is the drug of choice for severe, life-threatening situations. Whereas topical preparations are available for the treatment of allergic conjunctivitis, allergic dermatitis and pruritus resulting from a sting, oral therapy yields better results. Long-term topical antihistamine use may cause sensitization.

Antihistamines are often ineffective in the treatment of hypersensitivity reactions to drugs, foods and allergens. The serious manifestations of hypersensitivity reactions, such as hypotension and bronchoconstriction, also fail to respond to antihistamines. The flushing, urticaria and pruritus of transfusion reactions are usually reduced by antihistamine treatment.

Antihistamines are used for a number of indications that appear unrelated to their ability to block H_1 receptors. Their sedative effects have made them popular drugs in over-the-counter sleeping preparations. Hydroxyzine (Atarax, Vistaril) and promethazine (Phenergan) are used for preoperative sedation. Cyproheptadine (Periactin) is used as an appetite stimulant. It is claimed to stimulate both linear growth and weight gain in children. Unfortunately, this effect is transient and disappears when the drug is stopped. Several antihistamines are used for their antiemetic effects, and these are discussed in Chapter 25.

Adverse Effects

The adverse effects of antihistamines are rarely serious and usually disappear within a few days of stopping treatment. Sedation is the most frequently encountered effect, and patients should be warned about the dangers of working around moving machinery or driving a car. They should also be informed of the additive effects of taking antihistamines with other central nervous system depressants such as ethanol, benzodiazepines and barbiturates. Other adverse effects attributable to central nervous system depression are dizziness, lassitude, incoordination, fatigue, tinnitus and diplopia. Three newer antihistamines, astemizole (Hismanal), loratadine (Claritin) and terfenadine (Seldane), produce minimal central nervous system

depression and are generally considered to be extremely valuable drugs. Paradoxic adverse effects of antihistamines include euphoria, irritability, insomnia and increased tendency to convulsions.

Loss of appetite is a common adverse effect of most antihistamines. Nausea and vomiting are also experienced by some patients. Other adverse effects include abdominal discomfort, constipation and diarrhea. Their anticholinergic effects cause dry mouth, throat and nasal passages. Tightness of the chest, headache, palpitations, and urinary retention or dysuria can also occur.

Nursing Process

Assessment

Prior to administering antihistamines, nurses should be familiar with the patient's history. The presence of asthma, convulsive disorders, glaucoma, hyperthyroidism, circulatory or cardiovascular disease, or diabetes should be the signal for particularly stringent nursing evaluation following antihistamine administration.

When the goal of therapy is the treatment of allergic reactions, an appropriate time should be chosen for careful assessment of any recent deviations from usual habits which might have precipitated the allergic reaction. Together, the nurse and patient should attempt to identify any recent changes in diet, drugs, environment or stressful life events.

Administration

Giving antihistamines with food or milk may reduce adverse gastrointestinal effects. Capsules can be emptied and mixed with food or drink to facilitate swallowing. If the goal of therapy is to treat motion sickness, antihistamines should be given thirty minutes before the trip, before meals, and at bedtime during travel. Oral preparations should be stored in tightly covered containers at room temperature. Elixirs and parenteral preparations should be stored in light-resistant containers in the dark.

The intramuscular route is preferred for parenteral administration. The injection should be given in a large muscle rather than subcutaneously because of the irritating effects.

Antihistamine dosage should be reduced in elderly or debilitated patients.

Evaluation

Nurses should evaluate the therapeutic response to the antihistamine, and its adverse effects. Patients with circulatory or cardiovascular conditions should be the subject of rigorous monitoring of their vital signs, including blood pressure.

Nurses should be alert for the adverse effects listed above and check closely for additive effects if antihistamines are used concomitantly with other drugs having central nervous system depressant effects.

Teaching

Patients should be told that antihistamines can cause drowsiness. They should be cautioned to avoid driving or using power equipment while taking these drugs. Nurses should tell patients that the depressant effects of antihistamines on the central nervous system can be compounded when other CNS depressants (such as sedatives, alcohol, hypnotics or anxiolytics) are used concurrently. Advise patients that antihistamines thicken bronchial secretions and dry mucus membranes; therefore, patients should increase fluid intake and use a vaporizer. Store this and all medications out of the reach of children.

Further Reading

Ciprandi, G., Scordamaglia, A., Buscaglia, S., Passalcqua, G. and Canonica, G.W. (1989). Antihistamines in atopic dermatitis. *Allergy 44* (Suppl. 9):114-116.

Davies, R.J., Ollier, S. and Cundell, D.R. (1989). Drug treatment for nasal allergy. *Clin. Experimental Allergy 19* : 559-568.

Histamine and antihistamines (1986). *AMA Drug Evaluations,* 6th ed., pp. 1041-1048.

Table 53
Antihistamines.

Pharmacologic Classification: Antihistamines

Generic Name (Trade Name)	Use (Dose)	Action	Adverse Effects	Drug Interactions	Nursing Process
Astemizole (Hismanal)	For allergic react'ns (**Oral:** Adults and children > 12 years - 10 mg od; 6-12 years - 5 mg od; < 6 years - 2 mg/10 kg/day)	Antihistamines block H₁ receptors. They prevent histamine from contracting smooth muscle, dilating blood vessels, increasing capillary permeability, inducing tissue edema, and stimulating mucus secret'n. Antihistamines do not inhibit histamine-induced bronchiolar constrict'n, nor prevent histamine from stimulating gastric acid secret'n (an H₂ receptor-mediated effect)	Drowsiness, dizziness, dryness of mouth, nausea, nervousness, palpitat'ns, and (rarely) allergic react'ns. Astemizole, terfenadine and loratadine are less likely to produce CNS depress'n.	**CNS depressants** (e.g., ethanol, hypnotics, anxiolytics): Have additive depressant effects w. most antihistamines. This interact'n is prob. not seen w. astemizole, terfenadine and loratadine.	**Assess:** Hx for asthma, convulsive disorders, glaucoma, hyperthyroidism, circulatory or CV disease, diabetes; for recent deviat'ns in habits which might have precipitated allergic react'n, e.g., diet, environment, drugs, stressful life events. **Administer:** With food or milk to reduce GI effects; empty capsules, mix w. food or drink to facilitate swallowing. *For mot'n sickness:* Give 30 min ac, and hs during travel; store in light-resistant containers at room temp. IM route preferred for parenteral administrat'n; inject deep into large muscle. Dosage should be reduced in elderly or debilitated pts. **Evaluate:** For tx response; for adv. effects; VS, incl. BP. Be alert for adv. or additive effects. **Teach:** To avoid driving or using power tools; risk of synergism when taken w. other CNS depressants; that antihistamines thicken bronchial secret'ns and dry mucous membranes. Incr. fluid intake and use vaporizer. Store this and all medicat'ns out of reach of children.
Azatadine maleate (Optimine)	For allergic react'ns (**Oral:** Adults - 1 mg a.m. and p.m. In refractory or more severe cases, 2 mg bid may be used. Children 6-12 years - 0.5-1 mg bid)	As for astemizole	As for astemizole	As for astemizole	
Brompheniramine maleate (Dimetane)	For allergic react'ns (**Oral:** Adults - 4-8 mg tid-qid, or 1 sustained-release 8- or 12-mg tablet q8-12h. Children > 6 years - 4 mg tid-qid, or 1 sustained-release 8- or 12-mg tablet q12h; 3-6 years - 2 mg tid-qid. **IM/IV/SC:** Adults - 5-20 mg q6-12h. Max. dose, 40 mg/day. Children < 12 years - 0.5 mg/kg/day, divided into 3-4 doses)	As for astemizole	As for astemizole	As for astemizole	
Cyclizine (Marezine, Marzine)	For postoperative vomiting (**IM:** Adults - 50 mg 15-30 min before end of operat'n; may be repeated tid prn during first postop. days. Children < 6 years - 25% adult dose; 6-10 years - 50% adult dose. *For mot'n sickness:* **Oral:** Adults - 50 mg 30 min before depar-	As for astemizole	As for astemizole	As for astemizole	As for astemizole

ture, then q4-6h prn. Max. dose, 200 mg/day. Children 6-10 years - 3 mg/kg, divided into 3 doses in a 24-h period)				
Cyproheptadine (Periactin) For weight gain (**Oral:** Adults - 4 mg tid w. meals for 6 months max. Children 6-14 years - Initially, 2 mg tid-qid, depending on age; maint. dose, 4 mg tid. 2-6 years - Initially, 2 mg tid; max. dose, 8 mg/day)	As for astemizole	As for astemizole	As for astemizole	As for astemizole
Dexchlorpheniramine maleate (Polaramine) For allergic react'ns (**Oral:** Adults and children >12 years - 2 mg tid-qid, or 1 sustained-release 6-mg tablet bid; 6-12 years - 1 mg tid-qid)	As for astemizole	As for astemizole	As for astemizole	As for astemizole
Dimenhydrinate (Dramamine, Gravol) Prevent'n and tx of vertigo, incl. that assoc. w. Meniere's disease and mot'n sickness (**Oral:** Adults - 50-100 mg q4h. Children - 1-1.5 mg/kg q6h. Max. dose, 300 mg/day. **IV:** Adults - 50 mg in 10 mL of NaCl inject'n over 2 min. **IM:** Adults - 50 mg q3-4h prn. Children - 1-1.5 mg/kg q6h. Max. dose, 300 mg/day)	As for astemizole	As for astemizole	As for astemizole	As for astemizole
Diphenhydramine (Benadryl) For allergic react'ns (**Oral:** Adults - 25-50 mg tid-qid. Children < 12 years - 5 mg/kg/day, in 4 divided doses over 24 h. **IV/IM:** Adults - 10-50 mg. Max. dose, 400 mg/day. Children - 5 mg/kg/day, in 4 divided doses. Max. dose, 300 mg/day)	As for astemizole	As for astemizole	As for astemizole	As for astemizole
Chlorpheniramine maleate (Chlor-Trimeton, Chlor-Tripolon) For allergic react'ns (**Oral:** Adults - 2-4 mg tid-qid, or 1 time-release 8- or 12-mg capsule bid. Children < 12 years - 0.35 mg/kg/day, divided into 4 doses)	As for astemizole	As for astemizole	As for astemizole	As for astemizole

Generic Name (Trade Name)	Use (Dose)	Action	Adverse Effects	Drug Interactions	Nursing Process
Clemastine fumarate (Tavist)	For allergic react'ns (**Oral:** *Adults and children > 6 years - 1-6 mg/day in divided doses; 2-5 years - 0.5-1.5 mg/day in divided doses*)	As for astemizole	As for astemizole	As for astemizole	As for astemizole
Hydroxyzine (Atarax, Vistaril)	Urticaria and other dermatological disorders (**Oral:** *Adults - 25 mg tid; incr. prn to 100 mg qid. Children > 6 years - 50-100 mg/day in 3-4 doses; < 6 years - 50 mg/day, divided into 3-4 doses*)	As for astemizole	As for astemizole	As for astemizole	As for astemizole
Loratadine (Claritin)	For allergic react'ns (**Oral:** *Adults and children > 12 years - 10 mg od*)	As for astemizole	As for astemizole	As for astemizole	As for astemizole
Meclizine (Antivert, Bonamine, Bonine)	For mot'n sickness (**Oral:** *Adults - 25-50 mg od, 1 h prior to departure. For labyrinth/vestibular disturbances: Adults - 25-100 mg/day in divided doses, depending on clin. response. For radiat'n sickness: Adults - 50 mg administered 2-12 h prior to radiat'n tx*)	As for astemizole	As for astemizole	As for astemizole	As for astemizole
Methdilazine (Tacaryl)	For pruritus (**Oral:** *Adults - 16-32 mg/day, divided into 2-4 doses. Children > 3 years - 4 mg bid-qid*)	As for astemizole	As for astemizole	As for astemizole	As for astemizole
Promethazine (Phenergan)	For allergic react'ns (**Oral:** *Adults - 25 mg hs, or 12.5 mg qid. Children - 25 mg hs, or 6.25-12.5 mg tid.* **IM/IV/Rectal:** *Adults - 25 mg repeated in 2 h prn. Children - No more than 50% adult dose.*)	As for astemizole	As for astemizole	As for astemizole	As for astemizole

Drug	Dose				
	For tx of nausea, vomiting: **IM/Rectal:** Adults - Initially, 25 mg; then 12.5-25 mg prn q4-6h. Children < 12 years - Adjust dose on basis of age/weight of pt and severity of condit'n; no more than 50% suggested adult dose. *Selected high-risk postoperative:* Adults - Initially, 12.5 mg. *For mot'n sickness:* **Oral/rectal:** Adults - 25 mg bid, given 30-60 min prior to travel. Children - 12.5-25 mg bid)				
Terfenadine (Seldane)	For allergic react'ns (**Oral:** Adults and children > 12 years - 60 mg bid or 120 mg od, pref. in a.m.; 7-12 years - 30 mg a.m. and p.m.; 3-6 years - 15 mg a.m. and p.m.)	As for astemizole	As for astemizole	As for astemizole	As for astemizole
Trimeprazine tartrate (Panectyl)	Relief of pruritus; control of cough and asthma-like symptoms (**Oral:** Adults - 2.5 or 5 mg bid pc and 5 mg hs; or 5-10 mg hs. Children 2-12 years - 2.5 or 5 mg hs)	As for astemizole	As for astemizole	As for astemizole	As for astemizole
Tripelennamine (PBZ, Pyribenzamine)	For allergic react'ns (**Oral:** Adults - 25-50 mg q4-6h, or 1 time-release 100-mg tablet bid-tid. Children - 5 mg/kg/day, divided into 4-6 doses)	As for astemizole	As for astemizole	As for astemizole	As for astemizole
Triprolidine (Actidil)	For allergic react'ns (**Oral:** Adults - 2.5 mg bid-tid. Children > 6 years - 1.25 mg bid-tid; < 6 years - 0.3-0.6 mg tid-qid, depending on age)	As for astemizole	As for astemizole	As for astemizole	As for astemizole

SECTION 10

Ophthalmic and Otic Pharmacology

Section 10 discusses the local application of drugs to treat disorders of the eye or ear. The information provided in Chapters 36 to 39 is particularly relevant to nurses who are often involved in the management of patients with ocular or otic disorders. Beginning first with a discussion of mydriatics and cycloplegics, the section proceeds to a presentation of drugs used to treat glaucoma. The last two chapters deal with the local application of drugs to treat inflammations and/or infections of the eye and ear.

CHAPTER 36

Mydriatics and Cycloplegics

Teaching Objectives

Following completion of this chapter, the reader should be able to:

1. Describe autonomic nervous system innervation of the iris and ciliary body.
2. Define miosis and explain how drugs may produce miosis.
3. Define mydriasis and explain the mechanisms of action of mydriatics.
4. Discuss the therapeutic uses and adverse effects of mydriatics and the nursing process precipitated by their use.
5. Define cycloplegia and explain the mechanism of action of cycloplegics.
6. Discuss the therapeutic uses and adverse effects of cycloplegics and the nursing process precipitated by their use.

Autonomic Innervation of the Eye

Before discussing the mechanisms of action of mydriatics and cycloplegics, it is essential to review autonomic innervation of the eye. To understand the material presented below, it may be necessary to review briefly the information provided in Chapter 4 dealing with the neurochemical transmission of autonomic nerves.

Both parasympathetic and sympathetic nerves innervate the iris (Figure 24). The circular smooth muscles receive parasympathetic innervation; stimulation, accompanied by the release and action of acetylcholine on muscarinic receptors, constricts the pupil. This is called **miosis** and drugs that produce miosis are called **miotics.** Drugs produce miosis either by stimulating muscarinic receptors on the circular muscle of the iris or inhibiting sympathetic stimulation of the radial muscle.

The action of parasympathetic nerves on circular muscles is counteracted by sympathetic innervation of the radial muscles. Stimulation of alpha$_1$ receptors by norepinephrine, released by the sympathetic nerves, or epinephrine, secreted by the adrenals, dilates the pupil. Dilatation of the pupil is called **mydriasis** and drugs that produce mydriasis are known as **mydriatics.**

The ciliary muscle is innervated only by parasympathetic nerves. Cholinergic stimulation constricts the ciliary sphincter, releasing tension on the suspensory ligaments holding the lens. When this occurs the lens becomes more round and accommodates for near vision. **Cycloplegia** is the inability of the eye to accommodate for near vision. Drugs that produce cycloplegia are called **cycloplegics.**

Figure 24
Autonomic innervation of the iris and ciliary body.

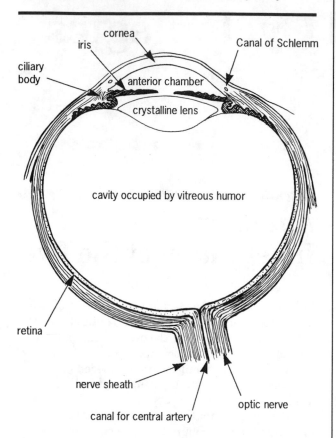

Table 54 provides a summary of the autonomic innervation of the eye.

Table 54
Summary of the autonomic innervation of the eye.

	Innervation	Receptor	Effects
Iris	Parasympathetic to circular muscles	Muscarinic	Constricts pupils (miosis)
	Sympathetic to longitudinal muscles	Alpha$_1$	Dilates pupils (mydriasis)
Ciliary Body	Parasympathetic to circular muscle	Muscarinic	Constricts sphincter, permitting accommodation

Mydriatics and Cycloplegics

Mechanism of Action and Pharmacologic Effects

Mydriatics dilate pupils by either blocking muscarinic receptors on the circular muscle (anticholinergics) or stimulating alpha$_1$ receptors on the radial muscle (adrenergics). Cycloplegics are anticholinergics. They prevent accommodation for near vision by blocking muscarinic receptors on the ciliary body.

Therapeutic Uses

Cycloplegics and mydriatics are used in estimating errors of refraction. Cycloplegia prevents accommodation during refraction, and mydriasis simplifies the retinoscopic estimation of the refractive error. Atropine has a slow onset and long duration of action. The duration of action of scopolamine (Isopto Hyoscine) is shorter than that of atropine, but is still too long for refraction in adults. Homatropine (Homatrocel, Isopto Homatropine), cyclopentolate (Ak-Pentolate, Cyclogyl) and tropicamide (Mydriacyl) are often preferred because they have a rapid onset and short duration of action. If tropicamide is used, the examination should be conducted within twenty to twenty-five minutes of instilling the drug. Complete recovery occurs within two to six hours.

Mydriatics are also used for intraocular examination. Because cycloplegia is not required, adrenergic drugs or anticholinergics with minimal cycloplegic effects are used. Phenylephrine (Neo-Synephrine) or hydroxyamphetamine (Paredrine) are adrenergics often employed. They may be used alone or combined with an anticholinergic, such as cyclopentolate or tropicamide, to facilitate wider mydriasis. Eucatropine may also be used. Although its anticholinergic effects last longer than those of tropicamide and cyclopentolate, it has little cycloplegic action.

Mydriatics can be instilled in the provocative test for angle-closure glaucoma. Tropicamide, eucatropine, phenylephrine and hydroxamphetamine are used for this purpose. The results are positive if the pressure increases by 8 mm Hg within one hour and the angle is gonioscopically closed at the time of elevation. The effects of these drugs can be easily reversed.

Mydriatics are employed in intraocular surgery. They are used to facilitate round-pupil cataract extraction and to locate retinal break during retinal detachment operations. Atropine is usually used alone or with phenylephrine before the operation. If its long duration of action is a problem, shorter-acting anticholinergics can be instilled. Anticholinergics may also be used regularly to prevent synechiae (adhesions) following intraocular surgery. Phenylephrine may also be used. Mydriatics are used until slit-lamp examination shows minimal iritis.

Atropine or scopolamine is applied locally in the nonspecific treatment of anterior uveitis and in glaucoma secondary to ocular inflammation. Phenylephrine may be added to assist in mydriasis. Anticholinergics assist in anterior uveitis by (1) relaxing the intraocular muscles, (2) reducing abnormal vascular permeability and (3) dilating the pupil.

Adverse Effects

Mydriatics can precipitate an attack of acute angle-closure glaucoma in eyes with anatomically narrow angles. If mydriatics, particularly long-acting drugs, are used for prolonged periods to treat inflammation of the anterior segment, posterior synechiae may form. The drug should be stopped for a short time if slit-lamp examination reveals formation of synechiae.

Systemic reactions (including dryness of the mouth and skin, flushing, tachycardia, irritability, thirst, fever, ataxia, confusion, somnolence, hallucinations and delirium) can occur following instillation of an anticholinergic in the eye. They are more common in children with fair skin, patients with Down's syndrome, and in individuals with brain damage. On rare occasions, convulsions, coma and death have been reported.

Adrenergic drugs instilled in the eye can rarely cause hypertension, ventricular arrhythmias, angina, myocardial infarction, cardiac arrest, hyperhidrosis, blanching, tremors, agitation, subarachnoid hemorrhage and confusion.

Nursing Process

The drugs discussed in this chapter are locally applied anticholinergics or adrenergics used to accomplish a specific purpose: mydriasis or cycloplegia. Readers are advised to review Chapters 6 and 7 for detailed discussion of the nursing process associated with systemic use of anticholinergics and adrenergics, respectively.

Assessment

Prior to administering a mydriatic or cycloplegic, nurses must check the patient's history for documentation of glaucoma, hypertension, coronary artery disease, chronic gastrointestinal conditions, asthma or pulmonary disease. Mydriatics reduce aqueous humor drainage and are contraindicated in patients predisposed to narrow-angle glaucoma. Their use in this condition may lead to an abrupt increase in the intraocular pressure and an attack of acute glaucoma.

Physical assessment should focus on the patient's cardiovascular status. Baseline measures of vital signs should be carefully documented, particularly the cardiovascular parameters.

Administration

When instilled in the eye, these drugs should be placed in the lower conjunctival sac and followed by compression of the nasal-lacrimal duct for one minute to prevent systemic absorption. Wait five minutes prior to the use of other drops. Ensure that the patient does not blink more than usual.

Evaluation

Nursing evaluation should consider drug effectiveness. The major focus of nursing evaluation should be the early detection of systemic anticholinergic or adrenergic effects that might occur as a result of absorption. Discontinue use of drug if eye pain occurs. Report any changes in vision, blurring, loss of sight, trouble breathing, sweating or flushing to the physician.

Teaching

Patient safety is the paramount concern following ocular instillation. Patients who receive these drugs for purposes of eye examinations should be cautioned to use great care in navigating stairs or other uneven surfaces until the effects of the drug have worn off. They should also be warned not to drive after an eye examination using these drugs. Instruct the patient that blurred vision will decrease with repeated use of the drug.

Further Reading

Brown, C. and Hanna, C. (1978). Use of dilute drug solutions for routine cycloplegia and mydriasis. *Amer. J. Ophthalmol. 8* : 820-824.

Fruanfelder, F.T. (1976). *Drug-Induced Ocular Side Effects and Drug Interactions*. Philadelphia: Lea and Febiger.

Table 55
Mydriatics and cycloplegics.

Pharmacologic Classification: Anticholinergic Mydriatics/Cycloplegics

Generic Name (Trade Name)	Use (Dose)	Action	Adverse Effects	Drug Interactions	Nursing Process
Atropine sulfate (Atropine Care, Atropisol, BufOpto Atropine, Isopto Atropine)	For pre- and postoperative mydriasis, in anterior uveitis, and in some 2° glaucomas (**Instill:** *For refract'n:* Infants <1 year - 1 drop 0.125% solut'n. Children 1-5 years and all children w. blue irides - 0.25% solut'n. Children > 5 years - 0.5% solut'n. Children w. dark irides - 1% solut'n. Use tid 3 days before refract'n and 1x on a.m. of refract'n. *For preop. mydriasis:* 1 drop 1% solut'n tog. w. 1 drop phenylephrine before surgery. *For anterior uveitis or postop. mydriasis:* 1 drop 1-2% solut'n od)	Anticholinergic drugs produce mydriasis by blocking muscarinic receptors on the circular muscles of the iris. By preventing parasympathetic stimulat'n to the iris, anticholinergics upset the balance normally present bet. parasympathetic stimulat'n of the circular muscles (tending to produce miosis) and sympathetic stimulat'n to the radial muscles (tending to cause mydriasis). As a result, the sympathetic system acts unopposed on the iris, and mydriasis ensues. The ciliary body is innervated only by the parasympathetic nervous system. When the eye accommodates for near vision the ciliary body constricts, releasing tension on the suspensory ligaments holding the lens, and allowing the lens to become rounder. Anticholinergics	*Local:* Acute angle-closure glaucoma, contact dermatitis, allergic conjunctivitis, posterior synechiae. *Systemic:* Dryness of mouth and skin, flushing, tachycardia, irritability, thirst, fever, ataxia, confusion, somnolence, hallucinat'ns, delirium	See Table 4	**Assess:** Hx glaucoma, hypertens'n, coronary artery disease, chronic GI condit'ns, asthma or pulmonary disease. VS. **Administer:** From light-resistant container. After instilling, compress canaliculi and nasal-lacrimal duct for 1 min and wait 5 min before using other drugs. Instruct pt not to blink more than usual. **Evaluate:** Effectiveness for purpose for which it was administered; for atropine toxicity; fluid balance and electrolyte status prn for pts on long-term tx. Discontinue use of drug if eye pan occurs. Report any change in vision, blurring, loss of sight, dyspnea, diaphoresis or flushing to physician.
Homatropine HBr (Homatrocel, Isopto Homatropine)	For ophthalmoscopy and refract'n (**Instill:** *For refract'n:* 1 drop 2-5% solut'n. May be repeated prn in 5-10 min. For *mild anterior uveitis:* 1 drop 2-5% solut'n bid or tid)		As for atropine sulfate	See Table 4	As for atropine sulfate
Scopolamine HBr (Isopto Hyoscine)	As for atropine sulfate (**Instill:** *For postop. mydriasis:* 1 drop 0.25% solut'n od. *For anterior uveitis:* 1 drop 0.25% solut'n od, more frequently in severe inflammat'n. To break posterior synechiae: 1 drop 0.25% solut'n prn. May be alternated w. 10% phenylephrine. *For malignant glaucoma:* 1 drop 0.25% solut'n and 1 drop 10% phenylephrine tid-qid or prn,		As for atropine sulfate	See Table 4	As for atropine sulfate

Name	Uses / Dosage	Action	Side Effects / Adverse Reactions	Interactions	Nursing Considerations
Cyclopentolate HCl (Ak-Pentolate, Cyclogyl)	For ophthalmoscopy and refract'n (**Instill:** *For ophthalmoscopy:* 1 drop 0.5% solut'n. For wider mydriasis in older children and adults - 1 drop solut'n containing 0.5% cyclopentolate and 2.5% phenylephrine solut'n. *For refract'n:* 1 drop 1% solut'n [2% in dark irides] or 1 drop 0.5% solut'n, repeated in 5 min) followed by maint. tx of 1 drop 0.25% solut'n od)	prevent the ciliary body from constricting, thus the eye cannot accommodate for near vision. This effect is called cycloplegia.	As for atropine sulfate	See Table 4	As for atropine sulfate
Tropicamide (Mydriacyl)	For ophthalmoscopy and refract'n (**Instill:** *For refract'n:* 1 drop 1% solut'n. *For ophthalmoscopy:* 1 drop 0.5% solut'n. Wider mydriasis can be obtained w. 1 drop 0.5% solut'n and 2.5% phenylephrine)	As for atropine sulfate	As for atropine sulfate	See Table 4	As for atropine sulfate

Mydriasis without cycloplegia

Pharmacologic Classification: Adrenergic Mydriatics

Name	Uses / Dosage	Action	Side Effects / Adverse Reactions	Interactions	Nursing Considerations
Phenylephrine HCl (Ak-Dilate, Efricel, Mydfrin, Neo-Synephrine HCl)	for examinat'n of intraocular structure; to facilitate ocular surgery; as adjunct in tx of anterior uveitis, postop. inflammat'n and some 2° glaucomas; occ. for provocative testing for acute angle-closure glaucoma (**Instill:** *For ophthalmoscopy:* 1 drop 2.5% solut'n. *For preop. mydriasis:* 1 drop 2.5% solut'n q15min for 2-4 doses. *For postop. mydriasis after iridectomy:* 1 drop 10% solut'n od-bid)	By stim. alpha1 receptors on radial muscles of the iris, alpha-adrenergic stimulants cause radial muscles to contract, resulting in mydriasis.	*Local:* Transient pain; transitory incr. in intraocular pressure. *Systemic:* Hypertens'n, anginal pain, ventricular arrhythmias, myocardial infarct, cardiac arrest, subarachnoid hemorrhage	**Antidepressants, tricyclic:** May potentiate pressor responses to adrenergic drugs. **Beta blockers** (nonselective): May potentiate pressor responses to adrenergic drugs. **MAOIs:** If used concurrently with, or up to 21 days before phenylephrine, may exaggerate pressor response to phenylephrine. Such use requires careful supervis'n.	**Assess:** Pt hx of coronary disease, hypertens'n, glaucoma, diabetes mellitus, bradycardia; establish baseline BP, pulse (rate, rhythm). **Administer:** From light-resistant container into lower conjunctival sac; compress nasal canaliculi for 1 min.

To produce mydriasis for ophthalmoscopy; to localize

Generic Name (Trade Name)	Use (Dose)	Action	Adverse Effects	Drug Interactions	Nursing Process
Hydroxyamphetamine HBr (Paredrine)	lesion in Horner's syndrome; for provocative testing for acute angle-closure glaucoma (**Instilled:** *For ophthalmoscopy:* 1 drop 1% solut'n. *To localize lesion in Horner's syndrome:* 1 drop 1% solut'n in each eye, repeated in 5 min)	As for phenylephrine HCl	As for phenylephrine HCl	As for phenylephrine HCl	As for phenylephrine HCl

CHAPTER 37

Antiglaucoma Drugs

Teaching Objectives

Following completion of this chapter, the reader should be able to:

1. Define glaucoma and explain its cause.
2. Describe the primary goal in the treatment of glaucoma.
3. List the means by which drugs may decrease intraocular pressure.
4. Discuss the mechanisms of action, pharmacologic effects, therapeutic uses and adverse effects of miotics, as well as the nursing process precipitated by their use.
5. Describe the mechanism of action, pharmacologic effects, therapeutic uses and adverse effects of epinephrine when instilled in the eye, and the nursing process associated with its ocular application.
6. Discuss the mechanism of action, pharmacologic effects, therapeutic uses and adverse effects of osmotic agents when they are administered in the treatment of glaucoma, and the nursing process precipitated by their administration.
7. Discuss the therapeutic uses and adverse effects of beta blockers when they are applied to the eye, and the nursing process precipitated by their ocular use.
8. Describe the mechanism of action, pharmacologic effects, therapeutic uses and adverse effects of acetazolamide when it is administered in the treatment of glaucoma, and the nursing process associated with its use.

Glaucoma

Glaucoma refers to a group of eye diseases characterized by an increase in the intraocular pressure of the aqueous humor, which causes pathologic changes in the optic disc and defects in the field of vision. The primary goal in the treatment of glaucoma is to reduce intraocular pressure and prevent extension of the damage to the optic nerve. Aqueous humor is formed by the ciliary body, flows around the iris, and drains through the Canals of Schlemm (see Figure 24, Chapter 36). Drugs are used to decrease aqueous formation or increase its drainage. Patients often receive both types of drugs simultaneously.

Drugs That Increase Aqueous Humor Drainage

Miotics

Mechanism of Action and Pharmacologic Effects

Miotics are cholinergic drugs that constrict the circular muscle of the iris, thereby facilitating drainage of the aqueous humor through the trabecular meshwork. (Please see Chapter 5 for detailed information on the pharmacology of cholinergic drugs.) Cholinergic drugs may act directly, by stimulating muscarinic receptors on the circular muscles, or indirectly, by inhibiting acetylcholinesterase, allowing acetylcholine to accumulate around the receptors. Pilocarpine and carbachol act directly, and physostigmine (Eserine), demecarium bromide (Humorsol), echothiophate iodide (Echodide, Phospholine Iodide), and isoflurophate (DFP, Floropryl) are cholinesterse inhibitors. With the exception of physostigmine, which produces a reversible inhibition of cholinesterase and short-term effects, all anticholinesterase drugs have long durations of action.

Therapeutic Uses

Miotics are often used to increase aqueous drainage in the treatment of chronic open-angle glaucoma. They are also employed in angle-closure glaucoma because miosis pulls the iris away from the trabeculum, thereby relieving the pupillary block.

Pilocarpine is a short-acting miotic often preferred as a first-line drug because it is better tolerated than many other agents. If resistance or intolerance to it develops, carbachol or physostigmine, both short-acting drugs, may be tried. Concern over their cataractogenic properties and other toxicities has relegated the long-acting cholinesterase inhibitors demecarium, echothiophate and isoflurophate to patients who have either not responded to the short-acting miotics (pilocarpine, carbachol and physostigmine), or who have become refractory to them.

Adverse Effects

The adverse effects of miotics include ciliary spasm, brow ache, headache, false myopia and poor night vision (fixed small pupil). Patients should be warned about driving at night. Following prolonged use, particularly with long-acting cholinesterase inhibitors, miosis may persist when the drug is discontinued. Long-acting cholinesterase inhibitors may also hasten cataract formation, especially in individuals over the age of sixty.

Absorption of long-acting cholinesterase inhibitors into the general circulation can cause abdominal cramps, diarrhea, rhinorrhea, lacrimation and upper respiratory congestion. If toxic amounts are absorbed, ataxia, confusion, convulsions, coma and muscular paralysis can ensue, with the patient dying of respiratory failure.

Nursing Process

Readers are advised to refer to Chapter 5, which contains detailed discussion of the nursing process associated with systemic use of cholinergic drugs.

Assessment
Prior to the initial administration of a directly acting cholinergic drug, the nurse should review the patient's history for evidence of asthma, peptic ulcers, hypotension, vasomotor instability, coronary artery disease, epilepsy or parkinsonism. If any of these conditions are documented in the patient's history the physician should be contacted to verify the order. It is imperative that baseline measures of vital signs be established for later use in evaluating the patient for possible adverse effects.

Administration
Cholinergic miotics should be instilled in the lower conjunctival sac and the canaliculi, and nasal-lacrimal ducts immediately compressed against the bridge of the nose for one minute. This will prevent excess medication from draining with the tears into the nasopharynx. Pilocarpine is light sensitive; therefore, it should be stored in a dark place in a light-resistant container.

Evaluation
Evaluation of drug efficacy following local ocular instillation of either pilocarpine or carbamylcholine is accomplished by measuring the intraocular pressure with a tonometer. This is generally done by a physician or under the direction of a physician.

Patients should be monitored for cholinergic crisis (flushing of the skin, headache, sudden drop in blood pressure, decreased pulse rate and altered rate, depth or rhythm of respiration) precipitated by inadvertent systemic absorption of the miotic. Abdominal cramping or bronchial asthma should be reported to the physician immediately.

Teaching
Patients should be warned about the dangers of driving or working with power tools (e.g., circular or band saws, lathes, grinders) immediately following the instillation of these drugs because they can produce blurred vision and difficulty in focusing.

Epinephrine

Mechanism of Action and Pharmacologic Effects

It may seem unusual at first glance to consider using epinephrine to treat glaucoma because it might be expected that stimulation of alpha$_1$ receptors by the drug should lead to mydriasis and a decrease in aqueous humor drainage. Whereas the pharmacological rationale for this view is sound, epinephrine, in the low concentrations used to treat glaucoma, causes only a brief mydriasis in some patients. This is not sufficient to increase intraocular pressure. The mechanism of action of epinephrine is not clear. The drug may decrease intraocular pressure by vasodilating the conjunctival blood vessels and increasing aqueous drainage.

Epinephrine is available as epinephrine bitartrate (Epitrate, Mytrate), epinephrine HCl (Epifrin, Glaucon) and epinephryl borate (Epinal, Eppy/N) for the treatment of glaucoma. Dipivefrin HCl (Propine) is a dipavalyl epinephrine (a pro-drug) converted to epinephrine by esterase in the cornea and anterior chamber. It is claimed to produce less burning and irritation and fewer allergic reactions than epinephrine.

Therapeutic Uses

Epinephrine is often used with either miotics or acetazolamide to treat patients with primary open-angle glaucoma because the combination is more effective than either drug used alone. Patients should be monitored regularly because epinephrine can sometimes cause a paradoxic increase in intraocular pressure. Considerable variability exists in patient response to epinephrine. Individuals with dark irides are generally more resistant to the drug.

Adverse Effects

The local adverse effects of epinephrine include brow ache, headache, blurred vision, ocular irritation, lacrimation and conjunctival adrenochrome deposits. Epinephryl borate may be less toxic than epinephrine HCl or bitartrate, and dipivefrin HCl may produce less irritation and burning. Reactive hyperemia, allergic conjunctivitis and contact dermatitis may occur following repetitive use of epinephrine. Epinephrine can induce cystoid macular edema in aphakic eyes. Because of the possibility of mydriasis, epinephrine is contraindicated preoperatively in the treatment of angle-closure glaucoma.

The systemic effects of epinephrine are tachycardia, premature ventricular contractions (PVCs), headache, hypertension, disorientation, blanching and tremors. Epinephrine should be used with care in patients with arrhythmias, recent myocardial infarction, arteriosclerotic heart disease, hypertension and hyperthyroidism. Epinephrine can sensitize the heart to halothane, resulting in PVCs, tachycardia and fibrillation.

Nursing Process

The nursing process associated with the use of epinephrine is discussed in detail in Chapter 7. Readers should refer to this chapter.

Osmotic Agents

Mechanism of Action and Pharmacologic Effects

When used in hypertonic solutions, glycerin, urea and mannitol increase the osmolarity of the blood, withdrawing fluid from the eyeball and producing an immediate fall in intraocular pressure and reduction in vitreous volume.

Therapeutic Uses

Osmotic agents are effective in patients who do not respond to miotics or acetazolamide. They are used to reduce intraocular pressure rapidly in patients with acute angle-closure glaucoma before iridectomy. Osmotic drugs also help to open the angle by reducing the volume of the posterior segment of the eye, thereby decreasing pressure behind the iris. Patients with chronic glaucomas may also be treated with osmotic agents both pre- and postoperatively.

Adverse Effects

Headache, nausea and vomiting are adverse effects common to all osmotic agents. Glycerin may also cause hyperglycemia and should be used with caution in diabetics. Mannitol will cause massive diuresis. It has also been associated with chills, dizziness and chest pains. Invert sugar solutions containing fructose are often used to reconstitute urea. Fructose can cause hypoglycemia, nausea, vomiting, tremors, coma and convulsions in patients with hereditary fructose intolerance (aldolase deficiency).

Nursing Process
Osmotic agents are diuretics and are discussed in detail in Chapter 16. Readers wishing to review the nursing process associated with the use of osmotic agents should refer to this previously presented information.

Drugs That Decrease Aqueous Humor Formation

Beta Blockers (Timolol Maleate, Levobunolol HCl, Betaxolol HCl)

Mechanism of Action and Pharmacologic Effects

Timolol (Timoptic) and levobunolol (Betagan) are nonselective beta blockers. Betaxolol (Betoptic) is a cardioselective beta blocker. The pharmacology of beta blockers is presented in several other chapters of this text, including Chapter 8. Their mechanism of action in the eye is not clear, but these drugs decrease aqueous humor production.

Therapeutic Uses

Timolol, levobunolol and betaxolol are indicated for the reduction of elevated intraocular pressure in patients with chronic open-angle glaucoma.

Adverse Effects

Locally, beta blockers can cause irritation, conjunctivitis, blepharitis and keratitis. Their systemic effects include bradycardia, hypotension, syncope and bronchospasm.

Nursing Process

As indicated above, timolol, levobunolol and betaxolol are beta blockers. Discussion of the nursing process associated with the use of beta blockers is presented in Chapters 8, 12 and 14. Readers requiring further information should refer to the previously presented material.

Acetazolamide (Diamox)

Mechanism of Action and Pharmacologic Effects

Acetazolamide inhibits carbonic anhydrase, an enzyme responsible for the production of bicarbonate in the body. Bicarbonate, formed in the ciliary body, is secreted by this tissue into the aqueous humor bathing the lens and iris. This process is important to the subsequent formation of aqueous humor because the secreted bicarbonate draws fluid after it, giving rise to more aqueous humor production. By inhibiting carbonic anhydrase, acetazolamide decreases bicarbonate production and, accordingly, aqueous humor formation.

Therapeutic Uses

Acetazolamide is of greatest value in the treatment of primary open-angle glaucoma and other chronic glaucomas. It is usually added to a patient's regimen when a miotic alone has proven inadequate. In the treatment of the phakic eye, acetazolamide is used before a weak miotic is replaced by a stronger one. Its value in the emergency treatment of acute glaucoma can be attributed to an opening of the angle as a result of a decrease in pressure behind the iris. The drug must be used only for a short period of time in angle-closure glaucoma before iridectomy. If surgery is delayed and miotics do not open the angle, peripheral anterior synchiae can develop and the angle may eventually close permanently.

Adverse Effects

The common adverse effects of acetazolamide include malaise, fatigue, anorexia, weight loss, impotence and loss of libido, gastric distress, nausea, vomiting and diarrhea. Less commonly seen are the adverse effects of sulfonamides (see Chapter 64).

Nursing Process

Assessment
Prior to the administration of acetazolamide, patients' histories should be reviewed for evidence of previous hypersensitivity to sulfonamides, chronic pulmonary disease, renal or hepatic disease, electrolyte imbalance or pregnancy. In the presence of any of these conditions the physician should be contacted to verify the order. In preparation for later evaluation for possible adverse effects, it is imperative that baseline measures of the patient's vital signs and body mass/weight be established. Baseline measures of intraocular pressure should be established in order to determine drug efficacy later.

Administration
This drug should be administered in the early
morning or at a time when it is least likely to interfere with the patient's daily routine. Reconstituted
parenteral solutions should be discarded after
twenty-four hours and syrup-based suspensions
should be discarded after one week. Tablets and
sustained-release tablets should be stored in
airtight, light-resistant containers. Potassium
replacement should be recommended for patients
with serum potassium less than 3.0.

Evaluation
Drug effectiveness is determined by reduced introc-
ular pressure as measured by tonometer. Evidence
of adverse effects includes paresthesia, drowsiness,
glucosuria, muscle weakness, respiratory distress,
cardiac irregularities, malaise, headache, vomiting
or dehydration. Nurses should advise patients to
drink two to three liters per day unless contraindicated, and to rise from a lying or sitting position
slowly.

Teaching
Patients should be advised of the diuretic effect of
this medication. They should be instructed to take
precautions related to drowsiness, especially while
driving or using power equipment. They should
also be alerted to the importance of a high-potassi-
um diet.

Further Reading

Chandler, P.A. and Grant, W.M. (1979). *Glaucoma*,
    2nd ed. Philadelphia: Lea and Febiger.
Drance, S.M. (1978). Use of miotics in management
    of intraocular pressure. In: R.P. Burns, ed.,
    Symposium on Ocular Therapy 11 : 1-9. New
    York: John Wiley and Sons.
Sears, M.L. (1976). Adrenergic therapy of open-
    angle glaucoma. In: R.P. Burns, ed.,
    Symposium on Ocular Therapy 8 : 67-78. New
    York: John Wiley and Sons.
Two new beta blockers for glaucoma (1986). *The
    Medical Letter 28* : 45-46.

Table 56
Antiglaucoma drugs.

Generic Name (Trade Name)	Use (Dose)	Action	Adverse Effects	Drug Interactions	Nursing Process
Pharmacologic Classification: Miotics — Directly Acting Cholinergic Drugs					
Pilocarpine HCl (Adsorbocarpine, Akarpin, Isopto Carpine, Pilocar, Pilocel), pilocarpine nitrate (PV Carpine), Ocusert Pilo-20/Pilo-40 Ocular Therapeutic System	Miotic of choice in 1° open-angle glaucoma and many other chronic glaucomas. Also used w. systemically administered ocular hypotensive drugs in emergency tx of acute angle-closure glaucoma (**Instill:** Initially, 1 drop 1-2% in solut'n q4-8h. *In 1° angle-closure glaucoma, before surgery:* Initially, 1% or 2% drops instilled frequently until angle opens and pressure decr. *Ocuserts:* 1 Pilo-20 or Pilo-40 system in upper or lower cul-de-sac hs, replaced q7days)	By stim. muscarinic receptors on circular muscles of iris, pilocarpine causes these muscles to constrict, resulting in miosis. Constrict'n of pupil opens Canals of Schlemm and permits better drainage of aqueous humor, plus fall in intraocular pressure.	Stinging, local irritat'n, ciliary spasm, allergic react'ns, miosis, poor night vision		**Assess:** Hx for asthma, peptic ulcers, bradycardia, hypotens'n, vasomotor instability, coronary artery disease, epilepsy, parkinsonism. **Administer:** From light-resistant container into lower conjunctival sac; compress lacrimal duct against bridge of nose to prevent absorpt'n of excess via nasopharynx. **Teach:** To avoid driving following administrat'n.
Carbachol (Carbacel, Isopto Carbachol)	Us. used when resistance or intolerance develops to pilocarpine (**Instill:** Initially, 1 drop 0.75-3% solut'n q8h)	As for pilocarpine	As for pilocarpine		As for pilocarpine
Pharmacologic Classification: Miotics — Short-Acting Anticholinesterase Drug					
Physostigmine sulfate, physostigmine salicylate (Eserine, Miocel, Isopto P-ES)	Tx 1° open-angle glaucoma and other chronic glaucomas (**Instill:** 1 drop 0.25% physostigmine sulfate or 0.5% physostigmine salicylate solut'n q4-6h or 0.25% physostigmine sulfate ointment hs)	By reversibly inhibiting acetylcholinesterase, physostigmine allows incr. am'ts of acetylcholine to stim. muscarinic receptors on circular muscles of iris. This produces miosis and opens wider the Canals of Schlemm to permit better drainage of	Hyperemia of conjunctiva and iris		As for pilocarpine

aqueous humor, plus fall in intraocular pressure.

Pharmacologic Classification: Miotics — Long-Acting Anticholinesterase Drugs

Drug	Action / Dosage	Side Effects / Adverse Reactions	Interactions	Nursing Considerations
Demecarium bromide (Humorsol)	Potent long-acting miotic used when other agents are inadequate (**Instill:** 1 drop 0.125% or 0.25% solut'n q12-48h). As for physostigmine, except effects of demecarium, echothiophate and isoflurophate are longer lasting. These drugs are also more potent than physostigmine.	Cataracts, spasm of accommodat'n, systemic parasympathomimetic effects, iris cysts	**Procaine:** Hydrolysis is reduced by isoflurophate and echothiophate because these drugs inhibit pseudocholinesterase, the enzyme responsible for inactivat'n of procaine. **Succinylcholine:** Action is prolonged in pts on prolonged isoflurophate or echothiophate tx, because these drugs inhibit pseudocholinesterase, the enzyme responsible for terminating the effects of succinylcholine.	**Assess:** Intraocular pressure (by physician); baseline VS. **Administer:** Initially by physician, due to need to monitor intraocular pressure w. tonometer, in light of risk of transient paradoxic incr. in intraocular pressure w. initial doses. Instill in lower conjunctival sac; blot excess from eyelid to prevent contact dermatitis; keep dry— do not touch tube to eye or wash tip of tube. **Teach:** S/s cholinergic crisis; proper technique of self-administrat'n.
Echothiophate (Echodide, Phospholine Iodide)	As for demecarium (**Instill:** 1 drop 0.03% or 0.06% solut'n q12-48h) As for demecarium		See above.	
Isoflurophate (DFP, Floropryl)	As for demecarium (**Apply:** One-quarter-in. strip 0.025% isoflurophate ointment q8-72h)			

Pharmacologic Classification: Adrenergic Drugs

Drug	Action / Dosage	Side Effects / Adverse Reactions	Nursing Considerations
Epinephrine bitartrate (Epitrate, Mytrate), epinephrine HCl (Epifrin, Glaucon), epinephryl borate (Epinal, Eppy/N)	Tx chronic simple open-angle glaucoma, alone or w. miotics (**Instill:** 1 drop 0.25-2% solut'n od-bid) May decr. intraocular pressure by vasodilating conjunctival blood vessels and incr. aqueous drainage.	Redness, transitory stinging, some pain following initial instillat'n; conjunctival adrenochrome deposits	**Assess:** Hx for glaucoma; CV, circulatory or cerebrovascular disease; prostatic hypertrophy; diabetes mellitus; hyperthyroidism; pregnancy. Establish baseline BP, rate/rhythm of pulse, color/temp. extremities. **Administer:** As for miotics. **Evaluate:** BP, pulse, color/temp. extremities. **Teach:** As for miotics.
Dipivefrin HCl (Dipivalyl Epinephrine, Propine)	As for epinephrine (**Instill:** 1 drop 0.1% dipivefrin HCl solut'n q12h) Prodrug converted to epinephrine in cornea and anterior chamber.	As for epinephrine but less likely to burn, irritate or cause allergic react'ns	

Pharmacologic Classification: Beta Blocker

Drug	Action / Dosage	Side Effects / Adverse Reactions	Nursing Considerations
Timolol maleate ophthalmic (Timoptic)	Reduct'n of elevated intraocular pressure in pts w. chronic open-angle glaucoma; ocular hypertens'n; aphakic pts having glaucoma, incl. those wearing contact lenses; pts w. narrow angles and hx of spontaneous or iatrogenically induced narrow. Timolol is a beta blocker. It decr. aqueous humor product'n, but its mechanism of action is unclear.	Ocular irritat'n, conjunctivitis, blepharitis, corneal anesthesia, keratitis. Bradycardia, hypotens'n, syncope, heart block, cerebrovascular. Refer to Tables 8, 13 and 15.	Refer to Tables 8 and 13.

Generic Name (Trade Name)	Use (Dose)	Action	Adverse Effects	Drug Interactions	Nursing Process
	angle-closure in opposite eye in whom reduct'n of intraocular pressure is nec. (**Instill:** Us. 1 drop 0.25% solut'n in affected eye bid. If nec., incr. to 1 drop 0.5% solut'n bid)		accident, cerebral ischemia, palpitat'ns and cardiac arrest are incl. in list of official adv. react'ns. Respiratory react'ns, incl. bronchospasm, have also been reported. In spite of this list, timolol maleate is us. well tolerated)		
Levobunolol HCl (Betagan)	Control of intraocular pressure in chronic glaucoma and ocular hypertens'n (**Instill:** 1 drop 0.5% levobunolol in affected eye[s] od-bid)	As for timolol	Blepharoconjunctivitis and decr. heart rate/BP have been reported occasionally.	Refer to Tables 8, 13 and 15.	Refer to Tables 8 and 13.
Betaxolol HCl (Betoptic)	Tx ocular hypertens'n or chronic open-angle glaucoma (**Instill:** 1 drop 0.5% betaxolol solut'n in affected eye[s] bid)	As for timolol	Gen. well tolerated. Occ. tearing.	Refer to Tables 8, 13 and 15.	Refer to Tables 8 and 13.

Pharmacologic Classification: Carbonic Anhydrase Inhibitor

Generic Name (Trade Name)	Use (Dose)	Action	Adverse Effects	Drug Interactions	Nursing Process
Acetazolamide (Diamox)	To decr. ocular aqueous humor secret'n in glaucoma [chronic, simple and secondary types] (**Oral:** Chronic simple [open-angle] glaucoma: 250 mg od-qid or 1 [500-mg] sustained-release capsule bid. Secondary glaucoma and preoperative tx of some cases acute congestive [closed-angle] glaucoma: 250 mg q4h)	Inhibits carbonic anhydrase, an enzyme responsible for bicarbonate product'n. Bicarbonate, formed in ciliary body, is secreted into aqueous humor. This is important to subsequent format'n of aqueous humor because secreted bicarbonate draws fluid after it, giving rise to more	Paresthesias, loss of appetite, polyuria, occ. instances of drowsiness and confus'n, urticaria, melena, hematuria, glycosuria, hepatic insufficiency, flaccid paralysis and convuls'ns. Adv. react'ns common to all sulfonamide derivatives, incl. fever, rash, crystalluria, renal calculus, bone	**Amphetamine:** Renal reabsorpt'n is decr. by acetazolamide. Thus acetazolamide may incr. effects of amphetamine. **Aspirin:** Interacts w. acetazolamide, which produces acidosis and incr. salicylate levels in brain. **Barbiturates:** Levels in brain are incr. by acetazolamide. **Digitalis:** Toxicity can incr. w. acetazolamide because acetazolamide can produce hypokalemia. **Diuretics:** Acetazolamide can incr. their hypokalemic effects. **Lithium carbonate:** Can have its	**Assess:** Hx for hypersensitivity to sulfonamides, chronic pulmonary disease, renal/hepatic disease, electrolytic imbalance, pregnancy. Establish baseline measures VS and weight, intraocular pressure. **Administer:** In early a.m. or at other time compatible w. pt's daily routine. Use reconstituted parenteral solut'ns within 24 h and syrup-based suspens'ns within 1 week. Store tablets and sustained-release capsules in airtight, light-resistant containers. K replacement recommended if serum K < 3.0. **Evaluate:** Drug efficacy by reduced

aqueous humor format'n. By inhibiting bicarbonate product'n, acetazolamide blocks above process and reduces aqueous humor format'n.

marrow depress'n, thrombocytopenic purpura, hemolytic anemia, leukopenia, pancytopenia and agranulocytosis. If such react'ns occur, discontinue tx and begin appropriate measures.

cardiotoxic/neurotoxic effects incr. by acetazolamide. **Quinidine:** Renal reabsorpt'n is incr. by acetazolamide, resulting in incr. quinidine serum levels.

intraocular pressure as measured by tonometer; adv. effects. **Teach:** Poss. diuretic effect; to avoid driving or using power equipment; importance of high-K diet. Advise pt to drink 2-3 L/day unless contraindicated; to rise from lying/sitting posit'n slowly.

Anti-Infective and Anti-Inflammatory Drugs for the Eye

Teaching Objectives

Following completion of this chapter, the reader should be able to:

1. Discuss the use of drugs to treat blepharitis and the related nursing process.
2. Discuss the use of drugs to treat conjunctivitis and the related nursing process.
3. Discuss the use of drugs to treat corneal infections and the related nursing process.
4. Discuss the mechanism of action, therapeutic uses and adverse effects of corticosteroids in the treatment of ocular inflammation, as well as the nursing process related to this use.
5. Discuss the use of nonsteroidal, anti-inflammatory drugs in the treatment of ocular inflammation.

Most of the drugs mentioned in this chapter are described in greater detail elsewhere in the book. Chapter 38 presents information pertaining to the use of these drugs only for eye infections or inflammation. Readers are encouraged to refer to the relevant chapters in this text if additional information is required.

Ocular Infections

Blepharitis, conjunctivitis, corneal ulcers and endophthalmitis should receive prompt and intensive antimicrobial therapy. Combined topical corticosteroid and antimicrobial products are popular but should be used cautiously because suppression of inflammation may convey the false impression that the infection is controlled.

Nursing Process

As indicated above, the systemic uses of drugs presented in this chapter are discussed elsewhere in this book. Readers are advised to refer to the appropriate sections for detailed information on each drug. The nursing process associated with the use of ocular anti-infective and anti-inflammatory drugs is primarily addressed to proper administration. Patients should be instructed in the appropriate methods of self-administration. Specialized information related to the more general aspects of nursing care for patients with these conditions is beyond the scope of this text. Readers should refer to an appropriate medical-surgical or ophthalmologic nursing source.

Blepharitis

Seborrheic blepharitis is usually associated with seborrheic dermatitis and often responds to antiseborrheic shampoos. The lids can be treated with a mild baby shampoo. Staphylococcal blepharitis can be treated with 10 – 30% sodium sulfacetamide solution or ointment (Sodium Sulamyd) or 0.5% chloramphenicol solution (Chloromycetin). Topical corticosteroids may also be applied if corneal hypersensitivity occurs. Angular blepharitis is often caused by the Morax-Axenfeld gram-negative bacillus (*M. lacunata*) and responds to sulfonamides, zinc sulfate or gentamicin (Garamycin).

Conjunctivitis

Acute bacterial conjunctivitis in children and adults is often due to *Staphylococcus aureus. Streptococcus pyogenes, Haemophilus influenzae* and *Neisseria gonorrhoeae* are other common causative organisms. Most cases of bacterial conjunctivitis in children and adults respond to topical sulfacetamide 10 – 30%, 0.5% chloramphenicol or combinations of bacitracin or gramicidin with polymyxin B and neomycin (Neosporin Ointment or Solution).

Neonatal conjunctivitis usually results from infection with *Chlamydia trachomatis, Staphylococcus aureus, Streptococcus pneumoniae* or *Neisseria gonorrhoeae. Pseudomonas* may also cause conjunctivitis in the neonate. Neonatal chlamydial infections are usually treated with topical sulfonamides or tetracycline. Treatment of gonococcal infections in the neonate should include both topical and systemic treatment. Either penicillin drops (10 000 U/mL) or tetracycline ointment (Achromycin) should be instilled every one or two hours, together with intramuscular penicillin G, ampicillin or amoxicillin.

Viral conjunctivitis is usually self-limiting. Patients may be treated with a topical sulfonamide to prevent secondary infections.

Chronic conjunctivitis can result from the use of antibiotics, antiseptics, preservatives and vasoconstrictors. All medication should be stopped for several days if progress is lacking to determine whether drugs are the cause.

Allergic conjunctivitis usually responds to sodium cromoglycate/cromolyn (Opticrom) instilled two or three times daily.

Corneal Infections

Bacterial keratitis is caused by *Pseudomonas aeruginosa,* beta-hemolytic streptococci, gonococci, pneumococci and *Staphylococcus aureus.* Treatment should be started immediately because corneal pathology is rapidly destructive, often leading to perforation and loss of sight despite intensive therapy. A variety of antibiotics may be administered subconjunctivally. Depending on bacterial sensitivity, ampicillin, bacitracin, carbenicillin, chloramphenicol, colistin, gentamicin, methicillin, neomycin, penicillin G, polymyxin B, tobramycin or vancomycin may be used. Chloramphenicol, sulfacetamide and Neosporin may also be used topically. Supportive therapy includes the use of cycloplegics to control uveitis and prevent synechiae.

Syphilitic keratitis is treated for seven to ten days with penicillin G. Hourly applications or daily subconjunctival injections of corticosteroids may be used to control severe keratitis and uveitis.

The treatment of fungal keratitis is disappointing because of the lack of effective, nontoxic drugs. Fungal keratitis is treated topically every two hours with natamycin (Natacyn), clotrimazole (Canesten) or amphotericin B (Fungizone).

Herpes simplex keratitis usually responds to idoxuridine (Dendrid, Herplex, Stoxil) instilled every two to three hours for one week. If this fails, vidarabine (Vira-A) or trifluridine (Viroptic) can be tried. Use of topical corticosteroids should be avoided for fear of spreading the infection.

In the absence of specific treatment for herpes zoster keratitis, inflammation is treated with topical corticosteroids, together with a cycloplegic to control uveitis. Secondary infection may be reduced by a topical sulfonamide.

Exogenous endophthalmitis is usually caused by *Staphylococcus aureus, Pseudomonas, Proteus* or *Escherichia coli.* After an aqueous and vitreous tap for smear and culture, direct intravitreal antibiotic(s) injections may be given. Systemic corticosteroids are warranted for the first forty-eight hours to reduce inflammatory damage to the retina and other tissues.

Ocular Inflammation

Corticosteroids

Mechanism of Action and Therapeutic Uses

Corticosteroids have a nonspecific anti-inflammatory action. They are used to control ocular inflammation, reduce scarring and prevent visual loss.

Corticosteroids are useful in ocular allergic disorders, Thygeson's superficial punctate keratopathy, sterile uveal tract inflammation, episcleritis, scleritis and temporal arteritis. Although they are often used in the treatment of ocular infections, they must be accompanied by therapy aimed at the specific causative organism. Corticosteroids are useful in treating postoperative iridocyclitis but delay healing and increase the susceptibility to, or the masking of, postoperative infections.

Topical corticosteroid treatment usually controls inflammation of the lids, conjunctiva, cornea and anterior sclera. Subconjunctival injections can be used to complement topical therapy in the treatment of resistant inflammations. Anterior uveitis may require systemic therapy. Treatment of the posterior segment of the globe may require both systemic and local injections.

Adverse Effects

Repeated use of corticosteroids can increase intraocular pressure, promote the development of posterior subcapsular cataracts, reduce the rate of wound healing and increase the risk of infections spreading. The concomitant use of antibiotics or antibacterials may reduce the risk of bacterial infection but increase the danger of fungal infections. The administration of a corticosteroid to treat herpes simplex, corneal stromal disease or uveitis should be accompanied by an antiviral drug to prevent reactivation of the epithelial infection.

Nonsteroidal Anti-Inflammatory Drugs

Nonsteroidal anti-inflammatory drugs (NSAIDs) have been studied for their ability to reduce ocular inflammation. Indomethacin (Indocid Ophthalmic Suspension) is indicated for prophylaxis of aphakic cystoid macular edema following cataract surgery. One drop is instilled in the operative eye four times daily on the day prior to surgery and one drop forty-five minutes before surgery. This is followed by one drop four times daily for ten to twelve weeks postoperatively. Its efficacy is still open to question. Flurbiprofen (Ocufen) is indicated for the treatment of postoperative and postlaser trabeculoplasty inflammation of the anterior segment of the eye. This drug is also approved for the inhibition of intraoperative miosis.

Further Reading

Furgiuele, F.P. (1978). Eye and eyelid infections. Treatment and prevention. *Drugs 15* : 310-316.

Table 57
Anti-infective and anti-inflammatory drugs for the eye.

Pharmacologic Classification: Ocular Anti-Bacterial Drugs

Generic Name (Trade Name)	Use (Dose)	Action	Adverse Effects	Drug Interactions	Nursing Process
Bacitracin (Baciguent)	Tx superficial staph, strep infect'ns (**Instill:** Drops [10 000 U bacitracin/mL] or ointment [400-500 U bacitracin/g] hourly or less frequently)	Polypeptide antibiotic. Active against many gram-positive organisms, incl. streptococci, staphylococci, anaerobic cocci and clostridia of gas gangrene group, corynebacteria, *T. pallidum* and certain gram-negative cocci, incl. gonococci and meningococci.	Few; 1° sensitivity in bacitracin is not often seen.		*Identical for all drugs in this chapter. Consult related material in chapters elsewhere in text.* **Assess:** Prior drug sensitivity. **Administer:** Using proper technique. **Evaluate:** Drug efficacy; monitor for adv. react'ns such as drug sensitivity. **Teach:** Proper methods of self-adminis-trat'n.
Chloramphenicol (Antibiopto, Chloromycetin, Chloroptic SOP, Econochlor, Ophthochlor)	Tx superficial conjunctival and/or corneal infect'ns (**Instill:** 2 drops solut'n [5 mg/mL] or small am't ointment [10 mg/g] in affected eye q3h or prn)	Antibiotic w. broad-spectrum activity. Effective against many gram-positive/-negative micro-organisms. Also effective against chlamydiae and rickettsia.	Rarely causes sensiti-zat'n.		
Colistin sulfate (Coly-Mycin S)	Effective against most gram-negative organisms (**Instill:** Drops hourly, or less frequently for milder infect'ns)	Activity only against gram-negative bacteria. *Enterobacter, E. coli,* klebsiella, salmonella, pasteurella, bordetella and shigella are most sensitive.	Low incidence of mild burning or painful sensat'n.		
Erythromycin (Ilotycin)	For conjunctival and/or corneal infect'ns, caused by many gram-positive organisms (**Instill:** Solut'n [5-10 mg/mL] or ointment [5 mg/g] od or more, depending on severity)	Most effective against gram-positive cocci, such as *Streptococcus pyogenese* and *Streptococcus pneumoniae.*	Use may be assoc. w. overgrowth of antibi-otic-resistant organ-isms.		

Drug	Indications/Dosage	Activity	Comments
Gentamicin sulfate (Garamycin, Genoptic)	For ocular infect'ns caused by S. aureus, P. aeruginosa, A. aerogenes, E. coli, P. vulgaris and K. Pneumoniae. (**Instill:** Solut'n [3-10 mg gentamicin sulfate/mL] or ointment [3 mg gentamicin sulfate/g] q15-30min for serious infect'ns. In milder cases, instill drops or ointment hourly or less frequently)	**Active against gram-positive bacteria commonly found in eye infect'ns; coagulase-positive/-negative staphylococci; group A beta hemolytic/nonhemolytic streptococci; and S. pneumoniae. Also active against gram-negative bacteria incl. P. aeruginosa, indole-positive/-negative Proteus, E. coli, K. pneumoniae, S. marcescens, H. influenzae, E. aerogenes, N. gonorrhoeae, providencia species and H. vaginocoli.**	Irritat'n
Tobramycin sulfate (Tobrex)	As for gentamicin sulfate (**Instill:** Solut'n [3-10 mg/mL] as described for gentamicin)		As for gentamicin sulfate
Neomycin sulfate	For gram-positive/-negative organisms, incl. proteus (**Instill:** Solut'n [2.5-5 mg/mL] or ointment [5 mg/g] q15-30min for serious infect'ns. Hourly or less frequently in milder cases)	Active against a broad spectrum of gram-positive/-negative bacteria.	Produces sensitizat'n more readily than any other topical antibiotic.
Polymyxin B sulfate (found in many combinat'n products)	For broad-spectrum activity (**Instill:** Drops or ointment hourly or less frequently for milder cases)	Active only against gram-negative bacteria. Spectrum sim. to colistin (see above).	
Sulfacetamide sodium (Ak-Sulf, Bleph-10 Liquifilm, Cetamide, Isopto Cetamide, Sulamyd, Sulfacel-15)	For superficial ocular infect'ns caused by H. aegyptium, S. pneumoniae and many strains of S. aureus (**Instill:** Solut'n [100-300 mg/mL] or ointment [100-300 mg/g] q2-3h or less frequently, acc. to severity of infect'n)	Broad-spectrum activity. Used extensively in management of ocular infect'ns.	Irritat'n

Generic Name (Trade Name)	Use (Dose)	Action	Adverse Effects	Drug Interactions	Nursing Process
Tetracycline HCl (Achromycin), chlortetracycline HCl (Aureomycin)	For superficial infect'ns caused by sensitive organisms (**Instill:** Solut'n [10 mg/mL] or ointment [10 mg/g] to infected eye at least q2h)	Wide range of antimicrobial activity against gram-positive/-negative bacteria. Also effective against rickettsiae, mycoplasma and chlamydia.			

Pharmacological Classification: Ocular Antifungal Drugs

Generic Name (Trade Name)	Use (Dose)	Action	Adverse Effects	Drug Interactions	Nursing Process
Amphotericin B (Fungizone)	For keratomycoses caused by fungi, particularly candida, coccidiodes, cryptococcus, histoplasma, blastomyces and sporotrichum (**Instill:** 1 drop 0.5-1.5 mg/mL every 30 min, then every 60 min)	Broad-spectrum antifungal activity	Strong concentrat'ns may cause severe local irritat'n.		
Natamycin (Natacyn)	Drug of choice for initial fungal keratitis, blepharitis and conjunctivitis (**Instill:** *For fungal keratitis* - For first 3-4 days, 1 drop 50 mg/mL hourly during day and q2h at night. Then 1 drop 6-8x/day for 14-21 days. *For fungal blepharitis and conjunctivitis* - 1 drop 4-6x/day)	Broad-spectrum antifungal activity, esp. against ocular pathogens	Allergic react'ns have been reported rarely.		
Nystatin	For external ocular infect'ns caused by candida or aspergillus (**Instill:** Initially, 1 drop 25 000 U/mL q15min)	Active against candida, cryptococcus, histoplasma, blastomyces, trichophyton, epidermophyton and *Microsporum audouini.*	Irritat'n		

Pharmacologic Classification: Ocular Antiviral Drugs

Generic Name (Trade Name)	Use (Dose)	Action	Adverse Effects	Drug Interactions	Nursing Process
Idoxuridine (Dendrid, Herplex, Stoxil)	Tx herpes simplex keratitis only (**Instill:** Ointment 5x/day q4h, w. last dose hs. Continue 3-5	Primary clinical use is herpes simplex keratitis. Epithelial	Irritat'n, pain, pruritus, inflammat'n, photophobia	**Boric acid:** Should not be administered during course of tx because it may irritate in	

Drug	Dosage	Action/Use	Side Effects/Precautions	Nursing Process/Comments
	days after healing appears complete. In deep lesions, continue prn. If steroids are being used, continue idoxuridine until after steroids have been w'drawn)	infect'ns, esp. initial attacks in which a dendritic figure is present, respond best. Total healing does not occur in all instances, even those w. the most superficial involvement. Herpes simplex type II does not respond to this drug.		presence of idoxuridine. Antibiotics may be used w. idoxuridine to control secondary infect'ns, and atropine preparat'ns may be employed adjunctively prn.
Trifluridine (Viroptic)	Herpes simplex infect'ns of conjunctiva and cornea (**Instill:** 1 drop 10 mg/mL q2h during day to max. 9 drops. Continue 1 week after healing appears complete, w. 1 drop q4h, to max. 3 weeks)	Active against herpes simplex types I and II, Varicella zoster, adenovirus and viccinia virus.	As for idoxuridine	
Vidarabine (Vira-A)	Herpes keratoconjunctivitis manifested by dendritic keratitis or geographic corneal ulcers (**Instill:** 1.5 cm ointment [30 mg/g] 5x/day until corneal re-epithelializat'n. Continue 7 days at reduced dose [e.g., bid] to prevent recurrence)	As effective against herpes simplex keratoconjunctivitis as idoxuridine and less irritating.	Lacrimat'n, foreign-body sensat'n, burning irritat'n, superficial punctate keratitis, pain, photophobia, punctal occlus'n, sensitivity	

Pharmacologic Classification: Ocular Anti-Inflammatory Drugs — Corticosteroids†

Drug	Dosage	Action/Use	Side Effects/Precautions	Nursing Process/Comments
Hydrocortisone, hydrocortisone acetate	Steroid-responsive inflammatory condit'ns of anterior segment of eye (**Instill:** 0.2-0.5% solut'n or 2.5% suspens'n q1-2h until response seen; then reduce frequency. Ointment 0.5-1.5% tid-qid or hs)	Possesses nonspecific anti-inflammatory effects that can be directed against immunologically mediated disorders, mechanical or chemical injury, or infect'ns. In infect'ns, tx must also incl. appropriate antibacterial, antifungal or antiviral medicat'n.	Glaucoma w. optic nerve damage, visual acuity and field defects, posterior subcapsular cataract format'n, 2° ocular infect'n from pathogens, perforat'n of globe	*Consult related material in chapters elsewhere in this text, as all Nursing Process comments for corticosteroids apply to ocular anti-inflammatory drugs.*

Generic Name (Trade Name)	Use (Dose)	Action	Adverse Effects	Drug Interactions	Nursing Process
Dexamethasone, dexamethasone sodium phosphate (Maxidex, Decadron Phosphate)	Indicat'ns and frequency of dose as for hydrocortisone	As above	As above		
Fluorometholone (FML)	Indicat'ns and frequency of dose as for hydrocortisone	As above	As above		
Medrysone (HMS)	Indicat'ns and frequency of dose as for hydrocortisone	As above	As above		
Prednisolone acetate, prednisolone sodium phosphate (Ak-Pred, Ak-Tate, Econopred, Hydeltrasol, Inflamase, Metretone, Pred Mild and Forte)	Indicat'ns and frequency of dose as for hydrocortisone	As above	As above		

†In addition to the products listed here, corticosteroids are combined with chloramphenicol; neomycin; neomycin, polymyxin B and bacitracin; and sodium sulfacetamide.

CHAPTER 39

Topical Otic Drugs

Teaching Objectives
Following completion of this chapter, the reader
should be able to:
1. Describe the use of acetic acid in the ear and its
adverse effects.
2. Describe the use of chloramphenicol to treat ear
infections and its adverse effects.
3. Discuss the otic use of neomycin and its adverse
effects.
4. Discuss the otic use of the polymyxins and their
adverse effects.
5. Describe the therapeutic use of combination
antibiotic/corticosteroid products in the ear and
their adverse effects.
6. Describe the topical antifungal drugs available
for the treatment of otic infections.
7. Discuss the use of topical otic analgesics.
8. Discuss the nursing process precipitated by the
use of topical otic drugs.

Otic Infection

A breakdown in the natural defenses of the ear
produced by trauma leaves it susceptible to infection. *Pseudomonas aeruginosa* and *Aspergillus* are
particularly common infections. Other common
pathogens include *Staphylococcus aureus*, streptococci, *Escherichia coli*, *Proteus* species, and
Candida.

Before beginning treatment, the ear canal
should be cleansed thoroughly with products such
as Burow's solution or Domeboro Otic Solution;
effective drug treatment often requires repeated
debridement of the ear canal. The effective delivery
of a topical medication may entail placement of a
"wick", at least until swelling is decreased. Severe
cases of external otitis may require systemic treatment.

Nursing Process
The systemic uses for many of the drugs discussed
in the remainder of this chapter are described
elsewhere in this book. Readers are advised to refer
to the appropriate sections for detailed information
on each drug.

The nursing process for all otic drugs is essentially the same. It is primarily addressed to assessment of prior drug sensitivity, proper drug administration, evaluation of drug efficacy and monitoring
for adverse reactions. Patient teaching involves
instruction on self-administration. Specialized
information related to the more general aspects of
nursing care for patients with these conditions is
beyond the scope of this text. Readers should refer
to an appropriate medical-surgical or specialty
nursing source.

Acetic Acid

Two- to five-per-cent solutions of acetic acid reduce swelling of the ear canal if it is infected by *Pseudomonas aeruginosa, Candida,* or *Aspergillus.* Acetic acid solutions also relieve the other signs and symptoms of external otitis (pain, pruritus, erythema and a foul-smelling discharge). Although usually well tolerated, acetic acid solutions can cause irritation and sensitization.

Chloramphenicol (Chloromycetin)

Chloramphenicol is effective against a wide range of pathogens causing external otitis. These include *Staphylococcus aureus, Escherichia coli,* and strains of *Pseudomonas* and *Proteus* species. If signs of drug-induced local irritation appear, chloramphenicol should be discontinued. Blood dyscrasias have been reported following topical use in the ear.

Neomycin Sulfate (Otobiotic)

Neomycin is effective against *Enterobacter aerogenes, Escherichia,* most species of *Klebsiella, Salmonella, Shigella* and *Proteus,* as well as many strains of *Staphylococcus aureus.* It has only weak activity against *Pseudomonas.*

Neomycin can cause skin sensitization. Unfortunately, the signs of skin sensitization often mimic the symptoms of external otitis. Although it may not be easy to differentiate between the two, inflammation caused by skin sensitivity usually spreads to the tragus, antetragus and ear lobule. Cross-sensitization can occur between neomycin and other aminoglycosides, such as gentamicin and tobramycin.

The Polymyxins

Polymyxin B and colistin (polymyxin E) are effective against *Pseudomonas aeruginosa, Escherichia coli,* and some other gram-negative organisms. Their clinical usefulness is limited by the fact that they have no activity against *Proteus* or gram-positive bacteria. The products Aerosporin Otic and Lidosporin Otic contain polymyxin B. Lidosporin Otic also contains lidocaine for the relief of pain. Coly-Mycin Otic contains both colistin and neomycin and it, too, is indicated for the treatment of acute and chronic otitis externa caused by susceptible bacteria and for the treatment or prophylaxis of recurrent "swimmer's ear."

Patients do not usually experience adverse reactions to the polymyxins. However, treatment should be stopped if irritation or sensitivity occurs.

Combination Products

Several products contain more than one antibacterial (Table 58). Fixed-ratio products have reasonable therapeutic success. However, they also have a greater likelihood of causing drug-induced adverse effects.

Corticosteroids may be added to an antibacterial to reduce inflammation and pruritus. Examples include Coly-Mycin S Otic with Neomycin and Hydrocortisone, Cortisporin Otic Solution and Suspension, Locacorten-Vioform, Otic Tridesilon, Otobione, Otocort, Pyocidin-Otic and VoSol HC. Corticosteroid-containing products are contraindicated in patients with herpes simplex, vaccinia and varicella.

Antifungal Drugs

Fungal infections in the ear canal are not so prevalent as bacterial infections. They occur most commonly in warm climates and require a warm, dark, damp environment with dead tissue for growth. Three products are available to treat fungal infections in the ear canal. These are Fungizone Lotion, VoSol Otic Solution and VoSol HC. They should be used along with thorough cleansing of the ear. Amphotericin B is the active ingredient in Fungizone and it is effective against many fungi — in particular, *Candida.* VoSol contains 2% acetic acid and propylene glycol. The latter chemical is dehydrating and may assist in fighting mycotic infections. VoSol HC contains acetic acid, propylene glycol and hydrocortisone.

Topical Otic Analgesics

Three products, all containing benzocaine, are used to relieve otitis externa or otitis media pain. These are Americaine Otic, Auralgan Otic Solution and Tympagesic Ear Drops. Their clinical effectiveness can be questioned. First, the absorption of benzocaine from the skin or tympanic membrane is poor; second, the effectiveness of benzocaine is unpredictable. As a result, patients are often treated with a systemic analgesic that is more effective and circumvents the problem of hypersensitivity reactions to the local anesthetic.

Further Reading

Farmer, H.S. (1980). Guide for treatment of external otitis. *Amer. Fam. Phys. 21* (June): 96-101.

Keim, R.J. (1977). Common ear disease: Recognition and management. *Postgrad. Med. J. 61* (May): 72-80.

Table 58
Topical otic drugs.

Generic Name (Trade Name)	Use (Dose)	Action	Adverse Effects	Drug Interactions	Nursing Process
Pharmacologic Classification: Antibacterial Drugs					
Chloramphenicol (Chloromycetin Otic)	Tx superficial gram-positive/-negative infect'ns of external auditory canal (**Instill:** 2-3 drops solut'n [5 mg/mL] tid-qid)	Effective against a wide range of pathogens.	Irritat'n. Blood dyscrasias have been reported following topical use in ear.		*Identical for all drugs in this chapter. Consult related material in chapters elsewhere in text.* **Assess:** Prior drug sensitivity. **Administer:** Using proper technique. **Evaluate:** Drug efficacy; monitor for adv. react'ns such as drug sensitivity. **Teach:** Proper methods of self-administrat'n.
Neomycin sulfate (Otobiotic)	Tx external otitis caused by many gram-negative bacilli and some strains of S. aureus (**Instill:** Several drops solut'n [5 mg/mL] in ear tid-qid)	Effective against E. aerogenes, escherichia, most species of klebsiella, salmonella, shigella and proteus, as well as many strains of S. aureus.	Topical sensitizat'n and cutaneous hyper-sensitivity react'ns.		
Polymyxin B (Aerosporin Otic, Lidosporin Otic [which contains polymyxin B and lidocaine])	Tx external otitis due to P. aeruginosa, E. coli and some other gram-negative organisms (**Instill:** 3-4 drops solut'n [10 000 U/mL] tid-qid)	Antibiotic effective against bacteria as listed, left.	Irritat'n, sensitivity.		
Colistin (found in Coly-Mycin S Otic with Neomycin and Hydrocortisone)	As for polymyxin B	As for polymyxin B	As for polymyxin B		
Pharmacologic Classification: Antibacterial Drugs with Corticosteroids					
Coly-S Otic with Neomycin and Hydrocortisone; Cortisporin Otic Solution/Suspension; Otobione; Otocort [all containing polymyxin B sulfate, neomycin sulfate and	External otitis, otitis media w. perforated tympanic membrane, infect'ns of mastoidectomy and fenestrat'n cavities (**Instill:** Us. 3-4 drops preparat'n tid-qid)	Antibacterial actions of drugs included in each product, plus anti-inflammatory effects of topical corticosteroid	Sensitizat'n to neomycin when present in product		

hydrocortisone];
Otic Tridesilon
[containing acetic
acid and desonide];
Pyocidin-Otic [contain-
ing polymyxin B and
hydrocortisone]

Pharmacologic Classification: Antifungal Drugs

Drug	Indication / Dosage	Comment	Adverse
Acetic acid (VoSol Otic Solution, Otic Domeboro Solution)	Prevent'n and tx of otitis externa caused by P. aeruginosa, candida and aspergillus (**Instill:** 4-6 drops of 2% solut'n in ear q2-3h prn)	Reduces swelling of ear canal if infected w. P. aeruginosa, candida or aspergillus.	Irritat'n
VoSol HC [containing acetic acid and hydrocortisone]	As for VoSol Otic plus anti-inflammatory effect of hydrocortisone (**Instill:** As for VoSol Otic)	As for VoSol Otic	Irritat'n
Amphotericin B (Fungizone Lotion)	Mycotic infect'ns of ear canal, particularly if caused by candida (**Instill:** 3% lotion prn)	Active against many fungi, particularly candida	Irritat'n

Pharmacology of the Integumentary System (Skin)

Section 11 is devoted to a discussion of the application of drugs to the skin. Unlike diseases of many other parts of the body that can, at least for a while, remain hidden from others, disorders of the skin are often all too obvious to even the most casual observer. As a result, patients are acutely aware of their skin problems and respond by applying all manner of ointments, creams, lotions and gels in an attempt to restore the appearance of healthy skin.

The first chapter in this section reviews the most important subject of topical corticosteroids. It is followed by a discussion of drugs to treat acne and psoriasis. Finally, no consideration of drugs and the skin would be complete without a chapter on the use of topical anti-infective drugs.

CHAPTER 40

Topical Corticosteroids

Mechanism of Action and Pharmacologic Effects

Corticosteroids reduce inflammation by causing vasoconstriction, impairing chemotaxis, reducing prostaglandin formation, stabilizing lysosomal membranes in neutrophils and diminishing the lymphocytic response to allergic stimuli. Because of these actions, corticosteroids are incorporated into lotions, gels, creams and ointments for the treatment of a variety of dermatologic conditions. Corticosteroids also suppress mitosis and are used in the treatment of psoriasis.

Potency of Different Corticosteroids

In using topical steroid therapy safely, it is important for nurses to recognize the differences in potency between the various products on the market. Corticosteroids range in potency from **low potency** through **moderately potent, very potent** to **most potent.** Representatives of each group are presented in Table 59. Although the more potent steroids will usually provide a rapid and profound response, the temptation to use these products should be resisted because they are also capable of causing severe local adverse effects. Drugs in the very potent and most potent categories should be used only when less potent products fail.

Role of the Vehicle

The choice of vehicle is important in determining steroid absorption. To exert an anti-inflammatory effect, a corticosteroid must penetrate the stratum corneum of the epidermis to reach the dermis. Occlusion of pores with dressings (e.g., saran wrap) has long been recognized as an effective way of increasing topical corticosteroid activity. The increased hydration of the stratum corneum, which accompanies occlusion, facilitates transport of a corticosteroid to deeper skin tissues. Ointments are the most occlusive vehicles and are most effective in

Table 59
Classification of topical corticosteroids.

Generic Name	Trade Name
Low-Potency Corticosteroids	
Hydrocortisone 1%	Aeroseb-HC, Alphaderm, Cetacort, Cort-Dome, Cortef, Cortril, Emo-Cort, Hydro-Cortilean, Hytone, Nutracort, Synacort, Unicort
Methylprednisolone 0.25%	Medrol
Moderately Potent - Potent Corticosteroids	
Betamethasone valerate 0.05%	Betnovate, Celestoderm-V/2, Valisone
Clobetasone butyrate 0.05%	Eumovate
Desoximetasone 0.05%	Topicort Mild, Topicort LP
Fluocinolone acetonide 0.01%	Fluoderm, Fluonid, Synalar, Synamol
Fluocinonide 0.01%	Lidemol, Lidex, Topsyn
Halcinonide 0.025%	Halog
Hydrocortisone valerate 0.2%	Westcort
Triamcinolone acetonide 0.025%	Aristocort, Aristocort D, Kenalog, Triacet, Triaderm
Potent - Very Potent Corticosteroids	
Amcinonide 0.1%	Cyclocort
Beclomethasone dipropionate 0.025%	Propaderm
Betamethasone benzoate 0.025%	Beben, Betnisone, Uticort
Betamethasone valerate 0.1%	Betaderm, Betnovate, Celestoderm-V, Valisone
Desonide 0.05%	Tridesilon
Desoximethasone 0.25%	Topicort
Diflurasone diacetate 0.05%	Fluoderm, Fluonide, Synalar, Synamol
Fluocinonide 0.05%	Lidemol, Lidex, Topsyn
Flurandrenolide 0.05%	Cordran, Drenison
Halcinonide 0.1%	Halciderm, Halog
Triamcinolone acetonide 0.1%	Aristocort, Aristocort R, Kenalog, Triacet, Triaderm
Very Potent Corticosteroid	
Betamethasone dipropionate 0.05%	Diprosone
Most Potent Corticosteroid	
Clobetasol propionate 0.05%	Dermovate
Fluocinolone acetonide 0.2%	Synalar HP
Triamcinolone acetonide 0.5%	Aristocort, Aristocort A, Aristocort C, Kenalog, Triacet

promoting steroid penetration. Creams are less occlusive and generally less effective in guaranteeing corticosteroid penetration. Lotions are least occlusive and so least effective. Gels usually contain alcohol and a jelling agent, such as propylene glycol. They are most suitable for hairy areas of the body and should not be used on mucous membranes because the alcohol may be severely irritating.

These comments must be weighed with the knowledge that creams, being oil in water vehicles, are more miscible with, and suitable for, wet or weepy dermatoses. Fortunately, wet or weepy skin problems offer less of a barrier to corticosteroid penetration; for these, creams provide adequate steroid penetration. Dry dermatoses offer greater impediment to corticosteroid penetration and usually require treatment with ointments. Lotions are often used in hairy areas of the body.

Regional differences exist with respect to the ease with which drugs penetrate the skin. The back, scalp, axillae, forehead, jaw angle and scrotum present little impediment to drug absorption. They are best treated with weaker steroids (e.g., hydrocortisone). Only hydrocortisone should be used on the face and in the groin and axillae. If diaper rash requires steroid use, only hydrocortisone should be applied. The plantar surface of the foot and the ankle present greater barriers to absorption and may require stronger corticosteroids.

Therapeutic Uses

Allergic contact dermatitis, primary irritant dermatitis, endogenous eczema (e.g.,atopic, neurodermatitis, cheiropompholyx), psoriasis (especially of the face and flexures), seborrheic eczema and varicose eczema usually respond well to topical corticosteroids. Alopecia areata, discoid lupus erythematosus, granuloma annulare, hypertrophic scars and keloids may respond to topical steroids but are treated faster with intralesional corticosteroids. The same statement can be made for necrobiosis lipoidica, nodular prurigo, pretibial myxedema and sarcoidosis.

Topical corticosteroids should not be used alone in skin infections; they reduce the host's defense mechanisms and permit the spread of infection. In addition, by reducing inflammation, they lull the patient, the physician and the nurse into the false belief that the condition is on the wane. In cases of impetiginized eczema, which are usually colonized by *Staphylococcus aureus,* corticosteroids should be combined with antimicrobials. Other indications for combination products include seborrheic eczema, diaper rash, otitis externa, and intertriginous eruptions. However, the use of a combination preparation can also produce problems, such as the emergence of resistant strains, contact sensitization (particularly to neomycin) and skin staining (with iodochlorhydroxyquin [Vioform]).

Adverse Effects

The major complications occurring after the repeated use of topical corticosteroid treatment involve the dermis. Dermal atrophy is a common adverse effect of topical steroids. Dermal collagen is damaged and striae appear. This is more likely to occur in children and adolescents. The more potent steroids cause thinning of the epidermis. Rebound pustulation can also be seen when a strong corticosteroid is discontinued.

Consistent with the effects of corticosteroids on the host defense mechanisms, their topical application may both mask and encourage skin infections. It is important to determine if a topical inflammatory condition is secondary to an infection. When it is impossible to differentiate between an inflammatory condition and inflammation secondary to an infection, the patient should be treated with a combination of a steroid and appropriate antibacterials and antifungals.

Nursing Process

Administration
Nurses must maintain sterile technique when applying topical corticosteroids to open areas because of the danger of infection. They must also be cautious to prevent applying it to their own hands or arms.

Evaluation
Nursing evaluation of patients receiving topical applications of corticosteroids should note the effectiveness of the medication. Skin conditions should be observed closely for any evidence of infection. The temperature of patients with large occlusive dressings should be taken every four hours and the dressings removed if it rises. The major complications for which nurses should evaluate patients following the repeated use of topical corticosteroid treatment involve damage to the dermis. Finally, nurses must evaluate patients receiving topical applications of corticosteroids for evidence of systemic absorption of the medication. It is not inconceivable that patients who receive treatment with a very potent or most potent corticosteroid over a large area of their bodies will absorb sufficient quantities of the drug to experience systemic toxicities. This is particularly true in the case of babies.

Teaching
Patient teaching should emphasize the proper application of topical corticosteroids. It should also include providing the same information given to patients receiving systemic therapy (see Chapter 29).

Further Reading

Giannotti, B. and Stuttgen, G. (1988). Symposium on topical corticosteroids, today and tomorrow. *Drugs 36* (Suppl. 5):1-61.

Miller, J.A. and Munro, D.D. (1980). Topical corticosteroids: Clinical pharmacology and therapeutic use. *Drugs 19* :119-134.

Sneddon, I.B. (1976). Clinical use of topical steroids. *Drugs 11* : 193-199.

Wilkinson, S.M., Cartwright, P.H. and English, J.S.C. (1991). Hydrocortisone: An important cutaneous allergen. *The Lancet 337* : 761-762.

Table 60
Topical corticosteroids.

Pharmacologic Classification: Topical Products Containing Only a Corticosteroid

Category	Use	Action	Adverse Effects	Drug Interactions	Nursing Process
1. Low-potency 2. Moderately potent to potent 3. Potent to very potent 4. Very potent 5. Most potent	Topical management of corticosteroid-responsive dermatoses, incl. psoriasis, endogenous eczema [atopic, cheiropompholyx, neurodermatitis], contact dermatitis [irritant, allergic], seborrheic eczema, stasis eczema, pruritus ani and vulvae (hydrocortisone), intertrigo (hydrocortisone).	Corticosteroids reduce inflammat'n by causing vasoconstrict'n, impairing chemotaxis, reducing prostaglandin format'n, stabilizing lysosomal membrane in neutrophils and diminishing lymphocytic response to allergic stimuli. Intensity of these effects correlates directly w. potency of the steroid concerned. The more potent the steroid, the greater its anti-inflammatory effects.	Miliaria, folliculitis, pyoderma, macerat'n of skin or localized cutaneous atrophy and striae, erythema, perioral dermatitis, masking tinea infect'n. Sensitizat'n us. due to base or preservative. Systemic effects may occur if strong preparat'ns are used on large body areas for extended periods. Incidence of adv. effects and their intensity correlates directly w. potency of steroid concerned.		**Assess:** Skin condit'n at site of applicat'n. **Administer:** Using sterile technique; without accidentally applying to the nurse. **Evaluate:** Efficacy of medicat'n; for evidence of development of overlying infect'n; for hyperthermia; for dermal atrophy, striae, thinning of epidermis, rebound pustulat'n; for systemic absorpt'n. **Teach:** Proper applicat'n; as for systemic corticosteroids (see Chapter 29).

Pharmacologic Classification: Topical Products Containing Neomycin Plus a Corticosteroid

Generic Name (Trade Name)	Use	Action	Adverse Effects	Drug Interactions	Nursing Process
Neomycin plus dexamethasone (Neodecadron) Neomycin plus fluocinolone (Neo-Synalar) Neomycin plus flurometholone (Neo-Oxylone)	Adjunctive tx of contact, endogenous and seborrheic eczema, pruritus ani and vulvae, and neurodermatitis when complicated by infect'n caused by organisms sensitive to antibiotics/antibacterials in ea. product. Products containing nystatin can also be used in tx of inflammatory disorders	Corticosteroids should not be used alone in skin infect'ns because they reduce the host's defense mechanisms and permit spread of infect'n. In these cases an appropriate antibacterial and/or	Neomycin can cause contact dermatitis. Hypersensitivity to nystatin, bacitracin and gramicidin is uncommon. Sensitivity react'ns include burning, itching, irritat'n, dryness, erythema,		As for topical corticosteroids. See also Chapter 63.

Generic Name (Trade Name)	Use	Action	Adverse Effects	Drug Interactions	Nursing Process
Pharmacologic Classification: Topical Products Containing Neomycin Plus a Corticosteroid					
Neomycin plus flurandrenolide (Cordran-N)	complicated by infect'n due to candida.	antifungal should be combined w. the corticosteroid to combat infectious component of inflammat'n.	folliculitis, hypertrichosis, acneform erupt'ns and hypopigmentat'n. Striae may occur. Damage to collagen. Delayed healing. Systemic effects may occur if strong preparat'ns are used on large body areas for extended periods.		
Neomycin plus hydrocortisone (Neo-Cortdome, Neo-Cortef)					
Neomycin plus methylprednisolone (Neo-Medrol Acetate Topical)					
Neomycin plus prednisolone (Neo-Deltacortef)					
Pharmacologic Classification: Oxytetracycline Plus a Corticosteroid					
Oxytetracycline plus hydrocortisone (Terra-Cortril)	See combination products, above	See combination products, above	See combination products, above		As for topical corticosteroids. See also Chapter 62.
Pharmacologic Classification: Iodochlorhydroxyquin Plus a Corticosteroid					
Iodochlorhydroxyquin plus hydrocortisone (Racet, Vioform-Hydrocortisone, Vytone)	See combination products, above	See combination products, above	See combination products, above		As for topical corticosteroids. See also Chapter 70.
Pharmacologic Classification: More Than One Antibiotic/Antifungal Plus a Corticosteroid					
Neomycin, nystatin and halcinonide (Halcicomb)	*For all products in this classif-cat'n:* See combination products, above	*For all products in this classificat'n:* See combination products, above	*For all products in this classificat'n:* See combination products, above		*For all products in this classificat'n:* As for topical corticosteroids. See also Chapters 62, 63 and 67.

Neomycin, bacitracin, polymyxin B and hydrocortisone acetate (Cortisporin Ointment)

Neomycin, gramicidin, polymyxin B and hydrocortisone acetate (Cortisporin Cream)

Neomycin, gramicidin, nystatin and fluocinonide (Lidecomb)

Neomycin, gramicidin, nystatin and triamcinolone acetonide (Kenacomb, Kenacomb Mild, Mycolog, Mytrex, Viaderm KC)

CHAPTER 41

Antiacne Drugs

Teaching Objectives

Following completion of this chapter, the reader should be able to:

1. Explain the etiology of acne vulgaris.
2. List the aims of drug therapy in the treatment of acne.
3. Discuss the mechanism of action, pharmacologic effects, therapeutic uses, adverse effects and nursing process related to the use of benzoyl peroxide.
4. Describe the mechanism of action, therapeutic uses, adverse effects and nursing process for antibiotics used in the treatment of acne.
5. Discuss the mechanism of action, therapeutic use and adverse effects of retinoic acid, and the nursing process related to its use.
6. Describe the mechanism of action, therapeutic use and adverse effects of isotretinoin, and the nursing process related to its use.
7. Discuss briefly the use of corticosteroids in the treatment of acne.

Acne Vulgaris

Acne vulgaris is caused by an exaggerated response of the pilosebaceous gland to the secretion of androgens. Sebum production increases and epithelial cells lining the duct adhere to each other to form a plug that blocks the follicular channel. The resulting impaction and distention of the sebaceous glands lead to the formation of comedones and the disruption of the follilcular epithelium. Discharge of the follicular contents into the dermis produces an inflammatory reaction. The presence of the anaerobic diptheroid *Propionibacterium acnes* contributes to the problem. By secreting a variety of enzymes, including hyaluronidase, it may disrupt the follicular epithelium and increase inflammation.

Drug therapy of acne vulgaris is aimed at promoting peeling and comedolysis, reducing sebum production, increasing epidermal cell mitosis and turnover, and eradicating *Propionibacterium acnes*.

Benzoyl Peroxide

Mechanism of Action and Pharmacologic Effects

Benzoyl peroxide is both keratolytic and bacteriostatic. It removes keratin plugs sealing the follicular channels and reduces the involvement of *Propionibacterium acnes*.

Therapeutic Uses

Benzoyl peroxide is available in 2.5%, 5%, 10% and 20% creams, lotions and gels for the treatment of mild to moderate acne. The drug can be very irritating, particularly on fair-skinned individuals;

lower concentrations should be used by these patients. To minimize irritation, benzoyl peroxide should be applied for only fifteen minutes the first night before washing it off. The duration of exposure may be lengthened thereafter until the drug can be left on the face overnight. It may be necessary to apply a second daily dose in the morning.

Adverse Effects

Irritation, ranging from mild to severe, is the major adverse effect of benzoyl peroxide. One per cent to three per cent of individuals applying the drug experience contact sensitivity. Irritation is often the result of the base used. Alcohol-based products are most irritating, with acetone and water bases following, in that order. Fair-skinned, blue-eyed patients may be able to tolerate only the water-based benzoyl peroxide products.

Nursing Process

Assessment
Prior to use of this medication nurses should ensure that patients have no previous hypersensitivity to benzoyl peroxide or to benzoic acid derivatives. Use on inflamed, denuded or highly sensitive skin is contraindicated.

Administration
The medication should not come into contact with the eyes, eyelids, lips, inside of nose, and sensitive skin areas on the neck. Treatment should be initiated with a fifteen-minute application in the evening followed by thorough washing with soap and water, thorough rinsing and careful drying. The duration of the application should be extended by fifteen minutes each evening until it is tolerated without irritation or evidence of skin sensitivity for two hours. It can then be applied and left on overnight. Patients must wash their hands immediately following application to avoid irritation of skin on the hands.

Teaching
Advise patients of the expected therapeutic benefits, i.e., dryness and mild peeling of skin. Patients should also be told that benzoyl peroxide can produce temporary redness of the skin and mild stinging. If these effects are excessive the medication should be immediately washed off, rinsed and gently dried. The next application should use less medication for a shorter period of time. If these effects increase in severity, use of benzoyl peroxide should be discontinued.

Preparations containing benzoyl peroxide should not be used in combination with harsh soaps, vigorous scrubbing or other acne preparations. Alert patients that products containing benzoyl peroxide will bleach hair and colored fabrics.

General nursing measures related to the teaching of patients with acne are beyond the scope of this text. Readers seeking such information should refer to a medical-surgical or dermatological nursing text.

Antibiotics

Mechanism of Action and Pharmacologic Effects

Antibiotics eradicate *Propionibacterium acnes*. For moderate acne the topical use of clindamycin phosphate, erythromycin, meclocycline sulfosalicylate and tetracycline HCl may suffice. Applied to the skin, these drugs penetrate the sebaceous follicle and suppress *Propionibacterium acnes*. Oral tetracycline HCl, minocycline (Minocin), erythromycin and trimethoprim plus sulfamethoxazole (Bactrim, Septra) are usually required for severe acne.

Therapeutic Uses

Long-term antibiotic therapy is often required for the treatment of inflammatory acne with pustules and cysts. Several antibiotic preparations are available for topical use. These include clindamycin phosphate (Cleocin T, Dalacin T), erythromycin (A/T/S, EryDerm, Staticin), meclocycline sulfosalicylate (Meclan) and tetracycline HCl (Topicycline). It is not yet clear whether topical antibiotics offer any advantage over benzoyl peroxide. They are useful if patients experience contact dermatitis from benzoyl peroxide. Neo-Medrol Acne Lotion contains neomycin and methylprednisolone. Enthusiasm for it must be tempered by concern for the skin-sensitizing effects of the antibiotic. If the topical antibiotic use is not adequate, systemic antibacterial therapy may be required.

Oral tetracycline HCl can be taken in an initial dose of 250 mg four times daily for severe inflammation. Later, the dose may be reduced slowly over a period of months. If tetracycline is not effective, minocycline (Minocin), 100 mg twice daily, may be tried. Oral erythromycin may be used as a substitute for tetracycline in patients in whom tetracycline is either contraindicated or not effective. As indicated earlier, trimethoprim plus sulfamethoxazole (Bactrim, Septra) is also an alternate form of treatment for severe acne.

Adverse Effects

The systemic adverse effects of antibiotics are presented in Section 14. Applied topically, the adverse effects of the drugs and their vehicles include erythema, desquamation, tenderness, excessive dryness, pruritus, urticaria, oiliness, and fissuring around the mouth. Topical tetracycline can cause a slight yellowing of the skin, which can be removed with soap and water.

Nursing Process

The nursing process related to the systemic use of antibiotics is discussed in detail in Section 14. Readers should refer to the appropriate chapters in that section for further information.

Retinoids

Mechanism of Action and Pharmacologic Effects

Retinoids are derivatives of vitamin A. Two are employed in the treatment of acne. These are vitamin A acid, given the generic names of tretinoin or retinoic acid (Retin-A, Stei VAA, Vitamin A Acid) and isotretinoin (Accutane). Applied topically, tretinoin increases the proliferation rate of epithelial cells lining comedones and loosens and disrupts the stratum corneum. The drug unseats existing comedones in eight to twelve weeks and prevents the formation of new lesions.

Isotretinoin is taken orally. It inhibits sebum production and alters the lipid film on the surface of the skin. The drug also has anti-inflammatory, antibacterial and desquamative effects on poral occlusion.

Therapeutic Uses

Tretinoin is used topically to treat mild to moderate acne. Within three to four months seventy-five per cent of patients experience good to very good results, with the most marked improvement being in the number of comedones, papules or pustules. The drug has less effect on nodules or cysts. Because of its ability to enhance stratum corneum sloughing, epidermal cell mitosis and cell turnover, tretinoin may aggravate acne during the first six weeks of treatment.

Isotretinoin is usually effective in severe, resistant acne. A period of transient exacerbation is occasionally seen during the initial treatment period. Isotretinoin should be taken with food. A complete course of therapy lasts for twelve to sixteen weeks. Fear of adverse effects restricts its use to the treatment of (1) cystic acne, (2) conglobate acne or (3) severe acne that has failed to respond to an adequate course of systemic antimicrobial therapy.

Adverse Effects

Tretinoin irritates the skin, which may become erythematous, edematous, blistered or crusted. Temporary hyper- or hypopigmentation can occur with repeated application of the drug.

Isotretinoin is a teratogen. *Patients must not become pregnant during therapy and for at least one month after stopping the drug.* The most common adverse effects are of the mucocutaneous type and include cheilitis, facial dermatitis, dry nose, desquamation, pruritus, dry skin, conjunctivitis, alopecia, and irritation of the eyes. Other adverse effects are joint pain, transient elevations in sedimentation rate and serum levels of alanine and aspartate transaminase, increases in serum triglycerides, and a mild-to-moderate decrease in high-density lipoproteins (HDL).

Nursing Process

Assessment

Nurses should expect that the physician will order laboratory studies to establish baseline blood lipid levels, blood glucose for diabetics, and urinalysis weekly for protein and blood.

Administration

Isotretenoin capsules should be stored in a light-resistant container in a dark place. Isotretenoin should be taken with meals, usually once daily, or in a divided dose twice daily. The capsules should be swallowed whole and not crushed.

Before tretinoin is applied, the affected area should be thoroughly cleansed with a mild soap and gently dried. The drug can be applied using a cotton swab, gauze pad or finger tip. Hands should be thoroughly washed before and after treatment.

Evaluation

Nursing evaluation of patients taking isotretinoin is emphasized because of the severity of its adverse effects. Anticipate that regular blood lipid studies will be ordered. Evaluate patients for evidence of liver dysfunction such as jaundice, pruritus, tea-colored urine or light-colored stools. In the presence of visual disturbances accompanied by nausea, vomiting or headache, discontinue the medication immediately. Notify the physician, who will investigate the patient to eliminate the possiblity of benign intracranial hypertension (papilledema). Visual disturbances should also precipitate consultation with an ophthalmologist to rule out corneal opacities. Abdominal pain, rectal bleeding and/or severe diarrhea may indicate drug-induced bowel disorders and should be reported to the physician immediately.

Teaching
Alert patients to the desired therapeutic effect associated with both isotretinoin and tretinoin. These are decreased erythema, less tenderness, reduced oiliness of skin, decreased number of comedones and noncystic lesions. Patients should also be prepared for the temporary and transient increase in severity of acne often experienced during the first few weeks of therapy with these two medications.

Emphasize the teratogenic effects of isotretinoin to patients and ensure that they understand the importance of not taking isotretinoin for one month before a planned pregnancy. They must also recognize that *isotretinoin must definitely not be taken during pregnancy*. Patients who become pregnant during therapy with isotretinoin should immediately consult with their physician regarding continuing the pregnancy.

Instruct patients that multivitamin supplements usually contain vitamin A and that their use may increase the risk of vitamin A toxicity. Patients should also know that these drugs may cause photosensitivity; therefore, they should avoid sunlight or sunlamps, and should use a sunscreen and protective clothing when outdoors. Patients should be taught not to use other acne preparations concurrently with tretinoin.

General nursing measures related to the teaching of patients with acne are beyond the scope of this text. Readers seeking such information should refer to a medical-surgical or dermatological nursing text.

Corticosteroids

Corticosteroids are applied topically, usually with antibacterials, to reduce inflammation. The rationale for these "shotgun" preparations may be questioned but their popularity cannot. Corticosteroids, such as triamcinolone, are administered by intralesional injection to hasten the resolution of cysts and diminish scarring.

The nursing process related to the use of topical corticosteroids is discussed in Chapter 40. Readers should refer to that material for additional information.

Further Reading
Cunliffe, W.J. (1983). The conventional treatment of acne. *Seminars in Dermatology 2* :138-144.
Goodman, D.S. (1984). Vitamin A and retinoids in health and disease. *New Engl. J. Med. 310* :1023-1031.
Heel, R.C., Brogden, R.N., Speight, T.M. and Avery, G.S. (1977). Vitamin A acid: A review of its pharmacological properties and therapeutic use in the topical treatment of acne vulgaris. *Drugs 14* : 401-419.
Leyden, J.J. and Kligman, A.M. (1976). Acne vulgaris: New concepts in pathogenesis and treatment. *Drugs 12* : 292-300.
Reisner, R.M. and Puhvel, S.M. (1982). The acne syndromes. In: *Seminars of Dermatology 1* (No. 4). New York: Thieme-Stratton.

Table 61
Antiacne drugs.

Generic Name (Trade Name)	Use (Dose)	Action	Adverse Effects	Drug Interactions	Nursing Process
Pharmacologic Classification: Antibacterial/Keratolytic Drug					
Benzoyl peroxide (avail. in many creams, lotions and gels in concentrat'ns of 2.5%, 5%, 10% and 20%)	Tx of mild to moderate acne vulgaris (**Topical:** Benzoyl peroxide can be very irritating, particularly on fair-skinned pts; lower concentrat'ns should be used on these. To minimize irritat'n, apply for only 15 min on 1st night before thoroughly washing off w. soap and water. Durat'n of exposure can be lengthened by 15 min/night thereafter until drug can be left on face overnight. May be nec. to apply 2nd dose in a.m.)	Benzoyl peroxide is both keratolytic and bacteriostatic. It removes keratin plugs sealing follicular channels and reduces involvement of *Propionibacterium acnes.*	Irritant contact dermatitis (rarely allergic); severe erythema w. crusting		**Assess:** Previous hypersensitivity to benzoyl peroxide or to benzoic acid derivatives; avoid use on inflamed, denuded or highly sensitive skin. **Administer:** Avoid contact w. eyes, eyelids, lips, inside of nose, sensitive areas of neck. For administrative procedures, refer to Use. Wash hands immed. following applicat'n. **Teach:** Expected tx benefits (dryness, mild peeling of skin); to expect temporary redness of skin and mild stinging. If stinging is excessive, immed. wash off, rinse and gently dry; next time use less medicat'n for shorter durat'n; discontinue if discomfort severe. Avoid concurrent use w. harsh soaps, vigorous scrubbing or other acne preparat'ns that may bleach hair or colored fabrics.
Pharmacologic Classification: Antibiotics					
Tetracycline HCl	Tx of inflammatory acne (**Oral:** *For severe inflammat'n* - 250 mg qid, followed by 250-500 mg daily for prolonged maint. tx. **Topical:** Apply solut'n containing 2.2 mg tetracycline HCl/mL bid, a.m. and hs)	Antibiotics eradicate *P. acnes,* the anaerobic pathogen responsible for hydrolysis of sebum lipids to fatty acids. Fatty acids are irritating and responsible for inflammatory component of acne.	Nausea, vomiting, epigastric burning, stomatitis, glossitis, hepatotoxicity, nephrotoxicity; binding to bone, resulting in stained teeth, delayed bone growth; photosensitivity; superinfect'n in oral, anogenital and intestinal areas; pseudomembranous colitis.	Refer to Table 94	Refer to Chapter 63 and Table 94

Generic Name (Trade Name)	Use (Dose)	Action	Adverse Effects	Drug Interactions	Nursing Process
Minocycline HCl (Minocin, Vectrin)	As for tetracycline HCl (**Oral:** 50-200 mg daily)	As for tetracycline HCl	As for tetracycline HCl	Refer to Table 94	Refer to Chapter 62 and Table 94
Meclocycline sulfosalicylate (Meclan)	As for tetracycline HCl (**Topical:** Apply cream containing 1% meclocycline sulfosalicylate bid, a.m. and hs)	As for tetracycline HCl	As for tetracycline HCl	Refer to Table 94	Refer to Chapter 62 and Table 94
Clindamycin phosphate (Cleocin-T, Dalacin T)	Tx of mild to moderate inflammatory acne (**Topical:** Apply 1% clindamycin phosphate solut'n bid, a.m. and hs)	As for tetracycline HCl	Burning, pruritus, erythema, peeling	Refer to Table 92	Refer to Chapter 61 and Table 92
Erythromycin (A/T/S, EryDerm, Staticin)	Tx of mild to moderate inflammatory acne vulgaris; for use primarily in tx of inflammatory papular lesion of acne (**Topical:** Apply 1.5-2% erythromycin solut'n bid, a.m. and hs)	As for tetracycline HCl	Irritat'n, erythema, desquamat'n, tenderness, excess. dryness	Refer to Table 92	Refer to Chapter 61 and Table 92

Pharmacologic Classification: Vitamin A Derivatives

Generic Name (Trade Name)	Use (Dose)	Action	Adverse Effects	Drug Interactions	Nursing Process
Tretinoin, vitamin A acid (Retin-A, Stie VAA, Vitamin A Acid)	Tx acne vulgaris, primarily grades I, II and III in which comedones, papules and pustules predominate (**Topical:** Apply cream, gel or solut'n containing 0.01%, 0.025% or 0.05% daily, pref. hs, to skin where acne lesions appear, using enough to cover affected areas lightly)	Tretinoin incr. proliferat'n rate of epithelial cells lining comedones, loosening and disrupting stratum corneum. Drug unseats existing comedones in 8-12 weeks, prevents format'n of new lesions.	Skin may become erythematous, edematous, blistered or crusted. Temporary hyper- or hypopigmentat'n can occur.	**Peeling agents** (sulfur, resorcinol, salicylic acid): Should be used w. caution because of poss. interact'n w. tretinoin. **Medicated/abrasive soaps, cleansers, cosmetics:** Do not use products that contain alcohol or astringents, or have strong drying effects, concomitant w. tretinoin.	**Administer:** Thoroughly cleanse affected area w. mild soap, dry gently; apply using cotton swab, gauze pad or fingertip; wash hands thoroughly before and after. **Teach:** Not to use other acne preparat'ns concurrently w. tretinoin. Otherwise as for isotretinoin (see below).
Isotretinoin (Accutane)	Tx cystic acne, conglobate acne and severe acne that has failed to respond to adequate course of a systemic antimicrobial (**Oral:** Initially, 0.5 mg/kg/day for 2-4 weeks as	Inhibits sebum product'n and alters lipid film on surface of skin. Isotretinoin also has anti-inflammatory, antibacterial and	Cheilitis, facial dermatitis, dry nose, pruritus, dry skin, conjunctivitis, joint pain, alopecia, irritat'n of eyes, incr. in serum	**Vitamin A:** Should be avoided in pts taking isotretinoin. Because of relat'nship bet. vitamin A and isotretinoin, pts taking both may experience additive toxicity.	**Assess:** Expect physician to order lab. studies to establish baseline blood lipid levels, blood glucose for diabetics, and urinalysis weekly for protein and blood. **Administer:** Store in light-resistant container in dark place; w. meals us.

single dose or 2 divided doses w. food. Maint. dose, 0.1-1 mg/kg/day. In except'nal cases, up to 2 mg/kg/day may be needed. Complete course of tx, 12-16 weeks)

desquamative effects on poral occlus'n.

triglycerides, mild to moderate decr. in serum HDL.

1x/day or in divided doses bid. Capsules should be swallowed whole—do not crush.

Evaluate: Regular blood lipid studies; for evidence of liver dysfunct'n (jaundice, pruritus, tea-colored urine, light-colored stools); for visual disturbances accompanied by nausea, vomiting, headache (benign intracranial hypertens'n—papilledema); report visual disturbances (poss. corneal opacities); report abdom. pain, rectal bleeding and/or severe diarrhea (poss. drug-induced bowel disorders).

Teach: Desired tx effect (decr. erythema, less tenderness, reduced oiliness of skin, decr. no. comedones and noncystic lesions); to expect temporary and transient incr. in severity of acne during 1st few weeks of tx. *That drug has teratogenic effects: isotretinoin must not be taken for 1 month before planned pregnancy and definitely not during pregnancy. Those who become pregnant during tx should immed. consult physician.* That use of vitamin supplements may incr. risk of toxicity. To avoid sunlight, sunlamps; to use sunscreen, protective clothing when outdoors.

CHAPTER 42

Antipsoriatic Drugs

Psoriasis is characterized by chronically dry, scaling skin. Treatment is aimed at suppressing the disease. Once treatment is discontinued, the disease often returns. Three forms of therapy are available for the treatment of psoriasis. These are topical, systemic and photochemotherapy.

Topical Treatment of Psoriasis

Ultraviolet Light (UVB)

Ultraviolet light is sometimes effective in clearing psoriasis when used alone. It also forms an important part of a combined regimen involving tar and anthralin or etretinate.

Anthralin, Dithranol (Anthraforte, Anthra-Derm, Anthranol, Anthrascalp, Drithocreme, Lasan)

Mechanism of Action and Pharmacologic Effects

Applied to psoriatic plaques, anthralin reduces DNA synthesis and mitosis in the hyperplastic epidermis.

Therapeutic Uses

Anthralin, used either alone or combined with UVB treatment, is safe and effective. Its incorporation into Lasar Paste in products such as Lasan provides a stiff preparation that can be applied more easily to psoriatic plaques, and retained on them. Anthralin should be applied only to quiescent or chronic patches of psoriasis. It should not be used to treat acute eruptions or excessively inflamed areas. Anthralin should never be used on the face or intertriginous areas.

Adverse Effects

Anthralin stains skin, clothing and bedding. It irritates and can even burn the skin. The irritant effect is more common in fair-skinned individuals.

Nursing Process

Nonpharmaceutical nursing care measures for patients with psoriasis are beyond the scope of this text. Readers seeking such information should consult a medical-surgical or dermatological nursing text.

Assessment
Prior to the use of anthralin, the patient's history should be reviewed for evidence of previous hypersensitivity, renal disease or pregnancy. Patients should be assessed for acute eruptions or inflammatory areas; the medication should not be applied to such areas. A preliminary test for sensitivity on a small area is advisable, particularly for individuals with very fair complexions.

Administration
Anthralin should be carefully applied in a thin coating in the evening and left on the skin for the duration specified by the prescribing physician (usually between twenty minutes and twelve hours). Adjacent skin surfaces that are not involved may be protected with petroleum jelly or zinc oxide ointment. Often anthralin ointment is dusted with talcum powder and covered with a loose, well-ventilated dressing to protect bedding and night clothes. Treatment usually continues for two to four weeks. Cover with dressing to avoid staining clothing.

Ointments should be stored at room temperature in light-proof containers.

Nurses applying this medication must take care not to have it contact their own skin. Use of finger cot, plastic gloves or tongue depressor to apply anthralin is the best protection for healthy skin. Wash hands thoroughly after applying the medication.

Cleansing of the affected areas between treatments is imperative to promote drug effectiveness and prevent tissue damage. Of the various methods used, warm mineral oil is one of the most popular; it

is wise to consult the physician regarding his or her personal preference.

Anthralin must never come in contact with the eyes. It should not be used on the face, intertriginous areas or genitalia.

Evaluation
Unaffected skin surfaces should be inspected for erythema, an indication that frequency or strength of medication should be reduced. An increase in the number or size of lesions, the appearance of skin irritation or pustular folliculitis should result in treatment being terminated.

Nurses should expect that the physician will order weekly urine tests to permit early detection of renal irritation.

Teaching
Patients should be taught proper methods of application and self-evaluation for adverse effects. Nurses should warn patients that skin, nails or hair may turn brown-yellow if anthralin is applied to these areas and advise patients to discontinue use of the drug if a rash or irritation occurs.

Coal Tar

Like anthralin, coal tar also suppresses epidermal DNA synthesis. Although it may stain less, it is just as messy and has a worse smell. The choice between the two is largely a personal one. Newer "clean" coal tar products are often favored by patients and physicians. Alone or combined with UVB, coal tar is effective in chronic plaque psoriasis. The nursing process for coal tar is identical to that described above for anthralin.

Topical Corticosteroids

Potent corticosteroids may be applied topically to treat psoriasis. Corticosteroids may be applied when the skin is irritated or for limited periods when other topical preparations are cosmetically unacceptable or ineffective. Steroids may be rotated if tolerance develops to the products employed. Potent steroids should not be used on the face. A preparation of 1% hydrocortisone should be used on the groin or axillae. The adverse effects of topical corticosteroids and the nursing process related to their use are described in Chapter 40. Readers should refer to that material for detailed information.

Systemic Treatment of Psoriasis

Methotrexate, Amethopterin (Mexate)

Mechanism of Action and Pharmacologic Effects

DNA synthesis and cellular reproduction depend on the reduction of folic acid to tetrahydrofolic acid by the enzyme folic acid reductase. Methotrexate inhibits this enzyme.

Therapeutic Uses

Methotrexate is an effective antipsoriatic drug. However, because of the risk attending its use, the drug is indicated only in the symptomatic control of severe, recalcitrant, disabling psoriasis not responsive to other forms of therapy. Methotrexate should be prescribed only by dermatologists.

Adverse Effects

Methotrexate is an antineoplastic drug with acute toxicities on bone marrow, germ cells and liver.

Nursing Process

The nursing process associated with the use of antineoplastic drugs is discussed in Chapter 72. Readers should refer to that chapter for detailed information.

Etretinate (Tegison)

Mechanism of Action and Pharmacologic Effects

Etretinate is a retinoic acid derivative. It normalizes pathologic changes in epidermal and dermal skin, particularly by inhibiting hyperkeratinization and cell differentiation.

Therapeutic Uses

Etretinate is indicated in the treatment of severe intractable psoriasis, Darier's disease, ichthyosiform dermatoses, palmoplantar pustulosis and other disorders of keratinization. Despite long-term maintenance therapy, relapse occurs in some patients on stopping. Used with PUVA (see below) or UVB, etretinate lowers the required irradiation dose. Combined therapy is often successful in patients who fail to respond to etretinate or PUVA alone.

Adverse Effects

Etretinate causes a high incidence of adverse effects. These include cheilitis in about eighty per cent of patients. Other adverse effects often encountered are dry oral and nasal mucous membranes, skin desquamation and thinning of the skin. Hair loss is the major reason for stopping therapy. Hepatitis and liver necrosis have been reported rarely. *Etretinate is absolutely contraindicated in women of childbearing potential because of its severe teratogenic properties. Effective contraception must be instituted and maintained for at least twelve to eighteen months after stopping the drug.* Etretinate significantly elevates total triglycerides and cholesterol.

Nursing Process

Assessment
Nurses should expect that the physician will order laboratory studies to establish baseline blood lipid levels. Because etretinate is a major teratogen, expect the physician to order a pregnancy test for female patients.

Evaluation
Nursing evaluation of patients taking etretinate is emphasized because of the severity of its adverse effects. Anticipate that regular blood lipid studies will be ordered. Evaluate patients for evidence of liver dysfunction such as jaundice, pruritus, tea-colored urine or light-colored stools. Abdominal pain, rectal bleeding and/or severe diarrhea may indicate drug-induced bowel disorders and should be reported to the physician immediately. Excessive hair loss is subjectively evaluated by the patient and often precipitates termination of therapy. Discontinue the drug if visual problems of blurring, decreased night vision or poor visual acuity occur.

Teaching
Alert patients to the desired therapeutic effect. Emphasize the teratogenic effects and the importance of not taking etretinate for twelve to eighteen months before a planned pregnancy and definitely not taking it during pregnancy. Patients who become pregnant during therapy with etretinate should immediately consult their physician regarding continuing the pregnancy.

Instruct patients that use of vitamin supplements may increase the risk of toxicity.

General nursing measures related to the teaching of patients with psoriasis are beyond the scope of this text. Readers seeking such information should refer to a medical-surgical or dermatological nursing text.

Photochemotherapy — PUVA

Mechanism of Action and Pharmacologic Effects

Photochemotherapy involves the administration of a photosensitizing drug, usually psoralen (methoxsalen, 8-methoxypsoralen) by mouth, followed two hours later with exposure to long ultraviolet light (UVA at 320 – 400 nm). The combination of psoralen with UVA is known as PUVA therapy. In the presence of UVA, psoralens unite with DNA, forming cross-linkages and reducing epidermal cell turnover.

Therapeutic Uses

PUVA therapy is usually given three times a week. It is currently considered in chronic plaque psoriasis when anthralin has failed or relapse has occurred quickly. Plaque psoriasis is usually cleared within five weeks. PUVA therapy is also first-line treatment in patients over age sixty with extensive plaque psoriasis.

Adverse Effects

The adverse effects of PUVA therapy include increased risk of premature aging of the skin and possible skin cancer. The association with skin cancer is uncertain at this time.

The interaction of psoralen with oral anticoagulants is described in Table 62. In addition, psoralen may have photosensitivity effects with a variety of compounds, i.e., anthralin, coal tar, diuretics, griseofulvin, phenothiazines, sulfasalazine, sulfinpyrazone, sulfonylurea oral antihyperglyemics, sulfonamides and tetracyclines.

Nursing Process

Assessment

Prior to starting treatment with psoralen, nurses should review patients' histories for evidence of contraindications, such as sunburn, previous sensitivity to psoralens, diseases associated with photosensitivity (e.g., albinism, melanoma, lupus erythematosus), squamous cell carcinoma, pregnancy. Particularly stringent evaluation following therapy should be initiated if the patient's history reveals evidence of hepatic insufficiency, gastrointestinal disease, chronic infection, cardiovascular disease or immunosuppression.

Expect that the physician will order an ophthalmic examination for cataracts prior to starting therapy. Laboratory studies to establish baseline levels of white blood cells as well as renal and hepatic function will also be performed.

Administration

Administer orally with milk or food to minimize gastrointestinal distress. The drug is given on alternate days to accommodate the frequently delayed phototoxic reaction. Patients receiving systemic treatment must wear fully protective sunglasses (both indoors and outdoors during daylight hours) during and for twenty-four hours following UVA treatment.

The lotion is never dispensed to patients for self-care. Physicians apply the lotion using finger cots, disposable gloves or cotton swabs. Surrounding tissue is protected with petroluem jelly and sunscreen to prevent damage.

Both the lotion and oral dosage forms are stored at room temperature in light-proof containers.

Evaluation

Patients should be carefully monitored for treatment effectiveness. Nursing evaluation should emphasize early detection of adverse effects, including allergic reactions characterized by bronchial asthma. Nurses should expect the physician to order regular studies of renal and hepatic function, white blood cell levels and ophthalmic examination for cataracts.

Teaching

Patients must thoroughly understand the treatment regimen. A printed instruction sheet will facilitate remembering. Patients should be instructed to avoid sunlight or other sources of ultraviolet light for eight hours following oral administration of psoralen and UVA exposure. Following topical application of psoralen and UVA exposure, patients should not expose the skin to sunlight or other sources of ultraviolet light for twenty-four to forty-eight hours.

Further Reading

Farber, E.M., Abel, E.A. and Charuworn, A. (1983). Recent advances in the treatment of psoriasis. *J. Amer. Acad. Dermatol.* 8 : 311-321.

Marks, J.M. (1980). Psoriasis: Utilizing the treatment options. *Drugs 19* : 429-436.

Derbes, V.J. (1981). Psoriasis. *Rational Drug Therapy 15* (1):1-5.

Ward, A., Brogden, R.N., Heel, R.C., Speight, T.M. and Avery, G.S. (1983). Etretinate: A review of its pharmacological properties and therapeutic efficacy in psoriasis and other skin disorders. *Drugs 26* :9-43.

Table 62
Antipsoriatic drugs.

Generic Name (Trade Name)	Use (Dose)	Action	Adverse Effects	Drug Interactions	Nursing Process
Pharmacologic Classification: Coal Tar Preparations					
Anthralin, dithranol (Anthra-Term, Anthranol, Drithocream, Lasan)	Tx of psoriasis (**Topical:** Apply without a dressing hs and leave on lesions 8-12 h. Remove in a.m. with warm oil, followed by hot bath and poss. UVB tx. Repeat nightly. High-strength [1-3%] short-term [10-20 min] tx followed by wash, or as directed)	Applied to psoriatic plaques, anthralin reduces DNA synthesis and mitosis in hyperplastic epidermis.	Irritat'n, burning. Stains skin, clothing and bedding.		**Assess:** For hx of hypersensitivity, renal disease, pregnancy; for acute erupt'ns or inflammatory areas. Test for sensitivity on small area, particularly in fair-skinned pts. **Administer:** Carefully apply thin coating hs, leave on skin for specified time [us. 20 min - 12 h]. Protect adjacent uninvolved skin w. petroleum jelly or zinc oxide ointment; dust w. talcum powder; cover w. loose porous dressing to protect bedding and clothes. Store at room temp. in light-proof container. Protect nurse's fingers w. gloves, tongue depressor; wash hands thoroughly after applying. Cleanse affected areas bet. treatments w. warm mineral oil; never allow contact w. eyes, face, intertriginous areas or genitalia. **Evaluate:** Unaffected skin surface for erythema; if present, reduce frequency or strength of medicat'n. For incr. in no./size of lesions; for skin irritat'n or pustular folliculitis [in either case, stop tx]. Expect order for weekly urine tests. **Teach:** Proper method of applicat'n; self-evaluat'n for adv. effects. Warn pt that skin, nails, hair may turn brown-yellow if medicat'n is applied to these areas and to discontinue use if rash or irritat'n occurs.
Coal tar	Tx of chronic plaque psoriasis of palms, soles and scalp (**Topical:** Apply od-bid. "Clean" products are used almost exclusively)	As for anthralin	Has foul odor and may stain clothing.		
Pharmacologic Classification: Corticosteroids					
Topical corticosteroids	Tx of psoriasis when anthralin or coal tar are inappropriate or	Corticosteroids have antimitotic activity	Miliaria, folliculitis, pyoderma, macerat'n		Refer to Chapter 40 and Table 60

Drug	Action	Use / Dosage	Side Effects	Drug Interactions
	that enables them to reduce cell multipli-cat'n in psoriasis and decr. format'n of keratin cells.	when rapid effect is required. See Chapter 40 for list of topical steroids. Potent steroids should not be used on face. Use 1% hydrocortisone on groin or axillae (**Topical:** Apply od-bid)	of skin or localized cutaneous atrophy and striae, erythema, perioral dermatitis, masking tinea infect'n. For addit'nal adv. effects, see Table 60.	See Chapter 72

Pharmacologic Classification: Antineoplastic Drug

Drug	Action	Use / Dosage	Side Effects	Drug Interactions
Methotrexate (Amethopterin, Mexate)	Inhibits folic acid reductase, decr. DNA synthesis and cellular reproduct'n.	Symptomatic control of severe, recalcitrant disabling psoriasis not responsive to other forms of tx (**Oral/IM/IV:** Adult recommended starting doses - *Weekly single dose schedule,* 10-25 mg/week until adequate response is achieved. Should ordinarily not exceed 50 mg/week. *Divided oral dose schedule,* 2.5 mg at 12-h intervals for 3 doses or at 8-h intervals for 4 doses ea. week. Should not exceed 30 mg/week. Doses in ea. schedule may be adjusted to achieve optimal clinical response, but not to exceed max. stated for ea. schedule)	Most common are: ulcerative stomatitis, leukopenia, nausea and abdominal distress. Other effects: malaise, undue fatigue, chills and fever, dizziness and decr. resistance to infect'n.	**Chloramphenicol:** Decr. intestinal absorpt'n and interferes w. enterohepatic circulat'n of methotrexate. **Chlorpropamide:** Incr. toxicity of methotrexate. **Ethanol:** May enhance poss. methotrexate-induced hepatotoxicity. **NSAIDs:** May decr. renal tubular secret'n of methotrexate and enhance its toxicity. **Phenylbutazone:** May displace methotrexate from plasma protein binding, incr. its pharmacologic activity. **Probenecid:** Inhibits renal excret'n of methotrexate. **Salicylates:** Displace methotrexate from plasma protein binding and block renal secret'n of drug, incr. concentrat'n of methotrexate in body. **Sulfonamides:** May incr. toxicity of methotrexate. **Sulfonylurea oral hypoglycemics:** Can incr. toxicity of methotrexate. **Tetracyclines:** May incr. methotrexate toxicity. **Thiazides:** Incr. methotrexate toxicity. **Trimethoprim:** May incr. bone marrow suppress'n following methotrexate tx.

Generic Name (Trade Name)	Use (Dose)	Action	Adverse Effects	Drug Interactions	Nursing Process
Pharmacologic Classification: Vitamin A Derivative					
Etretinate (Tegison)	Tx of severe intractable psoriasis, Darier's disease, ichthyosiform dermatoses, palmoplantar pustulosis and other disorders of keratinizat'n (**Oral:** Initially, 0.75-1 mg/kg/day [max. 75 mg/day] taken in divided doses. Cutaneous areas us. respond within 2-4 weeks. If no tx response seen by 4 weeks and in absence of toxicity, incr. daily dose in increments of 10 mg at biweekly intervals until response is observed or total daily dose of 75 mg is given. Once response is seen, dose may be reduced to 0.3-0.6 mg/kg/day in divided doses)	Normalizes pathologic changes in epidermal and dermal skin, particularly by inhibiting hyperkeratinizat'n and cell differentiat'n.	Cheilitis, dry oral and nasal mucous membranes, skin desquamat'n, thinning of skin, hair loss. Occasionally, hepatitis and liver necrosis. Elevat'n of triglycerides and cholesterol.	**Milk:** Taken concomitantly, will incr. etretinate serum levels. **Phenytoin (Dilantin):** May have its effects incr. by etretinate, which can displace phenytoin from its plasma protein binding sites. **Vitamin A and retinoids:** Should not be taken by pts on etretinate to prevent risk of additive toxic effects (etretinate is a derivative of vitamin A).	**Assess:** Expect order for lab. studies for baseline blood lipid levels and pregnancy for female pts. **Evaluate:** Blood lipids; for liver dysfunct'n (jaundice, pruritus, tea-colored urine or light-colored stools); for drug-induced bowel disorders (abdom. pain, rectal bleeding and/or severe diarrhea); excess. hair loss. Discontinue drug if visual problems of blurring, decr. night vision or poor visual acuity occur. **Teach:** Desired tx effect; that use of vitamin supplements may incr. risk of toxicity; teratogenic effects, esp. importance of not taking etretinate for 18 mos. before a planned pregnancy and definitely not taking it during pregnancy. Pts who become pregnant should immediately consult physician.
Pharmacologic Classification: Photochemotherapy — PUVA					
Psoralen, methoxsalen (Oxsoralen, Ultra MOP)	Tx of psoriasis and atopic dermatitis in combinat'n w. high-intensity UVA light (**Oral:** 20 mg, taken 2 h before exposure. **Lotion:** Apply 1% 1x/week to a few depigmented areas and expose to UV light for max. 1 min)	In presence of ultraviolet light [UVA at 320-400 nm], psoralens unite w. DNA, forming cross-linkages and reducing epidermal cell turnover.	Occasionally, nervousness, insomnia or depress'n	**Anticoagulants:** And psoralen should be used together w. caution.	Refer to Chapter 42.

CHAPTER 43

Anti-Infective Drugs for Skin and Mucous Membranes

Antibacterial Drugs

Streptococcus pyogenes and *Staphylococcus aureus* are the most common causative bacteria in primary skin infections. Other common pathogens are *Escherichia coli, Pseudomonas aeruginosa,* and klebsiella, enterobacter, pasteurella and proteus species.

Aminoglycoside Antibiotics — Gentamicin (Garamycin), Framycetin (Soframycin) and Neomycin (Myciguent)

Therapeutic Uses

The mechanism of action and antibacterial spectra of aminoglycoside antibiotics are presented in Chapter 63. Used topically, these drugs are effective in the treatment of primary and secondary skin infections caused by sensitive strains of streptococci, *Staphylococcus aureus, Pseudomonas aeruginosa, Enterobacter aerogenes, Escherichia coli, Proteus vulgaris* and *Klebsiella pneumoniae.* Neomycin remains a popular drug. Unfortunately, it often causes hypersensitivity reactions, manifested primarily as skin rashes. Although available alone, neomycin is most often combined with polymyxin B and either bacitracin or gramicidin in the products Neosporin Ointment and Cream.

Framycetin is available alone in the product Soframycin or combined with dexamethasone in Sofracort. It is also impregnated in a lightweight paraffin gauze dressing (Sofra-Tulle).

Gentamicin is applied topically for infected severe burns when the causative bacteria is *Pseudomonas aeruginosa.*

Adverse Effects

Hypersensitivity reactions usually of the delayed type are the most common adverse effects of the aminoglycosides. If gentamicin is applied to a large denuded surface, it may be absorbed in sufficient quantity to produce systemic toxicity (see Chapter 63).

Nursing Process

Assessment
Prior to the initial application of this or any topical anti-infective agent, nurses should ensure that any cultures that have been ordered have been taken. Infected areas should be inspected for open wounds (e.g., burns, ulcers), which facilitate absorption and increase the risk of adverse effects. The extent of the affected area should be noted so that drug efficacy can be determined later.

Evaluation
Drug efficacy is determined by the patient's subjective reports of relief from symptoms of infection and by clinical observation of reduction in the extent of the infection. Sensitivity reactions (itching, burning, redness, swelling) should be reported to the physician immediately so that another treatment can be prescribed. Adverse effects from systemic absorption are discussed in Chapter 63. Readers should refer to that material for detailed information.

Teaching
Patients should be taught to evaluate the effectiveness of the treatment and to observe for adverse effects of systemic absorption.

Mafenide (Sulfamylon) and Silver Sulfadiazine (Flamazine, Silvadene)

Mechanism of Action, Therapeutic Uses and Adverse Effects

Mafenide is a sulfonamide that is used in conjunction with debridement for the prevention and treatment of infection, particularly by *Pseudomonas aeruginosa,* in second- or third-degree burns. In addition to typical sulfonamide-type allergic reactions, mafenide can produce pain or a burning sensation.

Silver sulfadiazine is effective in vitro against various strains of the following pathogens isolated from infected burn wounds: *Pseudomonas aerugi-*
nosa, Enterobacter aerogenes, Escherichia coli, Proteus mirabilis, Proteus vulgaris, Staphylococcus aureus, Klebsiella, Aerobacter niger and *Candida albicans*. The drug owes its activity to the formation of silver chloride, silver protein complexes and sodium sulfadiazine. Both sulfadiazine and silver exert bacteriostatic effects. Silver sulfadiazine is indicated for the treatment of leg ulcers, burns, skin grafts, incisions and other clean lesions, abrasions, minor cuts and wounds. It is particularly valuable in the treatment and prophylaxis of infections in victims of serious burns. Silver sulfadiazine does not penetrate so well as mafenide. However, it also does not produce the pain on application that characterizes mafenide. As well, the incidence of allergic reactions is also lower.

Nursing Process

The nursing process associated with topical use of mafenide or silver sulfadiazine is essentially the same as that previously identified in relation to the topical use of the aminoglycosides. Adverse effects of systemic absorption are discussed in Chapter 64. Readers should refer to that material for additional information.

Bacitracin (Baciguent)

Bacitracin is an excellent topical antibiotic. It is active against staphylococci and streptococci. Although severe allergic disorders have been seen when bacitracin is applied locally, these are very rare. The nursing process is essentially the same as that identified for the aminoglycosides.

Fusidic Acid, Sodium Fusidate (Fucidin Topical)

Mechanism of Action and Pharmacologic Effects

Fusidic acid inhibits bacterial protein synthesis by interfering with amino acid transfer from aminoacyl-sRNA to protein on the ribosomes. Fusidic acid may be bacteriostatic or bactericidal, depending on the inoculum size. Fusidic acid is virtually inactive against gram-negative bacteria. The differences in activity against gram-negative and gram-positive organisms are believed to be due to a difference in cell wall permeability.

Therapeutic Uses

Fusidic acid is indicated for the treatment of primary and secondary skin infections caused by sensitive strains of *S. aureus,* streptococcccus species and *C. minutissimum.* Primary skin infections that may be expected to respond to treatment with fusidic acid topical include impetigo contagiosa and erythrasma. Fusidic acid is used in secondary skin infections such as infected wounds and infected burns. Resistance to fusidic acid has readily been induced in vitro. The development of resistance has also been shown to occur in the clinical setting.

Adverse Effects

Mild irritation has occasionally been reported in patients with dermatoses treated with fusidic acid.

Nursing Process

As with any new medication, nurses administering this drug for the first time are advised to consult the pharmacist and to refer to the manufacturer's literature enclosed with the product before administering this drug.

Mupirocin (Bactroban)

Mechanism of Action and Pharmacologic Effects

Mupirocin exerts a bactericidal action against sensitive organisms by inhibiting bacterial protein synthesis. It reversibly and specifically binds to bacterial isoleucyl transfer-RNA synthetase.

Therapeutic Uses

Mupirocin is indicated for the topical treatment of impetigo caused by sensitive strains of staphylococcus and streptococcus species as well as for other superficially infected dermatoses and lesions that are moist and weeping. For abrasions, minor cuts and wounds, the use of mupirocin may prevent the development of infection by sensitive gram-positive organisms. No cross-resistance has been shown between mupirocin and other commonly used antibiotics.

Topical mupirocin compares well with fusidic acid for skin infections. Although both appear equally effective in the topical treatment of acute bacterial skin infections, mupirocin has been reported to be particularly effective against primary skin infections, impetigo, and against staphylococcal and streptococcal infections. In addition, fusidic acid is used systemically for severe staphylococcal infections; induction of resistant bacteria is therefore a concern. Mupirocin is unsuitable for systemic administration and its topical use cannot influence subsequent systemic treatment of severe infections.

Adverse Effects

Local adverse reactions have been reported with mupirocin. These include itching, burning, erythema, stinging and dryness.

Nursing Process

All areas affected should be inspected for continuing infection, increased size or increased number of lesions.

Administration
Apply topically, then cover with gauze if necessary. Store mupirocin at room temperature. Wash hands thoroughly after application. Children two to five days old require wound isolation restrictions.

Evaluation
Examine lesions for therapeutic response (reduction of size and number of lesions).

Teaching
Instruct patients to report irritation or extension of lesions. Tell them to trim fingernails to prevent scratching and to wash hands after applying the ointment.

Nitrofurazone (Furacin)

Nitrofurazone has antibacterial activity against a number of gram-positive and gram-negative bacteria. It is used topically for superficial wounds, burns, ulcers and skin infections. If applied continuously for five days or longer, nitrofurazone can cause generalized allergic skin reactions. The nursing process is essentially the same as that previously identified in relation to the topical use of aminoglycosides.

Miscellaneous Drugs

Gramicidin is effective against many gram-positive bacteria. It is often incorporated into creams, together with polymyxin B (Polysporin), neomycin (Spectrocin) and polymyxin B plus neomycin (Neosporin) for the treatment of superficial bacterial skin infections.

Iodochlorhydroxyquin, or Clioquinol (Vioform), has both antibacterial and antifungal activities. It is applied topically to treat dermatoses and infections in which a mild antibacterial and antifungal effect is desired. Unfortunately, the drug may stain fabrics and hair.

Polymyxin B has bactericidal action against most gram-negative bacilli except proteus species. It is particularly effective against *Pseudomonas aeruginosa, E. coli,* enterobacter and klebsiella species. Polymyxin B is not active against gram-positive bacteria or fungi.

Betadine contains 10% povidone-iodine USP (1% available iodine). It is available as a solution, ointment, shampoo and skin cleanser and is also impregnated into gauze pads. Povidone-iodine is bactericidal and fungicidal. Unlike iodine, it does not stain natural fabrics.

Antifungal Drugs

Dermatophytosis (fungal infections) may involve the skin, hair and nails. Dermatophytes show specificity for the type of keratin they invade. Microsporum usually attacks hair; trichophyton, the skin, hair and nails; and epidermophyton, the skin.

1. Topically Applied Antifungal Drugs

Amphotericin B (Fungizone)

Amphotericin B is active against candida species and can be used to treat cutaneous and mucocutaneous infections. Topical applications can cause local irritation, pruritus and skin rash.

Clotrimazole (Canesten, Lotrimin, Gyne-Lotrim, Mycelex, Myclo)

Therapeutic Uses and Adverse Effects

Clotrimazole is effective against a wide range of fungi, including microsporum and trichophyton species. Topical creams and solutions are used to treat tinea pedis, tinea cruris and tinea corporis caused by *Trichophyton rubrum, Trichophyton mentagrophytes* and *Epidermophyton floccosum,* as well as candidiasis caused by *Candida albicans,* and tinea versicolor produced by *Microsporum furfur.* Vaginal creams and tablets are used in the treatment of vaginal candidiasis and trichomoniasis.

Although skin reactions have been reported, clotrimazole is generally well tolerated.

Nursing Process

Assessment
Prior to the initial application of this or any topical antifungal agent, nurses should ensure that any cultures that have been ordered have been taken. Infected areas should be inspected for open wounds (e.g., burns, ulcers), which facilitate absorption and increase the risk of adverse effects. The extent of the affected area should be noted so that drug efficacy can be determined later.

Administration
Clean the area with soapy water before each application and dry well.

Evaluation
Drug efficacy is determined by the patient's subjective reports of relief and by clinical observation of reduction in the extent of the infection. Treated areas should be evaluated for indications of sensitivity reactions (erythema, stinging, blistering, localized edema, peeling, itching or urticaria).

Teaching
Patients should be taught to wear gloves when applying the drug to prevent further infection. They also need to know how to observe for the adverse effects of systemic absorption and to evaluate the effectiveness of the treatment.

Econazole (Ecostatin, Spectazole)

Therapeutic Uses and Adverse Effects

Econazole exhibits a broad spectrum of fungistatic activity in vitro against species of the genus candida. Vaginal ovules are used to treat vulvovaginal candidiasis (moniliasis). Topical creams are employed in the treatment of tinea pedis, tinea cruris, tinea corporis, tinea versicolor and cutaneous candidasis. Econazole may occasionally cause itching, burning or other local irritations.

Nursing Process

The nursing process is essentially the same as that presented above in relation to the topical use of clotrimazole.

Haloprogin (Halotex)

Therapeutic Uses and Adverse Effects

Haloprogin is used in the topical treatment of superficial fungal infections of the skin, such as tinea pedis, tinea cruris, tinea corporis and tinea manuum due to infection by *Trichophyton rubrum*, *Trichophyton tonsurans*, *Trichophyton mentagrophytes*, *Microsporum canus* and *Epidermophyton floccosum*. The drug is also useful in the treatment of tinea versicolor due to *Microsporum furfur* and for monilial infections of the skin caused by *Candida albicans*. Topical application occasionally causes irritation, burning, vesicle formation and pruritus.

Nursing Process

The nursing process is essentially the same as that presented above in relation to the topical use of clotrimazole.

Teaching

Teach the patient to avoid over-the-counter creams, ointments and lotions unless directed by the physician. Instruct the patient to use good asepsis and hand washing and to avoid contact with the eyes. Patients should be told to continue treatment even though the condition improves. They should also be advised to discontinue the drug if the condition worsens and notify the physician.

Miconazole (Micatin, Monistat-Derm, Monistat)

Therapeutic Uses and Adverse Effects

Miconazole is applied topically to inhibit epidermophyton, microsporum and trichophyton species, as well as candida. Infections often treated with miconazole include tinea pedis, tinea cruris, tinea corporis, tinea unguium and tinea versicolor. Rarely, mild pruritus, irritation and burning at the site of application have been reported.

Nursing Process

The nursing process is essentially the same as that presented above in relation to the topical use of clotrimazole.

Terconazole (Terazol)

Therapeutic Uses and Adverse Effects

Terconazole exhibits fungicidal activity in vitro against the genus candida. Both the yeast and mycelial form of *C. albicans* are sensitive to terconazole. Terconazole vaginal ovules and cream are indicated for the local treatment of vulvovaginal candidiasis (moniliasis). Both dosage forms of terconazole have been associated with a higher incidence of headache. However, the overall degree of safety of terconazole appears to be high.

Nursing Process

The nursing process for terconazole is essentially the same as that presented in relation to the use of clotrimazole.

2. Orally Administered Antifungal Drugs

Griseofulvin (Fulvicin-U/F, Fulvicin-P/G, Grifulvin V, Grisactin, Grisactin Ultra, Gris-PEG, Grisovin-FP)

Therapeutic Uses and Adverse Effects

Griseofulvin is effective orally against superficial infections caused by fungi responsible for dermatomycoses. It is useful in the treatment of fungal infections of the scalp and glabrous skin. Griseofulvin is less effective in chronic infections of the feet, palms and nails. Because these chronic infections tend to cause hyperkeratosis, concomitant topical keratolytic therapy is almost always necessary. Griseofulvin is absorbed over a prolonged period of time from the gastrointestinal tract. Its absorption is greatly increased by reducing the particle size of the drug. Once absorbed, griseofulvin is deposited in the stratum corneum of the skin, the keratin of the nails, and the hair, thus preventing fungal invasion of newly formed cells.

Its adverse effects include headache, skin rashes, dryness of the mouth and gastrointestinal disturbances. Griseofulvin can cause hepatotoxicity. It is contraindicated in patients with acute intermittent porphyria, a history of porphyria, or hepatocellular failure. The drug is also contraindicated in patients who are hypersensitive to it.

Nursing Process

Assessment

Prior to administering griseofulvin, nurses should review the patient's history for evidence of previous penicillin allergy, which can occasionally predict an allergic response to griseofulvin. Nurses should also look for evidence of liver disease, which predisposes the patient to increased risk of developing griseofulvin-induced hepatotoxicity. Renal studies and blood counts are recommended throughout therapy, as are blood counts, to provide a baseline for observations for blood dyscrasias.

Administration

Griseofulvin is usually self-administered on an outpatient basis. Patients should be advised that taking the drug with high-fat foods will enhance its absorption. Griseofulvin should be continued until three separate cultures prove negative for the infective organism.

Teaching

Patients should be taught that completion of the entire course of therapy is required to assure that recurrence of the fungal infection does not occur. Patients should also be instructed to avoid exposure to ultraviolet light because of the risk of photosensitivity. It is also important that they be familiar with the indicators of adverse effects. Tell patients to avoid alcohol.

3. Orally and Topically Administered Antifungal Drugs

Ketoconazole (Nizoral)

Therapeutic Uses and Adverse Effects

The use of oral ketoconazole to treat systemic fungal infections is described in Chapter 67. The drug can also be used orally to treat patients with dermatophyte or yeast skin infections, pityriasis versicolor, onychomycoses and oral or vaginal candidiasis. Transient elevated liver enzymes occur in about ten per cent of patients, gastrointestinal reactions in five per cent, and pruritus in two per cent.

Ketoconazole is also available in a 2% cream. Applied topically, ketoconazole is indicated for the treatment of tinea pedis, tinea corporis and tinea cruris by *Trichophyton rubrum*, *Trichophyton mentagrophytes* and *Epidermophyton floccusum*. It is also used in the treatment of tinea versicolor (pityriasis) caused by *Malassazeia furfur (Pityrosporum orbiculare)*, and in the treatment of seborrhoeic dermatitis caused by *Pityrosporum ovale*. Ketoconazole cream appears to be well tolerated by the skin.

Nursing Process

Administration

Ketoconazole requires an acid medium for dissolution. It should be administered with citrus or pineapple juice, coffee or tea. Antacids (or other agents that might elevate the pH of the gastrointestinal system) should not be given within two hours of administering ketoconazole.

Teaching

Patients should be advised to avoid driving or using power equipment until individual response to the drug is determined. Some patients experience dizziness or drowsiness in the initial period of treatment. Patients should be given careful instructions about proper self-administration. They should be advised that successful treatment will be determined by precise adherence to the prescribed dose and schedule of administration. Warn patients to avoid antacids, over-the-counter and alkaline products. They should also be told to notify the physician if gastrointestinal symptoms occur.

Nystatin (Candex, Mycostatin, Nilstat)

Therapeutic Uses and Adverse Effects

Nystatin is effective against candida species. Topical creams, ointments, powders and vaginal tablets are available for the treatment of mycotic infections caused by *Candida albicans*. Vaginal preparations may also be used during pregnancy to prevent thrush in the newborn. Because nystatin is not absorbed from the gastrointestinal tract, it is taken orally to prevent or treat candidal infections of the oral cavity or esophagus, for intestinal candidiasis, and for protection against candidal overgrowth during antimicrobial or corticosteroid therapy. Large oral doses occasionally cause gastrointestinal distress, diarrhea, nausea and vomiting.

Nursing Process

The nursing process is essentially the same as that presented above in relation to the topical use of clotrimazole and the oral use of griseofulvin.

Further Reading

Elewski, B.E. and Hazen, P.G. (1989). The superficial mycoses and the dermatophytes. *J. Am. Acad. Dermatol. 21* : 655-673.

Heel, R.C., Brogden, R.N., Carmine, A., Morley, P.A., Speight, T.M. and Avery, G.S. (1982). Ketoconazole: A review of its therapeutic efficacy in superficial and systemic fungal infections. *Drugs 23* : 1-36.

Leyden, J.J. and Kligman, A.M. (1978). Rationale for topical antibiotics. *Cutis 22* : 515-528.

Pegg, S.P. (1982). Role of drugs in the management of burns. *Drugs 24* :256-260.

Table 63
Anti-infective drugs for skin and mucous membranes.

Generic Name (Trade Name)	Use (Dose)	Action	Adverse Effects	Drug Interactions	Nursing Process
Pharmacologic Classification: Aminoglycoside Antibiotics					
Gentamicin sulfate (Garamycin)	Tx of infect'ns caused by pyogenic organisms, in part. *S. aureus, proteus spp., coliforms* and *P. aeruginosa* (**Topical:** Gently apply cream or ointment [1 mg gentamicin/g] to lesions tid-qid)	Aminoglycosides are effective in tx of primary and secondary skin infect'ns caused by sensitive strains of streptococci, *S. aureus, P. aeruginosa, E. aerogenes, E. coli, P. vulgaris* and *K. pneumoniae.*	Allergic react'ns, irritat'n	See Table 96 for drug interact'ns involving absorbed aminoglycosides.	**Assess:** Ensure that cultures have been taken; inspect infected areas for open wounds (burns, ulcers), which facilitate absorpt'n and incr. risk of adv. effects; note extent of affected area. **Evaluate:** Drug efficacy (subjective reports of relief from signs of infect'n and by clinical observat'n of reduced extent of infect'n); sensitivity react'ns (itching, burning, redness, swelling); adv. effects of systemic absorpt'n. **Teach:** Self-evaluat'n for drug efficacy and systemic absorpt'n.
Neomycin (Myciguent)	(**Topical:** Apply 0.5 mg/g ointment to affected area od-bid)	As for gentamicin	As for gentamicin	As for gentamicin	
Pharmacologic Classification: Sulfonamides					
Mafenide acetate (Sulfamylon)	Topical antibacterial agent for adjunctive tx in pts w. 2nd-/3rd-degree burns (**Topical:** Clean and debride wounds before applying cream [85 mg/g] w. sterile glove at least od-bid)	Mafenide is a sulfonamide used in conjunct'n w. debridement for prevent'n and tx of infect'n, part. by *P. aeruginosa*, in 2nd-/3rd-degree burns.	Pain, burning, allergic manifestat'ns		As for aminoglycosides. See Chapter 64 for systemic effects of sulfonamides.
Silver sulfadiazine (Flamazine, Silvadene)	Tx of leg ulcers, burns, skin grafts, incis'ns and other clean lesions, abras'ns, minor cuts and wounds; esp. indicated in tx/prophylaxis of infect'n in serious burns (**Topical:** Apply 3-5 mm layer 1% cream od for burns. At least 3x/week for other wounds and leg ulcers, or prn)	Effective against various strains of *P. aeruginosa, E. aerogenes, E. coli, P. mirabilis, P. vulgaris, S. aureus, A. niger, C. albicans* and *klebsiella* spp.	Sensitivity has been observed.		As for aminoglycosides. See Chapter 64 for systemic effects of sulfonamides.

Pharmacologic Classification: Miscellaneous Antibacterials

Bacitracin	Inhibits cell wall format'n and funct'n.	Against staphylococci and streptococci (**Topical:** Apply ointment [500 USP U/g] od or prn)	Occ. hypersensitivity react'ns	As for Chapter 38, Table 57
Fusidic acid, sodium fusidate (Fucidin Topical)	Inhibits bacterial protein synthesis by interfering w. amino acid transfer from aminoacyl-sRNA to protein on ribosomes.	Primary and secondary skin infect'ns caused by sensitive strains of *S. aureus, C. minutissimum* and streptococcus spp. (**Topical:** Apply small am't of ointment [2% sodium fusidate] or cream [2% fusidic acid] to lesion tid-qid until favorable results are achieved)	Mild irritat'n occ. reported	As w. any new drug, when administering for 1st time consult pharmacist and follow package insert.
Mupirocin (Bactroban)	Inhibits bacterial protein synthesis in sensitive micro-organisms.	Impetigo caused by sensitive strains of staphylococcus and streptococcus, as well as for other superficially infected dermatoses and lesions that are moist and weeping; for abras'ns, minor cuts and wounds (**Topical:** Apply small am't of 2% ointment to affected area tid)	Itching, burning, erythema, stinging, dryness	**Assess:** All areas affected for continuing infect'n, incr. size/no. of lesions. **Administer:** Apply topically, then cover w. gauze if nec. Store at room temp. Wash hands thoroughly after applicat'n. Children 2-5 days old require wound isolat'n precaut'ns. **Evaluate:** Examine lesions for tx response (reduct'n of size/no. of lesions). **Teach:** To report irritat'n or extens'n of lesions. To trim fingernails to prevent scratching; to wash hands after applying ointment.
Nitrofurazone (Furacin)	Antibacterial activity against many gram-positive/-negative strains.	Used locally for superficial wounds, burns, ulcers, skin infect'ns; for preparat'n of surfaces before skin grafting (**Topical:** Apply 0.2% nitrofurazone cream or soluble dressing bid-tid)	Sensitiza'n and gen. allergic skin react'ns may be produced by continuous applicat'n for > 5 days.	As for aminoglycosides

Generic Name (Trade Name)	Use (Dose)	Action	Adverse Effects	Drug Interactions	Nursing Process
Pharmacologic Classification: Topically Applied Antifungal Drugs					
Amphotericin B (Fungizone)	Tx of candidal cutaneous and mucocutaneous infect'ns **(Topical:** Apply 3% cream, ointment or lotion bid-tid prn. **Instill** [in eye]: Drops containing 0.5-1.5 mg/mL; 1 drop q30min, then q1h)	Active against candida spp.	Local irritat'n, pruritus, skin rash		**Assess:** Ensure that cultures have been taken; inspect infected areas for open wounds (burns, ulcers), which facilitate absorpt'n and incr. risk of adv. effects; note extent of infected area. **Evaluate:** Drug efficacy (pt's subjective reports of relief; clinical observat'n of extent of infect'rn); treated areas for sensitivity react'n (erythema, stinging, blistering, localized edema, peeling, itching or urticaria; for adv. systemic effects (see Chapter 67). **Teach:** To evaluate tx effectiveness; to observe for adv. effects of systemic absorpt'n.
Clotrimazole (Canesten, Lotrimin, Gyne-Lotrimin, Mycelex, Myclo)	Topical tx of tinea cruris and tinea corporis due to *T. rubrum*, *T. mentagrophytes* and *E. floccosum.* Candidiasis due to *C. albicans.* Tinea versicolor due to *M. furfur.* Vaginally for candidiasis and trichomoniasis **(Topical:** *Skin infect'ns* - 1% cream and solut'n. Apply to selected and surrounding areas bid, or gently spray and massage suff. 1% solut'n from atomizer into affected area and surrounding skin areas bid. *Vaginal trichomoniasis* - 1 [100-mg] tablet intravaginally for 6 consec. days, pref. hs. *Vaginal candidiasis* - 1 [200-mg] tablet intravaginally for 3 consec. days, pref. hs; or 1 [100-mg] tablet intravaginally for 6 consec. days, pref. hs. *Vaginal cream* - 1 full applicator 1% cream intravaginally for 6 consec. days, pref. hs; or 1 full applicator 2% cream for 3 consec. days, pref. hs)	Effective against wide range of fungi, incl. microsporum and trichophyton spp.	Erythema, stinging, blistering, edema, peeling, pruritus, urticaria, gen. skin irritat'n		
Econazole nitrate (Ecostatin, Spectazole)	Used topically against susceptible pathogenic organisms, incl. *C. albicans* and other candida spp., *T. rubrum, T. mentagro-*	Exhibits broad-spectrum fungistatic activity against candida spp.	Local skin irritat'n manifested by erythema, pruritus, burning and stinging		As for amphotericin B

Drug	Uses and Dosage	Action	Side effects/adverse reactions	Interactions	Nursing considerations
Miconazole nitrate (Micatin, Monistat-Derm, Monistat 7)	phytes, *E. floccosum* and *M. furfur*. Vaginally, to treat vulvo-vaginal candidiasis (**Topical:** Apply 1% cream bid, a.m. and hs. **Vaginal:** 1 ovule [150 mg] for 3 consec. days)	Effective against trichophyton, microsporum, epidermophyton, candida and *Pityrosporon orbiculare*.	As for econazole	As for amphotericin B	
Terconazole (Terzol)	Tx of dermatophytic infect'ns of intertriginous and glabrous skin, tinea versicolor and mucocutaneous candidiasis (**Topical:** Apply suff. 2% cream or lotion to cover infected area bid. Massage area gently until cream or lotion disappears)				
	Local tx of vulvovaginal candidiasis (**Vaginal:** 1 ovule [80 mg] od hs for 3 consec. days; 1 applicator [20 mg terconazole/5 g] od hs for 7 consec. days)	Pharmacologic mechanism of action is uncertain. Exhibits fungicidal activity in vitro against candida.	Headache, body pain, fever, chills, burning	As for amphotericin B	
Haloprogin (Halotex)	Tx of superficial fungal infect'ns, such as tinea pedis, tinea cruris, tinea corporis and tinea manuum due to infect'ns caused by *T. rubrum*, *T. tonsurans*, *T. mentagrophytes*, *M. canus* and *E. floccosum*. Also used for tinea versicolor caused by *M. furfur* and for fungal infect'ns caused by *C. abicans* (**Topical:** Apply cream or solut'n [10 mg/g or 10 mg/mL] bid)	Haloprogin exerts fungicidal action against various spp. of epidermophyton, pityrosporum, microsporum, trichophyton and candida.	Occ. irritat'n, burning, vesicle format'n and pruritus		**Teach:** To avoid OTC creams, ointments, lotions unless directed by physician; to use good asepsis, hand washing; to avoid contact w. eyes; to continue tx even though condit'n improves; to discontinue drug if condit'n worsens.

Pharmacologic Classification: Orally Administered Antifungal Drug

Drug	Uses and Dosage	Action	Side effects/adverse reactions	Interactions	Nursing considerations
Griseofulvin (Fulvicin U/F, Fulvicin P/G, Grifulvin V, Grisactin, Grisactin Ultra, Gris-PEG, Grisowin-FP)	Tx of ringworm infect'ns of skin, hair and nails, viz., tinea corporis, tinea pedis, tinea cruris, tinea barbae, tinea capitis, tinea unguium when caused by susceptible microsporum or epidermophy-	Effective orally against superficial infect'ns caused by fungi responsible for dermatomycoses.	Headache, skin rashes, dryness of mouth, GI disturbances	**Anticoagulants, oral:** May demonstrate reduced activity in presence of griseofulvin, which has been shown to incr. metabolism of oral anticoagulants. **Barbiturates:** Have same inter-	**Assess:** Hx for penicillin allergy, liver disease. Renal studies and blood counts are recommended throughout tx to provide baseline for observat'ns for blood dyscrasias. **Administer:** Us. self-administered on outpt. basis; w. fat foods. Continue drug

Generic Name (Trade Name)	Use (Dose)	Action	Adverse Effects	Drug Interactions	Nursing Process
ton	**(Oral:** *Microcrystalline form* - Adults, 500 mg/day in single or divided doses pc. Children, approx. 10 mg/kg/day in single or divided doses pc. *Ultramicrocrystalline form* - Adults, 330 mg/day in single or divided doses pc. *To eradicate more difficult fungal infect'ns* - 660 mg in divided doses. Children, 5.5 mg/kg/day)			act'ns as oral anticoagulants. **Contraceptives, oral:** May have decr. contraceptive effects if griseofulvin is taken.	until 3 separate cultures prove negative for infective organism. **Teach:** That complet'n of entire course of tx is essential; to avoid exposure to UV light; indicators of adv. effects. To avoid alcohol.

Pharmacologic Classification: Oral and Topically Administered Antifungal Drug

Generic Name (Trade Name)	Use (Dose)	Action	Adverse Effects	Drug Interactions	Nursing Process
Ketoconazole (Nizoral)	For serious or life-threatening systemic fungal infect'ns in normal, predisposed or immunocompromised pts where alternate tx is inappropriate or has been unsuccessful: systemic candidiasis, chronic mucocutaneous candidiasis, coccidioidomycosis and paracoccidioidomycosis, histoplasmosis and chromomycosis. May be considered for severe, recalcitrant dermatophytoses unresponsive to other forms of tx. Used topically for wide variety of superficial fungal infect'ns **(Oral:** Take ac. Adults - 200 mg od. Children > 40 kg - 200 mg od; 20-40 kg - 100 mg od; < 20 kg - 50 mg od. Length of tx should be based on clinical and mycologic response. See product monograph for more details. **Topical:** Apply 2% cream od for 4-6 weeks for tinea pedis; 3-	Ketoconazole has broad-spectrum antifungal activity. Given orally, it is used to treat a wide variety of superficial or "deep" fungal infect'ns. Effective in pts w. dermatophyte or yeast skin infect'ns, pityriasis versicolor, onychomycoses, and oral or vaginal candidiasis. In vitro studies suggest that ketoconazole's antifungal properties may be related to its ability to impair synthesis of ergosterol, a component of fungal and yeast cell membranes.	Nausea, pruritus, headache, dizziness, abdominal pain, constipat'n, diarrhea, somnolence, nervousness, poss. hepatotoxicity. *Warning: Cases of idiosyncratic hepatocellular dysfunct'n have been reported during ketoconazole tx. It is important to recognize that liver disorders can occur. These can be fatal unless properly recognized and managed. Monitor liver funct'n during ketoconazole tx.* Ketoconazole cream is well tolerated.	**Antacids:** May reduce bioavailability because absorpt'n of ketoconazole depends on gastric acidity. Antacids should be avoided or given no sooner than 2 h after ketoconazole. **Anticoagulants, oral:** May have incr. effects if ketoconazole is taken. **Histamine₂ (H₂) blockers:** Have same interact'ns as antacids. **Hypoglycemics, oral:** May produce severe hypoglycemia if ketoconazole is taken. **Phenytoin:** And ketoconazole, may affect each other's rate of metabolism. **Rifampin:** Can reduce blood levels of ketoconazole.	**Administer:** W. citrus or pineapple juice, coffee or tea. Antacids or other agents that elevate pH of GI system should not be given within 2 h. **Teach:** To avoid driving or using power equipment; proper self-administrat'n; that successful tx requires precise adherence to prescribed dose and schedule of administrat'n. To avoid antacids, OTC and alkaline products. Notify physician if GI symptoms occur.

Drug	Uses/Dosage	Adverse Effects	Remarks
4 weeks for tinea corporis; 2-4 weeks for tinea cruris; 2-3 weeks for tinea versicolor)			Topical form as for clotrimazole. Oral form as for griseofulvin.
Nystatin (Candex, Mycostatin, Nadostine, Nilstat)	Given *orally* for prevent'n/tx of candidal infect'ns of mouth and esophagus, for intestinal candidiasis, and for protect'n against candidal overgrowth during antimicrobial or corticosteroid tx; *topically* for tx of cutaneous or mucocutaneous mycotic infect'ns caused by candida spp.; *vaginally* for local tx of vaginal mycotic infect'ns caused by C. albicans and other candidal spp., and tx of pregnant pts to prevent thrush in newborn (**Oral:** [Tablets] Adults - 500 000-1 000 000 U tid. [Suspens'n] Adults/children - 400 000-600 000 U qid. Hold half of dose for some time in each side of mouth before swallowing. Infants - 200 000 U qid. Premature and low birth-weight infants - 100 000 U qid. **Vaginal:** 100 000-200 000 U/day for 2 weeks. **Topical:** Apply cream or ointment [100 000 U/g] to lesions bid. Use powder for moist lesions bid-tid)	Effective against candida spp. Topical creams, ointments and powders and vaginal tablets are avail. for tx of mycotic infect'ns caused by C. albicans. Because nystatin is not absorbed from GI tract, it can be taken orally. Large oral doses have occ. produced diarrhea, GI distress, nausea and vomiting. Local or intravaginal irritat'n occurs rarely.	

SECTION 12

Central Nervous System Pharmacology

The importance of drugs affecting the brain cannot be minimized. The brain controls mood, motor function and the appreciation of pain, to mention but three functions. Section 12 presents the various groups of drugs used to modify these activities. The importance of psychoactive drugs in our society today is reflected in our decision to discuss them first. Following upon our presentation of mood-modifiers, we discuss both general and local anesthetics. Strictly speaking, the latter group should not be placed in this section because they affect primarily peripheral nervous function. However, they are placed here because it seems only reasonable to discuss them immediately after a review of the pharmacologic properties of general anesthetics. Drugs for the treatment of epilepsy and parkinsonism have afforded relief to millions of patients, and these are discussed in Chapters 51 and 52. Finally, we turn our attention to the treatment of pain. The importance of this group of agents cannot be underestimated. More patients arrive in physicians' offices for the treatment of pain than for any other single problem. It is important that nurses recognize the therapeutic significance of narcotic and non-narcotic analgesics and antimigraine products. Accordingly, they are presented in Chapters 53, 54 and 55.

CHAPTER 44

Antipsychotic Drugs and Lithium

Teaching Objectives

Following completion of this chapter, the reader should be able to:

1. Discuss the mechanism of action, pharmacologic effects, therapeutic uses and adverse effects of antipsychotic drugs, as well as the nursing process related to their use.
2. Describe the pharmacokinetics, pharmacologic effects, therapeutic uses and adverse effects of lithium, and the nursing process related to its administration.

Antipsychotic Drugs

The appearance of chlorpromazine in France in the early 1950s heralded the introduction of antipsychotic drugs. Originally called major tranquilizers, these chemicals are now classified as antipsychotic drugs, a term that more adequately describes their therapeutic effects. Chlorpromazine was soon followed on the market by other antipsychotics and the number of patients in mental hospitals dropped sharply. The feeling pervaded that a cure for psychoses was at hand. However, this euphoria dissipated when the rates of readmission to hospitals increased and the toxicities of the drugs became better known. It is now recognized that antipsychotic drugs aid a great number of mentally ill patients. They do not, however, provide a cure. Indeed, not all patients respond to the drugs, and the possible benefits from their use must be weighed against their adverse effects.

Mechanism of Action and Pharmacologic Effects

The mechanism of action of antipsychotic drugs is not known with certainty. This is understandable because the neurochemical etiology of schizophrenia is still the subject of dispute. It is most difficult to explain how a drug helps a patient when the cause of the illness is not understood. It is known, however, that all antipsychotic drugs block dopamine receptors in the brain. An approximate correlation exists between the ability of an antipsychotic to inhibit the actions of dopamine in the brain and the dose required to treat psychoses. This has led to the suggestion that schizophrenia may be due, in part, to an increased activity of dopamine in the brain, and antipsychotics work by blocking the actions of this neurotransmitter. This is likely a

Table 64
Properties of some antipsychotic drugs.

Drug	Usual Oral Dose[1] (mg/day)	IM Dose[2] (mg)	Extrapyramidal Effects	Sedative Effects	Hypotensive Effects
Phenothiazines					
Chlorpromazine (Largactil, Thorazine)	300 – 800	25 – 50	Moderate	High	Moderate
Thioridazine (Mellaril)	200 – 400	–	Low	Moderate	Moderate
Fluphenazine (Moditen)	2.5 – 10 [3]	12.5 – 100 [4]	High	Low	Low
(Modecate)	–	2.5 – 50 [5]	High	Low	Low
Perphenazine (Trilafon)	6 – 24	5 – 10	High	Low	Low
Trifluoperazine (Stelazine)	15 – 20	1 – 2 [6]	High	Low	Low
Thioxanthene					
Chlorprothixene (Tarasan)	30 – 400	25 – 50	Moderate	Moderate	Moderate
Butyrophenone					
Haloperidol (Haldol)	12 – 18	2.5 – 5 [7]	High	Low	Low
Dibenzoxazepine					
Loxapine (Loxapac, Loxitane)	60 – 100	–	Moderate	Low	Low

[1] Approximate dose only. Dosage should be adjusted carefully to meet each patient's needs.
[2] Approximate doses only. Dosage should be adjusted carefully to meet each patient's needs. Unless otherwise indicated, these doses may be repeated approximately q.i.d.
[3] Refers to use of fluphenazine hydrochloride (Moditen) orally.
[4] Refers to use of fluphenazine enanthate (Moditen Enanthate). During maintenance therapy, dose may be repeated q. 1 - 3 weeks.
[5] Refers to use of fluphenazine decanoate (Modecate). During maintenance therapy, dose may be repeated q. 2 - 3 weeks.
[6] Dose may be given q.4 h p.r.n.
[7] Dose may be repeated q. 4-6 h p.r.n.

gross oversimplification of the situation and overlooks the fact that antipsychotics have other actions in the brain. For example, these drugs also block $alpha_1$ and muscarinic receptors, and these actions may also play a role in their therapeutic effects.

Chemically, antipsychotics may be classified as phenothiazines, thioxanthenes, butyrophenones, dibenzoxazepines and dibenzodiazepines. Regardless of chemical differences, all antipsychotics are pharmacologically similar. Table 64 lists some of the more important antipsychotic drugs. In addition to their antipsychotic actions, these drugs can produce extrapyramidal effects, sedation and hypotension. The likelihood of each effect occurring varies from drug to drug.

Dopamine is essential for normal motor function. By blocking its actions in the basal ganglia, antipsychotics modify motor activity and produce extrapyramidal adverse effects. The hypotensive effects of antipsychotics result from vasodilation secondary to a block of adrenergic $alpha_1$ receptors on blood vessels. Antipsychotics can also lower body temperature because they decrease heat production and increase heat loss. The decrease in heat production is secondary to the central nervous system depression, and the increase in heat loss results from vasodilatation. Body temperature is affected most in patients who are exposed to low environmental temperatures.

Antipsychotics block muscarinic receptors, producing dry mouth, constipation, urinary retention and cycloplegia.

Therapeutic Uses

Psychoses are the major indications for the use of these drugs. Antipsychotic drug therapy is the most effective treatment for the acute onset phase in schizophrenia or schizophreniform disorder. These drugs also may be very helpful in the prevention or recurrence of acute schizophrenic disturbances. Antipsychotic agents are less effective in the chronic phase of schizophrenia, particularly when negative symptoms such as anergia, low motivation and flat affect are part of the symptoms. These drugs are also used to treat other psychoses, including mania and paranoia.

Usually three weeks or more of treatment are required in the hospitalized schizophrenic before significant effects are seen. The question of duration of therapy is still controversial. Although discontinuing the drug to minimize or abolish adverse effects is appealing, many patients relapse when this is done and may require life-long therapy. For others, intermittent therapy may be a means of managing the condition while reducing drug-related toxicities. Each patient must be managed on a protocol that best meets the clinical problem.

The question of drug selection is very important. Despite differences in potency, all antipsychotic drugs are equally effective in equivalent doses. The drug of choice is usually the one the patient can best tolerate. High-potency drugs are more likely to produce extrapyramidal adverse effects, and low-potency agents sedation and hypotension. Patients should receive the lowest possible dose to maintain therapeutic response.

With regard to the treatment of schizophrenia, the newest antipsychotic drug, clozapine (Clozaril) deserves special note. This drug is indicated for the management of treatment-resistant schizophrenia. Unlike other antipsychotics, clozapine has not been reported to cause tardive dyskinesia. However, a major drawback of clozapine is its potential to induce agranulocytosis, a serious and potentially fatal decrease in white blood cells. Agranulocytosis occurs in approximately one to two per cent of patients and can be minimized by discontinuing the drug when critical white blood cell levels are reached. Because of this serious side effect, clozapine is usually distributed through a strict monitoring program. The drug is dispensed weekly, contingent upon satisfactory weekly hematology results.

For patients with bipolar affective disorders, antipsychotic drugs are often combined with lithium, both to treat the acute manic episode and to prevent recurrences. Chlorpromazine or haloperidol are used most often.

Organic mental syndromes, manifested as either delirium or dementia, can be treated with antipsychotic drugs. In delirium, short-term antipsychotic therapy is used in patients with specific, identifiable behavioral problems until the medical cause for the delirium can be diagnosed and treated. Chronic intermittent therapy is warranted in patients with dementia in whom structural brain changes cannot be rectified but behavioral symptoms can be modified.

Anxiety is normally not an indication for the use of antipsychotics. The adverse effects dictate that they be used only when safer drugs, notably the benzodiazepines, have failed.

Nausea and vomiting resulting from the use of anticancer drugs, radiation, estrogens, tetracyclines and narcotics, and from uremia, can be treated with antipsychotic drugs. Only thioridazine seems devoid of antiemetic effects. Antipsychotics do not appear effective in controlling motion sickness. Chapter 25 discusses in some detail the treatment of nausea and vomiting and the place of antipsychotic drugs in these situations.

Hiccough may be treated with chlorpromazine. Its mechanism of action in this condition is not known.

Adverse Effects

The adverse effects of antipsychotic drugs can be divided into those which manifest as motor disturbances and those which do not involve motor dysfunction. Because of the importance of the former, these will be discussed first.

Antipsychotic Drug-Induced Motor Dysfunctions
Dopamine and acetylcholine are physiological antagonists in the corpus striatum, with dopamine acting as an inhibitory and acetylcholine as an excitatory neurotransmitter. Because antipsychotic drugs block dopamine receptors, they disturb the normal neurotransmitter balance of the brain, and the effects of acetylcholine are seen unfettered by the inhibitory actions of dopamine. The consequences of this interaction can be divided into the direct and indirect effects of the block of dopamine receptors. Parkinsonism, dystonic reactions and akathisia fall into the first category, with tardive dyskinesia being attributed to the indirect effects of antipsychotic drugs blocking dopamine receptors.

Parkinsonian effects can appear within the first one to three weeks of treatment. Patients experience a decrease or slowing of voluntary movements associated with masked facies, tremor at rest and a decrease in reciprocal arm movements when walking. Reducing the dose of the antipsychotic or adding an anticholinergic-antiparkinsonian drug, such as benztropine or trihexyphenidyl, decreases the severity of the parkinsonian syndrome.

Dystonic reactions include facial grimacing, torticollis, oculogyric crisis and uncoordinated spastic movements of the body and limbs. Treatment involves the use of an anticholinergic-antiparkinsonian drug.

Akathisia occurs usually within the first six weeks of treatment. Patients fidget, pace constantly and continually move their lips and tap their feet. An anticholinergic-antiparkinsonian drug should reduce the symptoms.

Tardive dyskinesia occurs in ten to twenty per cent of patients receiving long-term antipsychotic therapy. It is characterized by involuntary movement, lateral jaw movements and fly-catching movements of the tongue. Choreiform-like movements, characterized by quick, jerky, purposeless movements of the extremities, may also occur. As stated earlier, tardive dyskinesia differs from the parkinsonian effects, dystonic reactions and akathisia caused by antipsychotic drugs in that it is not a direct result of dopamine-receptor blockade. Rather, it is believed to be caused by just the opposite — increased dopamine-receptor stimulation. To understand this view, it is necessary to recognize that the chronic block of dopamine receptors by antipsychotic drugs leads to a reflex increase in dopamine stores and turnover presynaptically, and the synthesis of new and supersensitive receptors postsynaptically. Because tardive dyskinesia results from the overstimulation of dopamine receptors, secondary to the initial block of the receptors, and is not, like the other extrapyramidal effects, a reflection of cholinergic predominance, it does not respond to anticholinergic-antiparkinsonian drugs.

Other Types of Antipsychotic Drug-Induced Adverse Effects
Orthostatic hypotension can occur within the first few days of treatment. Tolerance may develop to this effect. It is more prevalent with high-dose (low-potency) antipsychotics, such as chlorpromazine, thioridazine and chlorprothixene. Potent, low-dose phenothiazines are less prone to induce orthostatic hypotension, but more likely to produce extrapyramidal effects.

Anticholinergic effects of antipsychotics include dry mouth, constipation, urinary retention, decreased tears, nasal congestion and blurred vision.

Hyperprolactemia may be seen following antipsychotic drug treatment. By blocking dopamine receptors in the anterior pituitary, antipsychotic drugs prevent the effects of the prolactin-releasing inhibitory hormone. As a result, prolactin release is increased, producing galactorrhea and amenorrhea in women and gynecomastia and loss of libido in men.

Hypersensitivity reactions to antipsychotic drugs include obstructive jaundice in two to four per cent of patients. Blood dyscrasias, manifested as leukopenia, leukocytosis and eosinophilia, are also classified as hypersensitivity reactions.

Skin pigmentation, seen most often with chlorpromazine and other low-potency drugs, is apparently the result of the accumulation of the antipsychotic and its metabolites in the skin. In extreme cases, involving the deposition of pigments in the lens and cornea, vision can be impaired. Pigment deposits tend to disappear slowly once drug treatment is stopped. Photosensitivity, most common with long-term chlorpromazine treatment, usually appears in the form of hypersensitivity to the sun and severe sunburn.

The ability of clozapine to induce agranulocytosis has already been mentioned. This effect must never be forgotten in the use of this drug.

Nursing Process
Assessment
Prior to the initial administration of an antipsychotic, dilute the drug in fruit juice, tea, coffee or semisolid food. Nurses should review the patient's history for evidence of previous drug hypersensitivity, bone marrow depression, myasthenia gravis, glaucoma, epilepsy, chronic respiratory disease, prostatic hypertrophy and diabetes mellitus. Nurses should also review the patient's history for evidence of cardiovascular, cerebrovascular, kidney, liver or chronic respiratory disease. The presence of any one of these conditions in the patient's history warrants confirmation of the drug order.

Nursing assessment should establish baseline measures for later use in evaluating drug efficacy or identifying adverse effects. Measurements of temperature, pulse, respirations, standing and reclining blood pressures, fluid intake and output, and body mass/weight should precede initial treatment. In addition, the patient's sleep pattern should be described in detail. Because of the teratogenic potential of antipsychotics, nurses should not administer these drugs to pregnant women.

In collaboration with the pharmacist, nurses should review the patient's current drug regimen for potential drug interactions. It is essential to identify any concurrent use of barbiturates, alcohol or other central nervous system depressants. If such concurrent use exists, withhold the antipsychotic and inform the attending physician.

Administration
When administering one of these medications orally, nurses should remain with the patient until they are certain that the drug has been swallowed. This will prevent hoarding of the drug for later use in suicide attempts. Parenterally, antipsychotics are injected either intramuscularly or intravenously. Nurses who frequently prepare antipsychotics for parenteral administration to large numbers of patients should wear disposable plastic gloves to

reduce drug-induced irritation and contact dermatitis. Antipsychotics should never be administered in the same syringe with other drugs because of the possibility of chemical interactions. Parenteral solutions of antipsychotics should be stored in a cool, dark place in a light-resistant container to prevent deterioration. Solutions that are discolored should be discarded.

Patients often experience discomfort when antipsychotics are administered intramuscularly. This can be reduced by diluting commercially available preparations with saline. Intramuscular injections should be given deeply and slowly into the gluteus maximus and the injection site massaged to reduce the pain of injection.

Intravenous infusions of antipsychotics must be given slowly, at the rate ordered by the physician, to minimize their hypotensive effects. Care must be taken to guard against extravasation of intravenous infusions because of tissue irritation.

Evaluation
Nursing evaluation of patients in whom antipsychotic medications have been effective should reveal decreased emotional and psychomotor activity; less paranoia; relief from, or reduction in, the number of hallucinations or delusions; reduced hostility; increased interpersonal interaction by patients who were withdrawn prior to therapy; more purposeful behavior; and logical and rational thought processes.

Simultaneously, nurses must be alert for early evidence of drug-related adverse effects. Observation of the patient's posture and movement patterns is important in identifying extrapyramidal effects. Nursing observation of the standing and lying blood pressures will reveal orthostatic hypotension. Anticholinergic effects are marked by dry mouth, decreased tears, nasal congestion, blurred vision, urinary retention or constipation. Nursing evaluation of fluid intake and output, body mass/weight, frequency and characteristics of bowel movements, and the presence and degree of abdominal distention will permit early detection of anticholinergic effects. Nurses must evaluate their patients for subjective reports of alterations in menstrual pattern or sexual activity due to hyperprolactemia.

Hypersensitivity reactions to antipsychotics have also been reported. These have taken the form of obstructive jaundice and blood dyscrasias, such as leukopenia, leukocytosis and eosinophilia. For this reason, nursing observations indicating blood dyscrasias (fever, sore throat, mucosal ulceration in the mouth, fatigue, upper respiratory infections) or

jaundice (fever, abdominal pain, rash, pruritus, clay-colored stools, tea-colored urine, yellowing of skin or sclera) should be reported to the attending physician immediately. The jaundice is usually mild. If it does not progress, therapy is usually continued. However, the presence of severe jaundice or blood dyscrasias requires that the drug be discontinued. Skin pigmentation is disturbing to the patient but usually does not warrant stopping the drug. If vision becomes impaired, the drug is stopped.

Finally, metabolic alterations have occurred in diabetics or prediabetics given antipsychotics. These patients must be subjected to rigorous nursing evaluation for glucosuria, acetonuria, polydipsia, polyphagia and weight loss.

Teaching
Orthostatic-induced falls can be reduced by instructing patients to remain prone for one hour following parenteral administration and then to move slowly from a reclining to a standing position. Dry mouth and oral candidiasis can be minimized if nurses tell patients to rinse their mouth regularly, drink large amounts of fluid and practise good oral hygiene.

Nurses should alert patients that antipsychotics might turn the urine a pink to reddish-brown color. Constipation, resulting from the anticholinergic effects of these drugs, can be reduced by a diet that is high in both bulk and fluids. Caution patients against operating power tools, driving or using industrial machinery until they are fully aware of their individual response to the sedative effects of the drugs. Antipsychotic drugs can interact with a large number of other agents (see Table 65). Therefore, warn patients not to take any other drugs, including over-the-counter products, that have not been prescribed by the physician. Patients who develop respiratory infections unrelated to blood dyscrasias should be instructed to establish consciously a deep-breathing and coughing routine, because antipsychotics diminish the cough reflex. Nurses should warn patients to take precautions in hot weather, to stay cool, and to use a sunscreen.

Lithium

Manic attacks are characterized by an increase in psychomotor activity, emotional lability and grandiosity. These are easily recognized. Milder forms of mania, called **hypomania,** are less easily diagnosed. Mania or hypomania may be seen repetitively, interspersed with normal or depressive intervals.

Mechanism of Action and Pharmacologic Effects

The mechanism of action of lithium is not known. Therapeutic concentrations of the drug have no noticeable effects in normal individuals. Lithium differs from other psychotropic drugs in that it is not a sedative, euphoriant or depressant. It corrects sleep patterns in the manic patient but has no primary action on sleep itself, other than perhaps a small decrease in REM phases.

Lithium carbonate is well absorbed from the intestine, producing sharp peaks in serum concentrations. The use of a sustained-release lithium carbonate preparation can reduce the frequency of absorption-related side effects in selected individuals who are particularly sensitive to rapid increases in serum lithium concentrations. However, sustained-release lithium carbonate preparations should not be used routinely instead of a standard product because of concern that lithium's nephrotoxicity may be due to continual exposure of the kidneys to effective levels of the drug. Although standard preparations of lithium produce serum peaks, they also produce valleys and afford the kidneys periods when the concentration of the drug perhaps falls below nephrotoxic levels.

Lithium is excreted by the kidney, with a half-life of seventeen to thirty-six hours. In patients with renal impairment, the elimination of lithium is reduced. A reduction in sodium intake increases the renal reabsorption of lithium; therefore, patients taking lithium carbonate should not be placed on a low-sodium diet.

Lithium has a low therapeutic index. It is easy to reach toxic levels quickly. Serum lithium levels are measured routinely to prevent this from occurring. The usual range of therapeutic concentrations is 0.8 – 1.2 mEq/L (0.8 – 1.2 mmol/L) of serum. Toxicity generally appears at levels over 2 mmol/L. A typical schedule calls for drawing blood for analysis before the first dose of the morning on the seventh, fourteenth, twenty-first and twenty-eighth days of treatment and every three to six weeks thereafter.

Therapeutic Uses

Manic and hypomanic patients are treated routinely with lithium carbonate. When mania is mild, lithium alone may be effective. In more severe cases, it is almost always necessary to give an antipsychotic drug (usually haloperidol or chlorpromazine). Once mania is controlled with antipsychotic medication, lithium can be added. After adequate serum levels of lithium have been reached, the antipsychotic may be withdrawn carefully.

Prophylactic lithium treatment is considered the therapy of choice to prevent recurrences of manic-depressive disorders. The drug is effective in sixty to seventy per cent of patients treated. The decision to use lithium prophylactically is based on the number and severity of attacks suffered by a patient and the patient's ability to understand and comply with the treatment regimen.

Lithium therapy is contraindicated in patients with significant cardiovascular or renal disease. It is also contraindicated in patients with evidence of severe debilitation or dehydration, sodium depletion, brain damage and in conditions requiring low sodium intake.

Adverse Effects

Mild neurologic effects, including general and muscular fatigue, lethargy, and fine tremor of the hands are common, especially during initial treatment. If these pose a risk to patient compliance, it may be possible to reduce the dose of lithium or administer a small dose of propranolol. As the concentration of lithium increases, the fine tremor may become coarse and ataxia, dysarthria, loss of coordination, difficulty in concentration, and mild disorientation are established. Other signs of neurological toxicity include muscle twitching and fasciculations in the limbs, hands and face, together with nystagmus, dizziness and visual disturbances. The signs of severe toxicity are restlessness, confusion, nystagmus, epileptic convulsions, delirium and eventually, coma and death.

Polyuria and polydipsia occur in fifteen to forty per cent of patients treated with lithium. These effects do not bother most patients. Occasionally, severe polyuria may occur. Disturbing reports have appeared in the literature on the possible long-term nephrotoxicity of lithium. Further studies are needed to clarify this point. As previously explained, the nephrotoxic effects of lithium appear greater if a sustained-release product is used.

Lithium can cause euthyroid goiter, hypothyroidism with or without goiter, and abnormal endocrine test results. The incidence of lithium-induced goiters is about five per cent. Hypothyroidism may begin weeks or years after starting therapy.

Nursing Process

Assessment

As with all other drugs, nursing assessment of the patient should occur before the first administration of lithium. The patient's history should be reviewed for evidence of organic brain syndrome or an existing cardiovascular, cerebrovascular, thyroid or renal condition. In the presence of any of these conditions, withhold the drug and clarify the order. The discovery of the concurrent use of diuretics (including the "natural" diuretics sold in health food stores) or a low-salt diet should be reported to the physician.

Nursing assessment prior to the first administration of lithium should also establish baseline measures of body mass/weight and fluid intake/output ratios. As well, sleep and behaviour patterns should be identified. These will assist in determining later the efficacy or adverse effects of the drug. Nurses should consult the laboratory reports of lithium blood levels before administering the drug. This is particularly important during the initial period of treatment. Blood levels above 1.5 mmol/L warrant withholding lithium until the physician is consulted. Similarly, if physical assessment of the patient reveals dehydration, malnutrition, pregnancy or lactation, the medication should be withheld until the physician is consulted.

Administration

Lithium should be administered with meals to reduce gastric upset. Nurses should check to determine whether the patient is using a contraceptive because lithium can harm the fetus.

Evaluation

Nursing evaluation is essential in determining the efficacy of lithium. Blood levels alone are inadequate for this purpose. The desired therapeutic effects of lithium are reduced aggressiveness, increased attention span and reduced flight of ideas, less irritability, reduced euphoria, improved judgment and problem-solving ability, rational decision making and normalization of sleep patterns.

The nephrotoxic effects of lithium are identified by nursing evaluation that reveals polydipsia, polyuria, high urine specific gravity, edema and/or sudden weight gain. Nursing observations of tremor, ataxia, dysarthria, severe lack of coordination, severe disorientation, muscle twitching, nystagmus, dizziness and/or visual disturbances suggest central nervous system toxicity. These symptoms should be reported to the physician at once. The patient's diet should be monitored for adequate salt intake. Fluid intake should be maintained at 2500 – 3000 mL/day. Nurses should report to the physician the development of any condition that has the potential to alter the patient's fluid and electrolyte balance. Diarrhea, vomiting, diaphoresis or prolonged hot spells all have the potential to precipitate severe lithium toxicity.

Nursing evaluation that identifies chronic fatigue, gradual weight gain, cold intolerance or facial edema suggests the myxedematous effects of lithium. This should be reported immediately to the physician.

Teaching

Nurses should instruct patients and their families in the evaluation of the efficacy and adverse effects of lithium. They should be made aware of the danger of driving a car, using power tools or working with heavy machinery because of the drowsiness and lack of coordination that are frequent adverse effects of the drug. Patients and their families should be advised of the importance of regular blood tests to determine lithium levels. They should also understand the significance of maintaining adequate fluid and salt intake as a means of preventing toxicity. Finally, patients and their families should be instructed to contact the physician at the first evidence of diarrhea, vomiting, diaphoresis, poor coordination, fine motor tremors or weakness.

Further Reading

Drugs for psychiatric disorders (1991). *The Medical Letter 33* : 43-50.

Drugs for psychiatric disorders (1989). Drugs of choice. *The Medical Letter 31* :13-20 and 32-45.

Farmer, A.E. and McGuffin, P. (1988). The pathogenesis and management of schizophrenia. *Drugs 35* : 177-188.

Harris, E. (1982a). Antipsychotic medication. *Amer. J. Nurs. 81* : 1316-1323.

Harris, E. (1982b). Extrapyramidal effects of antipsychotic medicines. *Amer. J. Nurs. 81* : 1324-1328.

Harris, E. (1982c). Lithium. *Amer. J. Nurs. 81* : 1310-1315.

Hollister, L.E. (1983). Drugs of schizophrenia. *Rational Drug Therapy 16* : No. 8.

Kane, J.M. (1989). The current status of neuroleptic therapy. *J. Clin. Psychiatry 50* : 322-328.

Lobeck, F. (1988). A review of lithium dosing methods. *Pharmacotherapy 8* : 248-255.

Shaw, D.M. (1988). Drug alternatives to lithium in manic-depressive disorders. *Drugs 36* : 249-255.

Table 65
Antipsychotic drugs and lithium.

Pharmacologic Classification: Low-Potency Antipsychotic Phenothiazines

Generic Name (Trade Name)	Use (Dose)	Action	Adverse Effects	Drug Interactions	Nursing Process
Chlorpromazine HCl (Largactil, Thorazine)	Tx of psychotic disorders; to prevent nausea and vomiting [except thioridazine] (**Oral: Adults** - 30-75 mg/day [mild cases] or 75-150 mg/day [severe cases] in divided doses. Elderly/debilitated pts - In lower dose range. Children - 0.5 mg/kg; repeat q4-6h prn. **Rectal:** 100-300 mg/day. Elderly/debilitated - In lower dose range. Children - 1 mg/kg; repeat q4-6h prn. **IM: Adults** - 25-50 mg; repeat tid-qid. Elderly/debilitated - In lower dose range. Children - 0.5 mg/kg; repeat q4-6h prn)	Regardless of pharmacologic classificat'n, all antipsychotics owe much of their action to their ability to block dopamine receptors in the brain. Antipsychotic effects result from blockade of dopamine receptors in mesolimbic and mesocortical areas of the brain. By blocking dopamine receptors in nigrostriatum and tuberinfundibulum, these drugs produce extrapyramidal effects and incr. prolactin secret'n, respectively. Antiemetic effects can be attributed to blockade of dopamine receptors in chemoreceptor trigger zone of medulla. Antipsychotic drugs also block muscarinic, alpha$_1$ adrenergic and histaminergic$_1$ receptors, thereby inhibiting parasympathetic funct'n, lowering BP and inducing sedat'n, respectively.	CNS depress'n [particularly prevalent w. low-potency phenothiazines]. *Extrapyramidal effects* - Parkinsonism, dystonic react'ns, akasthisia, tardive dyskinesia [more prevalent w. high-potency phenothiazines and thioxanthenes]. *Anticholinergic actions* - Hyperprolactinemia [galactorrhea/amenorrhea in women; gynecomastia/loss of libido in men]; skin pigmentat'n and impairment of vision; photosensitivity [particularly prevalent w. chlorpromazine]; cutaneous allergic react'ns [urticarial, maculopapular or petechial lesions]; cholestatic jaundice. *Hematologic effects* - Depress'n of leukopoiesis and agranulocytosis [particularly prevalent w. chlorpromazine and thioridazine].	**Antacids:** May inhibit absorpt'n of phenothiazines given orally. When nec. to give both oral phenothiazines and antacids, their times of administrat'n should be spaced to minimize interact'n. **Anticholinergics:** May decr. phenothiazine absorpt'n by reducing gastric motility. **Barbiturates:** Particularly phenobarbital, may incr. metabolism of chlorpromazine by inducing hepatic microsomal enzymes. If phenobarbital is used, be alert for evidence of reduced phenothiazine effect. **CNS depressants** (e.g., gen. anesthetics, opiates, barbiturates, alcohol): Antipsychotic drugs may incr. their effects. **Hypotensives:** May have additive effects w. phenothiazines. Use special care in those pts in whom hypotensive crisis would be undesirable, such as those w. arteriosclerosis or other CV disease. **Levodopa:** Has its effects reduced by antipsychotic drugs because of latter agents' ability to block dopamine receptors.	**Assess:** For hx alcoholism, drug hypersensitivity, bone marrow depress'n, myasthenia gravis, glaucoma, epilepsy, chronic resp. disease, prostatic hypertrophy, diabetes, CV or cerebrovascular disease, kidney or liver disease; current pregnancy, lactat'n. For concurrent use of barbiturates, alcohol, CNS depressants. Establish baseline measures of temp., pulse, respirat'n, standing/reclining BP, fluid intake/output ratio, weight, sleep pattern. **Administer:** *Oral* - Stay w. pt until drug is swallowed. Dilute in fruit juice, tea, coffee, semisolid food prn. *Parenteral* Wear plastic gloves to prepare solut'n for inject'n; dilute w. saline; do not mix w. other medicat'ns; store in cool dark place in light-resistant containers; discard discolored solut'ns; inject deeply and slowly; massage inject'n site; prevent extravasat'n of IV infus'ns. Physician must specify rate of IV infus'n. **Evaluate:** Tx effectiveness (decr. emot'nal/psychomotor activity; less paranoia; relief or reduct'n of hallucinat'ns or delus'ns; less hostility; incr. interpersonal interact'n by w'drawn pts; purposeful behavior; logical, rat'nal thought processes); for adv. effects (sore throat, oral ulcers, upper resp. infect'ns, abd. pain or distent'n, or by changes in standing/lying BP, fluid intake/output, weight, frequency/characteristics of BMs, menstrual pattern, sexual activity, temp., skin color, urine/stool color, visual acuity.
Thioridazine (Mellaril)	As for chlorpromazine HCl (**Oral: Adults** - 30-400 mg/day, depending on severity of condit'n. Elderly/debilitated - 33-50% adult dose. Children - 20-40 mg/day)				
Triflupromazine HCl (Vesprin)	As for chlorpromazine HCl (**Oral: Adults** - 50-150 mg/day in divided doses. Children - 2 mg/kg/day in divided doses. **IM: Adults** - Initially, 60-150 mg/day. Elderly/debilitated - 10-75 mg/day. Children over 30 months - 0.2-0.25 mg/kg [max. 10 mg daily])				

Pharmacologic Classification: Mid/High-Potency Antipsychotic Phenothiazines

Generic Name (Trade Name)	Use (Dose)	Action	Adverse Effects	Drug Interactions	Nursing Process
Fluphenazine HCl (Moditen, Permitil, Prolixin)	As for chlorpromazine (**Oral:** Adults - 2.5-10 mg/day in divided doses q6-8h. Elderly pts - 1-2.5 mg/day)	As for chlorpromazine HCl	As for chlorpromazine HCl	As for chlorpromazine HCl	**Teach:** Self-evaluat'n for tx effectiveness and adv. effects; that adv. effects are reversible if promptly reported to physician; to stay prone for 1 h after parenteral administrat'n; to change posit'n slowly; to lie down promptly if dizzy; to rinse mouth regularly; to maintain fluid intake; importance of good oral hygiene; nec. for compliance w. prescribed regimen to achieve tx response; poss. that urine may be discolored [pink to red-brown]; imp. of high-bulk food intake and high fluid intake to prevent constipat'n; imp. of gradual w'drawal of drug rather than stopping abruptly; caution against driving, using power tools or working w. industrial machinery until extent of sedat'n identified; to take only those medicat'ns prescribed by physician; establish deep-breathing/coughing routine if resp. infect'n develops. Warn pts to take precautions in hot weather, to stay cool and use sunscreen.
Fluphenazine decanoate (Modecate)	As for chlorpromazine (**IM:** Initially, 2.5-12.5 mg. Except particularly sensitive pts, a 2nd dose of 12.5-25 mg may be given in 4-10 days. Symptoms can us. be controlled w. 25 mg or less q2-3weeks)				
Fluphenazine enanthate (Moditen Enanthate)	As for chlorpromazine (**IM:** Us. 25 mg q2weeks. Dose may range from 12.5-100 mg q1-3weeks)				
Perphenazine (Trilafon)	As for chlorpromazine (**Oral:** Adults - 8-32 mg/day in divided doses. Elderly/debilitated pts - 33-50% adult dose. **IM:** For acute psychoses - 5-10 mg initially; 5 mg q6h thereafter. Total am't should not exceed 15 mg/day in ambulatory pts or 30 mg daily in hospitalized pts. Elderly/debilitated pts - 33-50% adult dose)	As for chlorpromazine HCl	As for chlorpromazine HCl	As for chlorpromazine HCl	
Prochlorperazine (Stemetil)	As for chlorpromazine (**Oral:** Adults - Initially, 10 mg tid-qid; incr. gradually by 5-10 mg q2-3 days until symptoms controlled. **IM:** 10-20 mg initially, repeated q2-4h until control obtained)	As for chlorpromazine HCl	As for chlorpromazine HCl	As for chlorpromazine HCl	As for chlorpromazine HCl
Trifluoperazine HCl (Stelazine)	As for chlorpromazine (**Oral:** Adults - Initially, 2-5 mg bid-tid;	As for chlorpromazine HCl	As for chlorpromazine HCl	As for chlorpromazine HCl	As for chlorpromazine HCl

incr. gradually to 15-20 mg/day. Some pts may require as much as 40 mg/day. Elderly/debilitated pts - 33-50% adult dose. Hospitalized children 6-12 years - 1 mg od-bid. **IM:** Adults - Initially, 1-2 mg)

Pharmacologic Classification: Thioxanthene Antipsychotics

Chlorprothixene (Taractan, Tarasan)	As for chlorpromazine (**Oral:** Adults - 30-400 mg/day. Initial dose, 15-50 mg tid-qid)	As for chlorpromazine HCl	As for chlorpromazine HCl	As for chlorpromazine HCl
Thiothixene (Navane)	As for chlorpromazine (**Oral:** 15-30 mg/day. In most cases, initially 5-10 mg/day)	As for chlorpromazine HCl	As for chlorpromazine HCl	As for chlorpromazine HCl

Pharmacologic Classification: Butyrophenone Antipsychotics

Haloperidol (Haldol)	As for chlorpromazine (**Oral:** Adults - 1-2 mg bid-tid, initially. Incr. prn. Generally, doses > 4-6 mg tid are not required. Children and debilitated/geriatric pts - Initially, 0.25-0.5 mg bid-tid. Upward adjustment of dose should be made gradually. **IM:** Adults - Initially, 2.5-5 mg q4-6h)	As for chlorpromazine HCl	As for chlorpromazine HCl	As for chlorpromazine HCl
Haloperidol decanoate (Haldol-LA)	As for chlorpromazine (**IM:** A ratio of 20:1 haloperidol decanoate to oral haloperidol appears to produce comparable steady-state plasma levels of haloperidol. Haloperidol decanoate should be administered q4weeks)	As for chlorpromazine HCl	As for chlorpromazine HCl	As for chlorpromazine HCl

Generic Name (Trade Name)	Use (Dose)	Action	Adverse Effects	Drug Interactions	Nursing Process

Pharmacologic Classification: Dibenzoxazepine Antipsychotic

| Loxapine (Loxitane, Loxapac) | As for chlorpromazine (**Oral:** Initially, 10 mg bid; incr. rapidly over next 7-10 days until symptoms controlled. Us. maint. dose, 60-100 mg/day. **IM:** 12.5-50 mg q4-6h) | As for chlorpromazine HCl | As for chlorpromazine HCl | As for chlorpromazine HCl | As for chlorpromazine HCl |

Pharmacologic Classification: Dibenzodiazepine Antipsychotic

| Clozapine (Clozaril) | Management of tx-resistant schizophrenia (**Oral:** Initially, 300-600 mg/day in divided doses, w. largest fract'n given hs. Once tx response obtained, dose may be reduced in many pts to 150-300 mg/day in divided doses. If dose is not > 200 mg/day, drug may be given od hs. Max. daily dose, 900 mg) | Atypical antipsychotic. Appears to have minimal effects on dopamine receptors. Possesses anticholinergic, adrenolytic, antihistaminic and antiserotonergic effects. | As for chlorpromazine, except has not been reported to produce tardive dyskinesia. *Can induce potentially fatal agranulocytosis. Weekly hematology tests are essential.* | As for chlorpromazine | As for chlorpromazine. However, pts must be taught s/s agranulocytosis and importance of weekly blood tests. |

Pharmacologic Classification: Antimanic-depressive Drug

| Lithium carbonate (Carbolith, Eskalith CR, Lithane, Lithotabs, Lithobid, Lithonane) | Prophylaxis of bipolar [manic-depressive] disorders and tx of mania [manic episodes] (**Oral:** For acute mania - Adults - Initially, 600-900 mg/day, reaching 1200-1800 mg/day on day 2. Give drug tid. After acute episode subsides, reduce dose rapidly to achieve serum levels bet. 0.6-1.2 mEq/L. Av. sugg. dose at this stage, 900 mg/day divided into 3 doses, w. range us. bet. 500-1200 mg/day. Elderly pts - Use Li cautiously and in reduced doses, beginning range 600-1200 mg/day) | Mechanism of action not known. Tx concentrat'ns have no noticeable effects in normal individuals. Li differs from other psychotropics in that it is not sedative, euphoriant or depressant. It corrects sleep patterns in manic pts but has no primary action on sleep itself. Li has a low tx index. It is easy to reach toxic levels quickly. Serum Li levels are | Gen. and muscular fatigue, lethargy; fine tremor of hands, coarse tremor, ataxia, dysarthria, loss of coordinat'n; difficulty in concentrat'n, mild disorientat'n; nystagmus, muscle twitching, fasciculat'n in limbs, hands, face; dizziness, vis. disturbances; restlessness, confus'n, epileptic convuls'ns, delirium, death; nephrogenic diabetes-like | **Diuretics:** Should be administered cautiously w. Li₂CO₃ because excret'n of Li decreases w. Na deplet'n. More frequent serum Li determinat'ns may be required. **Potassium iodide:** And Li₂CO₃ may have synergistic hypothyroid activity. **Sodium bicarbonate:** May incr. renal excret'n of Li. Monitor pts on combined tx for decr. Li₂CO₃ effect. **Sodium chloride:** Affects Li excret'n, which appears to be proport'nal to NaCl intake. Pts on salt-free diets who receive Li₂CO₃ | **Assess:** Hx for CV, cerebrovascular or renal disease, organic brain syndrome; for dehydrat'n, malnutrit'n, concurrent use of diuretics or low-salt diet; current pregnancy or lactat'n. Establish sleep pattern, baseline weight, fluid intake/output ratio; Li blood levels. **Administer:** W. meals. Check that pt is using contraceptive because Li may harm fetus. **Evaluate:** For reduced aggressiveness, flight of ideas; incr. attent'n span; less irritability or euphoria; improved judgment; normalizat'n of sleep patterns; for adv. CNS effects, nephrotoxicity and hypothyroidism; diet for adequate salt intake; maintain fluid |

	monitored to prevent this from occurring.	syndrome, euthyroid goiter, hypothyroidism w. and without goiter, dry mouth, anorexia, nausea and vomiting, diarrhea, incontinence, abd. pain.	are prone to Li toxicity. Increased Na intake has been assoc. w. reduced tx response to Li$_2$CO$_3$. **Succinylcholine:** May have its effects prolonged by Li$_2$CO$_3$.
Lithium carbonate sustained-release (Duralith)	As above (**Oral:** Adults - Initially, 600-900 mg/day, reaching a level of 1200-1800 mg/day on day 2, divided into 2 doses at 12-h intervals. After acute manic episode subsides, reduce dose rapidly to achieve serum levels bet. 0.6-1.2 mEq/L. Av. sugg. dose at this stage, 900 mg/day divided into 2 doses, given at 12-h intervals, w. range us. bet. 600-1200 mg/day. Elderly pts - Use cautiously and in reduced doses, beginning range 600-1200 mg/day or less, starting w. smaller doses)	As above	Polyuria, glycosuria, proteinuria, albuminuria, polydipsia, edema; drying of hair, alopecia, rash, pruritus, hyperkeratosis. *May harm fetus.*	As above

intake at 2500-3000 mL; for condit'ns that alter fluid and electrolyte balance. **Teach:** Self-evaluat'n for drug efficacy and/or adv. effects; to avoid use of power tools, heavy machinery, or driving vehicles during tx; imp. of regular blood tests for Li, maintaining adequate fluid and salt intake and reporting to physician any condit'n causing diarrhea, vomiting or other electrolyte loss. Teach pt and family to contact physician at 1st sign of adv. effects.

CHAPTER 45

Antidepressant Drugs

Teaching Objectives

Following completion of this chapter, the reader should be able to:
1. Describe endogenous and reactive depression.
2. Discuss the possible involvement of norepinephrine and 5-hydroxytryptamine in the etiology of endogenous depression.
3. Discuss the mechanism of action, pharmacologic effects, therapeutic uses and adverse effects of heterocyclic antidepressants, and the nursing process related to their use.
4. Describe the mechanism of action, pharmacologic effects, therapeutic uses, adverse effects and drug interactions of monoamine oxidase inhibitors, as well as the nursing process precipitated by their use.

Depression

Everyone feels depressed from time to time. You strut proudly into a clothing store after two months of rigorous dieting and are asked to step into the stout section. That is depressing. However, as profound as **secondary or reactive** depression is, it must not be confused with the affective disorder called **primary, endogenous or psychotic** depression. In the latter situation, depression may be reflected in feelings of self-reproach or guilt, recurrent thoughts of death or suicide, and a low opinion of one's own worth. Endogenous depression may also be accompanied by disturbances in appetite with changes in body mass/weight, inability to sleep, agitation or retardation, reduced ability to concentrate, loss of interest or pleasure in usual activities, and decreased sexual drive.

Drug treatment of depression has changed significantly in the past thirty years. Prior to 1957, amphetamine was often used. Although it produces central nervous system excitation and abolishes depression, its use created serious problems of drug dependence and profound depression upon drug withdrawal. The introduction of imipramine in 1957 provided the first of a new group of antidepressants called the **tricyclic antidepressants.** It was rapidly followed on the market by other drugs with three rings in their structure, all appropriately called "tricyclics". The subsequent introduction of maprotiline, trazodone and fluoxetine, drugs which do not have three rings in their chemical structure, led to the creation of a group of drugs called **heterocyclic antidepressants.** As explained below, heterocyclic antidepressants comprise the tricylic antidepressant drugs and those compounds whose pharmacologic properties are similar to those of the tricyclics. Heterocyclic antidepressants, together with the monoamine oxidase inhibitors (MAOIs), are used to treat patients suffering from endogenous depression. They are also given to patients with nagging reactive depression, but they are not as effective in this condition.

Heterocyclic Antidepressants

Mechanism of Action and Pharmacologic Effects

Amitriptyline (Elavil, Endep, Enovil), amoxapine (Asendin), desipramine (Norpramin, Pertofrane), doxepin (Adapin, Sinequan), imipramine (Imavate, Tofranil), nortriptyline (Aventyl, Pamelor), protriptyline (Vivactil, Triptil) and trimipramine (Surmontil) have three rings in their chemical structure and are accordingly called tricyclic antidepressants. As explained above, maprotiline (Ludiomil), trazadone (Desyrel) and fluoxetine (Prozac) are not structurally tricyclic antidepressants and, therefore, cannot be called tricyclics. However, their pharmacologic properties are quite similar to those of the tricyclic antidepressants. Together, the tricyclic antidepressants plus maprotiline, trazadone and fluoxetine are called the heterocyclic antidepressants. Fluvoxamine maleate (Luvox) is at this time the newest antidepressant on the market. This drug is chemically unrelated to any existing antidepressant. However, its pharmacologic properties and therapeutic indications are very similar to those of the heterocyclic antidepressants. For this reason, it is appropriate to present it here.

Little is known about the cause(s) of depression or the means by which drugs relieve it. It has been speculated that depression is caused by reduced release and action of norepinephrine or 5-hydroxytryptamine (serotonin), or both, in the brain. If that is the case, then increasing norepinephrine and/or 5-hydroxytryptamine concentrations acting on brain receptors should reverse depression. Neuronal reuptake is the major physiological mechanism for removing neurotransmitters from their receptors and terminating their actions. Some heterocyclic antidepressant drugs are believed to relieve depression by reducing reuptake, thereby increasing the actions of norepinephrine and/or 5-hydrox-ytryptamine in the brain.

However, there are some holes in this hypothesis. First, there is a problem with the time sequence of events. Although the block of neuronal reuptake occurs soon after drug treatment begins, the antidepressant effects of these drugs require several weeks of treatment. Second, some heterocyclic agents, such as doxepin and iprindole, have little or no effect on neuronal reuptake.

An alternate suggestion is that heterocyclic antidepressants may reduce the number of presynaptic alpha$_2$ receptors, thereby increasing norepinephrine release in the brain. It is argued that the resulting increase in norepinephrine release may account, at least in part, for the clinical effectiveness of some and perhaps all tricyclic antidepressants.

Both theories postulate an increase in norepinephrine levels around brain receptors. It is furthermore suggested that as a result of the increased norepinephrine levels a down regulation of brain beta receptors occurs, and this may account for the antidepressant effects. The expression **down regulation** indicates a decrease in the number of receptors in the brain capable of interacting with neurotransmitters. Down regulation is not an uncommon physiological response if receptors continue to be bombarded with high levels of neurotransmitters. If relief from depression is the result of a decrease in the number of brain beta receptors, it may be inferred that depression itself is due to excessive receptor stimulation. This concept is exactly opposite to the view expressed previously above, where it was postulated that depression results from inadequate stimulation. Now we are suggesting that depression results from too much stimulation. Students cannot be blamed if they find this confusing; some of the world's sharpest scientific minds are still trying to unravel this mystery.

Heterocyclic antidepressants also sedate patients and block cholinergic (muscarinic) receptors. The sedative effects are attributed to their antihistaminic actions. Table 66 summarizes the effects of several tricyclic antidepressants. It is apparent from the table that the sedative and anticholinergic actions differ among the drugs.

It may seem unusual that antidepressant drugs sedate patients. One might have expected them to stimulate individuals. One of the paradoxes of these drugs is that they sedate patients while they relieve depression. Doxepin and amitriptyline are the most potent antihistamines as well as the best sedatives. Sedation is seen after administration of the first dose or two, but the antidepressant effects require two or three weeks of continuous treatment.

Table 66
Properties of some tricyclic antidepressants.

Generic Name (Trade Name)	Usual Oral Dose[1]	Sedation[2]	Anticholinergic Effects[2]
Imipramine (Janimine, Tofranil)	Initially, 25 mg tid; incr. prn to 150 mg/day.	++	++
Desipramine (Norpramin, Pertofrane)	Initially, 75-150 mg/day in divided doses. More severe cases may require up to 200 mg/day.	+	+
Amitriptyline (Elavil, Endep)	Initially, 25 mg tid; incr. prn to 150 mg/day.	+++	+++
Nortriptyline (Aventyl, Pamelor)	30-100 mg/day in divided doses.	++	++
Doxepin (Adapin, Sinequan)	Initially, 25 mg tid; incr. prn to 150 mg/day.	+++	+++
Protriptyline (Vivactil, Triptil)	15-30 mg/day in divided doses.	0	++

[1] Approximate doses for adult outpatients. Smaller doses are required for the young or elderly. Seriously ill, hospitalized patients may require higher doses.
[2] 0 = none; + = slight; ++ = moderate; +++ = high.

The anticholinergic effects of heterocyclic antidepressants include blurred vision, dry mouth, constipation and urinary retention. Amitriptyline and doxepin are the most potent anticholinergics and desipramine and protriptyline the weakest.

Heterocyclic antidepressants have marked effects on the cardiovascular system. Orthostatic hypotension is the most frequent and troublesome adverse effect seen with therapeutic doses. At normal doses, heterocyclic antidepressants are antiarrhythmic. However, at high doses they block norepinephrine reuptake by cardiac sympathetic nerves and increase the risk of tachycardia or cardiac arrhythmias, or both. Maprotiline, trazadone and fluoxetine have minimal effects on the cardiovascular system.

Therapeutic Uses

Heterocyclic antidepressants are used to treat major depression. They are most effective in patients suffering from more severe depression, particularly with greater vegetative disturbance and melancholia. A period of two to three weeks may be required before patients improve significantly. Little evidence can be found to demonstrate that one drug is more effective than the others. Usually, the more sedative drugs (amitriptyline and doxepin) are preferred for anxious or agitated depressives, while the less sedative drugs (protriptyline) are better for patients with psychomotor withdrawal.

Imipramine, in a dose of 2.5 mg/kg or 50 mg total per day, is used in children over the age of six to treat enuresis.

Amitriptyline is combined with perphenazine in the products Elavil Plus, Etrafon 2-10, Etrafon-A, Etrafon-D, Etrafon-F and Triavil. They have been recommended for the treatment of patients with depression who also have marked anxiety, agitation or tension, and for the treatment of schizophrenic patients who have associated symptoms of depression. The therapeutic rationale for these products has been questioned. Endogenous depression should be treated with amitriptyline or another heterocyclic. The addition of perphenazine is usually not recommended, since it possesses poor sedative properties and limits the upper dose of amitriptyline in many patients.

Adverse Effects

Autonomic effects constitute the majority of adverse reactions to heterocyclic antidepressants. Orthostatic hypotension is the most common cardiovascular effect. Other effects seen with increasing doses are palpitation, tachycardia, cardiac arrhythmias and electrocardiographic abnormalities. Ventricular arrhythmias cause great concern. Ventricular tachyarrhythmias can be produced, and ventricular fibrillation is a cause of death in overdoses. As stated previously, maprotiline, trazadone and fluoxetine have minimal cardiovascular effects.

The anticholinergic actions of heterocyclic antidepressants produce dry mouth, decrease in sweating, constipation, urinary hesitancy and delayed ejaculation.

Confusion, seen most often in patients over the age of forty, is particularly likely to occur if the patient is receiving concomitant treatment with drugs that also possess anticholinergic effects, such as antipsychotics or antiparkinsonian agents. Tremors may also occur. The involvement of the sympathetic nervous system is suggested by the fact that propranolol, a beta-adrenergic blocker, has been used with some success to reduce them.

Weight gain may be seen in patients receiving heterocyclic antidepressant therapy. Depending on the original status of the patient, this may or may not be an adverse effect. In contrast to the other drugs, fluoxetine causes weight loss. The other adverse effects of fluoxetine include headache, nervousness, insomnia, drowsiness, fatigue or asthenia, anxiety, tremor, and dizziness or light-headedness. Patients may also experience gastrointestinal complaints, including nausea, diarrhea, dry mouth and anorexia. Fluoxetine can also produce excessive sweating. Controversy has swirled around fluoxetine. Both the professional and lay press have carried articles claiming that the use of fluoxetine may increase the risk of suicide. At this time, the issue is still subject to debate.

Trazodone has been associated with the development of priapism. In approximately one-third of the cases reported, surgical intervention has been required and, in a portion of these cases, permanent impairment of erectile function or impotence has resulted.

Treatment of Acute Heterocyclic Antidepressant Poisoning

The quantities of heterocyclic antidepressants prescribed are quite capable of killing. For example, 1 g of amitriptyline, imipramine or doxepin produces severe toxic reactions in adults, and 2 g can be fatal. The consequences of taking large single doses are due to many of the basic actions of the drugs described earlier. The symptoms of acute heterocyclic antidepressant overdose include coma, seizures, cardiac arrhythmias and conduction abnormalities. These last two are caused by increased sympathetic stimulation, due to the block in norepinephrine neuronal reuptake, and decreased parasympathetic activity, as a result of the anticholinergic actions of the drugs.

Supportive measures should be instituted, including correction of acidosis to increase protein binding of the heterocyclic. Gastric lavage is recommended for six to eight hours after drug ingestion. Activated charcoal can be given via nasogastric tube (following endotracheal intubation) in the comatose patient to reduce enterohepatic recycling of the heterocyclic antidepressant and its active metabolites. Hyperpyrexia can be handled by physical cooling and cardiac arrhythmias by lidocaine, propranolol and phenytoin. Quinidine, procainamide and disopyramide are contraindicated because of their additive effects on cardiac conduction.

Physostigmine (Antilirium) is a reversible inhibitor of acetylcholinesterase. It allows acetylcholine to accumulate in both the brain and peripheral tissues and thus overcomes the anticholinergic effects of the heterocyclic antidepressant. Physostigmine is preferred over neostigmine or pyridostigmine because it will cross the blood-brain barrier and reverse some of the central effects of the antidepressants. The other two drugs will not enter the brain in sufficient concentrations to affect the actions of the heterocyclics. Physostigmine, 1 – 2 mg intravenously administered at a rate of 1 mg/min, can help control myoclonus, choreoathetosis, delirium, coma and some cardiotoxic reactions. Repeat injections may be required. Physostigmine must be used cautiously because it can produce severe cholinergic effects, including excessive salivation, bronchoconstriction and convulsions.

Nursing Process

Assessment

Assessment of the patient prior to administration of these medications is the initial nursing responsibility. Nurses should review the patient's history for evidence of conditions that contraindicate heterocyclic antidepressant administration. These drugs should be withheld pending confirmation by the attending physician if the patient has a history of liver disease, urinary retention, cardiovascular disease, glaucoma, suicidal tendencies, epilepsy or hyperthyroidism. If the prescription is affirmed in spite of these conditions, the patient should be subject to particularly vigilant nursing evaluation for evidence of adverse effects. Patients with suicidal tendencies have an additional risk factor, and should be especially carefully monitored. They are also not strong candidates for self-administration of heterocyclics.

Baseline measures for later use in detecting therapeutic effectiveness or adverse reactions should include standing and lying blood pressures; radial and apical pulses, with descriptions of rate, rhythm and quality; fluid intake/output ratios; documentation of pretherapy bowel habits, body mass/weight and sleep pattern; and behavioral manifestations of the depression.

Administration
The nurse must be certain that the patient swallows the drug. This is essential to prevent hoarding of medication for future use in a suicide attempt. Store the drug in a tight container at room temperature. Give with food or milk to reduce gastrointestinal symptoms. Administer the drug at night if oversedation occurs during the day. Elderly patients may not tolerate single-dose therapy at night. Nurses should have gum, candy and sips of water available to alleviate dry mouth.

Evaluation
Therapeutic effectiveness is established by a nursing evaluation that reveals increased responsiveness of the patient to the environment, greater attention to personal appearance, more physical activity, change in eating and sleeping patterns, and increased frequency of positive interpersonal interactions. Other therapy must be maintained for a prolonged period of time before these therapeutic benefits are seen.

Nurses should be alert for early signs of hypersensitivity. These include allergic dermatitis (itchy, raised rash), blood dyscrasias (sore throat, fever, weakness, purpura), or cholestatic jaundice (abdominal pain, nausea, yellowing of skin or sclera, tea-colored urine or clay-colored stools). Patients may also suffer from orthostatic hypotension. Nurses should assist ambulation during the early stages of therapy, if necessary.

Adverse anticholinergic effects of heterocyclics are reflected by changes in the rate, rhythm or quality of the apical and/or radial pulses, due to cardiac irregularities; the fluid intake/output ratio, indicative of urinary retention, together with abdominal distention; and the frequency and/or characteristics of bowel movements, accompanied by abdominal distention and the absence of bowel sounds, symptoms of paralytic ileus. Gynecomastia, testicular swelling, galactorrhea, weight gain, glucosuria or acetonuria are indicators of adverse endocrine effects. Altered sleep patterns, confusion and disorientation suggest central nervous system effects. Use safety measures and side rails as necessary.

The final goal of nursing evaluation is to observe patients carefully for suicidal tendencies or behavior. Patients should be asked directly whether or not they have suicidal tendencies.

Teaching
In patient teaching, nurses must emphasize the signs of both beneficial and adverse drug effects. These should be reported to the physician. Patients and their families should be taught that therapeutic effectiveness is achieved only after several weeks' compliance with the prescribed regimen of therapy. Patients should be taught to move gradually from reclining to standing positions; to use power tools, industrial machinery and motor vehicles with caution, especially during the initial phase of therapy; to keep adequate supplies of the drug on hand; and to rinse their mouth, maintain high fluid intake, and practise good oral hygiene because of the anticholinergic effects of heterocyclic antidepressants. Patients can be reassured that adverse effects, especially those which are sex linked, are reversible when the medication is discontinued.

Nurses should alert patients to the danger of using alcohol or over-the-counter drugs concurrently with heterocyclic antidepressants. Patients should also be advised to use a sun shade and sunscreen, as necessary.

Monoamine Oxidase Inhibitors

Mechanism of Action and Pharmacologic Effects

Monoamine oxidase is a term used to refer to a group of enzymes widely distributed throughout the body that oxidatively deaminates and inactivates norepinephrine, dopamine and 5-hydroxytryptamine (5-HT, serotonin). Inhibition of monoamine oxidase increases brain levels of these neurotransmitters. The monoamine oxidase inhibitors (MAOIs) currently available for use in North America are phenelzine (Nardil) and tranylcypromine (Parnate). It is generally believed that these drugs relieve depression by increasing brain norepinephrine or 5-hydroxytryptamine levels, or both. This belief is complicated, however, by the fact that enzyme inhibition appears after a few doses of the drug but the antidepressant effects are seen only after two to four weeks of treatment.

In contrast to the sedative effects of heterocyclic antidepressants, monoamine oxidase inhibitors stimulate normal individuals. They also suppress REM sleep and are used to treat narcolepsy. Monoamine oxidase inhibitors may produce orthostatic hypotension.

Therapeutic Uses

Monoamine oxidase inhibitors are used as second-line drugs to heterocyclic antidepressants for the treatment of endogenous depression. Most physicians prefer heterocyclic agents because they are usually more effective and less toxic. Patients receiving monoamine oxidase inhibitors must be placed on tyramine-free diets and refrain from using sympathomimetic drugs to prevent the occurrence of a hypertensive crisis (see discussion following, on Interaction of Drugs and Foods with Monoamine Oxidase Inhibitors). This ban extends to include the topical application of nasal vasoconstrictors.

Because monoamine oxidase inhibitors suppress REM sleep, they may be used to treat narcolepsy. When used to treat depression, monoamine oxidase inhibitors correct the concomitant sleep disorder.

Adverse Effects

Monoamine oxidase inhibitors stimulate the central nervous system to produce tremors, insomnia and agitation. Convulsions have been reported occasionally, along with hallucinations and confusion.

Autonomic adverse effects include orthostatic hypotension. This can be treated immediately by having the patient lie down. If hypotension is severe, it may be necessary to reduce the dose of the drug or withdraw it entirely. Monoamine oxidase inhibitors can also decrease cholinergic stimulation, resulting in dry mouth, constipation, difficulty in urination, delayed ejaculation and impotence.

A low incidence of hepatotoxicity is reported with the currently used drugs. Its incidence does not appear to be related to the duration of therapy or dose of the drug.

Acute overdose presents very serious problems to both the patient and the medical team. Symptoms may be absent for several hours after the ingestion of a large number of tablets and then proceed suddenly to severe fever, agitation, hyperexcitable reflexes, hallucination and increase or decrease in blood pressure. Treatment is largely symptomatic.

Interaction of Drugs and Foods with Monoamine Oxidase Inhibitors

Monoamine oxidase inhibitors decrease the inactivation of sympathomimetic amines, leading to a potentiated adrenergic effect. The classical example of this type of interaction involves the ingestion of foods containing the chemical tyramine. Foods containing tyramine include cheese, beer, wine, pickled herring, snails, chicken liver and large quantities of coffee. Tyramine is normally inactivated quickly by monoamine oxidase in the liver. When monoamine oxidase is inhibited, tyramine is not destroyed. Instead, it enters sympathetic nerves and releases norepinephrine, which produces a generalized vasoconstriction. The resulting hypertensive crisis may be characterized by severe headache. Death can occur from intracranial hemorrhage.

Under normal circumstances, the concomitant use of a monoamine oxidase inhibitor and a heterocyclic antidepressant is contraindicated. Monoamine oxidase inhibitors should be used only in a few specific situations in combination with a heterocyclic antidepressant, under careful psychiatric and medical supervision.

Monoamine oxidase inhibitors decrease the hepatic metabolism of many drugs. As a result, the actions of a large number of drugs, such as narcotics, barbiturates, many anesthetics and anticholinergics are increased. In the absence of an emergency, it is advisable to delay surgery for a few weeks to withdraw the patient from monoamine oxidase inhibitor treatment.

Nursing Process

Assessment

Prior to the first administration of a monoamine oxidase inhibitor, nursing assessment should review the patient's history. Patients with histories of hyperthyroidism, cardiovascular or cerebrovascular disease, hepatic or renal impairment, hypertension, glaucoma, or alcohol or drug abuse should be evaluated most rigorously for adverse effects. *In view of the lack of information regarding teratogenic effects, these medications should be withheld from women who are pregnant.* Concurrent use of a monoamine oxidase inhibitor with other drugs is contraindicated because of the vast number of possible drug interactions (see above and Table 67).

Administration

Nurses who administer a monoamine oxidase inhibitor to an individual should remain with the patient until they are certain that the medication has been swallowed. This will prevent suicide attempts later using hoarded medication. Nurses should also assist ambulation or use side rails, particularly at the beginning of therapy, when this is indicated.

Evaluation

Evaluation of the therapeutic effectiveness of MAOIs is accomplished using the same criteria previously described for heterocyclic antidepressants.

Nurses caring for patients receiving these medications should be alert for evidence of adverse effects. Changes in standing or lying blood pressure, in association with dizziness on standing, indicate orthostatic hypotension. Elevated blood pressure in combination with headache and palpitations suggests hypertensive crisis. An alteration in the fluid intake/output ratio, weight gain and peripheral edema reflect either cardiovascular or renal consequences. Nursing observations of mental status and mood that reveal exaggerated feelings and/or ideas or excessive activity are symptomatic of hypomania. Hepatotoxicity is indicated by nursing observations of rash, pruritus, abdominal pain, yellowing of skin or sclera, tea-colored urine and/or clay-colored stools.

Teaching

Patient teaching in relation to self-administration of MAOIs should stress the importance of looking for evidence of drug efficacy and adverse effects.

The severe consequences of concomitant ingestion of a monoamine oxidase inhibitor and tyramine-containing foods should be emphasized. Patients and their families must be supplied with a list of foods to be avoided. These include beer, broad beans, cheese, wine, chicken liver, coffee, tea, cola drinks, figs, licorice, pickled herring, yogurt and chocolate.

Other aspects of patient teaching are the same as outlined previously for heterocyclic antidepressants.

Further Reading

Baldessarini, R.J. (1989). Current status of antidepressants. Clinical pharmacology and therapy. *J. Clin. Psychiatry 50* :117-126.

Drugs for psychiatric disorders (1991). *The Medical Letter 33* :43-50.

Drugs for psychiatric disorders (1989). Drugs of choice. *The Medical Letter 31* :13-20 and 32-45.

Food interacting with MAO inhibitors (1989). *The Medical Letter 31* :11-12.

Pollock, B.G. and Perel, J.M. (1989). Tricyclic antidepressants: Contemporary issues for therapeutic practice. *Can. J. Psychiatry 34* :609-617.

Problems when withdrawing (1986). *Drug and Therapeutics Bulletin 24* (8):29-30.

Table 67
Antidepressant drugs.

Pharmacologic Classification: Heterocyclic Antidepressants

Generic Name (Trade Name)	Use (Dose)	Action	Adverse Effects	Drug Interactions	Nursing Process
Amitriptyline HCl (Elavil, Endep)	Tx of major depress'n w. melancholia, or major depress'n w. psychotic manifestat'ns. Heterocyclic antidepressants can be used in major depress'n assoc. w. organic disease, depressive phase of bipolar affective disorder [manic-depressive psychosis] and major depress'ns assoc. w. dementia [Alzheimer's or multi-infarct demential, schizophrenia, alcoholism, mental deficiency **(Oral:** Initially, 25 mg tid; incr. prn to 150 mg/day. Elderly and adolescent pts - 10 mg tid w. 20 mg hs may be satisfactory. *For enuresis -* Children under 6 years - 10 mg)	Although heterocyclic antidepressants are known to affect norepinephrine, 5-hydroxytryptamine or dopamine-secreting neurons, their mechanisms of action are unclear. Some heterocyclics reduce neuronal reuptake of norepinephrine and/or 5-HT, thereby increasing their concentrat'ns around receptors, leading to speculat'n that these drugs work by blocking neurotransmitter reuptake. However, not all heterocyclics reduce neuronal reuptake. Regardless of their mechanisms of action, heterocyclic antidepressants are used to treat major depress'n, and are most effective in pts suffering from more severe depress'n, particularly w. greater vegetative disturbance and melancholia. Heterocyclic antidepressants also block cholinergic	*Anticholinergic and alpha-adrenergic blocking activities -* Flushing, diaphoresis, dryness of mouth, blurred vision, constipat'n, tachycardia, hypotens'n. Refer to Table 66 for descript'n of sedative and anticholinergic properties of indiv. heterocyclic antidepressants. *Other adv. effects* - Allergic skin react'ns and photosensitivity; agranulocytosis, cholestatic jaundice, leukopenia, leukocytosis, eosinophilia and thrombocytopenia; fine tremor, speech blockage, anxiety, insomnia. Incr. risk of suicide has been reported.	**Alcohol:** Plus a heterocyclic antidepressant, may produce greater than expected CNS depress'n and impairment in psychomotor skills. **Amphetamines:** Release norepinephrine and have enhanced effect in pts taking heterocyclic antidepressants. **Anticholinergics:** May show incr. effects, such as hyperpyrexia and paralytic ileus, in presence of heterocyclic antidepressant. **Antihistamines:** May show enhanced CNS depress'n in presence of heterocyclic antidepressant. **Antipsychotics:** May show enhanced CNS depress'n in presence of heterocyclic antidepressant. **Barbiturates:** May potentiate CNS-depressant effects of heterocyclic antidepressants. Chronic use of barbiturates, particularly phenobarbitol, may stim. metabolism of heterocyclic antidepressants. **Benzodiazepines:** May show enhanced effects in presence of heterocyclic antidepressants w. pronounced sedative properties, such as amitriptyline. **Clonidine:** Plus desipramine, may incr. BP. **Epinephrine, norepinephrine:** Given by IV infus'n to subjects	**Assess:** For hx liver disease, urinary retent'n, CV disease, glaucoma, suicidal tendencies, epilepsy, hyperthyroidism; for pregnancy or lactat'n; for concurrent use of alcohol or other medicat'ns. Establish baseline measures of standing/lying BP, radial/apical pulses, fluid intake/output ratios; document pre-tx bowel habits, weight, sleep pattern, manifestat'ns of depress'n. **Administer:** W. care to ensure that drug is swallowed, esp. w. suicide risk. Store in tight container at room temp. Give w. food or milk to reduce GI effects. Give hs if oversedated during day, but do this cautiously in elderly. Have gum, candy, sips of water available for dry mouth. **Evaluate:** Effectiveness as indicated by incr. response to environment, greater attent'n to personal appearance, more physical activity, change in eating and sleep patterns, incr. frequency of positive interpersonal interact'ns; for such adv. effects as allergic dermatitis (rash, itching), sore throat, fever, weakness, purpura, abd. pain, nausea, yellowing of skin or sclera, tea-colored urine, clay-colored stools, change in standing/lying BP. (Assist ambulat'n or use side rails prn.) For change in apical/radial pulses (rate, rhythm, quality), change in fluid intake/output ratio, abd. distent'n, change in frequency and/or characteristics of BMs, altered sleep pattern, weight gain, presence of gynecomastia, testicular swelling, galac-
Amoxapine (Asendin)	As for amitriptyline **(Oral:** Adults - Initially, 50 mg bid. Incr. to 50 mg tid prn as early as 3rd day of tx. In severely depressed, hospitalized pts or pts under close medical supervis'n, 50 mg tid may be used; this can be incr. to 100 mg bid-tid. Once effective dose is established, total daily dose may be given in single dose [not to exceed 300 mg]. Elderly/debilitated pts - Initially, 12.5 mg tid; incr. gradually prn to 50 mg bid-tid)				

Drug	Dosage	Adverse Effects	Drug Interactions	Nursing Considerations
Clomipramine HCl (Anafranil)	As for amitriptyline (**Oral:** Adults - Initially, 25 mg tid; incr. to 150 mg/day or more prn. Elderly/debilitated - Initially, 20-30 mg/day in divided doses, w. very gradual increments, depending on tolerance and response)	(muscarinic) receptors and may sedate pt. These drugs can have marked effects on CV system, resulting in orthostatic hypotens'n and incr. risk of tachycardia and/or cardiac arrhythmias.	receiving imipramine, can result in 2- to 4-fold incr. in pressor response. These drugs should be used only w. great caution in pts receiving heterocyclic antidepressants. **Guanethidine:** Has reduced antihypertensive effect in presence of heterocyclic antidepressants because heterocyclic agents inhibit uptake of guanethidine into adrenergic neurons. **Lithium carbonate:** And a heterocyclic antidepressant can produce hyperpyrexia. **MAOIs:** Are us.contraindicated w. heterocyclic antidepressants. Hyperpyretic crises or severe convulsive seizures may occur in pts when such drugs are combined. Potentiat'n of adv. effects can be serious or even fatal. **Narcotics:** May show enhanced CNS-depressant effects in presence of heterocyclic antidepressants w. pronounced sedative properties, such as amitriptyline.	torrhea, glucosuria, acetonuria; for suicidal tendencies. **Teach:** Self-evaluat'n for drug efficacy and adv. effects; that tx effectiveness requires several weeks; to change posit'n gradually; to lie down immediately if dizziness occurs; to use power tools, industrial machinery and motor vehicles w. caution; to keep adequate supplies of medicat'n on hand; to rinse mouth, maintain high fluid intake and practise good oral hygiene; *not* to take other drugs or consume alcohol during tx; that adv. effects are reversible when tx is completed and drug discontinued. Advise use of sun shade and sunscreen prn.
Desipramine HCl (Norpramin, Pertofrane)	As for amitriptyline (**Oral:** Adults - Initially, 25 mg tid; incr. gradually prn to 150 mg/day. Elderly/adolescents - Initially, 25-50 mg/day in divided doses, w. very gradual increments prn)	As for amitriptyline HCl	As for amitriptyline HCl	As for amitriptyline HCl
Doxepin (Adapin, Sinequan)	As for amitriptyline (**Oral:** Adults - Initially, 25 mg tid; incr. prn to 150 mg/day. Elderly/adolescents - 25-50 mg/day; incr. to 100 mg/day in divided doses)	As for amitriptyline HCl	As for amitriptyline HCl	As for amitriptyline HCl
Fluoxetine (Prozac)	As for amitriptyline (**Oral:** Adults - Initially, 20 mg od in a.m.; incr. gradually only after trial period of several weeks prn. Max. dose, 80 mg/day. Elderly and pts w. renal and/or hepatic impairment - A lower or less frequent dose is recommended)	As for amitriptyline HCl	As for amitriptyline HCl	As for amitriptyline HCl
Fluvoxamine maleate (Luvox)	As for amitriptyline (**Oral:** Adults - Initially, 100 mg od hs. Effective daily dose is us. bet. 100-200 mg. Adjust gradually in 50-mg increments to indiv. needs. Max. daily dose, 300 mg. Doses > 150 mg/day should be divided so that a max. of 150 mg is given hs)	As for amitriptyline HCl	As for amitriptyline HCl	As for amitriptyline HCl

Generic Name (Trade Name)	Use (Dose)	Action	Adverse Effects	Drug Interactions	Nursing Process
Imipramine (Janimine, Tofranil)	As for amitriptyline (**Oral:** Adults - Initially, 25 mg tid; incr. prn to 150 mg/day. Elderly/adolescents - Initially, 30-40 mg/day; incr. by 10 mg/day to a max. of 100 mg/day in divided doses. *For enuresis* - Children 5-15 years - 10-25 mg/day; incr. to 75 mg/day prn in children over 12)	As for amitriptyline HCl	As for amitriptyline HCl	As for amitriptyline HCl	As for amitriptyline HCl
Maprotiline (Ludiomil)	As for amitriptyline (**Oral:** Adults - Initially, 75 mg/day in 2-3 divided doses. After 2 weeks, incr. gradually in 25-mg increments prn. Max. outpatient dose - 150 mg. Elderly/debilitated - Initially, 10 mg tid, w. very gradual increments prn to 75 mg/day in divided doses)	As for amitriptyline HCl	As for amitriptyline HCl	As for amitriptyline HCl	As for amitriptyline HCl
Nortriptyline HCl (Aventyl, Pamelor)	As for amitriptyline (**Oral:** Adults - 30-100 mg/day in divided doses. Children - 10-75 mg/day in divided doses. Elderly - 10 mg tid-qid)	As for amitriptyline HCl	As for amitriptyline HCl	As for amitriptyline HCl	As for amitriptyline HCl
Protriptyline HCl (Triptil, Vivactil)	As for amitriptyline (**Oral:** Ambulatory pts - 15-30 mg/day in divided doses. Hospitalized pts - 30-60 mg/day in divided doses. Elderly/adolescents - Initially, 10-15 mg/day in 1-2 divided doses; incr. gradually prn. Monitor CV system closely in elderly if dose > 20 mg/day)	As for amitriptyline HCl	As for amitriptyline HCl	As for amitriptyline HCl	As for amitriptyline HCl
Trazadone HCl (Desyrel)	As for amitriptyline (**Oral:** Adults - Initially, 150-200 mg/day in 2-3 divided doses; incr. gradually prn by incre-	As for amitriptyline HCl	As for amitriptyline HCl	As for amitriptyline HCl	As for amitriptyline HCl

Drug	Use / Dosage	Action	Adverse Effects	Drug Interactions	Nursing Implications
(…ments of 50 mg, us. to 300 mg/day in divided doses. Elderly - Do not exceed 50% recomm. adult dose) **Trimipramine maleate (Surmontil)**	As for amitriptyline (**Oral:** Adults - Initially, 75 mg/day in 2-3 divided doses; incr. gradually to 150 mg/day. Elderly - Give test dose of 12.5-25 mg and after 45 min examine pt sitting and standing for orthostatic hypotens'n. Initial dose should be not > 50 mg/day in divided doses, w. weekly increments of not > 25 mg/week, leading to a us. dose range of 60-150 mg/day)	As for amitriptyline HCl	As for amitriptyline HCl	As for amitriptyline HCl	As for amitriptyline HCl

Pharmacologic Classification: Monoamine Oxidase Inhibitors (MAOIs)

Drug	Use / Dosage	Action	Adverse Effects	Drug Interactions	Nursing Implications
Phenelzine sulfate (Nardil)	Symptomatic tx of moderate to severe depress'n, particularly major depress'n assoc. w. high level of anxiety; panic disorder; and atypical depress'n w. hypersomnolence, lack of energy, and incr. appetite. These drugs are less effective in tx of major depress'n w. melancholia and psychotic depress'n. They may also serve a useful purpose in tx of panic disorder without major evidence of depress'n (**Oral:** Adults - Initially, 15 mg tid. If no response seen after 2 weeks, and in absence of adv. effects, dose may be incr. to 75 mg/day. After max. benefit is attained [4-6 weeks], reduce dose gradually over several weeks. Maint. dose may be as low as 15 mg/day or every other day)	Monoamine oxidase is an enzyme that inactivates norepinephrine, dopamine and 5-HT in the brain. One theory holds that MAOIs relieve depress'n by increasing brain levels of these neurotransmitters. MAOIs are used as 2nd-line drugs to heterocyclics for tx of endogenous depress'n. Heterocyclics are us. more effective and less toxic. In pts being transferred to an MAOI from a heterocyclic, allow a medicat'n-free interval of at least 1 week, then initiate the MAOI using half the normal dose for at least 1st week of tx.	Restlessness, insomnia, weakness, drowsiness, episodes of dizziness, dry mouth, nausea, diarrhea or consti-pat'n, abd. pain, tachycardia, anorexia, edema, palpitat'ns, blurred vision, chills, urinary retent'n, sweating, impotence, tinnitus, muscle spasm and tremors, paresthesias, skin rash, mild jaundice and habituat'n, serious hypertensive crises, overstimulat'n resulting in incr. activity, agitat'n and manic symptoms.	**Antidepressants, heterocyclic:** Refer to Actions of MAOIs and Drug Interactions for heterocyclics, both in this table. **Antidiabetic agents:** Can have enhanced or prolonged hypoglycemic actions in presence of an MAOI. This interact'n applies to both insulin and oral hypoglycemics. **Barbiturates:** May have their metabolism reduced by MAOIs. **CNS depressants** (e.g., morphine, meperidine, barbiturates, alcohol): Can have their effects potentiated by MAOIs. **Doxapram:** Can have its adv. CV effects (hypertens'n, arrhythmias) potentiated by MAOIs. **Food:** May interfere w. MAOI action; see discuss'n in Chapter 45. **Meperidine:** Plus an MAOI, may lead to excitat'n, sweating, rigidity and hypertens'n. Some pts may develop hypotens'n and	**Assess:** Pt hx for hyperthyroidism, CV or cerebrovascular disease, hepatic or renal impairment, hypertens'n, glaucoma, alcohol or drug abuse; for pregnancy or lactat'n; for use of alcohol or other drugs. Establish baseline measures of standing/lying BP. **Administer:** W. caution. Assist ambulat'n and use side rails prn, particularly at beginning of tx. **Evaluate:** Tx effectiveness as for heterocyclic antidepressants; for s/s adv. effects, such as changes in BP, dizziness, headache, palpitat'ns, fluid intake/output ratio, weight gain, peripheral edema, exaggerat'n of feelings, ideas or activity; rash, abd. pain, pruritus, yellowing of skin and sclera. **Teach:** Self-evaluat'n for drug efficacy and adv. effects; imp. of tyramine-free diet. Foods high in tyramine. Avoidance of exert'n; as for heterocyclic antidepressants.

Generic Name (Trade Name)	Use (Dose)	Action	Adverse Effects	Drug Interactions	Nursing Process
Tranylcypromine (Parnate)	As for phenelzine (**Oral:** Adults - 10 mg bid [morning and afternoon]. If no response in 2-3 weeks, incr. to 30 mg/day, 20 mg on arising and 10 mg in afternoon. Continue for at least 1 week. If no improvement, continued administrat'n is unlikely to help)	As for phenelzine sulfate	As for phenelzine sulfate	coma. Concomitant use of meperidine should be avoided. **Phenothiazines:** May have additive hypotensive effects when administered w. an MAOI. **Reserpine:** Given subsequently to an MAOI, can cause excitat'n and hypertens'n. **Succinylcholine:** May have prolonged effects in presence of phenelzine because the MAOI may decr. plasma levels of pseudocholinesterase, the enzyme responsible for inactivating succinylcholine. **Sympathomimetics:** Must not be used concomitantly w. an MAOI because combined use may cause severe hypertensive react'ns.	As for phenelzine sulfate

CHAPTER 46

Anxiolytics, Sedatives and Hypnotics

Teaching Objectives

Following completion of this chapter, the reader should be able to:

1. Define the terms anxiolytic, sedative and hypnotic.
2. Discuss the mechanism of action, pharmacologic effects, pharmacokinetics, therapeutic uses and adverse effects of the benzodiazepines, and the nursing process related to their use.
3. Describe the mechanism of action, pharmacologic effects, therapeutic uses and adverse effects of buspirone, and the nursing process related to its use.
4. Discuss the mechanism of action, pharmacologic effects, therapeutic uses and adverse effects of zopiclone, as well as the nursing process associated with its administration.
5. Describe the mechanism of action, pharmacologic effects, pharmacokinetics, therapeutic uses and adverse effects of the barbiturates, as well as the nursing process related to their use.
6. Discuss briefly the actions and uses of chloral hydrate.

Thirty years ago the expression anxiolytic, or minor tranquilizer, was unknown. Brain depressants were called either sedatives or hypnotics. A sedative was generally agreed to be a drug that calmed the patient and allayed anxiety. A hypnotic produced greater brain depression and was used to induce sleep in the patient suffering from insomnia. It is important to recognize that there is nothing qualitatively different in the actions of sedatives and hypnotics. They differ only in the quantitative sense. Often, sedative drugs were given in large doses when it was desired to produce a hypnotic effect.

In the late 1950s the so-called minor tranquilizers made their appearance in North America. Touted as being able to reduce our emotional reactions to pressure situations, they became popular very quickly. Soon the term sedative began to slip into the background and the expressions tranquilizer and anxiolytic became fashionable. It became most unpopular to consider giving a patient a drug that would "depress" the brain when one could use a tranquilizer that would, at least in the mind of the public, excommunicate that part of the brain responsible for emotion. Over the years the fallacy of this concept has become very evident. "Tranquilization" occurs only because brain function is depressed. Like the earlier sedative drugs, tranquilizers in higher doses can be used to produce sleep. When used this way, they are called hypnotics.

The Benzodiazepines

The introduction of chlordiazepoxide (Librium) in 1960 for the treatment of anxiety was the answer to a marketing man's dream (particularly if he worked for Hoffman-LaRoche, the drug company that first marketed it). Here for the first time was a drug that reduced anxiety without sedating the patient — or at least, that was the public's view of the drug. Chlordiazepoxide was soon followed by diazepam and oxazepam, and the race was on. It is almost impossible to keep track of all the benzodiazepines available for consumption at the present time. Some are marketed in lower doses for their antianxiety effects, and others in higher doses as hypnotics. They do offer some definite advantages over barbiturates. In contrast to barbiturates, benzodiazepines in lower doses may offer some antianxiety benefits without producing significant sedation. Taken in overdoses, they are much safer than barbiturates. Death is rare if a patient takes an overdose of a benzodiazepine. This contrasts with the acute toxicity of barbiturates. Both barbiturates and benzodiazepines can, on chronic administration, produce psychological and physical dependence. However, dependence is greater and the withdrawal effects far more severe with barbiturate use.

Mechanism of Action and Pharmacologic Effects

Benzodiazepines modify behavior. Regardless of what else is said to camouflage this point, nurses must never lose sight of the fact that the patient encased in a benzodiazepine bubble is not a normal individual — at least, not in the behavioral sense.

Benzodiazepines reduce anxiety by depressing the limbic system. The limbic system, composed of the septal region, the amygdala, the hippocampus and the hypothalamus, plays an important role in the emotional and autonomic responses to situations. The hypnotic effects of benzodiazepines can be attributed to depression of the limbic, neocortical and mesencephalic systems.

Diazepam is often used as a skeletal muscle relaxant in the injured athlete or the driver who has suffered whiplash. It has been contended that this action is due to an inhibition of brain stem and spinal cord function. However, it is also possible that patients fare better on the drug because they are sedated and do not move the damaged muscles.

The biochemical basis of these actions is still unclear. It is suggested that they calm the patient, relax skeletal muscles, and in high doses produce sleep by potentiating the actions of the inhibitory brain transmitter gamma-aminobutyric acid (GABA).

Pharmacokinetics

Benzodiazepines are absorbed rapidly. Their half-lives range from two to three hours, for triazolam, to approximately fifty to one hundred hours, for diazepam (Valium) and flurazepam (Dalmane) (Table 68). Chlordiazepoxide (Librium), ketazolam (Loftran) and diazepam are active in their own right and are also metabolized to active compounds. The half-lives given for these drugs take into account the durations of action of both the metabolites and the parent compounds. Flurazepam is rapidly converted to an active metabolite with a long half-life. Clorazepate is inactive. In stomach acid, it is converted to desmethyldiazepam, which is responsible for the effects produced by clorazepate.

Because benzodiazepines are often prescribed for lengthy periods of time, their long-term pharmacokinetic characteristics are important. When a drug is taken chronically, approximately five half-lives are required from the time of the first dose for concentrations of the drug in the body to reach steady state. Therefore, drugs with long half-lives, such as diazepam, require two to three weeks before they reach plateau levels, and patients may not experience the full effects of these drugs until treatment has continued for two to three weeks. Benzodiazepines with shorter half-lives, such as oxazepam, reach plateau concentrations within one to three days; for these agents, maximum effects are seen shortly after treatment is started.

Once a drug is stopped, it is eliminated from the body in relation to its half-life. Thus, the effects of chronic diazepam treatment last long after the drug is stopped. Lorazepam has a half-life of twelve to fifteen hours. Its effects disappear faster than those of diazepam, once treatment is stopped. The rapid elimination of a benzodiazepine from the body following prolonged treatment can be a mixed blessing. Although the patient may not be bothered with the "hangover" effects of the drug, rapid elimination of the benzodiazepine often causes rebound excitation and a request for another prescription. Patients on shorter-acting benzodiazepines are thus more likely to become dependent on the drugs (see Tolerance and Dependence, later in this chapter).

There is considerable misunderstanding of the importance of half-life to duration of benzodiazepine action. The relationship of drug half-life to the termination of drug effects, following single or

Table 68
Properties of some benzodiazepines.

Generic Name (Trade Name)	Usual Dose[1]	Peak Time of Effect (Hours)	Biologic Half-life (Hours)	Therapeutic Use(s)[3]
Triazolam (Halcion)	0.25-0.5 mg	2	2 – 3	Hypnotic
Oxazepam (Serax)	30-120 mg/day in divided doses	1 – 4	4 – 13	Anxiolytic
Temazepam (Restoril)	30 mg hs	0.8 – 1.4	8 – 10	Hypnotic
Bromazepam (Lectopam)	6-30 mg/day in divided doses	1 – 4	12	Anxiolytic
Alprazolam (Xanax)	0.25 mg bid-tid; incr. prn in 0.25-mg increments	1 – 2	6 – 20	Anxiolytic
Lorazepam (Ativan)	2 mg/day in 2-3 divided doses	1 – 6	12 – 15	Anxiolytic
Chlordiazepoxide (Librium)	10-40 mg/day in divided doses	2 – 4	20 – 24 [2]	Anxiolytic
Nitrazepam (Mogadon)	5-10 mg hs	2	26	Hypnotic
Clorazepate (Tranxene)	30 mg/day in divided doses	1 – 2	48 [2]	Anxiolytic
Ketazolam (Loftran)	15 mg od-bid; later, total daily dose can be given hs	?	50 [2]	Anxiolytic
Diazepam (Valium)	4-40 mg/day in divided doses	1.5 – 2	50 – 100 [2]	Anxiolytic
Flurazepam (Dalmane)	15 or 30 mg hs	1	50 – 100 [2]	Hypnotic

[1] Refers to usual adult dosage. Dosage for elderly or debilitated pts should be halved.
[2] Refers to half-life of drug plus active metabolites.
[3] Refers to anxiolytic and hypnotic uses only.

repeat doses, is best illustrated by referring to the two hypnotics triazolam and flurazepam. Triazolam has a much shorter half-life than the active metabolite of flurazepam. However, this does not mean that triazolam, given once or twice, has a shorter duration of action than flurazepam. During the initial nights of therapy with either drug, diffusion out of the brain and into other body tissues, not rate of elimination from the body, is the major factor responsible for terminating drug effect. As a result, flurazepam's duration of action is considerably shorter at this time than would be predicted on the basis of the long half-life of its active metabolite.

There is, however, a finite capacity for tissues to take up a drug like the active metabolite of flurazepam and remove it from the brain. The more frequently the drug is given, the less able are these tissues to take up more of subsequent doses. When this happens, diffusion out of the brain and into other body tissues stops being a major factor in terminating drug effect. At this point, the removal of flurazepam's active metabolite from the brain depends on its metabolism and elimination from the body. Now, if we compare flurazepam and triazolam, their respective rates of inactivation become progressively more important in determining duration of action. As a result, during chronic treatment, flurazepam has a long duration of action and triazolam short-term effects. Patients taking flurazepam night after night may experience daytime hangover, as significant residual concentrations remain in the brain during waking hours. If triazolam is taken on a nightly basis, its concentration in the brain during the day should be low and hangover should not be a problem. The other side of the coin is that patients may awaken in the early hours of the morning when the concentration of triazolam in the brain falls below the hypnotic level.

Half-life should also be considered when benzodiazepines are used as antianxiety drugs. The advantage of a benzodiazepine such as oxazepam

(Serax), which has a relatively short half-life, is minimal hangover once the drug is stopped. However, drugs with shorter half-lives should be given several times a day to ensure adequate concentrations in the brain. Long-acting drugs, such as diazepam, produce more sustained blood levels. Although divided doses are recommended, diazepam can be taken once daily at bedtime. If patients follow this regimen, they should sleep well during the night and benefit from the antianxiety actions of the drug throughout the day. The disadvantage of longer-acting antianxiety drugs is a more prolonged hangover when they are stopped.

The decision to sell a benzodiazepine either as an anxiolytic or a hypnotic is in many cases a marketing one. Obviously, it would make little sense to sell a lower dose of triazolam as an anxiolytic. With a half-life of two to three hours, it would be necessary to take many doses each day. However, oxazepam and temazepam have half-lives similar to each other. Oxazepam is sold mainly for the treatment of anxiety and temazepam as a hypnotic. It would have made just as much sense to reverse the indications and use a lower dose of temazepam, three times daily, as an anxiolytic. Likewise, diazepam and flurazepam are very similar drugs. Presumably Hoffman-LaRoche could have marketed a lower dose of flurazepam as a daytime anxiolytic. However, at the time they introduced this drug Roche already had diazepam on the market. It would have made no sense to have diazepam and flurazepam compete for the same market. Therefore, flurazepam was packaged in hypnotic strengths and sold for the treatment of insomnia.

Tolerance and Dependence

Tolerance is not uncommon with benzodiazepines. This is recognized by the need for increased doses to obtain the same pharmacologic effect. In addition, concern is mounting about the dependence liability of benzodiazepines, especially those with short half-lives. These drugs are more likely to leave the patient with rebound insomnia once the drug is discontinued. The danger of inducing drug dependence by yielding to requests for repeat prescriptions is obvious. It would be well to remember that under normal circumstances hypnotic drugs should not be used for more than fourteen to twenty-one nights consecutively. Patients also should be told to expect a few nights of relatively poor sleep once drug treatment is stopped. This is the price that must be paid for earlier drug-induced hypnosis.

Dependence can also be a problem with antianxiety drugs, particularly those with shorter half-lives. Once therapy is discontinued with one of these drugs, the patient may experience daytime anxiety and return to the physician for a repeat prescription.

Therapeutic Uses

Anxiety disorders, including panic and generalized anxiety disorders, are the main indications for benzodiazepine use. They may also be utilized for brief periods in stress-related conditions, but this must be done with some caution. A nonpharmacologic technique should be tried first. It should be emphasized that the use of a "benzodiazepine crutch" to allay anxiety should be employed for short periods of time only.

Alprazolam (Xanax) and bromazepam (Lectopam) are second-generation benzodiazepines, claimed by some to provide better antianxiety effects with minimal sedation. Alprazolam is indicated for the short-term symptomatic relief of excessive anxiety in patients with anxiety neurosis. The indications for bromazepam are for short-term, symptomatic relief of manifestations of excessive anxiety in patients with anxiety neurosis.

Insomnia is the second major use for benzodiazepines. The relative merits of short- and long-acting drugs have been discussed. Ideally, a hypnotic should produce sleep quickly and have no hangover effects the next day. The perfect hypnotic benzodiazepine has yet to be developed. Nitrazepam and flurazepam are long-acting and may produce daytime hangover. Temazepam is an effective hypnotic with a half-life of eight to ten hours. Triazolam works quickly and is less likely to produce morning hangover, but with a half-life of two to three hours may allow the patient to awaken after just a few hours of sleep.

It is well to reiterate that hypnotics should not be used for more than fourteen to twenty-one days. To ignore this is to predispose the patient to the danger of drug dependence, as discussed earlier. Upon withdrawal there may be periods of rebound insomnia. This is to be expected. If one depresses the central nervous system night after night with any drug, rebound excitation is usually seen once the agent is withdrawn. As mentioned before, this effect is more prevalent with short-acting drugs. For example, if flurazepam is administered on a regular basis, the body stores active metabolites. Once flurazepam treatment is stopped, the active metabolites leave their storage sites and enter the brain in ever-decreasing amounts over a period of several days or even weeks. In this way the patient is weaned off the medication and rebound insomnia is not so prevalent. On the other hand, daytime sedation may continue for a week or more.

Benzodiazepines can be used to reduce the central nervous system excitation that accompanies acute alcohol withdrawal. Once the patient is stabilized on the benzodiazepine, its dose can be reduced gradually and normal neuronal activity allowed to return slowly. Diazepam has been used for this purpose. Other benzodiazepines may also be appropriate.

Adverse Effects

Central nervous system depression is the major adverse reaction of benzodiazepines. Patients complain of fatigue, drowsiness and a feeling of detachment. Elderly patients are particularly prone to headache, dizziness, ataxia, confusion and disorientation.

Benzodiazepine use may also cause psychological impairment. This may be difficult to diagnose in the anxious patient because anxiety itself interferes with psychological performance. Relieving anxiety with a benzodiazepine may improve function and more than offset any direct action of the drug. Hostility is reported after benzodiazepine use.

Although overdosage is common with benzodiazepines, few patients die. Unless consumed with another central nervous system depressant such as alcohol, a barbiturate, a tricyclic antidepressant or a narcotic, benzodiazepines rarely kill. In this regard they are much safer than barbiturates or other hypnotics.

The problems of benzodiazepine dependence have been described but warrant repeating. Psychological dependence is probably common with benzodiazepines, as evidenced by the continuing demand for repeat prescriptions. Physiological dependence is characterized by anxiety, agitation, restlessness, insomnia and tension following drug withdrawal. Although the symptoms of withdrawal are not as severe as those following cessation of alcohol or a barbiturate, one should not be deceived into believing that benzodiazepines do not produce physical dependence.

Nursing Process

Regardless of the benzodiazepine prescribed, the implications for nursing care are identical.

Assessment

The nursing process begins with the assessment of the patient's history for evidence of previous hypersensitivity to benzodiazepines, or a history of allergies or asthma, which suggest a tendency to hypersensitivity reactions. If present, these conditions indicate a need for particularly rigorous nursing evaluation following drug administration. Benzodiazepines should be withheld from patients who have a history of glaucoma because of their potential to affect adversely the autonomic nervous system.

Nursing assessment should also stress the establishment of baseline measures of vital signs and blood pressure, both lying and standing, as objective physiological measures of anxiety. In addition, the patient's pretherapeutic fluid intake/output ratio should be noted as a means of determining later whether fluid retention occurs. The patient's employment and hobbies should also be considered. Those individuals who regularly work with power tools or industrial machinery, or who drive a car, must be thoroughly informed of the effects of the drugs.

Administration

Benzodiazapines should be given with food or milk to reduce gastrointestinal distress. Patients should also have hard candy or gum available to reduce the effects of dry mouth. Benzodiazepines are usually self-administered at home. Therein lies one of the greatest causes of concern. Benzodiazepine abuse by the public, which conceives of them as "harmless", has reached epidemic proportions. The societal ethos that anxiety and emotional stress are to be totally avoided has produced a large number of people who have failed to develop adequate mechanisms for coping with mild to moderate emotional stress or anxiety. These unhappy souls use benzodiazepines as a crutch in their daily lives. Nurses in physicians' offices should be alert for patients who believe that "pills will cure everything". These people are actual or potential benzodiazepine abusers.

Evaluation

Following administration of benzodiazepines, nursing evaluation should consider the patient's subjective reports of reduced anxiety. Objective observation of physiological responses suggestive of reduced anxiety, i.e., lower blood pressure, pulse rate and respirations, should also be made.

Nurses evaluating patients using benzodiazepines should be alert for the adverse effects outlined before. Patients who exhibit uncoordinated movements, slurred speech, jaundice, a rash, fever, altered level of consciousness or who report dizziness, falling, headache or sore throats should be considered to be suffering adverse effects from the medication. These observations should be immediately reported to the attending physician.

Teaching

Nurses should teach patients and families the criteria for determining benzodiazepine effectiveness and adverse effects. The patient's employment and hobbies should also be considered. Patients and families should be alerted to the dangers involved in driving cars or using machinery, as dizziness or drowsiness at the wrong time can result in injury or death for the patient and those around him. Patients should also be taught to move slowly from the reclining to the standing position to avoid dizziness. Nurses should caution patients to get assistance with ambulation and to use side rails at night as necessary.

Nurses should emphasize the synergistic action between alcohol and benzodiazepines. They should also caution the patient to avoid over-the-counter preparations unless approved by the physician. Under no circumstances should alcohol and a benzodiazepine be used concurrently. Patients should also be counseled that the abrupt termination of benzodiazepine use following prolonged administration can result in withdrawal effects. Finally, a warning should be given that these drugs produce dependency. Any benzodiazepine should be taken only in the amounts and at the times specified by the physician.

Buspirone (Buspar)

Mechanism of Action and Pharmacologic Effects

Buspirone is a psychotropic drug with antianxiety properties. It belongs chemically to the class of compounds known as azaspirodecanediones. Buspirone shares some of the properties of the benzodiazepines and neuroleptics but is devoid of anticonvulsant and muscle relaxant properties. The mechanism of action of buspirone remains to be fully elucidated. Buspirone does not bind to the benzodiazepine GABA-receptor complex.

Therapeutic Uses

Buspirone is indicated for the short-term symptomatic relief of excessive anxiety in patients with generalized anxiety disorder. Patients who have previously taken benzodiazepines may be less likely to respond to buspirone than those who have not. Interestingly, in controlled studies in healthy volunteers, single doses of buspirone up to 20 mg

had little effect on most tests of cognitive and psychomotor function, although performance on a vigilance task was impaired in a dose-related manner.

Adverse Effects

The most common adverse reactions encountered with buspirone are dizziness, headache, drowsiness and nausea. During premarketing clinical trials, approximately ten per cent of patients discontinued treatment due to an adverse event.

Nursing Process

The nursing process for buspirone is similar to the nursing care outlined for the benzodiazepine drugs previously presented in this chapter. The following precautions are to be added.

Assessment

Patients should be assessed for changes in mental status and mood, sleeping patterns, and for drowsiness and dizziness. Nurses should also check fluid intake and output for indications of renal dysfunction.

Evaluation

Nurses should evaluate patients for physical dependency and withdrawal symptoms, as well as for possible suicidal tendencies.

Teaching

Patients should be told that one to two weeks of therapy may be required before therapeutic effects are achieved.

Zopiclone (Imovane)

Mechanism of Action and Pharmacologic Effects

Zopiclone is a short-acting hypnotic. It belongs to a novel chemical class, the cyclopyrrolones, which is structurally unrelated to existing hypnotics. However, the pharmacologic profile of zopiclone is similar to that of the benzodiazepines.

Zopiclone is rapidly and well absorbed following oral administration. The drug is extensively metabolized and it has an elimination half-life of approximately five hours. In elderly subjects, the absolute bioavailability of zopiclone is increased from approximately seventy-seven per cent in young subjects to ninety-four per cent. The elimination half-life in elderly patients exceeds seven hours. In view of the fact that zopiclone is extensively metabolized in the liver, it is not surprising that its half-life is prolonged (nearly twelve hours) in patients with hepatic insufficiency.

Therapeutic Uses

Zopiclone is useful for the short-term management of insomnia characterized by difficulty in falling asleep, frequent nocturnal awakenings and/or early morning awakenings. As with all hypnotics, long-term continuous treatment is not recommended; a course of treatment should be no longer than four weeks in duration. Zopiclone is contraindicated in patients with myasthenia gravis or severe impairment of respiratory function, as well as those who have suffered acute cerebrovascular accidents.

Adverse Effects

The most common adverse reaction seen with zopiclone is a bitter taste. Severe drowsiness and impaired coordination are signs of drug intolerance or excessive doses. Patients may also experience somnolence, asthenia, dizziness, confusion, anterograde amnesia or memory impairment, feeling of drunkenness, euphoria, nightmares, agitation, anxiety or nervousness, hostility, depression, decreased libido, coordination abnormality, hypotonia, muscle spasm, paresthesia and speech disorder. These effects are completely consistent with a drug that depresses brain function, and can be expected with any of the medications discussed in this chapter.

Nursing Process

Zopiclone is a relatively new drug and nursing experience with it is limited. Readers are advised to consult information produced by the manufacturer and also to discuss the drug with the pharmacist for the latest information and clinical practice advice before administering this drug.

The Barbiturates

Barbiturates warrant only brief discussion. Many barbiturates remain on the market. However, with the exception of thiopental, used in anesthesia, and phenobarbital, administered for epilepsy, no justification can be found for their continued use. The availability of safer drugs (see previous discussion) for daytime sedation or nighttime hypnosis has made barbiturate use for these purposes inappropriate. Barbiturates are more toxic on acute overdosage and can produce severe drug dependence.

Mechanism of Action and Pharmacologic Effects

Barbiturates depress the central nervous system. By potentiating GABA-mediated inhibitory processes in the central nervous system, barbiturates exert muscle relaxant, anticonvulsant, sedative and hypnotic effects. Barbiturates also alter psychological functions. Psychomotor performance and complex tasks are most affected, especially those involving fine points of judgment. Increased doses lead to progressive impairment of brain function, culminating with respiratory failure.

Therapeutic Uses

Although amobarbital (Amytal), butabarbital sodium (Butisol), pentobarbital sodium (Nembutal) and secobarbital sodium (Seconal) are still prescribed by a few physicians, the availability of the safer benzodiazepines has removed any need for the continued use of barbiturates as sedatives or hypnotics.

Adverse Effects

Central nervous system depression is the major adverse effect of barbiturate use. Patients may experience drowsiness, confusion, wandering and perhaps even psychosis. Other signs of central nervous system depression include nystagmus, dysarthria and motor incoordination. The elderly are particularly at risk for ataxia and confusion. It is difficult to avoid many of these effects because satisfactory symptomatic control with barbiturates often requires oversedation.

Overdosage can cause respiratory failure. The concomitant use of a barbiturate with another central nervous system depressant, such as alcohol or a narcotic, compounds the problem. Treatment of overdosage is outlined below.

Paradoxic excitation is difficult to explain. It is not known why certain patients become restless, excited and may proceed to delirium when given a barbiturate. This is particularly prevalent in the elderly.

Psychological and physical dependence is a very serious problem with barbiturates, and withdrawal effects can be particularly severe.

Microsomal enzyme induction can occur following chronic barbiturate use. This is more likely to occur if phenobarbital is used. Stimulation of microsomal enzymes may mean that the durations of action and therapeutic effects of many drugs are reduced.

Nursing Process

The nursing process related to use of barbiturates is similar to that previously described for benzodiazepines.

Assessment

Nursing assessment prior to initial administration should begin with a review of the patient's history for evidence of previous sensitivity reactions or paradoxic excitation, chronic respiratory disease, hypotension, liver disease, blood dyscrasias, porphyria or thyroid disease. Nurses who discover documentation of any of these conditions should clarify the barbiturate order with the physician.

Physical assessment of the patient before the initial barbiturate dose should establish baseline measures of respiration and temperature for later use in determining the presence of adverse effects. Similarly, pretherapeutic descriptions of sleep patterns are essential. Physical assessment of patients prior to any administration of a barbiturate should emphasize identification of pain. Patients experiencing pain should be given a barbiturate only if it is administered with an analgesic. When barbiturates are given alone in acute and intense pain, patients frequently experience anxiety, restlessness and heightened awareness of, and response to, pain. In collaboration with the pharmacist, the current drug regimen should be reviewed for concurrent use of other medications that might react synergistically with the barbiturate.

Administration

When nurses are responsible for administering barbiturates to patients, they must do so in accordance with institutional policies and procedures developed in compliance with legal regulations governing the use of controlled substances (see Chapter 73). Nurses administering these drugs orally must be assured that the medication has been swallowed and not hoarded by the patient. Nurses should also remove cigarets and take necessary safety measure at bedtime as required.

Parenteral administration of barbiturates requires that the physician clearly specify the dosage and flow rate. Nurses must carefully monitor these to prevent accidental overdose. Accidental extravasation of an intravenous injection, while not life threatening, is serious because of the danger of necrosis accompanying interstitial subcutaneous administration.

Evaluation

Nursing evaluation of drug efficacy focuses on the purpose for which it was administered. Generally, its hypnotic or sedative effects are evaluated by noting relief from insomnia, anxiety or agitation. Patient requests for stronger prescriptions, or for more frequent administration of the barbiturate, in combination with complaints of decreased drug effectiveness suggest tolerance and drug dependency. They should be drawn to the physician's attention immediately.

Adverse effects resulting from central nervous system depression are suggested by nursing observations of drowsiness, confusion, psychoses, ataxia and confusion. Overdose or acute toxicity is manifested by extensive cortical and respiratory depression, shock (pallor, rapid and thready pulse, hypotension), hypothermia and stupor progressing to coma.

Teaching

Patient teaching should begin by instructing the individual to move slowly from the reclining to the standing position to prevent falling as a result of dizziness. If the patient taking barbiturates experiences dizziness or drowsiness while driving or using machinery, serious injury or death could result for the patient or innocent bystanders. Therefore, patients and their families should be strongly warned of the danger of performing these activities while taking barbiturates. Occupational health nurses in factories who are aware of workers taking barbiturates while operating machines should arrange for these patients to be assigned temporarily to another task or granted sick leave until their use of barbiturates is discontinued.

Patients and their families should be warned that the concomitant consumption of alcohol or other central nervous system depressants such as antihistamines or benzodiazepines is exceedingly dangerous and often fatal. Women taking oral contraceptives should be counseled to use other methods of birth control because the microsomal enzyme induction produced by barbiturates, particularly phenobarbital, can rarely reduce the efficacy of estrogens and progestins.

Patients should be instructed *not* to store the barbiturate at their bedside at home. Accidental overdose has occurred when patients have taken additional medication during the drowsiness of stage I sleep.

A responsible family member should be taught to observe for the symptoms of adverse effects. Both patient and family should be alerted to the dangers of barbiturate dependency. They should know that abrupt drug withdrawal following prolonged use can result in tremor, convulsions and delirium.

Chloral Hydrate (Noctec)

Chloral hydrate is available in capsule or elixir form. It works quickly and has a relatively short duration of action. Chloral hydrate is better suited for putting people to sleep rather than keeping them asleep. The drug is used often in pediatrics and geriatrics. The adverse effects of chloral hydrate include gastric irritation. It should be given with milk or water to reduce the possibility of nausea or vomiting. The therapeutic ratio of chloral hydrate is similar to that of barbiturates. If large doses are taken, death can occur as a result of respiratory depression.

Nursing Process
The nursing process is the same as the previous process outlined for barbiturates.

Further Reading
Baker, M.I. and Oleen, M.A. (1988). The use of benzodiazepine hypnotics in the elderly. *Pharmacotherapy 8* : 241-247.

Choice of benzodiazepines (1988). *The Medical Letter 30* :26-28. Drugs for psychiatric disorders (1991). *The Medical Letter 33* :43 -50.

Drugs for psychiatric disorders (1989). Drugs of choice. *The Medical Letter 31* :13-20 and 32-45.

Gillin, J.C. and Byerley, W.F. (1990). The diagnosis and management of insomnia. *New Engl. J. Med. 322* :239-248.

Hershey, L.A. (1988). Diagnosis and treatment of anxiety in the elderly. *Rational Drug Therapy 22* (3):1-6.

Hollister, L.E. (1986). Anxiety: Drug treatments for biologically determined disorders. *Rational Drug Therapy 20* (4):1-6.

Kales, A., Manfredi, R.L., Vgontzas, A. N., Bixler, E.O., Vela-Bueno, A. and Fee, E.C. (1991). Rebound insomnia after only brief and intermittent use of rapidly eliminated benzodiazepines. *Clinical Pharmacology and Therapeutics 49* :468-476.

Lader, M.H. (1987). Rational use of antianxiety drugs. *Rational Drug Therapy 21* (9):1-5.

Nicholson, A.N. (1986). Hypnotics. Their place in therapeutics. *Drugs 31* :164-176.

Oral hypnotic drugs (1989). *The Medical Letter 31* :23-24.

Sullivan, J.T. and Sellers, E.M. (1986). Treating alcohol, barbiturate and benzodiazepine withdrawal. *Rational Drug Therapy 20* (2):1-8.

Tiller, J.W.G. (1989). The new and newer antianxiety agents. *Med. J. Australia 151* :697-701.

Table 69
Anxiolytics, sedatives and hypnotics.

Pharmacologic Classification: Anxiolytic Benzodiazepines

Generic Name (Trade Name)	Use (Dose)	Action	Adverse Effects	Drug Interactions	Nursing Process
Alprazolam (Xanax)	*Gen'l indicat'ns for all anxiolytic benzodiazepines:* Tx of anxiety disorders, panic disorders, insomnia and delirium tremens rel. to alcohol w'drawal (**Oral:** Adults - 0.25-0.5 mg bid-tid. Elderly or debilitated pts - 0.125 mg bid-tid)	Benzodiazepines act on limbic system to reduce anxiety. They may exert their effects by potentiating actions of inhibitory neurotransmitter gamma-aminobutyric acid (GABA). Anxiety disorders, incl. panic and gen'l anxiety disorders, are the main indicat'ns for use of benzodiazepines. They may also be used w. caution for brief periods in stress-related condit'ns. Benzodiazepines can be used in tx of alcohol w'drawal syndrome. Diazepam is most often used for this purpose.	Drowsiness, ataxia, fatigue, dizziness, nausea, blurred vision, diplopia, vertigo, headache, slurred speech, tremors, hypoactivity, dysarthria, euphoria, impairment of memory, confus'n, depress'n, retrograde amnesia, rebound insomnia, leukopenia, jaundice, hypersensitivity and paradoxical react'ns.	**Antidepressants, heterocyclic:** Can potentiate actions of benzodiazepines. **Carbamazepine:** Can potentiate actions of benzodiazepines. **CNS depressants** (e.g., antipsychotics, anesthetics, barbiturates, hypnotics, narcotics): Have at least additive depressant effects on CNS w. benzodiazepines. Therefore, these agents should be used together w. caution. **Ethanol:** Has additive CNS-depressant effect w. benzodiazepines. Ethanol may also incr. absorpt'n of diazepam. Pts taking benzodiazepines should be warned against ingest'n of moderate to large am'ts of ethanol. **MAOIs:** May potentiate action of diazepam and us. should not be given concurrently.	**Assess:** For hx hypersensitivity to this drug; hx allergies/asthma, glaucoma; current pregnancy, lactat'n; employment involving machinery, power tools, driving. Establish baseline level of VS and standing/lying BP as objective measures of anxiety; note fluid intake/output levels. **Administer:** Us. self-administered at home. Give w. food or milk for GI symptoms. Have gum, candy available for dry mouth. **Evaluate:** Drug effectiveness (subjective reports of reduced anxiety; lower BP, pulse, respirat'ns); adv. effects (uncoordinated movements, slurred speech, dizziness or falling, headache, jaundice, rash, fever, sore throat, LOC, BP). **Teach:** Reliable family member to evaluate for adv. effects; to avoid power tools, industrial machinery and driving until dosage and pt response are stabilized; to move from reclining posit'n slowly, w. brief pause in sitting posit'n to avoid postural hypoten's'n; to get assistance w. ambulat'n, use side rails prn; to avoid use of alcohol; that abrupt terminat'n of use of this drug can result in w'drawal effects; that drug can produce dependency. Therefore, it should be taken in am't and at times specified. Caution pt to avoid OTC preparat'ns unless approved by physician.
Bromazepam (Lectopam)	As for alprazolam (**Oral:** Adults - 6-18 mg/day in equally divided doses. Max. dose, 30 mg/day. Elderly/debilitated - Initially, daily dose not > 3 mg, in divided doses)				As for alprazolam
Chlordiazepoxide (Librium)	As for alprazolam (**Oral:** Adults - 10-40 mg/day in divided doses. In severe cases, 25 mg tid-qid. Elderly/debilitated - 5 mg bid-qid. **IM:** *Acute anxiety -* Initially, 50-100 mg; then 25-50 mg tid-qid, prn. **IV/IM:** *Acute drug w'drawal -* Initially, 100 mg; then 50-100 mg q4-6h prn. Elderly/debilitated - Us. 25-50 mg. *Acute psychotic agitat'n -* Initially, 50-100 mg; repeat in 4-6 h prn. **IM:** *Preoperative anxiety -* 50-100 mg 1 h before surgery)		As for alprazolam	
Clorazepate dipotassium (Tranxene)	As for alprazolam (**Oral:** Adults - Us. 30 mg/day in divided doses. Elderly/debilitated -	As for alprazolam	As for alprazolam	As for alprazolam	As for alprazolam

Drug	Dosage				
	Initially, 3.75 mg od, preferably hs. Adjust carefully and gradually prn)	As for alprazolam	As for alprazolam	As for alprazolam	As for alprazolam
Diazepam (Valium)	As for alprazolam (**Oral:** Adults - For anxiety - 2-10 mg bid-qid. Elderly/debilitated [and those pts taking other CNS depressants] - Initially, 2-2.5 mg od-bid; incr. gradually prn. Children - Initially, 1-2.5 mg tid-qid; incr. gradually prn. Do not use in children < 6 months. **IV/IM:** *For severe anxiety or severe muscle spasm, spasticity, akathisia or tetanus* - Adults - Initially, 5-10 mg repeated in 3-4 h prn. Tetanus may need larger doses. Children - 0.04-0.2 mg/kg initially, repeated in 3-4 h prn. Max. dose, 0.6 mg/kg/8 h)	As for alprazolam	As for alprazolam	As for alprazolam	As for alprazolam
Halazepam (Paxipam)	As for alprazolam (**Oral:** Adults - 20-40 mg tid-qid. Elderly/ sensitive - 20 mg od-bid)	As for alprazolam	As for alprazolam	As for alprazolam	As for alprazolam
Ketazolam (Loftran)	As for alprazolam (**Oral:** Adults - 15 mg od-bid. Incr. should be made in 15-mg increments prn. Elderly/debilitated - 50% lowest adult dose)	As for alprazolam	As for alprazolam	As for alprazolam	As for alprazolam
Lorazepam (Ativan)	As for alprazolam (**Oral:** Adults - Initially, 2 mg/day in divided doses of 0.5 + 0.5 + 1 mg; or 1 mg + 1 mg. Adjust carefully by 0.5 mg prn. Elderly/debilitated - Initial dose not > 0.5 mg. Adjust carefully prn)	As for alprazolam	As for alprazolam	As for alprazolam	As for alprazolam
Oxazepam (Serax)	As for alprazolam (**Oral:** Adults - 30-120 mg daily in divided doses. Elderly/debilitated - 5 mg od-bid prn. Initiate tx at lower doses and incr. slowly prn as tolerated)	As for alprazolam	As for alprazolam	As for alprazolam	As for alprazolam

Generic Name (Trade Name)	Use (Dose)	Action	Adverse Effects	Drug Interactions	Nursing Process
Prazepam (Centrax)	As for alprazolam (**Oral:** Adults - Initially, 20 mg in single dose; incr. to 40-60 mg/day prn in divided am'ts or single dose, us. hs. Elderly/debilitated - 10-15 mg)	As for alprazolam	As for alprazolam	As for alprazolam	As for alprazolam

Pharmacologic Classification: Hypnotic Benzodiazepines

Generic Name (Trade Name)	Use (Dose)	Action	Adverse Effects	Drug Interactions	Nursing Process
Flurazepam (Dalmane)	*Gen'l indicat'ns for all hypnotic benzodiazepines:* Tx of insomnia, characterized by difficulty in falling asleep, frequent nocturnal awakenings and/or early a.m. awakenings. For short-term and intermittent use in pts w. recurring insomnia and poor sleeping habits. Safety of long-term use not established (**Oral:** Adults - 30 mg hs [some pts may find 15 mg adequate]. Elderly/debilitated - 15 mg hs)	Hypnotic actions of benzodiazepines can be attributed to depress'n of limbic, neocortical and mesencephalic reticular systems. Effect likely due to potenti-at'n of actions of inhibitory neurotransmitter GABA. Refer to Chapter 46 for discuss'n of relative merits of short/long half-life hypnotics.	Dizziness, drowsiness, lightheaded-ness, ataxia, severe sedat'n, lethargy, disorientat'n, depress'n, blurred vision, irritability, anterograde amnesia, rebound insomnia (particularly prevalent w. short-acting benzo-diazepines, e.g., triazolam)	As for anxiolytic benzodiazepines	As for anxiolytic benzodiazepines
Nitrazepam (Mogadon)	As for flurazepam (**Oral:** Adults - 5 or 10 mg hs. Elderly/debili-tated - Initially, 2.5 mg until response determined; doses > 5 mg not us. recommended)	As for flurazepam	As for flurazepam	As for anxiolytic benzodiazepines	As for anxiolytic benzodiazepines
Quazepam (Dormalin)	As for flurazepam (**Oral:** Adults - Initially, 15 mg until response determined. In some pts dose may be reduced to 7.5 mg. Elderly/debilitated - Attempt to reduce dose)	As for flurazepam	As for flurazepam	As for anxiolytic benzodiazepines	As for anxiolytic benzodiazepines
Temazepam (Restoril)	As for flurazepam (**Oral:** Adults - 30 mg hs. In some pts 15 mg may be adequate. Elderly/debili-tated - 15 mg hs)	As for flurazepam	As for flurazepam	As for anxiolytic benzodiazepines	As for anxiolytic benzodiazepines

Drug	Indications / Dose	Action	Side/Adverse Effects	Interactions	Nursing Considerations
Triazolam (Halcion)	As for flurazepam (**Oral: Adults** - Initially, 0.25 mg hs. Titrate bet. 0.25-0.5 mg prn. Elderly/debilitated - Initially, 0.125 mg hs)	As for flurazepam	As for flurazepam	As for anxiolytic benzodiazepines	As for anxiolytic benzodiazepines

Pharmacologic Classification: Azaspirodecadedione Anxiolytic

Drug	Indications / Dose	Action	Side/Adverse Effects	Interactions	Nursing Considerations
Buspirone (Buspar)	Short-term symptomatic relief of excess. anxiety in pts w. gen'l anxiety disorder (**Oral: Adults** - Initially, 5 mg bid-tid. Titrate prn by incr. daily dose of 5 mg q2-3days to max. of 45 mg/day in divided doses. Us. dose, 20-30 mg/day in 2-3 divided doses. Elderly - Max. dose, 30 mg for not > 4 weeks.	Mechanism of action not known. Shares some properties of benzodiazepines but is devoid of anticonvulsant and muscle relaxant properties.	Dizziness, headache, drowsiness, nausea	**Food:** Incr. bioavailability of buspirone. **MAOIs:** And buspirone, should not be used concomitantly because elevated BP has been reported in pts receiving both.	As for anxiolytic benzodiazepines, w. the following addit'ns: **Assess:** For changes in mental status, mood, sleeping patterns; for drowsiness, dizziness. For fluid intake/output; indica'rns of renal dysfunct'n. **Evaluate:** For physical dependency and w'drawal symptoms; for poss. suicidal tendencies. **Teach:** That tx effects may require 1-2 weeks.

Pharmacologic Classification: Cyclopyrrolone Hypnotic

Drug	Indications / Dose	Action	Side/Adverse Effects	Interactions	Nursing Considerations
Zoplicone (Imovane)	Short-term management of insomnia characterized by difficulty in falling asleep, frequent nocturnal awakenings and/or early a.m. awakenings (**Oral: Adults** - 7.5 mg hs. Dose should not be exceeded. Depending on clinical response and tolerance, dose may be lowered to 3.75 mg)	Mechanism of action not known. Pharmacological profile sim. to that of benzodiazepines.	Most commonly, bitter taste. Adv. effects attributable to CNS depress'n incl. somnolence, asthenia, dizziness, confus'n, anterograde amnesia or memory impairment, anxiety or nervousness, hostility, depress'n, decr. libido, coordinat'n abnormality, hypotonia, muscle spasms, paresthesia, speech disorder.	**Alcohol or other CNS depressants:** Have poss. additive effects w. zoplicone.	This is a rel. new drug; nurses are advised to consult pharmacist and read manufacturer's info. before administering.

Generic Name (Trade Name)	Use (Dose)	Action	Adverse Effects	Drug Interactions	Nursing Process
Pharmacologic Classification: Chloral Hydrate Hypnotic					
Chloral hydrate (Noctec)	Tx of insomnia (**Oral/rectal**: Adults - 500 mg - 1 g 15 min before retiring)	Depresses CNS. Better suited for putting pts to sleep than keeping them asleep.	Resp. depress'n, apnea, circulatory collapse, pain, skin rash. Allergic react'ns, CNS depress'n, nausea, vomiting, paradoxical excitement.	As for benzodiazepines	**Assess:** Pt hx for previous sensitivity react'ns or paradoxic excitat'n, resp. disease, hypotens'n, liver disease, blood dyscrasias, porphyria or thyroid disease. Establish baseline measures of respirat'n, temp., sleep patterns, pain for later determinat'n of tx/adv. effects. **Administer:** Ensure that medicat'n has been swallowed. Remove cigarets. **Evaluate:** For adv. effects, overdose; subjective reports of relief from insomnia, anxiety, agitat'n. Pt requests for stronger prescript'n or more frequent dosage suggest tolerance/dependency and should be reported to physican. **Teach:** Move from reclining to standing posit'n carefully; dangers of driving or using power equipment; dangers of concomitant use of alcohol or other CNS depressants. Not to store drug by bedside. A responsible family member the s/s of adv. effects.

Anorexiants and Other Central Nervous System Stimulants

Teaching Objectives

Following completion of this chapter, the reader should be able to:

1. Discuss the mechanism of action, pharmacologic effects, therapeutic uses and adverse effects of anorexiant drugs, as well as the nursing process related to their use.
2. Describe the mechanism of action, pharmacologic effects, therapeutic uses and adverse effects of dextroamphetamine, methylphenidate and pemoline, and the nursing process related to their administration.

Anorexiants

The anorexiants currently in use include diethylpropion (Tenuate, Tepanil), fenfluramine (Ponderal, Pondimin), mazindol (Sanorex) and phentermine (Fastin, Ionamin).

Mechanism of Action and Pharmacologic Effects

Anorexiants are central nervous system stimulants. Anorexia is only one manifestation of central nervous system stimulation. Other effects include euphoria, nervousness, irritability, insomnia, decreased fatigue, increased alertness and ability to concentrate. These actions are particularly prevalent with benzphetamine, dextroamphetamine, methamphetamine, chlorphentermine and phenmetrazine. Fenfluramine is the exception. Low doses of this drug may depress brain function. As with sympathomimetics, anorexiants cause dryness of the mouth, blurred vision, mydriasis, dizziness, lightheadedness, tachycardia, palpitations, hypertension and sweating.

Therapeutic Uses

Anorexiants should be used for short periods of time in adults to supplement dietary measures. They should never be used to treat obesity in growing children. The generally preferred drugs are diethylpropion, mazindol and phentermine. Fenfluramine is an alternative drug.

Adverse Effects

The adverse effects of anorexiants result mainly from their ability to stimulate both the central and sympathetic nervous systems (see preceding discussion). In addition, these drugs may cause nausea and vomiting. Overdosage causes nystagmus and tremor that can proceed to convulsions and coma. Anorexiants can induce both psychological and physical dependence. Drug withdrawal is often accompanied by depression and fatigue.

Nursing Process

Assessment

Prior to administering amphetamines, nurses should review the patient's history for documentation of previous hypersensitivity, drug abuse, hyperthyroidism, diabetes mellitus, severe agitation, depression, renal or cardiovascular disease, or parkinsonism. The order should be verified with the physician in the presence of any of these conditions.

Baseline measures must be established for body mass/weight and cardiovascular status, including blood pressure, pulse rate and rhythm.

Administration

Generally, anorexiants are given one-half to one hour before meals. The last daily dose should be administered at least six hours before bedtime to avoid insomnia.

Teaching

Patients must be informed that tolerance to the anorexic effects of these drugs frequently occurs within a few weeks. Thus, weight reduction cannot depend on anorexiants alone. They must be accompanied by a complete weight reduction program including dietary changes, increased exercise levels and behavioral change.

The long-term effect of these drugs on the growth of children has not been established.

Anorexiants stimulate the brain and may temporarily revitalize the tired user. However, this effect ends with even greater fatigue and depression. Patients using anorexiants must be told to maintain regular sleeping patterns.

Patients must be alerted to the fact that judgment of distance and rate of motion may be impaired. They should therefore be cautious in driving or using power equipment.

Patients who experience dry mouth should be instructed to maintain scrupulous mouth care to prevent the consequences of lack of saliva. They should also be told that rinsing the mouth with water, increasing fluid intake, or chewing sugarless gum can relieve dry mouth.

Anorexiants can produce physical dependence. Patients must be told that stopping the drug suddenly can cause withdrawal symptoms. These include lethargy, depression or psychotic behavior. Patients using these drugs for prolonged periods must be told to reduce their consumption gradually to avoid withdrawal effects. Medical assistance may be necessary.

Other Central Nervous System Stimulants

Dextroamphetamine (Dexedrine), Methylphenidate (Ritalin) and Pemoline (Cylert)

Mechanism of Action and Pharmacologic Effects

Although dextroamphetamine and methylphenidate increase dopamine release in the brain, their mechanism of action in attention-deficit disorders is not known. Similar to the anorexiants presented above, these drugs produce euphoria, nervousness, irritability, insomnia, decreased fatigue, increased alertness and increased ability to concentrate. They also cause dryness of the mouth, blurred vision, mydriasis, dizziness, lightheadedness, tachycardia, palpitations, hypertension and sweating.

Therapeutic Uses

Methylphenidate, dextroamphetamine and pemoline are used mainly in the management of children with attention-deficit disorders. Central nervous system stimulants may improve classroom behavior in the short term, but there are few data to demonstrate that they improve learning over long periods of time. In fact, some authorities contend that (1) there is virtually no research evidence to justify use of these drugs for treatment of learning disorders or behavioral disorders, and (2) there is no indication of sufficient benefit to outweigh potential risks associated with the use of these drugs in these contexts. Many feel that time and money would be better spent teaching parents and teachers better coping skills. If a decision is made to use one of these drugs, treatment should be stopped periodically to determine whether continued drug therapy is required.

Methylphenidate and dextroamphetamine are also used to treat narcolepsy. Unfortunately, tolerance is a major problem when these drugs are used for long periods of time.

Adverse Effects

Nervousness and insomnia are the most common adverse effects. Prolonged therapy can lead to weight loss and growth retardation. These drugs may occasionally cause dizziness, rash, abdominal pain, hypertension, hypotension, palpitations, change in pulse rate, tachycardia, arrhythmias and headache.

Treatment of Acute Overdosage

Acute overdosage causes pronounced central and sympathetic nervous system stimulation characterized by excitation, agitation, hypertension, tachycardia, mydriasis, slurred speech, ataxia and tremor. Patients may also experience chills, hyperreflexia, tachypnea, fever, headache and toxic psychoses. In severe cases, these drugs can cause hyperpyrexia, chest pain, acute circulatory failure, convulsions and death. Treatment involves lavage, sedative drugs, psychotherapy and custodial care. Chlorpromazine or haloperidol can be used to manage agitation or psychosis. Convulsions can be treated with diazepam. Cardiac arrhythmias may respond to propranolol, and hypertension can be treated with chlorpromazine. If hypertension is severe or sustained, sodium nitroprusside or diazoxide can be administered. The excretion of dextroamphetamine can be increased by acidification of the urine.

Nursing Process

The nursing process for these medications is essentially the same as that identified above in relation to the anorexiants. Readers should refer to that information.

Further Reading

Gugenheim, F.G. (1977). Basic considerations in the treatment of obesity. *Med. Clin. North Am. 61* :781-796.

Soldatos, C.R., Kales, A. and Cadieux, R.J. (1983). Treatment of sleep disorders: II. Narcolepsy. *Rational Drug Therapy 17* : No. 3.

Wolraich, M.L. (1977). Stimulant drug therapy in hyperactive children: Research and clinical implications. *Pediatrics 60* :512-518.

Table 70
Anorexiants and other central nervous system stimulants.

Generic Name (Trade Name)	Use (Dose)	Action	Adverse Effects	Drug Interactions	Nursing Process
Pharmacologic Classification: Anorexiants					
Diethylpropion HCl (Tenuate, Tepanil)	Adjunct in short-term [i.e., a few weeks] management of exogenous obesity in conjunct'n w. medically supervised regimen of weight reduct'n based on caloric restrict'n (**Oral:** 25 mg tid 1 h ac. An addit'nal 25 mg in evening prn to overcome night hunger, or 1 time-release Tenuate Dospan capsule taken midmorning)	CNS stimulant. Effects incl. anorexia, euphoria, nervousness, irritability, insomnia, decr. fatigue, incr. alertness, incr. ability to concentrate.	Insomnia, nervousness, dizziness, anxiety, jitteriness, tachycardia, precordial pain, arrhythmia, palpitat'n, incr. BP, diarrhea, constipat'n, nausea, vomiting, abd. discomfort	**Antidiabetics:** Doses may be altered by use of an anorexiant. **Antihypertensives:** May have reduced effectiveness in presence of anorexiants. Pts should be monitored closely. **MAOIs:** Should not be given w. an anorexiant. Do not give anorexiants w. MAOIs or within 14 days following w'drawal of these agents to avoid hypertensive crisis.	**Assess:** Hx for previous hypersensitivity, drug abuse, hyperthyroidism, severe agitat'n, depress'n, renal or CV disease, parkinsonism. Establish baseline measures of weight, BP, pulse rate and rhythm. **Administer:** 30 min - 1 h ac; last daily dose at least 6 h before bedtime. **Teach:** That tolerance to anorexic effects of amphetamines frequently occurs within a few weeks; that weight reduct'n must be accompanied by complete weight reduct'n program, incl. dietary changes, incr. exercise levels and behavioral change; to maintain regular sleeping patterns; to be cautious in driving or using power tools or machinery; to rinse mouth w. water, incr. fluid intake or chew sugarless gum or candy; to maintain scrupulous mouth care; that sudden terminat'n of drug may result in lethargy, depress'n or psychotic behaviors; to reduce consumpt'n gradually after prolonged use.
Mazindol (Mazanor, Sanorex)	As for diethylpropion (**Oral:** 1-2 mg in single dose 1 h before main meal or 1 mg tid. Can be taken w. meals to avoid GI discomfort)	As for diethylpropion	As for diethylpropion	**Sympathomimetics (vasoconstrictors):** Produce exaggerated pressor effect if given w. anorexiants. If nec. to administer a pressor amine to a pt in shock who has recently taken an anorexiant, exercise extreme caution in giving such agents (beginning w. low initial doses and careful titrat'n). As well, monitor BP.	
Phentermine (Adipex-P, Fastin, Ionamin Phentrol)	As for diethylpropion (**Oral:** 30 mg approx. 2 h after breakfast; 15-30 mg phentermine resin 10-14 h before bedtime)	As for diethylpropion	As for diethylpropion		
Fenfluramine (Pondomin)	As for diethylpropion (**Oral:** Initially, 20 mg tid 1 h ac, prn. Incr. to 40 mg tid 1 h ac, prn. 1 Extentab containing 60 mg daily when use of divided doses is not convenient)	As for diethylpropion	As for diethylpropion		
Pharmacologic Classification: Other Central Nervous System Stimulants					
Dextroamphetamine (Dexedrine)	Management of children w. attent'n-deficit disorders; tx of narcolepsy (**Oral:** For attent'n-deficit disorder - Children ≥ 6	Although dextroamphetamine and methylphenidate are CNS stimulants, their	Nervousness, insomnia, anorexia, weight loss, growth retardat'n, dizziness, dyski-	**Acetazolamide:** May incr. renal reabsorpt'n of dextroamphetamine. **Anticoagulants, oral:** Serum	As for diethylpropion, w. these added precaut'ns: **Assess:** For s/s overdose, pain, fever, dehydrat'n, insomnia, hyperactivity.

Drug	Dosage		Side Effects	Drug Interactions	Nursing Implications
	years - Initially, 2.5 mg tid, us. 30 min ac; incr. by 2.5 mg/dose q3-4days prn [max. dose, 40 mg/day]. For *narcolepsy* - Adults and children > 6 years - 5-60 mg/day in divided doses)	mechanism of action in attent'n-deficit disorders is not understood. As CNS stimulants, they have all the effects of the anorexiants presented earlier in this table.	nesia, rash, nausea, abd. pain, hypertens'n, hypotens'n, palpitat'ns, changes in pulse rate, arrhyth-mias, headache, psychic and physical dependence	levels may incr. if methylphenidate is administered. **Anticonvulsants** (e.g., pheny-toin, phenobarbital, primidone): Serum levels may incr. if methylphenidate is administered. **Antidepressants, heterocyclic:** May incr. pressor effects of amphetamine. Methylphenidate inhibits metabolism of hetero-cyclics and may incr. hetero-cyclic-induced effects. **Furazolidone:** May incr. pressor effect of amphetamines. **Guanethidine:** May have its effects reduced by amphetamines and methylphenidate. **MAOIs:** Should not be given to pts on amphetamines, methylphenidate or pemoline for fear of acute hypertensive crisis. **Phenothiazines:** May decr. effect of amphetamines, methylphenidate or pemoline. **Phenylbutazone:** Concurrent use of methylphenidate can incr. serum levels of phenylbutazone. **Sodium bicarbonate:** Can incr. renal reabsorpt'n of amphetamines.	As for dextroamphetamine
Methylphenidate HCl (Ritalin)	As for dextroamphetamine (**Oral:** *Attent'n-deficit disorder* - Children ≥ 6 years - Initially, 5-10 mg tid w. weekly increments of 5-10 mg in daily dosage. For *narcolepsy* - Adults - 10 mg bid-tid [range, 10-60 mg/day])	As for dextroam-phetamine	As for dextroam-phetamine		
Pemoline (Cylert)	As for dextroamphetamine (**Oral:** *Attent'n-deficit disorder* - Children ≥ 6 years - Initially, 37.5 mg od given in a.m.; incr. by 18.75 mg at 1-week inter-vals prn [effective range is us. 56.25-75 mg/day]. Improvement may not be observed for 3-4 weeks)	As for dextroam-phetamine	As for dextroam-phetamine		As for dextroamphetamine, with added teaching that tx effect may take 2-4 weeks.

CHAPTER 48

The Alcohols — Ethanol and Methanol

Teaching Objectives

Following completion of this chapter, the reader should be able to:

1. Describe the immediate effects of ethanol on the body.
2. Discuss the consequences of chronic ingestion of ethanol.
3. Discuss the pharmacokinetics of ethanol.
4. Explain the interaction of ethanol with other drugs.
5. Discuss the nursing process related to the use of ethanol.
6. Discuss briefly the pharmacology of methanol.
7. Explain the mechanism of action, therapeutic use and nursing process for disulfiram.

Ethanol

Ethanol, or ethyl alcohol, is a simple alaphatic alcohol. It is found in varying concentrations in alcoholic beverages such as whiskey, wine, beer and liqueurs. Ethanol has found great favor with the masses because it is relatively cheap and can modify brain function. In moderate amounts, it makes you feel good, and has become almost a universal solvent in some households. There is nothing like a drink at the end of a hectic day to smooth ruffled feathers and mend ravelled nerves. The effects of ethanol are, however, dose dependent. Small quantities may put a nice glow on the world but larger amounts carry a good thing just a bit too far.

Mechanism of Action and Pharmacologic Effects (Immediate Effect)

Ethanol depresses neuronal function in the central nervous system. It may be difficult to convince someone who feels like a giant that alcohol is depressing him. However, such is the case. Initially, as low concentrations of ethanol begin to wash over the brain, higher centers are depressed and the mind is unfettered from its learned inhibitions. Confidence abounds, your boss's spouse looks better all the time and life just couldn't be more enjoyable. At the same time, motor and intellectual functions that depend on polysynaptic pathways are impaired and finer grades of discrimination and concentration slip away.

As the concentration of ethanol in the brain increases, so does the degree of central nervous system depression, and the fortunes of our victim decline. Operating a motor car becomes difficult and perhaps even illegal. An initial boisterous mood gives way to general depression as the effects of ethanol percolate further down the brain stem. Mood swings, and perhaps even fist swings, become more prominent. Fights, facial rearrangements, loss of beloved teeth are not uncommon.

If our victim continues to imbibe, profound brain depression ensues. Sleep is the usual and most humane result. However, if the concentration of ethanol is sufficiently high, respiratory failure and death can occur and that really takes the fun out of a party.

The nice warm glow produced by ethanol is due to moderate vasodilatation in the skin. This leads to an increase in heat loss. Ethanol also decreases heat production. Individuals in cold climates should be warned not to expose themselves (drunks are often prone to do this) lest they run the danger of freezing all, or parts of, their tender bodies. Ethanol depresses the secretion of the antidiuretic hormone, producing a well-known renal response.

Anyone who has interviewed a toilet bowl at close quarters after a drinking bout will attest to the fact that ethanol can irritate the stomach. Although it may be of only academic interest to them at the time, you can always inform such individuals that concentrations of forty per cent or more of ethanol cause congestive hyperemia and inflammation of the stomach. Food dilutes the concentration of ethanol in the stomach and reduces gastric irritation.

Mechanism of Action and Pharmacologic Effects (Chronic Effect)

Given the fact that some lost souls find ethanol appealing enough to return for more, and more, and more, we must consider the consequences of bathing the body tissues in it over long periods of time. Chronic excessive ethanol use produces serious neurological and mental disorders. These include brain damage, memory loss, sleep disturbances and psychoses. In addition, many alcoholics replace food with ethanol and as a result suffer from vitamin deficiencies. Evidence for this is found in the development of Wernicke's encephalopathy, polyneuritis, nicotinic acid deficiency encephalopathy and Korsakoff's psychosis.

The liver bears much of the brunt of long-term, high-dose ethanol consumption. Ethanol increases hepatic fat synthesis. Protein also collects in the liver. Eventually, the accumulation of both fat and protein in the liver leads to hepatic cirrhosis.

Ethanol may be the most common teratogen in North America. The fetal alcohol syndrome is well recognized and occurs with a frequency of four to seven per one thousand live births. Women should be advised to refrain from drinking even moderate amounts of ethanol during pregnancy. Fetal alcohol syndrome is characterized by low I.Q. and microcephaly, both reflections of central nervous system damage. Other characteristics are a group of facial abnormalities that include a hypoplastic upper lip, a short nose, short palpebral fissures and slow growth.

Pharmacokinetics

Ethanol is absorbed from both the stomach and duodenum, with absorption occurring faster from the latter site due to its larger surface area. Often the rate-limiting factor in the absorption of ethanol is the speed with which it is passed to the duodenum. Suitably diluted and given to a person with an empty stomach, ethanol is passed quickly to the duodenum and absorbed within fifteen to thirty minutes. Food closes the pyloric sphincter. Ethanol taken with food is trapped in the stomach and absorbed more slowly.

Once absorbed, ethanol is distributed in the total body water before being metabolized to acetaldehyde by the enzyme alcohol dehydrogenase. Acetaldehyde is subsequently metabolized by acetaldehyde dehydrogenase. The inactivation of ethanol proceeds at a constant rate of 100 mg/kg of body mass/hour. Blood ethanol levels fall at the rate of approximately 0.015 g/100 mL/h. Under normal circumstances about two per cent of ethanol is eliminated unchanged by the kidneys. The fact that ethanol can be expired has enabled scientists to develop the Breathalyser. Because the concentration of ethanol in alveolar air is in equilibrium with its level in blood and brain, it is possible to measure alveolar ethanol concentrations and calculate blood levels. In most parts of North America 0.08 g of ethanol per 100 mL of blood has been established as the legal limit for driving a motor vehicle.

Interactions of Ethanol with Other Drugs

Ethanol is often consumed by patients on other medications. It is important for nurses to recognize the consequences of such actions. Psychopharmacological drugs, particularly the benzodiazepines, are used widely. They also depress the central nervous system. Taken together with ethanol, they can produce profound brain depression and even death. Nurses should warn patients of these interactions and caution against the operation of machinery, power tools or motor vehicles while under the influence of ethanol and other central nervous system depressants.

Nursing Process

A lengthy discussion of the nursing actions and responsibilities related to alcohol abuse and alcoholism is beyond the scope of this text. However, we would be remiss if we failed to identify the autonomous teaching responsibilities that devolve to nurses because of their greater awareness of the pharmacologic effects of ethanol. These responsibilities fall on all nurses to some extent; however, a greater onus lies upon nurses practising in community settings as opposed to those practising in hospitals. Community health nurses must regularly include among their programs educational sessions to increase public awareness of the importance of the moderate use of alcohol in promoting and protecting individual health and safety; the chronic effects of long-term abuse; the teratogenic effects of alcohol use during pregnancy; and the dangers of alcohol consumption concurrently with the use of psychopharmacological drugs. Because prevention is usually more effective than cure, one of the primary target groups for these programs is the preteen and early teenage group. Therefore, school health nurses have a particularly strong obligation to provide these types of information programs. In planning nursing care, it is important to promote family support. This can be done by referral of the family to community family support programs.

Methanol

Methanol's actions on the brain are similar to those of ethanol. Concern over its acute toxicity results from the metabolism of methanol by alcohol dehydrogenase to formaldehyde, which in turn is converted to formic acid. Formaldehyde and formic acid are toxic to the retina and the optic nerve and can produce permanent blindness. In addition, formic acid produces metabolic acidosis which, if severe, can be fatal.

Treatment involves the administration of ethanol, which competes with methanol for the available alcohol dehydrogenase. This reduces the formation of formaldehyde and formic acid, and methanol is slowly eliminated unchanged in the urine. Methanol may also be eliminated by hemodialysis. It is also usual to treat the metabolic acidosis with intravenous sodium bicarbonate solutions.

Disulfiram (Antabuse)

Disulfiram inhibits the enzyme acetaldehyde dehydrogenase. In the presence of disulfiram, ethanol ingestion causes large quantities of acetaldehyde to accumulate, producing intense flushing, tachycardia, nausea, vomiting and circulatory collapse.

Disulfiram is used as a deterrent to drinking. If the alcoholic knows that he is taking the drug, he is motivated to refrain from using ethanol lest he incur the unpleasant effects mentioned above. On the other hand, the individual must have the will to stop drinking or he will not take disulfiram. The drug takes two to four hours to begin to act and reaches its maximum effect in twelve to twenty-four hours.

Disulfiram is not devoid of other toxicities. It blocks the enzyme dopamine-ß-hydroxylase and thereby reduces catecholamine synthesis. This may explain the weakness, dizziness and cardiac arrhythmias seen in patients. Disulfiram may also produce a toxic psychosis or skin allergies on occasion.

Nursing Process

Assessment

In caring for patients receiving disulfiram, the nursing process is initiated at the patient assessment phase. First, the patient's history is reviewed for conditions that contraindicate disulfiram administration. Under no circumstances should nurses give disulfiram to patients having a history of hypersensitivity to this drug, cardiac disease, epilepsy, hypothyroidism, liver disease or psychosis. Nurses who discover previously undisclosed evidence of any of the preceding conditions should withhold the drug and immediately contact the physician. Nurses should also withhold the medication and contact the physician immediately if the physical or psychological assessment reveal a current pregnancy, alcohol intoxication, or inadequate intellectual capacity to understand the purpose and consequences of disulfiram use.

Administration

Disulfiram is administered only to cooperating patients who fully comprehend the effects of the medication. There must be at least a twelve-hour period, and preferably a forty-eight hour interval, of abstinence from alcohol preceding the first administration of disulfiram. Usually the patient's resolve to maintain abstinence from alcohol is strongest in the morning. Consequently, disulfiram should be offered to the patient in the morning with breakfast. Should disulfiram produce marked drowsiness, however, it can be administered at bedtime. Following the initial brief period of hospitalization, patients are usually discharged. Therapy is continued on an outpatient basis with disulfiram being self-administered by the patient at home. Disulfiram tablets can be crushed and mixed with a beverage.

Evaluation

Nursing evaluation of patients receiving disulfiram must focus on compliance with the therapeutic regimen. This usually includes psychotherapy in conjunction with the use of the drug. Patients should also be evaluated for both abstinence from alcohol use and the adverse effects of disulfiram. Nurses should evaluate for signs of hepatotoxicity, such as jaundice, dark urine, clay-coloured stools and abdominal pain.

Teaching

Nurses must teach the patient's family that disulfiram must *never* be given to the patient secretly. This is dangerous because the unsuspecting patient may consume a large volume of alcohol, without knowing that he has taken disulfiram, resulting in a severe or potentially fatal disulfiram-alcohol reaction. This can occur as quickly as fifteen minutes after drinking. Patients should be advised that adverse effects of disulfiram which occur in the absence of alcohol usually subside within two to three weeks of therapy. Patients should also be advised to wear or carry medical-alert identification while taking disulfiram. This will facilitate prompt medical treatment should a disulfiram-alcohol reaction occur. They should also be instructed that the effects of the drug persist for up to two weeks following the last dose. The sensitivity of the body to alcohol increases as the use of disulfiram is prolonged. Patients should be advised to read the labels on over-the-counter medications since many contain alcohol, e.g., cough syrups. Similarly, flavorings (such as wine, vinegar or vanilla), flamed desserts and food cooked with alcohol should also be avoided.

Finally, nurses should counsel patients receiving disulfiram to avoid driving, the use of power tools, or industrial machinery during this initial period of treatment, because of the danger of dizziness or drowsiness.

Further Reading

Lieber, C.S. (1985). Interaction of ethanol with drugs and vitamin therapy. *Rational Drug Therapy 19* (11).

Holt, S. (1981). Observations on the relation between alcohol absorption and the rate of gastric emptying. *Can. Med. Assoc. J. 124* :267-277.

CHAPTER 49

General Anesthetics

Anesthesia is the loss of sensation. General anesthesia is a state of unconsciousness with the absence of pain. General anesthetics produce, in varying degrees, the following effects:
1. amnesia;
2. loss of consciousness;
3. analgesia;
4. loss of reflexes;
5. muscle relaxation.

General anesthesia is usually produced by the inhalation or intravenous administration of drugs. This chapter concentrates on the pharmacology of inhalation anesthetics. Mention is also made of intravenous anesthetics.

Inhalation Anesthetics

Mechanism of Action and Pharmacologic Effects

Inhalation anesthetics depress central nervous system function, beginning with the cerebral cortex and moving down the central nervous system, with increasing concentrations, to inhibit the basal ganglia, cerebellum, spinal cord and medulla oblongata, in that order. It is fortunate that spinal function is affected before medullary activity because this allows the anesthetic to paralyze both the sensory and motor functions of the cord before it stops respiration. Complete central nervous system paralysis is apparent when the respiratory and cardiovascular centers in the medulla oblongata are completely depressed. Although many theories have been advanced to explain the means by which inhalation anesthetics work, their exact mechanism of action is not known.

Two factors control the degree of central nervous system depression: the concentration of the drug and its intrinsic activity. The latter is expressed as the **minimal alveolar concentration (MAC)** necessary to prevent movement in fifty per cent of individuals subjected to a painful stimulus.

Pharmacokinetics

Understanding the pharmacokinetics of inhalation anesthetics is not easy. The induction of anesthesia involves the following steps:

1. inhalation of the anesthetic and mixing it with gas already present in alveoli;
2. diffusion of the anesthetic into the pulmonary circulation;
3. transport of the anesthetic in blood throughout the body; and
4. diffusion of the anesthetic from blood into brain.

Inhalation anesthetics are administered as gases. They exist under pressure in the gas machine, lungs and blood. Although these truths are self-evident, they bear mentioning because this is the first time that we have discussed gaseous drugs.

Once absorbed through alveoli, anesthetics are held in solution in the blood under pressure. The partial pressure of an anesthetic determines the rate at which it leaves the blood and enters the brain. The higher the partial pressure of the gas in blood, the greater the force pushing it into the brain. For its part, the partial pressure of the gas is determined by its concentration and solubility in blood. Gases with poor solubility in blood attain high partial pressures rapidly and are forced into the brain quickly.

From the preceding discussion, it is logical to conclude that anesthetic gases differ in their blood solubility. This is true. The importance of blood solubility to the onset and duration of action of an anesthetic can be illustrated by referring to two agents that differ markedly in this regard. Nitrous oxide is poorly soluble in blood. As a result, when nitrous oxide is inhaled and passes from alveoli into blood, its partial pressure increases rapidly, reflecting the inability of blood to dissolve and hold large amounts of the gas. The high partial pressure of the gas in blood quickly drives the anesthetic into the brain, giving the drug a rapid onset of action.

Ether is very soluble in blood. When ether is inhaled, its partial pressure rises very slowly. Keeping in mind that it is the partial pressure of the gas in blood that drives the anesthetic into the brain, the reader can readily understand why ether enters the brain slowly. As a result, induction of anesthesia with ether proceeds over a longer period of time. Most gaseous anesthetics have blood solubilities and partial pressures between the extremes of ether and nitrous oxide.

Once the operation is complete and the anesthetist turns off the gas machine, the rates of recovery from nitrous oxide and ether differ markedly. In the case of nitrous oxide, recovery is very rapid. The high partial pressure of this gas in blood rapidly drives the drug back into the alveoli, from whence it is expired. The resulting fall in nitrous oxide levels in blood quickly draws the gas out of the brain. The capacity of blood to dissolve and hold ether is much greater. As a result, it is not cleared as quickly by the lungs. Because it continues to circulate through the body, perfusing the brain, ether's recovery time is longer. From this discussion we can derive a principle: *Anesthetic gases with low solubility in blood accumulate quicker in the brain during inhalation and leave more rapidly once administration of the anesthetic is stopped.*

Other factors that influence the onset of anesthesia are (1) the inspired concentration, (2) the alveolar ventilation and (3) the cardiac output.

Inspired concentration is important in determining the uptake of gas by blood and brain. The principle is: *The higher the inspired concentration, the more rapid will be the rate of increase of the partial pressure of the anesthetic in blood.* This is particularly true for gases readily soluble in blood. If the initial inspired anesthetic tension is set higher than required for the maintenance of anesthesia, the concentration and partial pressure of the gas in blood will rise more rapidly and the drug will enter the brain more quickly. This technique is called **overpressure.**

If the patient breathes more rapidly, increased quantities of anesthetic enter the blood, saturating it quickly and raising the partial pressure of the gas. The principle is: *Improving alveolar ventilation increases the rate of anesthetic uptake by blood.* Again, the effect is greater for agents readily soluble in blood.

Increasing cardiac output improves blood flow through the lungs. Because a greater volume of blood is exposed to the gas in the alveoli per unit of time, it becomes more difficult to saturate it with anesthetic. Thus, the principle is: *Increasing cardiac output reduces the rate at which partial pressure increases, thereby delaying induction of anesthesia.* Here too, the effect is greatest with those anesthetics possessing good blood solubility.

Excitement, fever and other hypermetabolic states, all conditions that increase cardiac output, delay anesthetic induction. Conversely, shock reduces cardiac output. As a result, anesthetic induction occurs very quickly in a patient in shock.

Stages of Anesthesia

Over sixty years ago, anesthetists recognized four stages of anesthesia as they related to the effects of ether. These reflect increasing concentrations of the anesthetic in the central nervous system and the progressive deterioration of neuronal function. The stages are still used today to describe the depth of anesthesia, even though they may be somewhat obscured in the newer anesthetics.

Stage I (Stage of Analgesia) begins at the time of drug administration and lasts until the patient loses consciousness. The patient starts stage I with normal memory and sensation and leaves with amnesia and analgesia.

Stage II (Stage of Delirium or Excitement) starts with loss of consciousness and continues to the point where the patient is ready for surgery. Excitement and involuntary activity may be present. At this time the patient may shout, sing, laugh or attempt to fight. Sympathetic nervous system activity is high. The pupils may be dilated, the heart rate fast, and the blood pressure raised. These effects are due to the release of lower and more primitive areas of the brain from the overriding influence of higher inhibitory centers, which have just been depressed. As a result, basic emotional reactions appear unfettered by learned inhibitions. Anesthetists try to pass patients through stage II as quickly as possible.

Stage III (Stage of Surgical Anesthesia) starts when the patient passes through stage II and continues until the cessation of spontaneous respiration. At one time stage III was divided into four planes to delineate the extent of muscular relaxation and respiratory depression. Today, this has little meaning, as drugs such as tubocurarine or succinylcholine (see Chapter 9) are used for the specific purpose of relaxing muscles. As the name indicates, this is the stage during which surgery is performed.

Stage IV (Stage of Respiratory Paralysis) begins with respiratory failure and concludes with complete circulatory collapse.

Nursing Process

Anesthetics are administered by anesthetists, usually physicians (nurses in some legal jurisdictions) who have had advanced training in the process of administering anesthetics (i.e., assessment, planning, administration and evaluation). It is beyond the scope of this text to present detailed information regarding the process of administering anesthetics. Rather, our focus is to provide information to facilitate knowledgeable nursing care for patients who are emerging from anesthesia. Obviously, emergence from anesthesia is only one aspect of immediate postoperative nursing care. Readers are referred to a medical-surgical nursing text for detailed information related to other aspects of postoperative nursing care.

Nursing responsibilities related to the care of patients receiving anesthetics begin with preoperative teaching and preparation for the anesthetic and surgery. The preoperative check for blood work and electrocardiographic abnormalities is always an important nursing responsibility. Postoperative care includes monitoring the patient for adverse effects and promoting patient safety during emergence from anesthesia. Generally, the following parameters are monitored for deviations from the norm during this period: temperature, pulse (rate, rhythm and quality), blood pressure (as compared to a preoperative baseline measure), respirations (rate, depth, equality of bilateral chest expansion, regularity), color (particularly of nailbeds and lips), level of consciousness (orientation to place, time, person), urinary output, and the duration of emergence in relation to the anesthetic used.

Nurses promote patient safety during emergence from anesthesia by positioning the patient in a semiprone position to prevent aspiration of vomitus; installing and using side rails on the patient's bed; suctioning excessive secretions in the mouth, nose and nasopharynx; maintaining adequate ventilation; maintaining a low-stimulus environment (quiet, dim lighting, pastel colors, calm demeanor, soft voice); keeping the patient covered to prevent heat loss and hypothermia; and using analgesics cautiously. Additional specific nursing measures related to care of patients during emergence from specific anesthetic agents are included in Table 71.

Specific Inhalation Anesthetics

Ether

Ether, or diethyl ether to be correct, is a colorless, highly volatile liquid with a pungent odor. In contrast to most inhalation anesthetics, it has significant solubility in water. With the exception of nitrous oxide, ether is the oldest inhalation anesthetic in use. If was first used in 1842 and, although its popularity has dropped greatly over the past twenty years, ether is still used occasionally. Our interest in it, however, is largely historical.

Anesthesia with ether is characterized by prolonged induction and emergence. Patients suffer from a high incidence of postanesthetic nausea and vomiting. Ether is also very irritating and its use results in increased salivary, bronchial and gastric secretions. Laryngeal spasm is not uncommon with the drug. In addition, ether is flammable. All possibility of sparks in the operating room must be eliminated.

Nitrous Oxide

Nitrous oxide, with a low solubility in blood, has a rapid onset of action and a quick recovery. It is an excellent baseline anesthetic and is often used in conjunction with other anesthetics to allow for lower concentrations of the latter drugs. The main limitation to nitrous oxide use is its weak potency. The minimal alveolar concentration (MAC) for nitrous oxide is 100%. Obviously, it is impossible to give a patient 100% nitrous oxide, unless you want him to asphyxiate. Nitrous oxide should be administered with at least 30% oxygen during induction and maintenance.

Halothane (Fluothane)

Halothane was introduced in the mid 1950s. Since that time it has become one of the most popular inhalation anesthetics in North America. It is a potent anesthetic with a MAC of 0.76%, compared to 100% for nitrous oxide. Halothane induces anesthesia rapidly with little or no excitement but does not provide good muscle relaxation. As a result, neuromuscular blockers are often required.

Nitrous oxide is often used concomitantly to reduce the concentration of halothane required. Controlled ventilation may be required, particularly if deep anesthesia is indicated. Halothane can lower blood pressure and sensitize the myocardium to catecholamines.

Hepatitis, occurring three to ten days after operation and preceded by fever, is a rare complication. It is believed to be a hypersensitivity reaction and is unpredictable in its occurrence. A portion of the administered halothane is metabolized in the liver and it is believed that one of the metabolites is responsible for the hepatitis.

Enflurane (Enthrane)

Enflurane has a MAC of 1.68%. Its action is characterized by rapid onset and quick recovery. Enflurane produces better muscle relaxation and less myocardial sensitization to catecholamines than halothane. It also causes profound respiratory depression. Nitrous oxide is often used to enable the anesthetist to administer a lower concentration of enflurane. Episodes of tonic-clonic or twitching movements or *grand mal* seizures, particularly in children, have occurred with enflurane. Liver damage has also been reported, but no cause-and-effect relationship with enflurane has been established.

Methoxyflurane (Penthrane)

With a MAC of 0.16%, methoxyflurane is the most potent anesthetic available. Because of its high solubility in blood, methoxyflurane is rarely used for induction. Nitrous oxide or barbiturates are administered for induction. Awakening from methoxyflurane is slow because of its high solubility in blood. Methoxyflurane produces good muscle relaxation and minimal sensitization of the myocardium to catecholamines. The drug is also a good analgesic and patients often awake free of pain. The major deterrent to its use is the likelihood of renal failure. Methoxyflurane is metabolized, in part, giving rise to inorganic fluoride that can damage the kidneys. Although its nephrotoxicity is usually reversible, many anesthetists feel that this is too high a price to pay for the use of the drug.

Isoflurane (Forane)

A potent anesthetic with a MAC of 1.2%, isoflurane has a pungent odor that limits the concentration patients will accept without coughing or holding the breath. Induction is usually smooth if patients are premedicated and given nitrous oxide or intravenous agents. Isoflurane does not sensitize the myocardium to catecholamines.

Intravenous Anesthetics

The ideal intravenous anesthetic should provide smooth induction, have a predictable dosage and a large therapeutic index (high safety), produce minimal cardiovascular and respiratory depression, allow rapid and complete recovery, provide absence of pain or injury from injection, and be stable in solution.

Barbiturates

Thiopental (Pentothal) is a potent intravenous anesthetic used to provide rapid induction. Emergence, usually quick, may be delayed if large doses are given by continuous intravenous drip. Laryngospasm may occur during induction. Thiopental depresses both respiration and circulation. High doses are required to relax skeletal muscles. Thiopental decreases urine output by reducing perfusion pressure, constricting renal arteries and releasing the antidiuretic hormone (ADH).

Methohexital sodium (Brevital Sodium) is a short-acting barbiturate used for induction and in conditions such as electroconvulsive therapy, when loss of consciousness is required.

Thiamylal sodium (Surital) is similar to thiopental and has the same uses and adverse effects.

Benzodiazepines

Diazepam (Valium) can be used intravenously to induce anesthesia. However, it has a slower onset than thiopental and, except in patients with cardiovascular disease, is usually less satisfactory. Its therapeutic applications include basal sedation during regional analgesia, cardioversion, and endoscopic and dental procedures. Intravenous diazepam can produce superficial, painless venous thrombosis at the injection site and is associated with a high incidence of phlebitis.

Midazolam (Versed) is a short-acting, water-soluble benzodiazepine. Depending on the route of administration and dose used, midazolam can produce sedative-hypnotic effects or induce anesthesia. The administration of midazolam may often be followed by anterograde amnesia. Onset of sedative effects after intramuscular administration is about 15 min, with peak sedation occurring 30 – 60 min following injection. Sedation after intravenous injection is usually achieved within 3 – 6 min. When midazolam is used intravenously, induction of anesthesia can usually be achieved in 1.5 min when narcotic premedication has been administered and in 2 – 2.5 min without narcotic premedication.

Midazolam is indicated as an intramuscular premedication prior to diagnostic procedures. As an intravenous agent, midazolam can be used for patients requiring conscious sedation prior to and during short endoscopic diagnostic procedures and direct-current cardioversion. Midazolam can also be used intravenously as an induction anesthetic.

Propofol (Diprivan)

Propofol is an intravenous hypnotic agent that can be used for both induction and maintenance of anesthesia as part of a balanced anesthesia technique for inpatient and outpatient surgery. The drug is formulated in an oil-in-water emulsion. Intravenous injection of a therapeutic dose of propofol produces hypnosis rapidly and smoothly, usually within forty seconds from the start of an injection, although induction times of greater than sixty seconds have been observed.

Droperidol (Inapsine) and Fentanyl Citrate (Sublimaze)

Fentanyl is a narcotic with a very short half-life. Droperidol is a butyrophenone, with properties similar to those of the antipsychotic haloperidol (see Chapter 44). The two are often used together to produce **neuroleptanalgesia,** a state in which consciousness is not lost but the anxiety of the patient is allayed and the ability to perceive pain reduced or abolished. Neuroleptanalgesia may be valuable for diagnostic and therapeutic procedures.

Innovar is a fixed-ratio combination of fentanyl and droperidol. It is often used to premedicate patients or as an adjunct to inhalation anesthesia.

Ketamine (Ketalar)

Ketamine is a nonbarbiturate anesthetic that can be administered intravenously or intramuscularly. It is sometimes called a **dissociative** anesthetic because patients become unresponsive to pain and to the environment. Duration of anesthesia is short; ketamine is useful for repeated anesthesia in burn patients, for diagnostic studies, for sedating uncontrollable patients and for minor surgical procedures. An anticholinergic should be administered concomitantly to reduce salivary secretion.

The use of ketamine is limited because of its ability to produce elevated blood pressure, vivid dreams, hallucinations and other psychic disturbances after recovery. These effects may be reduced by oral premedication with 4 mg of lorazepam or 10 mg of diazepam. Alternatively, intravenous diazepam (0.15 – 0.30 mg/kg) can be administered at the end of anesthesia.

Further Reading

Attia, R.R. and Grogono, A.W. (1978). *Practical Anesthetic Pharmacology.* New York: Appleton-Century-Crofts.

Vickers, M.W., Wood-Smith, F.G. and Steward, H.C. (1978). *Drugs in Anesthetic Practice,* 5th ed. Toronto: Butterworths.

Table 71
General anesthetics.

Pharmacologic Classification: Inhalation Anesthetics

Generic Name (Trade Name)	Use (Dose)	Action	Adverse Effects	Drug Interactions	Nursing Process
Nitrous oxide	Inhalat'n anesthetic w. low anesthetic potency (*For sedat'n* - 25%. *For analgesia* - 25-50% w. O_2. *For induct'n* - 70% N_2O w. 30% O_2 for 2-3 min)	Low solubility in blood, rapid onset of action, quick recovery. Excellent baseline anesthetic.	Serious effects do not occur when adequate concentrat'n of O_2 and ventilat'n is maintained.		**Evaluate:** Level of postanesthesia dizziness, confus'n; monitor emergence from anesthesia; promote pt safety.
Enflurane (Enthrane)	Gen'l anesthetic that produces rapid induct'n and rapid recovery (*Surgical anesthesia in 7-10 min* - 2-4.5% enflurane. *Maintenance* - 0.5-3% enflurane)	MAC of 1.68%. Rapid onset, quick recovery. Better muscle relax at'n and less myocardial sensitizat'n to catecholamines than halothane.	Profound resp. depress'n, slight abnormalities in liver funct'n, tonic-clonic or twitching movements, *grand mal* seizures.	**Neuromuscular blocking agents:** Have their actions potentiated by halothane, enflurane and isoflurane. Dose of competitive blocker must be reduced to acc't for this potentiat'n.	**Evaluate:** Pulse rate, rhythm, quality; monitor emergence from anesthesia; promote pt safety.
Halothane (Fluothane)	Inhalat'n anesthetic that provides rel. rapid induct'n w. little or no excitement (*For induct'n* - 1-4%. *Maintenance* - 0.5-2%)	MAC of 0.76%. Rapid anesthesia w. little or no excitement. Poor muscle relaxat'n. Can lower BP and sensitize myocardium to catecholamines.	Depress'n of pharyngeal and laryngeal reflexes, tachypnea, dimin. sympathetic activity, depressed myocardial contractility, venodilat'n, circ. failure, arrhythmias.	*As for enflurane, plus:* **Catecholamines:** Have their effects potentiated by halothane.	**Assess:** Establish baseline measures of BP, respirat'ns and cardiac status. **Evaluate:** For hypotens'n, bradycardia, depressed respirat'ns; monitor emergence from anesthesia; promote pt safety.
Isoflurane (Forane)	Potent anesthetic that produces smooth induct'n (*For induct'n* - 3-3.5% in O_2 or in N_2O-O_2. *Maintenance* - 0.5-3%)	MAC of 1.2%. Smooth induct'n if pts premedicated and given N_2O or IV agents. Pungent odor limits concentrat'n pts will accept without holding breath.	Mental alertness depressed for 2-3 h after anesthesia.	*As for enflurane, plus:* **Baclofen:** Has its muscle-relaxant effects potentiated by isoflurane. **Cyclobenzaprine:** Has its muscle-relaxant effects potentiated by isoflurane. **Dantrolene:** Has its muscle-relaxant effects potentiated by isoflurane.	As for halothane

Generic Name (Trade Name)	Use (Dose)	Action	Adverse Effects	Drug Interactions	Nursing Process
Methoxyflurane (Penthrane)	Inhalat'n agent for use in gen'l anesthesia and/or analgesia. It is recomm. to be used in combinat'n w. N$_2$O (For analgesia - 0.3-0.8% in air. Maintenance - Tog. w. at least 50% N$_2$O)	MAC of 0.16%. Most potent inhalat'n anesthetic. Because of high solubility in blood, rarely used for induct'n. Awakening slow. Produces good analgesia, good muscle relaxat'n, min. sensitizat'n of myocardium to catecholames. Can be nephrotoxic.	Renal dysfunct'n, hepatic dysfunct'n, cardiac arrest, malignant hyperpyrexia, prolonged postop. somnolence, resp. depress'n, laryngospasm, bronchospasm, nausea, vomiting, postop. headache, hypotens'n and emergence delirium	As for enflurane, plus: **Aminoglycosides:** And methoxyflurane, have additive nephrotoxic effects. **Catecholamines:** Such as epinephrine and levarterenol, should be used cautiously. **Tetracyclines:** And methoxyflurane, may result in fatal renal toxicity.	As for halothane

Pharmacologic Classification: Injectable Anesthetics

Generic Name (Trade Name)	Use (Dose)	Action	Adverse Effects	Drug Interactions	Nursing Process
Thiopental sodium (Pentothal Sodium)	Sole anesthetic agent for brief surgical procedures; for induct'n of anesthesia; for control of convulsive states; for supplementat'n of reg'nal anesthesia or low-potency agents (**IV**: Adults - 50-100 mg intermittently q30-40s prn. Alternatively, a single inject'n of 3-5 mg/kg. Maintenance - 50-100 mg of 2.5% solut'n prn. Children 5-15 years - 2.5% solut'n injected slowly and intermittently at 30-s intervals. Total dose, 4-5 mg/kg. Maintenance - Children 30-50 kg - 25-50 mg intermittently. **Rectal:** Basal anesthesia in children - 30 mg/kg in 40% suspens'n)	Potentiates GABA-mediated inhibitory processes of brain, producing CNS depress'n, resulting in muscle-relaxant, anticonvulsant, sedative and hypnotic effects. Provides rapid induct'n.	Resp. depress'n, myocardial depress'n, cardiac arrhythmias, prolonged somnolence and recovery, bronchospasm, hypersensitivity	**CNS depressants:** Used concomitantly w. a barbiturate, will incr. brain depress'n.	**Assess:** For hx sensitivity to barbiturates or paradoxic excitat'n, chronic resp. disease, hypotens'n, liver disease, blood dyscrasias, porphyria, thyroid disorders, pregnancy, lactat'n; for pain; for dependence. Establish baseline measures of respirat'n and temp., sleep patterns. **Administer:** According to local policies and procedures for compliance w. legal regulat'ns regarding controlled substances. *IV:* Monitor flow rate carefully; guard against extravasat'n of IV. **Evaluate:** For adv. effects; for toxicity.
Diazepam (Valium)	Relief of anxiety states before surgical procedures, cardiovers'n; in endoscopic and dental procedures (**IV:** For	Used IV to induce anesthesia. Has slower onset than thiopental and is less	As for benzodiazepines (see Table 69). Superficial, painless venous	As for benzodiazepines (see Table 69)	As for benzodiazepines (see Chapter 46, Table 69)

Drug	Dosage	Action	Adverse Effects	Nursing Considerations
		satisfactory (except in pts w. CV disease).	thrombosis and phlebitis.	
Midazolam (Versed)	induct'n - 0.1-1.5 mg/kg. Basal sedat'n - 2.5 mg q30s) IM as premedicat'n before surgical or diagnostic procedures. IV for conscious sedat'n prior to and during short endoscopic and diagnostic procedures, DC cardiovers'n or induct'n of anesthesia (Dosage must be carefully individualized. Elderly/debilitated pts should receive lower doses. Consult manufacturer's informat'n for dosage schedules)	Short-acting, water-soluble benzodiazepine w. CNS-depressant effects. Depending on route of administrat'n and dose used, midazolam can produce sedative-hypnotic effects or induce anesthesia.	As for benzodiazepines (see Table 69). Sedative effects and fluctuat'ns in VS are most frequent adv. effects.	As for benzodiazepines (see Table 69) *As for benzodiazepines, plus:* **Assess:** Inject'n site for pain, redness, swelling. Monitor elderly for poss. incr. degree of amnesia.
Propofol (Diprivan)	Induct'n and maintenance of anesthesia as part of balanced anesthesia technique for in-pt/out-pt surgery (IV: *Induct'n -* Adults - 2-2.5 mg/kg. Elderly, debilitated and/or ASA III or IV pts - 1-1.5 mg/kg. *Maintenance -* Adults - Generally, 0.1-0.2 mg/kg/min. Elderly, debilitated and/or ASA III or IV pts - Generally, 0.05-0.1 mg/kg/min)	IV hypnotic agent. IV inject'n produces hypnosis rapidly and smoothly, us. within 40 s.	Hypotens'n, apnea, spontaneous movement, twitching, bucking, jerking, thrashing, hiccoughs, clonic-tonic movement, headache, dizziness, nausea, vomiting, abd. cramping	*As for benzodiazepines, plus:* **Administration:** By IV only. Give alone; do not mix w. other agents. Dilute w. D5W and use only glass containers. Not stable in plastic.
Droperidol (Inapsine)	(Adults - **IM:** *Premedicat'n -* 2.5-10 mg administered 30-60 min preop. *Diagnostic procedures [without a gen'l anesthetic] -* 2.5-10 mg 30-60 min before procedure. Addit'nal IV 1.25-2.5 mg may be given. **IV:** *Induct'n -* 2.5 mg/9-11 kg)	Butyrophenone w. properties sim. to those of haloperidol (antipsychotic).	As for haloperidol (see Table 65)	As for haloperidol (see Chapter 44, Table 65)
Fentanyl citrate (Sublimaze)	Analgesia of short durat'n during anesthetic periods, premedicat'n, induct'n and maintenance, and in immed. postop. periods (Adults - **IM/IV:** *For premedicat'n or induct'n -* 0.05-0.1 mg. For addit'nal details on dosage, consult manufacturer's monograph)	Narcotic w. very short half-life.	As for other narcotic analgesics (see Table 76)	As for other narcotic analgesics (see Table 76)

Generic Name (Trade Name)	Use (Dose)	Action	Adverse Effects	Drug Interactions	Nursing Process
Droperidol plus fentanyl citrate (Innovar)	Premedicat'n for anesthesia and as adjunct to N2O-O2 anesthetic techniques (For information on IM/IV doses consult manufacturer's monograph)	Droperidol and fentanyl are combined to produce neuroleptanalgesia, a state in which consciousness is not lost but anxiety is allayed and ability to perceive pain reduced or abolished.	Because Innovar contains both droperidol and fentanyl, consult Adverse Effects for both drugs [earlier in this table].	Because Innovar contains both droperidol and fentanyl, consult Drug Interactions for both drugs [earlier in this table].	As for narcotics and haloperidol
Ketamine (Ketalar)	Alone for diagnostic surgical procedures; for induct'n of anesthesia; to supplement low-potency agents such as N2O (**IV:** *For induct'n* - 2 mg/kg administered over 60 s. *Maintenance* - 50% induct'n dose repeated prn. **IM:** *For induct'n* - 6.5-13 mg/kg. *Maintenance* - 50% induct'n dose repeated prn. *Analgesia* - 2 mg/kg)	"Dissociative" anesthetic. Pts become unresponsive to pain and environment. Durat'n of anesthetic short. Useful for repeated anesthesia in burn pts, for diagnostic studies, for sedating uncontrollable pts and for minor surgical procedures.	Effects consistent w. CNS depress'n, plus elevated BP, vivid dreams, hallucinat'ns and psychic disturbances after recovery	*As for enflurane, plus:* **Barbiturates:** And ketamine, can form precipitate if mixed in same syringe. **CNS depressants:** May prolong recovery time if used concurrently w. ketamine.	As for enflurane

CHAPTER 50

Local Anesthetics

Teaching Objectives

Following completion of this chapter, the reader should be able to:

1. Explain why local anesthetics are used.
2. Discuss the mechanism of action, pharmacologic effects, pharmacokinetics and adverse effects of local anesthetics.
3. Discuss the basis for the availability of different concentrations of local anesthetic solutions and the rationale for the use of epinephrine.
4. List the methods of administering local anesthetics and explain the rationale behind the use of each technique.
5. Discuss the nursing process associated with use of local anesthetics.
6. List some commonly used local anesthetics and briefly describe their properties.

Local anesthetics block peripheral nerve function. Strictly speaking, they should not be discussed in this section, which deals with the effects of drugs on the central nervous system. However, we shall take poetic license here, because it seems most appropriate to present the pharmacologic properties and uses of local anesthetics immediately following the chapter on general anesthetics.

Mechanism of Action and Pharmacologic Effects

Local anesthetics are used to block pain sensation from discrete areas of the body. They either anesthetize nerve endings or prevent the subsequent conduction of impulses in the peripheral nerves leading to the brain. Local anesthetics prevent the nerve action potential from reaching the threshold necessary for the electrical transmission of impulses.

To understand how local anesthetics work it is essential to review quickly how nerves carry impulses. Impulses are transmitted by successive depolarizations of the neuronal membrane. Depolarization depends on the flux of potassium and sodium across the membrane. In the resting state, the neuronal membrane is largely impermeable to sodium. As a result, sodium concentrations outside the nerve are much higher than inside. By way of contrast, potassium is concentrated inside the nerve. When a nerve is stimulated and a wave of depolarization sweeps along it, the neuronal membrane becomes permeable to sodium and it enters the nerve. At the same time, potassium leaves. These ion changes are essential if a nerve is to transmit an impulse. Subsequently, the nerve repolarizes by pumping sodium out, allowing potassium to re-enter. It is then ready to accept the next impulse.

Local anesthetics exist in solution in the body in both the ionized and nonionized forms. The latter, being more lipid soluble, penetrate the nerve membrane. Once inside the nerve some of the molecules ionize, attach to the nerve membrane, and interfere with neuronal ion transport. They block nerve conduction by decreasing or preventing the large transient increase in the permeability of the membrane to sodium ions. Figure 25 demonstrates the effects of a local anesthetic on the intracellular nerve action potential.

Figure 25

Intracellular nerve action potential prior to and following exposure to lidocaine.

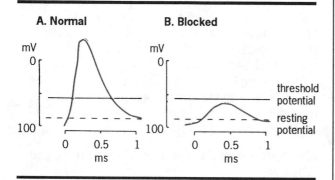

From: R.R. Attia and A.W. Grogono (1978), *Practical Anesthetic Pharmacology*. New York: Appleton-Century-Crofts. Reproduced with permission.

Pharmacokinetics

Local anesthetics are either applied to the surface of a mucous membrane or injected in the vicinity of the nerve(s) to be blocked. The extent of the nerve block produced depends on the ability of the drug to penetrate the nerve and its inherent ability to block the transmission of impulses along the cell membrane. The duration of activity of a local anesthetic is determined by the speed at which it diffuses away from the nerve and is absorbed by the blood.

Most local anesthetic solutions are prepared in at least two concentrations. They are also supplied with and without epinephrine. For example, procaine hydrochloride can be found in 1% and 2% solutions, with and without epinephrine. The higher concentration produces neuronal blockade for a longer period of time. It may also block more neurons. In light of these comments, it might seem reasonable to use the higher concentration each time. However, this is not true. The higher concentration is more likely to produce adverse effects and may not be required. For example, smaller nerves have larger surface areas relative to their size and

may be blocked by lower concentrations of a local anesthetic. Furthermore, nonmyelinated nerves are more readily paralyzed than myelinated neurons. Finally, nerves lying near the outside of a nerve bundle are blocked more easily than those inside. In each of these situations in which a block of a small nerve, a nonmyelinated neuron or nerves near the outside of a bundle may be required, it may be possible to use the lower concentration of the anesthetic.

Epinephrine is added to ensure that the local anesthetic stays local. Once the anesthetic leaves the site of administration, it loses its value to the patient. Large quantities of a local anesthetic entering the general circulation can produce systemic toxicity. Therefore, epinephrine is often added as a vasoconstrictor to prevent rapid absorption and ensure a longer duration of action.

There are situations when epinephrine is contraindicated. It can prove catastrophic if injected into a finger, toe, ear or nose. The reduction in blood flow to these areas can produce gangrene. Imagine the consequences of using a local anesthetic containing epinephrine to produce a ring block prior to performing a circumcision.

Once absorbed, epinephrine may produce systemic effects. For example, the cardiac palpitations encountered in a dentist's chair are not always due to the stark terror of the moment. They can also result from absorption of the epinephrine in the local anesthetic solution.

Following their absorption, local anesthetics are metabolized. Local anesthetic esters, procaine, chloroprocaine, tetracaine and cocaine are rapidly destroyed by cholinesterase in plasma. Ten to twelve per cent of a cocaine dose is excreted unchanged.

The amides, bupivicaine, etidocaine, lidocaine, mepivacaine and prilocaine are inactivated by hepatic mixed function oxidases. They have considerably longer half-lives than the esters, ranging from 96 min for lidocaine to 210 min for bupivacaine. The longer half-lives of the amides is a problem only if, as a result of an overdose or inadvertent intravenous administration, significant amounts reach the systemic circulation. Used properly, local anesthetics are absorbed slowly and differences in rates of metabolism have no clinical significance.

Therapeutic Uses

Topical anesthesia involves the application of a local anesthetic to mucous membranes for the purpose of anesthetizing the surface areas of the nose, mouth, throat, esophagus, tracheobronchial tree and genitourinary tree. Cocaine, tetracaine and lidocaine are used most often. Procaine and mepivicaine are not effective because they do not penetrate mucous membranes. The choice of drug depends on the site to be anesthetized. Cocaine can be used for the ear, nose and throat, but not the urethra, rectum or skin. Tetracaine is recommended for all sites except the urethra. Benzocaine can be used for the ear, nose, throat, urethra, rectum and skin, but not the eye.

Infiltration anesthesia is the injection of a local anesthetic directly into the tissues concerned. Epinephrine approximately doubles the duration of anesthesia. Lidocaine is used most frequently. Infiltration anesthesia offers the advantage of good anesthesia while maintaining normal physiological function. Unfortunately, it requires relatively large amounts of anesthetic and is appropriate only for minor surgery.

Nerve block anesthesia is used for larger areas of the body and is produced when a local anesthetic is injected in the vicinity of peripheral nerves or nerve plexuses. Nonmyelinated nerve pain fibers are blocked before myelinated motor neurons, making it possible to block pain without decreasing movement.

Intravenous regional anesthesia involves the injection of a local anesthetic, without a vasoconstrictor or preservatives, into a vein of a previously exsanguinated limb for operations of the elbow or areas distal to it. It may also be used to anesthetize the foot, but is not suitable for the entire leg because of the large amount of local anesthetic required. When the operation is finished, the tourniquet is released. If the tourniquet has been inflated for at least 15 min, only 15 – 30% of the original local anesthetic flows into the general circulation.

Spinal anesthesia is a safe and effective method for operations on the lower abdomen, extremities and perineum. It is produced when a local anesthetic is injected into the subarachnoid space usually between the second and fifth lumbar vertebrae. The major factors controlling the level of anesthesia are (1) site of injection, (2) specific gravity and volume of solution, (3) position of the patient and (4) volume of the spinal subarachnoid space. Isobaric, hyperbaric or hypobaric solutions may be injected, depending largely on the administrator's personal preference. The level of block can be kept low in the distal subarachnoid space by making the solution hypertonic with glucose and sitting the patient in a head-up position. Duration of anesthesia depends on the rate of drug absorption into blood. This can be reduced by adding epinephrine to the solution. Spinal anesthesia produces sympathetic denervation, causing a fall in peripheral resistance, venous return, cardiac output and blood pressure. Venous return can be guaranteed if sympathetically blocked areas are elevated above the level of the right atrium.

Epidural anesthesia is accomplished when a local anesthetic is injected into the epidural space. The anesthetic diffuses into the subarachnoid space, where it acts like a spinal anesthetic, and outside the spinal cord into the paravertebral area, where it produces multiple paravertebral blocks. Epidural anesthesia is usually subdivided into thoracic epidural, lumbar epidural and caudal epidural. Thoracic epidural anesthesia is useful in surgical procedures involving the thorax or upper abdomen. Lumbar epidural anesthesia is the most frequently employed and is useful in obstetrics and for surgical procedures involving the lower abdomen. Caudal anesthesia is usually reserved for interventions on the pelvis and perineum and for vaginal deliveries.

Adverse Effects

Local anesthetics can stimulate the central nervous system. Generally, the more potent local anesthetics are more likely to produce restlessness, tremors and, if the concentration is sufficiently high, clonic convulsions. The sequel to central stimulation is depression and death, as a result of respiratory failure.

Local anesthetics are potent myocardial depressants. If present in adequate concentrations they decrease electrical excitability, conduction rate and force of contraction. In the case of lidocaine, these properties are used to make the drug a very valuable agent for the treatment of ventricular arrhythmias (see Chapter 11). However, one should not confuse the deliberate, controlled use of lidocaine for this purpose with the consequences of inadvertently confronting the heart with large amounts of the drug. In the latter situation, patients experience bradycardia, hypotension and heart block, which can progress to cardiac and respiratory arrest. The cardiovascular symptoms usually begin after the signs of central nervous system intoxication.

Hypersensitivity reactions may occur following the use of local anesthetics. They appear as allergic dermatitis, asthma or fatal anaphylaxis. Hypersensitivity is seen mainly with the esters benzocaine, cocaine, procaine and tetracaine. Individuals allergic to one ester are usually allergic to the others. These patients should receive one of the amides.

Nursing Process

Normally, responsibility for determining the need for a local anesthetic, selecting the appropriate one from among those available, administering it and monitoring its effectiveness is the responsibility of a physician, dentist or anesthetist (either physician or nurse).

Evaluation

The responsibilities of the nurse who has no advanced training in anesthesiology are confined to the evaluation of the patient's generalized physiological response to the local anesthetic, so that any adverse reactions are promptly and accurately identified. Therefore, the nurse caring for the patient who has received a local anesthetic should monitor and evaluate the status of the patient's central nervous and cardiovascular systems, and be alert for evidence of local or generalized allergic reactions or anaphylaxis. Subjective reports by the patient of nervousness, dizziness or blurred vision, combined with nursing observations of tremors, high anxiety or drowsiness, suggest adverse central nervous system effects which, if untreated, may progress to respiratory distress, convulsions, unconsciousness and even death.

Preoperative teaching and preparation should always be part of the nursing care plan. Preoperative assessment of blood work and electrocardiographic results are a nursing responsibility.

Adverse cardiovascular effects of local anesthetics are identified by nursing observations of hypotension and bradycardia. If untreated, these signs may proceed to cardiac arrest. Nurses must report any of the preceding observations to the physician immediately and be prepared to initiate emergency measures or assist in whatever measures the physician deems necessary to reverse these medical emergencies.

Localized allergic reaction to local anesthetics is usually manifested by burning, tenderness, swelling and redness which may later proceed to tissue sloughing and necrosis. Generalized allergic responses to local anesthetics are signified by a rash, urticaria, edema or anaphylaxis. These effects should be reported immediately to the physician because anaphylaxis constitutes a medical emergency. In this situation, the nurse should stay with the patient and be prepared to initiate emergency measures or assist the physician in doing so.

Characteristics of Some Commonly Used Local Anesthetics

Cocaine is too toxic to be injected but provides excellent surface anesthesia when applied topically. It has good vasoconstrictor potency and promotes the shrinking of mucous membranes. Cocaine should not be used in the genitourinary areas because it is absorbed too quickly. Solutions range from one to ten per cent.

Procaine (Novocain) was the standard local anesthetic against which all others were compared. It has been replaced by lidocaine in this regard. Procaine penetrates mucous membranes poorly and should not be used for topical anesthesia. When procaine is injected, anesthesia begins quickly. Depending on the concentration used or the presence of a vasoconstrictor, the duration of anesthesia can last for an hour or longer.

Tetracaine (Pontocaine) is also a local anesthetic ester. Its onset of action (ten minutes or more) and duration of action are longer than procaine's. For injection purposes, the drug is available in 0.3% solution. Topically, it works well in 0.5 – 2% concentrations.

Lidocaine (Xylocaine) is more potent and versatile than procaine and can be used for infiltration and nerve block anesthesia, as well as topical anesthesia. It is prepared in concentrations ranging from 0.5 – 2%. Lidocaine is an amide and may be used in patients who are hypersensitive to local anesthetic esters.

Mepivicaine (Carbocaine) is an amide with essentially the same properties as lidocaine, with the exception that it has poor activity when used topically, and a longer duration of action when injected.

Bupivacaine (Marcaine) is another amide. Its properties are similar to those of the other drugs. Bupivacaine is used for infiltration, nerve block and peridural anesthesia. It is more potent and longer acting than mepivicaine. Bupivacaine is available in injection solutions of 0.25%, 0.5% and 0.75%.

Dibucaine (Nupercaine) is a very potent amide with a long duration of action. The concentrations available for injection usually range from 0.05 – 0.1%. Dibucaine is also used often for topical anesthesia.

Further Reading

Attia, R.R. and Grogono, A.W. (1978). *Practical Anesthetic Pharmacology*. New York: Appleton-Century-Crofts.

Concepcion, M. and Corino, B.G. (1984). Rational use of local anesthetics. *Drugs 27* :256-270.

Table 72
Local anesthetics.

Pharmacologic Classification: Local Anesthetic Esters

Generic Name (Trade Name)	Use (Dose)	Action	Adverse Effects	Drug Interactions	Nursing Process
Cocaine HCl	Local anesthesia in ear, nose and throat and in bronchoscopy (**Topical:** *For ENT/bronchoscopy* - 4% cocaine HCl. *For corneal anesthesia* - 0.25-0.5% solut'n)	Blocks nerve impulses; vasoconstrictor. If sufficient quantities absorbed, CNS excitat'n and incr. BP.	Euphoria, cortical stimulat'n, excitement, restlessness, tremors followed by *grand mal* seizures, tachycardia, elevated BP, psychic dependence, tolerance	**Antidepressants, heterocyclic; guanethidine; MAOIs:** Potentiate vasoconstrictor effects of cocaine.	**Evaluate:** CNS status; for local or gen'lized allergic react'ns or analphylaxis
Procaine HCl (Novocain)	For infiltrat'n and nerve block anesthesia (**Infiltrat'n:** Up to 100 mL of 0.25% or 0.5% solut'n w. or without epinephrine. **Nerve block:** Up to 50 mL of 1% or 25 mL of 2% solut'n w. or without epinephrine)	Blocks nerve impulses; may be used w. vasoconstrictors. Not effective if used topically.	CNS stimulat'n followed by depress'n; skin allergy	**Echothiophate iodide:** Used for prolonged periods in the eye, reduces pseudocholinesterase activity, resulting in reduced rate of inactivat'n of procaine.	As for cocaine
Tetracaine HCl (Pontocaine)	Spinal anesthesia; surface anesthesia of eye, minor burns, scalds, ulcers, operative wounds, hemorrhoids, mild sunburn (**Subarachnoid:** Dilute 1% solut'n w. equal volume of 10% dextrose. *For obstetric saddle block* - 2-4 mg. *For lower extremities and perineal operat'ns* - 3-6 mg. *For most cesareans and lower abdominal surgery* - 9-12 mg. *For upper abdominal surgery* - 12-15 mg. **Topical:** *Adults - Skin and anus:* Not > 30 g. *Children* - 7.5 g/24 h. *Nose and pharynx* - Up to 2 mL of 1% solut'n. *Esophageal and laryngeal reflexes* - 2 mL of 1% solut'n*)	Blocks nerve impulses; longer durat'n than procaine. Also effective if used topically.	CNS stimulat'n followed by depress'n; allergic rashes or urticaria	As for procaine	As for cocaine

Pharmacologic Classification: Local Anesthetic Amides

Generic Name (Trade Name)	Use (Dose)	Action	Adverse Effects	Drug Interactions	Nursing Process
Bupivacaine HCl (Marcaine, Sensorcaine)	Peripheral nerve block; infiltrat'n, sympathetic block-ade; caudal, epidural, paracervi-cal and pudendal block; spinal anesthesia **(Caudal/epidu-ral/peripheral nerve block:** *For incomplete motor block -* 0.25% solut'n. *Motor block but incomplete muscular relaxat'n -* 0.5%. *Complete motor block -* 0.75%. For detailed dosage, consult product literature)	Blocks nerve impuls-es; more potent than mepivicaine	Hypersensitivity react'ns; CNS stimu-lat'n, followed by depress'n and death; myocardial depress'n, bradycardia, hypotens'n, heart block, cardiac arrest	**Antidepressants, heterocyclic; MAOIs:** Incr. activity of epinephrine. Local anesthetic solut'ns should be used w. caution, if at all, in pts receiving heterocyclic antidepressants or MAOIs.	As for cocaine
Lidocaine HCl (Xylocaine)	Infiltrat'n, IV regional nerve block, epidural, spinal and topical anesthesia (See product literature for various formulat'ns available and recommended dosages)	Blocks nerve impulses	As for bupivacaine	**Phenytoin:** Administered IV tog. w. IV lidocaine, may produce excess. cardiac depress'n.	As for cocaine
Mepivicaine HCl (Carbocaine)	*(For nerve block -* 5-20 mL of 1% or 1.5% solut'n. *For epidural block -* 15-25 mL of 1% solut'n. *For infiltrat'n -* Up to 40 mL of 1% solut'n)	Blocks nerve impuls-es; longer action than lidocaine	As for bupivacaine	As for bupivacaine	As for cocaine

C H A P T E R 51

Antiepileptic Drugs

Teaching Objectives

Following completion of this chapter, the reader should be able to:

1. Describe the two major classifications of epilepsy.
2. Discuss the etiologies of primary and secondary epilepsy.
3. Discuss briefly the means by which antiepileptic drugs affect seizures.
4. Describe the mechanism of action, pharmacokinetics, pharmacologic effects, therapeutic uses, adverse effects and drug interactions of phenytoin, and the nursing process related to its use.
5. Discuss the pharmacokinetics, therapeutic uses and adverse effects of carbamazepine, and the nursing process associated with its use.
6. Describe the mechanism of action, therapeutic uses, adverse effects and drug interactions of phenobarbital, as well as the nursing process related to its use.
7. Discuss the mechanism of action, pharmacokinetics, pharmacologic effects, therapeutic uses and adverse effects of primidone, and the nursing process precipitated by its use.
8. Describe briefly the pharmacokinetics, therapeutic uses and adverse effects of ethosuximide, and the nursing process related to its administration.
9. Discuss briefly the pharmacokinetics, therapeutic uses and adverse effects of valproic acid and divalproex, and the nursing process related to their use.
10. Describe briefly the therapeutic uses and adverse effects of clonazepam and clobazam, as well as the nursing process associated with their administration.
11. Describe briefly the use of intravenous diazepam in the treatment of status epilepticus.

Classification of Epilepsy

Epilepsy (or more correctly, the epilepsies) is a group of disorders involving similar path~ ~hysiolog-ical mechanisms occurring in different a   of the brain. They have different causes and present different clinical symptoms. Although it is always difficult to define a disorder precisely, the definition of epilepsy we favor is "a symptom of excessive temporary neuronal discharge, due to intracranial or extracranial causes; it is characterized clinically by discrete episodes, which tend to be recurrent, in which there is a disturbance of movement, sensation, behavior, perception and/or consciousness." (From: J.M. Sutherland et al. [1974], *The Epilepsies, Modern Diagnosis and Treatment*, 2nd ed. New York: Churchill Livingstone.)

This definition stresses the intermittent nature of epilepsy. Whereas it is true that patients may suffer attacks caused by abnormal neuronal firing, they can also experience long seizure-free periods. It is important to re-emphasize that epilepsy can result from many different causes affecting various parts of the brain. The site of neuronal discharge and the extent to which it spreads in the brain determines the clinical effects seen in the patient.

Etiologically, epilepsy can be classified as either **primary** or **secondary.** The cause of primary epilepsy is not known and therefore it is also called **idiopathic.** Primary epilepsy is characterized by major seizures (*grand mal*) or minor seizures (*petit mal,* myoclonic seizures and akinetic seizures). Secondary epilepsy is also called **symptomatic epilepsy** because it is symptomatic of an underlying identifiable problem. It can result from either intracranial causes (such as cerebral tumors, cerebrovascular occlusive disease or head injury) or extracranial problems (such as anoxia, uremia or eclampsia).

It is also popular to classify epilepsy on the basis of seizure patterns. Table 73 presents the classification suggested in 1969 by the International League Against Epilepsy. **Generalized seizures** are characterized by an abnormal neuronal discharge that originates in the midbrain reticular formation. This part of the central nervous system acts much like a telephone system, connecting with all parts of the brain. Any neuronal discharge starting there or reaching there from another site may be transmitted to other areas of the brain. The extent of its propagation and the areas of the brain to which it is transmitted determine the nature of the epileptic attack. As a result, generalized seizures may vary in severity. They always involve a loss of consciousness and bilateral motor events, but they can range all the way from brief periods of unconsciousness (*petit mal*) to severe tonic-clonic seizures (*grand mal*). Generalized seizures may be due to genetic factors that make the midbrain reticular formation unstable, or to structural abnormalities or chemical causes (such as uremia, eclampsia or anoxia).

Partial seizures result from an excessive neuronal discharge anywhere in the cerebral hemispheres. The initial symptoms are determined by the anatomic site of the original discharge. The discharge may remain localized or it may spread to other anatomical areas of the brain. The farther it spreads, the greater will be its clinical effect. If the impulse reaches the midbrain reticular formation, it may be transmitted throughout the brain, producing a generalized seizure. If, for example, the neuronal discharge occurs in the motor cortex, unusual muscle movements will be seen. An illustration of this is the Jacksonian March, which begins with involuntary movements in the fingers of one hand and then moves to include the hand, arm and leg of the same side, if the impulse spreads to other motor neurons on the same side of the cerebral cortex. If the impulse reaches the midbrain reticular formation, it may be carried to all areas of the brain and a generalized seizure will occur. Etiologically, partial epilepsy is caused by pathology in a discrete area of the brain.

Table 73
Characteristics of generalized, partial and unclassified epileptic seizures.[†]

1. **Generalized seizures**
   Bilateral symmetrical seizures without local onset; clinically:
   (a) Absences
   (b) Bilateral myoclonus
   (c) Infantile spasms
   (d) Clonic seizures
   (e) Tonic seizures
   (f) Tonic-clonic seizures
   (g) Akinetic seizures

2. **Partial seizures**
   Seizures beginning locally with:
   (a) Elementary symptomatology
   • motor
   • sensory
   • autonomic
   (b) Complex symptomatology
   • impaired consciousness
   • complex hallucinations
   • affective symptoms
   • automatism
   (c) Partial seizures becoming generalized tonic-clonic seizures

3. **Unclassified seizures**
   Seizures that cannot be classified because of incomplete data

[†] As suggested by International League Against Epilepsy, 1969.

Antiepileptic Drugs — General Comments

Petit mal (absence) seizures are relatively uncommon and begin exclusively in childhood. Patients experience recurrent brief sudden interruptions of consciousness without falling and have minimal twitching around the face and eyes. The drugs of first choice are either valproic acid (Depakene), divalproex sodium (Depakote, Epival) or ethosuximide (Zarontin). Clonazepam (Klonopin, Rivotril) is an alternate drug.

Myoclonic seizures are characterized by bilateral myoclonic jerks of the limbs, face and trunk that, if severe, may throw the patient to the ground. There may be brief lapses of consciousness. Early treatment of myoclonic epilepsy in infancy (hypsarrhythmia) is imperative. Corticosteroids (e.g., prednisone, 10 mg three or four times daily) or corticotrophin (40 U daily) given for two weeks may stop these seizures and prevent mental deterioration. If these agents fail, clonazepam or valproic acid may control the seizures but are less likely to prevent mental retardation. Myoclonic epilepsy in children, adolescents or adults is best treated with clonazepam or sodium valproate.

Generalized tonic-clonic seizures may be a manifestation of primary generalized epilepsy or occur secondary to focal or myoclonic seizures. Carbamazepine (Tegretol) or phenytoin (Dilantin) are the drugs of first choice, with phenobarbital, primidone or valproic acid serving as second-line drugs. Phenobarbital is usually used for the prevention of febrile seizures in infants.

Partial or focal epilepsy may activate the deep central gray matter to produce a secondarily generalized tonic-clonic seizure. Phenytoin and carbamazepine are first-line drugs in the treatment of partial or focal epilepsy. Phenobarbital and primidone are second-line agents.

Status epilepticus is the only situation in which urgent treatment of seizures is essential. It is usually treated with intravenous diazepam. Alternatively, phenobarbital or phenytoin can be administered intravenously.

Drugs Effective Against Generalized Tonic-Clonic Seizures

Phenytoin (Dilantin)

Mechanism of Action, Pharmacokinetics and Pharmacologic Effects

Phenytoin is slowly absorbed from the gastrointestinal tract. Approximately ninety per cent of the drug in the blood is bound to plasma proteins. Phenytoin appears to prevent the spread of seizure activity in the cerebrum by reducing sodium transport across cell membranes. Elimination of phenytoin depends on hepatic metabolism. At low doses the drug has a half-life of twenty-four hours. However, as the dosages of phenytoin increase the metabolic pathways responsible for its inactivation become progressively more saturated and the half-life of the drug increases. Relatively small increases in dose can produce significant increases in plasma concentrations and drug-related toxicity. Measuring phenytoin plasma levels is valuable in adjusting the dose. Plasma concentrations of phenytoin between $10 - 20$ µg/mL ($39.6 - 79.2$ µmol/L) are often effective without causing undue toxicity.

Problems may be encountered if phenytoin is injected intramuscularly or intravenously. Phenytoin is soluble only in concentrated solutions at an alkaline pH. Dilantin injection solution has a pH of 12. If injected intramuscularly, body fluids rapidly change the pH of the drug solution to 7.35. Phenytoin is not soluble in a concentrated solution at this pH and precipitates in the muscle. Thereafter, its rate of absorption depends on slow dissolution in the muscle. Problems can also be encountered if phenytoin is placed in a glass intravenous bottle. In this environment the drug adheres to the glass. Using a glass container serves only to treat the inside of the bottle and not the inside of the patient.

Therapeutic Uses

Phenytoin capsules are indicated for the control of generalized tonic-clonic and psychomotor (*grand mal* and temporal-lobe) seizures and prevention and treatment of seizures occurring during or following neurosurgery. The pediatric formulations (Infatabs and suspension) are used for the control of generalized tonic-clonic (*grand mal*) and complex partial (psychomotor, temporal-lobe) seizures. When used parenterally, phenytoin is indicated for the treatment of status epilepticus of the *grand mal* type and the treatment of seizures occurring during or following neurosurgery.

Monotherapy is the preferred mode of therapy for most patients. If seizures continue and further increases in dosage appear inadvisable because of adverse effects or high serum concentrations of the drug, at least one and sometimes a second alternative drug should be tried before considering the use of two drugs at the same time. However, if multiple-drug therapy is required, phenytoin is often combined with phenobarbital, carbamazepine (Tegretol) and/or primidone (Mysoline) to manage difficult problems. Phenytoin may be combined with ethosuximide in the treatment of patients with both *petit* and *grand mal*.

Because of its effect on ventricular automaticity, intravenous phenytoin is contraindicated in sinus bradycardia, S-A block, second- and third-degree A-V block, and patients with Adams-Stokes syndrome. Phenytoin should be used with caution in patients with hypotension and severe myocardial insufficiency.

Adverse Effects

Phenytoin irritates the stomach, causing nausea and vomiting. Prolonged use can lead to gum hypertrophy, hirsutism, immunologic abnormalities, skin rashes and other hypersensitivity reactions. Gingival hyperplasia is the most common pediatric adverse effect, and can occur in up to twenty per cent of children. Although gingival hyperplasia can be reduced by good oral hygiene, it remains an embarrassing problem.

Overdosage produces nystagmus, ataxia, diplopia and drowsiness. Generally, concentrations above 20 µg/mL (80 µmol/L) are associated with nystagmus; above 30 µg/mL (120 µmol/L) with ataxia; and above 40 µg/mL (160 µmol/L) with lethargy.

Other adverse effects include hyperglycemia, osteomalacia (treated with high doses of vitamin D), lymphadenopathy, leukopenia, megaloblastic anemia (managed with folic acid) and aplastic anemia.

If given rapidly intravenously, phenytoin can produce hypotension. Cardiac arrhythmias, including ventricular fibrillation or arrest, can also occur.

Recent reports indicate a correlation between the use of anticonvulsant drugs and elevated incidence of birth defects in children born to epileptic women taking such medication during pregnancy. The increase is largely associated with specific defects (e.g., congenital malformations of the heart, cleft lip and/or palate). However, there is no justification for stopping the drug, particularly if it is very effective. The danger to the fetus is greater if the mother has a seizure than if the drug is continued.

Drug Interactions

Phenytoin may interact with numerous other drugs. Some, such as phenobarbital and carbamazepine, have been reported to increase the metabolism of phenytoin. Although it is recommended that plasma concentrations of phenytoin be followed carefully if other drugs are added to the patient's therapeutic regimen, examples of patients who have experienced increases in their abilities to metabolize phenytoin are the exception rather than the rule. Chronic ethanol ingestion may increase phenytoin metabolism. This fact should be borne in mind in treating a patient with a long history of enjoying the joyous juices of the grapes or hops.

Several drugs have been reported to inhibit phenytoin metabolism. These include chlorpromazine, prochlorperazine, chlordiazepoxide, phenylbutazone, propoxyphene, halothane, ethosuximide, estrogens, diazepam, disulfiram and isoniazid.

Phenytoin has a complex interaction with the oral anticoagulant dicumarol. Dicumarol increases serum phenytoin levels, possibly by inhibiting its metabolism. Phenytoin, for its part, stimulates the metabolism of dicumarol, while at the same time displacing it from plasma protein binding sites. Warfarin is less likely to interact with phenytoin and is the anticoagulant of choice in this situation. Additional phenytoin drug interactions are given in Table 74.

Nursing Process

Assessment

The nursing process is initiated with patient assessment, including review of the patient's history for evidence of asthma, allergies, kidney or liver disease, heart block, bradycardia, hypotension or alcohol abuse. Documentation of any of these conditions justifies withholding the initial dose until the physician has been consulted. The physician's affirmation of the drug order in the presence of these contraindications should alert the nurse to conduct a particularly rigorous evaluation of the patient's response to phenytoin.

Nursing assessment of the patient must include establishment of baseline measures of blood pressure, respirations, apical and radial pulses, as well as a thorough documentation of the frequency and type of seizures experienced by the patient.

Administration

The intravenous solution of phenytoin should be prepared for administration using only the diluent supplied by the manufacturer. It requires approximately ten minutes to dissolve completely and only clear solutions should be administered. Intravenous preparations of phenytoin should be used immediately and unused portions discarded. As pointed out earlier, this medication should *never* be added to an intravenous solution in a glass bottle for administration. Although most institutions now stock intravenous solutions in plastic bags, it is still the preferred practice to administer intravenous injections of phenytoin slowly (over 1 – 2 min) into the tubing of a running intravenous infusion and then flush the tubing with saline.

The administration of oral doses of phenytoin with meals may alleviate some of the gastric distress that often accompanies the use of this medication.

Evaluation

Nursing evaluation of patients who have received phenytoin is initially concerned with its efficacy. The number and type of seizures that the patient experiences should be included in the nursing record. The absence of seizures should also be noted.

Patients should also be observed for evidence of adverse effects. When phenytoin is injected intravenously, the possibility of adverse cardiovascular effects is of particular concern. Patients who receive intravenous phenytoin should be carefully monitored for evidence of bradycardia, myocardial depression and/or hypotension which suggest reduced A-V conduction and could progress to cardiac arrest.

Adverse hematological effects are demonstrated by sore throat, frequent nose bleeds, the appearance of contusions without remembered injury, and petechiae. The observation of jaundice, tea-colored urine, light-colored stools, anorexia or sudden acute abdominal pain indicates adverse hepatic effects. Any of the preceding observations warrants withholding phenytoin while the physician's advice is urgently sought.

Evidence of folic acid or vitamin D deficiency should be reported to the physician promptly; however, it is not a medical emergency and does not warrant withholding the drug. Patients receiving phenytoin should be observed for evidence of hypoglycemia and the physician informed if it occurs.

Teaching
Nurses should include families as well as patients in teaching programs related to the use of phenytoin. They should be advised that discontinuing the medication, alteration in its dosage or brand might precipitate seizure recurrence. Adequate supplies of medication must always be kept on hand, especially in anticipation of holidays or vacations. It is also advisable to refill prescriptions at the same pharmacy where a record is kept of the brand of medication dispensed.

Patients should also be taught the importance of good oral hygiene, including brushing, flossing and regular dental checkups to reduce the gingivitis and gingival hyperplasia that often accompany phenytoin use. Nurses should advise patients that excessive alcohol use may reduce phenytoin's effectiveness. Alerting the patient to the fact that phenytoin can color the urine pink or reddish-brown may prevent unnecessary concern. Phenytoin can interfere with folic acid metabolism and nurses must emphasize the importance of adequate folic acid and vitamin D intake. Patients should avoid driving cars or using power tools or industrial machinery during the initial period of dosage adjustment because high doses of phenytoin can cause nystagmus, vertigo, ataxia and diplopia.

Patients and families should be taught the adverse effects of phenytoin and instructed to seek medical advice immediately should any appear.

Providing a printed list facilitates recall and emphasizes their importance.

Other aspects of nursing care for patients with epilepsy are beyond the scope of this text. Readers requiring such information are advised to consult a medical-surgical nursing text.

Carbamazepine (Tegretol)

Pharmacokinetics and Therapeutic Uses
Carbamazepine's spectrum of activity is similar to that of phenytoin. It is considered a first-line drug for the treatment of generalized tonic-clonic seizures and partial seizures with complex symptomatology. Carbamazepine is ineffective in controlling *petit mal,* minor motor, myoclonic and predominantly unilateral seizures.

Carbamazepine is absorbed slowly from the gastrointestinal tract. Its half-life during chronic therapy may range from eight to over twenty-four hours. Carbamazepine's usual therapeutic range is 5 –12 ug/mL (21.1 – 50.8 umol/L) ; 15 – 17 ug/mL (63.3 –71.7 umol/L) may be necessary in some patients.

Adverse Effects
At usual therapeutic doses, carbamazepine has a low incidence of adverse effects. The most common include gastric irritation, dizziness, diplopia and blurred vision. Carbamazepine can also produce oculomotor disturbances, tinnitus, abnormal involuntary movements, peripheral neuritis, rashes, congestive heart failure, hypotension, syncope, and cholestatic and hepatocellular jaundice. Agranulocytosis, thrombocytopenia and leukopenia are recognized adverse effects of the drug. Fortunately, they are rare.

Nursing Process
Assessment
Nurses must contact the physician before administering carbamazepine if they uncover information in the patient's history that might contraindicate its use. Carbamazepine should be withheld pending consultation with the physician if the history reveals documentation of bone marrow depression; previous hypersensitivity to this drug; liver, kidney or cardiovascular disease; or glaucoma. Most physicians weigh the benefit/risk ratio for the fetus before administering carbamazepine during pregnancy; however, patients should be advised that the safe use of carbamazepine in pregnancy has not been established. Serum drug-level studies are important initially and during continuing therapy.

Evaluation

Nursing evaluation should include recording the frequency and type of seizures experienced. Although the incidence of carbamazepine-induced adverse effects is statistically very low, we remind readers that no patient likes to think of himself as a statistic; a patient either experiences adverse effects or he does not. Therefore, because of the rarely reported deaths due to irreversible blood dyscrasias, patients receiving carbamazepine must receive rigorous, meticulous and attentive nursing evaluation for evidence of dyscrasias. Nurses must be particularly vigilant for reports of sore throat, mucosal ulceration, petechiae, contusions of unknown origin or lethargy. Other previously identified adverse effects of this medication have less life-threatening outcomes, but nevertheless should not be overlooked. Eye problems require ophthalmic examinations before, during and after treatment.

Teaching

Nurses should instruct patients and their families how to evaluate the effectiveness of the medication, i.e., reduced frequency and/or severity of seizure activity. Both patient and family must also be familiar with the symptoms of blood dyscrasias and understand the importance of promptly seeking medical advice should any appear. Patients and families should also be advised of the importance of keeping regularly scheduled appointments for laboratory tests and physician evaluation. Instructions regarding driving, use of power tools and machinery, and maintaining adequate supplies of medication are the same as those previously discussed for phenytoin. Patients should be instructed to a carry medic-alert identification bracelet. They should also be told to avoid alcohol ingestion, as convulsions may result.

Phenobarbital

Mechanism of Action and Therapeutic Uses

Phenobarbital is a central nervous system depressant that may act as an antiepileptic by reducing sodium and potassium flux across cell membranes. It remains a popular drug for the treatment of tonic-clonic epilepsy, focal seizures and complex partial seizures. Phenobarbital is a long-acting barbiturate, with a half-life ranging from 60 – 120 h in adults. The plasma levels considered to be consistent with good therapeutic effect and minimal toxicity fall between 15 – 25 µg/mL (64.6 – 107.7 µmol/L). Phenobarbital is also employed prophylactically in young children when febrile seizures are feared.

Adverse Effects

Central nervous system depression is the major adverse effect of phenobarbital. This can be seen as either sedation or sleep and can be minimized by increasing the dose gradually. Fortunately, tolerance to the CNS-depressive effects of phenobarbital occurs when the drug is given chronically. Nevertheless, the first few weeks of treatment can be a problem.

Allergic rashes are reported in one to two per cent of patients taking phenobarbital. Prolonged therapy may be associated with folate deficiency, hypocalcemia and osteomalacia. These effects will respond to folic acid treatment and high doses of vitamin D. Hypoprothrombinemia with hemorrhage has been reported in babies delivered from mothers given phenobarbital. This can be treated with vitamin K injections.

Drug Interactions

Phenobarbital will produce at least an additive effect with other central nervous system depressants. Patients taking phenobarbital should be warned about the dangers of consuming other CNS depressants such as alcohol, antihistamines, narcotics, antianxiety drugs, etc.

Phenobarbital may induce hepatic drug-metabolizing enzymes. If this happens, the ability of the liver to metabolize a large number of drugs will increase. It was noticed several years ago that phenobarbital increased the metabolism of phenytoin. Although this can happen, it is not usual when both drugs are used concomitantly.

Phenobarbital has also been reported to increase the metabolism of oral anticoagulants. As a result, larger than normal doses may be required to decrease prothombin levels. If phenobarbital is discontinued later, the ability of the liver to metabolize the anticoagulants will decrease. Failure to make a corresponding reduction in the dose of the anticoagulant will result in hemorrhaging.

Phenobarbital can also increase the metabolism of antihistamines, griseofulvin, oral contraceptives, quinidine, steroids, methoxyflurane and vitamin D.

Nursing Process

The nursing process related to the use of barbiturates was discussed in detail in Chapter 46. We need only add the necessity for observing the frequency and type of seizures in both nursing assessment and evaluation.

Primidone (Mysoline)

Mechanism of Action, Pharmacokinetics and Pharmacologic Effects

Primidone is structurally similar to phenobarbital and has a spectrum of antiepileptic activity similar to that of the latter. Primidone is quickly absorbed from the gastrointestinal tract and metabolized to phenobarbital and phenylethylmalonamide, both having antiepileptic activity. The half-life of primidone is eight hours and the half-lives of phenobarbital and phenylethylmalonamide 60 – 120 h and 24 – 48 h, respectively. Therefore, patients treated with primidone accumulate its metabolites in their bodies. Effective plasma levels of primidone usually fall between 5 – 10 ug/mL (22.9 – 45.8 µmol/L). However, phenobarbital plasma levels frequently can be used to guide dosage.

Therapeutic Uses

Primidone is useful in the prevention of *grand mal* and psychomotor seizures. It may be used alone or in combination with other anticonvulsants. To avoid undue central nervous system depression, primidone should be taken at night and the dose increased gradually.

Adverse Effects

Primidone depresses the central nervous system and can cause sedation, vertigo, nystagmus, ataxia and diplopia. Other complaints include nausea and vomiting. Serious adverse effects are not common. However, leukopenia, thrombocytopenia, systemic lupus erythematosus and lymphadenopathy have been encountered. Similar to phenobarbital, primidone may cause maculopapular and morbilliform rashes, hemorrhage in the newborn, megaloblastic anemia and osteomalacia. The appearance of a rash is justification for stopping the drug. The other conditions may be treated as explained earlier for phenobarbital.

Nursing Process

Because of its similarity in structure and action to phenobarbital, the nursing implications for primidone are the same as those discussed in Chapter 46 for barbiturates. The only difference is that nurses caring for patients receiving primidone will also evaluate their patients for the previously identified adverse effects which differ from those of phenobarbital.

Drugs Effective Against Absence Seizures

Ethosuximide (Zarontin)

Pharmacokinetics and Therapeutic Uses

Ethosuximide is a first-line drug for the treatment of *petit mal* epilepsy. With a half-life of thirty hours in children, ethosuximide requires five to seven days of regular treatment to reach steady-state levels. Therapeutic effects are usually obtained with serum levels of 50 –100 µg/mL (354.2 – 708.3 µmol/L).

Adverse Effects

Gastric irritation is the most common adverse reaction to ethosuximide. This can be minimized by giving the drug in divided daily doses. Other drug-related problems include central nervous system depression and rashes. Eosinophilia is seen in about ten per cent of patients taking ethosuximide. Other blood problems that have occurred are pancytopenia and aplastic anemia. Systemic lupus erythematosus and the Stevens-Johnson syndrome have also been noted rarely in patients given ethosuximide.

Nursing Process

Nursing assessment includes a review of the patient's history for evidence of conditions that contraindicate ethosuximide use. These include previous hypersensitivity to the drug, and kidney or liver disease. Patient assessment by nurses will also incorporate documentation of the frequency and type of seizures.

Nursing evaluation must consider drug efficacy, as described for the preceding anticonvulsants, and adverse effects as outlined before.

Valproic Acid (Depakene)

Pharmacokinetics and Therapeutic Uses

Valproic acid, or sodium valproate, is indicated as sole or adjunctive therapy in the treatment of simple or complex absence seizures, including *petit mal,* and is useful in primary generalized seizures with tonic-clonic manifestations. Valproic acid may also be used adjunctively in patients with multiple seizure types, which include either absence or tonic-clonic seizures. With a half-life of six to sixteen hours, valproic acid should be administered three or four times daily. The therapeutic plasma window for valproic acid is 50 – 100 µg/mL (347 – 694 µmol/L).

Divalproex sodium (Depakote, Epival) is a derivative of valproic acid. Provided in enteric-coated tablets, it dissociates into valproic acid in the intestinal tract. The drug may produce less gastric distress than valproic acid.

Adverse Effects

Anorexia, nausea and vomiting are major deterrents to the use of valproic acid. Taking the drug with food may assist greatly. Sedation, ataxia, and incoordination occur very infrequently. Minor elevations of transaminases (e.g., SGOT and SGPT) and LDH are frequent and appear to be dose related. Occasionally, laboratory tests also show increases in serum bilirubin and abnormal changes in other liver function tests. These results may reflect serious hepatotoxicity. Hepatic failure resulting in fatalities has occurred in patients receiving valproic acid. This has usually occurred during the first six months of treatment with valproic acid. *Because children two years of age or younger have nearly a twenty-fold increase in risk of fatal hepatotoxicity, valproic acid should be used in this age group with extreme caution and as a sole agent.* Liver function tests should be performed on patients receiving valproic acid prior to therapy and at frequent intervals thereafter, especially during the first six months. However, physicians should not rely totally on serum biochemistry, since these tests may not be abnormal in all instances, but should also consider the results of a careful interim medical history and physical examination. Care should be observed when administering valproic acid to patients with a prior history of hepatic disease.

Reports have appeared implicating valproic acid as a teratogen. The incidence of congenital malformations in the general population may be increased two- to three-fold by valproic acid. The increase is largely associated with specific defects, e.g., congenital malformations of the heart, cleft lip and/or palate, and neural tube defects. Nevertheless, the great majority of mothers receiving anticonvulsant medication deliver normal infants.

Drug Interactions

Valproic acid interacts with other antiepileptic drugs. It increases the plasma levels of phenobarbital and primidone. The mechanism behind this effect is not clear but it can lead to phenobarbital or primidone toxicity.

Nursing Process

Assessment
The nursing process is initiated with patient assessment. This includes a review of the patient's history for documentation of liver disease. Female patients should undergo physical assessment for pregnancy or lactation. If the nursing assessment reveals either of these, the first dose should be withheld pending consultation with the physician. Nursing assessment should also document the frequency and type of seizures experienced by the patient prior to initiation of therapy.

Administration
Because valproic acid can irritate the stomach, it is administered with food.

Evaluation
Nursing evaluation of patients receiving valproic acid is similar to that previously described for other anticonvulsants. Nurses caring for patients who have both epilepsy and diabetes should be aware that valproic acid can cause a false positive test for acetonuria. Nurses should evaluate patients for respiratory dysfunction and withhold the drug if respirations are fewer than twelve per minute or the pupils dilated.

Teaching
Patient teaching in relation to the use of valproic acid is the same as that identified for other anticonvulsants.

Clonazepam (Klonopin, Rivotril)

Therapeutic Uses

Clonazepam is a benzodiazepine. It is indicated alone or as an adjunct in the management of myoclonic and akinetic seizures and *petit mal* variant. The drug may also be of some value in patients with absence spells (*petit mal*) who have failed to respond to succimides.

Adverse Effects

Sedation and drowsiness are the main complaints with clonazepam. In this regard it does not differ from other benzodiazepines (see Chapter 46). Ataxia may also be seen. Alterations in behavior include aggressiveness, argumentative behavior, hyperactivity, agitation, depression, euphoria, irritability, forgetfulness and confusion. These are particularly likely to occur in patients with a prior history of psychiatric disturbances and are known to occur in patients with chronic seizure disorders.

Nursing Process

The nursing process related to the use of the benzodiazepines is discussed in detail in Chapter 46 and Table 69. The only addition required for clonazepam is that the nurse must document the frequency and type of seizures experienced by the patient in both the assessment and evaluation phases.

Miscallaneous Antiepileptics

Clobazam (Frisium)

Clobazam is a new benzodiazepine introduced for epilepsy refractory to standard therapy. In most studies, clobazam has been added to current antiepileptic therapy in patients with refractory seizures and the drug appears to be a useful adjuvant medication in a variety of seizure types in adults and children. Clobazam has a rapid onset of action. Peak levels occur one to three hours after oral administration. Because it has a long half-life (10 – 30h for clobazam and 36 – 46 h for its main active metabolite, N-desmethylclobazam), clobazam may be given once daily. Combined use of clobazam and other antiepileptic drugs may result in serum level changes (increases or decreases) of either agent. Serum concentrations of other anticonvulsants should be monitored and drug dosage alterations instituted when necessary.

Some patients have developed tolerance to the antiepileptic effect of clobazam after weeks or months of therapy. This seems to occur sooner in patients started on a higher milligram-per-kilogram dose.

Clobazam appears to have a lower incidence of neurological adverse effects when compared to clonazepam. The adverse effects of clobazam are dose related. Most common are sedation, drowsiness, fatigue and dizziness. Ataxia, insomnia, depression, behavioral changes and weight gain have also been reported. As with other benzodiazepines, physical and psychological dependence have occurred. Clobazam must be discontinued slowly over several months to avoid withdrawal seizures.

Diazepam (Valium)

Intravenous diazepam is the recommended treatment of status epilepticus. Repeated injections are required to maintain the high brain levels necessary to terminate status epilepticus. Continued use of diazepam is not effective in the prevention of seizures. Detailed discussion of the nursing process related to the use of diazepam is presented in Chapter 46. Readers seeking detailed information are advised to consult that material.

Further Reading

Beghi, E., Di Mascio, R. and Tognoni, G. (1986). Drug treatment of epilepsy. Outlines, criticism and perspectives. *Drugs 31* :249-265.

Chadwick, D. (1988). Drug withdrawal and epilepsy. When and how? *Drugs 35* :579-583.

Drugs for epilepsy (1989). Drugs of choice. *The Medical Letter 31* :1-4 and 18-25.

Gal, P. (1985). Anticonvulsant therapy after neonatal seizures — How long and should it be continued? *Pharmacotherapy 5* :268-273.

Hodson, A. (1985). A case for long-term treatment with anticonvulsants. *Pharmacotherapy 5* :274-277.

Knudsen, F.U. (1988). Optimum management of febrile seizures in childhood? *Drugs 36* :111-120.

Oral benzodiazepines as prophylaxis for epilepsy (1986). *Drug and Therapeutics Bulletin 24* (12):45-46.

Pugh, C.B. and Garnett, W.R. (1991). Current issues in the treatment of epilepsy. *Clinical Pharmacy 10* :335-358.

Shinnar, S., Vining, E.P.G., Mellits, E.D., D'Souza, B.J., Holden, K., Baumgardner, R.A. and Freeman, J.M. (1985). Discontinuing antiepileptic medication in children with epilepsy after two years without seizures. A prospective study. *New Engl. J. Med. 313* : 976-980.

Table 74
Antiepileptic drugs.

Pharmacologic Classification: Drugs Effective Against Generalized Tonic-Clonic Seizures

Generic Name (Trade Name)	Use (Dose)	Action	Adverse Effects	Drug Interactions	Nursing Process
Phenytoin (Dilantin)	Tx of gen'lized tonic-clonic seizures in adults and children; tx of simple and complex partial seizures **(Oral:** Adults [pts who have rec'd no previous tx] - 100 mg tid. For most adults, satisfactory maint. dose will be 300-400 mg/day. Children - Initially 5 mg/kg/day in 2-3 divided doses w. subsequent dosage individualized to max. 300 mg/day. Recomm. daily maint. dose is us. 4-8 mg/kg. Children > 6 years - May require min. adult dose [300 mg/day]. **IV:** *For status epilepticus* - Adults - Loading dose of 10-15 mg/kg, admin. slowly at rate not > 50 mg/min, followed by maint. doses of 100 mg orally or IV q6-8h. Neonates or children - Loading dose of 15-20 mg/kg injected slowly at rate not > 1-3 mg/kg/min)	Decr. spread of ectopic electrical impulses in brain by reducing Na$^+$ transport across cell membranes. Slowly absorbed from GI tract. Eliminat'n rate depends on dose. At low doses, phenytoin has half-life of 24 h. As dosage incr., metabolic pathways for its eliminat'n become saturated. At this point relatively small incr. in dose can produce significant incr. in plasma concentrat'ns and dose-related toxicities.	Gastric irritat'n, nystagmus, ataxia, diplopia, drowsiness, gum hypertrophy, hirsutism, immunological abnormalities, skin rashes, hyperglycemia, osteomalacia, lymphadenopathy, leukopenia, megaloblastic anemia, teratogenicity	**Antidepressants, heterocyclic:** In high doses, may precipitate seizures; dosage of phenytoin may need adjustment. **Barbiturates:** May enhance metabolism of phenytoin. This effect is variable and unpredictable. **Carbamazepine:** Metabolism may be incr. by phenytoin. For its part, carbamazepine may alter the effect of phenytoin (both incr. and decr. phenytoin concentrat'ns have been reported). It is important to monitor both carbamazepine and phenytoin plasma concentrat'ns. **Chloramphenicol:** May inhibit metabolism of phenytoin, leading to incr. adv. effects. **Clonazepam:** Metabolism can be incr. by phenytoin and its effect decr. Clonazepam can have variable effect on concentrat'n of phenytoin. Monitor both clonazepam and phenytoin concentrat'ns. **Corticosteroids:** May experience enhanced metabolism in presence of phenytoin. **Coumarin anticoagulants:** May inhibit metabolism of phenytoin, leading to incr. adv. effects. **Disulfiram:** May inhibit metabolism of phenytoin, leading to incr. adv. effects. **Ethanol:** Abused chronically, can diminish effect of phenytoin. **Folic acid:** Replacement in	**Assess:** Pt hx for asthma, allergies, alcohol abuse, kidney or liver disease, heart block, bradycardia, hypotens'n. Establish baseline VS and no./type of seizures. **Administer:** Prepare IV solut'n w. diluent supplied by manufacturer; use only clear solut'ns. Complete dissolut'n requires approx. 10 min to prepare. Use immediately; do not add to IV solut'ns in glass bottles. Follow IV inject'n w. normal saline. Never add to running IV. Give oral doses w. meals. **Evaluate:** BP, pulse, respirat'n; for adv. CNS effects; for hepatic/hematological toxicity; for folic acid deficiency; for frequency/type of seizures; for hypoglycemia. **Teach:** *Not* to discontinue medicat'n or alter dosage/brand of medicat'n; importance of oral hygiene, dietary intake of vitamin D; to avoid excess. use of alcohol; that urine may change color; to avoid driving/use of power tools, industrial machinery during dosage regulat'n; to self-evaluate for adv. effects.

folate-deficient pts receiving phenytoin may incr. metabolism of phenytoin and decr. serum phenytoin levels. **Isoniazid:** Inhibits metabolism of phenytoin. Pts who are slow isoniazid acetylators may suffer from phenytoin intoxicat'n. **Lidocaine:** Combined IV w. IV phenytoin, can cause excess. cardiac depress'n. **Phenylbutazone:** May inhibit metabolism of phenytoin, leading to incr. adv. effects. **Primidone:** Phenytoin can incr. primidone's metabolism to phenobarbital. **Quinidine:** May undergo incr. rate of hepatic metabolism in presence of chronic phenytoin tx. **Thyroid hormones:** May be displaced from plasma proteins by phenytoin, thereby elevating free thyroxin levels. **Valproate:** Can incr. phenytoin effects by displacing phenytoin from its binding to plasma proteins. Monitor plasma phenytoin concentrat'n and clinical status of pt.

Drug	Uses/Dosage	Action	Adverse effects	Interactions	Nursing considerations
Carbamazepine (Tegretol)	Tx of simple partial, complex partial, and generalized tonic-clonic seizures (**Oral: Adults and children > 12 years -** Initially, 100-200 mg od-bid, depending on severity of case and previous tx hx. Incr. initial dose prn in divided doses. Us. optimal dose, 800-1200 mg/day. As soon as seizures have stopped and pt remains free of them, reduce dose very gradually until min. effective dose is reached. Children 6-12 years - Initially, 100 mg in divided doses on 1st day. Incr.	Reduces propagat'n of aberrant impulses in brain. Absorbed slowly from GI tract. Average half-life, 36 h	Nystagmus, drowsiness, dizziness, ataxia, nausea, diplopia	**Alcohol:** Tolerance may be reduced in pts taking carbamazepine. **Anticoagulants, oral:** Dosage should be readjusted to clinical requirements whenever carbamazepine is started or stopped. **Cimetidine:** Can incr. carbamazepine levels. **Contraceptives, oral:** May be less effective in presence of chronic carbamazepine tx. Pts should be advised to use alternative, nonhormonal methods of contracept'n. **Erythromycin; trolean-**	**Assess:** For hx bone marrow depress'n, previous hypersensitivity, liver, kidney or CV disease, glaucoma, pregnancy or lactat'n. Serum drug-level studies are important during initial and continuing drug tx. **Evaluate:** Frequency/type of convuls'ns; for adv. effects, esp. sore throat, mucosal ulcerat'n, petechiae, bruising, lethargy. Eye problems require ophthalmic exams. before, during and after tx. **Teach:** Self-evaluat'n for drug efficacy and adv. effects; to avoid driving/using power tools during initial tx; to maintain adequate supplies of drug at all times;

Generic Name (Trade Name)	Use (Dose)	Action	Adverse Effects	Drug Interactions	Nursing Process
	gradually by 100 mg/day prn. Dose should generally be not > 1000 mg/day. Reduce gradually to min. effective dose once seizures have stopped and pt has remained free of them)			**domycin:** Can incr. carbamazepine levels. **Isoniazid:** Can incr. carbamazepine levels. **Lithium:** And carbamazepine, may incr. risk of neurotoxic side effects. **MAOIs:** Should not be admin. immed. before, in conjunct'n w., or immed. after carbamazepine. **Phenytoin:** Incr. metabolism of carbamazepine. **Primidone:** Convers'n to phenobarbital is incr. Monitor primidone and phenobarbital concentrat'ns. Primidone can also decr. effect of carbamazepine. **Propoxyphene:** Can incr. carbamazepine levels. **Valproate:** Metabolism can be incr. and its effects decr. Monitor valproate concentrat'n. **Verapamil:** Can incr. carbamazepine levels.	importance of regular medical evaluat'n of blood for hematological disorders. Instruct pts to carry medic-alert ID and to avoid alcohol ingest'n, as convuls'ns may result.
Phenobarbital	Tx of generalized tonic-clonic, simple partial and complex partial seizures. Prevent'n of febrile seizures (**Oral:** Adults - 50-100 mg bid. Children - 15-50 mg bid. **IV:** For status epilepticus - Adults - Initially, 10-20 mg/kg given at rate of 25-50 mg/min. Repeat prn in doses of 120-240 mg q20min. Max. dose/24 h, 1-2 g. Children - Initially, 20 mg/kg, given at rate of 25-50 mg/min. Repeat prn in doses of 6 mg/kg q20min. Max. dose/24 h, 40 mg/kg)	Reduces propagat'n of aberrant impulses in brain. Decr. Na$^+$ and K$^+$ flux across cell membranes.	Sedat'n, nystagmus, ataxia, osteomalacia, hyperactivity in young children	**Anticoagulants, oral; anticonvulsants; antihistamines:** Phenobarbital may incr. their metabolism, resulting in decr. pharmacologic activity. **Clonazepam:** Phenobarbital incr. its metabolism, decr. its effects. Monitor clonazepam plasma concentrat'ns. **CNS depressants:** Admin. concomitantly w. phenobarbital, will result in additive CNS depress'n. **Contraceptives, oral:** Phenobarbital may incr. their metabolism, resulting in decr.	**Assess:** For hx sensitivity to barbiturates or paradoxic excitat'n, chronic resp. disease, hypotens'n, liver disease, porphyria, blood dyscrasias, pregnancy, lactat'n; for pain or dependency; for chronic toxicity; concurrent use of other medicat'ns. Establish descript'n of sleep patterns, baseline measures of respirat'ns and temp. **Administer:** Acc. to local policies and procedures for compliance w. legal regulat'ns regarding controlled substances. *Oral:* Be assured that drug is swallowed and not hoarded. *IV:* Monitor flow rate carefully; guard against extravasat'n of IV.

Drug	Action	Dosage / Use	Adverse effects	Interactions	Nursing considerations
Primidone (Mysoline)	Reduces propagat'n of aberrant impulses in brain.	Effective in tx of same types of seizures as phenobarbital (**Oral:** Adults and children > 8 years - 250 mg bid [week 1]; 250 mg bid, a.m. and hs [week 2]; 250 mg tid [week 3]; 250 mg qid [week 4]. Children < 8 years - 125 mg hs [week 1]; 125 mg bid, a.m. and hs [week 2]; 125 mg tid [week 3]; 125 mg qid [week 4])	Drowsiness, vertigo, nausea, vomiting, megaloblastic anemia and lupus erythematosus-like syndrome	pharmacologic activity. **Griseofulvin:** Phenobarbital may incr. its metabolism, resulting in decr. pharmacologic activity. **Methoxyflurane:** If given to pt on chronic phenobarbital tx, may experience incr. rate of metabolism, thereby giving rise to incr. quantities of its nephrotoxic metabolites. **Valproate:** Decr. metabolism and incr. toxicity of phenobarbital. Monitor phenobarbital plasma concentrat'n. **Vitamin D:** Metabolism may incr. in presence of phenobarbital.	**Evaluate:** For drug efficacy [reduced no./severity of convuls'ns]; for adv. effects; for dependence, toxicity. **Teach:** Dangers of abrupt cessat'n of use; not to use power tools, industrial machinery, drive vehicle during initial tx; not to use alcohol during tx; to use birth control measures other than oral contraceptives; to rise slowly and carefully from bed in a.m.; not to store barbiturates at bedside; indicators of adv. effects, chronic toxicity, dependence.

Pharmacologic Classification: Drugs Effective Against Absence Seizures

Drug	Action	Dosage / Use	Adverse effects	Interactions	Nursing considerations
Ethosuximide (Zarontin)	Reduces propagat'n of aberrant impulses in brain. Half-life of 30 h in children.	Tx of absence seizures (**Oral:** *Initial dose* - Children < 6 years - 250 mg/day. Older pts - 500 mg daily in divided doses. Individualize dose thereafter prn. Incr. daily dose by 250 mg q4-7days until control is achieved w. minimal adv. effects. Daily dosage of 1-1.5 g in divided doses frequently controls seizures)	GI distress, fatigue, lethargy, headache, dizziness, eosinophilia and leukopenia		**Assess:** For hx previous hypersensitivity, kidney or liver disease; establish frequency/type of seizures. **Evaluate:** Frequency/type of seizures; for adv. effects. **Teach:** As for phenobarbital.
Valproic acid (Depakene)	Reduces propagat'n of aberrant impulses in brain. Half-life of 6-10 h.	Tx of absence seizures (**Oral:** Initially, 15 mg/kg/day; incr. at 1-week intervals by 5-10 mg/kg/day until seizures are controlled or adv. effects prevent further increases. Max. recomm. dose, 60 mg/kg/day. When total daily dose > 250 mg, give in divided regimen)	Transient nausea, vomiting and diarrhea. Severe hepatic toxicity rarely.	**Carbamazepine:** Incr. metabolism and decr. effects of valproate. Monitor valproate plasma concentrat'ns. **Clonazepam:** Used concomitantly w. valproic acid, may produce absence attacks. **Diazepam:** Admin. IV, may show incr. toxicity in presence of valproate. **Drugs affecting coagulat'n** (e.g., ASA, warfarin): Should be used w. caution w. valproic acid because valproic acid affects 2nd	**Assess:** For hx liver disease; for pregnancy or lactat'n. **Administer:** W. food. **Evaluate:** Frequency/type of seizures; diabetics for false-positive test for acetonuria. **Teach:** As for other anticonvulsants.

Generic Name (Trade Name)	Use (Dose)	Action	Adverse Effects	Drug Interactions	Nursing Process
Divalproex sodium (Depakote, Epival)	As for valproic acid **(Oral:** Initially, 15 mg/kg/day; incr. at 1-week intervals by 5-10 mg/kg/day until seizures are controlled or side effects preclude further increases. Max. recomm. dose, 60 mg/kg/day. When daily dose > 125 mg, give in divided doses)	As for valproic acid	As for valproic acid	stage of platelet aggregat'n. **Ethanol:** May have its CNS-depressant actions potentiated by valproic acid. **Phenobarbital:** Serum levels may be incr. by valproic acid. Monitor pts on phenobarbital for neurologic toxicity.	As for valproic acid
Clonazepam (Klonopin, Rivotril)	Tx of absence seizures; particularly used for myoclonic and akinetic seizures that resist tx w. other anticonvulsants **(Oral:** Adults - Initially, not > 1.5 mg/day in 3 divided doses; incr. by 0.5-1 mg q3days prn. Doses > 20 mg/day should be given w. caution. Infants and children ≤ 10 years or 30 kg - Initially, 10-30 µg/kg/day; not > 50 µg/kg/day given in 2-3 divided doses. Doses should be incr. by not > 250-500 µg q3rd day until maint. dose of 100-200 µg/kg has been reached, unless seizures have been controlled or adv. effects preclude further increases. Wherever poss., daily dose should be divided into 3 equal doses. If doses are not divided equally, largest dose should be given hs)	Benzodiazepine drug that reduces propagat'n of aberrant impulses in brain.	Drowsiness, ataxia, behavioral changes	**CNS depressants:** May potentiate action of benzodiazepines. **Valproic acid:** And clonazepam, may produce absence seizures.	Refer to Table 69 for Nursing Process common to all benzodiazepines.

Pharmacologic Classification: Miscellaneous Drug in Treatment of Epilepsy

Drug				
Clobazam (Frisium)	Valuable adjuvant tx in pts not adequately controlled by current drugs (**Oral: Adults -** Initially, 5-15 mg/day; incr. gradually prn up to 80 mg/day. Children < 2 years - 0.5-1 mg/kg/day. 2-16 years - 5 mg/day; may incr. at intervals of 5 days up to max. dose of 40 mg/day. Daily dose ≤ 30 mg may be taken od hs. If dose is divided, larger portion should be taken hs)	Benzodiazepine drug. Its action may be related to its ability to potentiate action of GABA in brain. This action may explain ability of drug to incr. seizure control when added to existing medicat'ns.	Appears to have lower incidence of neurological adv. effects than clonazepam. Adv. effects are dose related and include sedat'n, drowsiness, fatigue, dizziness, ataxia, insomnia, depress'n, behavioral changes and weight gain.	**Antiepileptic drugs:** May show incr. or decr. in serum levels if clobazem is added to tx regimen. Monitor serum concentrat'ns of these agents.	Refer to Table 69 for Nursing Process common to all benzodiazepines.

Pharmacologic Classification: Drug Effective Against Status Epilepticus

Drug				
Diazepam (Valium)	Tx of status epilepticus (**IV:** *Status epilepticus -* Adults - 5-10 mg infused at rate of 5 mg/min; repeat at 10-15 min intervals. Max. dose, 30 mg. This dose may be repeated in 2-4 h prn. Children ≥ 5 years - 1 mg q2-5min; repeat in 2-4 h prn. Max. dose, 10 mg. Infants > 30 days and children < 5 years - 0.2-0.5 mg q2-5min. Max. dose, 5 mg)	Reduces propagat'n of aberrant impulses in brain.	See Table 69	See Table 69	See Chapter 46 and Table 69

CHAPTER 52

Antiparkinsonian Drugs

Parkinsonism

Parkinsonism refers to two main disorders that present with similar clinical symptoms. The first is called **paralysis agitans** or **idiopathic Parkinson's disease.** It accounts for at least ninety per cent of the cases of parkinsonism and, as the name idiopathic implies, its cause is unknown. The second condition is **secondary** or **symptomatic parkinsonism,** caused by a past infection with the virus of lethargic encephalitis. Both Parkinson's disease and postencephalitic parkinsonism occur usually after the age of forty and are seen most often for the first time in patients between age fifty and sixty. The symptoms of parkinsonism can also be produced by drugs that either deplete dopamine stores in the brain or block dopaminergic receptors in the central nervous system.

The most prominent symptoms of parkinsonism are akinesia, tremor and rigidity. **Akinesia** is difficulty in initiating movements or modifying ongoing motor activity. The patient may show slowness and loss of dexterity, as well as problems with speech, manual skills and gait. Tremor is seen at rest and usually disappears when the affected limb is moved. Rigidity is due to an abnormal increase in muscle tone, producing cogwheel resistance to passive movement of an extremity. In addition, the patient may suffer from a stoop when standing or walking and a characteristic posturing of the hands and feet. Perspiration, excessive salivation, seborrhea and difficulty in swallowing may also be seen. The occurrence and severity of the symptoms vary from patient to patient.

A discussion of parkinsonism centers on the function of the basal ganglia. This area of the brain is responsible for the smooth control of skeletal muscle movement and contains high concentrations of the neurotransmitters dopamine and acetylcholine. The two appear to function as physiological antagonists, with dopamine acting as an inhibitory and acetylcholine as an excitatory neurotransmitter. Normal control of muscle movements depends on a delicate balance between these two. In patients with parkinsonism this balance is destroyed, as the levels of dopamine in the basal ganglia are reduced and acetylcholine acts unopposed. Drug treatment of parkinsonism is based on either stimulating dopamine receptors and/or blocking cholinergic receptors in the basal ganglia.

Dopaminergic Drugs

Levodopa (Dopar, Larodopa)

Mechanism of Action and Pharmacological Effects

Levodopa is the immediate precursor of dopamine. When administered to patients, a small portion of the dose enters the brain and is converted to dopamine by the enzyme dopa decarboxylase. (If this statement needs further explanation, the reader is asked to review the biosynthesis of dopamine in Chapter 4.) Dopamine cannot be administered itself for the treatment of parkinsonism because, in contrast to levodopa, it will not cross the blood-brain barrier.

Levodopa is given orally. In spite of the fact that attention is directed to its effects on the brain, only one per cent of the administered dose reaches the central nervous system. Ninety-nine per cent is converted to dopamine, norepinephrine and their metabolites in peripheral tissues. As a result, very large doses of levodopa must be given for the drug to produce significant changes in dopamine levels in the basal ganglia. The obvious consequence of administering very large doses is a high incidence of drug-related adverse effects.

Therapeutic Uses

Levodopa, alone or combined with a dopa decarboxylase inhibitor (see later discussion), is the most useful drug for the treatment of Parkinson's disease. Although treatment may be started with an anticholinergic or amantadine, the disease usually progresses to the point where levodopa is required within one year. Treatment with levodopa relieves the symptoms of parkinsonism and improves functional capacity in about seventy-five per cent of patients. In fifty per cent of patients the quality of life is markedly improved for many years. Patients with postencephalic parkinsonism are also treated with levodopa. However, these individuals appear to tolerate only small doses of the drug and are more susceptible to its adverse effects.

The combination of levodopa and an anticholinergic may benefit patients who are not adequately treated by either drug alone. By increasing dopamine levels in the basal ganglia and blocking excessive cholinergic stimulation, these drugs, taken in combination, often afford greater relief than either used alone. Patients may also benefit from the combined use of amantadine and levodopa.

Levodopa is contraindicated in patients with parkinsonism secondary to the use of antipsychotic drugs because it will reverse the therapeutic benefits provided by phenothiazines and butyrophenones. Levodopa should not be administered to patients in whom sympathomimetic amines are contraindicated. Levodopa is contraindicated in patients with dementia accompanied by a significant degree of memory defect. It is also contraindicated in patients having episodic mental confusion, hallucinations or paranoid ideation. The drug should be used with caution in individuals with severe dizziness or fainting due to postural hypotension. It is contraindicated in patients with serious endocrine, renal, hepatic, cardiovascular or pulmonary disease. Patients with an existing or previously excised malignant melanoma must not be given levodopa because the drug can cause the disease to recur or lead to its progression or dissemination.

Adverse Effects

Up to eighty per cent of patients taking levodopa complain of anorexia, nausea, vomiting or epigastric pain. These effects can be reduced by taking the drug with food. About thirty per cent of patients experience mild postural hypotension. An increase in cardiac arrhythmias is also a recognized adverse effect of levodopa.

Abnormal involuntary movements occur in about fifty per cent of patients taking levodopa. Beginning approximately two to four months after starting therapy, they include faciolingual tics, grimacing, head bobbing and various rocking and rotating movements of the arms, legs or trunk.

Levodopa can also produce behavioral changes. Many patients with parkinsonism are elderly and may suffer from impairment of memory or dementia.

Given to these individuals, levodopa can stimulate the central nervous system, resulting in hallucinations, paranoia, mania, insomnia and nightmares. It can also cause depression. Levodopa is perhaps best noted for its ability to stimulate the sexual interests of elderly patients, leading to additional behavioral changes.

Drug Interactions

Dopa decarboxylase is a pyridoxine-dependent enzyme. Patients should be advised not to take pyridoxine (Vitamin B$_6$) because it will increase the extracerebral conversion of levodopa to dopamine and reduce its therapeutic effectiveness. Even marginal increases in pyridoxine consumption above the normal dietary requirements may have a detrimental effect.

Monoamine oxidase inhibitors, such as phenelzine (Nardil) or tranylcypromine (Parnate), impair dopamine and norepinephrine metabolism and increase both the central and peripheral effects of levodopa. As a result, patients may suffer a hypertensive crisis and/or hyperpyrexia. Monoamine oxidase inhibitors should be withdrawn at least fourteen days before starting levodopa treatment.

Antipsychotic drugs block dopamine receptors in the brain and reduce or abolish the effects of levodopa. Phenothiazines should not be used to reverse the emetic action of levodopa. If tricyclic antidepressants are used with levodopa, postural hypotension can occur. Administering the tricyclic once daily, at bedtime, will minimize this effect.

Nursing Process

Assessment

Nursing assessment prior to the administration of the initial dose of levodopa begins with a review of the patient's history for the diagnosed cause of the parkinsonian symptoms. Nurses should not administer levodopa to patients whose parkinsonian symptoms are secondary to the use of an antipsychotic drug. Similarly, confirmation of the order from the physician should be sought if the patient's history reveals evidence of psychological problems, dementia, memory loss, confusion, hallucinations or paranoia; postural hypotension; tachycardia, ventricular fibrillation; diabetes; hypothermia; endocrine, renal, hepatic or pulmonary impairment; or malignant melanoma.

The patient's drug-use profile should be reviewed in consultation with the pharmacist. Concurrent use of pyridoxine, recent or concurrent use of MAO inhibitors, antipsychotics or tricyclic antidepressants is contraindicated with levodopa because of the drug interactions presented before.

Physical assessment of the patient should establish baseline physiological measures. Of particular importance are standing and reclining blood pressures, apical and radial pulses, and color and temperature of extremities. Descriptive documentation of the type and extent of the parkinsonian effects in the individual is necessary for later determination of drug efficacy.

Administration

Levodopa should be administered with food to prevent gastric distress. Give assistance with ambulation during initiation of drug therapy and as necessary throughout therapy.

Evaluation

Nursing evaluation following administration should stress documentation of therapeutic effectiveness; that is, the reduction in severity of the parkinsonian symptoms.

Simultaneously, nurses should evaluate the patient for drug-related adverse effects. These include postural hypotension, cardiac arrhythmias, poor peripheral circulation and urinary retention. Therefore, nursing observations of standing and reclining blood pressures, apical and radial pulses, color and temperature of extremities, and urinary output are essential to the early identification of levodopa's adverse effects.

Furthermore, nursing observation of the patient's mentation and psychological behavior is essential for the prompt identification of undesirable emotional stimulation or depression.

Teaching

Nursing instruction related to the use of levodopa should be conducted with both the patient and the family. They should be taught the indicators of drug efficacy and adverse effects. Patients and their families should also be advised of the impact of pyridoxine (vitamin B$_6$) on levodopa's effectiveness and counseled to avoid vitamin supplements, fortified cereals and antinauseants containing pyridoxine supplements.

An informed patient complies better with drug therapy. Therefore, nurses should tell the patient and family that urine and perspiration might darken. They should also know that the full effects of the drug may require several months of treatment. This information provides reassurance and enhances compliance. Instruct the patient to report side effects of twitching and eye spasms, as these may indicate overdose.

Levodopa plus Carbidopa (Sinemet) and Levodopa plus Benserazide (Prolopa)

Carbidopa and benserazide are two drugs capable of inhibiting dopa decarboxylase. Because they do not cross the blood-brain barrier, these drugs reduce only the peripheral metabolism of levodopa to dopamine. The formation of dopamine in the brain is not affected. A higher percentage of the administered levodopa is converted to dopamine in the brain. By using either carbidopa or benserazide, it is possible to administer lower doses of levodopa, thereby reducing its peripheral adverse effects. As a result, the products Sinemet and Prolopa have replaced levodopa as the most useful agents for parkinsonism. The nursing process related to the use of either carbidopa or benserazide is the same as previously identified for levodopa.

Bromocriptine (Parlodel)

Bromocriptine stimulates dopaminergic D_2 receptors in the brain and has been found to be clinically useful as an adjunct to levodopa (usually with carbidopa or benserazide) in the symptomatic management of selected patients with Parkinson's disease who experience prominent dyskinesia or "wearing-off" reactions on long-term levodopa therapy. The best results with the drug have been seen early in the treatment of parkinsonism when it was given with Sinemet. Doses of bromocriptine below 30 mg/day, combined with Sinemet, can ameliorate the "on-off" and wearing-off effects encountered after long-term levodopa therapy.

The adverse effects of bromocriptine include nausea, vomiting, transient dizziness, abdominal pain, constipation and blurred vision, with or without diplopia. Digital vasospasm in response to cold, erythromelalgia, mental disturbances and dyskinesias may also be experienced. Bromocriptine, especially in higher doses, can produce mental disturbances. These include nightmares, mild agitation, hallucinations and paranoid delusions and are most common in elderly patients.

The nursing process related to the use of bromocriptine for the treatment of parkinsonism is the same as that previously outlined for levodopa.

Pergolide (Permax)

Pergolide is a long-acting dopamine agonist. Like bromocriptine, pergolide is effective when given with Sinemet. Pergolide and bromocriptine appear similar in their therapeutic and adverse effects. However, some patients respond to one and not to the other.

Nursing Process

Pergolide is a relatively new drug, and nursing experience with it is limited. Readers are advised to consult the manufacturer's literature and the pharmacist for the latest advice on information and clinical practice before administering this drug.

Selegiline (Eldepryl)

Mechanism of Action and Therapeutic Use

Selegiline, formerly known as l-deprenyl, is a selective monoamine oxidase type-B (MAO-B) inhibitor. It is a most interesting new compound, and one that has stimulated a great deal of interest. Inhibition of MAO-B may block the metabolism of dopamine and increase the amount of dopamine available. Selegiline may also block dopamine neuronal reuptake, and this effect would also increase the amount of dopamine available to stimulate receptors. The next few years will determine whether this drug is the breakthrough product that many feel it is at the present time. Selegiline has been found to be of value as an adjunct to the management of some patients with Parkinson's disease when added to levodopa/carbidopa (Sinemet) therapy.

Adverse Effects

Monoamine oxidase inhibitors (MAOIs) are not new to medicine. At least two MAOIs, phenelzine and tranylcypromine, are currently used as antidepressants (see Chapter 45). These agents interact with foods containing tyramine and sympathomimetics to produce significant, and sometimes dangerous, increases in blood pressure. However, these drugs inhibit monoamine oxidase type A (MAO-A), an enzyme that is found in the intestine and liver. Selegiline inhibits MAO-B, which is found in the brain but not in the liver or intestine. It would not be expected, therefore, to interact with tyramine and sympathomimetics. At this point, clinical observations with selegiline appear to confirm this hypothesis. It must be emphasized, however, that doses above 10 mg/day result in a loss of selectivity of selegiline towards MOA-B and an increase in the inhibition of MAO-A. At this point, patients are at increased risk of experiencing reactions with tyramine-containing foods or sympathomimetics.

The adverse effects of selegiline are those usually associated with an excess of dopamine. The drug may potentiate the adverse effects of levodopa/carbidopa, and adjustments of drug dosages may be required. Hallucinations and confusion have been seen with the combined use of selegiline and levodopa/carbidopa. Other adverse effects associated with selegiline include nausea, depression, loss of balance, insomnia, orthostatic hypotension, increased akinetic involuntary movements, arrhythmia, bradykinesia, chorea, delusions, hypertension, angina pectoris and syncope.

Nursing Process

The nursing process for selegiline is the same as that previously described for levodopa. Doses of selegiline should not exceed 10 mg/day because of the risk associated with the nonselective inhibition of monoamine oxidase (see Adverse Effects, above).

Amantadine (Symmetrel)

Amantadine was first introduced as an antiviral agent for the prophylaxis of A_2 influenza. Because amantadine releases dopamine from the remaining intact dopaminergic nerves in the basal ganglia, it is also used to treat parkinsonism. Although less effective than levodopa, amantadine produces a more rapid response and fewer adverse effects, and its dosage is easier to adjust. Amantadine is indicated for the treatment of Parkinson's syndrome and in the short-term management of drug-induced extrapyramidal symptoms. Unfortunately, the initial clinical improvement may not be sustained. Performance deteriorates over three to six months. Therefore, amantadine is used most often with levodopa where it often improves the effects of the latter drug. However, amantadine usually has little effect in patients receiving near-maximal therapeutic benefits from levodopa.

The more important adverse effects with amantadine are orthostatic hypotensive episodes, congestive heart failure, depression, psychosis and urinary retention. Rarely, convulsion, reversible leukopenia and neutropenia, and abnormal liver function test results have been seen. Patients may also experience hallucinations, confusion or nightmares if high doses are used. These effects are more common if the patient is also receiving an anticholinergic.

In spite of the fact that the mechanism of action of amantadine is different from that of levodopa, its ultimate effect is the same. Amantadine increases the amount of endogenous dopamine available for use in the central nervous system. Therefore, the nursing process accompanying the use of amantadine is the same as that identified for levodopa.

Central Anticholinergic Drugs

Mechanism of Action and Pharmacologic Effects

Anticholinergic drugs have been used for more than a century in the treatment of parkinsonism. As explained earlier, the deficiency of dopamine in basal ganglia exposes patients to excessive cholinergic stimulation. By administering an anticholinergic, it is possible to reduce the effects of acetylcholine and hopefully restore neurotransmitter balance.

Atropine and hyoscine, two classical anticholinergics, are no longer used because of their generalized effects on the body. In their place, newer agents have been synthesized with preferential effects on the brain. These include trihexyphenidyl hydrochloride (Artane), benztropine mesylate (Cogentin), procyclidine hydrochloride (Kemadrin) and biperiden hydrochloride (Akineton). The antihistamines diphenhydramine (Benadryl) and orphenadrine (Disipal) and the phenothiazine ethopropazine (Parsidol) have antiparkinsonian activity because they, too, block cholinergic receptors in the basal ganglia.

Therapeutic Uses

The introduction of levodopa has reduced the use of anticholinergic drugs. They have remained in use for patients at the early stage of disease, for those with minor symptoms, and in individuals who cannot tolerate levodopa. In addition, anticholinergic drugs are often used in conjunction with levodopa. Trihexyphenidyl, biperiden or benztropine are usually preferred for initial therapy. Levodopa, amantadine or an anticholinergic from another chemical class may be added if required. If therapy is started with levodopa, an anticholinergic may be added to achieve maximal response. Ethopropazine and diphenhydramine are often used in this situation. Patients often become refractive to anticholinergics during long-term therapy. This may be caused by progression of the disease.

Anticholinergics are also used to reduce drug-induced parkinsonism. This practice has been questioned, with the suggestion that anticholinergics may increase the probability of phenothiazines or butyrophenones causing tardive dyskinesia.

Adverse Effects

The adverse effects of these drugs can be attributed, in the main, to a reduction of peripheral cholinergic stimulation. Although more selective than atropine, the drugs can still produce cycloplegia, urinary retention and constipation. Because of their mydriatic effects, they can precipitate an attack of acute-angle glaucoma in patients predisposed to angle closure. The decrease in salivation that accompanies their use benefits the patient who experiences sialorrhea. Confusion and excitement can occur with large doses or in susceptible patients such as the elderly, patients with existing mental disorders, and those taking other drugs with anticholinergic properties. Care must be taken in using anticholinergic therapy in patients over the age of seventy or any individual with dementia. Drowsiness and dizziness are common with the antihistamines diphenhydramine and orphenadrine and the phenothiazine ethopropazine.

Nursing Process

The nursing process precipitated by the prescription of anticholinergic drugs is discussed in detail in Chapter 6 and summarized in Table 75 at the end of this chapter.

Further Reading

Drugs for parkinsonism (1989). Drugs of choice. *The Medical Letter 31* :99-103.

Drugs for parkinsonism (1988). *The Medical Letter 30* :113-115.

Ho, K.Y. (1988). Therapeutic applications of bromocriptine in endocrine and neurological diseases. *Drugs 36* :67-82.

Langtry, H.D. and Clissold, S.P. (1990). Pergolide: A review of its pharmacological properties and therapeutic potential in Parkinson's disease. *Drugs 39* :399-437.

Marsden, C.D. (1990). Parkinson's disease. *Lancet 335* :948-952.

Pergolide and selegiline for Parkinson's disease (1989). *The Medical Letter 31* :81-83.

Table 75
Antiparkinsonian drugs.

Pharmacologic Classification: Dopaminergic Drugs

Generic Name (Trade Name)	Use (Dose)	Action	Adverse Effects	Drug Interactions	Nursing Process
Levodopa (Dopar, Larodopa)	Tx of mod. to severe parkinsonism (**Oral:** Initially, 500 mg - 1 g/day bid-qid; incr. gradually in increments of 125-250 mg q3-4 days over 6-8 weeks. Give in divided doses w. small meals to minimize GI symptoms. Us. maint. dose, 4-6 g/day; max. dose, 8 g/day)	Levodopa is precursor of dopamine. When administered, a small port'n of dose enters brain and is converted to dopamine.	Nausea, vomiting, anorexia, abd. pain, diarrhea, constipat'n, activat'n of peptic ulcer, abnormal involuntary movements, severe gen'lized choreoathetoid movements, psych. disturbances, orthostatic hypotens'n, transient flushing of skin, palpitat'ns	**Antidepressants, heterocyclic:** If used w. levodopa, can produce postural hypotens'n. **Antihypertensives:** Can have their effects potentiated by levodopa. Monitor pts carefully on methyldopa and reserpine. **Antipsychotics:** Block dopamine receptors in brain and will reduce or abolish effects of levodopa. **MAOIs:** Reduce rate of dopamine and norepinephrine metabolism and incr. both central and peripheral effects of levodopa. Stop at least 2 weeks before levodopa. **Pyridoxine:** Incr. extracerebral metabolism of levodopa, thus decr. amt. available to brain. Pyridoxine should be avoided in pts receiving levodopa, unless levodopa is combined w. peripheral dopa decarboxylase inhibitor such as benserazide (in Prolopa) or carbidopa (in Sinemet). **Sympathomimetics:** Interact w. levodopa. Administer levodopa w. extreme caution to pts w. bronchial asthma or emphysema who may require tx w. sympathomimetic.	**Assess:** For hx parkinsonism 2º to use of antipsychotic drugs; dementia, memory loss, confus'n, hallucinat'ns, paranoia; postural hypotens'n; endocrine, renal or hepatic impairment; glaucoma; malignant melanoma; tachycardia, ventr. fibrillat'n; diabetes; hypothermia. Establish baseline BP (standing, reclining), pulse (apical, radial), color and temp. of extremities. **Administer:** W. food. Assist ambulat'n during initiat'n of tx and throughout tx prn. **Evaluate:** For sympathomimetic effects: BP (standing, reclining), pulses (apical, radial), color and temp. of extremities, urinary output. For mentat'n, psych. behavior; for tx effect (reduct'n in parkinsonian symptoms). **Teach:** To change posit'n slowly; to avoid fortified cereals, vitamin supplements and antinauseants containing pyridoxine (vitamin B6); that urine and perspirat'n may darken in color; that drug efficacy may not occur for several months. Instruct pt to report side effects of twitching and eye spasms, as these may indicate overdose.
Levodopa 50 mg + benserazide 12.5 mg; levodopa 100 mg + benserazide 25 mg; levodopa 200 mg + benserazide 50 mg (Prolopa Oral Capsules)	As for levodopa (**Oral:** *For pts not on levodopa tx* - Initially, 1 capsule of 100/25 mg od-bid; incr. by 1 capsule q3rd/4th day until optimal effect obtained. Opt. dosage for most pts is us. 4-8 capsules of 100/25 mg/day. *Initiat'n in pts on levodopa tx* - Allow 12 h or more bet. last dose of levodopa and 1st dose of Prolopa. Dosage of Prolopa should provide approx. 15% of previous levodopa daily dosage)	Benserazide inhibits dopa decarboxylase, enzyme responsible for convers'n of dopa to dopamine. Because it does not cross blood-brain barrier, it reduces only peripheral metabolism of dopa. Format'n of dopamine in brain is not affected. It is thus poss. to use lower doses of levodopa without sacrificing clinical efficacy, while reducing peripheral adv. effects.	As for levodopa but w. reduct'n in peripheral adv. effects (see comments under Action)		

Generic Name (Trade Name)	Use (Dose)	Action	Adverse Effects	Drug Interactions	Nursing Process
Levodopa 100 mg + carbidopa 10 mg; levodopa 100 mg + carbidopa 25 mg; levodopa 250 mg + carbidopa 25 mg (Sinemet Oral Tablets)	As for levodopa (**Oral:** *For pts not on levodopa tx* - Initially, 1 tablet of 100/25 mg tid; incr. by 1 tablet q3days until optimal effect obtained, or unacceptable adv. effects preclude further incr. *Initiat'n in pts on levodopa tx* - Levodopa should be discontinued at least 12 h before initiating tx w. Sinemet. Initial daily dose should provide approx. 20% of previous daily dose of levodopa)	Carbidopa, like benserazide (above), also inhibits dopa decarboxylase without crossing blood-brain barrier.	As for levodopa but w. reduct'n in peripheral adv. effects	As for levodopa	As for levodopa
Bromocriptine (Parlodel)	As alternative to levodopa if that drug is not effective, is contraindicated or not tolerated; combined w. levodopa in pts w. significant fluctuat'ns in tx response, end-of-dose dystonia and painful muscle cramps (**Oral:** Initially, 1.25 mg hs w. food to establish tolerance; thereafter, 2.5 mg daily in 2 divided doses w. meals. Incr. very gradually prn in increments of 2.5 mg/day q2-4weeks, to be taken always in divided doses w. meals)	Stims. dopamine receptors in brain.	Nausea, vomiting, transient dizziness, abd. pain, constipat'n, blurred vision w. or without diplopia, digital vasospasm in response to cold, erythromelalgia, mental disturbances, dyskinesias	As for levodopa w. respect to heterocyclic antidepressants, antihypertensives, antipsychotics, clonidine and sympathomimetics	As for levodopa
Pergolide (Permax)	As for bromocriptine (**Oral:** Initially, 0.1 mg/day; incr. by 0.1-0.4 mg/day to max. 5 mg/day)	Long-acting dopamine agonist.	As for bromocriptine	As for bromocriptine	This is a new drug. Nurses are advised to consult pharmacist and review manufacturer's informat'n before administering.
Selegiline (Eldepryl)	As adjunct to management of pts w. Parkinson's disease when added to levodopa-carbidopa tx (**Oral:** 10 mg/day, given as 5 mg at breakfast + 5 mg at lunch. Doses higher than 10 mg/day should not be used.	Inhibitor of MAO-B; thus blocks metabolism of dopamine and incr. am't of dopamine available to stim. its receptors in brain.	Hallucinat'ns and confus'n seen w. combined use of selegiline and levodopa-carbidopa. Other adv. effects incl. nausea,		*Follow Nsg Process for levodopa, w. the following changes:* **Administer:** Doses should not exceed 10 mg/day because of risks assoc. w. nonselective inhibit'n of MAO. **Teach:** To check w. physician concerning poss. need to adjust diet.

Drug / Dose	Action	Side effects	Interactions	Nursing considerations
When selegiline is added to existing levodopa-carbidopa (Sinemet) tx, a reduct'n in dose of levodopa-carbidopa, us. of 10-30%, may be required during period of adjustment of tx)	Selegiline may also block dopamine neuronal reuptake; this effect would also incr. amt of dopamine available to stim. receptors.	depress'n, loss of balance, insomnia, orthostatic hypotens'n, incr. akinetic involuntary movements, arrhythmia, bradykinesia, chorea, delus'ns, hypertens'n, angina pectoris, syncope		As for levodopa
Amantadine (Symmetrel) Tx of parkinsonism (**Oral:** Initially, 100 mg/day for pts w. serious assoc. illnesses or those who are receiving high doses of other antiparkinsonian drugs. After 1 to several weeks at 100 mg od, dose may incr. to 100 mg bid. When amantadine and levodopa are used concurrently, dose of amantadine should be held constant at 100 mg od-bid while daily dose of levodopa is gradually incr. to optimal dose. When used alone, us. dose of amantadine is 100 mg bid)	Releases dopamine from remaining intact dopaminergic nerves in basal ganglia.	Hallucinat'ns, confus'n, nightmares, lethargy, drowsiness, slurred speech, dizziness, insomnia	**Amphetamine; dexamphetamine; methamphetamine; methylphenidate; pemoline**: Should be used w. caution w. amantadine. **Anticholinergics**: May demonstrate potentiated effects when amantadine is administered. Confus'n and hallucinat'ns have been reported. Reduce dose of anticholinergic prn.	

Pharmacologic Classification: Central Anticholinergic Drugs

Drug / Dose	Action	Side effects	Interactions	Nursing considerations
Benztropine mesylate (Cogentin) Tx of all forms of parkinsonism, as well as prevent'n or control of drug-induced extrapyramidal effects (**Oral:** For arteriosclerotic and idiopathic parkinsonism - Initially, 0.5-1 mg hs; gradually incr. to 4-6 mg/day prn. For postencephalitic parkinsonism - Initially, 2 mg/day in 1 or more doses. In highly sensitive pts, start w. 500 µg hs and incr. prn. For drug-induced parkinsonism - 1-4 mg od-bid)	Anticholinergic w. preferential effects on brain. Reduces excess. cholinergic stimulat'n in basal ganglia that occurs in face of lowered dopamine levels.	Dry mouth, blurred vision, dizziness, mild nausea, nervousness, constipat'n, drowsiness, urinary hesitancy/retent'n, tachycardia, mydriasis, incr. intraocular tens'n, weakness, vomiting, headache	**Amantadine:** May potentiate anticholinergic adv. effects of this agent. Confus'n and hallucinat'ns that characterize excess. anticholinergic activity have been reported when amantadine is added to dosage regimen. If poss., reduce high-dose anticholinergic tx before administering amantadine.	**Assess:** For hx glaucoma, hypertens'n, coronary artery disease, chronic GI condit'n, asthma or pulmonary disease. **Administer:** From light-resistant container. **Evaluate:** For effectiveness; for adv. effects, incl. fluid balance and electrolyte states. **Teach:** Pt and family s/s of anticholinergic toxicity; to use hard candy, gum for dry mouth.

Generic Name (Trade Name)	Use (Dose)	Action	Adverse Effects	Drug Interactions	Nursing Process
Biperiden HCl (Akineton)	As for benztropine (**Oral:** *Idiopathic and postencephalic parkinsonism* - 2 mg tid-qid; incr. grad. to 20 mg/day prn. *Drug-induced extrapyramidal symptoms* - 2 mg od-tid)	As for benztropine mesylate	As for benztropine mesylate	As for benztropine mesylate	As for benztropine mesylate
Diphenhydramine HCl (Benadryl)	As for benztropine (**Oral:** *Idiopathic and postencephalic parkinsonism* - Initially, 25 mg tid; incr. grad. to 50 mg qid prn.	Antihistamine that also blocks cholinergic receptors in basal ganglia.	As for benztropine mesylate	As for benztropine mesylate	As for benztropine mesylate
Ethopropazine HCl (Parsitan, Parsidol)	As for benztropine (**Oral:** *Idiopathic and postencephalic parkinsonism* - Initially, 50 mg tid; incr. from 50-100 mg daily q2-3 days prn. *Drug-induced extrapyramidal react'ns* - 100 mg bid)	Phenothiazine that also blocks cholinergic receptors in basal ganglia.	As for benztropine mesylate	As for benztropine mesylate	As for benztropine mesylate
Orphenadrine HCl (Disipal)	As for benztropine (**Oral:** Initially, 50 mg tid. Subsequent adjustments prn)	As for benztropine mesylate	As for benztropine mesylate	As for benztropine mesylate	As for benztropine mesylate
Procyclidine (Kemadrin)	As for benztropine (**Oral:** *Idiopathic and postencephalic parkinsonism* - Initially, 2.5 mg tid pc; incr. [if well tolerated] to 5 mg tid, and occas'nally 5 mg hs. *Drug-induced extrapyramidal symptoms* - Initially, 2.5 mg tid pc; may incr. by 2.5-mg daily increments until pt obtains relief, us. w. 10-20 mg/day)	As for benztropine mesylate	As for benztropine mesylate	As for benztropine mesylate	As for benztropine mesylate
Trihexyphenidyl HCl (Artane, Tremin)	As for benztropine (**Oral:** *Idiopathic and postencephalic parkinsonism* - 1 mg on day 1; incr. by 2 mg/day q3-5days, up to 6-10 mg/day. Best tolerated in divided doses at mealtime. *Drug-induced parkinsonism* - Us. 5-15 mg/day)	As for benztropine mesylate	As for benztropine mesylate	As for benztropine mesylate	As for benztropine mesylate

C H A P T E R   5 3

Narcotic Analgesics

edited by Sheila Rankin Zerr, R.N., M.Ed.

Teaching Objectives

Following completion of this chapter, the reader should be able to:

1. Divide analgesics into two major groups.
2. Describe the mechanism of action, pharmacologic effects, therapeutic uses and adverse effects of narcotics.
3. Explain the nursing process associated with the assessment and management of pain and the appropriate use of analgesics.
4. Describe briefly the distinguishing pharmacologic properties, therapeutic uses and adverse effects of Pantopon, morphine, codeine, hydromorphone, oxymorphone, hydrocodone, oxycodone, meperidine, alphaprodine, levorphanol, methadone, propoxyphene, pentazocine, butorphanol and nalbuphine.
5. Discuss briefly the mechanism of action and therapeutic use of naloxone, and the nursing process related to its administration.

General Properties of Narcotics

Pain is a useful sensation when it protects the body from damage. Pushed to the extreme, however, or continued over long periods of time, pain is counterproductive and steps must be taken to alleviate it. Drugs used to relieve pain are called analgesics. They are divided into narcotic and non-narcotic analgesics. The latter group is also called the analgesic-antipyretics. This chapter discusses narcotic analgesics. Chapter 54 presents the non-narcotics.

In 1680 the English physician Thomas Sydinham wrote, "Among the remedies which it has pleased Almighty God to give man to relieve his sufferings, none is so universal and so efficacious as opium." That statement is as true today as it was more than three hundred years ago. Morphine, the major narcotic contained in the opium plant, still serves as the ultimate standard of analgesic effectiveness. No analgesic has proven to be so effective as morphine.

Narcotic analgesics may be classified according to their source. These are:

1. opium preparations;
2. purified alkaloids of opium;
3. semisynthetic modifications of morphine or codeine;
4. synthetic compounds that resemble morphine in many of their actions.

Mechanism of Action and Pharmacologic Effects

All narcotics, regardless of their origin, reduce pain by stimulating opiate receptors in the central nervous system. In doing this they mimic the analgesic effects of naturally occurring brain opiates — the endorphins. Not all endogenous chemicals with opioid activity have been identified. However, two pentapeptides, leucine-enkephalin and methionine-enkephalin, have been found, which have properties similar to those of narcotics. By mimicking the actions of endogenous enkaphalins, opiates probably inhibit the release of excitatory transmitters from terminals of nerves that carry pain impulses.

At least four types of opioid receptors are found in the central nervous system. These are:

1. μ (Mu) receptors, which are thought to mediate supraspinal analgesia, respiratory depression, euphoria and physical dependence. These receptors are associated with morphine-like analgesia and euphoria.
2. K (Kappa) receptors, which mediate analgesia, miosis and sedation. These receptors are associated with pentazocine-like analgesia, sedation and miosis.
3. ∂ (Delta) receptors, which are associated with alterations in affective behavior.
4. Σ (Sigma) receptors, which are associated with dysphoria and psychotomimetic effects.

Pain can be classified as either productive or nonproductive. The difference between productive and nonproductive pain is best illustrated by an example. Suppose a man puts his hand on a hot object. The pain he feels is productive because he can take his hand away from the object. The same man may experience the pain of a myocardial infarct. This pain is nonproductive because it does not allow the man to stop its cause. Narcotics are more effective in relieving nonproductive pain. Nonproductive pain usually emanates from the viscera, productive pain from skeletal muscles. Thus, it may also be stated that narcotics are more effective in reducing visceral pain.

All narcotic analgesics have the same major pharmacologic properties. In addition to analgesia, their effects include euphoria, drowsiness, depressed respiration, nausea and vomiting, miosis, altered gastrointestinal activity and dependence. If narcotics are given chronically, tolerance occurs to many of these effects and larger doses must be given to provide satisfactory pain relief.

Opiate receptors are found in high concentrations in the limbic system, that part of the brain responsible for emotion. All potent narcotics cause **euphoria.** This effect must not be minimized because the **analgesia** produced by narcotics depends, to a great degree, on their ability to induce euphoria. The emotional reaction to pain is very important. If a feeling of well-being can be produced in patients, the perception of, and reaction to, pain is reduced. Nurses have often heard patients state after receiving a narcotic that they can still feel pain but it no longer bothers them.

Drowsiness is a characteristic feature of stronger narcotics and plays a role in their analgesic effects. The word narcosis means a condition of stupor or insensitivity. Following the administration of a narcotic, patients may experience drowsiness, apathy and even sleep.

Respiratory depression occurs with even small doses of narcotics because they reduce the sensitivity of the brain-stem respiratory centers to increases in carbon dioxide tension. Therapeutic doses of morphine, for example, will depress the respiratory rate, minute volume and tidal exchange. As the dose is increased, respiratory depression deepens. Death from an overdose is due to respiratory failure.

Nausea and vomiting may occur because narcotics stimulate the chemoreceptor trigger zone in the medulla of the brain. Some patients never experience these effects. Others are bothered every time. The more potent phenothiazine drugs (see Chapters 25 and 44) may block narcotic-induced nausea and vomiting.

Miosis is a constriction of the pupil. Most narcotics produce miosis by stimulating the autonomic segment of the nucleus of the oculomotor nerve.

Gastrointestinal effects are prominent during chronic narcotic use. Constipation is most noticeable. This is due to (1) a delayed emptying time of the stomach as a result of the constriction of the pyloric sphincter and increased tone of the antral portion of the stomach and duodenum, (2) a decrease in the propulsive contractions of the small intestine, together with an increase in nonpropulsive contractions and increased tone of the colon, and (3) increased tone of the anal sphincter. The result of this triple-threat attack is constipation that can, when severe, proceed to **obstipation** (constipation severe enough to produce a serious obstruction).

Therapeutic doses of most narcotics increase biliary tract pressure. This can result in symptoms that vary from epigastric distress to typical biliary colic.

Physiological and psychological dependence develop during chronic administration. These effects are one of the main reasons for caution in narcotic use. If a dependent subject is suddenly deprived of his narcotic, a withdrawal effect (absence syndrome) occurs quickly. The signs of physical withdrawal are autonomic hyperactivity, including diarrhea, vomiting, lacrimation, rhinorrhea, chills and fever. Patients may also suffer from abdominal cramps, pain and tremors. As serious as these effects may seem, they are usually not life threatening, and the patients can be weaned off their drugs, at least as far as the physiological requirements of the body are concerned. Psychological dependence is a far more vexing problem. It is difficult to understand why an individual who has been weaned off narcotics still feels a psychological compulsion to take the medication. Yet this does happen and is the major reason why people return to old habits.

Tolerance occurs to the analgesic, euphoric and respiratory-depressant effects of narcotics. If a narcotic is used on a daily basis over a prolonged period of time, larger and larger doses must be given to maintain the same degree of analgesia. Once a patient develops tolerance to one narcotic he or she will show tolerance to all other narcotics. This is known as **cross-tolerance.** Cross-tolerance does not extend to other groups of central nervous system depressants, such as alcohol or barbiturates. Tolerance does not develop to the gastrointestinal or miotic effects of narcotics.

Therapeutic Uses

Pain is the major reason for the use of narcotics. They should be used only when non-narcotic analgesics prove ineffective. On the other hand, narcotics should not be withheld from seriously ill patients because of fear of dependence. It matters little to the terminally ill patient that a narcotic can produce dependence. Narcotics should not be used in the treatment of chronic pain from nonmalignant causes. It is also important to use a narcotic in an effective dose. Often patients receive inadequate doses.

Narcotics are often used in severe pain resulting from trauma, surgery, obstetrics, renal and biliary colic, and carcinoma. Caution should be exercised in obstetrics because narcotics cross the placenta and can depress respiration in the newborn. Narcotics are not recommended while the cause of a patient's pain is being diagnosed lest analgesia interfere with the diagnosis.

Dyspnea produced by acute left-ventricular failure and pulmonary edema may be treated with a narcotic. This effect is caused by a decrease in preload secondary to vasodilatation.

Diarrhea responds to narcotic treatment. This topic is discussed in Chapters 23 and 24. Diphenoxylate (Lomotil) or loperamide (Imodium) are the narcotics of choice because they are poorly absorbed and have minimal systemic effects.

Cough relief is afforded by some narcotics (see Chapter 34). By suppressing the cough center in the medulla of the brain, many narcotics serve as excellent antitussives. The narcotics used most often are codeine and hydrocodone.

Narcotics are contraindicated in patients hypersensitive to the drugs. In addition, they are contraindicated in respiratory insufficiency or depression, in severe CNS depression, during an attack of bronchial asthma, in heart failure secondary to chronic lung disease, and in cardiac arrhythmias. Additional contraindications include increased intracranial or cerebrospinal fluid pressure, head injuries, brain tumor, acute alcoholism, delirium tremens, convulsive disorders, post biliary tract surgery, suspected surgical abdomen, and surgical anastomosis. Patients taking monoamine oxidase inhibitors should also not receive narcotics either concomitantly or within fourteen days of monoamine oxidase inhibitor treatment (see Drug Interactions, Table 76).

Adverse Effects

The major adverse effects of narcotic analgesics are respiratory depression, dependence, constipation, nausea and vomiting. Concern over these effects has led to the use of non-narcotic analgesics in conditions in which they provide adequate relief of pain.

Although one must not minimize the danger of inducing narcotic dependence in a patient during chronic therapy, *this concern should not serve as the basis for withholding treatment in the terminally ill patient.* Often patients are denied the relief of a narcotic analgesic because physicians and nurses do not want them to become addicted. This is nonsense. If a patient has only a short time to live, why worry about addiction?

A more appropriate reason to show caution in the terminally ill patient is the ability of most narcotics to produce severe constipation, bordering on obstipation. Even terminally ill patients must clear their intestines. If the narcotic binds the bowels, this can represent a serious medical/ nursing problem.

The nausea and vomiting effects of narcotics can be minimized by the use of antinauseant drugs, such as the phenothiazines or diphenhydramine.

Because of their ability to depress the respiratory center, decrease ciliary activity, reduce the cough reflex, and increase bronchomotor tone, narcotics must be used with caution in patients with excessive respiratory secretions or decreased ventilation.

Narcotics can cause hypoventilation and hypercapnia, resulting in cerebrovascular dilatation and increased intracranial pressure. Therefore, they must be used very cautiously, if at all, in patients with head injuries, delirium tremens, and conditions in which intracranial pressure is increased.

Narcotics can produce hypotension and shock and should be given in reduced doses, if at all, to patients in shock or with decreased blood volume. If it is absolutely necessary to administer a narcotic to a patient in shock, it should be given intravenously to circumvent poor uptake following intramuscular or subcutaneous injection.

The spasmogenic effects of narcotics on the urinary bladder can lead to urinary retention in patients with prostatic hypertrophy or urethral stricture. Narcotics should be used in lower doses in patients with myxedema, hypothyroidism or hypoadrenalism.

Nursing Process

Over the years many authorities have addressed the problem of pain management. In discussing the nursing process related to the relief of pain we have drawn from the work of many of these writers. Each work cited will be found in the Further Reading list at the end of this chapter.

Pain probably affects, and even disables, more individuals than any other disease. Assessing, diagnosing and managing the patient in pain can be a daily challenge to the clinical nurse. The ability to diagnose pain accurately is critical to its management, and each patient's experience and expression of pain is unique. Often the nurse's subjective judgments about the reality or intensity of a patient's pain, coupled with exaggerated fears about addiction, result in the withholding of pain relief measures (Meinhart and McCaffery, 1983). But pain is "whatever the experiencing person says it is, existing whenever [he or she] says it does" (McCaffery, 1979).

The responsibility for the pharmacologic control of pain rests with the entire health care team: the physician, the nurse and the patient (McCaffery and Beebe, 1989). The nurse's assessment of the patient's response to pain is critically important to the physician and to the patient. The nurse must constantly assess pain and establish the effectiveness of its management by:

- choosing the appropriate analgesic;
- determining whether to give it;
- evaluating its effectiveness; and
- obtaining a change in analgesic prescription if needed (McCaffery and Beebe, 1989).

Recognition of the need for effective treatment and treatment facilities for the person experiencing pain has resulted in better pain management programs. Numerous pain clinics, established across the country since the early 1970s, are now available to those experiencing chronic pain. The future should see further variety in treatment modalities for inpatient and outpatient management. Presently, the clinical nurse has access to a wide variety of options for pain assessment and management.

Assessment

Many factors contribute to the nurse's assessment of an individual patient's pain. Obtaining a thorough history provides essential neurophysiological information, as well as pertinent social or cultural background. The nurse must be able to distinguish between acute and chronic pain, and should be familiar with current pain theories — endorphins and nonopiod pathways, gate control and multiple opioid theories, etc. (McCaffery and Beebe, 1989).

To assist the nurse's assessment, a variety of pain assessment tools are available in current nursing literature. The "Initial Pain Assessment Tool" by McCaffery and Beebe (1989) gives a comprehensive guide to pain assessment. Other well-known methods include the *McGill Pain Questionnaire* (Melzack, 1983) and various pain-intensity numerical scales and visual analog scales. The use of daily pain flow sheets and diaries is helpful in patient/family teaching plans.

In any assessment of pain and its management, nurse and patient must consider the risk factors associated with pain medications. While fears of drug dependency may be reasonable in managing chronic long-term pain, they may not be justifiable in a palliative care situation. The nurse must therefore possess sound knowledge of physical dependency, tolerance and addiction (McCaffery and Beebe, 1989). Understanding the risk/benefit ratio helps both nurse and patient to establish realistic, attainable goals in pain control, and to accept any necessary limitations in treatment.

Diagnosis

Nursing diagnosis of pain is critical to its management. A widely accepted definition of **nursing diagnosis** is: "... a statement of a patient response which is actually or potentially unhealthful and which nursing intervention can help change in the direction of health" (Mundinger and Jauron, 1975). The National Conference Groups, now the North American Nursing Diagnosis Association (NANDA), have been working since the early 1970s to identify categories of problems that should be considered elements of nursing diagnoses. As of 1989, NANDA had approved 98 diagnoses. These include Chronic Pain and many diagnoses that may be appropriate to the patient with pain, such as Anxiety, Constipation, Fear, and Sleep Pattern Disturbances. For the patient living with pain, the nursing diagnosis has been qualified to include:

- type of pain;
- factors that influence the existence and characteristics of the pain sensation;
- patient's behavioral responses to the pain experience;
- factors that influence the patient's pain sensation (McCaffery, 1979).

A commonly accepted diagnostic statement format is known as the P-E-S format (Gordon, 1987). In this format, the problem, the etiology, and the signs and symptoms that led to determination of the problem are listed. The nurse is advised to use McCaffery's diagnostic pain criteria as a guide when developing a nursing diagnostic statement, with the P-E-S elements as the basic structural format.

At this point, the nursing process (diagnosis, planning and interventions, evaluation) involved in the treatment of a patient in pain can be explained best by creating a clinical example:

Ms R., 21 years old, suffers from severe, recurrent, right-sided, migraine headaches. The headaches occur each month with her period and last 48-72 h. She is taking Fiorinal with Codeine No. 3 (acetylsalicylic acid 352 mg, butalbital 50 mg, caffeine 40 mg, and codeine phosphate 30 mg) q 6 h. The medication reduces the pain but does not relieve it completely. Ms R. is completely dysfunctional and sleeps in a dark room as she moves in and out of bouts of excruciating pain. On a scale of 0-10, with 10 being the most severe, the patient rates her pain at 10 at the peak of the migraine, and at 6-7 one hour after taking her medication. She is nauseated, unable to eat, and has bouts of vomiting when pain is at the most severe point.

The nursing diagnosis is severe pain in the right side of the head, accompanied by nausea and vomiting. Having established the diagnosis, it is now appropriate to plan a course of action by carrying out the steps of the nursing process.

Planning and Interventions

When planning goals and interventions for the management of the patient in pain, the nurse will consider each patient as an individual. The plan is best arrived at by mutual agreement between patient and nurse, in consultation with the physician and pharmacist. Figure 26 highlights some of the factors to be considered. A fuller explanation of each of the approaches suggested can be found in McCaffery and Beebe (1989).

Evaluation

Evaluation of pain medication begins with observations for the therapeutic effect of the drug. The nurse will also observe for any side effects and/or adverse effects. It is important to check for patient compliance and knowledge of the plan for pain control. If the patient has been involved in the plan, there is a much greater chance for success.

Evaluation is a process that helps to measure the patient's progress or lack of progress toward mutually set goals. The question that now must be asked is, What happens if those mutually set goals are not met? Let us refer back to our clinical example:

Ms R. states that her headache is "out-of-control". As her nurse, you have administered her medication as ordered, and assessed that none of the drug therapies or nonpharmaceutic interventions have helped to give her relief. She tells you she feels "hysterical" because the pain is so bad and she seems to have little hope of relief from it.

When attempts to relieve pain have failed, the suggested nursing approach is to:

- listen and acknowledge that it still hurts;
- acknowledge the reasons you cannot provide further pain relief measures;
- provide continued contact, concern and support;
- offer reasonable hope that the migraine cycle will complete itself and that Ms R.'s periods will be pain-free.

Success in pain management depends on all members of the health care team cooperating to find the most effective treatment regime. The nurse's ability to assess and monitor pain and pain management is a vital link to patient comfort and successful pain control.

Figure 26
Nursing care plan.

Diagnosis	Possible Inverventions	Action
Severe pain in Ⓡ side of head with accompanying nausea and vomiting related to acute migraine	Pharmacological choices: • Non-narcotic • Narcotic • Antimigraine • Combinations for adjuvant and potentiating effects	With drug administration, observe • Safety factors • consider ATC • consider controlled analgesia • consider titrating dose to effect
	Non-pharmacological choices	• cutaneous stimulation • distraction • relaxation • imagery
	Patient/family teaching	• pain flow sheet with pain rating/analgesic effect • daily diary

Individual Narcotic Analgesics

In view of the preceding discussion, a review of individual narcotic analgesics can be kept to a minimum. Only particular aspects relating to the pharmacokinetics, relative potency and therapeutic uses for individual drugs will be discussed. The use of combination tablets, containing both a narcotic and a non-narcotic analgesic, is discussed in Chapter 54.

Opium Preparations (Pantopon)

Pantopon is a mixture of purified opium alkaloids in solution as hydrochloride salts. Pantopon has the same indications as morphine and is used most commonly for postoperative pain. The analgesic effect of Pantopon is the same as would be expected from its morphine content (50%). It has no proven advantage over an equivalent amount of morphine.

Purified Alkaloids of Morphine

Morphine Sulfate

Morphine remains the standard against which all other narcotics must be compared. Although the drug is best administered parenterally, orally effective preparations are available. As for most narcotics, the half-life of morphine is about three to four hours. The major use of morphine is in the treatment of moderate to severe pain. In addition to the adverse effects of narcotics previously discussed, morphine can release histamine from mast cells, resulting in itching and skin rashes. Barbiturates, alcohol, heterocyclic antidepressants, monoamine oxidase inhibitors and phenothiazines increase the central nervous depression produced by morphine and should not be used with the drug.

Codeine Phosphate

Codeine is similar to morphine in its effects but much weaker. Administered orally in doses of 30 – 60 mg, codeine is effective in the treatment of mild to moderate pain. Sixty-five milligrams of the drug are equal in effectiveness to 650 mg of either aspirin (acetylsalicylic acid) or acetaminophen. Codeine is often administered in combination with aspirin or acetaminophen; the analgesia produced is usually greater than if either narcotic or non-narcotic is used alone.

Semisynthetic Modifications of Morphine or Codeine

Hydromorphone (Dilaudid)

Hydromorphone is a semisynthetic derivative of morphine. It is approximately eight times more potent than morphine and relatively more effective when given orally. Hydromorphone has the same actions and uses as morphine. It is indicated for the relief of moderate to severe pain.

Oxymorphone (Numorphan)

Oxymorphone is another semisynthetic morphine derivative that is closely related to hydromorphone. The drug is indicated for the relief of moderate to severe pain. It is similar to both hydromorphone and morphine but is devoid of antitussive activity.

Oxycodone

Oxycodone is available only in combination with aspirin (Percodan) or acetaminophen (Percocet) for the treatment of pain. Oxycodone is effective orally and is more potent than codeine. As might be expected, its dependence liability is also greater than that of codeine. The doses for oxycodone in combination with either aspirin or acetaminophen can be found in Chapter 54.

Synthetic Narcotics

Meperidine HCl, Pethidine HCl (Demerol)

Meperidine or pethidine is eight to ten times less potent than morphine. Oral meperidine is one-third to one-quarter as effective as parenteral meperidine. Meperidine's duration of action is two to four hours. A common mistake with meperidine is to give the drug every six hours. Often this leaves the patient with two hours of pain before the next dose. Meperidine is indicated for the relief of moderate to severe pain in many medical, surgical, obstetric and dental situations. It has less effect on the gastrointestinal tract than morphine and no antitussive properties.

Alphaprodine (Nisentil)

Alphaprodine is related chemically to meperidine but has a more rapid onset and shorter duration of action than meperidine. It may be more suitable for short procedures, such as in obstetrics and urological examinations.

Levorphanol (Levo-Dromoran)

Related both chemically and pharmacologically to morphine, levorphanol is four to five times more potent than morphine. Given orally, it is a more effective drug. Levorphanol may also be administered subcutaneously or by slow intravenous injection.

Methadone (Dolophine)

Methadone is a synthetic narcotic with a half-life of twenty-five hours. Its long duration of action and excellent analgesic effects make it a good drug for the treatment of cancer. Methadone is also useful orally in narcotic detoxification programs. In this situation its long half-life is an advantage because patients may be treated once daily in a heroin clinic. Although methadone is similar to morphine and other potent narcotics, its long duration of action ensures less intense, but more prolonged, withdrawal symptoms.

Propoxyphene (Darvon)

Propoxyphene HCl or napsylate (Darvon-N) is effective for the relief of mild to moderate pain. Sixty-four milligrams of propoxyphene HCl and 100 mg of propoxyphene napsylate contain equivalent amounts of propoxyphene and are as effective as 650 mg of aspirin. Propoxyphene owes its popularity over codeine and aspirin to the fact that it does not irritate the stomach or constipate the patient.

Agonist-Antagonist Narcotics

Most narcotics, such as morphine, codeine, meperidine and levorphanol, are agonists. They stimulate both μ (mu) and K (kappa) receptors. A few narcotics, such as pentazocine, butorphanol and nalbuphine, are called agonist-antagonist drugs. In the absence of agonists they produce analgesia. In the presence of pure agonists, they block many of the actions of the latter drugs. This action can be explained by the fact that they competitively block μ receptors, which are responsible for most of the analgesic effects of agonists such as morphine, while serving as agonists of K and Σ (sigma) receptors.

Individual Mixed Agonist-Antagonist Narcotics

Pentazocine (Talwin)

Pentazocine is an agonist-antagonist drug. As just explained, in the presence of other narcotics, it acts as a narcotic antagonist, blocking their actions on μ receptors. In the absence of other narcotics, the ability of pentazocine to stimulate K receptors becomes apparent and the drug produces analgesia. Pentazocine is claimed to cause less respiratory depression than morphine, but it is also less effective.

Pentazocine is indicated for relief of moderate to severe pain. It is also used as a preoperative or preanesthetic medication, and as a supplement to surgical anesthesia. The drug has the same adverse effects as other narcotics. Particular attention should be paid to the psychotomimetic effects of large doses. Pentazocine should not be given to patients who are dependent on narcotics because its antagonist properties on μ receptors may precipitate a withdrawal effect. In the United States, Talwin tablets contain naloxone, an opioid antagonist (see below), to reduce abuse potential. Naloxone is not absorbed from the gastrointestinal tract and will not affect the analgesic effects of orally administered pentazocine. If, however, Talwin tablets reach the "street trade" and are dissolved and injected, the naloxone will block the effects of the pentazocine.

Butorphanol Tartrate (Stadol)

Butorphanol is more potent than either morphine or meperidine, with 2 – 3 mg parenterally producing analgesia equal to 10 mg of morphine or 80 mg of meperidine. It is ineffective if given by mouth. Butorphanol is indicated for relief of moderate to severe pain, including preoperative and postoperative pain and renal colic. The drug may also be used for analgesia during balanced anesthesia. Butorphanol is claimed to produce less respiratory depression than morphine. Its major side effects are drowsiness, weakness, sweating, nausea and a feeling of floating. Like pentazocine, it should not be given to patients who are dependent on narcotics because it will act as an antagonist and cause withdrawal effects.

Nalbuphine HCl (Nubain)

Nalbuphine is about as potent as morphine and three times more active than pentazocine. Its adverse effects are similar to those of the stronger narcotics. Similar to pentazocine and butorphanol, nalbuphine should not be given to patients dependent on narcotics. Nalbuphine is indicated for relief of moderate to severe pain. It may also be used for preoperative analgesia, as a supplement to surgical anesthesia, and for obstetrical analgesia during labor.

Narcotic Antagonists

Narcotic antagonists competitively block opiate receptors and are used to treat narcotic overdoses. Naloxone (Narcan) is the narcotic antagonist most frequently used in North America. When administered parenterally to a patient who has overdosed on a narcotic, it rapidly reverses the effect of the latter drug.

The nursing process for naloxone begins with an assessment of the extent of narcotic-induced respiratory depression and a determination of any existing addiction. Because the drug is used in a medical emergency, it is usually administered by, or under the direct supervision of, a physician. Nursing evaluation following the administration of this medication focuses on monitoring the patient's vital signs (particularly respiration) and observing the level of consciousness, euphoria or analgesia. Unconscious patients should be protected from the adverse effects of narcotics on the gastrointestinal system, specifically the possibility of aspiration of vomitus, by positioning them on their side.

Detailed discussion of the nursing process related to the treatment of patients experiencing narcotic overdose is beyond the scope of this text. Readers seeking such information should consult a medical-surgical or psychiatric nursing text.

Further Reading

Copolov, D.L. and Helme, R.D. (1983). Enkephalins and endorphins: Clinical pharmacology and therapeutic implications. *Drugs 26* :503-519.

Friedman, D.P. (1990). Perspectives on the medical use of drugs of abuse. *J. Pain and Symptom Management 54* (1):S2-3.

Gordon, M. (1987). *Nursing Diagnosis: Process and Application,* 2nd ed. New York: McGraw-Hill.

Health and Welfare Canada (1987). *Pain Relief: Information for People with Cancer and Their Families.* Ottawa: Minister of Supply and Services, Cat. No. 311578.

Health and Welfare Canada (1984). *Cancer Pain: A Monograph on the Management of Cancer Pain.* Ottawa: Minister of Supply and Services Canada, Cat. No. H42-2/4-1984.

Hoskin, P.J. and Hanks, G.W. (1991). Opioid agonist-antagonist drugs in acute and chronic pain states. *Drugs 41* :326-344.

Houde, R.W. (1980). Rational use of narcotic analgesics for controlling cancer pain. *Drug Ther. Hos. 5* :41-47.

Houde, R.W. (1979). Analgesic effectiveness of narcotic agonist-antagonists. *Brit. J. Clin. Pharmacol. 7* (Suppl. 3):297-308.

Loan, W.B. and Morrison, J.D. (1973). Strong analgesics: Pharmacological and therapeutic aspects. *Drugs 5* :108-142.

Logan, M. and Fothergill-Bourbonnais, F. (1990). Continuous subcutaneous infusion of narcotics. *Canadian Nurse 86* (4):31-32.

McCaffery, M. and Beebe, A. (1983). *Pain: Clinical Manual for Nursing Practice.* St. Louis: C.V. Mosby.

McCaffery, M. (1979). *Nursing Management of the Patient with Pain,* 2nd ed. Toronto: J.B. Lippincott.

Meinhart, N. and McCaffery, M. (1983). *Pain: A Nursing Approach to Assessment and Analysis.* New Haven, CT: Appleton-Century-Crofts.

Melzack, R. and Wall, P. (1983). *The Challenge of Pain.* New York: Basic Books.

Morgan, J.P. (1986). American opiophobia: Customary underutilization of opioid analgesics. In: *Controversies in Alcoholism and Substance Abuse,* pp.163-173. New York: The Haworth Press.

Mundinger, M.O. and Jauron, G.D. (1975). Developing a nursing diagnosis. *Nursing Outlook 23* (2):94-98.

North American Nursing Diagnosis Association (1989). *Classification of Nursing Diagnosis: Proceedings of the Eighth Conference.* St. Louis, MO: J.P. Lippincott.

Table 76
Narcotic analgesics and antagonists.

Pharmacologic Classification: Narcotic Analgesics

Generic Name (Trade Name)	Use (Dose)	Action	Adverse Effects	Drug Interactions	Nursing Process
Morphine sulfate	Symptomatic relief of pain (**IM/SC**: Adults - 10 mg/70 kg [range, 5-20 mg]. Children - [SC] 0.1-0.2 mg/kg [max, 15 mg]. **IV**: Adults - 2.5-15 mg in 4-5 mL water for inject'n over 4-5 min. **Oral**: Adults - Us. 20-25 mg. Some may require 75 mg or more q4h)	Reduces pain by mimicking actions of enkephalins. Produces analgesia and euphoria. Decr. resp. rate, minute volume and tidal exchange. Stims. chemoreceptor trigger zone, leading to nausea and vomiting. Produces constipat'n by (1) delaying emptying of stomach; (2) decr. propulsive contract'ns of sm. intestine, tog. w. incr. in nonpropulsive contract'ns and colonic tone; and (3) incr. tone of anal sphincter. Most narcotics incr. biliary pressure.	Respiratory and circulatory depress'n, respiratory and cardiac arrest, shock, lightheadedness, dizziness, sedat'n, nausea, vomiting, sweating, euphoria, dysphoria, weakness, headache, agitat'n, tremor, uncoordinated muscle movements, transient hallucinat'ns, disorientat'n, visual disturbances, dry mouth, constipat'n, biliary tract spasm, flushing of face, tachycardia, bradycardia, palpitat'ns, faintness, syncope, urinary retent'n, allergic skin react'ns. **Note:** Reduced dosage is indicated in pts w. renal dysfunct'n or w. resp. problems, in very young or elderly pts, and in pts receiving CNS depressants.	*The following drug interact'ns apply to all narcotics unless otherwise stated:* **CNS depressants:** Incr. central depressant effects of narcotics. Narcotics should be used cautiously and in reduced dosage in pts currently receiving other narcotic analgesics, gen'l anesthetics, phenothiazines, other tranquilizers, sedative-hypnotics, heterocyclic antidepressants and other CNS depressants (incl. alcohol). Resp. depress'n, hypotens'n and profound sedat'n or coma may result. **MAOIs:** And meperidine, can give rise to serious adv. effects. When meperidine is given to a pt receiving an MAOI, severe react'ns may occur, gen'lly immediate, w. excitat'n, sweating, rigidity and hypertens'n. Some pts develop hypertens'n and coma. Several deaths have been reported from this interact'n. Meperidine should be avoided in pts receiving MAOIs. Although this interact'n is perhaps greater than w. other narcotics, there is gen'l concern relating to use of morphine and other narcotics, either concomitantly w. or within 14 days of discontinuing MAOI tx. **Rifampin:** Stims. hepatic metabolism of methadone.	**Assess:** (Use a pain assessment tool to guide your initial assessment.) For concurrent use of barbiturates, alcohol, antidepressants; hx chronic respiratory/liver disease, convulsive disorders, Addison's disease, myxedema, physiological status for diabetic acidosis, head injury or elevated intracranial pressure, very young or very advanced age, gen'l debilitat'n, hemorrhage, prostate hypertrophy, severe obesity; pain as indicated by elevated pulse, respirat'ns, facial express'n, restlessness, posture, color. **Administer:** Prior to development of severe pain; acc. to local policies and procedures for compliance w. legal regulat'ns regarding controlled substances; IV in highly dilute solut'n by slow infus'n; IM or SC only after aspirating carefully on barrel of syringe; without mixing w. other drugs. **Evaluate:** By use of pain flow sheets throughout drug administrat'n; for relief of pain; for durat'n of analgesic effects; for incr. dosage or too-frequent administrat'n; for hypersensitivity react'ns; for developing dependence. **Teach:** To refrain from smoking and to walk only w. assistance; that side rails are for safety; to cough, breathe and change posit'n regularly; that flushing, sweating and sensory distort'ns are temporary.
Codeine phosphate	As for morphine (**Oral/SC/IM:** Adults - 30-60 mg q4-6h prn. Children - 0.5 mg/kg q4-6h)				
Hydromorphone HCl (Dilaudid)	As for morphine (**IM/SC:** Adults - 2 mg q4-6h prn. **IV:** 3-4 mg q4-6h prn. **Oral:** Adults - 2-4 mg q4h prn. **Rectal:** Adults - 3 mg q6-8h)	As for morphine	As for morphine		As for morphine
Oxymorphone HCl (Numorphan)	As for morphine (**IV:** Adults - Initially, 0.5 mg. **SC/IM:** Adults - 1-1.5 mg q4-6h. **Rectal:** 5 mg q4-6h. *For analgesia during labor* - **IM:** 0.5-1 mg)	As for morphine			
Meperidine HCl (Demerol)	As for morphine (**IM/SC/Oral:** Adults - 50-100 mg. For pts in severe pain, 150 mg. May be repeated q3-4h prn. Children - 1-1.5 mg/kg q3-4h. Max. dose, 100 mg)	As for morphine	As for morphine		As for morphine
Alphaprodine HCl (Nisentil)	As for morphine (*Obstetrical analgesia* - **SC:** 40-60 mg after cervical dilatat'n has begun;	As for morphine	As for morphine		As for morphine

Drug	Dosage and Indications				
Levorphanol tartrate (Levo-Dromoran)	repeat q2h prn. *For major or minor surgery* - **SC:** 20-40 mg. **IV:** 10-20 mg. *Max. SC/IV dose, 240 mg/24 h. For cytoscopy -* **IV:** 20-30 mg) ⟶ As for morphine (**SC/Slow IV:** *Severe acute pain or rapid relief of pain* - 1-4 mg. **SC:** *Premedicat'n* - 1-2 mg w. atropine or scopolamine 1.5 h before operat'n. **Oral:** *Severe chronic pain* - 1-3 mg prn)	As for morphine	As for morphine	As for morphine	As for morphine
Methadone (Dolophine)	As for morphine (**IM/SC:** 2.5-10 mg; repeat prn. **Oral:** Adults - 2.5-10 mg in tablet form or 5-20 mg in solut'n q6-8h)	As for morphine	As for morphine	As for morphine	As for morphine
Propoxyphene (Darvon)	As for morphine (**Oral:** Adults - 65 mg propoxyphene HCl or 100 mg propoxyphene napsylate tid-qid)	As for morphine	As for morphine	As for morphine	As for morphine
Purified opium alkaloids (Pantopon)	As for morphine (Use 20 mg in place of 10-15 mg morphine. **SC/IM:** Adults - Av. single dose, 20 mg. Max. dose, 40 mg. Max./day, 120 mg. Children > 2 years - 1 mg for each year of age in single dose)	As for morphine	As for morphine	As for morphine	As for morphine

Pharmacologic Classification: Mixed Agonist-Antagonist Narcotic Analgesics

Drug	Dosage and Indications				
Pentazocine (Talwin)	As for morphine (**Oral:** Adults - 50 mg q4h pc, adjusted within a range of 50-100 mg q3-4h [max., 600 mg/day]. **IM/SC/IV:** Adults[excl. pts in labor] - Av. dose, 30 mg; repeat q3-4h. Pts in labor - 30 mg IM or 20 mg IV)	Most narcotics stim. μ and K receptors. Mixed agonist-antagonist analgesics are competitive antagonists of μ receptors but agonists of K receptors. Thus when administered alone they stim. K receptors and produce analgesia. However, if given	As for morphine, plus incr. incidence of dysphoria and psychotomimetic effects.	As for morphine	As for morphine, w. requirement for addit'nal assessment of narcotic addict'n
Butorphanol tartrate (Stadol)	As for morphine (**IM:** Adults - 1-2 mg q3-4h prn. **IV:** Adults - 0.5-2 mg q3-4h prn)	As for pentazocine	As for pentazocine	As for morphine	As for pentazocine

Generic Name (Trade Name)	Use (Dose)	Action	Adverse Effects	Drug Interactions	Nursing Process
Nalbuphine HCl (Nubain)	As for morphine **(SC/IM/IV: Adults** - 10 mg/70 kg; repeat q3-6h prn. Recomm. dosage range, 10-20 mg; max. dose, 160 mg/day)	to a pt taking a pure agonist (such as morphine), agonist-antagonist drugs block effects of the pure agonist by competitively antagonizing effects on μ receptors. Because mixed agonist-antagonist narcotics also stim. Σ receptors, they produce dysphoria and psychotomimetic effects.	As for pentazocine	As for morphine	As for pentazocine

Pharmacologic Classification: Narcotic Antagonist

Generic Name (Trade Name)	Use (Dose)	Action	Adverse Effects	Drug Interactions	Nursing Process
Naloxone HCl (Narcan, Narcan Neonatal)	Narcotic antagonist for complete or partial reversal of narcotic depress'n **(IV: Adults -** *Narcotic overdose* - 0.4-2 mg; repeat prn at 2-3 min intervals. *Postop. narcotic depress'n* - 0.1-0.2 mg; repeat IV, IM or SC at 2-3 min intervals prn. Children - *Narcotic overdose* - **IV:** 0.01 mg/kg. If desired degree of improvement is not obtained, 0.1 mg/kg may be given. Naloxone may be diluted w. sterile H₂0 for inject'n. *Postop. narcotic depress'n* - 0.005-0.01 mg; repeat prn at 2-3 min intervals. Neonates - *Narcotic-induced depress'n* - **IV/IM/SC:** 0.01 mg/kg; repeat prn at 2-3 min intervals)	Competitively blocks opiate receptors.	Abrupt reversal of narcotic depress'n may result in nausea, vomiting, sweating, tachycardia, incr. BP, tremulousness. In postop. pts, excess. dosage of naloxone may result in significant reversal of analgesia and excitement; in some cardiac pts, resultant hypertens'n and tachycardia may lead to left-ventr. failure and pulmonary edema. In absence of narcotics, naloxone is essentially devoid of side effects.		**Assess:** Extent of narcotic-induced resp. depress'n; for narcotic addict'n. **Evaluate:** Ameliorat'n of resp. depress'n.

CHAPTER 54

Non-Narcotic Analgesics

Teaching Objectives

Following completion of this chapter, the reader should be able to:

1. Discuss the mechanism of action, pharmacokinetics, pharmacologic effects, therapeutic uses and adverse effects of aspirin, as well as the nursing process associated with its administration.
2. Describe briefly the therapeutic uses and advantages of diflunisal.
3. Discuss the pharmacologic properties, therapeutic uses, adverse effects and related nursing process for ketorolac.
4. Discuss the mechanism of action, pharmacologic effects, therapeutic uses and adverse effects of acetaminophen, as well as the nursing process related to its use.
5. Explain the rationale for the combination of a narcotic and a non-narcotic analgesic in the same tablet and the nursing process related to the use of these combination products.

Non-narcotic analgesics are also called **analgesic-antipyretics** because they relieve pain and reduce fever. In contrast to narcotics, analgesic-antipyretics do not produce euphoria and drug dependence. Generally speaking, their analgesic activity is less than that of narcotics and they are used in pain of mild to moderate intensity. In progressive diseases, analgesic-antipyretics are often used first to treat pain and as the condition worsens, the patient is switched to a narcotic.

Single-Ingredient Products

Aspirin, Acetylsalicylic Acid, ASA

For years aspirin has been the standard analgesic-antipyretic used in North America. In the United States, aspirin is a generic name, with many companies using it. In Canada, Aspirin is a trade name. The generic name for the drug in Canada is acetylsalicylic acid, often shortened to ASA. In this book, aspirin will be used as a generic name to indicate all manufacturers' brands.

Mechanism of Action and Pharmacologic Effects

Aspirin acts both peripherally and within the brain to produce analgesia. Peripherally, it interferes with the production of prostaglandins in various organs and tissues. Prostaglandin E_2 sensitizes pain receptors to noxious substances, such as histamine and bradykinin. By reducing the synthesis of prostaglandin E_2, aspirin diminishes pain. Centrally, aspirin acts in the hypothalamus to reduce pain perception. The antipyretic actions of aspirin also result from its action in the hypothalamus. Acting through the hypothalamus, aspirin improves heat loss by dilating small skin vessels and increasing sweating.

The other effects of aspirin include gastric irritation, an inhibition of platelet aggregation, and a prolongation of bleeding time. The drug also affects kidney function. Small doses (1 –2 g daily) decrease renal uric acid secretion. Larger amounts (5 g daily or more) increase uric acid excretion by reducing its renal reabsorption. Aspirin, in large doses, can also increase sodium, chloride and water reabsorption by the kidneys.

Pharmacokinetics

Aspirin can be absorbed from both the stomach and the duodenum. However, its absorption proceeds faster from the latter site. Taking aspirin with food slows absorption of the drug because food closes the pyloric sphincter, trapping aspirin in the stomach.

Shortly after its absorption, aspirin is metabolized to salicylate. Approximately 90% of the salicylate is metabolized in the liver. A glycine conjugate, called salicyluric acid, accounts for 75% of the metabolites. The capacity of the liver to furnish enough glycine to inactivate salicylate is limited. If the daily dose of aspirin exceeds the capacity of the liver to provide glycine, serum salicylate levels rise sharply and the patient may become toxic. About 10% of the salicylate in the body is eliminated unchanged by the kidney. If the urine is alkalinized, this can be increased three- to five-fold.

Therapeutic Uses

Aspirin is an effective analgesic and antipyretic for the relief of mild to moderate pain. It is more effective in the relief of skeletal muscle pain than visceral pain and is often given to patients with headaches, neuralgias, myalgias or primary spasmodic dysmenorrhea. Aspirin is also a popular anti-inflammatory drug for the treatment of rheumatoid arthritis and osteoarthrosis. This aspect of its use is discussed in Chapter 57. Six hundred and fifty milligrams of aspirin are as effective as 30 mg of codeine or 100 mg of propoxyphene napsylate.

Concern over a possible correlation between the use of aspirin as an antipyretic in children with varicella or influenza virus infection and the development of Reye's syndrome has led to the recommendation that it not be used in these conditions.

Aspirin is also contraindicated in patients allergic to the drug, in patients who have had a bronchospastic reaction, or in generalized urticaria, angioedema, severe rhinitis, laryngeal edema, or shock precipitated by aspirin or nonsteroidal anti-inflammatory drugs (NSAIDs). In addition, because of its irritant effects on the gastric mucosa, aspirin is contraindicated in patients with active peptic ulcer.

Adverse Effects

Gastric irritation, ranging from discomfort to gastric ulceration and hemorrhage, is a common adverse effect of aspirin. Aspirin has direct irritant effects on the gastric mucosa, and also reduces prostaglandin formation. Prostaglandins promote the secretion of protective gastric mucous. Although enteric-coated tablets will minimize the initial irritant effects of aspirin on the gastric mucosa, they will not prevent damage to the mucosa from drug carried back to the stomach in the circulation.

Aspirin is rapidly metabolized in the body. Its primary product is salicylate, a vitamin K antagonist. Large doses of aspirin taken for several days can cause hypoprothrombinemia. This effect is usually only significant in patients taking oral anticoagulants or suffering from liver disease.

Aspirin can cause serious allergic reactions, including acute asthmatic attacks, hives and hypotension. Patients allergic to aspirin should not be given the drug nor any other nonsteroidal anti-inflammatory drug.

Mild toxicity is usually seen with serum salicylate levels of 500 µg/mL (3620 µmol/L). Hepatitis has been reported rarely in patients with systemic lupus erythematosus and juvenile rheumatoid arthritis with serum salicylate levels above 250 µg/mL (1810 µmol/L).

Large doses of aspirin can be very toxic. Beginning with tinnitus and decreased hearing, the symptoms of acute poisoning can proceed to respiratory alkalosis. In response to the increased loss of CO_2, renal excretion of bicarbonate rises and systemic pH returns to normal — but at the cost of a reduced bicarbonate reserve. If sufficient aspirin is consumed, metabolic rate increases and metabolic acidosis ensues. The final stage in salicylate intoxication is respiratory depression and death.

Four steps can be taken to treat patients who have overdosed on aspirin. First, patients can be gavaged or induced to vomit to remove any unabsorbed drug. Second, Ringer's solution and isotonic sodium bicarbonate can be infused to restore normal electrolyte balance and pH. Third, the urine can be alkalinized with sodium bicarbonate to increase salicylate elimination. Hemodialysis may also be tried to eliminate the drug.

Drug Interactions

Aspirin must not be given to patients receiving oral anticoagulants. Drugs such as warfarin and bishydroxycoumarin are extensively bound to plasma albumin, similarly to salicylate. If aspirin is taken, it will displace some of the bound oral anticoagulant, which will then enter the liver and inhibit prothrombin formation. The result is an increase in anticoagulant activity. Aspirin should not be given to patients receiving uricosuric drugs, such as probenecid, because it will reduce their effects.

Nursing Process

The majority of aspirin tablets consumed in North America are purchased on a nonprescription basis and self-administered for self-diagnosed illnesses. Therefore, the primary nursing process lies in patient teaching. Patients should be advised that although it is a commonly used household remedy, aspirin must be used judiciously. Nurses, particularly those whose practice is based in the community, should make certain that patients are familiar with the adverse effects of aspirin. These are manifested by dizziness, tinnitus, dimness of vision, confusion, diaphoresis, thirst, nausea, vomiting and diarrhea. Patients who experience mild dyspepsia with aspirin should be advised to take the drug with milk or food. If this fails to prevent gastric irritation, they should be advised to use acetaminophen. As with all medications, aspirin (especially the flavored variety) should be kept out of the reach of children, preferably in a locked cupboard or drawer. Nurses in doctors' offices should regularly remind patients who are on anticoagulant therapy, are using uricosuric drugs or have ulcerative conditions of the gastrointestinal tract, that they should *not* take aspirin-containing products.

Diflunisal (Dolobid)

Diflunisal is, like aspirin, a salicylate derivative. The indications for the use of diflunisal are the relief of mild to moderate pain accompanied by inflammation in conditions such as musculoskeletal trauma, postdental extraction or postepisiotomy and symptomatic relief of osteoarthritis. Diflunisal's mechanism of action is not known precisely but it appears to act peripherally by inhibiting the synthesis of prostaglandins. A major advantage for diflunisal is its relatively long half-life, eight to twelve hours, making it possible to treat patients twice daily. Diflunisal is not recommended for use as an antipyretic agent.

Nursing Process

Assessment
Nurses should review the patient's history for documentation of prior hypersensitivity to diflunisal, aspirin or other salicylates prior to administering diflunisal. Documentation of gastrointestinal bleeding, active gastric ulcer, renal or cardiovascular disease accompanied by edema, or prolonged clotting times contraindicates the use of diflunisal. Withhold the medication pending consultation with the physician. *Under no circumstances should diflunisal be administered to women in the third trimester of pregnancy because it is known to cause premature closing of the ductus arteriosus in the fetus.*

The physical assessment of the patient should establish the location and intensity of the pain.

Administration
Tablets should be administered whole. They should not be crushed or chewed prior to swallowing. Those patients who experience gastric irritation with diflunisal might find relief by taking it with food or milk.

Evaluation
Drug efficacy is determined by the relief or reduction of pain. Nurses caring for patients receiving diflunisal should be alert for evidence of adverse effects including ophthalmic complications (blurred vision, reduced visual acuity, changes in color vision, and corneal deposits or retinal disturbances), hepatic disorders (jaundice, tea-colored urine, clay-colored stools and pruritus); gastric effects (black or tarry stools, hematemesis and severe abdominal pain).

Teaching
Nurses should advise patients taking diflunisal for chronic inflammatory pain that full anti-inflammatory benefits of the drug are often not experienced for several weeks. Patients should be instructed to take diflunisal only in the amount and at the times specified. Nurses should alert patients to the adverse effects of the drug. In addition, nurses should warn patients that diflunisal may cause drowsiness or dizziness. Patients should avoid driving or using power tools or machinery until their individual response to diflunisal has been determined.

Ketorolac Tromethamine (Toradol)

Ketorolac is a nonsteroidal anti-inflammatory drug that exhibits analgesic activity. Its mechanism of action is to inhibit the cyclo-oxygenase enzyme system, thereby inhibiting the synthesis of prostaglandins. Ketorolac is considered to be a peripherally acting analgesic. At analgesic doses, it has minimal anti-inflammatory and antipyretic activity. Oral ketorolac is indicated for the short-term management of mild to moderately severe pain, including postsurgical pain (such as general, orthopedic and dental surgery), acute musculoskeletal trauma pain and postpartum uterine cramping. Intramuscular injection of ketorolac is also indicated for the short-term management of moderate to severe pain, including pain following major abdominal, orthopedic and gynecological operative procedures.

The adverse effects of both oral and parenteral ketorolac include dyspepsia and gastrointestinal pain. Patients taking the drug orally have also occasionally reported nausea, headache and dizziness. Parenteral ketorolac has been associated with drowsiness.

Nursing Process

The nursing process for ketorolac is similar to that for aspirin, with the following additions.

Assessment
Prior to administration, review the patient's history and blood work for evidence of contraindications, such as hypersensitivity to the drug, liver or kidney disease.

Administration
Ketorolac is best taken on an empty stomach but may have to be taken with food if gastrointestinal symptoms occur. Store at room temperature.

Evaluation
Nurses should evaluate patients for the therapeutic effect of decreased pain, stiffness and swelling in joints. They should evaluate the patient for blurred vision and tinnitus because these symptoms may indicate drug-induced toxicity.

Teaching
Nurses should teach both patient and family to report the signs of toxicity listed above. Patients should be cautioned to avoid driving or other hazardous activities if dizziness or drowsiness occur. Tell patients to report changes in urine patterns, weight increase, edema, pain increase in joints, fever, or blood in urine. Also warn patients that therapeutic effects may take up to one month to occur.

Other Nonsteroidal Anti-inflammatory Drugs

Like aspirin, nonsteroidal anti-inflammatory drugs inhibit the formation of the various prostaglandins and can be used as analgesic-antipyretics. Drugs such as ibuprofen (Motrin, Rufen), naproxen sodium (Anaprox) and fenoprofen (Nalfon) are sold as analgesics. Their availability has decreased the need to use weaker narcotics. The pharmacology of these agents and the nursing process related to their use are discussed in detail in Chapter 57.

Acetaminophen, Paracetamol (Tylenol)

Mechanism of Action and Pharmacologic Effects
The analgesic and antipyretic actions of acetaminophen are similar to those of aspirin. Acetaminophen has no anti-inflammatory activity and does not affect platelet aggregation or irritate the stomach.

Therapeutic Uses
The major use for acetaminophen is as an analgesic-antipyretic in patients who cannot tolerate aspirin. This applies to patients who experience gastric discomfort with aspirin or who are allergic to the drug. Acetaminophen should also be used in place of aspirin in patients taking oral anticoagulants. The drug is valuable in relieving the pain of osteoarthritis. Because it is devoid of anti-inflammatory effects, it is less effective in rheumatoid arthritis.

Acetaminophen has proven popular in pediatrics because of its availability in liquid formulations. In addition, the previously mentioned concern over the connection between the use of aspirin in children with varicella or influenza virus infection and the development of Reye's syndrome has led to the recommendation that acetaminophen be used in these conditions. Nurses should warn parents of the potential lethal effects of the drug. It should be stored in a safe place in a child-proof container.

Adverse Effects

Taken in the recommended doses, acetaminophen is well tolerated. Skin rash, drug fever and mucosal lesions have been reported occasionally. A few cases of neutropenia, pancytopenia and leukopenia have also been found.

Hepatic necrosis can occur if overdoses of acetaminophen are taken. Single doses of 10 – 15 g in adults may cause hepatotoxicity and 25 g or more can kill. The first signs of toxicity occur about 12 – 24 hours after acute overdose and include nausea, vomiting, diarrhea, diaphoresis, pallor and abdominal pain. Hepatic damage is seen 24 – 48 hours after an overdose and is manifested by increased serum transaminases, lactic dehydrogenase, prothrombin time and serum bilirubin concentrations. Severe hepatic damage can subsequently proceed to liver failure, encephalopathy, coma and death. The culprit is an acetaminophen metabolite that binds to the liver producing necrosis, primarily in the centrolobular region.

Acetylcysteine (Mucomyst) is used as an antidote for severe acetaminophen poisoning. Because of the low incidence of adverse effects associated with acetylcysteine, therapy should be initiated immediately without waiting for determination of plasma acetaminophen levels. The decision to continue therapy may then be guided by the laboratory results.

When serum determinations of acetaminophen are above 990 µmol/L (150 µg/mL) at 4 h, or above 260 µmol/L (40 µg/mL) at 12 h after the estimated time of ingestion, the patient is at risk of liver damage and therapy is required immediately. Ipecac-induced emesis or gastric lavage should, when possible, commence within four hours of drug ingestion. Activate charcoal is effective only when given within one to two hours of the alleged overdose. Prior to antidotal treatment with acetylcysteine, residual charcoal must be removed by gastric lavage with water.

Acetylcysteine is effective orally. A loading dose of 140 mg/kg is given as a single dose. A maintenance dose of 70 mg/kg is then given every four hours for 17 doses. If nausea and vomiting occur within one hour of the loading or maintenance dose, the entire dose should be repeated. If nausea and vomiting persist, a nonphenothiazine antiemetic (e.g., dimenhydrinate) may be administered. Acetylcysteine, 20% solution, may be diluted to a 5% concentration with a soft drink to make it more palatable. This mixture should be consumed within one hour of preparation. The use of intravenous acetylcysteine is recommended when oral therapy is not feasible or practical. A loading dose, 150 mg/kg of acetylcysteine, is infused in 200 mL of 5% dextrose in water (D5W) over 15 min, followed by an infusion of 50 mg/kg in 500 mL D5W over 4 h, and finally 100 mg/kg in 1000 mL D5W during the next 16 h. The total dose is 300 mg/kg administered over 20 h.

Nursing Process

The nursing process for acetaminophen is similar to that for aspirin. However, because of the irreversible consequences of an overdose, greater emphasis must be placed on keeping acetaminophen out of the reach of children.

Analgesic Products Containing Both a Narcotic and a Non-Narcotic Drug

Mechanism of Action and Pharmacologic Effects

Narcotic analgesics stimulate opiate receptors in the brain. Non-narcotic analgesics block the formation of prostaglandin E_2. Their different mechanisms of action make their combination rational. It is often possible, for example, to provide greater pain relief with aspirin plus codeine than with either drug alone. The nursing process for these products is identified by combining the information previously provided in relation to each of the component substances.

In the United States, caffeine and phenacetin are also incorporated into the mixtures. In Canada, only caffeine finds its way into the tablets. These ingredients serve no therapeutic value. The amount of caffeine in an analgesic tablet is usually about 30 mg. This is equivalent to one-third of a cup of coffee. It may take three cups of coffee in the morning to relieve the pain of awakening but one-third of a cup is useless as an analgesic! Phenacetin acts similarly to salicylate. Tablets containing phenacetin usually have lower doses of aspirin. Nothing is accomplished by replacing a portion of the dose of one analgesic-antipyretic with a few milligrams of another drug with the same actions. This is particularly true when the second drug is phenacetin, which has been removed from sale in most parts of the world because of concern over its nephrotoxicity.

Mixtures Containing Codeine

Aspirin plus codeine preparations (e.g., Empirin/ Codeine, 222s, 282s, 292s) or acetaminophen plus codeine products (e.g., Tylenol/Codeine, Phenaphen/ Codeine) are most popular. In the United States, these products also contain phenacetin. The tablets contain either 15 mg, 30 mg or 60 mg of codeine, together with 325 mg of aspirin or acetaminophen. Fifteen milligrams of codeine is, at best, minimally effective and it is not clear whether combinations containing this amount of narcotic are more effective than the analgesic-antipyretic alone. The preparations with 30 mg of codeine in combination with either aspirin or acetaminophen are most popular and more effective than either ingredient used alone.

Mixtures Containing Propoxyphene

The rationale for combining propoxyphene with an analgesic-antipyretic is the same as that for similar combinations containing codeine. Control studies with propoxyphene combinations have been limited, but available results suggest that the analgesic effects of the individual components are additive. However, since propoxyphene is less effective than codeine, these combinations may be less effective than comparable codeine-containing preparations.

Mixtures Containing Oxycodone (Percodan, Percocet)

Oxycodone combined with non-narcotic analgesics is available as Percodan and Percocet. Each Percodan tablet contains oxycodone hydrochloride, 5 mg, and aspirin, 325 mg. Percodan-Demi tablets contain 2.5 mg of oxycodone HCl and 325 mg of aspirin. Percocet and Percocet-Demi tablets contain acetaminophen in place of aspirin. Oxycodone is more potent than codeine and its dependence liability is also greater. Whereas the Percodan-Demi and Percocet-Demi tablets are indicated for the relief of mild to moderate pain, the full-strength Percodan

and Percocet tablets are used in the treatment of moderate to moderately severe pain, including conditions accompanied by fever.

Mixtures Containing Codeine and Butalbital (Fiorinal-C)

Fiorinal preparations have been popular for many years. They contain aspirin, caffeine and the barbiturate butalbital. Fiorinal-C products also contain either 15 mg or 30 mg of codeine. These products are indicated for the relief of acute and chronic pain of mild, moderate or severe degree, which is accompanied by tension or anxiety, and in all cases in which a simultaneous sedative and analgesic action is required, such as tension headache, musculoskeletal pain, postoperative pain, dysmenorrhea and pain associated with dental procedures, neoplastic disease or trauma.

Butalbital has a longer half-life than the analgesics and the chronic use of Fiorinal-C will lead to barbiturate accumulation. In addition, there is the possibility that a preparation containing a barbiturate may induce dependence in the patient. Therefore, these products are not recommended for the routine or chronic management of pain.

Further Reading

Brenner, B.E. and Simon, R.R. (1982). Management of salicylate intoxication. *Drugs 24* :335-340.

Lasagna, L. and Prescott, L.F. (1986). Non-narcotic analgesics today. Benefits and risks. *Drugs 32* (Suppl. 4):1-208.

MacMillian, K. (1990). Pain corner: Equivalent analgesic dose. *AARN Newsletter 46* (3):25.

Parkhouse, J. (1975). Simple analgesics. *Drugs 10* :366-393.

Prescott, L.F. (1983). Paracetaminol overdosage: Pharmacological considerations and clinical management. *Drugs 25* : 290-314.

Wyant, G.M. (1983). Chronic pain: Principle and treatment. *Drugs 26* : 262-267.

Table 77
Non-narcotic analgesics

Pharmacologic Classification: Single-Ingredient Non-Narcotic Analgesics

Generic Name (Trade Name)	Use (Dose)	Action	Adverse Effects	Drug Interactions	Nursing Process
Aspirin, acetylsalicylic acid, ASA	Relief of mild to moderate pain, fever and inflammation. For reducing risk of recurrent TIA or stroke in men who have had transient ischemia of the brain due to fibrin platelet emboli (**Oral:** *For analgesia and antipyresis* - Adults - 650 mg 4-6x/day. Children - 10-15 mg/kg q4-6h, to max. 65 mg/day)	Aspirin works both peripherally and within brain to produce analgesia. Peripherally, it interferes w. production of prostaglandins in various organs and tissues. Prostaglandin E$_2$ sensitizes pain receptors to noxious substances, such as histamine and bradykinin. In the brain, aspirin acts in the hypothalamus to reduce pain perception. The antipyretic actions of aspirin also result from its action in the hypothalamus, improving heat loss by dilating small skin vessels and incr. sweating.	Nausea, vomiting, diarrhea, gastritis, GI bleeding and/or ulcerat'n, tinnitus, vertigo, hearing loss, leukopenia, thrombocytopenia, purpura, urticaria, angioedema, pruritus, skin erupt'ns, asthma, anaphylaxis, reversible hepatotoxicity, mental confus'n, drowsiness, sweating, thirst	**Ammonium chloride; ascorbic acid:** Acidify urine and reduce renal excret'n of salicylates. In this situat'n, 3 g aspirin may produce toxicity. **Antacids, systemic:** Alkalinize urine and incr. renal excret'n of salicylates. **Anticoagulants, oral:** May have incr. effects in presence of aspirin. Large doses of aspirin reduce plasma prothrombin levels and displace oral anticoagulants from plasma proteins. Aspirin can also produce GI bleeding. Avoid concomitant use of aspirin and oral anticoagulants. **Antidiabetic agents:** May demonstrate incr. effects in presence of aspirin because aspirin decr. hyperglycemia of diabetes and displaces tolbutamide and chlorpropamide from binding to plasma proteins. Give salicylates cautiously to pts receiving hypoglycemics. Large doses may affect insulin requirements. **Corticosteroids:** Can enhance salicylate excret'n. **Dipyridamole; heparin:** Incr. risk of bleeding in pts taking aspirin. **Methotrexate:** Renal excret'n is reduced by salicylate administrat'n. **Spironolactone:** May have its	**Assess:** Hx for allergy or sensitivity; anticoagulant tx or use of uricosuric drugs; dyspepsia or GI ulcerat'n; kidney or liver disease; asthma; bleeding tendencies. Establish baseline descript'n of pain and inflammat'n. **Administer:** W. meals. **Evaluate:** Relief of pain, level of inflammat'n; for rash, GI distress/bleeding, dizziness, incr. bleeding tendencies, salicylism. **Teach:** Self-evaluat'n for side effects and toxicity; to take w. food, milk or antacids. Keep out of reach of children.

Generic Name (Trade Name)	Use (Dose)	Action	Adverse Effects	Drug Interactions	Nursing Process
				ability to incr. Na excret'n reduced by salicylates. **Uricosurics:** Incr. uric acid excret'n. Smaller doses of salicylates decr. uricosuric effects of probenecid, sulfinpyrazone, oxyphenbutazone and phenylbutazone.	
Diflunisal (Dolobid)	Relief of pain, inflammat'n and fever (**Oral:** *Mild to moderate pain* - 1000 mg initially, followed by 500 mg q12h. A lower dose may be appropriate depending on such factors as pain severity, pt response, weight or advanced age; for example, 500 mg initially, followed by 250 mg q12h. *Osteoarthritis* - 500-1000 mg daily in 2 divided doses according to pt response. Maint. doses > 1000 mg not recommended)	Salicylate derivative. Mechanism of action similar to aspirin's.	Nausea, dyspepsia, GI pain and diarrhea, edema and tinnitus	**Acetaminophen:** Administered concomitantly w. diflunisal, may result in incr. plasma acetaminophen levels. **Antacids:** Can reduce bioavailability of diflunisal. **Anticoagulants, oral:** May interact w. diflunisal. In some normal volunteers, concomitant administrat'n of diflunisal and warfarin resulted in prolongat'n of prothrombin time. This may occur because diflunisal competitively displaces coumarins from plasma protein binding sites. Monitor prothrombin time closely for several days after concomitant drug administrat'n. **Furosemide:** May have its hyperuricemic, but not its diuretic, effect reduced by diflunisal. **Indomethacin:** May have reduced renal clearance and incr. plasma levels in presence of diflunisal. Fatal GI-tract hemorrhage has occurred. Do not administer these agents concurrently. **Thiazide:** Plasma levels may be incr. by diflunisal. Diflunisal may decr. hyperuricemic effects of thiazides.	**Assess:** Hx for hypersensitivity to diflunisal, aspirin or other salicylates; GI bleeding or active gastric ulcer; renal or CV disease accompanied by edema; prolonged clotting times. *Under no circumstances administer in 3rd trimester of pregnancy.* Document locat'n and intensity of pain. **Administer:** Whole tablets, w. milk or food. **Evaluate:** Drug efficacy; for adv. effects, incl. eye complicat'ns (blurred vision, reduced acuity, changes in color vision, corneal deposits or retinal disturbances); hepatic disorders (jaundice, tea-colored urine, clay-colored stools, pruritus); GI effects (black or tarry stools, hematemesis, severe abd. pain). **Teach:** That full analgesic effects not seen for several weeks; to take only in am't and at times specified; indicators of adv. effects; to avoid driving or using power equipment until response to drug is determined.

Drug	Action and Use / Dose	Side Effects	Interactions	Nursing Considerations
Ketorolac tromethamine (Toradol)	Inhibits cyclo-oxygenase enzyme system, thereby inhibiting synthesis of prostaglandins. Considered a peripherally acting analgesic. At analgesic doses it has minimal anti-inflammatory/antipyretic activity. — Orally for short-term management of mild to moderate pain, e.g., acute musculoskeletal trauma, postpartum uterine cramping. IM for short-term management of moderate to severe pain, incl. pain following major abd., orthopedic and gyn. operative procedures (**Oral:** 10 mg q4-6h prn. Doses > 40 mg/day not recomm. **IM:** Initially, 30 mg. Subsequently, 10-30 mg q4-6h prn. Lower dose may be suitable for pts > age 65)	Dyspepsia, GI pain. Oral preparat'n may also cause nausea, headache and dizziness. Parenteral use has been assoc. w. drowsiness.	**Anticoagulants, oral:** May interact w. ketorolac. Monitor prothrombin time carefully in pts receiving both an oral anticoagulant and ketorolac. **Furosemide:** May have its diuretic effects reduced slightly by ketorolac.	**Assess:** Hx for drug sensitivity, liver or kidney disease. **Administer:** Preferably on an empty stomach, but w. meals if GI symptoms occur. Store at room temp. **Evaluate:** For tx effect of decr. pain, stiffness and joint swelling. Be alert for s/s toxicity, such as blurring of vision and tinnitus. **Teach:** Pt and family to check for s/s toxicity. Caution to avoid driving and hazardous activities if dizzy or drowsy. Report changes in urine patterns, fever, blood in urine. Tx effects may take up to 1 month.
Acetaminophen (Tylenol)	Analgesic and antipyretic actions are similar to aspirin's. No anti-inflammatory activity. Does not affect platelet aggreg'n or irritate stomach. — Relief of mild to moderate pain and reduct'n of fever (**Oral: Adults** - 650-1000 mg q4-6h, not > 4000 mg/24 h. **Children** - 10-15 mg/kg q4-6h, not > 65 mg/kg/24 h)	Hepatotoxicity w. overdosage	**Phenobarbital:** Incr. activity of microsomal enzymes, which produce a toxic metabolite and enhance toxicity of acetaminophen.	**Assess:** Hx for allergy. Establish baseline descript'n of pain and fever. **Administer:** Orally. **Evaluate:** Relief of pain and fever. **Teach:** Dangers of overdose. Keep out of reach of children.

Pharmacologic Classification: Combination Non-Narcotic + Narcotic Analgesic Products

Drug	Action and Use / Dose			
Aspirin or acetaminophen + caffeine and codeine	Relief of mild to moderate pain, fever and inflammat'n (**Oral:** 1-2 tablets containing 15 or 30 mg codeine q4h prn; or 1 tab containing 60 mg codeine q4h prn)	The narcotic relieves pain by stim. opiate receptors in CNS. Aspirin and acetaminophen are analgesic-antipyretics. Because narcotics and analgesic-antipyretics reduce pain by different mechanisms, a combinat'n of both often provides better pain relief than either drug used alone. There is little justificat'n for incorporating caffeine into these products.	As for narcotics (see Table 76) and either aspirin or acetaminophin, above	As for narcotics (see Table 76) and either aspirin or acetaminophin, above

Generic Name (Trade Name)	Use (Dose)	Action	Adverse Effects	Drug Interactions	Nursing Process
Aspirin + oxycodone (Percodan); acetaminophen + oxycodone (Percodet)	Relief of mild to moderate pain [Percodan-Demi, Percocet-Demi] or moderate to severe pain [Percodan, Percocet] (**Oral:** *Percodan and Percocet Tablets* - Adults - 1 tab q6h prn for pain. *Percodan-Demi and Percocet-Demi Tablets* - Adults - 1-2 tabs q6h. Children ≥ 12 years - $^1/_2$ tab q6h. Children 6-12 - $^1/_4$ tab q6h. Not indicated for children < 6 years)	As for aspirin/ acetaminophen tablets containing codeine	As for narcotics (see Table 76) and either aspirin or acetaminophin, above	As for narcotics (see Table 76) and either aspirin or acetaminophin, above	As for narcotics (see Table 76) and either aspirin or acetaminophin, above
Aspirin + caffeine and propoxyphene HCl (Darvon Compound-65); Acetaminophen + propoxyphen napsylate (Darvocet-N)	Relief of mild to moderate pain present alone, or when pain is accompanied by fever (**Oral:** 1 tablet or capsule tid-qid)	As for aspirin/ acetaminophen tablets containing codeine	As for narcotics (see Table 76) and either aspirin or acetaminophin, above	As for narcotics (see Table 76) and either aspirin or acetaminophin, above	As for narcotics (see Table 76) and either aspirin or acetaminophin, above
Aspirin + caffeine, codeine and butalbital (Fiorinal-C)	Relief of acute or chronic pain of mild, moderate or severe degree, accompanied by tension or anxiety (**Oral:** 1-2 capsules containing 15 mg or 30 mg of codeine; thereafter, 1 cap q3-4h. Max., 6 caps/day)	As for aspirin tablets containing codeine. The barbiturate is used to relieve muscle spasms or anxiety. Its use can be questioned. Chronic Fiorinal use leads to butalbital accumulat'n and CNS depress'n.	As for narcotics (see Table 76), barbitu-rates (see Chapter 46) and aspirin, above	As for narcotics (see Table 76), barbiturates (see Chapter 46) and aspirin, above	As for narcotics (see Table 76), barbitu-rates (see Chapter 46) and aspirin, above

CHAPTER 55

Antimigraine Drugs

Migraine

Migraine headaches are associated with a dilatation of the arteries of the scalp and face. However, although migraine attacks are characterized by an abnormal reactivity of blood vessels to stimuli, vasodilatation alone cannot entirely explain the pain. Exercise and heat exposure will dilate scalp arteries without producing pain. Other factors must be involved in migraine headaches.

It is now recognized that migraine headaches are caused by dilatation of the arteries of the scalp, together with the release of 5-hydroxytryptamine (5-HT, serotonin), histamine, bradykinin, substance P and prostaglandins that sensitize pain receptors in the scalp vessel wall and adjoining tissue. Pulsation in scalp arteries, together with sensitization of pain receptors, leads to the pain of migraine.

Migraine headaches may be divided into two major groups —**common migraine** and **classic migraine.** Both groups tend to be severe, characterized by a throbbing, sharp pain that is made worse by movement. Common migraine has a high incidence, reputedly affecting ten to twenty per cent of the population. In common migraine the patient may experience a prodromal period before an attack. The prodromal symptoms involve changes in mood, activity, appetite or fluid balance. The patient may experience depression, lethargy or elation, a craving for unusual food, or the accumulation of edema. These symptoms give way to headache pain as blood vessels in the scalp and face dilate.

Classic migraine is much rarer, occurring about one-tenth as often as common migraine. It is characterized by the presence of an aura, lasting for periods of five to thirty minutes, between the prodromal period and the headache. The aura causes visual disturbances, often characterized by the presence of bright or colored lights, or holes in the visual field. Complex visual disturbances or hemiparesis may occur. The aura is due to pronounced vasoconstriction, with an accompanying cerebral ischemia.

Drugs are used either to prevent attacks (by inhibiting vasodilatation) or to terminate an attack (by producing analgesia or by constricting the already-dilated vessels).

Drugs to Prevent Migraine Attacks

Beta blockers, antidepressants, 5-HT antagonists and calcium channel blockers are used to prevent migraine headaches. The disparity in their mechanisms of action reflects our lack of understanding of the multifactorial etiology of migraine headaches and our willingness to try many types of drugs in an attempt to prevent attacks. In addition, nonsteroidal, anti-inflammatory drugs (NSAIDs) have been used to prevent migraine attacks.

Beta Blockers

Propranolol is the beta blocker most commonly used for migraine prevention. Other beta blockers that have shown antimigraine effectiveness include timolol (Blocadren), atenolol (Tenormin), nadolol (Corgard) and metoprolol (Betaloc, Lopresor, Lopressor). Because propranolol is the only beta blocker officially recommended for migraine prophylaxis in North America, it will be the only agent presented in this chapter. Propranolol reduces the number of moderately severe attacks in more than fifty per cent of cases. Its clinical effectiveness does not differ markedly from that of pizotyline (see below). Like pizotyline, propranolol is often ineffective in patients with severe migraine.

The adverse effects of propranolol, and the related nursing process, are described in Chapters 8, 12 and 14. It is less toxic than methysergide (see below) and warrants a trial before patients are placed on the latter compound. Nurses should warn patients not to stop propranolol abruptly for fear of "backlash headaches". The withdrawal period should extend over two weeks.

Tricyclic Antidepressants

Tricyclic antidepressants can prevent migraine in some patients and may be given concurrently with other prophylactic agents. Amitriptyline (Elavil) has been used most frequently. Its pharmacology and related nursing process are discussed in Chapter 45. The mechanism of amitriptyline's anti-migraine action is not clear. Amitriptyline appears to be an effective prophylactic in approximately fifty-five to sixty per cent of migraine patients.

5-Hydroxytryptamine Antagonists

1. Pizotyline (Sandomigran)

Pizotyline blocks 5-hydroxytryptamine receptors but it is not clear whether this mechanism explains the drug's ability to prevent migraine attacks. Approximately one-third to two-thirds of patients respond to the drug after three to four weeks of treatment. Compared to methysergide (see below), pizotyline has fewer adverse effects. The adverse effects of pizotyline include central nervous system depression which may disappear after a few days of treatment, and an increase in appetite with weight gain. Other adverse effects that occur less frequently included fatigue, nausea, dizziness, headache, confusion, edema, hypotension, depression, weakness, epigastric distress, dry mouth, nervousness, impotence and muscle pain. In normal doses pizotyline has minimal anticholinergic effects. Nevertheless, because of its anticholinergic potential, pizotyline is contraindicated in patients taking monoamine oxidase inhibitors, as well as in patients with pyloroduodenal obstruction or stenosing pyloric ulcers. Other aspects of the nursing process related to the use of pizotyline are similar to those identified for methysergide (see below).

2. Methysergide (Sansert)

Mechanism of Action and Pharmacologic Effects
Methysergide is also a 5-hydroxytryptamine antagonist. It is not clear whether this action explains or is just coincidental to its ability to prevent migraine attacks. If the aura associated with classic migraine is due to a 5-hydroxytryptamine-mediated vasoconstriction, methysergide may prevent attacks by blocking the initial vasoconstrictive phase.

Therapeutic Uses

With a seventy-to-eighty per cent success rate, methysergide is more effective than most other drugs, but also more toxic. Methysergide's adverse effects have limited its use to patients who do not respond to other drugs. The useful effects of methysergide may begin within a few days or may take two to three weeks to occur. The drug is indicated in the prophylactic treatment of severe recurring vascular headaches occurring one or more times weekly, or vascular headaches that are so severe or uncontrollable that preventative therapy is indicated regardless of frequency. Methysergide has proven effective in reducing or eliminating the pain and frequency of attacks of classical migraine, common migraine and cluster headache (histaminic cephalgia).

Adverse Effects

Methysergide may produce retroperitoneal fibrosis, as well as fibrosis in the pleura and heart valves. Because the risk of these adverse effects increases with the length of treatment, methysergide should not be taken continuously for longer than six months. Methysergide should be discontinued for at least one month before beginning treatment again. Other adverse effects of methysergide include nausea, vomiting, heartburn, abdominal discomfort and diarrhea. These occur more frequently than the serious adverse effects described above and can be avoided by giving the drug with food. Methysergide can also produce insomnia. These effects can be minimized by starting treatment with small doses.

Methysergide is contraindicated in a wide range of conditions. These include peripheral vascular disease (because on rare occasions methysergide can produce pronounced vasoconstriction), coronary artery disease, severe arteriosclerosis, moderate to severe hypertension, and valvular heart disease. The drug is also contraindicated in pulmonary or collagen disease, impaired liver or renal function, urinary tract disease, and cachectic or septic states.

Nursing Process

Assessment

Nurses charged with the clinical management of patients receiving methysergide should assess their patients for contraindications to the drug as indicated above. In addition, a description of the physiological aspects of the patient's migraine headache should be documented by the nurse prior to administering the first dose. *Assess for pregnancy, because this drug must not be given for fear of possible harm to the fetus.*

Evaluation

The effectiveness of methysergide is determined by a reduction in the frequency or severity of migraine headaches. Patients must also be evaluated for adverse effects, as identified above.

Administration

Give methysergide at the beginning the headache, and titrate the dose to the response of the patient.

Teaching

Patients should be taught to report indicators of adverse effects; to move slowly from the recumbent position to the sitting or standing position because of the possibility of postural hypotension; and to avoid abrupt withdrawal of the drug because of the danger of rebound headaches. Warn patients to avoid foods containing tyramine or food additives.

Flunarizine (Sibelium)

Mechanism of Action and Pharmacologic Effects

Flunarizine is a calcium channel blocker. Structurally different from other commercially available calcium channel blockers, flunarizine has no direct effects on the heart. Flunarizine selectively blocks the entry of calcium into cells when calcium is stimulated to enter cells in excess, thereby preventing cell damage caused by calcium overload in various tissues. It inhibits the contraction of vascular smooth muscle mediated by the entry of extravascular calcium, and it protects endothelial cells against damage from calcium overload and brain cells from the effects of hypoxia.

It has been postulated that migraine pathogenesis involves an initial decrease in cerebral blood flow leading to ischemia and hypoxia. Hypoxia causes an excessive influx of calcium into cells, resulting in cerebral cellular dysfunction. The fact that calcium plays a role in this process may explain the reason why flunarizine is effective in preventing both classic and common migraine.

Therapeutic Effects

Flunarizine is at least as effective in preventing migraine attacks as the other drugs discussed in this chapter, i.e., beta blockers, antidepressants, pizotyline and methysergide. Furthermore, it is at least as well tolerated as the other drugs, and better tolerated than methysergide. Flunarizine is most beneficial for reducing migraine frequency. It appears to have less effect on the severity and duration of attacks.

Adverse Effects

Flunarizine is usually well tolerated. Its adverse effects include drowsiness, weight gain, headache, insomnia, nausea, gastric pain and dry mouth. The most serious adverse effect reported during clinical trials was depression. Long-term therapy in the elderly has produced extrapyramidal effects. These effects are usually reversible when the drug is stopped. Flunarizine is contraindicated in patients with a history of depression or pre-existing extrapyramidal disorders.

Nursing Process

Because flunarizine appeared on the market as this text was being prepared for press, nursing experience with it is limited. Nurses caring for patients receiving flunarizine should read the latest information provided by the manufacturer and discuss the drug with the pharmacist.

Nonsteroidal Anti-inflammatory Drugs (NSAIDs)

The pharmacology of NSAIDs, together with their associated nursing process, is presented in Chapter 57. These drugs are effective in both terminating attacks (see below) and preventing attacks. In one trial, naproxen (Naprosyn) was found effective in preventing attacks in fifty-one per cent of patients, compared to nineteen per cent for placebo therapy.

Drugs to Treat Migraine Attacks

Analgesics

Analgesics, such as aspirin with codeine, may relieve migraine pain. They are best taken early in the attack before the pain has had an opportunity to become established. Narcotics stronger than codeine are not recommended because of the danger of dependence. Nonsteroidal anti-inflammatory drugs can be quite effective in the treatment of migraine attacks. Naproxen (Naprosyn; 825 mg at the onset and 275 mg 30 min later, p.r.n.) has been shown to be as effective as ergotamine (2 mg at the onset, with 1 mg 30 min later p.r.n.) in relieving the pain of migraine attacks, and more effective in relieving nausea and motor symptoms.

There has been a tendency to couple analgesic use with the administration of barbiturates. The products Fiorinal, which contains aspirin and a barbiturate, or Fiorinal-C, which also contains codeine, are popular. There is little evidence to support the contention that barbiturates increase the analgesic effects of these products. Nurses should be aware of the danger of dependence if they are used chronically. The patient's consumption of the medication should be monitored closely.

Ergotamine (Ergomar, Ergostat, Gynergen, Medihaler-Ergotamine)

Mechanism of Action and Pharmacologic Effects

Ergotamine is a vasoconstrictor that reduces migraine-induced vasodilatation. The drug should not be used in patients with pre-existing vascular disease, such as atherosclerosis, hypertension, Raynaud's phenomenon and Buerger's disease, because its vasoconstrictor properties can lead to ischemia.

Therapeutic Uses

Ergotamine is an effective drug to abort a migraine attack. It should be taken as soon as the patient feels an attack starting. Ergotamine is poorly absorbed if taken orally or sublingually. Rectal absorption may be better and suppositories can be used in patients who fail to absorb adequate amounts of oral or sublingual ergotamine. Suppositories are also used in the nauseated or vomiting patient.

Ergotamine can be given by inhalation from a pressurized nebulizer. Administered this way, ergotamine may be rapidly and completely absorbed. This route of administration is useful to treat patients whose severe headaches occur without warning. However, many patients have difficulty mastering the technique of inhaling the drug. In addition, the opportunity to administer an overdose is great. One can sympathize with the patient who feels that if one puff is good, two will be better. However, this philosophy can lead to ergotamine toxicity because larger than recommended amounts of the drug may be taken.

Ergotamine, or its analogue dihydroergotamine, may be given by injection. This is a procedure used only in Emergency departments of hospitals or physicians' offices. It is the most effective means to terminate an attack, but caution should be taken to ensure that an overdose is not given.

Caffeine is often incorporated into ergotamine tablets and suppositories (Cafergot and Cafergot-PB) on the belief that it increases ergotamine absorption. Antinauseant drugs are also combined with ergotamine (Megral, Migral) to reduce nausea and vomiting. There seems little rationale for the incorporation of either barbiturates (Cafergot-PB) or anticholinergics (Cafergot, Bellergal, Wigraine) into ergotamine-containing products.

Adverse Effects

Ergotamine's major adverse effects are generalized vasoconstriction and stimulation of the vomiting center in the brain. Patients may experience nausea and vomiting, weakness in the legs, muscle pains in the extremities, numbness and tingling of fingers and toes, precordial distress and pain, and transient tachycardia or bradycardia.

Ergotamine is metabolized in the liver and also eliminated unchanged by the kidneys. It is contraindicated in patients with hepatic or renal disease because it may accumulate to toxic levels. Ergotamine is also contraindicated in the presence of sepsis, occlusive vascular tissues, hypertension, peptic ulcer, infectious states, malnutrition, severe pruritus, pregnancy or lactation.

Nursing Process
Assessment
Nurses should review the patient's history for evidence of contraindications. These have been listed above and include cardiovascular, hepatic or renal disorders, and pregnancy.

Administration
Ergotamine may be taken orally, sublingually, rectally and by inhalation. Nurses should be aware that ergotamine is not well absorbed, regardless of the route of administration. The variability in individual-to-individual response can be explained, in part, by the ability of some patients to absorb the drug better than others, making it necessary to titrate the dose to patient response. Most patients prefer to take a drug orally. However, this may be difficult if nausea and vomiting accompany the attack. This problem is compounded further by the fact that ergotamine itself can cause vomiting by stimulating the vomiting center in the brain.

Although sublingual administration may assist nauseated patients, this route may still cause emesis because absorbed ergotamine stimulates the vomiting center.

Rectal ergotamine administration has long been important in the treatment of migraine headaches. Administered to nauseated and vomiting patients, rectal ergotamine may provide sufficient drug to terminate an attack.

Although ergotamine administered by inhalation may often afford rapid relief, many patients have difficulty mastering the technique of drug administration (as discussed, above).

Evaluation
Nurses caring for patients taking this drug should request information from the patient with regard to his perceptions of relief or reduced intensity of migraine attacks. Nurses should be alert for patients' reports of coldness, numbness or tingling of the extremities.

Teaching
Nurses should instruct patients to report coldness, numbness or tingling of the extremities to their physician at once. Nurses should also be aware that patients may feel they need ergotamine on a daily basis, claiming that stopping the drug for even one day precipitates a migraine attack. These patients should be taught that these headaches, although vascular in nature, are not migraines. If a patient takes ergotamine constantly the blood vessels are maintained in a state of constriction. Upon discontinuing the drug, the vessels may overdilate and produce the headache. If the patient remains off ergotamine for a period of time, the blood vessels will return to normal diameters and the headaches will subside. If patients will not wait for this to occur and resume ergotamine treatment, it may be necessary to hospitalize them while gradually reducing the dose of ergotamine. During this time it may be necessary to treat patients with analgesics and sedatives. Alert patients to avoid over-the-counter drugs, food containing tyramine and food additives while taking ergotamine.

Further Reading
Andersson, K.E. and Vinge, E. (1990). ß-Adrenoreceptor blockers and calcium antagonists in the prophylaxis and treatment of migraine. *Drugs 39* :355-373.

Diamond, S. and Solomon, G.D. (1988). Pharmacologic treatment of migraine. *Rational Drug Therapy 22* (10):1-5.

Drugs for migraine (1989). Drugs of choice. *The Medical Letter 31* :95-98.

Drugs for migraine (1984). *The Medical Letter 26* :95-96.

Peatfield, R. (1983). Migraine: Current concepts of pathogenesis and treatment. *Drugs 26* :364-371.

Table 78
Antimigraine drugs.

Generic Name (Trade Name)	Use (Dose)	Action	Adverse Effects	Drug Interactions	Nursing Process
Pharmacologic Classification: Beta Blocker to Prevent Migraine Attacks					
Propranolol (Inderal)	Prophylaxis of migraine headaches (**Oral:** Initially, 40 mg bid; incr. gradually prn [range, 80-160 mg/day])	Blocks beta$_1$ and beta$_2$ receptors in body. Block of latter may acc't for reduced dilatat'n of arteries in scalp. Reduces no. of moderately severe attacks in > 50% of pts.	Bronchoconstrict'n in asthmatics; potentiates effect of insulin; asystole, A-V block, bradycardia, heart failure; nausea, vomiting, constipat'n, diarrhea; depress'n, sleep disturbances; allergies	Refer to Table 8	Refer to Chapters 8, 12 and 14; Tables 8, 13 and 15.
Pharmacologic Classification: Tricyclic Antidepressant to Prevent Migraine Attacks					
Amitriptyline (Elavil)	Prophylaxis of migraine headaches (**Oral:** Initially, 25 mg hs; incr. prn by 25 mg q1-2 weeks to 100-200 mg/day prn)	Tricyclic antidepressant. Mechanism of antimigraine action unknown. Appears effective in 55-60% of pts.	Flushing, diaphoresis, dryness of mouth, blurred vision, constipat'n, tachycardia, hypotens'n, sedat'n. For addit'nal effects, refer to Table 67.	Refer to Table 67.	Refer to Chapter 45 and Table 67.
Pharmacologic Classification: 5-Hydroxytryptamine Antagonists to Prevent Migraine Attacks					
Pizotyline hydrogen maleate (Sandomigran)	Prophylaxis of migraine headaches (**Oral:** Initially, 0.5 mg hs; incr. gradually to 0.5 mg tid. Range, 1-6 mg/day)	Blocks 5-HT receptors; this may reduce dilatat'n of scalp arteries. About 75% of pts respond after 3-4 weeks' tx.	Incr. appetite, weight gain, CNS depress'n, nausea, dizziness, headache, weakness, dry mouth	**CNS depressants** (incl. antihistamines, ethanol, hypnotics, sedatives and psychotherapeutic agents): May potentiate CNS-depressant effects of pizotyline.	**Assess:** For pt hx of peripheral vascular disease, coronary artery disease, arteriosclerosis, hypertens'n, valvular disease. Check for pregnancy. Provide thorough descript'n of migraine. Establish baseline weight. **Administer:** At beginning of headache; w. meals; titrate dose to pt response. Give from airtight, light-resistant container. **Evaluate:** For tx effectiveness; for evidence adv. effects. **Teach:** To report indicators of adv.
Methysergide maleate (Sansert)	Prophylactic tx of severe vascular headaches 1-2x weekly; vasc. headaches so severe or uncontrollable that preventive tx is indicated regardless of frequency (**Oral:** 2 mg hs; incr.	5-HT antagonist. This may reduce dilatat'n of scalp arteries. Most effective prophylactic, but also most toxic.	Retroperitoneal fibrosis, fibrotic complicat'ns of pleural pulmonary tract, fibrotic thickening of aortic route and of		

effects; to move from recumbent to upright posit'n slowly; to avoid abrupt drug w'drawal. Warn pts to avoid foods containing tyramine or food additives.

Nurses caring for pts receiving flunarizine should read latest informat'n provided by manufacturer and discuss drug w. pharmacist.

Assess: For pt hx vascular disease, hepatic/renal disease, evidence of current pregnancy or infect'n. **Administer:** At beginning of headache; titrate dose to pt response. If GI symptoms occur, give w. meals. **Teach:** Proper dosage; to report coldness, numbness or tingling of extremities. Warn pts to avoid OTC drugs and foods containing tyramine or food additives.

Anticonvulsants: May reduce steady-state serum levels of flunarizine. This effect, seen when flunarizine is coadministered w. 2 or more anticonvulsants, is considered a result of enhanced 1st-pass metabolism of flunarizine as a consequence of liver enzyme induct'n by anticonvulsant medicat'ns.

Alpha-adrenergics: Plus ergotamine, may cause hypertens'n.
Dopamine: And ergotamine should not be given tog. because concomitant use of these 2 vasoconstrictors may result in excess. vasoconstrict'n.
Erythromycin: Used concomitantly w. ergotamine, may lead to elevated plasma concentrat'n of ergotamine, thereby causing

aortic/mitral valves; nausea, vomiting, heartburn, abd. discomfort, diarrhea; insomnia, excess. dreaming; weight gain; neutropenia, eosinophilia; weakness, arthralgia, myalgia; alopecia

Us. well tolerated. Adv. effects incl. drowsiness, weight gain, headache, insomnia, nausea, gastric pain, dry mouth. Most serious adv. effect is depress'n. Long-term tx in elderly may produce extrapyramidal effects. Contraindicated in pts w. hx depress'n or pre-existing extrapyramidal disorders.

Nausea, vomiting; pain and weakness in extremities; numbness and tingling of fingers, toes; precordial distress and pain; transient tachycardia or bradycardia

Selectivity blocks entry of Ca$^+$ into cells when Ca$^+$ is stimulated to enter in excess, thereby preventing Ca$^+$ overload in various tissues. Inhibits contract'n of vascular smooth muscle and protects endothelial cells against damage from Ca$^+$ overload and brain cells from effects of hypoxia. For more complete explanat'n, see Chapter 55.

Vasoconstrictor; reduces migraine-induced vasodilatat'n. Contraindicated in sepsis, occlusive vascular disease, impaired renal/hepatic function, severe hypertens'n, angina pectoris, infectious states, malnutrit'n, severe pruritus,

gradually to 2 mg tid w. meals. There must be medicat'n-free interval of 3-4 weeks after every 6-month course of tx)

Pharmacologic Classification: Calcium Channel Blocker to Prevent Migraine Attacks

Flunarizine (Sibelium)

To prevent both classic and common migraine in adults and children (**Oral:** Adults - 10 mg/day, given hs. Pts who experience side effects may be maintained on 5 mg hs)

Pharmacologic Classification: Drugs to Terminate Migraine Attack — Ergotamine-Containing Products

Ergotamine tartrate (Ergomar, Ergostat, Gynergen)

Tx to abort migraine and similar vascular attacks (**Oral:** Adults - 2 mg at 1st sign of attack and 1 mg q30min prn to max. 6 mg/day [10 mg/week]. **Sublingual:** Adults - 2 mg at 1st sign of attack and 2 mg q30min prn [max., 6 mg/day; 10 mg/week]. **Inhalat'n:** Adults - 1 inhalat'n [0.36 mg] at 1st sign of attack; repeat in 5 min prn. Any addit'nal inhalat'ns

Generic Name (Trade Name)	Use (Dose)	Action	Adverse Effects	Drug Interactions	Nursing Process
	should be spaced at intervals not < 5 min. Max., 6 inhalat'ns/24 h. Do not use > 5 consecutive days/7-day period)	pregnancy/lactat'n, hypersensitivity to ergotamine.		untoward peripheral vasocon-strict'n.	
Dihydroergotamine mesylate	As for ergotamine (**IM:** *Acute migraine attack* - 1 mg at 1st warning sign, repeated at 30-60 min intervals prn, to total of 3 mg/attack. **IV:** *Cluster headache [Horton's syndrome]* - 0.5 mg by slow inject'n. Max., 6 mg/week)	As for ergotamine	As for ergotamine	As for ergotamine	*As for ergotamine, w. these added precautions:* Store in dark area; do not use discolored solut'ns. Keep out of reach of children as death may occur.
Ergotamine + caffeine (Cafergot)	As for ergotamine (**Oral:** Adults - 2 tablets initially; then 1 tab q30min prn. Max. dose, 6 tabs/day, 10/week. Children 6-12 years - Initially, 1 tab; addit'nal doses of 1 tab may be given 2x only. Max., 3 tabs/day; 5/week. *Cafergot must not be adminis-tered prophylactically to adults or children*)	As for ergotamine. Caffeine may incr. ergotamine absorpt'n.	As for ergotamine	As for ergotamine	As for ergotamine
Ergotamine + caffeine, belladonna and pentobarbital (Cafergot-PB, Bellergal)	As for ergotamine (**Oral:** *Cafergot-PB Tablets* - As for Cafergot, above. *Bellergal Tablets* - Adults - 3-4 tabs/day; max., 6/day prn. Reduce gradu-ally after some days to lowest effect. dose. Max., 33 tabs/week. *Bellergal Spacetabs* - 1 in a.m. and 1 hs. Max., 16 tabs/week. **Rectal:** *Cafergot-PB Suppositories* - Adults - 1 supp. initially; repeat in 1 h prn. Max., 3 supps./day; 5/week. Children 6-12 years - Initially, 1/2 suppository; additional	As for ergotamine. For belladonna, see Table 4 (Anticholinergics). For pentobarbital, see Chapter 46.	As for ergotamine. For belladonna, see Table 4 (Anticholinergics). For pentobarbital, see Chapter 46.	As for ergotamine. For belladon-na, see Table 4 (Anticholinergics). For pentobarbital, see Chapter 46.	As for ergotamine. For belladonna, see Table 4 (Anticholinergics). For pentobar-bital, see Chapter 46.

Drug				
Ergotamine + caffeine and belladonna (Wigraine)	doses of $1/2$ supp. may be given 2x only prn in course of attack. Max., 1.5 supps./attack or day; or 2.5/week) As for ergotamine (**Oral/Rectal:** 1-2 tablets or suppositories at 1st sign of attack, followed by 1-2 tabs or supps. q20-30min until pain subsides. Max., 6 tabs or supps./attack [12 tabs or supps./week])	As for ergotamine. For belladonna, see Table 4 (Anticholinergics).	As for ergotamine. For belladonna, see Table 4 (Anticholinergics).	As for ergotamine. For belladonna, see Table 4 (Anticholinergics).
Ergotamine + cyclizine HCl (Megral, Migral)	As for ergotamine (**Oral:** Initially, $1/4$-1 tablet at 1st warning of attack; then $1/2$-1 tab q30min. Max., 3 tabs/attack; 6 tabs/week. Children - $1/4$-$1/2$ tab)	As for ergotamine. Cyclizine is an antinauseant to counteract nausea that accompanies migraine attacks and nauseant properties of ergotamine.	As for ergotamine. For cyclizine, an antihistamine, see Table 36 (Antinauseants).	As for ergotamine. For cyclizine, an antihistamine, see Table 36 (Antinauseants).

SECTION 13

Pharmacology of the Musculoskeletal System

Patients are often plagued with problems involving
the musculoskeletal system. These may range from
relatively minor, time-limited strains following
athletic insult to such serious, life-threatening
conditions as multiple sclerosis, spinal cord injuries
and myasthenia gravis. Rheumatoid arthritis,
osteoarthritis and gout are also considered musculoskeletal problems. Although not life-threatening,
these conditions can cause great pain and loss of
mobility. Chapters 56, 57 and 58 discuss the use of
drugs to alleviate the pain and discomfort of
patients afflicted with problems of the musculoskeletal system.

C H A P T E R   5 6

Drugs for the Treatment of Skeletal Muscle Disorders

Teaching Objectives

Following completion of this chapter, the reader should be able to:

1. Describe briefly the cause of spasticity.
2. Discuss the mechanism of action, pharmacologic effects, therapeutic uses and adverse effects of baclofen, as well as the nursing process associated with its use.
3. Discuss the administration of diazepam to treat spasticity, including its mechanism of action, therapeutic use, adverse effects and nursing process.
4. Describe the mechanism of action, pharmacologic effects, therapeutic uses and adverse effects of dantrolene, as well as the nursing process related to its administration.
5. Describe briefly the etiology of spasm.
6. List the central skeletal muscle relaxants available to treat spasm, explain their mechanism of action and adverse effects, and describe the nursing process associated with their use.
7. Discuss briefly the etiology of myasthenia gravis.
8. List the cholinesterase inhibitors available to treat myasthenia gravis, explain their mechanism of action, therapeutic uses and adverse effects, and describe the nursing process related to their administration.
9. Discuss the administration of adrenal corticosteroids to treat myasthenia gravis, including their mechanism of action, therapeutic uses, adverse effects and nursing process.

Spasticity

Spasticity involves a velocity-dependent increase in tonic stretch reflexes that cause hyperactive reflexes, flexor or extensor spasms, and loss of dexterity. The three major drugs used to treat spasticity are baclofen (Lioresal), diazepam (Valium) and dantrolene (Dantrium).

Baclofen (Lioresal)

Mechanism of Action, Pharmacologic Effects and Therapeutic Uses

Baclofen inhibits mono- and polysynaptic pathways in the spinal cord and depresses the tonic stretch reflex. It has no peripheral muscle relaxant activity. Baclofen relieves involuntary flexor and extensor spasms and resistance to passive movements. The drug is indicated to alleviate the signs and symptoms of spasticity resulting from multiple sclerosis. It may also be of some value in the treatment of patients with spinal cord injuries and other spinal cord diseases.

Adverse Effects

Baclofen is well tolerated by many patients. At full therapeutic doses, patients may initially experience drowsiness, dizziness, weakness and fatigue. Nausea, mild gastrointestinal upset, constipation or diarrhea, confusion, hypotension and urinary frequency are other reported adverse effects. Caution must be exercised if the drug is withdrawn. Abrupt withdrawal has, on occasion, led to severe reactions including visual and auditory hallucinations, status epilepticus, dyskinesia and confusion. Therefore, unless there are severe adverse effects, baclofen should be discontinued slowly over a period of one to two weeks.

Nursing Process

Assessment

Nurses should begin the nursing process by reviewing the patient's history. Documentation of renal or hepatic disorders, epilepsy, diabetes mellitus, neurological or psychiatric disorders, or upper gastrointestinal conditions should alert the nurse to the need for particularly rigorous evaluation and monitoring of the patient following baclofen administration.

Physiological assessment should begin with a description of the type, degree and extent of the spasticity. Baseline measures of vital signs and weight should be established for later comparison.

Administration

Baclofen is administered orally with food to reduce gastric distress. The drug should be stored in a tight container at room temperature. Titrate the dose to the individual response of the patient.

Evaluation

Therapeutic effectiveness is determined by decreased frequency of spasms, reduced severity in knee and ankle clonus, and greater range of motion. Patients' daily self-care activities should improve.

Nurses must evaluate patients receiving baclofen for early evidence of adverse effects. Specifically, these include: central nervous system effects (ataxia, drowsiness, dizziness, confusion, depression, hallucinations), cardiovascular changes (hypotension, edema accompanied by weight gain), and ocular alterations (blurred vision, diplopia, nystagmus).

Nurses caring for diabetic patients receiving baclofen should be alert for elevation of blood glucose levels as indicated by changes in urine and blood tests. These should be drawn to the attention of the physician.

Nurses should anticipate that the physician will order regular electroencephalograms for epileptic patients receiving baclofen because of its tendency to inhibit seizure control in these patients.

Teaching

Patients should be taught to seek assistance with ambulation until their individual responses to the medication are established. They should also be informed that full therapeutic benefits are often not experienced for several weeks. Caution patients taking baclofen to avoid driving and using power tools or heavy machinery until individual responses are established because of the risk of dizziness and drowsiness. Warn patients to abstain from using alcohol while taking baclofen. Taken concomitantly, the two drugs produce additive central nervous system depression. For the same reason, caution patients not to take over-the-counter medications without consulting the physician or pharmacist concerning possible drug interactions.

Patients and their families should be thoroughly briefed about the anticipated benefits and adverse effects of baclofen. A printed instruction sheet will help them remember the information and contribute to drug compliance.

Diazepam (Valium)

Mechanism of Action, Pharmacologic Effects and Therapeutic Uses

Diazepam is a polysynaptic inhibitor in the brain stem and spinal cord. The drug also has secondary sedative effects. Diazepam assists patients with spasticity associated with spinal cord lesions, multiple sclerosis and other central nervous system lesions. It is also used adjunctively in acute, localized, severe traumatic disorders associated with painful muscle spasms.

Adverse Effects

The adverse effects of diazepam are presented in Chapter 46. The dose of the drug that relieves spasticity usually produces sedation and some incoordination.

Nursing Process

The nursing process associated with the prescription and use of diazepam is discussed in Chapter 46. Readers should refer to that chapter for detailed information.

Dantrolene Sodium (Dantrium)

Mechanism of Action, Pharmacologic Effects and Therapeutic Uses

Dantrolene inhibits muscle contraction by acting directly on skeletal muscles to suppress calcium release from the sarcoplasmic reticulum. It is valuable in the treatment of spasticity induced by spinal cord injury, cerebral palsy, multiple sclerosis and stroke, whenever such spasticity results in a decrease in the functional use of residual motor activity. The drug not indicated in the relief of skeletal muscle spasms due to rheumatic disorders.

Adverse Effects

The most common adverse effects of dantrolene are muscle weakness, drowsiness, diarrhea, malaise and fatigue. Anorexia, nausea, vomiting, along with an acne-like rash, are also caused by dantrolene. Dizziness, headache, nervousness, insomnia and depression may also be produced by the drug.

Dantrolene has a potential for hepatotoxicity and should not be used in conditions other than those recommended here. Idiosyncratic or hypersensitivity-mediated hepatocellular injury (which occurs rarely, but has been fatal) is the most serious adverse reaction. The risk appears to be greatest in patients over age thirty-five and in women, especially those receiving estrogen therapy. Hepatotoxicity occurs most frequently between three and twelve months after starting therapy. Therefore, routine baseline hepatic function studies should be performed prior to therapy, and alanine transaminase (ALT) or aspartate transaminase (AST) and alkaline phosphatase (AP) levels should be determined at appropriate intervals during therapy. The lowest effective dose (preferably no more than 400 mg daily) should be prescribed. Therapy should be continued for more than sixty days only if symptoms are relieved and there is no evidence of hepatic injury. Dantrolene is contraindicated in patients with active hepatic disease.

Nursing Process

Assessment

Prior to administering the first dose of dantrolene, review the patient's history for evidence of active hepatic, cardiac or pulmonary disease. In their presence, withhold the drug pending consultation with the physician. Identification of pregnancy should also result in the medication being withheld. Physical assessment should emphasize documentation of the patient's gait, range of motion, coordination, reflexes, muscle strength and tone, and posture, as well as baseline measures of vital signs.

Administration

If patients are unable to swallow the capsules, they can be opened and mixed with liquid. Multiple-dose suspensions can be prepared by a pharmacist. Suspensions should be stored in a refrigerator, shaken well to ensure even distribution, and used within the time specified by the pharmacist.

Evaluation

Therapeutic effectiveness is determined by lessening of spasticity. Vital signs should be monitored for evidence of adverse cardiac or pulmonary effects. Jaundice, tea-colored urine, clay-colored stools and pruritus are early clinical assessments indicating hepatotoxicity. Nurses should assess patients for central nervous system depression, dizziness, drowsiness and psychiatric symptoms.

Teaching

Patients should be taught to seek assistance with ambulation until their individual responses to dantrolene are established. They should also be informed that dantrolene's full therapeutic benefits are often not experienced for several weeks. Caution patients taking dantrolene to avoid driving and using power tools or heavy machinery until individual responses are established because of the risk of dizziness and drowsiness. Patients should be alerted to the potential for photosensitivity. For this reason they should use a sunscreen and wear a hat when outdoors. Dantrolene should not be discontinued quickly. Nurses should caution patients not to take the drug with alcohol or other CNS depressants, and to avoid over-the-counter medications.

Spasm

Spasm involves the involuntary contraction of a muscle or groups of muscles, usually accompanied by pain and limited function. Reflex spasm may be a protective mechanism in response to injury of a local nature. Most muscle strains and minor injuries respond rapidly to rest and physical therapy. Some, however, appear to benefit from additional use of a central skeletal muscle relaxant.

Central Skeletal Muscle Relaxants: Carisoprodol (Rela, Soma), Chlorzoxazone (Paraflex), Cyclobenzaprine (Flexeril), Methocarbamol (Delaxin, Robaxin), Orphenadrine (Disipal, Norflex)

Mechanism of Action, Pharmacologic Effects and Therapeutic Uses

Central muscle relaxant drugs sedate patients and depress the facilitative and inhibitory neuronal activity affecting muscle stretch reflexes, primarily in the lateral reticular area of the brain stem. Most of them have been shown to be more effective than a placebo in treating localized muscle spasms. None has been demonstrated to be more effective than analgesic, anti-inflammatory drugs in relieving the pain of acute or chronic localized muscle spasm. There seems little reason to select one drug over the others. All are approximately equally effective and have similar adverse effects. Some are combined with analgesics. These include methocarbamol with aspirin (Robaxisal), chlorzoxazone plus acetaminophen (Parafon Forte), acetaminophen plus codeine (Parafon C8) and orphenadrine with aspirin and caffeine (Norgesic, Norgesic Forte). The FDA has classified these combinations as possibly effective. Central skeletal muscle relaxants are not recommended for the treatment of spastic disorders induced by cerebrospinal trauma, cerebral palsy or demyelinating disorders.

Adverse Effects

All central skeletal muscle relaxants produce drowsiness, light-headedness and dizziness. Central nervous system depression is particularly pronounced for cyclobenzaprine, a drug that also causes dryness of the mouth.

Nursing Process

Evaluation of therapeutic effectiveness of these drugs is determined by reduction in spasm and relief of pain. Central skeletal muscle relaxants are used for relatively short term-treatment (two to three weeks) of muscle spasm. Patient teaching should emphasize use of these drugs for only the minimum amount of time necessary because of the risks associated with prolonged use. Patients should be cautioned against driving and using power equipment or heavy machinery because of the possibility of dizziness or drowsiness associated with the use of these drugs. The central nervous system depressive effects of these drugs are increased when alcohol is consumed concurrently. Therefore, warn patients to abstain from using alcohol while taking any of these medications.

Myasthenia Gravis

Myasthenia gravis is an autoimmune disorder, caused by a deficiency of skeletal muscle cholinergic (nicotinic) receptors as a result of antireceptor antibodies. Patients experience impaired neuromuscular transmission and demonstrate rapid fatigability of skeletal muscles. Not all muscle fibers are equally involved, some being in a borderline condition and quickly paralyzed by activity, while others remain above threshold for some time. Myasthenic patients may be treated with reversible cholinesterase inhibitors and/or adrenal corticosteroids.

Cholinesterase Inhibitors: Pyridostigmine Bromide (Mestinon, Regonol), Neostigmine Bromide (Prostigmin), Ambenonium Chloride (Mytelase), Edrophonium Chloride (Tensilon)

Mechanism of Action and Pharmacologic Effects

By inhibiting acetylcholinesterase, these drugs prolong the survival of acetylcholine, permitting not only more receptor interactions but also a cooperative effect of several acetylcholine molecules on one receptor site. Unfortunately, cholinesterase inhibitors affect all cholinergic nerves, resulting in an increase in both nicotinic and muscarinic effects. Nurses wishing to review the consequences of a generalized cholinergic stimulation are referred to Chapter 5 in this book.

Therapeutic Uses

The primary indication for anticholinesterase therapy alone is to treat mild myasthenia, such as ocular myasthenia or mild residual involvement following thymectomy. More often, they are used with corticosteroids to treat patients with moderate to severe disease. Although anticholinesterase drugs improve many patients, muscle strength remains below normal in others. Pyridostigmine is usually the drug of choice because it produces fewer adverse effects than either neostigmine or ambenonium. Edrophonium has a more rapid onset and shorter duration of action. It is used exclusively for the diagnosis of myasthenia gravis.

Anticholinesterase drugs are contraindicated in patients with mechanical obstruction of the intestinal or urinary tracts and should be used with caution in individuals with bronchial asthma.

Adverse Effects

Excessive cholinergic stimulation accounts for the majority of adverse effects. Muscarinic stimulation produces abdominal cramps, nausea, vomiting, diarrhea, hypersalivation, increased bronchial secretion, lacrimation, miosis and diaphoresis. Although these effects can be counteracted by atropine, neither this drug nor any other anticholinergic should be routinely incorporated into the patient's therapeutic regimen. Masking the signs of increased muscarinic stimulation may lead to cholinergic crisis (see below). The effects of nicotinic stimulation include muscle cramps, fasciculations and weakness.

A cholinergic crisis may be difficult to differentiate from a myasthenic crisis. Both present with muscle weakness, the former as a result of an excessive accumulation of acetylcholine leading to a depolarizing skeletal muscle block, the latter because of the inability of acetylcholine to stimulate sufficient nicotinic receptors. Edrophonium may be used to differentiate between the two, but only after patients have first been intubated and controlled ventilation has been instituted. One to two milligrams of edrophonium given intravenously may improve strength in the patient with a myasthenic crisis but aggravate weakness in a cholinergic crisis.

Nursing Process

The nursing process associated with the prescription and use of anticholinesterases is discussed in Chapter 5. Readers should refer to that material for detailed information.

Adrenal Corticosteroids

Mechanism of Action and Therapeutic Uses

The pharmacology of adrenal corticosteroids is presented in detail in Chapter 29. Nurses wishing to review the effects of these drugs on the body are encouraged to read that chapter. With respect to the treatment of myasthenia gravis, adrenal corticosteroids suppress antireceptor antibody formation. They are used in patients not adequately managed with anticholinesterase therapy alone. The indications for corticosteroids also include older adults (usually over age forty) with moderate to severe involvement, whether or not they have undergone thymectomy. Corticosteroids should also possibly be used for an interim period following thymectomy because of the delayed response often associated with this procedure. Other indications for the use of corticosteroids include the possible preparation of patients for thymectomy and the treatment of patients who refuse to undergo, or fail to respond to, thymectomy. They can also be administered as maintenance therapy after surgical removal of an invasive thymoma.

Prednisone is the most frequently used corticosteroid. When given in a high-dose, alternate-day dose regimen, it usually improves muscular strength with reduced adverse effects. Treatment may be required indefinitely. Anticholinesterase therapy should be continued during the initial months of steroid treatment. Later, as the patient improves on corticosteroid treatment, the need for anticholinesterase therapy may decrease.

Adverse Effects

The adverse effects of corticosteroids are presented in Chapter 29 and Tables 45 and 46.

Nursing Process

The nursing process associated with the prescription and use of corticosteroids is discussed in Chapter 29. Readers should refer to that material for detailed information.

Further Reading

Drugs used to treat skeletal muscle disorders (1986). *AMA Drug Evaluations,* 6th ed., pp. 221-237.

Gyory, A.N. (1980). The rational use of muscle relaxants in rehabilitation medicine. *Drugs 20* :309-318.

Havard, C.W.H. and Fonseca, V. (1990). New treatment approaches to myasthenia gravis. *Drugs 39* : 66-73.

Hofmann, W.W. (1979). The treatment of myasthenia gravis. *Rational Drug Therapy 13* (2).

Table 79
Drugs for the treatment of skeletal muscle disorders.

Generic Name (Trade Name)	Use (Dose)	Action	Adverse Effects	Drug Interactions	Nursing Process
Pharmacologic Classification: Antispastic Drugs					
Baclofen (Lioresal)	Alleviat'n of s/s spasticity resulting from MS. May also be valuable in pts w. spinal cord injuries and diseases (**Oral:** 5 mg tid for 3 days; then 10 mg tid for 3 days; then 15 mg tid for 3 days; followed by 20 mg tid for 3 days. Thereafter, addit'nal incr. may be nec., but total daily dose should not > 80 mg [20 mg qid])	Inhibits mono- and polysynaptic pathways in spinal cord; depresses tonic stretch reflex. Relieves involuntary flexor and extensor spasms and resistance to passive movements.	Transient drowsiness, dizziness, weakness, fatigue, headache, insomnia, hypotens'n, nausea, constipat'n, urinary frequency	**Alcohol or other CNS depressants:** May have additive CNS-depressant effects w. baclofen.	**Assess:** Review hx for renal/hepatic disorders, epilepsy, diabetes mellitus, neurological or psych. disorders, or upper GI condit'ns; type, degree and extent of spasticity; VS and weight. **Administer:** Orally, w. food to reduce gastric distress. Titrate dose to indiv. response. **Evaluate:** Effectiveness; adv. effects incl. CNS, CV (hypotens'n, edema, weight gain), ocular (blurred vision, diplopia, nystagmus). Diabetics for incr. blood glucose; anticipate EEG orders for epileptics. **Teach:** To seek help walking until response established; that full effects often not seen for several weeks; to avoid driving or using power tools/machinery until effect established; not to take alcohol or OTC drugs without asking physician or pharmacist; benefits and adv. effects.
Diazepam (Valium)	For condit'ns as follows (*Adjunctively, for relief of skeletal muscle spasms* - **Oral:** 2-10 mg tid-qid. *For muscle spasm assoc. w. cerebral palsy, athetosis, stiff-man syndrome, or adjunctively in tetanus* - **IV/IM:** Initially, 5-10 mg; then 5-10 mg in 3-4 h prn. For tetanus, larger doses may be required)	Polysynaptic inhibitor in brain stem and spinal cord. Secondary effects from its sedative action.	Drowsiness, ataxia, fatigue, dizziness, nausea, blurred vision, diplopia, vertigo, headache, slurred speech, tremors, hypoactivity, dysarthria, euphoria, impairment of memory, confus'n, depress'n. For addit'nal adv. effects, see Table 69.	For Drug Interact'ns involving CNS depressants, ethanol, levodopa and MAOIs, see Table 69.	See Table 69.

Generic Name (Trade Name)	Use (Dose)	Action	Adverse Effects	Drug Interactions	Nursing Process
Dantrolene sodium (Dantrium Oral)	To control manifestat'ns of chronic spasticity of skeletal muscle resulting from spinal cord injury, cerebral palsy, MS, stroke, etc. (**Oral: Adults -** Initially, 25 mg od; incr. to 25 mg bid-qid and then by increments of 25-100 mg bid-qid prn. As most pts will respond to doses ≤ 400 mg/day, higher doses should be given only rarely. **Children -** Initially, 0.5 mg/kg bid; incr. to 0.5 mg/kg tid-qid and then by increments of 0.5 mg/kg up to 3.0 mg/kg bid-qid prn. Maintain dose level for 4-7 days depending on pt's tolerance; incr. only if tx goal has not been attained. Do not use doses > 100 mg qid in children)	Inhibits muscle contract'n by suppressing Ca^+ release from sarcoplasmic reticulum.	Most common are muscle weakness, drowsiness, diarrhea, anorexia, nausea, vomiting, acne-like rash, dizziness, headache, nervousness, insomnia, depress'n.	**CNS depressants:** May interact w. dantrolene. Although primary pharmacologic effect of dantrolene is exerted directly on skeletal muscle, an apparent transient CNS effect also may exist. Therefore, caution should be exercised in using dantrolene tog. w. tranquilizing agents or other CNS depressants. **Estrogens:** May interact w. dantrolene to incr. risk of liver damage.	**Assess:** Review hx for active hepatic, cardiac or pulmonary disease; pregnancy; pt's gait, ROM, coordinat'n, reflexes, muscle strength/tone, posture. Establish baseline VS. **Administer:** Orally; if unable to swallow, open capsules and mix w. liquid. Shake suspens'ns well; store in fridge and use in time specified. **Evaluate:** Tx effectiveness; adv. cardiac/pulmonary effects; for hepatotoxicity (jaundice, tea-colored urine, clay-colored stools, pruritus). Assess for CNS depress'n, dizziness, psych. symptoms. **Teach:** To seek help walking until response established; that full benefits often not experienced for several weeks; caution to avoid driving, using power tools/machinery until response established; potential for photosensitivity. Do not discontinue drug abruptly. Caution not to take w. alcohol or other CNS depressants, and to avoid OTC drugs.

Pharmacologic Classification: Antispasm Drugs — Central Muscle Relaxants

Generic Name (Trade Name)	Use (Dose)	Action	Adverse Effects	Drug Interactions	Nursing Process
Carisoprodol (Rela, Soma)	Tx of localized muscle spasm (**Oral: Adults -** 350 mg tid and hs. Use not recomm. in pts < age 12)	These drugs sedate pts and depress facilitative and inhibitory neuronal activity affecting muscle stretch reflexes, primarily in laterial reticular areas of brain stem.	Drowsiness, light-headedness, dizziness, mild nausea	**CNS depressants:** May have additive CNS-depressant effects w. skeletal muscle relaxants. **MAOIs:** May interact w. cyclobenzaprine, which is sim. in structure to tricyclic antidepressants. Hyperpyretic crises, severe convuls'ns and death have occurred in pts receiving tricyclic antidepressants and MAOIs.	**Evaluate:** Tx effectiveness (reduct'n in spasm, relief of pain). **Teach:** To use for only minimum am't of time nec.; to avoid driving, using power equipment/heavy machinery; to abstain from alcohol.
Chlorzoxazone (Paraflex)	As for carisoprodol (**Oral: Adults -** 500 mg qid)		As for carisoprodol	As for carisoprodol	
Cyclobenzaprine HCl (Flexeril)	As for carisoprodol (**Oral: Adults -** 10 mg tid, w. range of 20-40 mg/day in divided doses. Dosage should not be > 60 mg/day)		As for carisoprodol		As for carisoprodol

Drug	Dosage	Action/Use	Adverse Effects	Drug Interactions
Methocarbamol (Delaxin, Robaxin)	As for carisoprodol (**Oral:** Adults - 6 g/day for 1st 48-72 h of acute skeletal muscle spasm. Severe condit'ns, 8 g/day. Thereafter, reduce to 4 g/day)	As for carisoprodol	As for carisoprodol	As for carisoprodol
Orphenadrine (Disipal, Norflex)	As for carisoprodol (**Oral:** Adults - 100 mg bid)	As for carisoprodol	As for carisoprodol	As for carisoprodol

Pharmacologic Classification: Antimyasthenic Drugs — 1. Adrenal Cortical Steroid

Drug	Dosage	Action/Use	Adverse Effects	Drug Interactions
Prednisone	Tx of myasthenia gravis (**Oral:** Initially, 25 mg/day for 2 days; incr. by 5 mg q2days until optimum response occurs. Us. dose, 50-60 mg/day. To begin alternate-day program, add 10 mg to 1st day's dose [60 mg] and subtract 10 mg from 2nd day's dose [40 mg] each week until improvement reaches plateau or until 100 mg is given qod. Reduce dosage if poss. gradually over many months to establish minimum maint. alternate-day dose)	Adrenal corticosteroid; suppresses antibody format'n, thereby reducing product'n of cholinergic nicotinic antireceptor antibodies. Used in pts not adequately managed w. anticholinesterase tx alone and in place of cholinesterase inhibitors when 1 drug alone will suffice)	Na^+ and H_2O retent'n; hypokalemic alkalosis, hyperlipidemia, redistribut'n of fat, myopathy, osteoporosis, growth failure, psych. disorders, impaired wound healing, pituitary-adrenal suppress'n, incr. susceptibility to infect'ns. For addit'nal adv. effects, see Table 46.	For Drug Interact'ns involving amphotericin B, oral anticoagulants, antidiabetic agents, barbiturates, oral contraceptives, diuretics, indomethacin, phenytoin, rifampin and salicylates, see Table 46.

See Table 46.

Pharmacologic Classification: Antimyasthenic Drugs — 2. Reversible Cholinesterase Inhibitors

Drug	Dosage	Action/Use	Adverse Effects	Drug Interactions
Pyridostigmine bromide (Mestinon, Regonol)	Tx of myasthenia gravis (**Oral:** Adults - 60-180 mg bid-qid; more prn in severe cases. Children - 7 mg/kg/day in divided doses. For exacerbat'n of myasthenia gravis or when oral dosage is not practical - Adults - **IV:** Approx. $1/_{30}$th oral dose. For newborn infants of myasthenic mothers - 0.05-0.15 mg/kg)	By inhibiting acetyl cholinesterase, cholinesterase inhibitors prolong survival of acetylcholine, permitting not only more receptor interact'ns but also a cooperative effect of several acetylcholine molecules on 1 receptor site. Unfortunately, choline-sterase inhibitors affect all cholinergic nerves, resulting in an incr. in both nicotinic and muscarinic effects.	Nausea, vomiting, diarrhea, abd. cramps, incr. peristalsis, incr. salivat'n, incr. bronchial secret'ns, miosis, diaphoresis, bradycardia, hypotens'n, muscle cramps, fasciculat'n, weakness	**Drugs that depress neuromuscular transmiss'n** (aminoglycosides, tetracyclines, antiarrhythmic drugs [procainamide, quinidine, propranolol], chlorpromazine, lithium, phenytoin, thyroid hormones and methoxyflurane): Are known to aggravate or unmask myasthenia gravis. These drugs should be used w. caution in pts w. myasthenia gravis, esp. those already receiving anticholinesterase drugs.

See Table 3

Generic Name (Trade Name)	Use (Dose)	Action	Adverse Effects	Drug Interactions	Nursing Process
Neostigmine bromide (Prostigmin)	As for pyridostigmine bromide (**Oral:** Adults - 75-300 mg spaced over 24 h prn. **IM:** Occas'nally, up to 1 mg qh prn in myasthenic crisis)	As for pyridostigmine bromide	As for pyridostigmine bromide	As for pyridostigmine bromide	See Table 3
Ambenonium chloride (Mytelase)	As for pyridostigmine bromide (**Oral:** Adults - Initially, 5 mg tid-qid; incr. prn. Dosage should be adjusted at intervals of 1-2 days to avoid accumulat'n. Children - Initially, 0.3 mg/kg/day in divid-ed doses; incr. prn to 1.5 mg/kg/day in divided doses)	As for pyridostigmine bromide	As for pyridostigmine bromide	As for pyridostigmine bromide	See Table 3
Edrophonium chloride (Tensilon)	Differential diagnosis. Adjunct in evaluat'n of tx requirements in this disease. Also used for evaluating emergency tx in myasthenic crises. Because of short durat'n of action, edropho-nium is not recomm. for maint. tx (**IV:** Consult manufacturer's monograph)	As for pyridostigmine bromide	As for pyridostigmine bromide	As for pyridostigmine bromide	See Table 3

CHAPTER 57

Antiarthritic Drugs

Teaching Objectives

Following completion of this chapter, the reader should be able to:

1. Describe the etiology of the inflammation seen in rheumatoid arthritis.
2. Discuss the mechanism of action, pharmacologic effects, therapeutic uses and adverse effects of nonsteroidal anti-inflammatory drugs.
3. List the nonsteroidal anti-inflammatory drugs currently in use and briefly describe their pharmacologic properties, therapeutic uses and adverse effects, and nursing processes.
4. Describe the therapeutic uses, adverse effects and nursing process for chloroquine and hydroxychloroquine in the treatment of arthritis.
5. Describe the therapeutic uses, adverse effects and nursing process of aurothioglucose, gold sodium thiomalate and auranofin.
6. Discuss the mechanism of action, therapeutic uses and adverse effects of penicillamine in the treatment of arthritis, as well as the nursing process related to its administration.
7. Discuss the use and adverse effects of adrenal corticosteroids in the treatment of arthritis, and the nursing process associated with this use.
8. Describe the therapeutic use of azathioprine in the treatment of arthritis, together with its adverse effects and the nursing process related to this use.
9. Discuss the use of methotrexate in the treatment of arthritis, as well as its adverse effects and nursing process.

In recent years many new drugs have been introduced for the treatment of arthritis. Before discussing the pharmacotherapy of arthritis, it is important to separate first-line nonsteroidal anti-inflammatory, or symptomatic, drugs from second-line agents, such as the antimalarials, gold and penicillamine. The latter are remittive, slow acting and potentially much more toxic than the nonsteroidal anti-inflammatory drugs (NSAIDs). As result, they are only used after NSAIDs have proven unsatisfactory.

Before beginning a discussion of antiarthritic drugs, it is important to point out that acetaminophen is often the drug of choice for the treatment of osteoarthritis, a chronic degenerative disease characterized by variable degrees of inflammation. The significant analgesic relief and relative lack of serious adverse effects of acetaminophen have made it the first-line therapy for many osteoarthritic patients. Although acetaminophen differs from the NSAIDs in lacking anti-inflammatory action, this fact does not seem to hamper its ability to provide relief in osteoarthritis, probably because osteoarthritis often does not involve significant inflammation. The pharmacology of acetaminophen is described in Chapter 54.

First-Line Drugs: Nonsteroidal Anti-inflammatory Drugs (NSAIDs)

The number of nonsteroidal anti-inflammatory drugs has increased dramatically in the past fifteen years. Drugs such as naproxen, tolmetin, fenoprofen, ketoprofen, flurbiprofen, diclofenac, sulindac and piroxicam were not available at that time. The drugs are called nonsteroidal to differentiate them from the corticosteroids which are also used to alleviate inflammation in arthritis.

Nonsteroidal anti-inflammatory drugs are used to treat rheumatoid arthritis, osteoarthritis, and ankylosing spondylitis, conditions marked, to a greater or lesser degree, by pain and inflammation. Drug therapy is aimed at reducing both pain and inflammation. NSAIDs are better agents for the treatment of inflammatory arthritic conditions than standard analgesics, such as acetaminophen and narcotics, which are devoid of anti-inflammatory effects.

Mechanism of Action

Nonsteroidal anti-inflammatory drugs inhibit prostaglandin synthesis. To understand the significance of this it is essential to discuss briefly inflammation and the role played by prostaglandins. Inflammation is a reaction of both blood vessels and cells to a stimulus from infecting micro-organisms, physical trauma or immunological attack. In the first century A.D. the Roman writer Cornelius Celsus described the major signs of inflammation as *rubor et tumor cum calore et dolore* (redness and swelling with heat and pain). To these four signs Rudolph Virchow added a fifth in 1858: disturbed function. Although these signs apply to all forms of inflammation, and not solely to rheumatoid arthritis, they describe the agonies of the arthritic patient, and the processes against which therapy is aimed.

Rheumatoid arthritis is a chronic inflammatory disease of connective tissue, especially within the joints. About three per cent of women and one per cent of men are affected. It is generally believed to be caused by an antigen-antibody reaction. Whether the antigen is introduced directly into the body or formed within the body is not known. It is clear, however, that the body reacts to the presence of the antigen by producing antibodies specific to the antigen. The initial, or acute, response to the antigen-antibody reaction is vasodilatation (*rubor*), increased blood flow (*calore*) and increased vascular permeability. As a result of the increase in vascular permeability, plasma water, protein and blood cells, notably neutrophilic leukocytes and monocytes, escape into the tissues to produce a swelling (*tumor*).

Prostaglandins are involved in acute inflammation. Shortly after the antigen-antibody interaction and the attempts by neutrophils to phagocytose the immune complex, two important endogenous mediators of inflammation are released into the affected tissues. These are bradykinin, formed in blood, and histamine, released from mast cells. Both chemicals dilate blood vessels, increase vascular permeability and produce pain (*dolore*). Prostaglandin E_2 (PGE_2) and prostaglandin F_{2alpha} (PGF_{2alpha}) are formed from arachadonic acid in neutrophils by the enzyme cyclo-oxygenase. Released into tissues when neutrophils are destroyed in their attempt to digest the antigen-antibody complex, PGE_2 and PGF_{2alpha} increase the biological activities of both bradykinin and histamine. In the absence of normal quantities of PGE_2 and PGF_{2alpha}, the abilities of histamine and bradykinin to dilate blood vessels, increase vascular permeability and produce pain are reduced.

If not resolved, the acute phase of arthritic inflammation may proceed to a chronic stage as the synovial membrane changes into a granulomatous tissue called **pannus.** The invasion of joint cartilage and subchondrial bone at the synovial attachment by pannus results in the destruction of cartilage and erosion of bone. Over time, pannus may be gradually transformed into fibrous or even osseous tissue leading to ankylosis (stiffening). Because of this, it is important to reduce acute inflammation to minimize the development of chronic inflammation.

Although much will be said of the beneficial effects of nonsteroidal anti-inflammatory drugs, it is also important to recognize their limitations. They do not block all manifestations of inflammation. They neither block antibody production, nor diminish the roles played by the complement and clotting systems in inflammation. NSAIDs fail to modify the chemotactic actions of T-lymphocytes which attract neutrophils from blood and reduce the migration of macrophages away from inflamed tissues. Finally, NSAIDs neither reduce the release of destructive lysosomal enzymes by neutrophils nor diminish the production of hydrogen peroxide, nor of other toxic oxygen products, by leukocytes. Thus, it is not surprising that these drugs fail to arrest the disease process of rheumatoid arthritis or, in some cases, even to provide adequate relief of pain.

As previously mentioned, osteoarthritis is a degenerative joint disease, generally chronic and noninflammatory. Little is known of its etiology. It is characterized by deterioration of articular cartilage and bony outgrowths at joint margins. About five per cent of persons past age fifty are affected. If inflammation is present in osteoarthritis, it is usually less severe than is seen with rheumatoid arthritis. Although acetaminophen is often used to treat osteoarthritis, nonsteroidal anti-inflammatory drugs are also used.

Pharmacologic Effects

Pharmaceutical companies are quick to point out the differences between their nonsteroidal anti-inflammatory drugs and those of their competitors. It would be more appropriate to describe their similarities because they share most of their effects. As we indicated in Chapter 3, to know one drug well in a classification is to know all well, particularly in this case.

Other effects of nonsteroidal anti-inflammatory drugs that depend on their ability to block prostaglandin synthesis include:

1. **Analgesia:** PGE_2 and PGF_{2alpha} sensitize nerve endings to pain.
2. **Antipyresis:** Nonsteroidal anti-inflammatory drugs lower elevated body temperatures by dilating the small vessels in the skin of the patient with a fever. This action may depend on the inhibition of PGE_2 and PGI_2 formation in the hypothalamus. Prostaglandins are necessary for pyrogen-induced fever.
3. **Gastric irritation:** Nonsteroidal anti-inflammatory drugs can irritate the stomach locally. Following absorption, they can also damage the stomach. The latter effect is due to an inhibition of PGE_2 and PGI_2 synthesis in the gastric mucosa. PGE_2 and PGI_2 inhibit gastric acid secretion and promote the secretion of cytoprotective mucus in the intestine.
4. **Reduced platelet aggregation:** Some nonsteroidal anti-inflammatory drugs inhibit platelet aggregation. Thromboxane A_2, which is similar in structure to prostaglandins, is formed in platelets from arachadonic acid and promotes platelet aggregation. The inhibition of cyclo-oxygenase by NSAIDs reduces thromboxane A_2 synthesis.
5. **Decreased renal function:** PGE_2 increases the renal excretion of sodium, chloride and water. Inhibition of its formation results in salt and water reabsorption. Renal prostaglandins reduce the vasoconstriction produced by norepinephrine and angiotensin II. In patients with reduced renal function, prostaglandins are important in maintaining renal blood flow. In these patients, nonsteroidal anti-inflammatory drugs can significantly affect renal function (see Adverse Effects, below).

Therapeutic Uses

Nonsteroidal anti-inflammatory drugs are first-line therapy for the treatment of rheumatoid arthritis, osteoarthritis and ankylosing spondylitis. They can also be used to treat acute attacks of gout (see Chapter 58). Aspirin (acetylsalicylic acid) is still the drug of first choice for many clinicians. If it fails to achieve the desired therapeutic effects, or produces an unacceptable degree of gastric distress, one of the newer NSAIDs may be given.

The newer nonsteroidal anti-inflammatory drugs constitute a major advance. These include ibuprofen (Motrin, Rufen), fenoprofen (Nalfon), ketoprofen (Orudis), naproxen (Naprosyn), flurbiprofen (Ansaid), tolmetin (Tolectin), sulindac (Clinoril), diclofenac (Voltaren), piroxicam (Feldene) and tiaprofenic acid (Surgam). Many patients who were not treated effectively with the older drugs aspirin, indomethacin or phenylbutazone, or who demonstrated untoward effects with these agents, have been helped by the newer compounds.

There is considerable patient-to-patient variability in response to any particular drug. The appropriate nonsteroidal anti-inflammatory drug for any patient is the one that works on that patient at that particular time. Evidence would also suggest that patients who initially respond favorably to any particular drug may become tolerant to it later. The variability in patient-to-patient response, together with the often-encountered development of tolerance, provides some justification for the large number of drugs currently on the market. Nursing evaluation is invaluable in establishing drug efficacy and tolerance for individual patients.

Nonsteroidal anti-inflammatory drugs should not be used in patients who have previously exhibited a hypersensitivity reaction. They are also contraindicated in patients with nasal polyps, angioedema and bronchospastic reactivity to aspirin or other NSAIDs. Anaphylactoid reactions have occurred in patients with known aspirin hypersensitivity.

Adverse Effects

PGE_2 synthesis in the stomach protects the gastric mucosa. Because of their ability to inhibit PGE_2 synthesis, all nonsteroidal anti-inflammatory drugs can irritate the stomach and produce peptic ulceration and gastric bleeding. This is one of the two major reasons, along with lack of effect, for switching from one drug to another. On an individual basis, one drug may cause considerable distress while another produces little discomfort.

Nonsteroidal anti-inflammatory drugs can cause marked central nervous system toxicity, including headache, dizziness, nervousness, confusion, insomnia and drowsiness. These effects are particularly prevalent with indomethacin.

Most nonsteroidal anti-inflammatory drugs reduce platelet aggregation and adhesiveness. Their use with coumarin-type anticoagulants or heparin may cause bleeding and should be approached with caution. This interaction is definite with aspirin, meclofenamate and phenylbutazone, and possible with fenoprofen, indomethacin, ketoprofen, piroxicam and choline magnesium salicylate. It is unlikely with ibuprofen, naproxen, sulindac and tolmetin.

All nonsteroidal anti-inflammatory drugs should be administered cautiously to patients at risk of reduced renal function. As explained before, prostaglandins are important in maintaining renal blood flow in these individuals, who include patients with advanced age, renal dysfunction, atherosclerosis, hepatic cirrhosis, concomitant diuretic treatment, low serum sodium, hyperkalemia and acute gouty arthritis. The adverse effects of NSAIDs include renal insufficiency, the nephrotic syndrome with interstitial nephritis, hyperkalemia, hyponatremia and papillary necrosis.

Nonsteroidal anti-inflammatory drugs frequently cause dermatologic reactions. Urticaria, exanthema, photosensitivity and pruritus are the most often reported reactions.

Aspirin (Acetylsalicylic Acid, ASA)

Aspirin remains a first-line drug for the treatment of arthritis. The direct irritation of aspirin on the gastric mucosa can be reduced by the use of enteric-coated tablets or by taking the drug with meals. However, enteric-coated tablets may not prevent completely the adverse effects of aspirin on the stomach because once the drug is absorbed and carried back to the stomach in the circulation it can prevent prostaglandin synthesis, thereby damaging the gastric mucosa.

High doses of aspirin can saturate the capacity of the body to eliminate salicylate. When this happens, small increases in dose produce an abrupt increase in blood and tissue salicylate levels. Patients may suddenly experience salicylate poisoning. Determinations of serum salicylate levels can assist in titrating the proper dose for the patient. Anti-inflammatory therapeutic serum levels are 15-30 mg of salicylate/dL (1.1 - 2.2 mmoles/L).

Choline magnesium trisalicylate (Trilisate) and choline salicylate (Arthropan) are two nonacetylated salicylates that are claimed to produce less gastric irritation than aspirin. They do not appear to have been compared well against enteric-coated aspirin tablets, and their place in therapy should be reserved for patients who cannot tolerate aspirin.

Nursing Process

Assessment
Prior to administering aspirin, the nurse must assess the patient's history for any indication of aspirin allergy or sensitivity, liver or kidney disease, intestinal lesions, or anticoagulant therapy. Aspirin should be withheld until the physician is contacted if any of these factors are present in the patient's history.

Administration
Patients receiving large doses of aspirin for the treatment of rheumatoid arthritis should be given the drug with food or antacids, plus copious quantities of water to reduce gastric irritation.

Evaluation
Nursing evaluation of patients on long-term aspirin therapy should include observation for tarry stools, petechiae, bruising and hematemesis because reduced prothrombin levels, decreased platelet adhesiveness and gastric irritation can predispose patients to these effects. Salicylism (mild salicylate poisoning) is manifested by headache, dizziness, tinnitus, dimness of vision, confusion, sweating, thirst, nausea, vomiting and diarrhea. Evaluate patients for signs of hepatotoxicity such as dark urine, clay-colored stools, yellowing of skin and sclera, itching, diarrhea, abdominal pain or fever.

Teaching
Patients and their families must be alerted to aspirin's adverse effects on the blood and gastrointestinal system as well as to the symptoms of salicylism. They should be taught to self-evaluate for the indicators of these adverse effects. Nurses

must emphasize to patients the importance of taking the medication regularly. Patients should also be told to avoid alcohol ingestion because it may increase gastrointestinal bleeding.

Propionic Acid Derivatives (Profens): Ibuprofen (Motrin, Rufen), Fenoprofen (Nalfon), Flurbiprofen (Ansaid), Ketoprofen (Orudis), Naproxen (Naprosyn) and Tiaprofenic Acid (Surgam)

The propionic acid derivatives (**profens**) differ little from each other. Naproxen has a half-life of ten to seventeen hours and may be given twice daily. All profens are appropriate for the treatment of rheumatoid arthritis and osteoarthritis. Because of interpatient variability, there appears to be little basis for arbitrarily selecting one over the others.

Among the profens, fenoprofen is most likely to produce dizziness, lightheadedness, drowsiness, headache and confusion. This drug is also more commonly associated with renal adverse effects than the other profens.

Nursing Process

The nursing process associated with the prescription and use of the propionic acid derivatives is essentially the same as that identified above in relation to aspirin. Readers should consult that material for detailed information.

Indolacetic Acids: Indomethacin (Indocid, Indocin), Tolmetin (Tolectin) and Sulindac (Clinoril)

Indomethacin is an effective anti-inflammatory drug for the treatment of rheumatoid arthritis, osteoarthritis of the hip, ankylosing spondylitis, psoriatic arthritis and arthritis associated with enteropathic disease. Unfortunately, it often produces severe gastric distress. Indomethacin use is also associated with a high incidence of headaches, dizziness and lightheadedness, particularly in the elderly. Indomethacin capsules should be administered two to three times daily. The sustained-release product (Indocid-SR) may be

given twice daily. Indocid suppositories are usually inserted prior to retiring.

Tolmetin is indicated for the treatment of rheumatoid arthritis. Although less effective than indomethacin, tolmetin is also less irritating on the stomach. Nevertheless, it causes gastrointestinal adverse effects in about thirty per cent of patients.

Sulindac is an effective nonsteroidal anti-inflammatory drug, indicated for the treatment of rheumatoid and osteoarthritis. It is also approved in some countries for the treatment of ankylosing spondylitis, acute painful shoulder and acute gouty arthritis. Inactive in its own right, sulindac is converted to its active sulfide metabolite within the body. The half-life of the sulfide is eighteen hours, and sulindac may be given twice daily. Gastrointestinal adverse effects (constipation, epigastric pain, nausea) occur in about twenty-five per cent of patients.

Nursing Process

Assessment
Nurses should review the patient's history prior to administration for contraindications to the use of the indolacetic acids. These include allergy, intestinal lesions or ulcerogenic medications, impaired liver or kidney function, and pregnancy. Preliminary nursing assessment of the inflammatory process will provide an objective baseline against which to measure later the efficacy of these drugs.

Administration
The indolacetic acids deteriorate in light and should be stored in a dark container. Because of gastric irritation, these drugs should always be administered with food, milk or antacids.

Evaluation
Drug efficacy is determined by a reduction in the degree of inflammation and level of pain as compared to pretreatment assessment of the inflammatory process.

Patient evaluation following the administration of an indolacetic acid derivative should focus on the gastrointestinal system, central nervous system, blood and skin. These are the most common sites for adverse effects. Gastrointestinal effects include nausea, vomiting, anorexia, dyspepsia, abdominal pain, epigastric distress, diarrhea and peptic ulcer. Central nervous system adverse effects, seen mainly with indomethacin, include headache, dizziness, tinnitus, drowsiness, confusion, irritability, hallucinations and depression. Blurred vision and tinnitus may indicate toxicity. Aplastic anemia, agranulocytosis, leukopenia and anemia have been reported with indomethacin but a cause-and-effect relationship has not been established. Pruritus, urticaria and rashes are dermatologic adverse effects of indomethacin.

Teaching
Patient teaching should include alerting both patient and family to the possible toxicities of these drugs. Special emphasis should be placed on the drowsiness and confusion encountered with indomethacin. Patients should be warned of the potential danger of driving or working with mechanical equipment during initial treatment until the effects of indomethacin are recognized.

Fenamates: Diclofenac (Voltaren) and Meclofenamate Sodium Monohydrate (Meclomen)

Both diclofenac and meclofenamate are effective nonsteroidal anti-inflammatory drugs for the treatment of rheumatoid and osteoarthritis. Gastrointestinal effects are the most frequent adverse reactions of either drug.

Nursing Process
The nursing process associated with the prescription and use of the fenamates is essentially the same as that identified above in relation to aspirin. Readers should consult that material for detailed information.

Piroxicam (Feldene)

Piroxicam owes its popularity to its half-life of thirty-eight hours, enabling once-daily dosing. Some patients who previously had not been adequately treated have responded to piroxicam. However, the same statement can be made for any nonsteroidal anti-inflammatory drug. Gastric distress can be severe with piroxicam, particularly if more than the recommended dose of 10 – 20 mg/day is used.

Nursing Process
The nursing process associated with the prescription and use of piroxicam is essentially the same as that identified above in relation to aspirin. Readers should consult that material for detailed information.

Phenylbutazone (Butazolidin) and Oxyphenbutazone (Tanderil)

Phenylbutazone is a very effective anti-inflammatory drug and may be used for the symptomatic treatment of acute superficial thrombophlebitis, acute attacks of gout, rheumatoid arthritis and ankylosing spondylitis. Because of its toxicities, however, which include nausea, vomiting, peptic ulceration (sometimes with hemorrhage and perforation), agranulocytosis and aplastic anemia, it should be reserved until the other nonsteroidal anti-inflammatory drugs have failed. Agranulocytosis occurs soon after the onset of therapy in young patients and is rarely fatal. Aplastic anemia may appear after months of therapy in older patients and has a very high mortality rate. Oxyphenbutazone is the metabolite of phenylbutazone. Little evidence can be found to support the contention that it causes less gastric irritation than phenylbutazone.

Nursing Process
Assessment
Prior to treatment, nurses should review the results of renal and liver studies for evidence of existing problems. Recording the patient's weight prior to the initiation of drug therapy is essential because both phenylbutazone and oxyphenbutazone cause sodium, chloride and fluid retention. This effect can increase circulatory volume and produce congestive heart failure and pulmonary edema.

Evaluation
Daily monitoring of the patient's weight provides early indication of fluid retention. Nurses must also evaluate the patient's hands, feet and legs for evidence of peripheral edema. In some cases, a low-sodium diet will reduce or prevent fluid retention in patients receiving phenylbutazone therapy.

A nursing evaluation that reveals dermatitis, bruising, epistaxis, bleeding gums or a sore throat is justification for withholding the drug until the physician is contacted. These are signs of blood dyscrasias resulting from bone marrow depression. Nurses should evaluate patients for blurred vision or tinnitus because these symptoms may indicate drug-induced toxicities.

Teaching
Patients should be cautioned about the adverse effects of these drugs and strongly advised to keep scheduled laboratory appointments to have complete blood counts performed.

Second-Line Drugs: Antimalarials

Chloroquine Phosphate (Aralen) and Hydroxychloroquine Sulfate (Plaquenil Sulfate)

Therapeutic Uses

Although their mechanism of action is not understood, both chloroquine phosphate and hydroxychloroquine sulfate are used in rheumatoid arthritis, in juvenile arthritis, and for the arthritic and skin manifestations of systemic lupus erythematosus. About seventy per cent of patients with rheumatoid arthritis are provided with moderate relief.

Adverse Effects

Although gastric intolerance may occur with either drug, the most common adverse effect is eye damage. This may involve either (1) corneal infiltration, which is reversible on discontinuation of the drug; or (2) retinopathy, which can cause irreversible visual loss. The risk of retinopathy is small if doses less than 400 mg of chloroquine or 250 mg of hydroxychloroquine are taken daily. The importance of regular ophthalmologic monitoring must be stressed. Chloroquine or hydroxychloroquine should not be administered in the presence of retinal or visual field changes.

Nursing Process

The nursing process associated with the prescription and use of chloroquine and hydroxychloroquine is discussed in Chapter 69. Readers should consult that material for detailed information.

Second-Line Drugs: Gold Compounds

Aurothioglucose (Solganol) and Gold Sodium Thiomalate (Myochrysine)

Therapeutic Uses

Both the oil-based aurothioglucose and the water-based gold sodium thiomalate (aurothiomalate) are injected intramuscularly. Although the mechanism of action of gold is not known, it is useful and may even alter the course of arthritis in patients with active adult or juvenile rheumatoid arthritis or psoriatic arthritis. It may be used in patients who have failed to respond to nonsteroidal anti-inflammatory treatment, rest and physical therapy. Because of its slow onset of action (up to three or four months before possible benefit), gold should be added to a background of maintenance nonsteroidal anti-inflammatory drug therapy. Treatment with gold should be instituted before irreversible changes occur in the affected joints. Unfortunately, there is no convincing evidence that gold prevents joint damage.

Adverse Effects

Approximately thirty per cent of patients discontinue gold therapy because of its adverse effects, the most common being skin rashes and mucous membrane lesions. Gold can also cause irreversible aplastic anemia, agranulocytosis and thrombocytopenia. Proteinuria, resulting from a membranous glomerulonephritis, is seen in 2 – 10% of patients on gold therapy. Patients receiving gold should undergo regular laboratory monitoring. Gold preparations are contraindicated in the presence of renal or hepatic disease, history or presence of pernicious anemia, thrombocytopenia or other blood dyscrasias, or acute disseminated lupus erythematosus. They should also not be used in pregnancy, lactation or in diabetes mellitus, eczema, chronic dermatitis, advanced cardiovascular disease or hemorrhagic diathesis.

Nursing Process

Assessment

Accurate description of the patient's physical condition provides an essential baseline for later determination of the therapeutic effectiveness of aurothioglucose and gold sodium thiomalate.

Before each injection, the nurse should thoroughly assess the patient for evidence of developing adverse effects. Nurses should anticipate that the physician will order urinalysis, serum immunoglobulin, hematocrit, complete white blood count and platelet count before every injection.

Nurses should assess respiratory status before and throughout therapy. If dyspnea or wheezing occur, discontinue the drug and contact the physician.

Administration

The vial should be thoroughly shaken to ensure an even suspension of gold. Slightly warming the vial to body temperature will assist in drawing the contents into the syringe. Aurothioglucose is administered deeply into a large muscle mass, preferably the gluteus maximus, using a 1.5 – 2 inch 18- or 20-gauge needle. *Nurses must carefully aspirate on the syringe because under no circumstances must aurothioglucose be inadvertently administered intravenously.*

Evaluation

Therapeutic effectiveness is indicated by reduced pain, less stiffness and swelling in the affected joints, greater mobility and stronger grip.

Patients must be closely watched for anaphylactic shock or angioedema for 30 – 45 min following each injection. Throughout the course of treatment the patient must be carefully and rigorously evaluated for adverse effects. Renal damage is indicated by change in color of the urine, or alteration in fluid intake/output pattern, volume or ratio. Agranulocytosis (excessive fatigue, weakness, malaise, chills, fever, sore throat) and thrombocytopenia (unusual bleeding tendencies, including bleeding gums, nose bleeds, hematuria, petechiae, increased bruising tendencies) are of grave concern and should be drawn to the attention of the physician for immediate action.

Diarrhea is a common side effect. Nurses should check stools for blood. If blood is present, the physician should be notified immediately.

Teaching

Patients must be aware of the dangerous adverse effects of treatment with gold. They must thoroughly understand the importance of laboratory studies in the early detection of adverse effects and the necessity of keeping scheduled appointments for laboratory tests. Patients should be thoroughly briefed about potential adverse effects that must be immediately reported to the physician. They should also be given a printed instruction sheet to aid in recall.

Auranofin (Ridaura)

Auranofin is an oral gold preparation that appears as effective, and perhaps better tolerated, than gold sodium thiomalate. Patients with rheumatoid arthritis improve within three to four months of starting therapy. The most frequent adverse effects of auranofin are gastrointestinal disturbances (changes in bowel habits, loose stools, diarrhea). Like parenteral gold, auranofin can cause skin reactions. Patients may demonstrate proteinuria. Auranofin has the same contraindications and precautions as parenteral gold. Blood dyscrasias including leukopenia, granulocytopenia and thrombocytopenia have all been reported with injectable gold and auranofin. These reactions may occur separately or in combination at any time during treatment. *Because they have potentially serious consequences, blood dyscrasias should be constantly watched for, through monitoring of the formed elements of the blood, every two weeks for the first three months of treatment and at least monthly thereafter.*

Nursing Process

The nursing process associated with the prescription and use of auranofin is identical to that presented above for parenteral gold. Readers should refer to that material for detailed information.

Second-Line Drugs: Penicillamine (Cuprimine, Depen)

Mechanism of Action and Therapeutic Uses

Penicillamine may have an immunosuppressive action on T-cells. It is as effective as gold or azathioprine in the treatment of rheumatoid arthritis but of little value in ankylosing spondylitis or psoriatic arthritis. Penicillamine should be reserved for patients who have not responded adequately to nonsteroidal anti-inflammatory drug treatment.

Adverse Effects

Skin rashes and gastrointestinal disturbances are the most common adverse effects, but renal damage or bone marrow depression are the major reasons for stopping the drug. Other toxicities of penicillamine include autoimmune diseases such as systemic lupus erythematosus, myasthenia gravis, polymyositis and a syndrome similar to Goodpasture's. It can also cause painful breast engorgement in females and congenital abnormalities in infants born to patients taking the drug. Because of its potential for causing renal damage, penicillamine should not be administered to rheumatoid arthritis patients with a history or other evidence of renal insufficiency.

Nursing Process

Assessment

Nurses caring for patients for whom penicillamine has been prescribed should review the patient's history for evidence of previous penicillin allergy or hypersensitivity, kidney disease or blood dyscrasias. Nurses should anticipate that the physician will order urinalysis, liver function tests, serum immunoglobulin, hematocrit, complete white blood count and platelet count, as well as an ophthalmological examination.

Physical assessment that reveals pregnancy justifies withholding the medication. A detailed description of the clinical condition will provide an essential baseline for later determination of drug effectiveness.

Administration

Penicillamine should be administered on an empty stomach either one hour before or two hours after meals. Vitamin B_6 daily is recommended, as depletion occurs with this drug.

Evaluation

Therapeutic effectiveness is indicated by reduced pain, less stiffness and swelling in the affected joints, greater mobility and a stronger grip.

Throughout the course of treatment the patient must be carefully and rigorously evaluated for adverse effects. Renal damage is indicated by change in color of the urine; alteration in fluid intake/output pattern, volume or ratio. Agranulocytosis (excessive fatigue, weakness, malaise, chills, fever, sore throat) and thrombocytopenia (unusual bleeding tendencies, including bleeding gums, nose bleeds, hematuria, petechiae, increase in bruising tendencies) are of grave concern and should be drawn to the attention of the physician for immediate action. Early evidence of adverse liver effects is manifested as jaundice, tea-colored urine, clay-colored stools and pruritus.

Teaching

Patients must be aware of the dangerous adverse effects of treatment with penicillamine. They must thoroughly understand the importance of laboratory studies in early detection of adverse effects and the necessity of keeping scheduled appointments for laboratory tests. Patients should be thoroughly briefed about potential adverse effects to be reported immediately to the physician and given a printed instruction sheet to aid in recall.

Second-Line Drugs: Adrenal Corticosteroids

Therapeutic Uses

The pharmacology of adrenal corticosteroids is presented in detail in Chapter 29. Corticosteroids may be administered systemically when more conservative measures fail or during the hiatus between the initiation of second-line therapy and its onset of action in a patient whose condition cannot be controlled by rest, physical measures, analgesics and nonsteroidal anti-inflammatory drugs.

Prednisone is the steroid used most frequently. Long-acting corticosteroids, such as prednisolone tebutate (Hydeltra TBA), betamethasone sodium phosphate and acetate (Celestone Soluspan), triamcinolone acetonide (Kenalog), triamcinolone hexacetonide (Aristospan) and methylprednisolone (Depo-Medrol) may be used intra-articularly. The indications for intra-articular therapy include (1) the patient with otherwise well-controlled arthritis in whom a single joint is particularly resistant, (2) the individual in whom one or two particularly active joints are impeding ambulation or physiotherapy, or (3) the patient with one active joint, in whom nonsteroidal anti-inflammatory drugs are contraindicated.

Adverse Effects

The adverse effects of corticosteroids are presented in Chapter 29. Readers are urged to consult that chapter for this information.

Nursing Process

The nursing process associated with the prescription and use of corticosteroids is discussed in Chapter 29. Readers should refer to that material for detailed information.

Second-Line Drugs: Azathioprine (Imuran)

The immunosuppressant azathioprine should be used only in severe, active, progressive rheumatoid arthritis that has failed to respond to conventional treatment. It should be given together with nonsteroidal anti-inflammatory drugs. Gold, antimalarials and penicillamine should be discontinued. Azathioprine can cause nausea and vomiting, leukopenia, thrombocytopenia and anemia. Complete blood counts, including platelet counts, should be performed periodically.

The nursing process associated with the prescription and use of azathioprine is discussed in Chapter 23. Readers should refer to that material for detailed information.

Second-Line Drugs: Methotrexate (Rheumatrex)

Methotrexate is a competitive inhibitor of the enzyme folic acid reductase. In rheumatoid arthritis, the mechanism of action of methotrexate is unknown, but it may affect immune function. In patients with rheumatoid arthritis, the effects of methotrexate on articular swelling tenderness can be seen as early as three to six weeks. Although the drug clearly ameliorates symptoms of inflammation, there is no evidence that it induces remission of rheumatoid arthritis. No beneficial effect been demonstrated on bone erosions and other radiologic changes that result in impaired joint use, functional disability and deformity. Most studies of methotrexate in patients with rheumatoid arthritis are relatively short-term (three to six months). Data from long-term studies indicate that an initial clinical improvement is maintained for at least two years with continued therapy.

Methotrexate should be used only by physicians whose knowledge and experience includes the use of antimetabolite therapy. It is indicated in the management of selected adults with severe, active or definite rheumatoid arthritis who have had an insufficient therapeutic response to, or were intolerant to, an adequate trial of first-line therapy, including full-dose nonsteroidal anti-inflammatory drug treatment and usually a trial of a least one or more disease-modifying antirheumatic drugs. Methotrexate is contraindicated in pregnancy, blood dyscrasias, liver disease and active infectious disease; during immunization procedures; in nursing mothers; and when there is overt or laboratory evidence of immunodeficiency syndromes. The most common adverse reactions include nausea, stomatitis, gastrointestinal discomfort, diarrhea, vomiting and anorexia. Clinical laboratory findings include elevation of liver enzymes and occasionally, decreased white blood cell counts. In general, the incidence and severity of side effects are considered to be dose related.

Nursing Process

The nursing process for methotrexate is the same as that given in Chapter 72 for antineoplastic drug therapy. Although dosages may differ, all precautions and observations apply. Patient teaching will be directed toward observations for therapeutic effects, for arthritis, and for side effects.

Further Reading

Arnold, M., Schrieber, L. and Brooks, P. (1988). Immunosuppressive drugs and corticosteroids in the treatment of rheumatoid arthritis. *Drugs 36* :340-363.

Al-Arfag, A. and Davis, P. (1991). Osteoarthritis 1991: Current drug treatment regimens. *Drugs 41* :193-201.

Baker, D.G. and Rabinowitz, J.L. (1986). Current concepts in the treatment of rheumatoid arthritis. *J. Clin. Pharmacol. 26* :2-21.

Day, R.O., Graham, G.G., Williams, K.M. and Brooks, P.M. (1988). Variability in response to NSAIDs: Fact or Fiction? *Drugs 36* :643-651.

Drugs for rheumatoid arthritis (1989). Drugs of choice. *The Medical Letter 31* :61-64 and 104-111.

Furst, D.E. (1990). Rational use of disease-modifying antirheumatic drugs. *Drugs 36* :19-37.

Kremer, J.M. (1989). Methotrexate 1989 — The evolving story. *J. Rheumatology 16* :261-263.

McCormack, K. and Brune, K. (1991). Dissociation between the antinociceptive and anti-inflammatory effects of the nonsteroidal anti-inflammatory drugs: A survey of their analgesic efficacy. *Drugs 41* :533-547.

Nunes, D., Kennedy, N.P, and Weir, D.G. (1989). Treatment of peptic ulcer disease in the arthritic patient. *Drugs 38* :451-461.

Panayi, S.G. and Roth, S.H. (1990). Symposium on NSAIDs: Reducing the risk. *Drugs 40* (Suppl. 5).

Pelletier, J.-P. and Martel-Pelletier, J. (1989). The therapeutic effects of NSAIDs and corticosteroids in osteoarthritis: To be or not to be. *J. Rheumatology 16* :266-269.

Roth, S.H. (1988). Salicylates revisited: Are they still the hallmark of anti-inflammatory therapy? *Drugs 36* :1-6.

Wilken, R.F. (1989). New perspectives of secondary and tertiary therapy for rheumatoid arthritis. *Drugs 37* :739-754.

Wolfe, C.S. and Hughes, G.R.V. (1988). The optimum management of arthropathies. *Drugs 36* :370-381.

Table 80
Antiarthritic drugs.

Generic Name (Trade Name)	Use (Dose)	Action	Adverse Effects	Drug Interactions	Nursing Process
Pharmacologic Classification: Nonsteroidal Anti-inflammatory Drugs (NSAIDs)					
Aspirin, acetylsalicylic acid, ASA	All NSAIDs are indicated for relief of s/s osteo- and rheumatoid arthritis, spondylitis, bursitis and other forms of rheumatism and musculoskeletal disorders. Right drug is the one that works on that pt at that time (**Oral: Adults** - 3.6-5.4 g/day. Children weighing ≤ 25 kg - Up to 120 mg/kg/day. Children weighing > 25 kg - 2.4-3.6 g/day)	All NSAIDs reduce synthesis of prostaglandins E_2 and F_{2alpha} (PGE$_2$ and PGF$_{2alpha}$), chemicals normally released into tissues during inflammat'n, which incr. the activities of 2 endogenous mediators of inflammat'n, histamine and bradykinin. Reduced quantities of PGE$_2$ and PGF$_{2alpha}$ thus reduce ability of histamine and bradykinin to dilate blood vessels, incr. vascular permeability and produce pain. All NSAIDs are analgesic-antipyretics and can irritate stomach.	All NSAIDs have essentially the same adv. effects (see Table 77 for adv. effects of aspirin). Adv. effects for indiv. drugs can be obtained from product brochures.	**ACE inhibitors:** Their ability to dilate blood vessels may be reduced by NSAIDs. **Ammonium chloride; ascorbic acid:** Acidify urine and reduce salicylate excret'n. In presence of either of these drugs, doses > 3 g of salicylate may produce toxicity. **Antacids:** That alkalinize urine, may incr. salicylate excret'n. **Anticoagulants:** And aspirin used tog. may result in bleeding. **Antidiabetics** (chlorpropamide, tolbutamide): Are displaced from plasma proteins by salicylates, resulting in incr. hypoglycemic effects. Give salicylates w. caution to pts receiving antidiabetics. Large doses may affect insulin requirements. **Corticosteroids:** Incr. salicylate excret'n. Incr. salicylate concentrat'ns and toxicity may occur when an interacting agent is w'drawn. **Ketoprofen:** And aspirin taken tog., result in decr. plasma protein binding and incr. clearance of ketoprofen from plasma. Do not use these drugs concomitantly. **Methotrexate:** Renal excret'n is reduced by salicylates. **Piroxicam:** And aspirin should not be used tog. because of danger of incr. adv. effects. **Spironolactone:** Salicylates may	**Assess:** Hx for allergy or sensitivity; intestinal lesions; anticoagulant tx or use of uricosurics; dyspepsia or gastric ulcerat'n; kidney or liver disease; asthma; bleeding tendencies. Establish baseline descript'n of joint pain, inflammat'n. **Administer:** W. meals and large quantities of water. **Evaluate:** Relief of pain of inflammat'n; for rash, GI distress/bleeding, dizziness, incr. bleeding tendencies, salicylism, hepatotoxicity. Blurred vision or tinnitus may indicate toxicity. **Teach:** Self-evaluat'n for side effects, toxicity; need for compliance in maintaining adequate blood levels to achieve tx benefits; to take w. food, milk or antacids. To avoid alcohol, as it may incr. GI bleeding.
Choline magnesium trisalicylate (Trilisate)	As follows (**Oral:** *Rheumatoid arthritis and severe osteoarthritis* - Adults - 1-1.5 g bid or 0.5-1 g tid. *Less severe osteoarthritis* - 1 g bid)		As for aspirin		
Fenoprofen (Nalfon)	As follows (**Oral:** *Rheumatoid arthritis* - Adults - Initially, 600 mg tid-qid. If poss., decr. in 300-mg decrements to min. effect. dose. *Osteoarthritis* - Adults - 300-600 mg tid-qid)		As for aspirin		
Flurbiprofen (Ansaid)	As follows (**Oral:** *Rheumatoid arthritis* - Adults - 150-200 mg/day in 3-4 divided doses. *Osteoarthritis* - Adults - Initially, 100-150 mg/day in 2-3 doses. *Ankylosing spondylitis* - Adults - 200 mg/day in 4 doses)	As for aspirin	As for aspirin		As for aspirin
Ibuprofen (Motrin, Rufen)	As follows (**Oral:** *Rheumatoid arthritis and osteoarthritis* - Adults - 1.2-2.4 g/day in 3-4 divided doses)	As for aspirin	As for aspirin		As for aspirin

Ketoprofen (Orudis)	As follows (**Oral:** *Rheumatoid arthritis and osteoarthritis spondylitis* - Adults - 150-200 mg/day in 3-4 doses. Elderly or renal-impaired pts - Reduce dose by 33-50%. **Rectal:** 100 mg a.m. and hs)	As for aspirin	reduce its ability to incr. Na excret'n. **Uricosurics:** Low doses of salicylates may reduce actions of these drugs. **ACE inhibitors:** Their ability to dilate blood vessels can be reduced by NSAIDs. **Anticoagulants:** And profens (fenoprofen, flurbifrofen, ibuprofen, ketoprofen, naproxen and tiaprofenic acid) used tog., may result in bleeding.	As for aspirin
Naproxen (Naprosyn)	As follows (**Oral:** *For rheumatoid arthritis, osteoarthritis and ankylosing spondylitis* - Adults - Initially, 500 mg/day in 2 doses; incr. gradually prn to 750-1000 mg/day. **Rectal:** 500 mg supp. can replace 1 oral dose in pts receiving 1000 mg/day. Supps. not recomm. in children < age 12. *For juvenile rheumatoid arthritis* - **Oral:** Approx. 10 mg/kg/day in 2 divided doses)	As for aspirin	As for fenoprofen	As for aspirin
Tiaprofenic acid (Surgam)	As follows (**Oral:** *For rheumatoid arthritis* - Adults - 600 mg/day in 3 doses. *For osteoarthritis* - Adults - 600 mg/day in 2-3 doses)	As for aspirin	As for fenoprofen	As for aspirin
Tolmetin (Tolectin)	As follows (**Oral:** *For rheumatoid arthritis and ankylosing spondylitis* - Adults - Initially, 400 mg tid; adjust to 600-1800 mg/day. *For osteoarthritis* - Initially, 800-1200 mg/day tid-qid. Maint. dose, us. bet. 600-1600 mg/day. *For juvenile rheumatoid arthritis* - Children >2 years - Initially, 20 mg/kg/day in 3-4 divided doses. Maint. dose, 15-30 mg/kg/day)	As for aspirin	As for fenoprofen	As for aspirin

Generic Name (Trade Name)	Use (Dose)	Action	Adverse Effects	Drug Interactions	Nursing Process
Sulindac (Clinoril)	As follows (**Oral:** *For rheumatoid arthritis, osteoarthritis and ankylosing spondylitis* - Adults - 150 mg bid w. food. *For acute painful shoulder and gouty arthritis* - Adults - 200 mg bid w. food)	As for aspirin	As for aspirin	As for fenoprofen	As for aspirin
Diclofenac (Voltaren)	As follows (**Oral:** *For rheumatoid arthritis* - Adults - 25-50 mg tid w. food. Max., 150 mg/day. *For osteoarthritis* - Adults - 75 mg/day in 3 divided doses. **Rectal:** 50-100 mg supp. may be given as substitute for last of 3rd oral daily doses, to max. 150 mg/day)	As for aspirin	As for aspirin	As for fenoprofen	As for aspirin
Meclofenamate sodium monohydrate (Meclomen)	As follows (**Oral:** *For rheumatoid arthritis and osteoarthritis* - Adults - 200-400 mg/day in 3-4 equal doses, taken w. meals or milk)	As for aspirin	As for aspirin	As for fenoprofen	As for aspirin
Piroxicam (Feldene)	As follows (**Oral:** *For rheumatoid arthritis, osteoarthritis and ankylosing spondylitis* - Adults - Initially, 20 mg in single dose, or 10 mg bid)	As for aspirin	As for aspirin	**Anticoagulants, oral; antidiabetics, sulfonylurea:** Are highly bound to plasma proteins. Piroxicam, also highly bound to plasma proteins, may displace these drugs from their binding sites and incr. their effects. **Aspirin:** And piroxicam should not be used together. **Lithium:** May have reduced rate of eliminat'n if piroxicam is given concomitantly. As a result, serum Li levels may rise. **Phenytoin:** Is highly bound to plasma proteins. Piroxicam, also highly bound to plasma proteins, may displace phenytoin from its binding sites and incr. its effects.	As for aspirin

Drug	Dosage	Remarks	Drug Interactions	Nursing Considerations
Indomethacin (Indocid, Indocin)	As follows (**Oral:** *For rheumatoid arthritis and ankylosing spondylitis* - Adults - Initially, 25 mg bid-tid; incr. by 25-50 mg/day at weekly intervals until max. 200 mg/day is reached. Always give w. food or immed. pc, w. milk or antacids. Sustained-release caps [containing 75 mg indomethacin] may be given od-bid. *For severe osteoarthritis and degenerative joint disease of hip* - Adults - Initially, 25 mg bid-tid. If response not adequate, incr. daily dose by 25 mg at weekly intervals until satisfactory response is obtained or a dosage of 150-200 mg/day is reached. **Rectal:** 100-200 mg [i.e., 100 mg hs and 100 mg next a.m.])	As for aspirin	As for aspirin. Incidence of adv. effects is higher and their severity greater when indomethacin is used. Headache/CNS effects are often prominent.	**ACE inhibitors:** Have the same interact'ns as other NSAIDs. **Diflunisal:** May decr. renal clearance of indomethacin. Fatal GI hemorrhage has been assoc. w. combined use of these 2 drugs. Do not use concomitantly. **Diuretics, K-sparing:** Given tog. w. indomethacin, may result in hyperkalemia and nephrotoxicity. **Lithium:** May have reduced rate of elimina't'n if indomethacin is admin. concomitantly. As a result, serum Li levels may rise. **Probenecid:** Inhibits renal transport of indomethacin, thereby incr. its plasma levels. Modify dose of indomethacin.	**Assess:** Hx for allergy/sensitivity, GI ulcerat'n, dyspepsia, kidney or liver disease, asthma, bleeding tendencies; concurrent use of uricosurics or anticoagulants. Establish baseline descript'n of locat'n, extent of inflammat'n. **Administer:** From light-resistant container. **Evaluate:** Relief of pain and inflammat'n; for rash, GI distress/bleeding; dizziness; incr. bleeding tendencies; CNS effects; blood dyscrasias. Blurred vision and tinnitus may indicate toxicity. **Teach:** Self-evaluat'n for adv. effects; danger of driving or working w. power tools/industrial machinery. To take w. food; to keep out of reach of children.
Phenylbutazone (Azolid, Butazolidin)	Tx of severe osteoarthritis, acute superficial thrombophlebitis, acute attacks of gout, rheumatoid arthritis, ankylosing spondylitis, severe cases of acute noninfective condit'ns such as peritendonitis, capsulitis, bursitis (**Oral:** *For ankylosing spondylitis* - Adults - Initially, 300-600 mg/day in 3-4 divided doses. Maint. dose, not > 400 mg/day. If favorable response not obtained, discontinue drug. If dose of 100-200 mg/day controls symptoms, drug can be given for longer periods of time under careful observat'n. Elderly [> 60 years] - Restrict use of drug to short-term tx [max. 1 week, if poss.])	Mechanism of action sim. to aspirin's. Phenylbutazone can be extremely effective but because of toxicities, it should be reserved until other NSAIDs have failed.	As for aspirin and ibuprofen; however, incidence of adv. effects is higher w. phenylbutazone and their severity greater. Phenylbutazone can affect bone marrow, producing leukopenia, agranulocytosis, thrombocytopenia, pancytopenia and aplastic anemia.	**Anticoagulants, oral:** Should not be used tog. w. phenylbutazone because latter may prolong prothrombin time. **Hypoglycemics, oral; insulin:** Phenylbutazone may incr. their hypoglycemic actions.	**Assess:** As for ASA. Establish baseline weight. **Administer:** W. food. **Evaluate:** For relief of pain, reduced inflammat'n; for fluid retent'n, dermatitis, bruising, epistaxis, bleeding gums, sore throat. **Teach:** Self-evaluation and monitoring for side effects; importance of compliance w. lab. attendance for monitoring CBCs; to take medicat'n w. food, milk or antacids; low-Na diet to reduce fluid retent'n.

Generic Name (Trade Name)	Use (Dose)	Action	Adverse Effects	Drug Interactions	Nursing Process
Pharmacologic Classification: Antimalarial Drugs					
Chloroquine phosphate (Aralen); hydroxychloroquine sulfate (Plaquenil Sulfate)	Tx of rheumatoid arthritis (**Oral:** Adults - *Chloroquine phosphate* - 250 mg od w. evening meal or hs. *Hydroxychloroquine sulfate* - 200 mg od-bid w. meals. Max., 6.4 mg/kg/day)	Mechanism of action in arthritis not understood.	GI intolerance, retinophathy, bone marrow supress'n		See Table 103
Pharmacologic Classification: Gold Compounds					
Aurothioglucose (Solganol); gold sodium thiomalate (Myochrysine)	Tx of active adult or juvenile rheumatoid arthritis or psoriatic arthritis (**IM:** *Aurothioglucose or gold sodium thiomalate; single weekly injections* - Adults - 10 mg 1st week; 25 mg 2nd week; 25-50 mg 3rd week and each week thereafter until a total dose of 800-1000 mg has been given. If no improvement, either discontinue drug or incr. dose by 10 mg q1-4weeks. Max., 100 mg/single inject'n. If pt has responded and there is no evidence of toxic effects, 25-50 mg may be given q2-3weeks and then monthly. Children - 1 mg/kg/week for 20 weeks. Continue same dose at 2-4 week intervals after initial 20 weeks for as long as tx appears successful and there are no signs of toxicity. No single dose should be > 50 mg [except for largest of adolescents]. **Oral:** *Auranofin* - Us. starting dose, 6 mg/day. Can be given bid [breakfast and evening meal] or od [either breakfast or evening meal])	Mechanism of action not known. Useful and may even after course of arthritis in pts w. active adult or juvenile rheumatoid arthritis or psoriatic arthritis. Use in pts who have failed to respond to NSAID tx, rest and physical therapy.	Rash, mucous membrane lesions, serious hematologic complicat'ns, proteinuria; GI disturbances from auranofin.		**Assess:** Respiratory status before and throughout tx. If dyspnea or wheezing occur, discontinue drug. Establish baseline physical condit'n and adv. effects before each inject'n. Anticipate order for urinalysis, immunoglobulin, hematocrit, complete WBC and platelet count before every inject'n. **Administer:** Shake well; warm slightly; give deep into large muscle; use 1.5-2 inch, 18- or 20gauge needle; aspirate on syringe. **Evaluate:** For effectiveness and adv. effects. **Teach:** Dangerous adv. effects; importance of lab. studies in early detect'n of adv. effects; nec. of keeping appointments for lab. tests. Diarrhea is a common side effect. Stools should be checked for blood and, if blood is present, physician should be notified immediately.
Auranofin (Ridaura)					

Pharmacologic Classification: Penicillamine

Penicillamine (Cuprimine, Depen)				
Tx of severe, active rheumatoid arthritis unresponsive to adequate trial of convent'nal tx (**Oral:** Adults - Initially, 125-250 mg od; incr. prn by 125-250 mg/day at 1- or 3-month intervals. If no improvement, and no s/s potentially serious toxicity are seen after 2-3 months of tx w. 500-750 mg/day, may incr. by 125-250 mg/day at 2- to 3-month intervals until satisfactory remiss'n occurs or signs of toxicity develop. If no improvement after 3-4 months of 1000-1500 mg/day, pt is unlikely to respond, and drug should be stopped. Children - Initially, 5 mg/kg/day. Incr. to 10-15 mg/kg/day after 2 months if response to lower dose fails to produce desired effect)	May have immunosuppressive action on T-cells. As effective as gold or azathioprine in rheumatoid arthritis, but of little value in ankylosing spondylitis or psoriatic arthritis.	Skin rashes, renal damage (involving membranous or mesangial changes) and bone marrow depress'n (involving primarily thrombocytopenia but also occas'nally fatal marrow depress'n), autoimmune diseases (SLE, myasthenia gravis, polymyositis and Goodpasture-like syndrome), painful breast engorgement in females, congenital abnormalities in infants.	**Gold tx, antimalarial or cytotoxic drugs, oxyphenbutazone or phenylbutazone:** Should not be given along w. penicillamine because these drugs are also assoc. w. similar serious hematologic and renal adv. effects. Pts who have had Au-salt tx and discontinued it because of a major toxic react'n may be at greater risk of serious adv. effects w. penicillamine, but not nec. of the same type.	**Assess:** Hx for penicillin allergy or hypersensitivity, kidney disease or blood dyscrasias; for pregnancy. Establish baseline condit'n. Anticipate order for urinalysis, liver function, serum immunoglobulin, hematocrit, complete WBC and platelet count, ophthalmologic exam. **Administer:** On empty stomach; 1 h ac or 2 h pc. Vitamin B$_6$ daily is recomm., as deplet'n occurs w. this drug. **Evaluate:** Effectiveness; adv. effects, incl. renal damage, agranulocytosis, thrombocytopenia and hepatotoxicity. **Teach:** Dangerous adv. effects; importance of lab. studies; nec. of keeping appointment for lab. tests.

Pharmacologic Classification: Folic Acid Reductase Inhibitor

Methotrexate (Rheumatrex)				
Management of selected adults w. severe, active or definite rheumatoid arthritis (**Oral:** 7-10 days after test dose [to detect liability to severe effects], give oral doses of 7.5 mg 1x/week, or divided doses of 2.5 mg at 12-h intervals for 3 doses given as a course once weekly. Pts us. begin to respond in 3-6 weeks, and may continue to improve for another 12 weeks or more. May incr. dosage to 15 mg/week after 6 weeks in nonresponsive pts. If nec., gradually incr. dose further to achieve opt. response, but total dose ordinarily should not be >	Competitive inhibitor of enzyme folic acid reductase. Mechanism of action in rheumatoid arthritis is unknown, but may affect immune funct'n in pts w. rheumatoid arthritis, effects of methotrexate on articular swelling and tenderness can be seen as early as 3-6 weeks. Although methotrexate ameliorates s/s inflammat'n, there is no evidence that it induces	Nausea, stomatitis, GI discomfort, diarrhea, vomiting, anorexia. Clinical lab. findings incl. elevat'n of liver enzyme levels and occas'nally decr. WBC counts. CBC w. platelet counts should be determined 7-10 days after initial test dose to determine any extreme liability to adv. effects.	**Antibiotics, oral** (e.g., tetracycline, chloramphenicol, nonabsorbable broad-spectrum antibiotics): May decr. intestinal absorpt'n of methotrexate, or interfere w. enterohepatic circulat'n by inhibiting bowel flora and suppressing metabolism of drug by bacteria. **Phenylbutazone; phenytoin:** May displace methotrexate from plasma protein binding sites. **Probenecid; weak organic acids** (e.g., NSAIDs): Decr. renal tubular transport of methotrexate. **Salicylates:** Decr. renal tubular transport of methotrexate; may displace methotrexate from	*The Nsg Process for methotrexate is the same as that given in Chapter 72 for antineoplastic drug tx, w. the following addit'ns:* **Assess:** Monitor blood studies, liver tests and bleeding tendencies closely. **Administer:** W. antacids. **Teach:** To observe for tx effectiveness and adv. effects.

Generic Name (Trade Name)	Use (Dose)	Action	Adverse Effects	Drug Interactions	Nursing Process
	20 mg/week. Once response is achieved, each schedule should be reduced to lowest effective dose w. longest poss. rest period)	remiss'n of rheumatoid arthritis.		plasma protein binding sites. **Sulfonamides:** May displace methotrexate from plasma protein binding sites. **Trimethoprim-sulfamethazole:** Has been reported to incr. bone marrow depress'n in a few pts receiving methotrexate.	

Pharmacological Classification: Adrenal Corticosteroids

See Chapter 57 and Table 46.

CHAPTER 58

Antigout Drugs

Gout

Gout is a disorder in uric acid metabolism. The normal range for serum urate concentrations is 190 – 490 µmol/L (3 – 8 mg/100 mL). People with serum urate concentration in this range have little risk of gout. Individuals at high risk have serum urate levels of 610 – 675 µmol/L (10 – 11 mg/100 mL). In the latter group the concentration of urate exceeds the capacity of the body fluids to hold it in solution, and sodium urate crystals may deposit in a joint. When neutrophils attempt to phagocytose the crystals, inflammation ensues and the patient experiences gout.

Drugs can act (1) in the joint to reduce inflammation, (2) in the tissues to decrease the production of uric acid, or (3) in the kidneys to increase uric acid excretion.

Drugs That Act in the Joint

Colchicine

Mechanism of Action and Pharmacologic Effects

As previously explained, sodium urate deposits in joints if its concentration in joint fluids exceeds its solubility. When neutrophils attempt to phagocytose urate crystals they are destroyed, freeing chemicals that not only cause inflammation but also attract more neutrophils from the blood. The newly arrived neutrophils in turn attempt to phagocytose the sodium urate crystals and they, too, are destroyed, freeing additional inflammatory and chemotactic chemicals. This process can repeat itself many times.

Colchicine is not an analgesic. Its ability to reduce pain is restricted to gout. Following absorption from the gastrointestinal tract, colchicine concentrates in the liver, spleen, gastrointestinal tract and neutrophils. Its ability to concentrate in neutrophils may be most important because colchicine reduces inflammation by decreasing the release of chemotactic factors from neutrophils, with the result that fewer neutrophils are subsequently attracted to the affected joint.

Therapeutic Uses

Colchicine is effective in all crystal-induced arthropathies, including gout and pseudogout. It reduces inflammation in the affected joint(s) and is used to terminate an acute attack. Oral treatment, early in an attack, usually provides relief of pain and inflammation within twenty-four to forty-eight hours. Colchicine can also be given in reduced doses to prevent attacks or diminish their severity. It should be administered until all visible or radiographically demonstrated tophi are dissolved. Colchicine has an important value as an aid in the diagnosis of acute gout, since response to the drug is very specific.

During the initial treatment period with allopurinol or uricosurics (see later discussion), patients often experience more attacks. Colchicine can be given at this time to reduce the number of attacks.

Treatment with colchicine is contraindicated in patients with serious gastrointestinal, renal or cardiac disease. Because in certain species of animals colchicine has produced teratogenic effects, if it used during pregnancy, or if a patient becomes pregnant while taking it, the woman should be told of the potential hazard to the fetus.

Adverse Effects

Diarrhea, nausea, vomiting and abdominal pain often occur with the use of colchicine. If these occur the drug should be stopped, regardless of the condition of the joint(s). Large doses of colchicine cause a burning sensation in the throat, bloody diarrhea, hematuria, oliguria, central nervous system depression and death. Extravasation of intravenous colchicine results in inflammation and necrosis of the skin and soft tissues.

Nursing Process

Assessment
Prior to administering the first dose of colchicine the nurse should review the patient's history for evidence of kidney, liver or heart disease and pre-existing ulcerative disease of the gastrointestinal system. A history of any of these is sufficient justification for withholding the medication pending clarification of the prescription with the physician.

Colchicine should not be given if physical assessment of the patient reveals either advanced age or extensive debilitation. Another, but no less important, purpose of nursing assessment is the establishment of baseline measures of fluid intake and output, as well as documentation of the location and extent of joint swelling and inflammation.

Administration
Oral administration of colchicine ideally should be on an empty stomach to facilitate absorption. However, it may be necessary to take the drug with food to reduce gastric irritation. If parenteral administration is required, colchicine must be injected intravenously only because of the tissue irritation and possible necrosis associated with its subcutaneous or intramuscular injection. The tissue irritation is so severe that the needle used to withdraw the medication from the vial should be removed and a new needle attached to the syringe before venapuncture is performed.

Evaluation
Patient evaluation following colchicine administration should determine the effectiveness of the drug in relieving joint pain and swelling. Nurses should be alert for any pain, redness or hard area, usually in the legs.

Patients should be monitored for evidence of sore throat, bleeding gums, fever of unexplained origin, fatigue or lethargy. These suggest blood dyscrasias associated with bone marrow depression. Nausea, vomiting, diarrhea and abdominal pain are early indicators of toxicity resulting from either excessive dosage or prolonged usage. Colchicine should be stopped if any of these are seen. Fluid intake and output should be evaluated to ensure that output is maintained at a minimum of two liters per day to prevent uric acid crystals forming in the ureters and bladder.

Teaching

Patient education should stress prompt initiation of therapy at the earliest indication of an acute attack. Nurses should instruct patients to allow at least three days between courses of treatment to avoid toxicity resulting from prolonged usage. Use of colchicine for an acute attack of gout should be discontinued when the pain is no longer present or when adverse gastrointestinal effects begin, whichever occurs first. If the drug is self-administered at home, patients should be taught self-evaluation of adverse effects.

Surgery often precipitates acute attacks of gout. Nurses should advise patients to take colchicine prophylactically for three days preceding and three days after dental treatment or other minor surgery.

Nurses must stress the importance of maintaining high fluid intake. Low-purine foods should be consumed and the family referred for dietary counseling.

Nonsteroidal Anti-Inflammatory Drugs

The pharmacology of nonsteroidal anti-inflammatory drugs is presented in Chapter 57. Indomethacin, phenylbutazone and oxyphenbutazone have been used for years to provide short-term treatment of acute attacks of gout. More recently, the newer nonsteroidal anti-inflammatory drugs have largely supplanted colchicine for acute attacks because of the latter's invariable tendency to produce gastrointestinal upset. To be effective for gout, however, nonsteroidal anti-inflammatory drugs should be used promptly and in optimal doses. The adverse effects and nursing process for these drugs are presented in Chapter 57. Readers should consult that material for detailed information.

Drugs That Reduce Uric Acid Synthesis

Allopurinol (Lopurin, Zyloprim)

Mechanism of Action and Pharmacologic Effects

Allopurinol is rapidly absorbed from the gastrointestinal tract. Peak plasma concentrations are obtained thirty to sixty minutes after drug ingestion. Allopurinol and its major metabolite, oxypurinol, inhibit xanthine oxidase, the enzyme responsible for the synthesis of uric acid. Both plasma and urine uric acid levels fall within a few days to two weeks of starting treatment.

Therapeutic Uses

Allopurinol is used to treat chronic tophaceous gout. Administered chronically, allopurinol inhibits the formation of tophi, mobilizes stored urates and decreases the size of tophi already formed. Because the drug does not depend on the kidney for its effects, allopurinol benefits patients who already have developed renal obstructions as a result of uric acid stones or individuals with excessively high urate excretion who have not responded to uricosuric drugs. Allopurinol is also used to reduce uric acid synthesis in patients with a variety of blood disorders, such as polycythemia vera or leukemia. The drug is contraindicated in nursing mothers and in children (except in those with hyperuricemia secondary to a malignancy).

Adverse Effects

Skin rashes, gastrointestinal upset, hepatotoxicity and fever are the most common adverse effects of allopurinol. Attacks of acute gout may occur more frequently during the first months of treatment with allopurinol. The number of attacks can be kept to a minimum by administering colchicine and increasing fluid consumption to ensure adequate diuresis.

Nursing Process

Assessment

Prior to starting treatment with allopurinol, nurses should assess female patients for evidence of pregnancy. The frequency, severity, location and extent of gout attacks must also be established. Nurses should review the patient's history for evidence of hepatic or renal dysfunction. Allopurinol should not be administered to patients who exhibit symptoms of these conditions.

Administration

Allopurinol is administered with food to reduce gastric distress.

Evaluation

Nursing evaluation of patients following allopurinol administration is the same as that previously identified for colchicine. In addition, nurses should be alert for the development of a rash, indicating a hypersensitivity reaction, and for the occasional drowsiness that accompanies allopurinol use. It is recommended that uric acid levels be measured every two weeks to maintain a concentration of 6 mg of uric acid per deciliter.

Teaching

In teaching patients using allopurinol, nurses should stress the need for perseverance during the early treatment phases. Drug effectiveness is often not experienced for several weeks following the start of therapy. There is often a transient increase in the frequency of attacks during this time. Patients who are aware of this are more likely to comply with the prescribed regimen.

Patients should be instructed in self-evaluation for adverse effects. The importance of maintaining a high fluid intake and output and of keeping regularly scheduled appointments for laboratory studies of blood, liver and kidney functions should be stressed. Allopurinol may cause drowsiness. Therefore, patients should also be advised to avoid driving and using power tools during the early phase of therapy.

Drugs That Increase Renal Excretion of Uric Acid (Uricosurics)

Probenecid (Benemid)

Mechanism of Action and Pharmacologic Effects

Uric acid undergoes filtration, reabsorption and secretion in the nephron as outlined below:

1. First, uric acid is filtered through the renal glomeruli.
2. Second, some of the filtered uric acid is reabsorbed back into the blood from the proximal convoluted tubules.
3. Finally, uric acid is secreted from the blood into the renal tubules.

Stated simply, the amount of uric acid cleared in the urine is a result of filtration + secretion − reabsorption, or $(1 + 3) - 2$.

Probenecid decreases uric acid reabsorption (see item 2, above). The resulting increase in uric acid excretion causes a substantial fall in plasma uric acid levels. However, even high doses of probenecid fail to prevent more than fifty per cent of the filtered uric acid from being reabsorbed.

Therapeutic Uses

Probenecid is indicated for the treatment of hyperuricemia in all stages of gout and gouty arthritis, except a presenting acute attack. It prevents or reduces joint changes and tophi that occur in chronic gout. Because acute attacks of gout may occur during the first months of therapy, treatment should include colchicine and an increase in fluid consumption.

In an action unrelated to its uricosuric effects, probenecid may be indicated as an adjunct to therapy with any penicillin product. This use is based on the fact that probenecid reduces the renal secretion of penicillin products, thereby increasing both their plasma levels and half-lives.

Adverse Effects

Probenecid's adverse effects include headache, anorexia, nausea, vomiting, urinary frequency, hypersensitivity reactions (dermatitis, pruritus and fever), sore gums, flushing, dizziness, anemia and anaphylactoid reactions. Hemolytic anemia has been reported. This may be related to a genetic glucose-6-phosphate dehydrogenase deficiency in red blood cells. Probenecid is contraindicated in patients with uric acid kidney stones. It is also contraindicated in persons with blood dyscrasias and in children under two years of age.

Nursing Process

Assessment

The nursing process for probenecid begins with an assessment of the patient's history for previous renal calculi. Increased uric acid clearance by uricosuric drugs increases stone formation. Therefore, uricosurics should not be used in patients with renal calculi. Nursing assessment should also attempt to identify previous hypersensitivity reactions.

Administration

In spite of the adverse effects presented above, probenecid is generally well tolerated. Gastrointestinal discomfort is the most common reaction and it can be minimized by giving the drug with food.

Evaluation

Nursing evaluation following probenecid treatment should emphasize observing for evidence of gastrointestinal disturbances (anorexia, nausea, vomiting, diarrhea, constipation and abdominal discomfort). Skin rash, fever, pruritus or dermatitis indicate hypersensitivity reactions. Any retroperitoneal pain may be a precursor of renal colic, indicating renal calculi, and must be monitored closely. Diabetics receiving oral hypoglycemics should be closely watched because probenecid enhances the effects of oral hypoglycemics and increases the incidence of hypoglycemic reactions. Nurses should monitor uric acid levels to maintain a concentration of 3 – 7 mg/dL.

Teaching

Patient teaching should stress the importance of drinking at least three liters (twelve eight-ounce glasses) of water daily. This is particularly important in preventing the formation of kidney stones in the early stages of treatment. Nurses should instruct patients to report the number and frequency of gout attacks to their physician so that additional treatment can be considered. Nurses should caution patients to take probenecid regularly, unless otherwise directed by the physician. Probenecid does not alter the basic course of hyperuricemia and patients usually require the drug continuously for many years. Irregular dosage will cause fluctuations in serum uric acid, reducing the prophylactic effect of the medication.

Nurses must alert patients and their families to the signs of hypersensitivity. They must be instructed to report these immediately to the physician. Nurses should also inform patients that low doses of salicylates will antagonize the effects of probenecid. Therefore, patients must not take aspirin or any other over-the-counter medications without first consulting the physician. Patients must be taught to maintain a low-purine diet which restricts organ meats, anchovies, sardines, meat, gravy, dried beans, meat extract and alcohol.

Sulfinpyrazone (Anturane)

Sulfinpyrazone is a potent uricosuric with the same mechanism of action and clinical uses as probenecid. It may be given with probenecid because it causes an additional uricosuric effect in subjects receiving maximally effective doses of probenecid. Gastric irritation is its most common adverse effect. The nursing process for sulfinpyrazone is identical to that for probenecid. Readers should consult that material for detailed information.

Further Reading

Baum, J. (1978). Modern concepts in treatment of gout. *Drug Ther. 8* :76-81.

Bennett, D.R., ed. (1986). Agents used in gout and hyperuricemia. *American Medical Association Drug Evaluations,* 6th ed., pp. 1079-1088.

Emmerson, B.T. (1978). Drug control of gout and hyperuricemia. *Drugs 16* :158-166.

Homes, E.W. Jr. (1981). Rational approach to gout. *Drug Ther. 11* :117-124.

Table 81
Antigout drugs.

Pharmacologic Classification: Drugs That Act in the Joint

Generic Name (Trade Name)	Use (Dose)	Action	Adverse Effects	Drug Interactions	Nursing Process
Colchicine	Tx of gout. Colchicine is (1) effective in relieving pain of acute attacks, esp. if tx is begun early in attack, and (2) valuable as maint. tx w. allopurinol during intercritical periods (**Oral:** Start at 1st warning of acute attack. Initially, 1-1.2 mg, followed by 0.5-0.6 mg q2h until pain is relieved, or toxic symptoms appear. Total am't us. required during course of tx ranges from 4-8 mg. As interval tx, 0.5-0.6 mg may be taken 1-4x/week for mild or moderate cases, od-bid in severe cases. Reduce dose if weakness, anorexia, nausea, vomiting or diarrhea occur)	Colchicine concentrates in neutrophils, reducing release of chemotactic chemicals.	GI upsets (nausea, vomiting, abd. pain, diarrhea), vascular and renal damage, muscular weakness, urticaria, dermatitis, purpura, agranulocytosis, aplastic anemia, peripheral neuritis, alopecia	**Vitamin B$_{12}$:** Absorpt'n can be reduced by colchicine.	**Assess:** For hx kidney, liver or heart disease; for advanced age or debilitated physical condit'n. Establish baseline fluid intake/output; locat'n and extent of swelling, inflammat'n. **Administer:** Orally on empty stomach, but if GI symptoms occur, w. food. **Evaluate:** Effect on joint pain, swelling; for sore throat, bleeding gums, fever, fatigue, lethargy; for nausea, vomiting, diarrhea, abd. pain; fluid intake/output. **Teach:** To initiate tx at earliest indicat'n of acute attack; to maintain high fluid intake; to self-evaluate for adv. effects; to allow at least 3 days bet. courses of tx; to discontinue tx for acute attacks when pain is relieved or GI effects appear, whichever occurs first; to seek dietary counseling; to initiate preventive tx 3 days before and 3 days following dental or other surgery.
Nonsteroidal anti-inflammatory drugs (NSAIDs)	Short-term tx for acute attacks of gout (For doses, consult Table 80).	See Table 80	See Table 80	See Table 80	See Table 80

Pharmacologic Classification: Drugs That Reduce Uric Acid Synthesis

Drug	Uses / Dosage	Mechanism	Adverse Effects	Drug Interactions	Nursing Considerations
Allopurinol (Lopurin, Zyloprim)	Tx of chronic tophaceous gout; tx of hyperuricemia assoc. w. excess. product'n of uric acid excess. **(Oral: For mild gout** - Adults - Min. effective dose, 100-200 mg; av. dose, 200-300 mg/day. *Moderately severe tophaceous gout* - 400-600 mg/day. *Severe gout* - 700-800 mg/day. Max. dose, 800 mg/day for pts w. normal renal funct'n. Divide total daily requirements into 1-3 doses. For daily doses ≤ 300 mg, take od pc. Max. single dose, 300 mg. *Reduced dose for renal insufficiency* - Creatinine clearance of 10-20 mL/min - daily dose, 200 mg. Creatinine clearance < 10 mL/min - dose not > 100 mg/day. Creatinine clearance < 3 mL/min - length-en interval bet. doses)	Allopurinol and its major metabolite, oxypurinol, inhibit xanthine oxidase, enzyme responsible for uric acid synthe-sis.	Skin rashes, GI upset, hepatotoxicity and fever are most common adv. effects.	**Anticoagulants, oral:** Metabolism may be inhibited by allopurinol. **Azathioprine:** Inactivat'n is reduced by allopurinol. Use 25-35% usual azathioprine dose. **Chlorpropamide:** Its renal excret'n may be reduced by allop-urinol. When renal funct'n is poor, risk of chlorpropamide's prolonged hypoglycemic activity may incr. if allopurinol is given concomitantly. **Cyclophosphamide:** May show incr. incidence of bone marrow depress'n in presence of allopurinol. **Mercaptopurine (6-MP):** Inactivat'n is reduced by allopuri-nol. Use 25-33% usual 6-MP dose. **Uricosurics:** May decr. oxypurine excret'n and incr. urate excret'n.	**Assess:** For pregnancy; hx hepatic/renal dysfunct'n. Establish frequency, severity of gout attacks. **Administer:** W. food. **Evaluate:** For skin rash, drowsiness; as for colchicine. Monitor uric acid levels q2weeks to maintain 6 mg/dL level. **Teach:** That transient initial incr. in frequency of attacks may occur; that drug effectiveness might require several weeks; to self-evaluate for adv. effects; importance of maintaining high fluid intake/output and to keep scheduled appointments for lab. studies of blood and liver funct'n; hazards of driving, using power equipment/industrial machinery during early phase of tx.

Pharmacologic Classification: Drugs That Increase Renal Excret'n of Uric Acid (Uricosurics)

Drug	Uses / Dosage	Mechanism	Adverse Effects	Drug Interactions	Nursing Considerations
Probenecid (Benemid)	Tx of hyperuricemia in all stages of gout and gouty arthri-tis, except presenting acute attack. As adjunct to tx w. penicillin for elevat'n and prolon-gat'n of penicillin plasma concentrat'n **(Oral:** *For gout* - 250 mg bid for 1 week, followed by 500 mg bid. May incr. dose prn by 500-mg incre-ments q4weeks within tolerance [and us. not > 2 g/day] if s/s gouty arthritis are not controlled or 24-h urate excret'n is not > 700 mg. Adjust dose in renal impairment. Drug may not be effective in chronic renal insufficiency)	Reduces renal reabsorpt'n of uric acid. Resulting incr. in uric acid excret'n causes substantial fall in plasma uric acid levels.	Headache, GI symptoms (anorexia, nausea, vomiting), urinary frequency; hypersensitivity react'ns incl. dermati-tis, pruritus and fever; sore gums, flushing, dizziness, anemia, anaphylactoid react'ns. Hemolytic anemia rel. to G-6-P dehydrogenase deficiency.	**Acetaminophen:** Peak plasma concentrat'n may be incr. by probenecid. **Cephalosporin:** Renal excret'n is inhibited by probenecid. **Dapsone:** Renal excret'n may be inhibited by probenecid. **Indomethacin:** Renal excret'n may be inhibited by probenecid, resulting in incr. plasma levels. **Methotrexate:** Renal excret'n may be reduced and its plasma concentrat'n incr. by probenecid. Use concomitantly w. caution. **Para-aminosalicylic acid:** Renal excret'n may be inhibited by probenecid.	**Assess:** For pt tx of renal calculi, hyper-sensitivity, kidney disease, use of oral hypoglycemics. **Administer:** W. meals. **Evaluate:** For adv. effects (GI distur-bances, hypersensitivity), retroperitoneal pain in light of renal colic, incidence of hyperglycemia in diabetics using oral hypoglycemics. Monitor uric acid levels to maintain 3-7 mg/dL level. **Teach:** To drink large volumes of fluids, at least 12 (8-oz.) glasses (3 L)/day; to report number and frequency of attacks to physician; to continue medicat'n unless otherwise instructed by physi-cian; s/s hypersensitivity; not to take aspirin or other OTC drugs without consulting physician.

Generic Name (Trade Name)	Use (Dose)	Action	Adverse Effects	Drug Interactions	Nursing Process
				Penicillin: Renal excret'n is inhibited by probenecid. See comments under Use (Dose). **Salicylates:** Either in small or large doses, are *contraindicated* because they antagonize uricosuric action of probenecid.	
Sulfinpyrazone (Anturane)	Chronic phases of gout, both intercritical or silent stage and gouty arthritis stage. Clinical stages in which abnormal platelet behavior is a causative or assoc. factor (**Oral:** *For gout* - Days 1-2, 100 mg bid or 200 mg od; days 3-4, 200 mg bid; days 5-6, 200 mg tid; from day 7 onward, 200 mg qid)	As for probenecid	GI disturbances, aggravat'n or reactivat'n of peptic ulcer	**Hypoglycemics, oral; insulin:** May have their actions potentiated by sulfinpyrazone. **Salicylates:** May cause unpredictable, and at times serious, prolongat'n of bleeding time; in combinat'n w. sulfinpyrazone, may cause bleeding episodes. **Sulfonamide:** Action may be potentiated by sulfinpyrazone. **Warfarin:** May have its actions incr. by sulfinpyrazone.	As for probenecid

Chemotherapy

Chemotherapy is defined as the treatment of disease by chemical agents. By this definition, chemotherapy could refer to all types of drugs. At the present time, however, the expression chemotherapy refers to the administration of drugs to eradicate pathogenic bacteria, fungi, viruses, protozoans, helminths and cancer cells from the body. Section 14 discusses chemotherapy, emphasizing the various groups of drugs used, their mechanisms of action, selective toxicities, therapeutic uses, adverse effects and nursing processes.

CHAPTER 59

The Penicillins

Teaching Objectives

Following completion of this chapter, the reader should be able to:

1. Describe the mechanism of action of the penicillins.
2. List the major limitations to the use of penicillin G.
3. Describe the antibacterial spectra of the narrow-spectrum, penicillinase-resistant and expanded-spectrum penicillins.
4. Discuss the pharmacokinetics of the penicillins used in North America.
5. Discuss the major therapeutic uses of penicillin G and its semisynthetic derivatives.
6. Describe the adverse effects of the penicillins.
7. Discuss the nursing process related to the use of the penicillins.

In 1928 Fleming noted the lysis of bacteria growing in the vicinity of a contaminating mold. Perhaps no discovery in pharmacology has had such an impact on subsequent therapy. Ten years later Florey and colleagues were able to isolate from cultures of *Penicillum notatum* a crude preparation of penicillin, capable of killing several important pathogenic bacteria.

Since the introduction of penicillin G (benzylpenicillin), several derivatives have been synthesized (Table 82). The obvious differences between the various penicillins should not obscure the fact that they also have many similarities. All penicillins have the same basic chemical structure, mechanism of action and major adverse effects. This chapter will discuss the pharmacology of penicillins and the related nursing processes, emphasizing both their similarities and differences.

Mechanism of Action

Bacterial cells are encased by both cell membranes and cell walls. The cell wall lies on the outside of bacteria and is essential to the survival of the microbe. The cell membrane, found just to the inside of the cell wall, encloses the bacterium.

Bacterial cytoplasm is hypertonic. It is important to recognize this fact because it explains the necessity for a healthy cell wall. Without a rigid wall, the cell membrane cannot withstand the internal hypertonic media. If the cell wall is damaged, the high pressure within the bacterium causes the membrane first to bulge and finally to rupture, killing the bacterium. Penicillins block cell wall formation. As the old walls gradually deteriorate and are not replaced by new material, they become thinner. Eventually, they are not strong enough to support the cell membranes, which then rupture, killing the bacteria.

Table 82
Properties of some commonly used penicillins.

Name	Stability in Acid	Spectrum of Action	Sensitivity to Penicillinase	Routes of Administration
Penicillin G (benzylpenicillin penicillin)	Poor	Narrow	Sensitive	Oral, parenteral
Penicillin V (phenoxymethyl penicillin)	Good	Narrow	Sensitive	Oral
Penicillinase-Resistant Penicillins				
Methicillin	Poor	Narrow	Resistant	Parenteral
Oxacillin	Good	Narrow	Resistant	Oral, parenteral
Cloxacillin	Good	Narrow	Resistant	Oral, parenteral
Dicloxacillin	Good	Narrow	Resistant	Oral, parenteral
Flucloxacillin	Good	Narrow	Resistant	Oral
Nafcillin	Variable	Narrow	Resistant	Parenteral
Expanded-Spectrum Penicillins				
Ampicillin	Fair	Broad	Sensitive	Oral, parenteral
Amoxicillin	Good	Broad	Sensitive	Oral
Carbenicillin	Poor	Broad	Sensitive	Parenteral
Ticarcillin	Poor	Broad	Sensitive	Parenteral
Piperacillin	Poor	Broad	Sensitive	Parenteral

Antibacterial Spectra of the Penicillins

Narrow-Spectrum Penicillins

Table 83 presents the antibacterial spectra of the major penicillin groups. A discussion of the penicillins must begin with a review of penicillin G. This drug is extremely effective for the treatment of nonpenicillinase-producing cocci, gram-positive bacilli and spirochetes. However, penicillin G has three major limitations:

1. Its instability in an acid medium. Much of an oral dose is destroyed in the stomach, reducing the percentage of the dose absorbed;

2. Its inactivation by penicillinase-producing (beta-lactamase-producing) staphylococci, eliminating its use in many staphylococcal infections; and

3. Its narrow spectrum of activity, covering mainly only cocci, gram-positive bacilli and spirochetes.

Newer semisynthetic penicillins have overcome some of penicillin G's limitations. Their rational use depends on understanding how they differ from penicillin G.

Penicillin V (phenoxymethyl penicillin) has the same antibacterial spectrum as penicillin G but is more stable in the stomach and is better absorbed. Penicillin V is recommended in place of penicillin G for oral administration. Like penicillin G, it is not resistant to penicillinase and does not have an expanded spectrum of activity.

Table 83
Antibacterial spectra of the various penicillin groups.

	Narrow-Spectrum Penicillins		Expanded-Spectrum Penicillins	
	Penicillin G Penicillin V (Penicillinase-Sensitive Penicillins)	Methicillin Oxacillin, etc. (Penicillinase-Resistant Penicillins)	Ampicillin Amoxicillin	Carbenicillin Ticarcillin Piperacillin
Staphylococcus aureus (Pen.-Sens.)	+	+	+	+
Staphylococcus aureus (Pen.-Resis.)	−	+	−	−
Streptococcus pyogenes	+	+	+	+
Streptococcus pneumoniae	+	+	+	+
Enterococcus	−	−	+	−
Clostridium perfringens	+	+	+	+
Neisseria gonorrhoeae	+	±	+	+
Neisseria meningitidis	+	±	+	+
Haemophilus influenzae	−	−	±	+
Escherichia coli	−	−	±	±
Klebsiella	−	−	−	±
Proteus spp. (indole-negative)	−	−	±	+
Proteus spp. (indole-positive)	−	−	−	±
Serratla	−	−	−	±
Salmonella	−	−	+	+
Shigella	−	−	±	+
Pseudomonas aeruginosa	−	−	−	+
Bacteroides fragilis	−	−	−	±
Other bacteroides spp.	+	±	+	±
Chlamydiae	−	−	−	−
Mycobacteria pneumoniae	−	−	−	−

Legend: + = Sensitive; − = Resistant; ± = Some strains resistant. Consult text for details on the use of each group of drugs.

Penicillinase-Resistant Penicillins

Methicillin (Celbenin, Staphcillin), nafcillin (Nafcil, Nalpen, Unipen), oxacillin (Bactocil, Prostaphlin), cloxacillin (Bactopen, Cloxapen, Orbenin, Tegopen), dicloxacillin (Dycill, Dynapen, Pathocil) and flucloxacillin (Fluclox) are usually resistant to *Staphylococcus aureus*-secreted penicillinase.

Although they are active against many penicillin G-sensitive bacteria, the penicillinase-resistant drugs are not as effective as penicillins G or V. They should be used primarily to treat staphylococcal infections.

Expanded-Spectrum Penicillins — I

Ampicillin (Ampicin, Ampilean, Omnipen, Polycillin, Penbritin, Principen) and amoxicillin (Amoxil, Larotid, Polymox, Trimox) have inhibitory activity at low concentrations for all strains of S. pyogenes, S. faecalis (enterococci), S. pneumoniae and penicillin-G-sensitive S. aureus. However, it is not this activity that sets these two drugs apart from the narrow-spectrum antibiotics. Rather, it is their activity against most strains of Escherichia coli, Haemophilus influenzae, Proteus mirabilis, salmonella and shigella. Neither drug is resistant to penicillinase secreted by Staphylococcus aureus.

Bacampicillin (Penglobe, Spectrobid) and pivampicillin (Pondocillin) are inactive esters of ampicillin. Once absorbed they are hydrolyzed to ampicillin.

Expanded-Spectrum Penicillins — II

Amoxicillin has been combined with potassium clavulanate (Augmentin, Clavulin) in 2:1 or 4:1 fixed-ratio dosage forms. Amoxicillin is susceptible to hydrolysis by beta-lactamase enzymes; therefore, bacteria that secrete beta-lactamases are resistant to the antibiotic. Potassium clavulanate, or clavulanic acid, inhibits beta-lactamases secreted by some micro-organisms. By inhibiting these beta-lactamases, clavulanic acid protects amoxicillin from hydrolysis and enables it to act against micro-organisms that would normally be resistant to the antibiotic. Thus, clavulanic acid increases the spectrum of activity of amoxicillin to include beta-lactamase-producing Haemophilus influenzae, Haemophilus ducreyi, Neisseria gonorrhoeae, Staphylococcus aureus, and Branhamella catarrhalis. Concentrations attained in the urine will inhibit many beta-lactamase-producing strains of Escherichia coli, klebsiella, proteus and citrobacter.

Although Augmentin or Clavulin is a good product, it is more expensive than amoxicillin, and it is reasonable to ask when it should be used in place of amoxicillin. The combination should not displace amoxicillin or penicillin G for the treatment of gonococcal urethritis in regions of the world in which beta-lactamase-producing Neisseria gonorrhoeae are nonendemic. In regions where the incidence of penicillinase-producing Neisseria gonorrhoeae reaches five to ten per cent, Augmentin or

Clavulin should be considered one of the alternatives to the penicillins. The penicillinase-resistant penicillins are still indicated for gram-positive soft-tissue infections, unless resistant gram-negative rods are also present. Augmentin or Clavulin is probably not indicated at this time for the treatment of simple urinary tract infections that will respond to single-dose amoxicillin therapy. The combination of amoxicillin and potassium clavulanate appears suitable for the treatment of complicated urinary tract infections, otitis media, sinusitis and respiratory tract infections caused by beta-lactamase-producing strains of the previously mentioned bacteria.

Expanded-Spectrum Penicillins: Group III — Anti-Pseudomonal Penicillins

Azlocillin (Azlin), carbenicillin (Geopen, Pyopen), mezlocillin (Mezlin), piperacillin (Pipracil) and ticarcillin (Ticar) are effective in higher concentrations against most strains of Pseudomonas aeruginosa and indole-positive and indole-negative proteus species, which is their primary use. However, their spectrum of activity also covers many other bacteria (Table 83). They should be used primarily with an aminoglycoside antibiotic such as gentamicin, tobramycin, amikacin or netilmicin to treat infections caused by pseudomonas and proteus.

Expanded-Spectrum Penicillins: Group IV — Amidino Penicillins

Amdinocillin or mecillinam (Coactin) has a different spectrum of activity from other beta-lactam antibiotics, in that it is active primarily against gram-negative organisms and relatively ineffective against gram-positive organisms. Amdinocillin pivoxil, also known as pivmecillinam (Selexid), is a prodrug of amdinocillin or mecillinam that is converted to the microbiologically active amdinocillin or mecillinam during absorption from the gastrointestinal tract. Amdinocillin pivoxil is indicated in the treatment of acute and chronic urinary tract infections caused by sensitive strains of E. coli, klebsiella species, enterobacter species and proteus species.

Pharmacokinetics of the Penicillins

Most penicillins are destroyed, at least in part, by stomach acid and are not completely absorbed following ingestion. Approximately one-third of an oral dose of penicillin G is absorbed from the gastrointestinal tract, primarily from the duodenum. For maximum absorption, it should be taken either one hour before or two to three hours after a meal to facilitate rapid transport from the stomach to the duodenum. Under these conditions, peak blood levels are reached in about forty-five minutes.

Because penicillin G is poorly absorbed from the gastrointestinal tract, it should normally be administered intramuscularly. Thus injected, penicillin G attains peak blood levels within fifteen minutes. Procaine penicillin G or benzathine penicillin G given intramuscularly are absorbed more slowly; peak blood levels are seen two to four hours after procaine penicillin G, with concentrations falling to almost zero twenty-four hours later. Benzathine penicillin G produces very low serum levels of the antibiotic for three to four weeks after administration and must be used only to treat extremely sensitive bacteria. Figure 27 compares the blood levels of penicillin G following its oral and intramuscular administration.

Penicillin V is more stable than penicillin G in an acid pH and is better absorbed from the

Figure 27
Schematic presentation of the blood concentration of various forms of penicillin G, plotted as a function of time after oral or intramuscular administration.

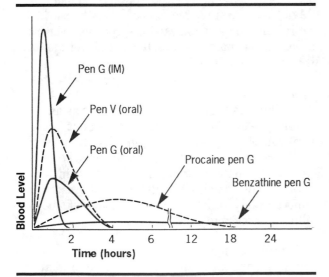

gastrointestinal tract. As it has the same antibacterial spectrum as penicillin G, penicillin V is preferred for oral administration. It should be given on an empty stomach.

The penicillinase-resistant penicillins vary in their absorption following oral administration. Methicillin is not stable in the stomach and must be injected. Nafcillin is absorbed quite erratically and should not be given orally. All other penicillinase-resistant penicillins can be taken orally. Cloxacillin has been the drug of choice for many physicians. It is prepared in both oral and parenteral dosage forms, provides effective therapeutic levels and is usually marketed at a reasonable cost. Although dicloxacillin and flucloxacillin produce higher blood levels following oral administration, they have not been shown to be clinically more effective than cloxacillin.

Both ampicillin and amoxicillin may be given orally. Ampicillin is not completely absorbed and should be taken on an empty stomach to reduce acid inactivation. Amoxicillin enjoys the major advantage of being stable in an acid pH. It is usually preferred because it is well absorbed when given orally, both in the presence and absence of food. As a result, amoxicillin is usually taken three times daily with meals, as opposed to ampicillin, which is ingested four times daily on an empty stomach. Because of its improved absorption, amoxicillin causes less severe diarrhea than ampicillin and is better accepted by many patients.

Carbenicillin, ticarcillin and piperacillin must be injected to produce a systemic effect. Although carbenicillin is not absorbed when given orally, its indanyl sodium derivative (Geocillin, Geopen Oral) can be given by mouth for the treatment of urinary tract infections caused by pseudomonas. The circulating levels of antibiotic following carbenicillin indanyl sodium are too low to treat a systemic infection.

The penicillins are distributed widely throughout the body but their passage into joint, ocular and cerebrospinal fluids is poor in the absence of inflammation. In the patient with inflamed meninges, however, they will enter the cerebrospinal fluid. It is this factor that enables penicillin G to treat meningitis caused by sensitive organisms.

All penicillins are rapidly excreted by the kidney. They undergo renal tubular secretion and, with renal clearance values of approximately 600 mL/min, have half-lives in the vicinity of one hour. Probenecid (Benemid) reduces penicillin excretion. The use of probenecid with either procaine penicillin or ampicillin for the treatment of gonorrhea is discussed later.

Therapeutic Uses

The preceding pages have considered the antibacterial activity of the penicillins. At this point it is appropriate to consider some of the more common clinical conditions that may be treated with these drugs. More complete dosing information can be obtained from Table 86.

Streptococcal Infections

Most beta-hemolytic group A streptococci and pneumococci are extremely sensitive to the penicillins. During the nearly forty years that penicillin G has been available, there has been no clinically significant development of resistance on the part of streptococci to this antibiotic. High doses of penicillin G are used to treat pneumococcal meningitis. Pharyngitis caused by group A streptococci usually responds rapidly to oral penicillin V. Penicillins G or V are effective for prophylaxis of rheumatic fever. Bacterial endocarditis, caused by streptococci of the viridans group, can be treated with intravenous penicillin G, given either alone or with streptomycin.

Staphylococcal Infections

Penicillin G, penicillin V, ampicillin and amoxicillin are sensitive to beta-lactamase (penicillinase) secreted by *Staphylococcus aureus* and should not be used to treat infections caused by this pathogen. In their place, penicillinase-resistant penicillins — methicillin, nafcillin, oxacillin, cloxacillin, dicloxacillin and flucloxacillin — should be given. Cloxacillin is usually the drug of choice for the treatment of staphylococcal-induced bacteremia, as well as tissue infections such as cellulitis, osteomyelitis and pneumonia.

Gonorrhea

Penicillin G is still the drug of choice for the treatment of gonorrhea. A currently recommended treatment for uncomplicated gonorrhea is one gram of probenecid administered at least thirty minutes before 4.8 million units of aqueous procaine penicillin G, intramuscularly. Alternatively, uncomplicated gonorrhea can be treated with a single one-gram dose of probenecid, given simultaneously with oral ampicillin (3.5 g) or amoxicillin (3.0 g). Gonococcal arthritis, disseminated gonococcal infections and those complicated by salpingitis, prostatitis or epididymitis should be treated with high doses of aqueous crystalline penicillin G.

Syphilis

Patients with primary, secondary, or latent syphilis of less than one year's duration can be treated effectively in a single visit with 2.4 million units of benzathine penicillin G, intramuscularly. For infections of more than one year's duration, patients can be treated weekly for three weeks with 2.4 million units of benzathine penicillin G, intramuscularly.

Anaerobic Infections

Penicillin G is active against several anaerobic bacteria. It has been used to treat anaerobic brain and lung abscesses. Actinomycosis and clostridial infections, such as tetanus and gas gangrene, also respond to penicillin G treatment. Abdominal infections are often caused by *Bacteroides fragilis,* which is resistant to penicillin G. It responds to clindamycin, metronidazole and cefoxitin. Fusobacterial infections produce trench mouth and usually respond to penicillin G treatment.

Haemophilus influenzae Infections

Haemophilus influenzae is not sensitive to penicillin G. Ampicillin or amoxicillin may be used to treat infections caused by this bacterium. In cases of meningitis, osteomyelitis, epiglotitis, pneumonia and septic arthritis, ampicillin may be given intravenously. *Haemophilus influenzae* resistance to ampicillin and amoxicillin is increasing. For resistant strains, cefaclor (Ceclor), trimethoprim plus sulfamethoxazole (Bactrim, Septra) or erythromycin-sulfisoxazole (Pediazole) may be used orally. If parenteral therapy is required, the second-generation cephalosporins cefamandole (Mandol) and cefuroxime (Zinacef) may be used. Third-generation cephalosporins, such as cefoperazone, may be more effective, but the cost of therapy is almost prohibitive.

Typhoid Fever

Ampicillin has been used for many years as an alternative to chloramphenicol for systemic infections caused by *Salmonella typhi*. Six grams daily of ampicillin for one to three months have been used to eliminate the typhoid carrier state in patients who do not have gall bladder disease. Unfortunately, resistance to ampicillin and amoxicillin is increasing.

Urinary Tract Infections

Ampicillin and amoxicillin are still used to treat acute urinary tract infections. However, *Escherichia coli, Proteus mirabilis* and enterococci are becoming increasingly resistant to these drugs. Urinary tract infections caused by *Pseudomonas aeruginosa* and indole-positive proteus can be treated with the indanyl ester of carbenicillin (Geocillin, Geocillin).

Adverse Effects

Allergic reactions are the major concern with the penicillins. They may occur in one to five per cent of patients. Patients allergic to one penicillin should be considered allergic to all penicillins. Allergic reactions vary from skin eruptions to anaphylactic shock and death. Anaphylaxis is more common when parenteral administration is used. Table 84 summarizes allergic reactions to the penicillins.

Table 84
Allergic reactions to penicillins.

Immediate Allergic Reactions
(occur 2 - 30 min after penicillin administration)

Urticaria
Flushing
Diffuse pruritus
Hypotension or shock
Laryngeal edema
Wheezing

Accelerated Urticarial Reactions (1 - 71 h)

Urticaria or pruritus
Wheezing or laryngeal edema
Local inflammatory reactions

Late Allergic Reactions (> 72 h)

Morbilliform eruptions (occasionally occur as early as 18 h
    after initiation of penicillin therapy)
Urticarial eruptions
Erythematous eruptions
Recurrent urticaria and arthralgia
Local inflammatory reactions

Some Relatively Unusual Late Reactions

Immunohemolytic anemia
Drug fever
Acute renal insufficiency
Thrombocytopenia

It is possible to test patients for their sensitivities to penicillin G or its semisynthetic derivatives. Benzylpenicilloyl-poly-L-lysine (BPO-PL) is a major antigenic determinant of benzylpenicillin. When used in a concentration of 6×10^{-5} M, together with 2×10^{-2} M of a benzylpenicillin minor determinant mixture (BP-MDM), it can predict about ninety-five per cent of penicillin IgE-mediated hypersensitivity reactions. BPO-PL and BP-MDM are safer and more reliable as a test for hypersensitivity than the alternate approach of injecting small doses of penicillin G. Nevertheless, prick tests should be performed intradermally before administering the test product to reduce the risk of anaphylaxis.

Given orally, the penicillins may produce gastrointestinal upset, nausea, vomiting and diarrhea. Ampicillin is particularly notorious for the burning diarrhea it causes. Amoxicillin is better tolerated. As troublesome as it may be, the diarrhea seen a few days after starting ampicillin should not be confused with the potentially fatal complication of pseudomembranous colitis. This condition is caused by the proliferation of *Clostridium difficile,* secondary to suppression of normal intestinal flora, and can occur later in a course of therapy.

Carbenicillin and ticarcillin are formulated as their disodium salts. Large doses can contribute significantly to the sodium load in patients with impaired sodium excretory mechanism (e.g., those with renal, cardiac or liver disease). Although azlocillin, mezlocillin (Mezlin) and piperacillin are prepared as the monosodium salts, they too can contribute significantly to the sodium load of patients. These drugs can also produce hypokalemia. In addition, they interfere with platelet function and may cause bleeding. The antipseudomonal penicillins are chemically incompatible with aminoglycoside antibiotics (such as amikacin, gentamicin, netilmicin and tobramycin) and must not be mixed in the same injection fluid with any of the latter drugs.

Nursing Process

The nursing process for patients receiving a penicillin is essentially the same regardless of the penicillin used or its route of administration. Penicillin G will be used here as the model for discussion of the nursing process initiated by the prescription and use of any penicillin. Unique features of the nursing care related to individual types of penicillin are included in Table 85 at the end of this chapter.

Assessment
Following the prescription of penicillin, nurses must review the patient's history for evidence of previous penicillin hypersensitivity and renal or liver pathology. Nurses should also review blood studies for red and white blood cell counts, hematocrit and hemoglobin, and bleeding time. If evidence of hypersensitivity is found, penicillin must *not* be given. A history of allergies (e.g., hayfever, asthma

or dermatitis) requires skin testing of the patient for sensitivity to penicillin prior to the administration of the first dose. Laboratory specimens for culture and sensitivity must be collected before administering the first dose. Physical assessment of the patient by the nurse must establish the baseline temperature and document observable indicators of the infection.

Administration
With the exception of amoxicillin, all commonly used oral forms of the penicillins must be given on an empty stomach, i.e., either one hour before eating or two to three hours following eating, to facilitate absorption. Oral suspensions of penicillin must be stored in a refrigerator to prevent deterioration. Regardless of the route of administration, penicillin must be administered at regular intervals around the clock to maintain adequate blood levels of the drug.

Parenteral administration is preferred during the early phases of treatment of severe infections. Preparations should be reconstituted according to the manufacturer's instructions and used before the expiry date. Intramuscular injections are given deep into the upper outer quadrant of the gluteus maximus and the procedure must include careful aspiration on the barrel of the syringe. Accidental intravenous injection of procaine penicillin G has resulted in pulmonary infarction and death. Injection of the solution into the muscle should be done slowly to reduce irritation and pain.

Long-acting forms of penicillin are administered *only* intramuscularly. Their injection sites must not be massaged because this hastens dispersal, increases the rate of absorption and contributes to the development of sterile abscesses at the injection site. Because of chemical incompatability with other drugs, parenteral penicillins are not normally mixed in the same injection or infusion fluid with other drugs without the advice of a pharmacist.

Evaluation
Following the administration of a penicillin nurses must observe the patient for improvement. This includes lowered body temperature.

Nurses must observe patients carefully for penicillin allergy. Nursing evaluation should stress observation for black furry tongue, nausea or diarrhea. These are symptoms of superinfections caused by the overgrowth of nonsensitive normal body flora in the gastrointestinal tract, particularly in the mouth and bowel.

Teaching
Patients taking penicillin at home should be advised of the indicators of drug efficacy and adverse effects. Patients should be told report any evidence of diarrhea.

They must be taught that failure to complete the entire course of therapy may lead to the development of resistant strains of bacteria. The resulting relapse may be difficult to treat. Therefore, even asymptomatic patients must continue to take the penicillin for the length of time specified. Patients should also be instructed to take penicillin at the prescribed times. Nurses should instruct patients to discard unused medication at the completion of the course of therapy so that they will not be tempted to self-medicate with outdated penicillin in the future.

Patients with identified penicillin allergies should be advised to wear or carry medical identification.

Further Reading
Choice of antimicrobial drugs (1986). *The Medical Letter 28* : 33-40.

Penicillin allergy (1988). *The Medical Letter 30* :79-80.

Rotschafer, J.C. and Scheife, R.T. (1988). Resistant staphylococci: Concern of the 1980s. *Pharmacotherapy 8* (No. 6, Part 2):1S-25S.

Todd, B. (1989). Antibiotics: Interactions with maintenance medications. *Geriatric Nursing 9* (6):364-365.

Todd, P.A. and Benfield, P. (1990). Amoxicillin/clavulanic acid: An update of its antibacterial activity, pharmacokinetic properties and therapeutic use. *Drugs 39* :264-307.

Treatment of sexually transmitted disease (1990). *The Medical Letter 32* :5-9.

Treatment of sexually transmitted diseases (1986). *The Medical Letter 28* :23-28.

Table 85
The penicillins.

Generic Name (Trade Name)	Use	Action	Adverse Effects	Drug Interactions	Nursing Process

Pharmacologic Classification: Antibiotics — Narrow-Spectrum Penicillins (for doses, consult Table 86)

Generic Name (Trade Name)	Use	Action	Adverse Effects	Drug Interactions	Nursing Process
1. Penicillin G, benzylpenicillin 2. Penicillin V, phenoxymethyl penicillin (Ledercillin VK, Pen-Vee K, Pfizerpen VK, Uticillin VK, V-Cillin K, Veetids)	Tx of infect'ns caused by susceptible strains of gram-neg. cocci, incl. groups A, B and nonenterococcal group D streptococci; S. viridans; S. pneumoniae. Drug of choice for sensitive gram-neg. cocci, incl. N. meningitidis and N. gonorrhœæ. Also preferred for infect'ns caused by certain gram-pos. bacilli, incl. B. anthracis and most strains of C. diphtheriæ and L. monocytogenes; some gram-neg. bacilli, incl. B. monilitrichia bucallis and Spirillum minor; certain anaerobic species such as Actinomyces israelii, most species of Bacteroides [except B. fragilis], clostridia, fusobacterium and peptostreptococcus; and various spirochetes, incl. Treponema pallidum, T. pertenue and leptospira.	The penicillins inhibit format'n of bacterial cell walls, w. preferential effects on crossseptum format'n. The result is a gradual reduct'n in the structural strength of the wall. A point is reached when the weakened wall is no longer able to protect the cytoplasmic membrane. Under stress from high internal osmotic pressure, the membrane first bulges and ruptures. Penicillin G should be injected to have max. effect. If taken orally, only 20-33% dose of penicillin G is absorbed. Penicillin V differs from penicillin G in that it is better absorbed when taken orally and is preferred over penicillin G when oral tx is desired.	See Table 84. Nausea, vomiting, diarrhea, suppress'n of normal bacterial intestinal flora; Na-overload w. carbenicillin, ticarcillin or piperacillin	**Aminoglycosides:** Cannot be mixed w. antipseudomonal penicillins. If any of these penicillins are mixed in the same IV infus'n as an aminoglycoside, they will impair the antibacterial activity of the latter. **Probenecid:** Reduces renal tubular secret'n of all penicillins. When given tog. w. a penicillin, it incr. the half-life of the penicillin.	**Assess:** For hx penicillin hypersensitivity, allergies (hayfever, asthma, atopic dermatitis), renal pathology. Gather specimens for culture and sensitivity tests prior to administering 1st dose. Establish baseline temp. and s/s infect'n. **Administer:** *Orally* - On empty stomach; at equal intervals ATC. Store oral suspens'ns in fridge. *Parenterally* - For severe infect'ns in acute phase from unexpired vial; deep IM into gluteus maximus; aspirate carefully; give long-acting forms *IM only*. Do not massage inject'n site of long-acting forms. **Evaluate:** For temp. reduct'n and alleviat'n of objective s/s infect'n; for allergic react'ns (see Table 84); for superinfect'n of nonsensitive normal flora of GI tract. **Teach:** To complete entire course of tx, even though asymptomatic; to discard unused medicat'n; to comply w. prescribed dosage schedule; pts w. penicillin allergies to wear or carry medical ID; to self-evaluate for drug efficacy and adv. effects.

Generic Name (Trade Name)	Use	Action	Adverse Effects	Drug Interactions	Nursing Process
Pharmacologic Classification: Antibiotics — Antistaphylococcal Penicillins (for doses, consult Table 86)					
1. Oxacillin (Bactocil, Prostaphlin)	These drugs are us. resistant to beta-lactamase [penicillinase] secreted by Staphylococcus aureus. Although they are effective against many penicillin-G-sensitive bacteria, the antistaphylococcal penicillins are not so effective as penicillins G or V, and should be used primarily to treat staphylococcal infect'ns.	As for penicillin G	As for penicillin G	As for penicillin G	As for penicillin G
2. Cloxacillin (Cloxapen, Orbenin, Tegopen)		As for penicillin G	As for penicillin G	As for penicillin G	As for penicillin G
3. Dicloxacillin (Dycill, Dynapen)		As for penicillin G	As for penicillin G	As for penicillin G	As for penicillin G
4. Flucloxacillin (Fluclox)		As for penicillin G	As for penicillin G	As for penicillin G	As for penicillin G
5. Nafcillin sodium (Nafcil, Unipen)	As for penicillin G	As for penicillin G	As for penicillin G	As for penicillin G	As for penicillin G
Pharmacologic Classification: Antibiotics — Expanded-Spectrum Penicillins, Group I (for doses, consult Table 86)					
1. Ampicillin (Amcill, Omnipen, Penbritin, Polycillin, Totacillin)	The narrow-spectrum and antistaphylococcal penicillins are inactive against most gram-negative bacilli. These expanded-spectrum penicillins are active against gram-pos. and many gram-neg. bacteria. They are not resistant to penicillinase secreted by S. aureus. Amoxicillin is the drug of choice; it is better absorbed than ampicillin and cheaper than bacampicillin and pivampicillin.	As for penicillin G	As for penicillin G, above. Diarrhea is a problem, particularly w. ampicillin. It is encountered less frequently and is not so severe w. the other expanded-spectrum penicillins.	As for penicillin G	*As for penicillin G, plus:* **Administer:** Reconstituted parenteral solut'n within 1 h; discard unused solut'n immediately.
2. Amoxicillin (Amoxil, Larotid, Polymox, Trimox, Wymox)		As for penicillin G	As for penicillin G	As for penicillin G	*As for penicillin G, plus:* **Administer:** May be given w. food.
3. Bacampicillin (Penglobe, Spectrobid)		As for penicillin G	As for penicillin G	As for penicillin G	As for amoxicillin
4. Pivampicillin (Pondicillin)	As for penicillin G	As for penicillin G	As for penicillin G	As for penicillin G	As for amoxicillin

Pharmacologic Classification: Antibiotics — Expanded-Spectrum Penicillin, Group II (for doses, consult Table 86)

Drug				
Amoxicillin + clavulanic acid (Augmentin, Clavulin)	An alternative to the penicillins. Appears suitable for complicated urinary tract infect'ns, otitis media, sinusitis and respiratory tract infect'ns caused by beta-lactamase-producing strains of bacteria (listed under Action).	Clavulanic acid is a potent inhibitor of many bacterial beta-lactamase enzymes. It incr. amoxicillin's spectrum to incl. beta-lactamase-producing *H. influenzae, H. ducreyi, N. gonorrhœæ, S. aureus* and *B. catarrhalis.* Concentrat'ns in urine will inhibit many beta-lactamase-producing strains of *E. coli,* klebsiella, proteus and citrobacter.	As for penicillin G and amoxicillin	As for penicillin G

Pharmacologic Classification: Antibiotics — Expanded-Spectrum Penicillins, Group III: Antipseudomonal Penicillins (for doses, consult Table 86)

Drug				
1. Carbenicillin disodium (Geopen, Geocillin)	These penicillins are effective in higher concentrat'ns against most strains of *Pseudomonas æruginosa* and indole-pos. proteus spp. They should be used primarily w. an aminoglycoside antibiotic.	As for penicillin G	As for penicillin G	As for *penicillin G, plus:* **Evaluate:** For electrolyte imbalance, peripheral edema, sudden weight gain, dyspnea.
2. Mezlocillin sodium (Mezlin)	As for carbenicillin	As for penicillin G	As for penicillin G	As for carbenicillin
3. Piperacillin sodium (Pipracil)	As for carbenicillin	As for penicillin G	As for penicillin G	As for carbenicillin
4. Ticarcillin disodium (Ticar)	As for carbenicillin	As for penicillin G	As for penicillin G	As for carbenicillin

Pharmacologic Classification: Antibiotics — Expanded-Spectrum Penicillins, Group IV: Amidino Penicillins (for doses, consult Table 86)

Generic Name (Trade Name)	Use	Action	Adverse Effects	Drug Interactions	Nursing Process
1. Amdinocillin mecillinam (Coactin)	These penicillins act primarily against gram-neg. organisms and are relatively ineffective against gram-pos. organisms.	As for penicillin G.	As for penicillin G.	As for penicillin G.	The Nsg Process for amdinocillin is the same as that for penicillin G, w. the following caution: **Assess:** Fluid intake/output ratio; report hematuria or oliguria; monitor BUN and creatinine to identify poss. nephrotoxicity.
2. Amdinocillin pivoxil, pivmecillinam (Selexid)	Amdinocillin pivoxil, also known as pivmecillinam, is a prodrug of amdinocillin or mecillinam that is converted to the microbiologically active amdinocillin during absorpt'n through the GI tract. Amdinocillin pivoxil is indicated in tx of acute and chronic urinary tract infect'ns caused by sensitve strains of E. coli, klebsiella spp., enterobacter spp. and proteus spp.				

Table 86
Doses of the penicillins.

(For reasons of space, it is not possible to provide dosages for patients with renal impairment. It is recommended that readers refer to the manufacturers' monographs to obtain that information.)

Generic Name (Trade Name)	Dose
Pharmacologic Classification: Antibiotics — Narrow-Spectrum Penicillins	
Penicillin G sodium, penicillin G potassium	**Oral:** Adults - 400 000 - 500 000 IU q 6-8 h; max. dose, 20 million IU/day. Children < 12 years - 25 000 - 90 000 IU/kg/day in 3-6 divided doses. (Note: Penicillin G is not recommended for oral administrat'n. When oral use is required, penicillin V should be used.) **IM/IV:** Adults - Min. 300 000 - 1.2 million IU/day. For IV infus'n, max. 20 - 30 million IU/day may be given. Children - For IV infus'n, min. 25 000 - 50 000 IU/kg/day; max. dose, 10 million IU/day. *For prophylaxis against recurrent Group A beta-hemolytic streptococcal infect'ns in pts who have had rheumatic fever and/or chorea:* **Oral:** 200 000 - 250 000 IU bid on continuing basis. (Note: If oral penicillin is preferred, penicillin V should be used.) *For prophylaxis of bacterial endocarditis in pts w. rheumatic or congenital heart lesions before dental or upper respiratory tract surgery or instrumentat'n:* **IM/IV:** Adults - 2 million IU aq. penicillin G 30-60 min prior to procedure and 1 million IU 6 h later. Children - 50 000 IU/kg aq. penicillin G 30-60 min prior to procedure and 25 000 IU/kg 6 h later.
Procaine penicillin G	**IM:** Adults - 900 000 - 1.2 million IU/day. Children - 600 000 - 900 000 IU/day. Dosage may be repeated at intervals of 48-72 h.
Penicillin V, phenoxymethyl penicillin	**Oral:** Adults - 125-500 mg q 4-6 h. Children - 25-50 mg/kg/day in divided doses q 6-8 h. Treat streptococcal pharyngitis for 10 days. *To prevent bacterial endocarditis in pts w. rheumatic or congenital heart lesions before dental surgery, upper respiratory tract surgery or instrumentat'n:* **Oral:** Adults - 2 g 1 h prior to procedure, then 1 g 6 h later. Children > 27 kg -Full adult dose; < 27 kg -1 g 1 h before procedure, then 500 mg 6 h later.
Pharmacologic Classification: Antibiotics — Antistaphylococcal Penicillins	
Cloxacillin (Bactopen, Cloxapen, Orbenin, Tegopen)	**Oral:** Adults - 250-500 mg q 6 h. Children ≤ 20 kg - 50-100 mg/kg/day in 4 equal doses q 6 h. **IM/IV:** Adults - 250-500 mg q 6 h. Children ≤ 5 kg - 125-250 mg/day divided equally into 4 doses; 5-40 kg - 25-50 mg/kg/day in 4 equal doses q 6 h. Incr. IV dosage in serious infect'ns.
Dicloxacillin (Dycill, Dynapen, Pathocil)	*For mild to moderate infect'ns:* **Oral:** Adults - 125 mg qid. Children - 12.5 mg/kg/day in equal doses qid. Larger doses (≥ 25 mg/kg/day) may be required for severe infect'ns. Children > 20 kg should be given adult dose. *For severe infect'ns:* **Oral:** Adults - 250 mg qid. Larger/more frequent doses may be required for very severe infect'ns.
Flucloxacillin (Fluclox)	**Oral:** Adults - 250-500 mg q 6 h. Children < 12 years and ≤ 40 kg - 125-250 mg q 6 h or 25-50 mg/kg/day in divided doses q 6 h; ≤ 6 months - 25 mg/kg/day in divided doses q 6 h. These dosages should not > recomm. adult dosage. (Note: Upper dosage levels should be reserved for use in serious infect'ns.)
Sodium nafcillin (Nafcil, Nallpen, Unipen)	Parenterally, initially, in severe infect'ns; institute oral antibiotic tx as soon as clinical situat'n warrants. **IV:** Adults - 500 mg q 4 h; double dose prn. **IM:** 500 mg by deep intragluteal inject'n q 4-6 h, depending on severity of infect'n. Infants and children - 24 mg/kg od-bid. Tx should be continued for at least 48 h after pt has become afebrile and asymptomatic, and cultures are negative.

Generic Name (Trade Name)	Use (Dose)	Action	Adverse Effects	Drug Interactions	Nursing Process
Pharmacologic Classification: Antibiotics — Expanded-Spectrum Penicillins, Group I					
Ampicillin (Amcil, Ampicin, Ampilean, Omnipen, Penbritin, Polycillin, Principen)	Give oral doses preferably 1 h ac. Adults and children > 20 kg - For ENT and respiratory tract infect'ns: **Oral/IM/IV:** 250 mg q 6 h. *For GU and GI infect'ns:* **Oral:** 500 mg q 6-8 h. **IM/IV:** 250-500 mg q 6-8 h. For more severe infect'ns, these doses should be incr. or doubled. IM form of ampicillin is not recomm. for severe infect'ns such as septicemia and meningitis, for which higher serum levels of drug are desirable. *For bacterial meningitis:* **IV:** 8-14 g/day divided equally and admin. q 4-6 h ATC. Children - *For respiratory, GU or GI infect'ns:* **Oral:** ≤ 5 kg - 250-500 mg/day; 5-20 kg - 25-100 mg/kg/day. **IM/IV:** ≤ 5 kg - 200 mg/day; 5-20 kg - 25-50 mg/kg/day. *For bacterial meningitis:* A total daily dose of 200-400 mg/kg given IV, divided equally and admin. q 4-6 h ATC until recovery is ensured. Dosage may then be given IM, depending on indiv. pt response.				
Amoxicillin (Amoxil, Larotid, Polymox, Trimox)	**Oral:** Adults - 250-500 mg q 8 h. *For urethritis due to nonbeta-lactamase-producing N. gonorrhœæ:* 3 g as single dose. Children - 25-40 mg/kg/day in divided doses q 8 h. Dosage should not > recomm. adult dosage.				
Bacampicillin (Penglobe, Spectrobid)	*For upper respiratory tract, urinary tract, skin and soft tissue infect'ns:* **Oral:** Adults - 400-800 mg bid. *For lower respiratory tract infect'ns:* **Oral:** Adults - 800 -1 600 mg bid.				
Pivampicillin (Pondocillin)	**Oral:** Adults and children > 10 years - 500 mg bid; double dose in severe infect'ns. *For gonococcal urethritis:* 1.5 g as single dose, w. 1 g probenecid concurrently. Children < 1 year - 40-60 mg/kg/day; > 1 year - 25 mg/kg/day.				
Pharmacologic Classification: Antibiotics — Expanded-Spectrum Penicillins, Group II					
Amoxicillin + potassium clavulanate (Augmentin, Clavulin)	*For upper respiratory tract, GU, skin and soft tissue infect'ns:* **Oral:** Adults - 1 Clavulin or Augmentin-250 tab to 1 Clavulin-500F or Augmentin-500 tab q 8 h. *For lower respiratory tract infect'ns:* **Oral:** Adults - 1 Clavulin-500F or Augmentin-500 tab q 8 h. Children - 25-50 mg/kg/day of Clavulin or Augmentin in equally divided doses q 8 h. *For otitis media and lower respiratory tract infect'ns:* 50 mg/kg/day of Clavulin or Augmentin in divided doses q 8 h.				
Pharmacologic Classification: Antibiotics — Expanded-Spectrum Penicillins, Group III (Antipseudomonal Penicillins)					
Carbenicillin disodium (Geopen, Pyopen)	**IV:** Adults - *For severe and overwhelming infect'ns:* 300-400 mg/kg/day by inject'n or infus'n, w. or without 1 g probenecid (orally) tid. *For moderately severe infect'ns, such as urinary tract infect'ns:* 1 g q 4 h for 5-10 days. Children - 100-300 mg/kg/day.				
Carbenicillin indanyl sodium (Geocillin, Geopen Oral)	Admin. oral doses ac or not < 2 h pc to maximize absorp'n. For tx acute and chronic infect'ns of upper and lower urinary tract and in asymptomatic bacteriuria due to susceptible bacteria: **Oral:** Adults - 0.5-1 g qid. *For acute E. coli urinary tract infect'ns:* 500 mg qid. If doses > 1 g qid are required, consider parenteral carbenicillin tx.				
Mezlocillin sodium (Mezlin)	**IM:** Adults - *For uncomplicated urinary tract infect'ns:* 1.5-2 g q 6 h. *For uncomplicated gonorrhea:* 1-2 g as single dose 30 min after administra'n of probenecid 1 g, orally. **IV:** Adults - *For severe lower respiratory tract, intra-abdominal, GYN, skin and skin-structure infect'ns or septicemia:* 4 g q 6 h or 3 g q 4 h. *For life-threatening infect'ns:* May incr. dosage to 4 g q 4 h.				

Piperacillin sodium (Pipracil)	**IV:** *For serious Infect'ns:* 3-4 g q 4-6 h as a 20- to 30-min infus'n. *For complicated urinary tract infect'ns:* 8-16 g/day, admin. q 6-8 h. **IM/IV:** *For uncomplicated urinary tract infect'ns and most community-acquired pneumonias:* 6-8 g/day, admin. q 6-12 h. *For uncomplicated gonorrhea:* 2 g IM as single dose 30 min after 1 g probenecid orally.
Ticarcillin disodium (Ticar)	**IV:** *For severe systemic infect'ns:* Adults - 200-300 mg/kg/day in divided doses q 3, 4 or 6 h. Children < 40 kg - 200-300 mg/kg/day by infus'n in divided doses q 4-6 h. *For severe urinary tract infect'ns:* Adults - 150-200 mg/kg/day in divided doses q 4-6 h. Children < 40 kg - 150-200 mg/kg/day by infus'n in divided doses q 4-6 h. *For uncomplicated urinary tract infect'ns:* **IM/IV:** Adults - 1 g q 6 h. Children < 40 kg - 50-100 mg/kg/day in divided doses q 6-8 h.

Pharmacologic Classification: Antibiotics — Expanded-Spectrum Penicillins, Group IV (Amidino Penicillins)

Amdinocillin (Coactin)	**IM/IV:** Adults - 10 mg/kg q 4-6 h.
Amdinocillin pivoxil, pivmecillinam HCl (Selexid)	**Oral:** *For uncomplicated cystitis and urethritis:* 400-800 mg daily in 2-3 equal divided doses. *For chronic recurrent urinary tract infect'ns:* 400 mg tid-qid.

CHAPTER 60

The Cephalosporins

Teaching Objectives

Following completion of this chapter, the reader should be able to:

1. List some of the desirable properties of cephalosporins.
2. Summarize the disadvantages of cephalosporins.
3. Describe the mechanism of action of cephalosporins.
4. Discuss the pharmacokinetics of cephalosporins.
5. Describe the antibacterial spectra of the first-, second- and third-generation cephalosporins.
6. Discuss the therapeutic uses and adverse effects of cephalosporins and the nursing process related to their administration.

Perhaps no group of drugs has had so mundane a beginning as the cephalosporins. Imagine a group of antibiotics springing out of a bed of sewage. Yet that is exactly the story. In 1945 the Italian scientist Guiseppe Brotzu isolated a strain of *Cephalosporium acremonium* from sea water near the sewage outlet in Cagliari, Sardinia. This strain secreted a substance that was inhibitory to a group of other organisms, including staphylococci, salmonellae, pasteurellae, brucellae, vibrios and shigellae. Over the next ten to fifteen years, scientists made the very long step from the septic tank to the patient's body and developed the cephalosporin antibiotics, capable of killing a wide range of pathogenic bacteria.

Before discussing the cephalosporins in greater detail, we should list some of their desirable properties.

1. They are bactericidal. In this respect, cephalosporins are similar to the penicillins.
2. They are relatively resistant to hydrolysis by beta-lactamases produced by *Staphylococcus aureus*. These are the enzymes most commonly called penicillinases when they attack penicillins. By withstanding their attack, cephalosporins are similar to penicillinase-resistant penicillins.
3. They possess an expanded spectrum of activity that includes both bacteria killed by penicillin G and several species of penicillin-G-resistant bacilli, including *Escherichia coli, Klebsiella pneumoniae* and *Proteus mirabilis*. Their spectrum of activity has been expanded further by the arrival of second- and third-generation cephalosporins.
4. They have a high therapeutic index. Allergic reactions are the most common adverse effects.
5. They have not been plagued by the development of resistance. Bacteria originally sensitive to cephalosporins have not become resistant.

From the preceding, it would appear that cephalosporins are ideal antibiotics, capable of eradicating most pathogens. This is not the case. Cephalosporins should be considered second-line antibiotics, used when other drugs, notably the penicillins, fail or are inappropriate. The reasons for this will become apparent in the next few pages. However, some of their disadvantages can be summarized at this time.

1. Cephalosporins are rapidly excreted by the kidneys and must be administered frequently to maintain adequate blood levels.
2. They do not penetrate into the cerebrospinal fluid well, even in patients with meningitis, and are useless in treating central nervous system infections.
3. First-generation cephalosporins lack activity against many bacteria, including enterococci, most strains of enterobacter species, indole-positive proteus species, providencia species, *Pseudomonas aeruginosa, Serratia marcescens,* and *Bacteroides fragilis.* Some of these bacteria are sensitive to second- and third-generation cephalosporins. However, our enthusiasm for these latter drugs is tempered somewhat by their cost, which is so high as to leave one with the impression that it must have been fixed by the Society for the Prevention of Cruelty to Bacteria (SPCB).

Mechanism of Action

Cephalosporins and penicillins have similar structures. Like the latter drugs, cephalosporins prevent sensitive bacteria from forming cell walls. As a result, the bacterial cell membrane, unable to withstand the pressure of the hypertonic liquid in the microbe, ruptures, killing the bacterium.

Pharmacokinetics

Most cephalosporins are destroyed in the acid medium of the stomach and must be administered parenterally. Cephalexin (Ceporex, Keflex), cephradine (Anspor, Velosef), cefadroxil (Duracef, Ultracef), cefaclor (Ceclor) and cefixime (Suprax) are sufficiently stable in the stomach to be administered orally.

Once absorbed, the cephalosporins penetrate most tissues well. Effective antibiotic concentrations can be attained in synovial, pleural, peritoneal and pericardial fluids in the presence of inflammation. Because cephalosporins do not penetrate well into the eye or prostate, therapeutic levels may not be attained in these tissues. First- and second-generation cephalosporins penetrate poorly into the cerebrospinal fluid, even when the meninges are

inflamed. Only third-generation cephalosporins reach therapeutic levels in the cerebrospinal fluid in the presence of inflammation.

Like the penicillins, cephalosporins are rapidly secreted by the kidneys. Probenecid can reduce their rates of excretion.

Based on their antibacterial spectra, they may be classified as first-, second- and third-generation cephalosporins (Table 87). They may also be divided into orally and parenterally administered cephalosporins.

Table 87
Some currently available cephalosporins.

First Generation	Second Generation	Third Generation
Cephalothin	Cefamandole	Cefoperazone
Cephapirin	Cefuroxime	Cefotaxime
Cefazolin	Cefoxitin	Ceftazidime
Cephalexin*	Cefaclor*	Ceftizoxime
Cephradine*	Cefonicid	Ceftriaxone
Cefadroxil	Ceforanide	Cefixime*

*Orally active drugs

Injectable Cephalosporins

First-generation cephalosporins are active against most gram-positive and many gram-negative organisms. Cephalothin (Ceporacin, Keflin, Seffin) is the most commonly used first-generation injectable cephalosporin. It can be accepted as the standard injectable cephalosporin against which all new cephalosporins should be compared. Table 88 presents the antibacterial spectrum of cephalothin.

Second-generation injectable cephalosporins differ little from cephalothin with respect to their activity against gram-positive bacteria. A major difference does exist, however, in their activities against gram-negative bacteria. Cefamandole (Mandol) and cefuroxime (Zinacef) have lower minimal inhibitor concentrations (MICs) against *Escherichia coli, Klebsiella pneumoniae, Haemophilus influenzae, Neisseria gonorrhoeae, Neisseria meningitidis,* salmonella species, shigella species and *Proteus mirabilis.* Furthermore, cefamandole and cefuroxime are active against strains of *Enterobacter aerogenes, Enterobacter cloacae,* and indole-positive proteus species that have traditionally been resistant to cephalosporins.

Cefoxitin (Mefoxin) is slightly less potent than cephalothin, cefamandole or cefuroxime against

Table 88
Antibacterial spectrum of first-generation injectable cephalosporins.

Micro-organism	Sensitivity
Staphylococcus aureus (both penicillin-sensitive and penicillin-resistant)	Highly sensitive but some resistant strains
Streptococcus pyogenes	Highly sensitive
Streptococcus pneumoniae	Highly sensitive
Streptococcus (viridans group)	Highly sensitive
Streptococcus faecalis	Some sensitivity but many resistant strains
Clostridium perfringens	Highly sensitive
Clostridium tetani	Very highly sensitive
Corynebacterium diphtheriae	Some sensitivity
Enterobacter cloacae	Resistant
Enterobacter aerogenes	Resistant
Escherichia coli	Moderate sensitivity but many resistant strains
Haemophilus influenzae	Moderate sensitivity but many resistant strains
Klebsiella pneumoniae	Highly sensitive
Neisseria gonorrhoeae	Moderate sensitivity but many resistant strains
Neisseria meningitidis	Highly sensitive but many resistant strains
Proteus mirabilis	Some sensitivity
Proteus morganii	Resistant
Proteus rettgeri	Resistant
Proteus vulgaris	Resistant
Pseudomonas aeruginosa	Resistant
Salmonella spp.	Moderate sensitivity but many resistant strains
Shigella spp.	Moderate sensitivity but many resistant strains

gram-positive bacteria. It is generally as effective against the same gram-negative bacteria as cefamandole but differs from the latter drug in its poor activity against enterobacter. Cefoxitin is more effective than cefamandole against indole-positive proteus and has some activity against *Serratia marcescens*. Most important is cefoxitin's activity against a range of strict anaerobes, including *Bacteroides fragilis*.

The medical world is currently witnessing the rapid development of third-generation cephalosporins as a distinct group of antibiotics. Because each drug differs somewhat from its counterparts, it is difficult to generalize in discussing the properties of the entire group. However, it is fair to say that the third-generation cephalosporins are less active against gram-positive bacteria than their first-generation counterparts. Their greatest activity is against aerobic gram-negative bacilli. Third-generation cephalosporins

have good to excellent activity against all members of the enterobacteriaceae family, including *Serratia marcescens*. Strains of enterobacteriaceae such as *Escherichia coli, Klebsiella pneumoniae*, enterobacter and proteus that are resistant to both first- and second-generation cephalosporins frequently respond to third-generation drugs.

Cefoperazone, ceftazidime and ceftizoxime have antipseudomonal activity; the activity of cefotaxime and ceftriaxone against *Pseudomonas aeruginosa* is variable.

Orally Effective Cephalosporins

Cephalexin (Ceporex, Keflex) is the standard against which all new orally effective cephalosporins must be compared. It is active against *Staphylococcus aureus*, viridans streptococci, group A streptococci, *Streptococcus pneumoniae, Neisseria meningitidis* and *Neisseria gonorrhoeae*. Salmonella, shigella, *Proteus mirabilis* and some strains of *Escherichia coli* are susceptible to cephalexin at clinically achievable concentrations. Cephalexin is inactive against *Streptococcus faecalis*, indole-positive proteus species, *Pseudomonas aeruginosa, Serratia marcescens* and *Haemophilus influenzae.*

Cefaclor (Ceclor) is a second-generation orally effective cephalosporin. It is equivalent or superior to cephalexin in activity against gram-positive cocci. Although it is highly active against *Escherichia coli, Klebsiella pneumoniae, Proteus mirabilis,* shigella and salmonella, cefaclor's major advantage over cephalexin is its activity, at low concentrations, against *Haemophilus influenzae.*

Cefixime (Suprax) an oral third-generation cephalosporin. The drug is at least as active in vitro as other oral cephalosporins against group A streptococci and pneumococci, but staphylococci, which are susceptible to other cephalosporins, are resistant to cefixime because the drug has a low affinity for a critical beta-lactam-binding protein. Cefixime is highly active against *Neisseria gonorrhoeae, Haemophilus influenzae* and *Branhamella catarrhalis,* including beta-lactamase-producing strains usually resistant to ampicillin, amoxicillin and, occasionally, to cefaclor. *Haemophilus influenzae* and branhamella are, with pneumococci, the most common pathogens in acute otitis media and sinusitis. The claim that cefixime is a third-generation cephalosporin is based on its resistance to plasmid-mediated beta-lactamases produced by many gram-negative bacteria, but the drug is not resistant to some chromosomal beta-lactamases found in certain gram-negative strains.

Cefixime is more active than other cephalosporins against many gram-negative bacilli, including *E. coli,* klebsiella, *Proteus mirabilis* and *Serratia marcescen.* It has, however, no useful activity against anaerobes, pseudomonas, or many strains of enterobacter and acinetobacter. It is less active against gram-negative bacteria than parenteral third-generation cephalosporins.

Therapeutic Uses

The cephalosporins have a broad antibacterial spectrum, including penicillinase-producing *Staphylococcus aureus.* In spite of this, the availability of equally effective and less expensive alternatives has often relegated cephalosporins to the position of second-line drugs.

Urinary tract infections caused by *Escherichia coli,* for example, may often be eradicated with cephalexin. However, ampicillin is usually equally effective and cheaper. Other drugs, notably trimethoprim plus sulfamethoxazole (Bactrim, Septra) and trimethoprim (Proloprim, Trimpex) alone, cost about the same as cephalexin but are more effective in treating acute urinary tract infections.

To select another example, it is uneconomical to use cephalexin to treat streptococcal pharyngitis when penicillins G or V are at least as effective and much cheaper.

A cephalosporin may be first-line therapy when resistance has developed to the drug normally used. For example, the resistance of *Haemophilus influenzae* to ampicillin and amoxicillin has created a need for other drugs. Cefaclor may well meet that need.

Cephalosporins reduce the incidence of surgical wound infections and are very effective if used properly after a wide variety of procedures.

The spectra of activity of the first- and second-generation cephalosporins are not sufficiently broad that they may be used alone in the treatment of gram-negative sepsis. They are usually administered with an aminoglycoside to treat serious infections suspected to be due to gram-negative organisms, before the results of bacteriologic tests are received.

Cefoxitin can be used to treat intra-abdominal infections resulting from disruption of the intestinal mucosa. These infections are usually caused by gram-negative bacilli and anaerobes, in particular *Bacteroides fragilis.* Cefoxitin is as effective as clindamycin (Dalacin C) plus gentamicin (Garamycin) for community-acquired infections. If the infection is nosocomial in origin, an aminoglycoside should be added to cefoxitin therapy.

Third-generation injectable cephalosporins have produced excellent results in gram-negative bacillary meningitis, particularly against *Escherichia coli,* klebsiella, proteus and *Haemophilus influenzae.* Third-generation injectable cephalosporins are also of value in the treatment of multiple resistant gram-negative infections. Other indications for these drugs include infections not responding to standard therapy, such as gram-negative pneumonia, urinary tract infections, osteomyelitis, pelvic or intra-abdominal infections, and suspected sepsis in the febrile neutropenic host. Whether the third-generation injectable drugs should be used alone in life-threatening infections caused by gram-negative bacilli remains to be determined.

Cefixime, administered orally, is indicated for the treatment of otitis media caused by *S. pneumoniae, H. influenzae* (beta-lactamase positive and negative strains), *B. catarrhalis* (beta-lactamase positive and negative strains) and *S. pyogenes.* It has been approved for acute uncomplicated cystitis and urethritis caused by *E. coli, P. mirabilis* and klebsiella species. Cefixime may also be used for pharyngitis and tonsillitis caused by *S. pyogenes*. Acute bronchitis caused by *S. pneumoniae, B. catarrhalis* (beta-lactamase positive and negative strains) and *H. influenzae* (beta-lactamase positive and negative strains) may also be treated with cefixime.

Adverse Effects

Cephalosporins are relatively safe drugs. Allergic reactions have been reported in as many as five per cent of patients receiving cephalosporins. Complaints include skin rash, urticaria, fever, serum sickness, hemolytic anemia and eosinophilia. Cephalosporins are often used to replace the penicillins in patients who are allergic to the latter drugs. Although this can often be done safely, some patients are allergic to both groups of drugs — not a surprising fact in view of their structural similarities.

Gastrointestinal adverse effects include nausea, vomiting and diarrhea. Pseudomembranous colitis can rarely occur with cephalosporin use. If this happens, the drug should be discontinued immediately and supportive measures instituted. Oral vancomycin or metronidazole can be used to eradicate the causative *Clostridium difficile*.

Other adverse effects include thrombophlebitis and pain at the site of intramuscular injection. Overgrowth of resistant organisms may occur after long-term cephalosporin administration. Patients receiving a third-generation drug should be observed for enterococcal superinfection. Finally, third-generation cephalosporins may suppress the gastrointestinal microflora, resulting in decreased vitamin K production and hypoprothrombinemia.

Nursing Process

Just as cephalothin and cephalexin provide the standards against which other cephalosporins are judged, they also serve as models for the nursing process related to the use of all cephalosporins. The nursing process that follows was developed for cephalothin and cephalexin, but applies to all cephalosporins.

Assessment
The nursing process begins immediately after the decision to administer a cephalosporin, with a review of the patient's history for evidence of allergies. Nurses should review the patient's history for evidence of nephrotoxicity, fluid intake and output imbalance and blood abnormalities. Particular

attention must be paid to previous hypersensitivity reactions to penicillins or cephalosporins. The patient's renal function should also be checked.

Nursing assessment incorporates a physical examination of the patient together with documentation of clinical observations related to the infection, including the patient's temperature. The collection of specimens for laboratory culture and sensitivity tests prior to the initial dose is also part of the initial physical assessment.

Administration
Cephalothin is administered parenterally. The intravenous route is preferred for initial treatment of serious infections. Reconstitute cephalothin according to the manufacturer's instructions. Unused and unrefrigerated reconstituted solutions should be discarded after twelve hours. Reconstituted solutions that have been refrigerated are stable for four days (ninety-six hours).

Cephalothin and other parenterally administered cephalosporins should be mixed with other drugs in the same syringe only after the advice of a pharmacist has been sought regarding the chemical compatibility of the substances involved.

Cephalothin irritates veins. For intravenous administration, insert a small needle (such as a scalp vein needle) into a large vein (such as the median cubital) to reduce the probability of thrombophlebitis. Intramuscular cephalothin should be injected slowly deep into a large muscle such as the gluteus maximus to reduce the pain associated with tissue irritation. Rotate the sites of injection or infusion with each dose.

Cephalexin is most effective when it is given on an empty stomach. However, if gastrointestinal distress occurs, it may be taken with food without a great loss of efficacy. Oral suspensions should be refrigerated to prevent deterioration and loss of effectiveness. Discard unused portions after two weeks.

Cephalosporins should be administered for ten to fourteen days to ensure death of the organism and to prevent superinfection.

Evaluation
Following the administration of a cephalosporin, the nurse should evaluate the patient for clinical improvement and adverse effects.

Patients can develop superinfections following prolonged cephalosporin administration. These are most commonly seen in the gastrointestinal and genitourinary tract. Black furry tongue, nausea, diarrhea, pruritus vulva and vaginal discharge are indicators of superinfections. Patients should also be monitored for reduced urinary output and proteinuria, which are early indicators of nephrotoxicity. Increased bleeding tendencies (petechiae, bleeding gums, epistaxis) suggest hepatic dysfunction. Tenderness and/or red streaking at the site of intravenous infusion indicates thrombophlebitis.

Teaching
Patients receiving these drugs should be taught the importance of completing the prescribed course of therapy even though they may have become asymptomatic. If the drug is taken at home, they should be told the indicators of drug efficacy and adverse effects. Patients must also be advised of the importance of contacting the physician immediately should adverse effects develop.

Further Reading

Choice of cephalosporins (1990). *The Medical Letter 32* :107-110.

Choice of antimicrobial drugs (1990). *The Medical Letter 32* :41-48.

Treatment of sexually transmitted diseases (1990). *The Medical Letter 32* :5-10.

Williams, J.D. (1987). The cephalosporin antibiotics. *Drugs 34* (Suppl. 2):1-258.

Table 89
The cephalosporins.

(* Signifies drug is orally effective)

Pharmacologic Classification: Antibiotics — First-Generation Cephalosporins (for doses, consult Table 90)

Generic Name (Trade Name)	Use	Action	Adverse Effects	Drug Interactions	Nursing Process
1. Cephalothin sodium (Ceporacin, Keflin)	Used parenterally, should be restricted to serious infect'ns caused by susceptible bacteria, incl. staphylococci, streptococci (except enterococci).	For all first-generat'n cephalosporins: Cephalosporins inhibit format'n of the bacterial cell wall and inactivate or remove an inhibitor of autolytic enzymes in the wall.	For all first-generat'n cephalosporins: Allergic react'ns incl. skin rash, urticaria, fever, hemolytic anemia and eosinophilia; neutropenia, leukopenia, thrombocytopenia, anorexia, nausea, vomiting, diarrhea, pseudomembranous colitis. Cephalothin may cause pain on inject'n.	Aminoglycosides: And cephalosporins, may have additive nephrotoxic effects. Combined use of these drugs should be undertaken w. caution. Pts w. normal renal funct'n receiving appropriate dosing and drug monitoring seldom develop nephrotoxic react'ns. Colistin: And cephalothin have been assoc. w. incr. incidence of renal toxicity. Pts should be monitored closely. Probenecid: Reduces renal excret'n of cephalosporins. As a result, cephalosporin levels will be higher than expected.	For injectable cephalosporins: **Assess:** For previous penicillin/cephalosporin allergy, hx allergies, renal dysfunct'n; fluid intake/output imbalance, blood abnormalities. Collect specimens for culture and sensitivity tests before first dose; document clinical observat'ns of infect'n, incl. temp. **Administer:** IM deep into large muscle; use small needles and large veins for IV infus'n; IV route preferred for serious systemic infect'ns; rotate inject'n/infus'n sites. Reconstitute according to manufacturer's instruct'ns; discard unrefrigerated solut'ns after 12 h, refrigerated solut'ns after 4 days. Not normally mixed w. other drugs. Give for 10-14 days to ensure death of organism and to prevent superimposed infect'n. **Evaluate:** For normalizat'n of clinical observat'ns of infect'ns noted during assessment; for allergic react'ns; for superinfect'ns of normal body flora; for reduced urinary output, proteinuria. **Teach:** Importance of completing prescribed course of tx even though asymptomatic.
2. Cephapirin sodium (Cefadyl)					
3. Cefazolin sodium (Ancef, Kefzol)					
4. Cephalexin* (Ceporex, Keflex)	*Effective orally against a range of gram-pos. and gram-neg. bacteria, incl. penicillinase-producing staphylococci. Used in tx of otitis media and bacterial infect'ns of respiratory tract, GU tract, bones and joints, skin and soft tissues if caused by susceptible organisms.				*For oral cephalosporins (cephalexin, cephradine, cefadroxil, cefaclor, cefixime) **Administer:** On empty stomach for greatest effect; give w. food if GI distress occurs. Refrigerate oral suspens'n; dispose of unused port'ns after 2 weeks.
5. Cephradine* (Anspor, Velosef)					
6. Cefadroxil* (Duricef, Ultracef)					

Pharmacologic Classification: Antibiotics — Second-Generation Cephalosporins (for doses, consult Table 90)

Generic Name (Trade Name)	Use	Action	Adverse Effects	Drug Interactions	Nursing Process
1. Cefamandole (Nafate, Mandol)	Used parenterally in tx of serious infect'ns caused by sensitive strains of E. coli, klebsiella, proteus, enterobacter or H. influenzae. As an alternative to ampicillin or chloramphenicol in pneumonias due to H. influenzae.	As for first-generat'n cephalosporins	As for first-generat'n cephalosporins	As for first-generat'n cephalosporins	
2. Cefuroxime sodium (Zinacef)		As for first-generat'n cephalosporins	As for first-generat'n cephalosporins	As for first-generat'n cephalosporins	
3. Cefoxitin sodium (Mefoxin)	As for cefamandole, plus tx of B. fragilis and other enteric anaerobes. Cefoxitin should not be used in tx of H. influenzae infect'ns.	As for first-generat'n cephalosporins	As for first-generat'n cephalosporins	As for first-generat'n cephalosporins	

Generic Name (Trade Name)	Use	Action	Adverse Effects	Drug Interactions	Nursing Process
4. Cefaclor* (Ceclor)	Administered orally. As for cephalexin, but particularly useful in tx of *H. influenzæ* infect'ns.	As for first-generat'n cephalosporins	As for first-generat'n cephalosporins	As for first-generat'n cephalosporins	**Teach:** Self-evaluat'n for drug efficacy and adv. effects.

Pharmacologic Classification: Antibiotics — Third-Generation Cephalosporins (for doses, consult Table 90)

Generic Name (Trade Name)	Use	Action	Adverse Effects	Drug Interactions	Nursing Process
1. Cefotaxime sodium (Claforan)	Tx of meningitis caused by *H. influenzæ*. Valuable in tx of multiple resistant gram-neg. infect'ns. Used in infect'ns not responding to standard tx, such as gram-neg. pneumonias, urinary tract infect'ns, osteomyelitis, pelvic or intra-abdominal infect'ns, and suspected sepsis in the febrile neutropenic host.	As for first-generat'n cephalosporins	As for first-generat'n cephalosporins. Third-generat'n cephalosporins may also cause enterococcal superinfect'ns or suppress the GI microflora, resulting in decr. vitamin K product'n and hypoprothrombinemia.	As for first-generat'n cephalosporins	As for first-generat'n cephalosporins
2. Cefoperazone sodium (Cefobid)	As for cefotaxime. Cefoperazone is more active against *P. aeruginosa.* May be particularly indicated for biliary tract sepsis.	As for first-generat'n cephalosporins	As for cefotaxime	As for first-generat'n cephalosporins	As for first-generat'n cephalosporins
3. Ceftazidime pentahydrate (Fortaz, Tazicef, Tazidime)	Tx of uncomplicated pneumonia or skin structure infect'ns; complicated or uncomplicated urinary tract infect'ns; bone infect'ns; peritonitis or septicemia.	As for first-generat'n cephalosporins	As for cefotaxime	As for first-generat'n cephalosporins	As for first-generat'n cephalosporins
4. Ceftizoxime sodium (Cefizox)	Tx of uncomplicated urinary tract infect'ns; infect'ns at other sites; severe or refractory infect'ns; life-threatening infect'ns.	As for first-generat'n cephalosporins	As for cefotaxime	As for first-generat'n cephalosporins	As for first-generat'n cephalosporins
5. Ceftriaxone disodium (Rocephin)	Tx of moderate and severe infect'ns; uncomplicated gonorrhea; serious miscellaneous infect'ns; meningitis.	As for first-generat'n cephalosporins	As for cefotaxime	As for first-generat'n cephalosporins	As for first-generat'n cephalosporins
6. Cefixime* (Suprax)	Orally effective. For otitis media, acute uncomplicated urinary tract infect'ns, urethritis, pharyngitis, tonsilitis and acute bronchitis.	As for first-generat'n cephalosporins	As for cefotaxime	As for first-generat'n cephalosporins	As for first-generat'n cephalosporins

Table 90
Doses of the cephalosporins.

Generic Name (Trade Name)	Dose
Pharmacologic Classification: Antibiotics — First-Generation Cephalosporins	
Cephalothin sodium (Ceporacin, Keflin, Seffin)	**IV:** Adults - 500-1000 mg q 4-6 h. Infants and children - 75-125 mg/kg/day in divided doses. For dosage adjustment in cases of impaired renal funct'n, consult product monograph.
Cephapirin sodium (Cefadyl)	**IM/IV:** Adults - 500-1000 mg q 4-6 h. Children - 40-80 mg/kg/day in 4 equal doses.
Cefazolin sodium (Ancef, Kefzol)	**IM/IV:** Adults - *For pneumococcal pneumonia:* 500 mg q12 h. *For mild gram-pos. infect'ns:* 250-500 mg q 8 h. *In acute uncomplicated urinary tract infect'ns:* 1 g q 12 h. *In moderate or severe infect'ns:* 500-1000 mg q 6-8 h. *In serious infect'ns such as endocarditis:* 6 g/day. Children - *For mild to moderately severe infect'ns:* 25-50 mg/kg/day in 3-4 equal doses. For pts w. renal impairment, consult product monograph.
Cephalexin (Ceporex, Keflex)	**Oral:** Adults - 1-4 g/day in divided doses. Us. adult dose, 250 mg q 6 h. Children - 25-50 mg/kg/day in 4 divided doses q 6 h.
Cephradine (Anspor, Velosef)	**Oral:** Adults - *For respiratory tract infect'ns other than lobar pneumonia:* 250 mg q 6 h or 500 mg q 12 h. *For pneumococcal lobar pneumonia:* 500 mg q 6 h or 1 g q 12 h. *For skin and soft tissue infect'ns:* 250 mg q 6 h or 500 mg q 12 h. *For urinary tract infect'ns:* 500 mg q 6 h or 1 g q 12 h. For pts w. renal impairment, consult product monograph.
Cefadroxil (Duricef, Ultracef)	**Oral:** Adults - *For urinary tract infect'ns:* 1-2 g/day as single dose hs or divided into 2 daily doses. *For acute pharyngitis/tonsillitis:* 1 g/day in single dose or 2 divided doses for 10 days. *For lower respiratory tract infect'ns:* 500-1000 mg bid. *For skin and soft tissue infect'ns:* 1 g daily in single dose. Children - *For tx of urinary tract and integumentary infect'ns, acute pharyngitis or tonsillitis, and lower respiratory tract infect'ns:* 30 mg/kg/day given q 12 h for 10 days. For pts w. renal impairment, consult product monograph.
Pharmacologic Classification: Antibiotics — Second-Generation Cephalosporins	
Cefamandole nafate (Mandol)	**IV/IM:** Adults - 500-1000 mg q 4-8 h. *For life-threatening infect'ns:* Up to 2 g q 4 h. *For uncomplicated pneumonia and soft tissue infect'ns:* 500 mg q 6 h. *For mild urinary tract infect'ns:* 500 mg q 8 h. *For moderate urinary tract infect'ns:* 1 g q 8 h. *For severe urinary tract infect'ns:* 1 g q 4-6 h. Children - 50-100 mg/kg/day in equal doses q 4-8 h. For pts w. renal impairment, consult product monograph.
Cefoxitin (Mefoxin)	**IV/IM:** Adults - 1-2 g q 6-8 h. *For uncomplicated pneumonia, urinary tract or soft tissue infect'n:* 1 g q 6-8 h. *For moderately severe or severe infect'ns:* 1 g IV q 4 h or 2 g q 6-8 h. *For infect'ns commonly needing antibiotics in higher dosages (e.g., gas gangrene):* 2 g IV q 4 h or 3 g q 6 h. Children - 20-40 mg/kg q 6-8 h. Infants,1 month - 2 years - 20-40 mg/kg q 6-8 h. Neonates (incl. premature infants) - **IV:** ≤1 week of age - 20-40 mg/kg q 12 h; 1-4 weeks of age - 20-40 mg/kg q 8 h. (Note: Solut'ns containing preservatives should not be used for inject'n or for flushing catheters in treating neonates.)

Generic Name (Trade Name)	Dose
Cefuroxime sodium (Zinacef)	**IM:** 750 mg tid. **IV:** 750 mg or 1.5 g tid. *For severe or life-threatening infect'ns or infect'ns of the lower respiratory tract caused by gram-neg. organisms:* 1.5 g IV tid. *For gonorrhea:* 1.5 g IM divided into 2 [750 mg] doses, 1 in each buttock. Probenecid 1 g is given orally at the same time. *For sole tx of bacterial meningitis:* 3 g IV q 8 h. Infants and children - 30-100 mg/kg/day divided into 3-4 doses. *For bacterial meningitis:* 200-240 mg/kg/day IV in 3-4 divided doses, then reduce to 100 mg/kg/day after 3 days or when clinical improvement occurs. Neonates - 30-100 mg/kg/day in 2-3 divided doses. For pts w. renal impairment, consult product monograph.
Cefaclor (Ceclor)	**Oral:** Adults - 250 mg q 8-12 h. Max. recomm. dose, 2 g/day. *For skin and soft tissue infect'ns:* 250 mg bid-tid. *For lower respiratory tract infect'ns:* 250 mg tid. Children - 20 mg/kg/day in divided doses q 8-12 h. *For more serious infect'ns (otitis media and those infect'ns caused by less susceptible organisms):* 40 mg/kg/day. For otitis media, administer dose q 12 h. For lower respiratory tract infect'ns, divide into 3 daily doses.

Pharmacologic Classification: Antibiotics — Third-Generation Cephalosporins

Generic Name (Trade Name)	Dose
Cefixime (Suprax)	**Oral:** Adults - 400 mg od. A dose of 200 mg may be given bid prn except for urinary tract infect'ns, for which once-daily dosing must be used. Children - 8 mg/kg/day od. A dose of 4 mg/kg may be given bid prn except for urinary tract infect'ns, for which once-daily dosing must be used.
Cefoperazone sodium (Cefobid)	**IM/IV:** Adults - *For mild to moderately severe infect'ns:* 1-2 g q 12 h. *For severe infect'ns or those caused by less sensitive organisms:* 2-4 g IV q 12 h. *For infect'ns commonly requiring antibiotics in higher dosage:* 3 g IV q 8 h. Because renal excret'n is not main route of eliminat'n, adult pts w. renal impairment us. require no adjustment in dosage, w. daily doses of 2-4 g. Children - Safety and efficacy of this drug in children have not been established.
Cefotaxime sodium (Claforan)	**IM/IV:** Adults - *For uncomplicated infect'ns:* 1 g q 12 h. *For moderately severe to severe infect'ns:* 1-2 g q 8 h. *For very severe infect'ns:* 2 g IV q 6-8 h. *For life-threatening infect'ns:* 2 g IV q 4 h. *For uncomplicated gonorrhea:* 1 g IM as single dose. Neonates up to 1 week of age - 50 mg/kg IV q 12 h; 1-4 weeks of age - 50 mg/kg IV q 8 h. Infants and children < 50 kg - 50-100 mg/kg/day IM or IV, divided into 4-6 equal doses, or up to 180 mg/kg/day for severe infect'ns. For pts w. renal impairment, consult product monograph.
Ceftazidime pentahy-drate (Fortaz, Tazicef, Tazidime)	**IM/IV:** Adults - *For uncomplicated pneumonia or skin-structure infect'n:* 0.5-1.0 g q 8 h. *For uncomplicated urinary tract infect'ns:* 250 mg q12 h. *For complicated urinary tract infect'ns:* 500 mg q 8-12 h. *For bone infect'ns:* 2 g IV q 12 h. *For peritonitis or septicemia:* 2 g IV q 8 h. Infants and children aged 1-2 months - 25-50 mg/kg/day IV in 2 equal doses; 2 months - 12 years - 30-100 mg/kg/day IV in 3 equal doses. For pts w. renal impairment, consult product monograph.
Ceftizoxime sodium (Cefizox)	**IM/IV:** Adults - *For uncomplicated urinary tract infect'ns:* 500 mg q 12 h. *For infect'ns at other sites:* 1 g q q 8-12 h. *For severe or refractory infect'ns:* 1 g q 8 h to 2 g q 8-12 h. Infants and children aged 6 months -12 years - 50 mg/kg q 6-8 h. For pts w. renal impairment, consult product monograph.
Ceftriaxone disodium (Rocephin)	**IM/IV:** Adults - *For moderate and severe infect'ns:* 1-2 g q 24 h or 0.5-1 g q 12 h. *For uncomplicated gonorrhea:* 250 mg IM as single dose. Infants and children aged one month - 12 years - *For serious miscellaneous infect'ns:* 25-37.5 mg/kg q12 h. Total daily dose should not > 2 g. If body mass is ≥ 50 kg, adult dose should be used. *For meningitis:* 50 mg/kg (w. or without loading dose of 75 mg/kg) q 12 h. Total daily dose should not > 4 g.

CHAPTER 61

Erythromycin and Clindamycin

Erythromycin and clindamycin are discussed together because they have similar mechanisms of action and antibacterial spectra. More attention will be given to erythromycin because this drug is used more extensively.

Erythromycin

Erythromycin was introduced in the early 1950s. In spite of the subsequent development of newer antibiotics, erythromycin remains a favorite of many prescribers.

Mechanism of Action

Erythromycin exerts its bacteriostatic effects by blocking protein synthesis in sensitive bacteria. It accomplishes this by binding selectively to the bacterial 50S ribosomal subunit and preventing elongation of the peptide chain. Because erythromycin does not bind to mammalian ribosomes, it has no effect on protein synthesis in the host. Erythromycin is bacteriostatic and not bactericidal. This fact has little clinical significance because once cell multiplication has stopped the defense mechanisms of the host usually kill bacteria.

Antibacterial Spectrum

The antibacterial spectrum of erythromycin is similar to that of penicillin G. It includes many strains of penicillin-resistant staphylococci, *Streptococcus pyogenes, Streptococcus pneumoniae,* viridans streptococci, anaerobic streptococci and many strains of *Streptococcus faecalis.*
Erythromycin is also effective against *Corynebacterium diphtheriae, Propionibacterium*

acnes, Clostridium tetani, Clostridium perfringens, Neisseria gonorrhoeae, Bordetella pertussis, and some species of brucella. *Haemophilus influenzae* is only moderately sensitive to the drug. Oropharyngeal strains of bacteroides are usually sensitive to erythromycin. The drug is also effective against *Mycoplasma pneumoniae, Treponema pallidum, Legionella pneumophilia,* and many species of rickettsia and chlamydia.

When used over short periods of time, resistance to erythromycin is not common. However, if erythromycin is used for long-term therapy or within a hospital environment, staphylococcal resistance often develops rapidly. Other bacteria that may become resistant to the drug are *Streptococcus pneumoniae, Streptococcus pyogenes,* the viridans streptococci and enterococci. This resistance is due to the ability of bacteria to produce an enzyme capable of destroying erythromycin.

Pharmacokinetics

Erythromycin is not stable in the stomach. It must be protected from gastric juices if it is to be absorbed from the intestine. This can be achieved by using enteric-coated tablets or capsules, or applying a protective film coating to the tablets. The product ERYC is formulated as a capsule containing enteric-coated pellets. Erythromycin can also be protected from stomach secretions by preparing the drug as an acid-resistant ester, as in erythromycin stearate, erythromycin ethylsuccinate or erythromycin estolate. Table 91 lists some of the available forms of erythromycin, together with some of their more common trade names.

Despite these steps, protection against acid destruction is often not complete. Therefore, with the exception of erythromycin ethylsuccinate and erythromycin estolate, all erythromycin products should preferably be taken on an empty stomach to speed their transit into the intestine. Unfortunately, erythromycin taken on an empty stomach often causes considerable gastric distress and food may be needed to reduce the patient's discomfort. Erythromycin ethylsuccinate and erythromycin estolate appear to be well absorbed when taken with food. In fact, maximum blood levels with erythromycin ethylsuccinate suspension or chewable tablets are obtained when the products are given immediately after meals. Both erythromycin estolate and erythromycin ethylsuccinate are hydrolyzed to erythromycin following absorption.

Once absorbed, erythromycin diffuses well throughout the body. It enters most tissue compartments, with the exception of the cerebrospinal fluid.

Erythromycin is concentrated in the liver and excreted in the bile. Little erythromycin is eliminated in the urine. Its half-life ranges from one to more than three hours.

Table 91
Forms of erythromycin currently available.

Orally Administered

Erythromycin
Enteric-coated tablets (E-Mycin, Ilotycin, Robimycin)
Film-coated tablets (Erythromid)

Erythromycin stearate
Tablets (Erythrocin, Bristamycin, Erypar, Ethril, Pfizer-E)
Liquid (Erythrocin)

Erythromycin estolate
Capsules (Ilosone)
Liquid (Ilosone)

Erythromycin ethylsuccinate
Tablets (EES, Pediamycin)
Liquid (EES, Pediamycin)

Parenterally Administered

Erythromycin gluceptate (Ilotycin Gluceptate)

Erythromycin lactobionate (Erythrocin Lactobionate)

Topically Administered

Erythromycin (Ilotycin)

Erythromycin + ethyl alcohol + Laureth 4 (Staticin — used for the treatment of acne)

Therapeutic Uses

Erythromycin is often used as a replacement for penicillin G or V in patients who are allergic to these drugs. Infections caused by group A streptococci, including tonsillitis, erysipelas and scarlet fever, often respond well to erythromycin. The drug can also be used as a penicillin substitute in the chemoprophylaxis of streptococcal infections. Pneumococcal infections can be treated with erythromycin. This agent can also be used as a substitute for penicillin in the treatment of the acute illness or the carrier state of diphtheria and the management of both early and late syphilis. Development of resistance has greatly restricted its value in minor staphylococcal infections.

Erythromycin is effective in the treatment of pneumonia caused by *Mycoplasma pneumoniae.* This is one of the few indications for which erythromycin is a first drug of choice. Erythromycin is effective for the treatment of Legionnaire's disease, caused by *Legionella pneumophilia.* Whooping cough, produced by *Bordetella pertussis,* may also be treated with erythromycin. However, evidence for its efficacy is not overwhelming. Erythromycin is a primary treatment for *Chlamydia trachomatis* infections in infants and children, and this agent is often used in conjunction with sulfisoxazole (Pediazole) to treat *Haemophilus influenzae* -induced otitis media in young children.

Erythromycin ophthalmic ointment is used in the treatment of superficial ocular infections involving the conjunctiva or cornea caused by organisms susceptible to erythromycin. For prophylaxis of ophthalmia neonatorum due to *N. gonorrhoeae* or *C. trachomatis,* 0.5% erythromycin ophthalmic ointment may be used.

Oral or topical erythromycin may be used in the treatment of acne vulgaris. The products are used, primarily in the treatment of the inflammatory papular lesions of acne. The rationale for this use lies in the fact that erythromycin can eradicate *Propionibacterium acnes,* the anaerobic diptheroid in pilosebaceous glands that secretes a variety of enzymes, including hyaluronidase, which are capable of disrupting follicular epithelium and increasing inflammation.

Adverse Effects

The incidence of adverse effects with erythromycin is low. The drug produces gastrointestinal upset with nausea, diarrhea and abdominal pain. Very rarely, erythromycin may cause reversible cholestatic hepatitis. This is characterized by fever, enlarged and tender liver, hyperbilirubinemia, elevated transaminase levels and dark urine. Previously believed to occur only with erythromycin estolate, it is now known to be produced by all forms of the drug.

Nursing Process

Assessment

Prior to the first dose of erythromycin, nurses must assess patients for previous adverse reactions to the drug, allergies (e.g., hayfever, asthma, dermatitis) or a history of renal or liver disease. Patients with histories of previous reactions to erythromycin should not be given the drug. Individuals with histories of allergies, liver or renal disease should be subject to particularly intense scrutiny following erythromycin administration. Prior to giving erythromycin, nurses should establish the clinical indicators of the infection and collect specimens for culture and sensitivity tests.

Administration

Erythromycin is normally administered orally. It should not be given with fruit juice. With the exception of erythromycin estolate and erythromycin ethylsuccinate, all forms of erythromycin ideally should be given with water on an empty stomach. This advice must, however, be counterbalanced with the knowledge that erythromycin can irritate the empty stomach. In that situation, if patients are taking either enteric-coated tablets of erythromycin or erythromycin stearate, it may be necessary to give the drug with a small amount of food. Patients should maintain adequate fluid intake.

To prevent thrombophlebitis, intravenous erythromycin should be given through small needles inserted in large veins. Intramuscular injections are performed slowly into large muscles to reduce irritation and pain. Both intravenous and intramuscular injection sites should be rotated for each dose.

Evaluation

The effectiveness of erythromycin should be apparent with the relief or reduction in the symptoms of the infection.

A sudden elevation in temperature, associated with an enlarged liver, tea-colored urine, clay-colored stools, jaundice, nausea and anorexia indicates cholestatic hepatitis. Erythromycin should be stopped immediately and the physician notified. Superinfections caused by overgrowth of nonsensitive, normal body flora are not uncommon and are evidenced by black furry tongue, nausea, diarrhea, pruritus vulva or perianal itching. As indicated earlier, gastrointestinal distress has been associated with oral erythromycin. Nurses should also be alert for pain, induration and red streaking at the site of intravenous infusions of erythromycin. These observations suggest thrombophlebitis.

Teaching

Patients taking erythromycin on an outpatient basis should be taught the indicators of drug efficacy and adverse effects. They should also be advised that failure to take erythromycin as directed and for the prescribed length of time may result in recurrence of the infection and development of resistant organisms. Patients should also be told to notify the nurse if diarrhea stools, dark urine, pale stools, or yellow discoloration of eyes or skin occurs.

Clindamycin (Cleocin, Dalacin C)

Mechanism of Action

Clindamycin binds to bacterial ribosomes and prevents protein formation. Similar to erythromycin, clindamycin is bacteriostatic.

Antibacterial Spectrum

Clindamycin is effective against many of the same bacteria that are inhibited by erythromycin. This includes many gram-positive cocci, including pneumococci, Group A streptococci and staphylococci. Clindamycin is also effective in the treatment of infections due to anaerobic bacteria, particularly *Bacteroides fragilis.*

Pharmacokinetics

Clindamycin is well absorbed from the gastrointestinal tract; food does not affect its absorption. Clindamycin penetrates tissues well, including bone, but does not readily cross normal or inflamed meninges. The drug is extensively metabolized in the liver and its dosage must be reduced in patients with liver disease. Clindamycin may also be given intramuscularly or intravenously for more severe infections.

Therapeutic Uses

Although clindamycin may be used for many of the same indications as erythromycin, it is more toxic than the latter drug and should not be used as a replacement for erythromycin. Because clindamycin can produce pseudomembranous colitis, its systemic use should be limited to the treatment of conditions for which other antibiotics are inappropriate or ineffective. Clindamycin should be reserved for the treatment of some staphylococcal infections in penicillin-allergic patients. It is also widely used in combination with an aminoglycoside for the treatment of mixed aerobic and anaerobic infections. A major justification for the continued availability of clindamycin is the sensitivity of the anaerobe *Bacteroides fragilis* to it.

Topical clindamycin (Cleocin-T, Dalacin-T) may be used to treat acne vulgaris. The rationale for its use is similar to that previously explained for erythromycin. Clindamycin can eradicate *Propionibacterium acnes* in pilosebaceous glands. This anaerobe secretes enzymes capable of disrupting follicular epithelium. By inhibiting *Propionibacterium acnes,* clindamycin reduces the inflammation of acne.

Adverse Effects

Rashes and diarrhea are the most common adverse reactions to clindamycin. Gastrointestinal intolerance, with abdominal pain, nausea and vomiting occurs infrequently. The greatest fear with clindamycin is the development of pseudomembranous colitis, secondary to the production of toxins by strains of *Clostridium difficile.* By inhibiting normal intestinal flora, clindamycin allows the proliferation of *Clostridium difficile.* Severe pseudomembranous colitis can prove fatal. Treatment usually involves the administration of vancomycin.

Nursing Process

Because of the similarity in action between erythromycin and clindamycin, the nursing process associated with their prescription and use is similar. Additionally, patients receiving clindamycin should be evaluated for diarrhea that contains mucus and blood, severe abdominal pain, changes in respiratory status and sudden high fever. These observations indicate the development of pseudomembranous colitis and should result in the immediate discontinuation of the medication and notification of the physician.

Further Reading

Choice of antimicrobial drugs (1990). *The Medical Letter 32* :41-48.

Choice of antimicrobial drugs (1986). *The Medical Letter 28* :33-40.

Gribble, M.J. and Chow, A.W. (1982). Erythromycin. *Med. Clin. North Am. 66* :79-89.

Oral erythromycins (1985). *The Medical Letter 27* :1-3.

Table 92
Erythromycin and clindamycin.

Pharmacologic Classification: Antibiotics — Erythromycin

Generic Name (Trade Name)	Use (Dose)	Action	Adverse Effects	Drug Interactions	Nursing Process
Erythromycin (Erythromycin Base Filmtab, Erythromid, E-Mycin, Ery-Tab, Ilotycin, Robimycin, ERYC); erythromycin stearate (Erythrocin Stearate Filmtab, Bristamycin, Pfizer-E, Erypar, Ethril); erythromycin estolate (Ilosone); erythromycin ethylsuccinate (EES, Pediamycin)	Often used as replacement for penicillins G or V in allergic pts. Tx of group A hemolytic streptococcal infect'ns, incl. tonsillitis, erysipelas, scarlet fever, chemoprophylaxis of streptococcal and pneumococcal infect'ns, acute illness or carrier state of diphtheria, and in early and late syphilis. Effective in tx of mycoplasma, *Legionnella pneumonophilia, Bordetella pertussis, Chlamydia trachomatis* and, tog. w. a sulfonamide, in tx of *H. influenzæ*. Systemically or topically to inhibit *Propionibacterium acnes* **(Oral:** Adults - 500 mg q12h or 250 mg q6h 1-1.5 h ac or pc. Erythromycin estolate and erythromycin ethysuccinate may be taken w. food. Children - 30-50 mg/kg/day or more, depending on severity of infect'n, admin. in 2-4 doses. All doses expressed as erythromycin base)	Bacteriostatic. Blocks protein synthesis by binding selectively to bacterial 50S ribosomal subunit and preventing elongat'n of peptide chain.	GI upset, nausea, diarrhea, abd. pain and occ. cholestatic jaundice.	**Anticoagulants, oral:** May demonstrate incr. anticoagulant effects if erythromycin is admin. IV. **Carbamazepine:** Blood levels may incr. when erythromycin lactobionate is given IV, resulting in potential carbamazepine toxicity. **Digoxin:** Blood levels may incr. if erythromycin lactobionate admin. IV. **Theophylline:** Administrat'n of erythromycin can incr. blood levels.	**Assess:** For previous erythromycin allergy, renal or liver disease; collect culture and sensitivity specimens, document clinical observat'ns of infect'n. **Administer:** IV into large vein using small needle; IM slowly, deep into large muscle mass; oral on empty stomach w. water only; topically after cleansing skin. **Evaluate:** Drug efficacy in relieving clinical manifestat'ns of infect'n; fever, enlarged liver, tea-colored urine, clay-colored stools, jaundice, superinfect'ns of nonsensitive normal body flora; GI distress, thrombophlebitis. **Teach:** Pts taking drug at home to recognize indicators of drug efficacy and adv. effects; importance of compliance w. prescribed regimen. To notify nurse or physician immed. if changes in stools, urine or skin occur.
Erythromycin lactobionate (Erythrocin Lactobionate-IV)	As for erythromycin **(IV:** 10-20 mg/kg/day. Larger doses may be given in very severe infect'ns [max. 4 g daily]. Although continuous infus'n is preferable, administrat'n in divided doses not < q6h is also effective)	As for erythromycin	As for erythromycin	As for erythromycin	As for erythromycin

Generic Name (Trade Name)	Use (Dose)	Action	Adverse Effects	Drug Interactions	Nursing Process
Erythromycin glucep-tate (Ilotycin glucep-tate)	As for erythromycin (**IV:** Adults and children - 15-20 mg/kg/day. Higher doses may be given in very severe infect'ns. Continuous infus'n is preferable, but administrat'n in divided doses no more frequently than q6h is also effective)	As for erythromycin	As for erythromycin	As for erythromycin	As for erythromycin

Pharmacologic Classification: Antibiotics — Clindamycin

Generic Name (Trade Name)	Use (Dose)	Action	Adverse Effects	Drug Interactions	Nursing Process
Clindamycin	Tx of serious infect'ns due to sensitive anaerobic bacteria such as bacteroides spp., peptostreptococcus, anaerobic streptococci, clostridium spp. and microaerophilic streptococci	Bacteriostatic. Binds to 50S ribosomal subunit of sensitive bacteria to inhibit protein synthesis. Effective against many bacteria inhibited by erythromycin. Clindamycin should not be used to replace erythromycin because it is more toxic. Should be reserved for tx of some staphylococcal infect'ns in penicillin-allergic pts. Used w. an aminoglycoside for tx of mixed aerobic and anaerobic infect'ns.	GI distress incl. abd. pain, nausea, vomiting, esophagitis and diarrhea or loose stools. Gen'lized mild to moderate morbilli-form-like skin rashes or urticaria can occur. Some cases of severe or persistent diarrhea have been reported. Some of these have involved pseudomembranous colitis. If significant diarrhea occurs during tx, stop drug. If colitis is suspected, endoscopy is recomm. If pseudomembranous colitis develops, treat appropriately. *Clostridium difficile* is us. sensitive to vancomycin.		As for erythromycin, plus: **Evaluate:** For diarrhea containing blood and mucus, severe abd. pain, high fever or changes in respiratory status.
Clindamycin HCl (Dalacin C, Cleocin HCl)	**(Oral:** Adults - *For serious infect'ns,* 150-300 mg q6h. *For more severe infect'ns,* 300-450 mg q6h. Children - *For serious infect'ns,* 8-16 mg/kg/day in 3-4 divided doses. *For more severe infect'ns,* 16-20 mg/kg/day in 3-4 divided doses)	As for clindamycin			As for clindamycin
Clindamycin palmitate HCl (Dalacin C Palmitate, Cleocin Pediatric)	As for clindamycin **(Oral:** Children > 1 month of age - Doses depend on severity of infect'n; give in 3-4 equal doses: 8-12 mg/kg/day; 13-16 mg/kg/day, or 17-25 mg/kg/day)				As for clindamycin

As for clindamycin

As for clindamycin

As for clindamycin

Clindamycin phosphate inject'n solut'n (Dalacin C Phosphate Sterile Solution, Cleocin Phosphate)

As for clindamycin (**IM:** Adults - 600 mg/day in 2 equal doses. *For moderately severe infect'ns,* 600-1200 mg/day in 2-3 equal doses. *For severe infect'ns,* 1200-2400 mg/day in 2-4 equal doses. **IV:** *For moderately severe infect'ns,* 900-1800 mg/day by continuous drip or in 2-3 equal doses, each infused over 20-min minimum. *For severe infect'ns,* 1800-2700 mg/day by continuous drip or in 3-4 equal doses, each infused over 20 min or longer. *For life-threatening infect'ns,* 2700-4800 mg/day by continuous drip or in 3-4 equal doses, each infused over 20 min or longer)

CHAPTER 62

The Tetracyclines

Teaching Objectives

Following completion of this chapter, the reader should be able to:
1. Describe the mechanism of action and antibacterial spectra of the tetracyclines.
2. Discuss the pharmacokinetics of the tetracyclines.
3. Discuss the therapeutic uses and adverse effects of the tetracyclines.
4. Compare the therapeutic uses of doxycycline and minocycline with other tetracyclines.
5. Describe the nursing process related to tetracycline use.

The drugs tetracycline HCl (Achromycin, Achromycin V, Sumycin, Tetracyn), oxytetracycline (Terramycin), demeclocycline (Declomycin), doxycycline (Vibramycin), methacycline (Rondomycin) and minocycline (Minocin) are collectively referred to as the tetracyclines. All tetracyclines have similar chemical structures and antibacterial spectra. Unless otherwise stated, the expression tetracycline or tetracyclines in this chapter refers to all of these drugs.

Mechanism of Action

Tetracyclines are concentrated within sensitive gram-positive and gram-negative bacteria by an energy-dependent process. Once inside bacteria, tetracyclines depress protein synthesis. Tetracyclines are bacteriostatic. Once bacterial cell multiplication is stopped, the host's defense mechanisms kill the pathogens. Because mammalian cells do not concentrate tetracyclines, protein synthesis in the host is not affected.

Antibacterial Spectrum

The tetracyclines have a wide spectrum of activity. Although they are more effective against gram-positive bacteria, the drugs are also active against gram-negative bacteria, rickettsiae, mycoplasmas and agents of the psittacosis-lymphogranuloma venereum group of conditions (Table 93). There are no major differences between the various tetracyclines. Doxycycline may be effective against some strains of *Bacteroides fragilis* that are resistant to other tetracyclines.

Development of bacterial resistance to the tetracyclines has been a particularly vexing problem. Strains of *Escherichia coli*, *Klebsiella pneumoniae*, pneumococci and streptococci (group A and pneumococci) that originally were sensitive to the tetracyclines have developed resistance.

Table 93
Sensitivities of some organisms to the tetracyclines.

Bacillus anthracis	Some sensitivity
Bacteroides spp.	Moderate sensitivity but many resistant strains
Clostridium perfringens	Moderate sensitivity
Clostridium tetani	Moderate sensitivity
Escherichia coli	Moderate sensitivity but many resistant strains
Haemophilus ducreyi	High sensitivity but many resistant strains
Haemophilus influenzae	High sensitivity but many resistant strains
Klebsiella pneumoniae	Moderate sensitivity but many resistant strains
Listeria monocytogenese	Moderate sensitivity
Mycoplasma pneumoniae	High sensitivity
Neisseria gonorrhoeae	Moderate sensitivity
Neisseria meningitidis	Moderate sensitivity
Salmonella	Moderate sensitivity but many resistant strains
Shigella	Moderate sensitivity but many resistant strains
Staphylococcus aureus (both penicillin-sensitive and penicillin-resistant)	Some sensitivity but tetracyclines not recomm. for tx
Streptococcus pneumoniae	Moderate sensitivity but some areas have many resistant strains
Streptococcus pyogenes	Moderate sensitivity but many resistant strains
Treponema pallidum	Sensitive; tetracycline is recomm. in penicillin-allergic pts

Pharmacokinetics

Tetracyclines are usually given orally, although formulations of tetracycline hydrochloride, tetracycline phosphate, oxytetracycline, minocycline and doxycycline are also available for parenteral administration. Absorption from the gastrointestinal tract ranges from 60 – 80% for oxytetracycline, tetracycline and demeclocycline, to 95 – 100% for minocycline and doxycycline. Most tetracyclines should not be taken with milk, nonabsorbable antacids or iron preparations because calcium, magnesium, aluminum and iron block tetracycline absorption. An exception is doxycycline, the absorption of which is not significantly influenced by the ingestion of food or milk.

Once absorbed, tetracyclines bind in varying degrees to plasma proteins. Oxytetracycline, tetracycline and minocycline are 35%, 65% and 76% bound, respectively. Methacycline, demeclocycline and doxycycline are approximately 90% bound to plasma albumin. Tetracyclines distribute throughout the body, penetrating tissues to varying degrees. High concentrations are usually found in bile. Tetracyclines cross the placenta but have difficulty crossing the blood-brain barrier. Concentrations in the cerebrospinal fluid are only 10 – 20% of those in plasma.

Lipid solubility is a major factor in determining tetracycline diffusion. Doxycycline and minocycline are more lipophilic and penetrate tissues and secretions better than the other tetracyclines. Doxycycline diffuses well into endometrial, myometrial, prostatic and renal tissues. Minocycline attains therapeutic concentrations in saliva and tears. The lipid solubility of minocycline can, however, be a disadvantage because it enables the drug to diffuse well into the highly lipid cells of the vestibular apparatus, leading to vestibular toxicity.

Tetracyclines bind to calcium and are retained in bones and growing teeth for long periods of time. Because they can damage developing teeth and delay the development of long bones, tetracyclines are usually contraindicated during pregnancy and in patients under eight to ten years of age (see Adverse Effects, below).

The half-lives of the tetracyclines range from eight to nine hours (for tetracycline HCl and oxytetracycline) to sixteen to eighteen hours (for minocycline and doxycycline). The differences in half-lives are reflected in the dosage intervals for minocycline and doxycycline. Whereas most tetracyclines are recommended on a three- or four-times-daily basis, minocycline is taken twice a day and doxycycline once daily.

Renal excretion is the major route of tetracycline elimination. Minocycline has a low renal clearance and less than ten per cent of a dose is recovered unchanged in urine. The drug undergoes enterohepatic circulation and may be metabolized to a considerable extent. Doxycycline elimination is independent of both renal and hepatic function. The drug is excreted in the feces, largely as an inactive chelated product. Thus, the dose does not require modification in patients with renal or hepatic insufficiency. Furthermore, the inactive product has relatively less impact on the intestinal microflora, resulting in lower incidence of irritative diarrhea and candidal overgrowth.

Therapeutic Uses

Despite their broad antibacterial spectrum, tetracyclines have relatively poor activity against most pathogens and are rarely considered drugs of first choice. They are considered first-line drugs for the treatment of *Mycoplasma pneumoniae,* Rocky Mountain spotted fever, endemic typhus, *Borrelia recurrentis* (relapsing fever), chlamydial disease, nonspecific brucellosis and infections caused by pasteurella. The use of tetracycline therapy to treat inflammatory acne is presented in Chapter 41.

For most infections, tetracyclines are second- or third-line drugs, falling behind more effective agents. Conditions for which tetracyclines are backup drugs are too numerous to mention. They are listed in *The Medical Letter 28* :33-40 (1986).

Doxycycline and minocycline warrant special note. For most clinical conditions they offer no advantage over tetracycline HCl and cost significantly more money. There are, however, a few situations in which they are superior to the other tetracyclines. Minocycline may be the preferred tetracycline for acne vulgaris. Minocycline is an effective alternative to rifampicin for the eradication of meningococci, including sulfonamide-resistant bacteria from the nasopharnynx.

As mentioned previously, doxycycline is eliminated unchanged in the feces. Consequently, it does not accumulate in patients with renal or hepatic impairment and is safer than other tetracyclines in these persons. Doxycycline is the tetracycline of choice for the treatment of sinusitis and acute exacerbations of chronic bronchitis caused by pneumococci, group A streptococci, and *Haemophilus influenzae.* Because it penetrates the noninflamed prostate better, doxycycline may be effective in chronic prostatitis. It is also preferred for the treatment of acute urethral syndrome because the most common causative bacteria, *Escherichia coli, Staphylococcus saprophyticus* and

chlamydia, are usually susceptible to the drug. Doxycycline has greater activity than the other tetracyclines against *Bacteroides fragilis*. It has been used successfully in the treatment of nongonococcal pelvic inflammatory disease produced by *E. coli,* other aerobic gram-negative coliforms and *B. fragilis.*

Tetracyclines are contraindicated in severe renal or hepatic disease. They are also normally contraindicated in pregnant or lactating women. Because of their ability to bind to calcium and affect the development of teeth and long bones, tetracyclines are contraindicated in children under eight years of age. Finally, tetracyclines should not be used in situations where bactericidal effect is essential, such as bacterial endocarditis.

Adverse Effects

Tetracyclines can cause nausea, vomiting, epigastric burning, stomatitis and glossitis when given orally. Administered intravenously, they can produce phlebitis. Tetracyclines can be hepatotoxic, particularly in patients with pre-existing renal or hepatic insufficiency. Hepatotoxicity does not occur frequently, but can be particularly severe during pregnancy. If given for long periods of time, tetracyclines can increase blood urea nitrogen (BUN) and occasionally cause nephrotoxicity. They should not be given with potentially nephrotoxic drugs.

As already stated, tetracyclines can stain teeth and retard bone growth if given to pregnant women after the fourth month of gestation or to children under the age of eight years.

Photosensitivity, manifested mainly as abnormal sunburn reactions, is particularly prevalent with demeclocycline therapy. Minocycline produces vertigo in a high percentage of patients taking the drug.

Superinfection is a recognized adverse reaction to many broad-spectrum antibiotics, including tetracyclines. By suppressing the normal bacterial flora, tetracyclines enable other bacteria, such as penicillinase-producing staphylococci and candida, to proliferate. Superinfections occur in the oral, anogenital and intestinal areas of the body. The consequences of the superinfection are determined by its site. When the superinfection occurs in the oropharynx, vagina and perirectal areas, itching and discomfort may occur. If overgrowth of bowel pathogenic bacteria occurs, diarrhea is observed.

Pseudomembranous colitis, secondary to the overgrowth of *Clostridium difficile,* can also occur, particularly in elderly or debilitated patients or in individuals being treated with several antibiotics, immunosuppressants or corticosteroids. If pseudomembranous colitis develops, the tetracycline should be stopped immediately, lost electrolytes replaced, and other supportive measures used as required. Oral vancomycin may be given, if necessary.

Nursing Process

Assessment

Nursing assessment related to tetracycline administration begins with a review of the patient's history for evidence of previous allergy, renal impairment or liver disease. Physical assessment should emphasize accurate determination of the patient's age, existence of a current pregnancy or lactation. As explained before, tetracyclines are contraindicated in young, pregnant or lactating patients.

Specimens for laboratory culture and sensitivity tests should be collected prior to the first administration of a tetracycline. Nurses should also document the clinical symptoms of the infection.

Administration

Tetracyclines should be administered before their expiry date. Outdated products can precipitate nephrotic syndrome, manifested by nausea, vomiting, acidosis, proteinuria, glucosuria, polydipsia, polyuria and hypokalemia. Because tetracyclines deteriorate more rapidly when exposed to heat, light or moisture, they should be stored in airtight, light-resistant containers, in a cool dark place.

Tetracyclines should be administered on an empty stomach, i.e., either one hour before or two hours after meals. Products or food containing calcium, magnesium, aluminum or iron (e.g., milk, antacids, iron supplements) should be avoided. If this is not possible, they should be withheld for at least two hours following oral administration of a tetracycline. Mild gastric irritation associated with tetracycline ingestion may be reduced by taking the drug with a small amount of food low in the four preceding elements. Milk must *never* be taken simultaneously with a tetracycline.

When administering a tetracycline intramuscularly, the needle should be inserted deep into a large muscle, with no more than 2 mL of drug injected at each site. Aspiration is essential because intramuscular preparations often contain local anesthetics which are harmful if injected intravenously. Inject the solution slowly into the muscle to minimize pain. When given intravenously, tetracyclines should be infused slowly into a large vein using a small needle to reduce the risk of phlebitis.

Evaluation

Nurses should evaluate patients for evidence of clinical improvement. At the same time, nurses should observe patients for allergic responses, characterized by fever, urticaria, angioedema, headache, papilloedema, pericarditis or anaphylaxis. The presence of severe gastritis may require switching tetracyclines or moving from oral to parenteral administration.

Nurses must be alert for evidence of uremia as manifested by nausea, vomiting, headache, dizziness, visual disturbances, stupor, stertorous respirations, reduced urinary output and elevated BUN. Adverse hepatotoxic effects are suggested by the presence of jaundice, including yellowing of the skin and sclera in association with tea-colored urine. Nurses must also monitor patients for the development of superinfections, as reflected by black furry tongue, pruritus ani, pruritus vulvae or diarrhea. Swelling, induration or redness at the site of intravenous infusions indicate phlebitis. Blood dyscrasias are indicated by sore throat, malaise and increased bleeding tendencies.

Teaching

Patients who take tetracyclines at home should be advised to avoid ultraviolet light because of the risk of photosensitivity. They should be told how to store the drug and warned against concomitant ingestion of products containing calcium, magnesium, aluminum or iron.

Outpatients should be reminded of the importance of completing the entire prescribed course of therapy to prevent recurrence of the infection. Individuals using doxycycline prophylactically for "Montezuma's revenge" should be advised upon returning home to discard any unused capsules. All patients should be reminded of the importance of maintaining good oral and perineal hygiene as a means of minimizing the development of superinfections. Nurses should warn diabetics to avoid the use of Clinistix, Diastix or Tes-Tape for urine glucose testing.

Further Reading

Advice for the travelers (1990). *The Medical Letter 32* :33-36.

Choice of antimicrobial drugs (1990). *The Medical Letter 32* :41-48.

Choice of antimicrobial drugs (1986). *The Medical Letter 28* :33-40.

Tetracyclines and chloramphenicol (1986). *AMA Drug Evaluations,* 6th ed., pp. 1409-1424. Chicago: American Medical Association.

Treatment of sexually transmitted siseases (1990). *The Medical Letter 32* :5-10.

Table 94
The tetracyclines.

Pharmacologic Classification: Antibiotics

Generic Name (Trade Name)	Use (Dose)	Action	Adverse Effects	Drug Interactions	Nursing Process
Tetracycline HCl (Achromycin, Achromycin V, Panmycin, Robetet, Sumycin, Tetracyn)	First-line drugs for tx of *Mycoplasma pneumoniae*, Rocky Mountain spotted fever, endemic typhus, *Borrelia recurrentis*, chlamydial diseases, nonspecific urethritis and cholera in adults. Also effective in brucellosis and infect'ns caused by pasteurella. Particular uses for doxycycline and minocycline are presented below **(Oral:** Adults - 250-500 mg q6h. Children > 8 years - 25-50 mg/kg/day in 2-4 divided doses. **IM:** Adults - 250 mg as single daily dose or 300 mg daily given as 2-3 divided doses. Children > 8 years - 15-25 mg/kg/day in 2-3 equal doses up to max. 250 mg/single daily inject'n. **IV:** Adults - 250-500 mg q12h w. max. 500 mg q6h. Max. dose, 2 g/day. Children > 8 years - 10-20 mg/kg/day in 2 divided doses prn. Refer to manufacturer's literature about dilut'n of IV solut'n. Inject'n rate not > 2 mg/min)	Bacteriostatic. Concentrated within sensitive gram-pos. and gram-neg. bacteria. Reduces protein synthesis by binding primarily at 30S ribosomal subunit to block attachment of aminoacyl transfer RNA to its receptor site. Wide spectrum of activity. Development of resistance has greatly reduced tx value of tetracyclines.	Nausea, vomiting, epigastric burning, stomatitis, glossitis, hepatotoxicity and nephrotoxicity. Binding to bone results in stained teeth and delayed bone growth. Photosensitivity. Superinfect'ns in oral, anogenital and intestinal areas of body. Pseudomembranous colitis.	**Antacids:** Containing Ca, Mg and Al impair absorpt'n of orally administered tetracyclines and should not be administered within an hour or so of tetracycline tx. **Antibiotics:** W. bacterICIDal action, such as penicillin and cephalosporins, may interact w. tetracyclines, which are bacteriostatic. Avoid giving tetracyclines in conjunct'n w. these agents. **Anticoagulants:** May require a downward adjustment in dosage because tetracyclines may depress plasma prothrombin activity. **Contraceptives, oral:** May demonstrate reduced efficacy and incr. incidence of breakthrough bleeding in presence of tetracycline. **Diuretics:** And tetracyclines may both incr. BUN levels. Avoid concomitant use if poss. **Foods:** Containing Ca and Mg reduce tetracycline absorpt'n. W. except'n of doxycycline, tetracyclines should be taken separately from milk and other dairy products. **Iron:** Binds to tetracycline, preventing its absorpt'n. **Methoxyflurane:** Used concurrently w. tetracyclines, has been reported to impair renal funct'n seriously, leading in some cases to death. Concomitant use of	**Assess:** Age < 12; pregnancy, lactat'n, renal impairment, liver disease, previous allergy. Collect specimens for culture and sensitivity before 1st dose; document clinical observat'n of infect'n. **Administer:** On empty stomach (1 h ac or 2 h pc); withhold Ca-, Mg-, Al- or Fe-containing substances (e.g., milk, antacids, Fe supplements) for 2 h following oral administrat'n. Gastric irritat'n may be alleviated by giving small am'ts of food. For IM inject'n, insert needle deeply into large muscle, aspirate carefully, inject slowly not > 2 mL at each site. Infuse IV slowly into large vein using small needle. **Evaluate:** Reduct'n/alleviat'n of clinical indicators of infect'n; for allergic response (fever, urticaria, angioedema, headache, papilloedema, pericarditis, anaphylaxis), gastric irritat'n; for uremia (nausea, vomiting, headache, dizziness, visual disturbances, stupor, stertorous respirat'ns, reduced urinary output, elevated BUN); jaundice (yellow skin/sclera, tea-colored urine); superinfect'ns (black, furry tongue, pruritus ani or vulvae, diarrhea); phlebitis at site of IV infus'n (swelling, indurat'n, redness); blood dyscrasias (sore throat, malaise, incr. bleeding tendencies). **Teach:** To avoid UV light; to store in airtight, light-resistant container in cool, dry place; to discard unused medicat'n; to maintain good oral and perineal hygiene; proper administrat'n practices. Warn diabetics to avoid use of Clinistix, Diastix or Tes-Tape for urine glucose testing.
Oxytetracycline (Terramycin)	As for tetracycline HCl **(Oral:** Adults - 250-500 mg qid; may be doubled in the severely ill. Children > 8 years - 25-50 mg/kg/day in 4 divided doses)	As for tetracycline HCl	As for tetracycline HCl		

Generic Name (Trade Name)	Use (Dose)	Action	Adverse Effects	Drug Interactions	Nursing Process
Demeclocycline (Declomycin)	As for tetracycline HCl (**Oral:** Adults - 150 mg qid or 300 mg bid. Children > 8 years - 6-12 mg/kg/day in 2-4 divided doses)	As for tetracycline HCl	As for tetracycline HCl	these agents is not recomm. **Milk:** May reduce absorpt'n of tetracyclines. See earlier discuss'n on food.	As for tetracycline HCl
Doxycycline (Vibramycin, Vibra-Tabs)	As for tetracycline HCl. For particular uses, see Chapter 62 (**Oral:** Adults - 200 mg on day 1, followed by maint. dose of 100 mg od at same time each day. For severe infect'ns such as lung abscesses or osteomyelitis, and in chronic urinary tract infect'ns, single daily dose of 200 mg may be used throughout. For tx acute gonococcal infect'ns - 200 mg stat, and 100 mg hs first day, followed by 100 mg bid for 3 days. For tx uncomplicated urethral, endocervical or vaginal infect'ns in adults assoc. w. C. trachomatis and ureaplasma infect'ns - 100 mg bid for at least 10 days)	As for tetracycline HCl	As for tetracycline HCl	As for tetracycline HCl	As for tetracycline HCl
Methacycline (Rondomycin)	As for tetracycline HCl (**Oral:** Adults - 600 mg/day in 2-4 divided doses. Children > 8 years - 6-12 mg/kg/day in 2-4 divided doses)	As for tetracycline HCl	As for tetracycline HCl	As for tetracycline HCl	As for tetracycline HCl
Minocycline HCl (Minocin)	As for tetracycline HCl. For particular uses, see Chapter 62 (**Oral:** Adults - 100-200 mg initially, followed by 100 mg q12h. Children ≥ 13 years - 4 mg/kg initially, followed by 2 mg/kg q12h. For inflammatory acne - 50-200 mg/day)	As for tetracycline HCl	As for tetracycline HCl	As for tetracycline HCl	As for tetracycline HCl

CHAPTER 63

The Aminoglycosides

Teaching Objectives

Following completion of this chapter, the reader should be able to:

1. Discuss the mechanism of action, antibacterial spectra, pharmacokinetics, therapeutic uses and adverse effects of aminoglycoside antibiotics.
2. Compare kanamycin, gentamicin, tobramycin, amikacin and netilmicin with respect to therapeutic uses and adverse effects.
3. Calculate dosage modifications for gentamicin, tobramycin, amikacin and netilmicin for patients with renal impairment.
4. Describe the nursing processes related to the use of kanamycin, gentamicin, tobramycin, amikacin and netilmicin.

The aminoglycoside antibiotics are a group of structurally related drugs. They derive their name from the fact that their structures contain at least one sugar attached to one or more amino groups. The aminoglycoside antibiotics in use today include neomycin and framycetin, which are used primarily on the skin (see Chapter 43), and streptomycin, which is used mainly in the treatment of tuberculosis (see Chapter 66). This chapter will consider the pharmacologic properties and therapeutic uses of the remaining aminoglycosides, kanamycin, gentamicin, tobramycin, amikacin and netilmicin. We will consider first the aminoglycosides as a group and then later the individual drugs.

Mechanism of Action

Aminoglycosides inhibit bacterial protein synthesis. They bind to the bacterial 30S ribosomal subunit of streptococci to cause a misreading of the genetic code. The proteins formed contain the wrong sequence of amino acids and have no biological value ("nonsense proteins"). Aminoglycosides block protein synthesis in other bacteria by inhibiting amino acid translocation.

Antibacterial Spectrum

Aminoglycosides are bactericidal. They are used almost principally to treat infections caused by sensitive strains of Enterobacteriaceae, including *Escherichia coli*, klebsiella, enterobacter, serratia and proteus species. With the exception of streptomycin and kanamycin, aminoglycosides are active against *Pseudomonas aeruginosa*. They have only limited activity against most gram-positive bacteria. They are active in vitro against certain species of streptococcus. Only minimal activity is usually found against *S. faecalis*, *S. pneumoniae* and streptococci of the viridans group. Although aminoglycosides inhibit staphylococci, safer drugs, such as the penicillins or cephalosporins, are usually used.

Aminoglycosides have little activity against anaerobic micro-organisms or facultative bacteria under anaerobic conditions.

Gentamicin, tobramycin, amikacin and netilmicin are extensively used for the treatment of systemic infections. Although their antibacterial spectra show few qualitative differences, the various aerobic gram-negative bacilli vary in their susceptibility to the four drugs. Table 95 describes the differing sensitivities of six gram-negative bacilli to tobramycin and gentamicin. The purpose of this table is not to suggest that tobramycin should always be used in place of gentamicin but instead to indicate that cultures should be performed, where practical, to determine the most appropriate aminoglycoside to treat a particular patient.

As a result of bacterial enzymatic inactivation, resistance has developed to some of the aminoglycosides, notably kanamycin and gentamicin. Cross-resistance can also occur. Organisms resistant to gentamicin are often insensitive to tobramycin, and possibly also to netilmicin. Bacterial inactivation is minimal with amikacin. Micro-organisms resistant to gentamicin and tobramycin are often sensitive to amikacin. On the other hand, if bacteria are resistant to amikacin, they are usually resistant to all aminoglycosides.

Table 95

In vitro activity of tobramycin and gentamicin against susceptible gram-negative organisms (percentage of isolates susceptible at 1.57 μg/mL).

	Number of Strains	Tobramycin	Gentamicin
Escherichia coli	100	93%	80%
Enterobacter spp.	52	94%	81%
Proteus mirabilis	38	92%	58%
Proteus spp. (indole-positive)	26	100%	85%
Klebsiella spp.	100	100%	98%
Serratia marcescens	41	86%	88%

Pharmacokinetics

The aminoglycosides are very polar (water-soluble) drugs and cannot diffuse across gastrointestinal membranes. Less than one per cent of an oral dose is absorbed. Aminoglycosides are absorbed rapidly from intramuscular injection sites, with peak concentrations appearing within one hour.

Aminoglycosides do not diffuse readily across body membranes. For example, concentrations of gentamicin in pleural and pericardial fluids are only one-quarter to one-half those in serum. Aminoglycoside levels in fetal serum are twenty to forty per cent of those in maternal serum. Aminoglycosides do not cross into the cerebrospinal fluid well, even in the presence of inflammation. If used to treat meningitis in adults, they must be given intrathecally. The poorly developed blood-brain barrier of the newborn presents little impediment to drug diffusion; therefore, systemic aminoglycoside administration can produce therapeutic levels of the antibiotic in the cerebrospinal fluid of neonates. Aminoglycosides enter the perilymph of the ear, where concentrations correlate with ototoxicity.

Aminoglycosides are eliminated by renal excretion. Their half-lives of two to three hours in patients with normal kidney function are extended in patients with renal impairment. Dosages must be decreased in the neonate or adult with reduced renal function. Although formulae are provided (see Therapeutic Uses, below) to assist in dosage calculations for patients with renal impairment, they should be used as guides only when it is impossible to measure serum levels of the drug.

Therapeutic Uses

Kanamycin (Kantrex, Klebcil)
Kanamycin is seldom used today because of bacterial resistance. Kanamycin capsules may be given orally to sterilize the bowel preoperatively, treat intestinal infections caused by susceptible organisms, or provide adjunctive treatment of neurologic manifestations associated with severe liver damage.

Gentamicin (Alcomicin, Cidomycin, Garamycin)
Gentamicin is still important in the treatment of many serious gram-negative bacillary infections (e.g., caused by *Escherichia coli, Proteus mirabilis,* indole-positive proteus, klebsiella, enterobacter, serratia and *Pseudomonas aeruginosa*), although resistance to the drug is developing. In addition to the foregoing, salmonella and shigella are often gentamicin-sensitive. Gentamicin can be considered for treatment of bacteremia, respiratory and urinary tract infections, infected wounds and bone and soft tissue infections, including peritonitis and burns complicated by sepsis. Peak serum levels should be at least 4 μg/mL (8.6 μmol/L), but should not exceed 10 μg/mL (21.6 μmol/L). Serious infections with *Pseudomonas aeruginosa* may require serum levels of 6 μg/mL (12.9 μmol/L) of gentamicin combined with carbenicillin (Geopen, Pyopen) or

ticarcillin (Ticar). The combination produces a synergistic effect with some strains and delays the emergence of resistant organisms. For patients with impaired renal function, the half-life of gentamicin in hours can be estimated by multiplying the serum creatinine (mg/100 mL) by four. The frequency of administration (in hours) may be approximated by doubling the half-life.

Gentamicin is also applied topically for use in the treatment of primary and secondary infections caused by sensitive strains of streptococci (group A beta-hemolytic, alpha-hemolytic), *S. aureus* (coagulase positive, coagulase negative and some penicillinase-producing strains), and the gram-negative bacteria *P. aeruginosa, Aerobacter aerogenes, E. coli, Proteus vulgaris* and *Klebsiella pneumoniae.* Gentamicin may also be used for ocular infections caused by *S. aureus, P. aeruginosa, A. aerogenes, E. coli, P. vulgaris* or *K. pneumoniae.*

Tobramycin (Nebcin)

Tobramycin has a similar antibacterial spectrum to that of gentamicin. It is usually active against most strains of the following organisms in vitro and in clinical infections: *P. aeruginosa;* proteus species (indole-positive and indole-negative) including *P. mirabilis, P. morganii, P. rettgeri* and *P. vulgaris; E. coli;* klebsiella-enterobacter-serratia group; citrobacter species; providencia species; and staphylococci, including *S. aureus* (coagulase-positive and coagulase-negative). Its minimal inhibitory concentration (MIC) against *Pseudomonas aeruginosa* is approximately one-quarter that of gentamicin. Tobramycin is considered by many to be the aminoglycoside of choice for *Pseudomonas aeruginosa* infections, in which case it is combined with carbenicillin or ticarcillin.

Tobramycin may be indicated for the treatment of the following infections when caused by susceptible organisms: septicemia, urinary tract infections, lower respiratory infections, serious skin and soft tissue infections (including burns and peritonitis), and central nervous system infections caused by organisms resistant to antibiotics usually considered efficacious in these infections.

Effective serum concentrations of tobramycin are similar to those previously presented for gentamicin. Prolonged serum concentrations above 12 μg/mL should be avoided. The dosage interval in hours can be calculated for adult patients with impaired renal function by multiplying the patient's serum creatinine (mg/100 mL) by six.

Like gentamicin, tobramycin can be used for ocular infections caused by *S. aureus, P. aeruginosa, A. aerogenes, E. coli, P. vulgaris* or *K. pneumoniae.*

Amikacin (Amikin)

Amikacin is indicated for the short-term treatment of serious infections due to amikacin susceptible strains of *Pseudomonas aeruginosa, E. coli, S. aureus,* as well as proteus, klebsiella-enterobacter-serratia, providencia, salmonella and citrobacter species. Among the aminoglycosides, it has the greatest resistance to bacterial aminoglycoside-inactivating enzymes. Amikacin is often considered to be the drug of choice for the initial treatment of serious gram-negative bacillary infections in hospitals, where gentamicin resistance is a problem. Amikacin's therapeutic serum concentrations range from 15 – 25 μg/mL (25.7 – 42.8 μmol/L). To obtain the dosage interval in hours for patients with impaired renal function, multiply the serum creatinine (mg/100 mL) by nine. This formula should not be used to calculate dosage for elderly patients.

Netilmicin (Netromycin)

Netilmicin has a similar spectrum of activity to that of gentamicin and tobramycin. However, because it is less sensitive to bacterial inactivation, netilmicin is effective against some gentamicin-resistant and tobramycin-resistant strains of Enterobacteriaceae. Netilmicin is indicated for the treatment of infections caused by susceptible strains of *E. coli,* proteus (indole-negative and some indole-positive), klebsiella, enterobacter, citrobacter and staphylococcus species. In using netilmicin, peak serum concentrations in excess of 16 μg/mL and trough levels below 4 μg/mL should be avoided. The dosage interval in hours can be calculated by multiplying the serum creatinine (mg/100 mL) by eight.

Adverse Effects

Aminoglycosides accumulate in the perilymph of the inner ear, destroying both the vestibular and cochlear sensory cells. The degree of permanent damage correlates with the number of destroyed sensory hair cells in the inner ear; this in turn relates to concentration of drug and length of exposure. Patients experience tinnitus and hearing loss (usually to high-frequency tones), dizziness and vertigo. Kanamycin and amikacin impair auditory functions preferentially, and gentamicin is more likely to damage vestibular function. Tobramycin causes auditory and vestibular damage with equal frequency. The diuretics ethacrynic acid (Edecrin) and furosemide (Lasix) potentiate aminoglycoside ototoxicity. Termination of drug treatment results in complete recovery, if hearing or balance loss, or both, are not extensive. However, if extensive damage has occurred, impairment may be permanent.

High concentrations of aminoglycosides accumulate in the renal cortex and urine. Five to seven days of therapy can cause dose-dependent damage to the proximal tubular epithelium, particularly in elderly or debilitated patients or in individuals with pre-existing renal impairment. Serum creatinine and blood urea nitrogen (BUN) increase and severe azotemia may occur. Tobramycin and netilmicin are claimed to be less nephrotoxic than the other aminoglycosides. Concomitant therapy with furosemide, ethacrynic acid, cephalosporins or methoxyflurane (Penthrane) increases the risk of nephrotoxicity.

Aminoglycosides can, rarely, reduce the release of acetylcholine from motor nerve terminals and cause a neuromuscular blockade, leading to a flaccid paralysis and respiratory failure. The risk is greatest in patients receiving an anesthetic or a neuromuscular blocker, or those suffering from myasthenia gravis or hypokalemia. It is speculated that aminoglycosides attach to calcium binding sites on the nerves and prevent calcium from participating in the release of acetylcholine. The neuromuscular blockade is treated by administering calcium gluconate, together with an anticholinesterase drug, such as neostigmine.

Allergic reactions characterized by pruritus, rash, urticaria, and (on very rare occasions) exfoliative dermatitis have occasionally been seen following aminoglycoside administration. Drug fever, hypotension and anaphylactic shock have also been reported.

Nursing Process

Assessment

Prior to administering an aminoglycoside antibiotic, nurses should determine whether the patient has previously experienced an allergic reaction to any member of the group. A previous allergy to one indicates generalized hypersensitivity to all aminoglycosides.

Nursing assessment should include a review of the patient's history for myasthenia gravis, hearing defects, ulcerative gastrointestinal conditions or renal impairment. Patients with a history of any of these must be evaluated more thoroughly following aminoglycoside administration.

Physical assessment prior to drug administration must include documentation of the patient's age and weight, as well as information on the fluid intake and output ratio, respirations, pulse and blood pressure, and hearing facility. As with all antibiotic usage, laboratory specimens for culture and sensitivity tests must be collected before the first administration of an aminoglycoside. The clinical observations related to the infection must be documented at this time. Nurses should anticipate that a complete urinalysis, blood urea nitrogen (BUN) and serum creatinine must also be performed. These baseline measures are essential to the later evaluation of the patient for adverse responses to the drug.

In consultation with the pharmacist, the nurse should review the patient's current drug regimen for the concurrent use of other ototoxic and nephrotoxic drugs.

Administration

Aminoglycoside antibiotics should be injected slowly, deep into a large muscle mass to minimize pain. Change injection sites every administration. If continued aminoglycoside therapy is required, physicians should provide a new order every ten days because of the increasing risk of adverse effects with prolonged treatment. This is not to say that these drugs should not be used for longer than ten days. In cases of particularly persistent infections, the physician may decide that the risk of adverse effects is outweighed by the benefits of continued therapy. Nurses should take vital signs during infusion and watch for hypotension, or change in the patient's pulse.

Evaluation

Following aminoglycoside treatment, nurses must document the patient's clinical performance. This will assist the physician in determining future doses and duration of therapy. Nurses must also be alert for early evidence of ototoxicity, such as dizziness, vertigo, nystagmus, tinnitus, roaring sounds and hearing loss. Casual conversational reference by the patient may provide the first clues of ototoxicity. Nurses should discuss with the attending physician the need for audiograms at regular intervals during the course of treatment and for one month thereafter.

Nephrotoxicity associated with aminoglycoside use is manifested by oliguria, proteinuria, decreased urine specific gravity, elevated BUN and serum creatinine. It is important, therefore, for the nurse to monitor the results of laboratory tests. Patients, particularly those with myasthenia gravis, are at risk of neuromuscular blockade following the administration of an aminoglycoside antibiotic. This is seen as depressed respirations which can proceed to apnea, reduced pulse rate, lowered blood pressure, ataxia, nystagmus, bladder distention due to urinary retention, as well as constipation and decreased bowel sounds due to intestinal atony. The appearance of any of these must be reported immediately to the physician.

Patients receiving topical aminoglycoside treatment should be observed for allergic dermatitis characterized by rash, itching, urticaria and/or angioneurotic edema. If the drug is applied on open wounds, such as burns, skin ulcerations, etc., nurses must be alert to the danger of systemic adverse effects.

Teaching
Patients should be instructed to report subjective effects relating to hearing and/or balance immediately. They should also be advised and regularly reminded to drink two to three liters per day in order to reduce the probability of nephrotic irritation. Patients applying one of these drugs topically on an outpatient basis must be told to seek medical advice if allergic dermatitis develops.

Further Reading

Burkle, W.S. (1981). Comparative evaluation of aminoglycoside antibiotics for systemic use. *Drug Intell. Clin. Pharm. 15* : 847-862.

Choice of antimicrobial drugs (1990). *The Medical Letter 32* :41-48.

Choice of antimicrobial drugs (1986). *The Medical Letter 28* :33-40.

Meyers, B.R. (1980). "Aminoglycosides." In: B.M. Kagan, ed., *Antimicrobial Therapy,* 3rd ed. Philadelphia: W.B. Saunders.

Table 96
The aminoglycosides.

Generic Name (Trade Name)	Use (Dose)	Action	Adverse Effects	Drug Interactions	Nursing Process

Pharmacologic Classification: Antibiotics — Aminoglycosides

Generic Name (Trade Name)	Use (Dose)	Action	Adverse Effects	Drug Interactions	Nursing Process
Gentamicin sulfate (Alcomicin, Cidomycin, Garamycin)	Tx of severe, complicated infect'ns caused by susceptible organisms. Aminoglycosides are active against aerobic gram-neg. bacilli, particularly E. coli, Pseudomonas aeruginosa, klebsiella, enterobacter, serratia and proteus spp. (**IM: For pts w. normal renal funct'n** - Adults - *For urinary tract infect'ns* - 160 mg od or 80 mg bid for 7-10 days. *For systemic infect'ns* - 3 mg/kg/day in 3 equal doses for 7-10 days. *For life-threatening infect'ns* - Up to 5 mg/kg/day in 3-4 equal doses; reduce to 3 mg/kg/day as soon as clinically indicated. Children - *For severe infect'ns* - 3-6 mg/kg/day in 3 equal doses q8h. If a dosage > 3 mg/kg/day is admin. initially, it should be reduced to 3 mg/kg/day when clinically indicated. Premature and full-term neonates ≤ 1 week of age - 6 mg/kg/day in 2 equal doses q12h; > 1 week of age - Give in 3 equal doses q8h. **For pts w. impaired renal funct'n** - Serum half-life can be estimated by multiplying serum creatinine level [in mg/100 mL] by 4. Frequency of administrat'n [in h] may be approximated by doubling serum half-life. **Topical:** Apply cream or	Bactericidal. Binds to bacterial 30S ribosomal subunit of streptococci to cause misreading of genetic code, resulting in incorrect sequencing of amino acids in format'n of proteins. For other bacteria it blocks protein synthesis by inhibiting amino acid translocat'n.	All aminoglycosides are potentially toxic to both auditory and vestibular funct'ns of 8th cranial nerve. Pts may have tinnitus or any degree of hearing loss, dizziness and vertigo. Can also produce nephrotoxicity w. dose-dependent damage to proximal tubular epithelium, beginning after 5-7 days of tx. Neuromuscular blockade can occur after aminoglycoside use that can progress to flaccid paralysis and potentially fatal respiratory arrest. Aminoglycosides can produce allergic or local hypersensitivity react'ns characterized by pruritus, rash, urticaria and (on occasion) exfoliative dermatitis.	**Aminoglycosides:** May incr. ototoxicity and nephrotoxicity of each other if admin. concomitantly. **Antibiotics, cephalosporin:** May incr. nephrotoxicity of aminoglycosides. **Anticoagulants, oral:** Aminoglycosides may incr. their activities by decreasing vitamin K product'n by bacteria in intestines. **Cisplatin:** May incr. nephrotoxicity of aminoglycosides. **Corticosteroids:** Reduce host defense mechanisms against infect'n. Prolonged tx w. an aminoglycoside and a corticosteroid should be undertaken w. caution owing to poss. of superinfect'n. **Dimenhydrinate:** May mask s/s ototoxicity caused by aminoglycosides. **Diuretics:** Such as ethacrynic acid and furosemide, have been assoc. w. dysfunct'n of 8th cranial nerve. Concomitant use of a potent diuretic w. an aminoglycoside should be avoided. It is believed that IV diuretics may cause rapid rise in aminoglycoside serum levels and potentiate nephrotoxicity. **Muscle relaxants:** May have their actions enhanced by aminoglycosides.	**Assess:** Pt hx of allergy to aminoglycosides, myasthenia gravis, hearing deficiency, ulcerative GI condit'ns, renal impairment. Establish age, baseline weight, fluid intake/output, respirat'ns, pulse and BP, hearing facility, complete urinalysis, BUN and serum creatinine levels. For concurrent use of other ototoxic or nephrotoxic medicat'ns. Send specimens for culture and sensitivity; document clinical observat'ns of infect'n. **Administer:** IM slowly and deeply into large muscle mass; take VS during infus'n and watch for hypotens'n or change in pulse. Give for max. 10 days without reconfirmat'n of order by physician. Administer only reduced dosages to pts w. renal impairment, premature or neonate infants and the elderly; topically w. caution on open wounds, e.g., burns, ulcers. **Evaluate:** Relief from or reduct'n in clinical observat'ns of infect'n; for early indicators of ototoxicity (dizziness, vertigo, nystagmus, tinnitus, roaring sounds, hearing loss); conduct audiogram at regular intervals; nephrotoxicity (oliguria, proteinuria, decr. specific gravity or incr. BUN or serum creatinine); for neuromuscular blockade (depressed respirat'ns, pulse, BP, ataxia, nystagmus, bladder distent'n, constipat'n and decr. bowel sounds); topical applicat'ns for localized allergic dermatitis (rash, itching, urticaria, angioneurosis). **Teach:** To report subjective percept'ns.

ointment containing 1 mg gentamicin/g to lesion tid-qid. **Ocular:** Instill 2 drops of solut'n containing gentamicin sulfate 5 mg/mL, or ophthalmic ointment containing gentamicin sulfate 5 mg/g, into affected eye tid-qid. Incr. dosage prn in severe infect'ns)	As for gentamicin sulfate	As for gentamicin sulfate	rel. to hearing or balance; to maintain fluid intake of 2-3 L/day; to seek medical advice if topical use produces allergic dermatitis.
Amikacin sulfate (Amikin)	As for gentamicin sulfate (**IM:** Adults, children and neonates - 15 mg/kg/day, admin. as 7.5mg/kg q12h. **IV:** Same dose may be admin. over a 30- to 60-min period. **For pts w. impaired renal funct'n -** Interval bet. doses can be calculated by multiplying serum creatinine [in mg/100 mL] by 9 to give dosage intervals [in h]. This formula should not be used to calculate dosage for elderly pts)	As for gentamicin sulfate	As for gentamicin sulfate	As for gentamicin sulfate
Kanamycin sulfate (Kantrex, Klebcil)	As for gentamicin sulfate (**IM/IV:** Rarely used parenterally because of bacterial resistance. For dosage, consult manufacturer's monograph. **Oral:** As adjunct in extended tx of hepatic coma - Adults - 8-12 g/day in divided doses. As adjunct in short-term mechanical cleansing of large bowel - 1 g qh for 4 h, followed by 1 g q6h for 36-72 h. Infants and children - For suppress'n of bowel flora - 150-250 mg/kg daily in divided doses q1-6h)	As for gentamicin sulfate	As for gentamicin sulfate	As for gentamicin sulfate

Generic Name (Trade Name)	Use (Dose)	Action	Adverse Effects	Drug Interactions	Nursing Process
Netilmicin sulfate (Netromycin)	As for gentamicin sulfate (**IM, IV: For pts w. normal renal funct'n** - Adults - For uncomplicated urinary tract infect'ns - 4 mg/kg/day in 2 equal doses, admin. q12h for 7-10 days. For systemic infect'ns - 4-6 mg/kg/day in 2-3 equal doses, admin. q8-12h. For serious/life-threatening systemic infect'ns - Up to 7.5 mg/kg/day IV, in 3 equal doses; reduce to 6 mg/kg/day as soon as indicated clinically, us. within 48 h. Children - 6-7.5 mg/kg/day IV, given in 3 equal doses q8h; reduce to 6 mg/kg/day as soon as indicated clinically. Infants and neonates > 1 week of age - 7.5-9 mg/kg/day IV, given in 3 equal doses q8h. Premature and full-term neonates < 1 week old - 6 mg/kg/day IV, given in 2 equal doses q12h. **For pts w. impaired renal funct'n** - Initial dose is same as that recomm. for pts w. normal renal funct'n. If serum concentrat'ns cannot be monitored, interval bet. the us. single dose given at 8-h intervals can be calculated by multiplying the pt's serum creatinine level [in mg/100 mL] by 8)	As for gentamicin sulfate	As for gentamicin sulfate	As for gentamicin sulfate	As for gentamicin sulfate
Tobramycin sulfate (Nebcin)	As for gentamicin sulfate (**IM/IV: For pts w. normal renal funct'n** - Adults - For mild to moderate infect'ns of lower urinary tract - 2-3	As for gentamicin sulfate	As for gentamicin sulfate	As for gentamicin sulfate	As for gentamicin sulfate

mg/kg/day od. When renal tissue is involved or in serious infect'ns, esp. when there are signs of systemic involvement, 2-3 equally divided doses are recomm. *For life-threatening infect'ns* - Up to 5 mg/kg/day in 3-4 equal doses; reduce to 3 mg/kg/day as soon as indicated clinically. Infants and children - 3-5 mg/kg/day in equal doses q8h. Neonates ≤ 1 week old - Up to 4 mg/kg/day in 2 equal doses q12h. **For pts w. impaired renal funct'n** - **IM:** After loading dose of 1 mg/kg, subsequent dosage must be adjusted, either w. lower doses admin. at 8-h intervals or w. normal doses at prolonged intervals. In latter situat'n, interval [in h] can be determined by multiplying pt's serum creatinine levels by 6. **Ocular:** Instill solut'n containing tobramycin sulfate 5 mg/mL, as described for gentamicin sulfate)

CHAPTER 64

The Sulfonamides, Trimethoprim and Trimethoprim Plus Sulfamethoxazole

Teaching Objectives

Following completion of this chapter, the reader should be able to:

1. Describe the mechanism of action and antibacterial spectrum of sulfonamides.
2. Discuss the pharmacokinetics, therapeutic uses and adverse effects of sulfonamides, as well as the nursing process related to their administration.
3. Describe the mechanism of action of trimethoprim and justify the combination of trimethoprim plus sulfamethoxazole.
4. Discuss the antibacterial spectrum, therapeutic uses and adverse effects of trimethoprim and trimethoprim plus sulfamethoxazole, and the nursing process associated with their use.

The Sulfonamides

When introduced in the 1930s, the sulfonamides provided a major breakthrough in the chemotherapy of infectious disease. Unfortunately, the development of bacterial resistance has reduced the number of sulfonamides on the market to a few. These include sulfisoxazole (Gantrisin), sulfamethoxazole (Gantanol) and sulfadiazine. Two topical sulfonamides, mafenide acetate and silver sulfadiazine, are valuable in the treatment of burn patients. These drugs are discussed in Chapter 43. Sodium sulfacetamide, presented in Chapter 38, is a very popular drug for ocular infections.

Mechanism of Action

Folic acid is an essential vitamin for both bacterial and mammalian cells. Human cells absorb folic acid from food. Bacteria, however, cannot absorb the vitamin and must synthesize it. One essential component of folic acid is para-aminobenzoic acid (PABA). Sulfonamides are structurally similar to PABA. By acting as competitive antimetabolites of PABA, sulfonamides block its incorporation into folic acid, thereby preventing folic acid synthesis and inducing bacteriostasis.

As previously mentioned, mammalian cells differ from those of bacteria. Whereas bacteria synthesize their own folic acid, mammalian cells do not. Humans require preformed folic acid, and we obtain this material in ample quantities from our diet. As a result, sulfonamides do not reduce folic acid levels in the human host. This accounts for the selective toxicity of sulfonamides on bacteria.

Unfortunately, bacterial resistance has developed to sulfonamides. Several mechanisms are involved in the development of resistance. At least some bacteria that were originally sensitive have developed the ability to synthesize large quantities of PABA. In the presence of an overwhelming concentration of PABA, the normal therapeutic dose of a sulfonamide is unable to inhibit competitively the incorporation of PABA into folic acid. For other organisms, the development of resistance may be explained by a decreased permeability of bacteria to sulfonamides, or a reduced affinity of the drugs for the enzyme that incorporates PABA into folic acid, or both.

Antibacterial Spectrum

When they were introduced, sulfonamides were effective against a wide range of gram-positive and gram-negative micro-organisms, as well as chlamydia. Bacteria originally sensitive included Group A streptococci, pneumococci, gonococci, meningococci, *Haemophilus influenzae, Haemophilus ducreyi, Escherichia coli,* brucellae, *Pasteurella pestis, Bacillus anthracis, Corynebacterium diphtheriae, Cholera vibrio* and shigellae. However, many of these bacteria are now resistant to sulfonamides. This is particularly true for many staphylococci, enterococci, clostridia and pseudomonas.

Pharmacokinetics

The sulfonamides discussed in this chapter are well absorbed from the gastrointestinal tract. They cross cell membranes freely and distribute to the brain, lung, liver, pancreas, muscle and nervous tissue. The concentrations of sulfonamides in the fetus are approximately equal to those in the mother.

Sulfonamides bind, in varying degrees, to plasma proteins. Given to a patient during the later stages of pregnancy, a sulfonamide will cross the placenta, enter the fetus and displace bilirubin from plasma albumin. In the absence of a developed blood-brain barrier, the newly freed bilirubin can enter the fetal brain to produce kernicterus. Therefore, the use of sulfonamides in pregnant women near term or in the nursing mothers is inadvisable. In addition, sulfonamides should not be given to infants less than two months old.

Some sulfonamides are extensively metabolized; others are mainly excreted unchanged by the kidneys. Only twenty per cent of sulfisoxazole is metabolized prior to excretion. Sulfadiazine and sulfamethoxazole are sixty to eighty-five per cent metabolized, respectively.

The pharmacokinetic characteristics of some commonly used sulfonamides are summarized in Table 97.

Table 97
Characteristics of some commonly used sulfonamides.

Drug	Pharmacokinetic Properties	Therapeutic Uses
Sulfadiazine Sulfamerazine Sulamethazine	All are rapidly absorbed and rapidly eliminated.	Often the 3 are combined and used in products that also contain penicillin G for tx of sensitive systemic infect'ns.
Sulfisoxazole (Gantrisin)	Rapidly absorbed; high concentrat'n of active drug in urine	Often used in tx of acute urinary tract infect'ns.
Sulfamethoxazole (Gantanol)	Rapidly absorbed; only 15% of dose found in urine unchanged	Often combined w. trimethoprim to form cotrimoxazole.
Sulfamylon (Mafenide) Silver sulfadiazine (Flamazine)	Topical use only; can be absorbed from burned skin.	Used in tx of burn pts.
Sulfacetamide sodium (Sodium Sulamyd)	Penetrates ocular fluids and tissues in high concentrat'ns.	Tx of conjunctivitis and corneal ulcers

Therapeutic Uses

The value of sulfonamides has been reduced greatly by the development of resistance. Sulfonamides have remained effective for the treatment of acute uncomplicated urinary tract infections, caused by sulfonamide-sensitive *Escherichia coli*.

Sulfisoxazole (Gantrisin) is a particularly appropriate sulfonamide because eighty per cent of the drug is excreted unchanged in the urine.

Sulfamethoxazole (Gantanol) is less suitable because only fifteen per cent of a dose of this drug is excreted in an unmetabolized active form.

The combination of phenazopyridine HCl (Pyridium) and sulfisoxazole is popular for the treatment of urinary tract infections. The two drugs can be taken as separate tablets or as the combination product Azo-Gantrisin. Phenazopyridine is a local analgesic on the inflamed mucosa of the urinary tract. Its use reduces discomfort during the first three or four days of treatment, before sulfisoxazole has had sufficient opportunity to work. Thereafter, as bacterial counts fall, phenazopyridine is not required and treatment may be continued with sulfisoxazole alone.

Sulfadiazine may be a drug of choice in nocardiosis. Although not a drug of first choice, it can also be used in the treatment of lymphogranuloma venereum and melioidosis. Sulfisoxazole can be employed for the long-term prophylaxis of rheumatic fever in penicillin-allergic patients. As mentioned in Chapter 61, the use of sulfisoxazole plus erythromycin (Pediazole) is recommended for haemophilus-induced otitis media in young children.

The topical use of sulfonamides (sulfamylon and silver sulfadiazine) in burn patients is discussed in Chapter 43. Sodium sulfacetamide is a very popular drug for ocular infections. Its use is discussed in Chapter 38.

Sulfonamides are contraindicated in patients with a history of hematologic, renal or hepatic dysfunction, allergic drug fever or skin eruptions due to sulfonamide derivatives, including antibacterial sulfonamides, oral hypoglycemics and thiazides. In addition, as indicated before, sulfonamides should not be given to premature and newborn infants, or pregnant women near partuition because of the possible occurrence of kernicterus. Other contraindications to the use of sulfonamides include uremia and a deficiency of erythrocytic glucose-6-phosphate dehydrogenase (G-6-PD). Patients with porphyria should not receive sulfonamides, because these drugs have been reported to precipitate an acute attack.

Adverse Effects

Nausea, anorexia and vomiting are seen in five to ten per cent of patients taking sulfonamides. Hypersensitivity reactions, beginning ten to twelve days after starting therapy or within hours in a previously sensitized patient, can cause generalized skin rashes, urticaria, photodermatitis or drug fever. Patients allergic to one sulfonamide should be considered allergic to all sulfonamides.

Blood dyscrasias are rare but they can be fatal. Acute or chronic hemolytic anemia, developing within two to seven days of starting therapy, or agranulocytosis, appearing between the second and sixth week of treatment in approximately 0.1% of patients, represent hypersensitivity reactions. All patients should know the symptoms of agranulocytosis and contact their physicians immediately if they occur.

Nursing Process

Assessment

Nursing assessment begins before the first dose of a sulfonamide is administered. Nurses must first document the clinical observations characterizing the infection. The patient's history is assessed for previous hypersensitivity to sulfonamides, allergies (drug or otherwise) or bronchial asthma. Patients with previous episodes of sulfonamide hypersensitivity should not be treated again with any member of the group. Individuals with other forms of allergy or asthma are at increased risk of developing a sulfonamide hypersensitivity. Patients with a history of liver or kidney disease are also at increased risk if treated with a sulfonamide. In such cases, nursing vigilance must be increased.

Sulfonamides are contraindicated in women who are pregnant or lactating because of the danger of kernicterus to the fetus or neonate. Although this admonition applies particularly to long-acting sulfonamides, which are extensively bound to plasma albumin, it should not be disregarded for drugs, such as sulfisoxazole, that are not bound appreciably to plasma proteins. Sulfisoxazole is very popular for the treatment of acute urinary tract infections which are very common in the latter weeks of pregnancy. Whereas it is true that many pregnant women have received sulfisoxazole for urinary tract infections without ill effects to the fetus, reports have appeared in the literature of the drug producing kernicterus.

Patients should not receive a sulfonamide concurrently with an oral anticoagulant, methotrexate, a sulfonylurea hypoglycemic, a thiazide diuretic or a uricosuric (see Table 98, Drug Interactions).

Administration

Administer sulfonamides orally with or following food at equally spaced intervals throughout a twenty-four-hour day. Each oral dose should be taken with a full glass of water.

Evaluation

Following treatment, nurses must evaluate patients for clinical improvement and adverse effects. Hypersensitivity reactions have already been described. Blood dyscrasias associated with the use of sulfonamides are usually characterized by high fever, prostration, necrotic ulcers of the mouth, rectum or vagina (agranulocytosis), or by lassitude, fatigue, dizziness, headache, jaundice, tarry stools and brownish urine (hemolytic anemia). The Stevens-Johnson syndrome associated with sulfonamide therapy is manifested by fever, headache, erythematous rash, rhinitis, conjunctivitis and stomatitis. Sulfonamides can produce a decrease in urinary output, proteinuria, hematuria and/or renal colic. This danger is reduced greatly if patients consume enough fluid to maintain a urine volume of at least 1500 mL per day. Fluid output should be 800 mL less than intake.

Teaching

Patient teaching is important. Nurses must alert patients to the importance of drinking large volumes of fluids. All patients, but particularly those treated at home, must be aware of the adverse effects of the drugs. They must understand the importance of seeking medical advice immediately should any appear. Patients should also be told that their urine might turn an orange shade and that this is not cause for alarm. Finally, nurses should inform patients of the danger of photosensitivity reactions and advise them to avoid, as much as possible, direct exposure to sunlight or other sources of ultraviolet light. Patients should be warned to avoid over-the-counter medications, especially those containing acetylsalicylic acid (Aspirin) or Vitamin C.

Trimethoprim (Proloprim, Trimpex) and Trimethoprim Plus Sulfamethoxazole/ Cotrimoxazole (Bactrim, Septra)

Trimethoprim was combined with sulfamethoxazole in the 1960s. In many parts of the world, including Canada, the combination product has the generic name of cotrimoxazole. In other areas, such as the United States, it is simply referred to as trimethoprim plus sulfamethoxazole. In this book we have shortened trimethoprim plus sulfamethoxazole to TMP/SMX. The addition of trimethoprim to sulfamethoxazole restored a credibility to the sulfonamides that had not been there since bacterial resistance to these drugs started to appear in the 1950s. Today, TMP/SMX (cotrimoxazole) is used to treat a variety of systemic infections, many of which were handled effectively by the sulfonamides alone in their early days.

Mechanism of Action of TMP/SMX (Cotrimoxazole)

Before folic acid can function as a vitamin it must be converted first to dihydrofolic acid, then to tetrahydrofolic acid. Trimethoprim competitively inhibits bacterial dihydrofolate reductase, the enzyme responsible for the conversion of dihydrofolic acid to tetrahydrofolic acid. In therapeutic doses it has no significant effect on the human form of the enzyme.

The TMP/SMX (cotrimoxazole) combination contains a 1:5 ratio of trimethoprim to sulfamethoxazole. In sensitive bacteria, it reduces both the formation of folic acid and its subsequent activation.

Antibacterial Spectrum of TMP/SMX (Cotrimoxazole)

TMP/SMX has a broad spectrum of activity. All strains of *Staphylococcus aureus, Streptococcus pneumoniae, Streptococcus epidermidis, Streptococcus pyogenes,* viridans streptococci, *Streptococcus faecalis, Escherichia coli, Proteus mirabilis, Proteus morganii, Proteus rettgeri,* enterobacter species, *Pseudomonas pseudomallei* and serratia are inhibited by TMP/SMX. Although many strains of shigella and salmonella remain sensitive to TMP/SMX, others have developed resistance to the antibacterial.

Pharmacokinetics of TMP/SMX (Cotrimoxazole)

Both sulfamethoxazole and trimethoprim are well absorbed from the gastrointestinal tract and distribute rapidly throughout the body, including the cerebrospinal fluid. High concentrations of both drugs are found in bile. The half-life of both drugs is approximately ten hours. Although most of the trimethoprim is eliminated unchanged in the urine, approximately eighty-fve per cent of sulfamethoxazole is inactivated prior to renal excretion.

Therapeutic Uses of TMP/SMX (Cotrimoxazole) and Trimethoprim

TMP/SMX (Bactrim, Septra) is used to treat a variety of systemic infections caused by gram-positive and gram-negative organisms, including infections of the upper and lower respiratory tract, urinary tract (acute, recurrent and chronic), genital tract, gastrointestinal tract, and skin and soft tissues; *Pneumocystis carinii* infections; and serious systemic infections, such as meningitis and septicemia caused by susceptible organisms.

Some of its more common uses include acute exacerbations of chronic bronchitis caused by *Haemophilus influenzae* and *Streptococcus pneumoniae* and the treatment of acute otitis media in children and acute maxillary sinusitis in adults. Acute gonococcal urethritis can also be managed with TMP/SMX. Gastrointestinal infections caused by shigellae, including ampicillin-resistant strains, can be treated with TMP/SMX. The combination is also effective for the treatment of typhoid fever and can be used in the management of carriers of *Salmonella typhi.* It is the treatment of choice for acute and chronic prostatitis. Trimethoprim is one of the few antibacterial agents that adequately penetrates into the uninflamed prostate.

Trimethoprim (Proloprim, Trimpex) is used in treating acute urinary tract infections due to susceptible strains of *E. coli* and *K. pneumoniae.* Limited clinical experience suggests the probability of therapeutic response in infections due to susceptible strains of *P. mirabilis* and enterobacter. The administration of trimethoprim alone is rational, given the fact that eighty-five per cent of sulfamethoxazole is inactivated before it reaches the bladder. As would be expected, trimethoprim is as effective as TMP/SMX for the treatment of acute urinary tract infections, but has a reduced incidence of adverse effects.

Adverse Effects of TMP/SMX (Cotrimoxazole)

The toxicities of sulfonamides have already been described. Trimethoprim has relatively few adverse effects. They include gastric distress (nausea and vomiting), rash, itching, and very rarely leukopenia, thrombocytopenia and methemoglobinemia.

Nursing Process

Assessment
Before administering either trimethoprim or trimethoprim plus sulfamethoxazole, nurses should review the patient's history for evidence of blood dyscrasias, renal impairment or liver disease. These conditions contraindicate the use of either product. Neither product should be used in pregnant or lactating patients. Physical assessment should also include the collection of specimens for culture and sensitivity tests. The clinical manifestations of the infection must also be recorded at this time.

Administration
Administer TMP/SMX or trimethoprim with a full glass of water. Maintain a fluid intake of 2 L/day to help decrease bacteria in bladder.

Evaluation
Once therapy with trimethoprim or TMP/SMX is started, nurses should evaluate patients for clinical improvement and adverse effects. With respect to the latter, nurses must be alert for the development of blood dyscrasias. These are indicated by reports of sore throat; fever; prostration; ulcerations of the mouth, rectum or vagina; headache; dizziness; pallor; bleeding gums; nose bleeds; unexplained bruising and petechiae. Skin rashes suggest the dermatological effects of trimethoprim and TMP/SMX.

Teaching

Trimethoprim and TMP/SMX are often self-administered at home. Nurses must inform patient that the drug must be taken in equal intervals around the clock to maintain blood levels. Patients should also be taught the indicators of drug efficacy and adverse effects. They must also be educated to the fact that laboratory studies may be essential for the early identification of adverse effects. It is therefore important for patients to keep scheduled laboratory appointments.

Further Reading

Advice for the travelers (1990). *The Medical Letter 32* :33-36.

Choice of antimicrobial drugs (1990). *The Medical Letter 32* :41-48.

Choice of antimicrobial drugs (1986). *The Medical Letter 28* :33-40.

Sulfonamides and trimethoprim (1986). *AMA Drug Evaluations,* 6th ed., pp. 1451-1467. Chicago: The American Medical Association.

Table 98
The sulfonamides and trimethoprim.

Pharmacologic Classification: Antibiotics — Sulfonamides

Generic Name (Trade Name)	Use (Dose)	Action	Adverse Effects	Drug Interactions	Nursing Process
Sulfadiazine	Agent of choice for tx of nocardiosis. For tx of other infect'ns as follows (**Oral:** Adults - Initially, 2-4 g; then 1 g q4-6h. Children and infants > 2 months of age - Initially, 75 mg/kg, then 150 mg/kg/day in 4-6 divided doses. Should not > 6 g/day. Durat'n for nocardiosis tx is 4-6 months or more. *For prophylaxis of rheumatic fever*, pts < 27 kg - 500 mg od; pts > 27 kg - 1 g od. *For prophylaxis of meningococcal disease* [only if *Neisseria meningitidis* isolate is known to be susceptible] - Adults - 1 g bid for 2 days. Children 1-12 years- 500 mg bid for 2 days. Infants 2 months- 1 year- 500 mg od for 2 days)	Bacteriostatic. Sulfonamides are structurally similar to PABA, from which bacteria synthesize folic acid essential for cell growth. By acting as antimetabolites to PABA, these drugs block its utilizat'n and inhibit folic acid synthesis. Originally, sulfonamides had a wide spectrum of activity, but resistance has developed in many bacteria to sulfonamides used alone.	Nausea, anorexia, vomiting, hypersensitivity react'ns, drug fever, hemolytic anemia, agranulocytosis	**Anesthetics, local:** Such as benzocaine, procaine, tetracaine and butacaine that are esters antagonize antibacterial activity of sulfonamides. **Anticoagulants, oral:** May demonstrate incr. activity because some sulfonamides may displace them from plasma protein binding. Pts should be monitored more closely, esp. when starting or stopping sulfonamide. **Diuretics** (particularly thiazides): May incr. incidence of thrombocytopenia w. purpura in elderly pts receiving a sulfonamide. **PABA:** Administrat'n antagonizes antibacterial effects of sulfonamides. Remember that PABA is sometimes combined w. ASA in proprietary analgesics. **Phenytoin:** Metabolism may be inhibited by sulfamethizole. Pts may experience incr. effect of phenytoin. **Tolbutamide:** Inactivat'n may be inhibited by sulfamethizole. Sulfamethoxazole has been reported to potentiate effects of tolbutamide.	**Assess:** For hx sulfonamide hypersensitivity, allergies, asthma, liver or kidney disease, blood dyscrasias; pregnancy or lactat'n; concurrent use of anticoagulants, methotrexate, sulfonylurea hypoglycemics, thiazides, uricosurics; document clinical observat'ns of infect'n. **Administer:** W. food or following meals w. full glass of water at equal intervals during day; cleanse open wounds prior to topical applicat'n. **Evaluate:** Reduct'n in or absence of clinical observat'ns characterizing infect'n; for hypersensitivity react'ns, blood dyscrasias (high fever, prostrat'n, necrotic ulcerat'ns of mouth, rectum or vagina); lassitude, fatigue, dizziness, headache, jaundice (tarry stools, brownish urine); Stevens-Johnson syndrome (fever, headache, erythematous rash, rhinitis, conjunctivitis, stomatitis); renal dysfunct'n (decr. urinary output, proteinuria, hematuria, renal colic). Maintain sufficient fluid intake to produce not < 1500 mL of output/day. Output should be 800 mL < intake. **Teach:** Importance of adequate fluid intake; indicators of adv. effects; importance of completing course of tx; that urine might become orange color; to avoid UV light. Warn pts to avoid OTC medicat'ns, particularly those containing ASA or vitamin C.
Sulfisoxazole (Gantrisin)	As for sulfadiazine (**Oral:** Adults - 2-4 g stat; then 4-8 g/24 h in 4-6 divided doses. Children > 2 months - 75 mg/kg stat, then 150 mg/kg/day in divided doses q4h; max. 6 g/day)	As for sulfadiazine	As for sulfadiazine		
Sulfamethoxazole (Gantanol)	As for sulfadiazine (**Oral:** Adults - 2 g stat, then 1 g q12h. Children > 2 months - 50-60 mg/kg stat, then 50% this am't q12h. *For severe infect'n* - Adults and children - Give maint. doses tid for 5-7 days or until asymptomatic for 48 h)	As for sulfadiazine	As for sulfadiazine		

Generic Name (Trade Name)	Use (Dose)	Action	Adverse Effects	Drug Interactions	Nursing Process
Pharmacologic Classification: Antibiotic — Trimethoprim					
Trimethoprim (Proloprim, Trimpex)	Tx of acute, uncomplicated urinary tract infect'ns due to susceptible strains of E. coli and K. pneumoniæ (**Oral:** Adults and children > 12 years - 100 mg q12h for 10 days)	Trimethoprim inhibits dihydrofolate reductase, the enzyme responsible for activat'n of folic acid.	Leukopenia, agranulocytosis, thrombocytopenia, methemoglobinemia, rash, pruritus, nausea, vomiting, abd. cramps, glossitis, stomatitis, headache, joint pain, apathy, muscle weakness, nervousness	As for sulfadiazine	**Assess:** Hx blood dyscrasias, renal impairment, liver disease; age < 12 years; pregnancy, lactat'n. Collect specimens for culture and sensitivity; document clinical observat'ns of infect'n. **Administer:** W. full glass water. Maintain fluid intake of 2 L to help decr. bacteria in bladder. **Evaluate:** For reduct'n in or absence of clinical manifestat'ns of infect'n; for blood dyscrasias (sore throat, fever, prostrat'n, ulcerat'ns of mouth, rectum, vagina, headache, dizziness, palor, bleeding gums, nose bleeds, unexplained bruising, petechiae); for skin rash. **Teach:** Indices of drug effectiveness and adv. effects; inform pts that drug must be taken at equal intervals ATC to maintain blood levels; to keep scheduled appointments for lab. studies of blood.
Pharmacologic Classification: Antibiotics — Trimethoprim Plus Sulfamethoxazole (Cotrimoxazole)					
Trimethoprim + sulfamethoxazole; cotrimoxazole (Bactrim, Septra)	Tx of condit'ns as follows (*For bacterial infect'ns* - **Oral:** Adults and children > 12 years - 2 adult tabs or 1 DS tab bid. *For severe infect'ns* - Incr. dosage to 3 adult or 1.5 DS tabs bid. Children < 12 years - 3 mg trimethoprim/kg + 15 mg sulfamethoxazole/kg bid for at least 5 days. *For prophylaxis and for salmonella carriers* - 1 adult tab or 0.5 DS tab bid. *For acute salmonellosis* - Tx should be continued for at least 7 days after defervescence. Carriers should continue tx until repeated stool cultures are negative. *For uncomplicated gonorrhea* - Adults and children - 2 adult or 1 DS tab qid for 2 days. *For Pneumocystis carinii pneumonitis* - Adults and children - 5 mg trimethoprim + 25 mg sulfamethoxazole/kg qid for at least 14 days)	Contains a 5:1 ratio of sulfamethoxazole to trimethoprim. In sensitive bacteria it reduces both format'n of folic acid and its subsequent activat'n.	As for sulfonamides and trimethoprim	As for sulfonamides	

Miscellaneous Antibiotics and Antibacterials

Teaching Objectives

Following completion of this chapter, the reader should be able to:

1. Describe the mechanism of action, therapeutic uses and adverse effects of chloramphenicol, as well as the nursing process related to its use.
2. Describe the mechanism of action, therapeutic uses, adverse effects and nursing process for nitrofurantoin.
3. Discuss the mechanism of action, therapeutic uses, adverse effects and nursing process for nalidixic acid.
4. Describe the mechanism of action, antibacterial spectrum, therapeutic uses, adverse effects and nursing process for norfloxacin.
5. Describe the mechanism of action, antibacterial spectrum, therapeutic uses and adverse effects of ciprofloxacin, as well as the nursing process related to its use.
6. Discuss the combination of imipenem plus cilastatin, including its mechanism of action, therapeutic uses, adverse effects and nursing process.

Chloramphenicol (Chloromycetin)

Mechanism of Action

Chloramphenicol penetrates readily into bacteria. It blocks protein synthesis by binding to the 50S subunit of the bacterial 70S ribosome and inhibiting the formation of peptide bonds between amino acids. Bacterial and mammalian ribosomes differ, and the ability of chloramphenicol to affect primarily the bacterial ribosomes accounts for its selective effect on protein synthesis in micro-organisms.

Antibacterial Spectrum

Chloramphenicol has a broad spectrum of activity. It is bacteriostatic against many gram-positive and gram-negative micro-organisms as well as chlamydia and rickettsia. In the United States and Canada, salmonella species, including *S. typhi*, generally are susceptible to chloramphenicol. Enterobacteriaceae are variable in their response to chloramphenicol. Most strains of *Escherichia coli*, *Klebsiella pneumoniae* and *Proteus mirabilis* are inhibited by chloramphenicol, but the majority of strains of serratia, providencia, *Proteus rettgeri* and *Pseudomonas aeruginosa* are resistant.

Therapeutic Uses

Chloramphenicol has severe toxicities (see later discussion). As a result it should only be used in those conditions for which it may be the antibiotic of choice. These would include (1) acute infections cause by *Salmonella typhi* (chloramphenicol is not recommended for routine treatment of the typhoid carrier state); (2) serious infections caused by susceptible strains of (a) salmonella species with systemic involvement, (b) *H. influenzae*, specifically meningeal infections, (c) rickettsia; psittacosis in children, (d) various gram-negative bacteria causing bacteremia, meningitis or other serious gram-negative infections, (e) other susceptible organisms that have demonstrated resistance to other appropriate antimicrobial agents; and (3) cystic fibrosis regimens.

Chloramphenicol is prepared in ocular formulations for use in the treatment of superficial conjunctival and/or corneal infections. It is also used topically in the ear because it is effective against a wide range of pathogens causing external otitis. These include *Staphylococcus aureus, Escherichia coli,* strains of pseudomonas and proteus species. If signs of drug-induced local irritation appear, chloramphenicol should be discontinued. Blood dyscrasias have been reported following topical use in the ear.

Adverse Effects

Chloramphenicol can cause a dose-dependent depression of bone marrow. Its therapeutic concentration in plasma ranges from $5 - 20$ µg/mL (approximately $15 - 62$ µmol/L). When its plasma concentration exceeds 25 µg/mL (77.3 µmol/L), anemia — sometimes with leukopenia or thrombocytopenia — can occur. This effect is reversible if the drug is discontinued. It should not be confused with choramphenicol-induced aplastic anemia, which is almost invariably fatal. Reported in one in 25 000 to one in 40 000 patients, aplastic anemia can occur after only one dose of chloramphenicol or several weeks or months after the drug is stopped.

Newborns, particularly premature infants, metabolize chloramphenicol slowly. The half-life of the drug is increased from four hours in the adult to twenty-six hours in babies less than two weeks of age. This fact must be taken into account in calculating dosage. Otherwise, toxic levels of the drug can accumulate, leading to the gray-baby syndrome, a condition characterized by abdominal distention, vomiting, cyanosis, irregular respiration, a fall in body temperature, and cardiovascular collapse.

Nursing Process

Assessment
Prior to the first dose of chloramphenicol, the nurse should review the patient's history for evidence of previous chloramphenicol allergy, blood dyscrasias, kidney or liver disease. These conditions contraindicate use of the drug without further consultation with the attending physician. Its concurrent use with other drugs known to have hematopoietic adverse effects is also contraindicated. Fear of the gray-baby syndrome should usually mitigate against the administration of chloramphenicol to nursing mothers or women in the last trimester of pregnancy.

Administration
Chloramphenicol should be administered only to hospitalized patients. It is difficult to envisage requiring the drug in patients who are not sick enough to be hospitalized. Capsules containing chloramphenicol should be stored in tight containers at room temperature. Chloramphenicol is usually administered orally on an empty stomach at equal intervals over a twenty-four-hour day. When required, it can be given intravenously. In this situation a ten per cent solution of the drug should be administered over a one- to two-minute time period through an established intravenous infusion.

Evaluation
Chloramphenicol's therapeutic effectiveness is evaluated by a reduction in the signs and symptoms of the infection. Nurses must concern themselves with the gray-baby syndrome when chloramphenicol is administered to neonates, particularly premature infants. Patients of all ages should be evaluated for drug-induced hematological toxicity.

Teaching
Warn patients to complete their entire course of medication (ten to fourteen days) to ensure eradication of the infecting micro-organism.

Nitrofurantoin (Macrodantin)

Mechanism of Action, Antibacterial Spectrum and Therapeutic Uses

Although nitrofurantoin inhibits many mammalian and bacterial enzymes, its mechanism of action isn't known. The basis for its selective effect in urinary tract infections lies in the fact that nitrofurantoin is concentrated in the urine. Therefore, bacteria residing in the urinary tract are exposed to very high levels of the drug. This is in contrast to the relatively low levels presented to most cells in the body.

Nitrofurantoin is indicated for the treatment of urinary tract infections (e.g., pyelonephritis, pyelitis, cystitis) that are due to susceptible strains of *E. coli,* enterococci, *S. aureus* and certain susceptible strains of klebsiella, enterobacter and proteus species. It is not indicated for the treatment of associated renal cortical or perinephric abscesses.

Anuria, oliguria or significant impairment of renal function (creatinine clearance under 40 mL/min) are contraindications to the use of nitrofurantoin, for two reasons. First, patients with renal impairment have difficulty eliminating the drug, and second, the drug may fail to achieve therapeutic concentrations in the bladder.

Adverse Effects

Nausea and vomiting are the most commonly observed adverse effects of nitrofurantoin. These can be minimized by the use of the macrocrystalline form of nitrofurantoin (Macrodantin) which is absorbed over a longer period of time.

Nitrofurantoin can cause allergic reactions, which include rashes, urticaria, angioneurotic edema, eosinophilia and fever. An acute pulmonary reaction, characterized by fever, myalgia, dyspnea, pulmonary infiltration and pleural effusion can also result from nitrofurantoin administration. A second type of pulmonary reaction involving pneumonic complications can be produced by nitrofurantoin. This involves shortness of breath on exertion and a cough. Both types of pulmonary reactions usually disappear when the drug is stopped.

A sensorimotor peripheral neuropathy has been associated with nitrofurantoin use. It is seen most often in patients with impaired renal function. Nitrofurantoin has also been reported to produce megaloblastic anemia and cholestasis. In patients deficient in glucose-6-phosphate dehydrogenase, the drug can produce hemolysis.

Nursing Process

Assessment
Nursing assessment of patients for whom nitrofurantoin has been prescribed must emphasize identification of impaired renal function, electrolyte imbalance, general debilitation, pregnancy or neonatal age, all of which contraindicate administration of the drug.

Administration
Nitrofurantoin is administered with food at equal intervals around the clock. It must be stored in a light-resistant container to prevent deterioration. Drug therapy should begin after urine culture and sensitivity studies are done.

Evaluation
Nurses should determine the therapeutic effectiveness of nitrofurantoin. This is done by monitoring relief of the symptoms of the infection. Nurses must also be alert for early identification of adverse effects.

Teaching
Patients should be taught to expect brown-colored urine and to rinse their mouths carefully with water after taking the oral suspension.

Nalidixic Acid (NegGram)

Mechanism of Action and Antibacterial Spectrum

Nalidixic acid inhibits DNA synthesis in sensitive bacteria. It is active against many gram-negative bacteria commonly found in urinary tract infections. One hundred per cent of the indole-positive proteus strains, ninety per cent of *Escherichia coli,* eighty per cent of *Proteus mirabilis,* and seventy per cent of klebsiella are killed by nalidixic acid in concentrations found in the urine. *Pseudomonas aeruginosa* is not sensitive to the drug.

Therapeutic Uses

Nalidixic acid is indicated for the treatment of acute or chronic urinary tract infections due to one or more species of nalidixic acid-sensitive gram-negative pathogenic organisms, in particular *E. coli,* proteus, aerobacter and klebsiella species. It is useful in mixed urinary tract infection when the nalidixic acid-sensitive gram-negative rods predominate. Because bacterial resistance may develop when nalidixic acid is used chronically, it is not recommended for long-term prophylaxis of urinary tract infections.

Adverse Effects

Nausea, vomiting, diarrhea and abdominal pain are the most commonly reported adverse effects of nalidixic acid. Other adverse effects include allergic reactions (rashes, urticaria, eosinophilia), photosensitivity and visual disturbances (blurring of vision, photophobia, changes in color vision). Its central nervous system adverse effects are drowsiness, weakness, dizziness, headaches and on very rare occasions, convulsions.

Nursing Process

Assessment
Before administering nalidixic acid, nurses must review the patient's history for evidence of convulsive disorders, hepatic or renal disease, pregnancy, or neonatal age under three months. Any of these conditions contraindicates administration of the drug. Specimens for laboratory culture and sensitivity studies should be collected before initial administration of nalidixic acid.

Administration
Nalidixic acid should be administered at equal intervals around the clock with food to prevent gastric irritation. The suspension must be protected from freezing and shaken well before administration.

Evaluation

Nursing evaluation of the patient following nalidixic acid administration emphasizes observation for reduction in, or absence of, the clinical manifestations of the infection. Nurses should also be alert for the early detection of gastric distress, allergic responses, photosensitivity, visual disturbances and central nervous system adverse effects.

Teaching

Patients should be taught to avoid exposure to ultraviolet light to prevent photosensitivity reactions.

Norfloxacin (Noroxin)

Mechanism of Action, Antibacterial Spectrum and Therapeutic Uses

Norfloxacin inhibits bacterial deoxyribonucleic acid (DNA) synthesis and is bactericidal. The drug is indicated for the treatment of upper and lower urinary tract infections, specifically complicated and uncomplicated cystitis, pyelitis and pyelonephritis caused by susceptible strains of *E. coli* and *K. pneumoniae;* unspecified klebsiella, enterobacter and citrobacter species; *P. mirabilis, S. aureus, S. faecalis* and *P. aeruginosa.*

Adverse Effects

The adverse effects of norfloxacin include a low incidence of gastrointestinal disturbances, headache, dizziness or lightheadedness, and hypersensitivity reactions involving the skin.

Nursing Process

Assessment

Before administering norfloxacin, nurses must review the patient's history for evidence of kidney or liver disease. The fluid intake and output ratio should be assessed and the urine pH should be less than 5.5.

Administration

Prior to administration of norfloxacin, a clean catch of urine should be obtained for culture and sensitivity studies. Norfloxacin should be taken one hour before or two hours after meals. Patients should limit their intake of alkaline foods, milk and dairy products.

Evaluation

Nurses should evaluate patients for evidence of the therapeutic effectiveness of norfloxacin (e.g., decreased pain, frequency, urgency, as well as the absence of infection in culture and sensitivity studies). Nurses should also be alert for central nervous system symptoms of insomnia, vertigo, headache, agitation or confusion. Patients should also be evaluated for evidence of allergic reactions, fever, flushing, rash, pruritus and urticaria.

Teaching

Patients should be taught to increase fluid intake to three liters a day to avoid crystallization in the kidneys. Nurses should teach the patient to be alert for allergic and central nervous system side effects. If these effects occur, they must be reported to the nurse immediately. Nurses must warn patients to take the full course of drug therapy.

Ciprofloxacin (Cipro)

Mechanism of Action, Antibacterial Spectrum and Therapeutic Uses

Ciprofloxacin, like norfloxacin, is a synthetic fluoroquinolone. It has a bactericidal mode of action. This action is achieved through inhibition of DNA gyrase, an essential component of the bacterial DNA replication system. It is also possible that ciprofloxacin acts by affecting RNA and protein synthesis.

Ciprofloxacin has a broad in vitro spectrum of activity covering common gram-positive and gram-negative pathogens, as well as a number of important intracellular bacterial pathogens, such as chlamydia, mycoplasma, legionella and brucella species, and *Mycobacterium tuberculosis.* Anaerobes are resistant to ciprofloxacin. The spectrum of activity of ciprofloxacin is greater than that of aminoglycoside antibiotics.

Taken orally, ciprofloxacin produces adequate serum levels for the treatment of systemic infections. Its clinical uses include urinary tract infections, sexually transmitted diseases, gastrointestinal diseases, respiratory infections, osteomyelitis and prophylaxis of neutropenic patients. Clinical trials have shown ciprofloxacin's effectiveness in improving clinical symptoms in cystic fibrotic patients infected with *Pseudomonas aeruginosa.* However, it does not eradicate this pathogen. Notwithstanding, the strength of ciprofloxacin may well lie in the treatment of serious gram-negative infections, particularly *P. aeruginosa.* Prior to the introduction of ciprofloxacin these infections, when found outside the urinary tract, were treated by parenteral antibiotic therapy. The availability of oral treatment, together with its relative lack of toxicity when compared with that of the aminoglycosides, would appear to make ciprofloxacin a reasonable replacement for aminoglycosides in the treatment of gram-negative infections. However, caution must still be advised because considerable work remains to be done to compare aminoglycosides with ciprofloxacin in clinical trials.

Adverse Effects

Ciprofloxacin is generally well tolerated and most adverse effects are only mild or moderate in severity. Its adverse effects include vomiting, dyspepsia, abdominal pain, anorexia, dizziness, lightheadedness, headache, nervousness, anxiety, agitation, restlessness, tremor, lethargy, drowsiness and somnolence. Skin hypersensitivity has also been reported.

Nursing Process

The nursing process for ciprofloxacin is similar to that of norfloxacin (above), with the following additions for patient teaching. This drug is not to be taken with antacids containing magnesium or aluminum. If antacids are to be taken, be sure there is a two-hour interval from drug administration. If gastrointestinal irritation occurs, the patient may take the drug with a little food.

Imipenem Plus Cilastatin Sodium (Primaxin)

Mechanism of Action and Therapeutic Uses

Imipenem inhibits cell wall synthesis in aerobic and anaerobic gram-positive and gram-negative bacteria. It is a bactericidal drug. Cilastatin blocks the metabolism and inactivation of imipenem in the kidney. By combining cilastatin with imipenem, it is possible to attain antibacterial concentrations of imipenem in the urine.

The combination of imipenem plus cilastatin is indicated in the treatment of serious infections when caused by sensitive bacteria. Lower respiratory tract infections, urinary tract infections, intra-abdominal and gynecological infections, and septicemia caused by susceptible bacteria may be treated with imipenem plus cilastatin. Endocarditis caused by *S. aureus* also may be treated with the combination, as can bone, joint and skin-structure infections produced by susceptible bacteria.

Adverse Effects

The combination of imipenem and cilastatin is generally well tolerated. The most common adverse effects include nausea, diarrhea and vomiting.

Nursing Process

Nurses are advised to consult the drug manufacturer's package insert, product monograph, and the pharmacist for information before administering this drug.

Further Reading

Bowen, R.C., Michel, D.J. and Thompson, J.C. (1987). Norfloxacin: Clinical pharmacology and clinical use. *Pharmacotherapy 7* :92-110.

Douidar, S.M. and Snodgrass, W.R. (1989). Potential role of fluoroquinolones in pediatric infections. *Rev. Infect. Dis. 11* :878-889.

LeBel, M. (1988). Ciprofloxacin: Chemistry, mechanism of action, resistance, antimicrobial spectrum, pharmacokinetics, clinical trials and adverse reactions. *Pharmacotherapy 8* :3-33.

Nitrofurantoin in pregnancy (1986). *The Medical Letter 28* :32.

Stein, G.E. (1988). The 4-quinolone antibiotics: Past, present and future. *Pharmacotherapy 8* :301-314.

Table 99
Miscellaneous antibiotics and antibacterials.

Generic Name (Trade Name)	Use (Dose)	Action	Adverse Effects	Drug Interactions	Nursing Process
Pharmacologic Classification: Antibiotic					
Chloramphenicol (Chloromycetin)	Tx of acute infect'ns caused by *S. typhi*; of serious infect'ns caused by susceptible strains of salmonella spp. w. systemic involvement; *H. influenzae*, specifically meningeal infect'ns; rickettsia; psittacosis in children; various gram-neg. bacteria causing bacteremia, meningitis or other serious gram-neg. infect'ns; other susceptible organisms demonstrated to be resistant to other appropriate antimicrobials; cystic fibrosis regimens **(Oral/IV:** Adults - 50 mg/kg/day in divided doses at 6-h intervals. Up to 100 mg/kg/day for moderately resistant organisms, but these doses should be decr. a.s.a.p. Pts w. hepatic or renal impairment may have reduced ability to metabolize or excrete drug; it may be nec. to reduce dosage. Children - 50 mg/kg/day in divided doses at 6-h intervals. Newborn infants [premature/full-term] - 25 mg/kg/day in 4 equal doses at 6-h intervals. After first 2 weeks of life, full-term infants may receive up to 50 mg/kg/day in 4 equal doses at 6-h intervals. *These dosage recommendat'ns are extremely important because blood concentrat'ns in*	Bacteriostatic. Blocks protein synthesis by binding to 50S subunit of bacterial 70S ribosome and inhibiting peptidyl transferase. Effective against many gram-pos. and gram-neg. micro-organisms, as well as chlamydia and rickettsia.	Blood dyscrasias (bone marrow depress'n, aplastic anemia, hypoplastic anemia, thrombocytopenia, granulocytopenia); neurotoxic react'ns (headache, mild depress'n, mental confus'n, delirium); hypersensitivity react'ns (fever, macular and vesicular rashes, angioedema, urticaria, anaphylaxis); gray-baby syndrome	**Anticoagulants, oral:** Can interact w. chloramphenicol. This antibiotic can inhibit metabolism of dicumarol. Chloramphenicol may also decr. vitamin K product'n by gut bacteria and product'n of prothrombin by liver cells. Therefore, concomitant use of chloramphenicol and dicumarol must be avoided. If chloramphenicol must be used, warfarin might be preferable. Test prothrombin times at more frequent intervals. **Bone marrow depressants:** Interact w. chloramphenicol and should not be used concomitantly. **Cephalosporins:** Bacteriostatic effects of chloramphenicol may interfere w. bactericidal effects of cephalosporins. If essential to use both drugs, give cephalosporin a few hours or longer before chloramphenicol and ensure that adequate am'ts of each agent are given. **Cyclophosphamide:** Metabolism may be inhibited by chloramphenicol, resulting in incr. in cyclophosphamide's effects. **Penicillins:** As for cephalosporins, above. **Phenytoin:** Metabolism may be inhibited by chloramphenicol, increasing the effect of phenytoin. May need to decr. phenytoin dosage in presence of chloramphenicol.	**Assess:** Pt hx of chloramphenicol allergy; concurrent use of other drugs that produce blood dyscrasias; pregnancy or lactat'n; kidney or liver disease. **Administer:** To hospitalized pts only. IV slowly (1-2 min) through tubing of established IV infus'n using syringe containing 10% solut'n. Oral route preferred; orally on empty stomach at equal intervals ATC. Oral capsules should be stored in tight containers at room temp. **Evaluate:** Tx effectiveness; adv. effects. **Teach:** Warn pts to complete entire course of drug tx (10-14 days) to ensure eradicat'n of infecting micro-organism.

all premature and full-term infants under 2 weeks of age differ from those of other infants)

Tolbutamide: Metabolism may be inhibited by chloramphenicol. Pts can expect enhanced hypoglycemic response. Reduct'n in tolbutamide dosage is prob. necessary.

Pharmacologic Classification: Urinary Antibacterials

Drug	Uses / Dosage	Action	Side Effects	Interactions	Nursing Considerations
Nitrofurantoin (Macrodantin)	Tx of pyelonephritis, pyelitis, cystitis caused by sensitive organisms, us. *E. coli*, *S. aureus*, enterococci, certain strains of proteus, enterobacter and klebsiella spp. (**Oral:** Adults - 50-100 mg qid. Children - 5-7 mg/kg/24 h, given in divided doses qid. Contraindicated in infants < 1 month old. Continue tx for at least 1 week and for at least 3 days after urine sterility is obtained)	Mechanism of action not known. Value of nitrofurantoin is its ability to inhibit *E. coli.*	Anorexia, nausea, vomiting. Fever, chills, cough, chest pain, dyspnea, pulmonary infiltrat'n, pleural effus'n and eosinophilia. Dermatologic react'ns. Hemolytic anemia, granulocytopenia, megaloblastic anemia. Peripheral neuropathy, headache, dizziness, nystagmus and drowsiness.	**Drugs that impair renal funct'n:** Should not be admin. concomitantly w. nitrofurantoin.	**Assess:** For impaired renal funct'n, pregnancy, neonatal age, electrolyte imbalance, debilitat'n. **Administer:** Orally w. food at equal intervals over 24 h from light-resistant container. Begin drug after urine culture and sensitivity studies have been done. **Evaluate:** For amelirat'n of s/s of infect'n; for adv. effects. **Teach:** To expect urine to become brown; to rinse mouth w. water after taking suspens'n.
Nalidixic acid (NegGram)	Tx of acute or chronic urinary tract infect'ns due to *E. coli,* proteus, aerobacter and klebsiella spp. (**Oral:** Adults - Initially, 1 g qid for 1-2 weeks. Max. 4 g/day. For prolonged tx, total dose/day may be reduced to 2 g after initial tx period. Children ≤ 12 years - Initially, 55 mg/kg/day, given in 4 divided doses. For prolonged tx, total daily dose may be reduced to 33 mg/kg/day)	Inhibits DNA synthesis in susceptible bacteria. Active in vitro against many gram-neg. bacteria commonly found in urinary tract infect'ns.	GI disturbances incl. abd. pain, nausea, vomiting and diarrhea. Allergic react'ns incl. rash, pruritus, urticaria, angioedema and eosinophilia. Reversible subjective visual disturbances.	**Anticoagulants, oral:** May be displaced from plasma protein binding sites by nalidixic acid. If this happens, oral anticoagulant may show incr. activity. **Nitrofurantoin:** May interfere w. antibacterial actions of nalidixic acid.	**Assess:** For hx convulsive disorders, hepatic or renal disease; pregnancy, neonatal age; collect specimens for culture and sensitivity. **Administer:** W. food at equal intervals during 24-h period. Protect suspens'n from freezing. Shake well before administrat'n. **Evaluate:** Reduct'n of clinical manifestat'ns for GU distress, allergic responses, photosensitivity, visual disturbances, CNS effects. **Teach:** To avoid exposure to sunlight.
Norfloxacin (Noroxin)	Tx of complicated and uncomplicated cystitis, pyelitis and pyelonephritis caused by susceptible strains of *E. coli, K. pneumoniae, P. mirabilis, S. aureus, S. faecalis, P. aeruginosa* and unspecified klebsiel-	Norfloxacin inhibits bacterial DNA synthesis and is bactericidal.	Low incidence of GI disturbances, headache, dizziness or lightheadedness, hypersensitivity react'ns involving skin.		**Assess:** Pt hx for evidence of kidney or liver disease. Fluid intake/output ratio; ensure urine pH < 5.5. **Administer:** Begin drug after clean catch of urine obtained for culture and sensitivity. Limit intake of alkaline foods, drugs, milk and dairy products. Drug to

Generic Name (Trade Name)	Use (Dose)	Action	Adverse Effects	Drug Interactions	Nursing Process
	la, enterobacter and citrobacter spp. **(Oral: Adults** - *For urinary tract infect'ns* - 400 mg bid for 7-10 days. *For women w. uncomplicated acute cystitis* - Durat'n of tx can be reduced to 3 days. *For pts w. impaired renal funct'n* - Pts w. GFR of < 30 mL/min/1.73m² but > 6.6 mL/min/1.73 m², 400 mg od)				be taken 1 h ac or 2 h pc. **Evaluate:** For tx response of decr. pain, frequency, urgency and absence of infect'n in culture and sensitivity studies. Be alert for CNS symptoms of insomnia, vertigo, headache, agitat'n, confus'n. Also look for evidence of allergic react'ns (fever, flushing, rash, pruritus, urticaria). **Teach:** Pts to incr. fluids to 3 L/day to avoid crystallizat'n in kidney. Pt to be alert for allergic and CNS side effects and to report them stat. Warn pt to take full course of drug.

Pharmacologic Classification: Fluoroquinolone Antibacterial

Generic Name (Trade Name)	Use (Dose)	Action	Adverse Effects	Drug Interactions	Nursing Process
Ciprofloxacin (Cipro)	For tx of wide variety of infect'ns, as follows **(Oral: Adults** - *For mild to moderate urinary tract infect'ns* - 250 mg q12h. *For severe or complicated urinary tract infect'ns* - 500 mg q12h. *For mild to moderate lower respiratory tract, bone and joint, skin and soft tissue infect'ns* - 500 mg q12h. *For severe or complicated lower respiratory tract infect'ns, bone and joint, skin and soft tissue infect'ns* - 750 mg q12h. *For mild, moderate or severe infectious diarrhea* - 500 mg q12h. Depending on severity of condit'n, average tx should be approx. 7-14 days. Continue 3 days past disappearance of clinical symptoms or until cultures are sterile. Pts w. osteomyelitis may require tx for min. 6-8 weeks, max. 3 months. W. acute cystitis, 5-day tx may suffice)	Bactericidal mode of action. Inhibits DNA gyrase, an essential component of bacterial DNA replicat'n system. Has broad spectrum of action, covering common gram-pos. and gram-neg. pathogens, plus many other important intracellular bacterial pathogens, such as *Mycobacterium tuberculosis*, *chlamydia*, *mycoplasma*, *legionella* and *brucella* spp.	Gen'ly well tolerated. most adv. effects are only mild or moderate in severity. These adv. effects incl. vomiting, dyspepsia, abd. pain, anorexia, dizziness, lightheadedness, headache, nervousness, anxiety, agitat'n, restlessness, tremor, lethargy, drowsiness and somnolence. Skin hypersensitivity has also been reported.	**Antacids:** Containing Al(OH)₃ or Mg(OH)₂, have been shown to reduce absorpt'n of ciprofloxacin. Avoid concurrent use of these agents. **NSAIDs:** Given concomitantly w. ciprofloxacin, incr. risk of CNS stimulat'n and convulsive seizures. **Probenecid:** Blocks renal secret'n of ciprofloxacin and has been shown to incr. serum levels of ciprofloxacin. **Theophylline:** Half-life and plasma levels can incr. if ciprofloxacin is given concurrently. If concomitant use cannot be avoided, plasma concentrat'ns of theophylline should be monitored and dosage adjustment made prn.	*As for norfloxacin, plus:* **Teach:** Pt that drug is not to be taken w. antacids containing Mg or Al. If antacids are to be taken, ensure 2-h interval from drug administrat'n. If GI irritat'n occurs, pt may take drug w. food.

Pharmacologic Classification: Combination Antibacterial Product

Imipenem + cilastatin (Primaxin)

Tx of serious infect'ns [lower respiratory tract, urinary tract, intra-abd. and GYN infect'ns, septicemia and endocarditis] when caused by sensitive bacteria (**IV: Adults - *Mild infect'ns - 250 mg q6h. Moderate infect'ns - 500 mg q8h. Severe (fully susceptible) infect'ns - 500 mg q6h. Severe infect'ns due to less susceptible organisms - 1000 mg q8h. Life-threatening condit'ns - 1000 mg q6h)***

Imipenem inhibits cell wall synthesis in aerobic and anaerobic gram-pos. bacteria. It is bactericidal. Cilastatin blocks metabolism and inactivat'n of imipenem in kidney.

Gen'ly well tolerated. Most common adv. effects incl. nausea, diarrhea and vomiting.

Nurses are advised to consult manufacturer's pkg. insert, product monograph and the pharmacist to obtain informat'n before administering this drug.

CHAPTER 66

Antitubercular Drugs

Tuberculosis can be a difficult disease to treat. First, *Mycobacterium tuberculosis* is often intracellular and relatively inaccessible to drugs. Second, drug resistance usually develops if only one agent is used. As a result, patients are frequently treated with several antimycobacterial drugs. Single-drug therapy is usually limited to the use of isoniazid for the prevention of tuberculosis.

First-line drugs for the treatment of tuberculosis include isoniazid, rifampin and ethambutol. Their pharmacologic properties and therapeutic uses are discussed in this chapter, together with those of the alternative drugs streptomycin, aminosalicylic acid, cycloserine, capreomycin and pyrazinamide.

Drugs of First Choice

Isoniazid (INH, Nydrazid)

Mechanism of Action

The mechanism of action of isoniazid (INH) is not known. However, it is speculated that the drug blocks the synthesis of mycolic acids by *Mycobacterium tuberculosis*. These acids are normal constituents of the bacterial cell wall. In their absence, the integrity of the cell wall is reduced and cell death occurs. Lower concentrations of isoniazid are bacteriostatic; higher levels are bactericidal.

Pharmacokinetics

Isoniazid is rapidly absorbed from the gastrointestinal tract and distributed throughout the body. Antacids reduce peak serum levels of the drug. Substantial concentrations of isoniazid are found in pleural effusions and the cerebrospinal fluid.

Figure 28

Distribution of the isoniazid (INH) half-lives of 336 experimental subjects.

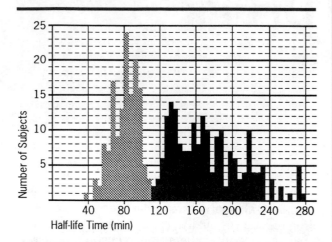

From: H. Tiitinen (1969), Isoniazid and ethionamide serum levels and inactivation in Finnish subjects. *Scand. J. Resp. Dis. 50*:110-124. Reproduced with permission.

Isoniazid crosses the placenta and can also be found in breast milk in concentrations equivalent to those in plasma.

Isoniazid is inactivated by acetylation. Patients can be characterized as either slow or rapid metabolizers of the drug. Approximately sixty per cent of Americans are slow acetylators and should receive lower doses of isoniazid. Rapid acetylators require more frequent dosing. Figures 28 and 29 present the bimodal distribution in isoniazid metabolism and the effects thereof on drug concentration in human serum.

Antibacterial Spectrum

The clinical usefulness of isoniazid is limited to the eradication of *Mycobacterium tuberculosis* and some atypical mycobacterial infections. Organisms of other generae and fungi are not affected unless extremely high concentrations of isoniazid are present. Unfortunately, *Mycobacterium tuberculosis* can become resistant to isoniazid.

Therapeutic Uses

Isoniazid is one of the safest and most effective drugs for the treatment of tuberculosis. Its ability to reach high concentrations in all body fluids, including the cerebrospinal fluid, combined with its antibacterial activity, makes isoniazid appropriate for the treatment of all types of tuberculosis infections. Isoniazid is included in first-line drug combi-

Figure 29

Serum isoniazid (INH) levels of 341 subjects at 180 min after IV injection of 5 mg/kg of INH.

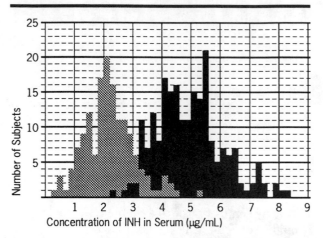

Gray columns refer to 143 rapid inactivators grouped according to their INH half-lives; black columns refer to 198 slow inactivators.

From: H. Tiitinen (1969), Isoniazid and ethionamide serum levels and inactivation in Finnish subjects. *Scand. J. Resp. Dis. 50*:110-124. Reproduced with permission.

nations. It is also considered a drug of choice when single-agent treatment is used prophylactically in patients who show positive skin reactions, but who are otherwise radiographically or clinically negative.

Adverse Effects

In spite of its wide acceptance, isoniazid can adversely affect both the central and peripheral nervous systems. Its most frequent adverse effect is a dose-related peripheral neuritis, characterized by numbness and tingling in the lower extremities. This is seen most often in undernourished or alcoholic patients or in slow acetylators. If the drug is withdrawn soon after the onset of the symptoms, the adverse effects usually reverse rapidly. However, if therapy is continued in the face of patient complaints, residual problems may persist for up to one year following cessation of treatment. The routine use of 15 – 50 mg/day of pyridoxine has been recommended to prevent peripheral neuritis, increased to 100 – 300 mg daily in patients with pre-existing neuritis.

The central nervous system adverse effects include symptoms of excitability, extending from irritability and restlessness to seizures. Hyperglycemia, metabolic acidosis and seizures can occur following isoniazid overdosage, and death or prolonged coma has occurred from persistent seizure activity, even when conventional doses have been given. The drug should be used with caution in patients with a known history of seizures.

Allergic reactions to isoniazid include fever and skin rashes. It can also cause a syndrome similar to systemic lupus erythematosus.

Isoniazid causes subclinical hepatic injury, with abnormal serum transaminase (SGOT) and bilirubin values, in ten to twenty per cent of patients. Although most patients can continue to take the drug and apparently recover, a few progress to clinically overt hepatitis. There does not appear to be a correlation between plasma isoniazid concentrations and drug-induced hepatotoxicity. Its incidence increases with age, being uncommon in patients under thirty-five.

Nursing Process

Assessment
Prior to administering the initial dose of isoniazid, the nurse should review the patient's history for evidence of seizure disorders, alcohol abuse, liver or kidney disease. The nurse should also physically assess the patient for general physical debilitation. These conditions indicate the need for particularly rigorous evaluation of the patient's response to isoniazid.

Administration
Oral doses of isoniazid should be administered from light-proof, moisture-resistant containers designed to prevent drug deterioration. Oral isoniazid should be given with meals to decrease gastrointestinal symptoms. Isoniazid solutions can crystallize at cool temperatures. To avoid this possibility, store intramuscular solutions at room temperature.

Evaluation
Nursing evaluation of patients receiving isoniazid should emphasize the early detection of adverse effects as identified in the preceding section. Nurses should be alert for early indications of central or peripheral nervous system toxicity, hepatotoxicity or allergic reactions. Patients must also be monitored for their mental status and mood changes.

Teaching
Patients receiving this or any other antitubercular drug must be instructed in the importance of taking the medication according to the prescribed regimen to achieve optimum drug efficacy. They should also be strongly advised to keep scheduled monthly appointments for evaluation of drug efficacy and adverse effects. Nurses must warn patients to avoid alcohol while taking isoniazid.

Rifampin (Rifadin, Rimactane)

Mechanism of Action and Antibacterial Spectrum
Rifampin forms a stable complex with DNA-dependent RNA polymerase to inhibit RNA synthesis. It is effective against most gram-positive bacteria, as well as many gram-negative microbes, such as *Escherichia coli,* pseudomonas, indole-positive and indole-negative proteus and klebsiella. It is particularly effective and bactericidal against *Mycobacterium tuberculosis.* Rifampin also increases the in vitro activity of streptomycin and isoniazid against *Mycobacterium tuberculosis.*

Pharmacokinetics
Rifampin is well absorbed when taken orally. Maximum serum concentrations are seen within two to three hours. Its absorption is reduced if the drug is taken immediately following a meal or together with aminosalicylic acid. Once absorbed, rifampin distributes widely in body tissue and fluids, reaching therapeutic levels in the cerebrospinal and pleural fluids. Rifampin is metabolized in the liver and excreted in the bile. Its metabolite is biologically active. Some unaltered drug is reabsorbed from the gastrointestinal tract following biliary excretion.

Therapeutic Uses
Resistance develops readily if rifampin is used alone. Thus, it is always used in combination with other agents for the treatment of tuberculosis. In combination with isoniazid or isoniazid and ethambutol, rifampin is effective in the initial treatment of moderate and advanced pulmonary tuberculosis. Rifampin should also be included in retreatment protocols for patients who have not received the drug during their initial therapy. It is also useful in treating extrapulmonary tuberculosis including miliary tuberculosis and tuberculosis meningitis.

Rifampin can be included in the treatment of *Mycobacterium leprae.* Its efficacy is increased by concomitant use of dapsone (Avlosulfon). Rifampin can also be used for short-term treatment of meningococcal carriers, but resistance can develop quickly, even when treatment is only two to three weeks. Because of this, rifampin is not usually used to treat clinical infections.

Adverse Effects
The most common adverse effects of rifampin are gastrointestinal disturbances and nervous system

complaints characterized by drowsiness, ataxia, dizziness, headache and fatigue. Liver damage is the most serious adverse effect.

The dosage interval is important with rifampin. If used once or twice weekly, as opposed to daily, it is more likely to produce fever, chills, aches, nausea and vomiting. Immune thrombocytopenia and hemolytic anemia, as well as acute renal failure, have also been reported in patients receiving intermittent therapy.

Rifampin can increase the metabolism of many other drugs (Table 100).

Nursing Process

Assessment
Nursing assessment prior to the first administration of rifampin should emphasize review of the patient's history for previous hepatic disorder which would contraindicate use of the drug. Renal studies and a blood workup for anemia should also be performed.

Administration
Rifampin should be given before meals and at different times than aminosalicylic acid. Nurses should administer rifampin on a daily basis. It should *not* be given on an intermittent basis for the reasons presented earlier.

Evaluation
Nursing evaluation of the patient receiving rifampin should focus on prompt identification of adverse effects. As with all other antitubercular drugs, patients must be taught the importance of compliance with the prescribed regimen. In addition, the prescription and use of rifampin requires warning the patient of the dangers of intermittent use of the drug. Female patients should be counseled to use birth control methods other than oral contraceptives because rifampin may increase estrogen and progestin metabolism. All patients should be advised that rifampin may give their body secretions and excretions, including saliva, tears, perspiration, sputum, feces and urine, a reddish discoloration. They should also be told that soft contact lenses may be permanently stained.

Ethambutol (Myambutol)

Mechanism of Action, Pharmacokinetics and Therapeutic Uses
Ethambutol interferes with protein metabolism in *Mycobacterium tuberculosis*. The drug is rapidly absorbed from the gastrointestinal tract. In patients with tuberculous meningitis, it enters the cerebrospinal fluid in therapeutic levels. Ethambutol is eliminated primarily by renal excretion and has a half-life of three hours in patients with normal kidney function. Its dose should be reduced in patients with renal impairment.

Resistance builds quickly if ethambutol is used alone. Therefore, it is used as an adjunct to isoniazid and rifampin in the conventional treatment of tuberculosis.

Adverse Effects
Generally, ethambutol is well tolerated. Its major adverse effect is unilateral or bilateral retrobulbar neuritis. Occurring after two or more months of treatment, this most commonly involves the central fibers of the optic nerve and is characterized by a loss of central vision and disturbances in color discrimination. Less often, the peripheral fibers of the optic nerve are affected, in which case there may be a constriction of the peripheral fields of vision with no loss of visual acuity. These effects are usually reversible if the drug is withdrawn. Nevertheless, patients should have a complete ophthalmologic examination before therapy is instituted to establish an accurate baseline for future reference. Because of difficulty in evaluating visual function in children, ethambutol is recommended only for adults.

Ethambutol can produce occasional mild gastrointestinal upset and allergic reactions, which include dermatitis, pruritus and, very rarely, anaphylaxis. The drug can also produce dizziness, mental confusion, fever, malaise and headache. Ethambutol can interfere with uric acid excretion. The precipitation of acute gout has been reported following its administration. Peripheral neuritis has also been reported, but this also occurs only rarely.

Nursing Process
The nursing process for ethambutol is similar to that previously detailed for rifampin with the following additions. Nursing assessment of patients for whom ethambutol has been prescribed should stress review of the patient's history for documentation of renal impairment or gout. The nurse should also establish baseline levels of visual function by arranging an ophthamological examination for the patient. Ethambutol is administered with food in an attempt to prevent gastrointestinal irritation. Nursing evaluation of patients following the administration of ethambutol focuses on identification of its adverse effects.

Alternative Drugs

Streptomycin

Streptomycin is an aminoglycoside antibiotic (see Chapter 63). It increases the activities of ethambutol and isoniazid and is most effective in the first weeks of treatment. Administered with intramuscular isoniazid, streptomycin immediately suppresses susceptible organisms and can be life-saving. Streptomycin is also useful in intermittent therapy. The adverse effects of streptomycin and its nursing process are discussed along with those of other aminoglycosides in Chapter 63.

Aminosalicylic Acid, PAS (Parasal Sodium, Teebacin Acid)

Aminosalicylic acid, or PAS, as it is often called, is structurally similar to para-aminobenzoic acid (PABA). By acting as an antimetabolite of the latter compound, PAS prevents the utilization of PABA in the synthesis of folic acid by *Mycobacterium tuberculosis*. PAS can be used as a substitute for ethambutol in children before adolescence. PAS may be incorporated into retreatment programs because it delays the emergence of resistance to first-line drugs.

Gastrointestinal irritation, sometimes leading to bleeding, is the most common adverse effect of aminosalicylic acid. The drug is used with caution when treating ulcer patients. Aminosalicylic acid can produce allergic reactions, including fever, rash, pruritus and hepatotoxicity. PAS should be used with caution in patients with renal or cardiac failure because larger doses of the sodium salt can cause sodium overload and fluid retention.

Nursing Process

Patients should undergo nursing assessment aimed at detecting conditions that contraindicate the use of PAS, e.g., a history of peptic ulcer, or renal or cardiac failure. PAS should be administered with food to minimize its gastrointestinal effects. To prevent deterioration, PAS should be stored in a light-proof and moisture-resistant container. Tablets that have turned a brownish-purple color should be discarded. Nursing evaluation of patients receiving this medication involves observing the patient for evidence of adverse effects.

Cycloserine (Seromycin)

Cycloserine is structurally similar to alanine. It competes with alanine to prevent cell wall formation by *Mycobacterium tuberculosis*. Because of central nervous system toxicity, cycloserine is usually restricted to urinary tract tuberculosis and difficult retreatment programs. Appearing within a few weeks of starting the drug, central nervous system adverse effects include headache, tremor, dysarthria, vertigo, confusion, somnolence, nervousness, irritability and psychotic states. Patients may also demonstrate catatonic and depressed reactions, hyperreflexia, visual disturbances, and *grand mal* seizures or absence attacks. These usually disappear if the drug is stopped.

Nursing Process

Patients whose nursing assessment prior to the first administration of cycloserine reveals a history of renal impairment should receive a smaller dose of cycloserine because of the increased risk of adverse effects. Evaluation of patients receiving cycloserine should emphasize close monitoring for early manifestations of central nervous system toxicity or signs of hepatic toxicity. Patient teaching should caution patients to avoid driving or using industrial machinery or power tools while taking cycloserine. Patients should also avoid alcohol because it increases the risk of adverse central nervous system effects.

Capreomycin (Capastat)

Intramuscular capreomycin is useful in streptomycin-resistant strains of *Mycobacterium tuberculosis*. When used with orally effective agents, it is rarely required on a regular daily basis. Capreomycin is both ototoxic and nephrotoxic. It should not be used with other antibiotics with similar properties.

Nursing Process

Assessment
Nurses caring for patients about to receive capreomycin should anticipate an order for bacterial sensitivity, hearing, complete blood count, serum potassium, liver function and renal status tests. Nurses must ensure that the ordered baseline studies are conducted prior to administering the first dose.

Administration

Dissolve capreomycin in either sterile normal saline or sterile water according to the manufacturer's directions. Although the solution may change color as it ages, this does not affect its activity. It may be used for up to fourteen days after dilution if stored in a refrigerator. Administer capreomycin intramuscularly deep into a large muscle mass and aspirate carefully to avoid inadvertant intravenous injection, which can cause neuromuscular blockade. Injection sites should be carefully documented and rotated.

Evaluation

Changes in the fluid intake/output ratio must be immediately reported to the physician. Nurses should observe patients for decreased hearing acuity and inquire about patients' perceptions of hearing changes. Patients should also be carefully observed for disturbances of balance. In addition, the hepatic status of the patient receiving capreomycin should be monitored.

Pyrazinamide

Pyrazinamide is an analogue of nicotinamide that can be used in retreatment programs. It may be valuable when short-term resistance to isoniazid is a problem and has been given with streptomycin, isoniazid and rifampin until the results of susceptibility studies are known.

A major factor limiting the use of pyrazinamide is a fourteen per cent incidence of hepatotoxicity. Deaths have occurred rarely. Before the drug is started, patients should undergo laboratory studies, including a complete liver function investigation. Once pyrazinamide is started, serum transaminases should be measured every two to four weeks. Patients receiving pyrazinamide should have a complete blood count, urinalysis and serum profile screen performed monthly. Pyrazinamide also increases serum uric acid levels. If gout develops, patients can be treated with a uricosuric drug.

Nursing Process

The major priority of the nursing process for patients receiving pyrazinamide is assessment for hepatotoxicity. Patients with a history of liver disease should not receive this medication. Patients who do receive pyrazinamide should be carefully evaluated for early evidence of hepatic damage — specifically, jaundice, increased bleeding tendencies and enlarged liver.

Further Reading

American Thoracic Society (1986). Treatment of tuberculosis and tuberculosis infections in adults and children. *Am. Rev. Respir. Dis. 134* :363-368.

Banner, A.S. (1979). Tuberculosis: Clinical aspects and diagnosis. *Arch. Intern. Med.139* :1387-1390.

Drugs for tuberculosis (1986). *The Medical Letter 28* :6-8.

Sbarbaro, J.A. and Iseman, M.D. (1981). Prophylactic treatment of tuberculosis. *Compr. Ther. 7* (June):14-19.

Stead, W.W. and Dutt, A.K. (1982). Chemotherapy for tuberculosis today. *Amer. Rev. Respir. Dis. 125* :94-101.

Youmans, G.P. (1979). *Tuberculosis.* Philadelphia: W.B. Saunders Co.

Table 100
Antitubercular drugs.

Pharmacologic Classification: First-line Antitubercular Drugs

Generic Name (Trade Name)	Use (Dose)	Action	Adverse Effects	Drug Interactions	Nursing Process
Isoniazid, INH (Nydrazid, Rimifon)	Used in conjunct'n w. other anti-TB drugs such as streptomycin, aminosalicylic acid and/or others in tx of pulmonary and extra-pulmonary TB, and alone in prophylaxis of TB **(Oral/IM: Adults** - *For prophylaxis* - 300 mg/day orally in a single dose. *For disseminated TB and pulmonary disease caused by atypical mycobacteria* - 10-20 mg/kg/day. Infants/children - *For active TB* - 10-20 mg/kg/day. *For preventative tx* - 10 mg/kg/day [max. 300 mg/day] in 1 dose)	Mechanism of action not known. May block format'n of cell walls by *M. tuberculosis*. One of safest and most effective drugs for tx of TB. Incl. in 1st-line drug combinat'ns; appropriate for tx of all types TB. Also drug of choice when single-agent tx is used prophylactically.	Peripheral neuropathy, convuls'ns, toxic encephalopathy, optic neuritis and atrophy, toxic psychoses, nausea, vomiting, epigastric distress, elevated SGOT and SGPT, bilirubinuria. Toxic effects are us. encountered only w. high doses of INH; their incidence is higher in slow inactivators.	**Antacids:** Containing Al, may inhibit INH absorp'n from GI tract. INH should be given at least 1 h before antacid. **Disulfiram:** And INH administered concomitantly, may result in behavioral changes. If poss., avoid disulfiram in pts already receiving INH. **Phenytoin:** Metabolism is inhibited by INH. May be nec. to reduce phenytoin dose to 100-200 mg/day to lower its toxicity while at same time controlling seizures.	**Assess:** For hx seizure disorders, alcohol abuse, liver/kidney disease, gen'l debilitat'n. **Administer:** Oral doses from light-proof, moisture-resistant containers; give w. meals to decr. GI symptoms; IM solut'ns at room temp. **Evaluate:** For numbness/tingling of extremities; irritability, restlessness, seizures, hyperglycemia, metabolic acidosis, coma; fever, skin rash, elevated SGOT and bilirubin, jaundice. Check mental status, mood changes. **Teach:** Importance of taking drug regularly and of monthly medical evalua't'n for adv. effects. Warn pts to avoid alcohol while taking drug.
Rifampin (Rifadin, Rimactane)	Tx of active pulmonary TB, whether in primary or chronic phase. Must be used in combinat'n w. at least 1 other effective anti-TB drug **(Oral: Adults** - Take on empty stomach [1 h ac] 600 mg in single daily dose. Should intolerance occur, daily dosage may be taken pc and/or reduced. In pts w. impaired liver funct'n, daily dose should not > 8 mg/kg. Frail/elderly pts - 10 mg/kg/day. Children > 5 years of age - ≤ 20 mg/kg; not > 600 mg/day)	Forms stable complex w. DNA-dependent RNA polymerase to inhibit bacterial RNA synthesis. Effective against most gram-pos. and many gram-neg. bacteria. Particularly effective against *M. tuberculosis*.	GI disturbances, CNS depress'n, headache, mental confus'n, muscle weakness, fever, pains in extremities, gen'l numbness, pruritus, urticaria, skin rashes, eosinophilia, sore mouth, sore tongue, thrombocytopenia, transient leukopenia and decr. Hgb, transient abnormalities in liver funct'n tests.	**Aminosalicylic acid (PAS):** Can reduce GI absorp'n of rifampin. Space doses 8-12 h apart, if poss. **Anticoagulants, oral; antidiabetic agents; contraceptives, oral; corticosteroids; digitalis; narcotics:** Rifampin can incr. their metabolism and thus decr. their effects. **Halothane:** Hepatotoxicity can incr. if rifampin is used after halothane. **Isoniazid:** Used concomitantly w. rifampin, should be approached w. caution because concomitant use incr. risk of hepatotoxicity.	**Assess:** For pre-existing hepatic or renal disease and anemia. **Administer:** ac and independently of PAS; on daily basis only. **Evaluate:** For nausea, vomiting, GI irritat'n, drowsiness, ataxia, dizziness, headache, fatigue; jaundice. **Teach:** Importance of compliance w. prescribed regimen; to use birth control measures other than oral contraceptives; to expect body excret'ns to become reddish-brown; that soft contact lenses may be stained permanently.

Generic Name (Trade Name)	Use (Dose)	Action	Adverse Effects	Drug Interactions	Nursing Process
Ethambutol HCl (Myambutol)	Adjunct to other anti-TB drugs in tx of primary TB. Should not be used as sole anti-TB drug (**Oral:** Initially in pts who have not rec'd previous anti-TB tx - 15 mg/kg as single oral dose 1x q24h. Re-tx in pts who have rec'd previous anti-TB tx - 25 mg/kg as single oral dose q24h. Concurrently administer at least 1 other anti-TB drug. After 60 days of ethambutol administrat'n, decr. dose to 15 mg/kg and give as single oral dose 1x q24h)	Interferes w. protein metabolism in *M. tuberculosis* by blocking synthesis of mycolic acids. Eliminated primarily by renal excret'n. Reduce dose in pts w. renal impairment. Resistance builds quickly if used alone; thus, use in conjunct'n w. other anti-TB drugs.	Decr. visual acuity, apparently due to optic neuritis and rel. to dose/durat'n of tx. Other adv. effects incl. anaphylactoid react'ns, headache, malaise, anxiety, anorexia, nausea, GI upset, dizziness, fever, bloody sputum, dermatitis, rash and pruritus, joint pain.	**Rifampin:** May incr. rate of elimi-nat'n of ethambutol. May be nec. to adjust ethambutol dosage in pts receiving concomitant rifampin tx.	**Assess:** For renal impairment, gout; establish baseline visual funct'n via ophthal. exam. **Administer:** W. food. **Evaluate:** For loss of central vision, disturbances of color discriminat'n, constricted peripheral vision, nausea, vomiting, dermatitis, pruritus, anaphylax-is, dizziness, confus'n, fever, malaise, headache, gout, numbness/tingling of extremities.

Pharmacologic Classification: Other Drugs Used in Tuberculosis

Generic Name (Trade Name)	Use (Dose)	Action	Adverse Effects	Drug Interactions	Nursing Process
Aminosalicylic acid, PAS (Parasal Sodium)	For use w. streptomycin and/or INH in tx of TB when due to susceptible strains of *M. tuber-culosis* (**Oral:** Adults - Administer [w. INH and/or strep-tomycin] 10-12 g/day in 2-3 divided doses. Children - 200-300 mg/kg/day in single dose or 3-4 divided doses. GI distur-bances may be minimized by taking pc or w. meals or w. Al(OH)₃ gel)	Acts as antimetabolite to PABA, preventing PABA utilizat'n in synthesis of folic acid by *M. tuberculosis*.	Nausea, vomiting, diarrhea, abd. pain. Hypersensitivity react'ns incl. fever, skin erupt'ns of various types, infectious mono-nucleosis-like syndrome, leukopenia, agranulocytosis, thrombocytopenia, hemolytic anemia, jaundice, hepatitis, encephalopathy, Löffler's syndrome, vasculitis. Goiter w. or without myxedema. Hypokalemia, acidosis.	**Anticoagulants, oral:** May require adjustment in dosage if given concomitantly w. PAS. **Diphenhydramine:** May impair absorpt'n of PAS. **PABA:** And PAS are competitive antagonists. Avoid PABA in pts receiving PAS. **Probenecid:** Inhibits renal excret'n of PAS. Pts receiving probenecid can prob. receive lower dose of PAS. **Rifampin:** May incr. rate of elimi-nat'n of PAS. May be nec. to adjust PAS dosage in pts receiv-ing concomitant rifampin tx.	**Assess:** For hx of peptic ulcers, renal or cardiac failure. **Administer:** W. food; from light-proof and moisture-resistant container; discard discolored tablets. **Evaluate:** For nausea, vomiting, hematemesis; fever, rash, jaundice; hepatitis; sore throat, bleeding gums, petechiae, unexplained bruising; periph-eral edema, sudden weight gain, altered fluid intake/output ratio.
Streptomycin	Tx of TB in conjunct'n w. other anti-TB agents (**IM only:** Adults - Active pulmonary TB, 1 g/day during early months of initial tx. Can reduce dose to 1 g 2-3x/week after disease is	Tog. w. INH, strepto-mycin immediately suppresses suscepti-ble organisms and can be life saving. Most effective during	As for aminoglycoside antibiotics, Table 96	For *Drug Interactions* involving oral anticoagulants, aminoglyco-side antibiotics, corticosteroids, dimenhydrinate, diuretics and skeletal muscle relaxants, see Table 96.	See Table 96

Drug	Dosage/Use	Action	Effects	Interactions	Nursing Considerations
	controlled. Elderly pts/pts w. auditory or renal funct'n impairment - Lower doses are recomm. For unusually severe pulmonary, meningeal, miliary or GU TB, 1-2 g streptomycin daily, tog. w. full doses of INH and/or PAS until remiss'n established; streptomycin dosage may then be 2x/week)	1st weeks of tx when it incr. activities of oral ethambutol and INH.			**Assess:** Renal or liver impairment. **Evaluate:** For headache, tremor, dysarthria, vertigo, confus'n, somnolence, nervousness, irritability, twitching, hyperreflexia, psychotic states, suicidal tendencies, paranoia, catatonia, depressive react'ns, *grand mal* seizures. Check for s/s hepatic toxicity. **Teach:** To avoid driving or using industrial machinery, power tools and alcohol.
Cycloserine (Seromycin)	Used primarily in urinary tract TB and problem re-tx programs (**Oral:** Initially, 250 mg bid q12h for 1st 2 weeks. Can incr. by 250 mg q few days [if tolerated] until tx serum levels obtained. Us. dose, 500 mg to max. 1 g/day in divided doses. Blood levels to be monitored during tx. Best results occur w. trough serum concentra'ns of 25-30 µg/mL. Serum levels > 30 µg/mL have been assoc. w. toxicity and should be avoided)	Competes w. alanine to prevent cell wall format'n by *M. tuberculosis*. CNS toxicity restricts use.	CNS toxicity, incl. both neurologic and psychic disturbances.	**Ethionamide:** Should not be given w. cycloserine because of additive CNS toxicity. **Isoniazid:** And cycloserine should be avoided, if poss., because of additive CNS toxicity.	
Capreomycin sulfate (Capastat)	In combinat'n w. other appropriate anti-TB agents, capreomycin is mod. effective for tx of pulmonary infect'ns caused by susceptible strains of *M. tuberculosis* when primary agents have been ineffective or cannot be used because of toxicity (**IM:** Adults - 15 mg/kg [approx. 1 g/day] for 2-4 weeks, followed by 1 g 2-3x/week for 6-12 months or longer prn. Most pts tolerate 1 g/day for 2-4 months and occ. for as long as 6 months. Daily dose should not > 20 mg/kg)	Useful in streptomycin-resistant strains of *M. tuberculosis*. Capreomycin is both ototoxic and nephrotoxic.	Elevat'n of BUN > 20 mg/dL observed in many cases. Toxic nephritis has been reported. Subclinical auditory loss, tinnitus, vertigo, pain and indurat'n at inject'n sites.	**Polymyxin, colistin, gentamicin, kanamycin, streptomycin, neomycin, paromomycin, vancomycin:** May either damage 8th cranial nerve funct'n or produce peripheral neuromuscular blocking action. Use of capreomycin w. any of these may have additive toxic effect.	**Assess:** Anticipate order for sensitivity, hearing, CBC, serum K, liver funct'n and renal status tests; complete tests before 1st dose. **Administer:** Dissolve in normal saline or water acc. to manufacturer's direct'ns. Deep into large muscle mass; aspirate carefully. Document and rotate inject'n sites. **Evaluate:** Changes in fluid intake/output ratio; hearing acuity, pt's percept'ns of hearing changes; observe for disturbances of balance. Monitor hepatic status.

Generic Name (Trade Name)	Use (Dose)	Action	Adverse Effects	Drug Interactions	Nursing Process
Pyrazinamide (Tebrazid)	May be administered after adequate course of tx w. primary drugs has failed; should be given only w. other effective anti-TB agents (**Oral:** Adults - 20-35 mg/kg, to max. 3 g/day. Should be given in 3-4 equally spaced doses)	May be valuable when short-term resistance to INH is a problem.	Hepatic toxicity; more serious react'ns involve clinical jaundice and rarely progressive fulminary acute yellow atrophy and death. Active gout, sideroblastic anemia, arthralgias, anorexia, nausea and vomiting, dysuria, malaise, fever, urticaria.		**Assess:** For hx liver disease. **Evaluate:** For early evidence of hepatic damage (jaundice, incr. bleeding tendencies, enlarged liver).

CHAPTER 67

Antifungal Drugs

Teaching Objectives

Following completion of this chapter, the reader should be able to:
1. State the difficulties in treating systemic mycotic infections.
2. Discuss the mechanism of action, therapeutic uses and adverse effects of amphotericin B, as well as the nursing process related to its administration.
3. Describe the mechanism of action, therapeutic uses and adverse effects of flucytosine, and the nursing process associated with its use.
4. Discuss the systemic use of ketoconazole, including its mechanism of action, therapeutic uses, adverse effects and nursing process.
5. Discuss the systemic use of miconazole, including its mechanism of action, therapeutic uses, adverse effects and nursing process.

Fungal Diseases

Fungal diseases can be either superficial or systemic. Systemic infections constitute a major therapeutic problem and can have a significant fatality rate. Systemic "opportunistic infections" occur commonly in debilitated and immunosuppressed patients. They include candidiasis, aspergillosis, cryptococcosis and phycomycosis. Other systemic infections, including blastomycosis, coccidioidomycosis, histoplasmosis and sporotrichosis, occur less frequently. This chapter discusses drugs used to treat systemic fungal infections. The treatment of fungal infections of the skin, hair, nails, gastrointestinal tract and vagina is discussed in Chapter 43.

The treatment of systemic fungal infections is unsatisfactory. At the present time only a limited number of drugs are available and their use is often associated with severe adverse effects. In addition, patients with systemic mycotic infections may be very ill with other diseases. Antibiotics or antibacterials are used on occasion to treat systemic mycotic infections. Penicillin G, for example, can be given intravenously for the treatment of actinomycosis. Patients allergic to penicillin can be given erythromycin, a cephalosporin, a tetracycline or clindamycin. Sulfonamides are the drugs of choice for nocardiosis. If they cannot be used, ampicillin, erythromycin or a tetracycline may be given. The pharmacology of these drugs is presented elsewhere in this text and will not be repeated here. Fluconazole (Diflucan) is a potent newer antifungal drug. Because of its importance in the treatment of patients with acquired immunodeficiency syndrome (AIDS), it is discussed in Chapter 68.

Amphotericin B (Fungizone)

Mechanism of Action and Therapeutic Uses

Amphotericin B increases membrane permeability of sensitive fungi. As a consequence, small molecules leak from the cells, causing a decrease in mass and termination of mycotic growth.

Amphotericin B has a broad-spectrum antifungal activity. Insoluble in water, the drug is provided as a sterile lyophilized powder, providing 50 mg of amphotericin B and approximately 41 mg of sodium deoxycholate, buffered with 25.2 mg sodium phosphate. The presence of sodium deoxycholate allows for solubilization of amphotericin B. Infused in a concentration of 100 µg/mL or less over a period of six hours to minimize irritation and reduce the high risk of thrombophlebitis, amphotericin B is used for the treatment of patients with progressive, potentially fatal disseminated mycotic infections. This potent drug should not be used to treat the common inapparent forms of fungal disease, which show only positive skin or serologic tests. Amphotericin B can also be used to treat opportunistic infections in immunosuppressed patients caused by candida, cryptococcus and torulopsis. Because amphotericin B does not diffuse well into the cerebrospinal fluid, intrathecal administration may be required for central nervous system infections.

Adverse Effects

Amphotericin B must be used with considerable care. The most common early adverse effect is an acute febrile reaction beginning about two hours after starting the infusion and peaking approximately one hour later. An antipyretic, such as aspirin, may reduce the fever.

A dose-dependent azotemia can also result from amphotericin B use. Although this is usually temporary, ceasing when the drug is stopped, permanent damage may be evident, particularly in patients with pre-existing renal impairment. More severe nephrotoxicity is manifested by hyponatremia, hypokalemia and renal tubular acidosis. If this occurs, the dose should be reduced, the patient hydrated, and serum electrolytes adjusted. Other nephrotoxic drugs should be discontinued. Renal function and serum electrolytes should be monitored twice weekly.

Hypersensitivity reactions are not usual. However, amphotericin B can produce generalized pain, seizures and anaphylactic shock. The drug can also cause headache, fever, chills, anorexia and vomiting.

Nursing Process

Assessment

Nursing assessment of patients for whom amphotericin B has been prescribed should focus on a review of the patient's history for evidence of previous allergy to amphotericin B or hematopoietic disorders.

Administration

Reconstitute amphotericin B according to the manufacturer's instructions using sterile distilled water with a bacteriostatic agent. The reconstituted solution is added to at least 500 mL of 5% dextrose in water for administration. Exposure to light causes the drug to deteriorate. Protect the solution with a paper bag or aluminum foil. Reconstituted solutions are stable for twenty-four hours if protected from light and for one week if stored in a refrigerator. Discard unused solutions after this time.

Administer amphotericin solutions intravenously using an in-line filter and distal vein. The infusion site should be inspected frequently for redness, swelling, induration and pain because of the danger of thrombophlebitis.

Vital signs should be monitored every fifteen to thirty minutes during the first infusion. Nurses should note any change in pulse and blood pressure. Fluid intake and output should monitored.

Evaluation

Patient evaluation should stress alertness for muscle weakness suggesting hypokalemia, altered fluid intake/output ratio, oliguria and hematuria, all of which indicate nephrotoxicity. Vital signs should be monitored at daily intervals because of the danger of allergic reactions.

Teaching

Nurses should teach patients to monitor for signs of allergic reactions, renal toxicity and ototoxicity.

Flucytosine (Ancotil, Ancobon)

Mechanism of Action and Therapeutic Uses

Flucytosine is a structural analog of cytosine, an essential component in body functions. Flucytosine is taken up into fungal cells where it acts as an antimetabolite of cytosine and blocks fungal thymidylate synthetase, an enzyme essential to the formation of DNA.

Administered orally, flucytosine is given for the treatment of serious infections caused by susceptible strains of candida or cryptococcus, or both. Flucytosine passes easily into the cerebrospinal fluid and enters the aqueous humor and bronchial secretions in concentrations adequate to inhibit sensitive fungi. Septicemia, endocarditis and urinary tract infections caused by candida have been treated effectively. Meningitis and pulmonary infections caused by cryptococcus have also responded to flucytosine. Limited trials in patients with candida pulmonary infections, cryptococcus septicemias, or cryptococcal urinary tract infections support the use of flucytosine in these conditions. Flucytosine also has been used in the treatment of chromomycosis caused by *Fonsecaea pedrosoi, Cladosporium carrioni,* or *Philaphora verrucosa.* Because resistance may develop to flucytosine during therapy, it is usually combined with amphotericin B. The administration of flucytosine often allows the use of lower doses of amphotericin B.

Flucytosine is excreted primarily by the kidneys. Its dosage schedule must be modified in patients with impaired renal function.

Adverse Effects

Reversible neutropenia, together with occasional thrombocytopenia, are the principal adverse effects of flucytosine. The drug can also cause nausea, eosinophilia and skin rashes. Flucytosine is capable of producing reversible hepatic dysfunction. Patients sometimes experience confusion, hallucinations, headache and vertigo. A few cases of irreversible bone marrow failure have been reported. Patients with a limited bone marrow reserve, such as individuals receiving cytotoxic drug treatment, may be prone to develop hematological adverse effects when treated with flucytosine.

Nursing Process

Assessment
Patients for whom flucytosine has been prescribed should undergo nursing review of their history for liver or kidney disease, or hematopoietic disorders. Simultaneously, in consultation with the pharmacist, nurses should review the patient's current drug regimen for the concurrent use of drugs that might interact with flucytosine. Patients undergoing treatment of a malignancy with either radiation or chemotherapy should not receive flucytosine. Laboratory specimens for culture and sensitivity must be collected prior to the first administration of this and all antifungal drugs.

Administration
The slow administration of flucytosine capsules over a twenty-minute period may reduce the nausea that often accompanies drug ingestion.

Evaluation
Patient evaluation during the course of flucytosine therapy includes complete blood counts every three days. Nurses should also be alert for evidence of confusion, hallucinations, headache and vertigo, which suggest central nervous system toxicity. The patient should also be observed for elevated BUN and SGOT levels, accompanied by jaundice, which indicate hepatic dysfunction. Nurses should warn patients that long-term therapy with flucytosine, possibly one to two months, may be needed to eradicate the infection.

Ketoconazole (Nizoral)

Mechanism of Action and Therapeutic Uses

The use of ketoconazole to treat superficial infections was discussed in Chapter 43. The drug is also effective in systemic fungal infections. Ketoconazole disrupts the plasma membrane of susceptible fungi by interfering with the biosynthesis of ergosterol. Its absorption is improved if ingested before meals. Drugs that reduce gastric acidity, such as antacids, histamine$_2$ blockers (see Chapter 22) or anticholinergics, reduce ketoconazole absorption and should be avoided. Ketoconazole is eliminated by hepatic metabolism and has a terminal half-life of approximately twelve hours.

Ketoconazole indicated for the treatment of serious life-threatening systemic fungal infections in normal, predisposed or immunocompromised patients in whom alternate therapy is considered inappropriate or has been unsuccessful: systemic candidiasis, chronic mucocutaneous candidiasis, coccidioidomycosis, paracoccidioidomycosis, histoplasmosis and chromomycosis. It is contraindicated in patients with hepatic dysfunction (see later discussion) and also in women of childbearing potential unless effective forms of contraceptive are employed.

Adverse Effects

The most common adverse effects of ketoconazole are nausea and pruritus. Patients may also experience headache, dizziness, abdominal pain, constipation, diarrhea, somnolence and nervousness. Concern is greatest over the possible hepatotoxic effects of ketoconazole. Cases of fatal massive hepatic necrosis have been reported. Liver function should be monitored periodically and the drug stopped if signs of hepatocellular dysfunction appear. Ketoconazole can block adrenal steroid synthesis. Approximately ten per cent of men on the drug experience gynecomastia.

Nursing Process

Assessment
Nurses should review the patient's history for evidence of liver disease. Laboratory specimens for culture and sensitivity tests must be collected prior to the first administration of this and all antifungal drugs.

Administration
Ketoconazole is best absorbed if taken before meals with citrus or other slightly acidic liquids. Drugs that reduce gastric acidity, such as antacids, histamine$_2$ blockers (see Chapter 22) or anticholinergics, reduce ketoconazole absorption and should be avoided.

Teaching
Ketoconazole can produce dizziness or drowsiness. Caution patients to avoid driving and using power tools or heavy machinery until their individual response to the medication has been determined. Patients must be advised to continue the drug in the dosage prescribed until laboratory and clinical tests indicate the absence of further fungal infection. Nurses must warn patients to avoid antacids, over-the-counter medications and alkaline products.

Miconazole Nitrate (Monistat IV)

Mechanism of Action and Therapeutic Uses

Miconazole disrupts plasma membranes of sensitive fungi. Miconazole does not cross the blood-brain barrier. If an effect in the cerebrospinal fluid is required, it must be injected intrathecally.

Administered intravenously, miconazole can be effective in the treatment of paracoccidioidomycosis and coccidioidomycosis. Although less reliable than amphotericin B, miconazole is also less toxic. It may be used as an alternative drug in patients with renal impairment.

Adverse Effects

The most common adverse effects of miconazole are thrombophlebitis, pruritus, rash, nausea and anorexia. Giving the drug over one hour in a volume of 200 mL or more reduces tachypnea, tachycardia and ventricular tachycardia.

Nursing Process

The intravenous administration of miconazole requires its dilution in at least 200 mL of 0.9% sodium chloride or 5% dextrose in water. This solution is administered over one hour. If the medication is diluted in a larger volume of fluid, its infusion should be correspondingly longer to prevent fluid overload of the circulatory system. Nurses should monitor the test dose and then be alert for systemic allergic reactions during infusion. The site of drug infusion should also be observed for the development of skin irritation to miconazole.

Further Reading

Bennett, J.E. (1990). Antifungal agents. In: G. L. Mandell et al. (eds.), *Principles and Practice of Infectious Diseases,* 3rd ed. New York: Churchill Livingstone, pp. 361-370.

Drugs for treatment of systemic fungal infections (1986). *The Medical Letter 28* :41-44.

Kowalsky, S.F. and Dixon, D.M. (1991). Fluconazole: A new antifungal agent. *Clinical Pharmacy 10* :179-194.

Table 101
Antifungal drugs.

Generic Name (Trade Name)	Use (Dose)	Action	Adverse Effects	Drug Interactions	Nursing Process

Pharmacologic Classification: Drugs for the Treatment of Systemic Fungal Infections

Generic Name (Trade Name)	Use (Dose)	Action	Adverse Effects	Drug Interactions	Nursing Process
Amphotericin B (Fungizone Intravenous)	Primarily intended for tx of progressive, potentially fatal disseminated mycotic infect'ns. Should not be used in common inapparent forms of fungal disease that show only positive skin or serologic tests (**Slow IV infus'n:** Us. 250 µg/kg/day initially; incr. gradually as tolerance permits. Opt. dose unknown. Total daily dose may range up to 1 mg/kg, or alternate-day dosages to 1.5 mg/kg. *Under no circumstances should total daily dose of 1.5 mg/kg be exceeded. Several months of tx are us. necessary*)	Incr. membrane permeability of sensitive fungi. Small molecules leak from cells, causing decr. mass and terminat'n of mycotic growth. Broad-spectrum antifungal activity.	Fever, sometimes accomp. by shaking, chills, headache, anorexia, nausea, vomiting, weight loss, dyspepsia, diarrhea, gen'lized pain incl. muscle and joint pain, cramping, epigastric pain and malaise. Renal damage is often accomp. by granular and hyaline casts, and sometimes by microhematuria. Renal dysfunct'n is us. reversible on discontinuat'n of tx, but serious and permanent damage has been reported in pts given large doses for prolonged periods, esp. when total dosage > 5 g.	**Antibiotics; antineoplastics:** May lead to emergence of deep fungal infect'ns. Therefore, these drugs should be avoided if poss. in pts taking amphotericin B. Antineoplastics may also incr. risk of renal damage. **Aminoglycoside antibiotics:** Are nephrotoxic and should not be administered concomitantly w. amphotericin B. **Corticosteroids:** May predispose pts to systemic mycotic infect'ns. Furthermore, they may enhance K deplet'n produced by amphotericin B. Pts should be monitored closely for electrolyte abnormalities and cardiac dysfunct'n. **Digitalis:** Toxicity is incr. by hypokalemia, which amphotericin B may produce. Observe pts receiving amphotericin B and digitalis very closely; treat K deficiency stat. **Skeletal muscle relaxants:** Have greater effect in presence of hypokalemia. Amphotericin B–induced hypokalemia may incr. effect of curare-like drug.	**Assess:** For previous allergy to amphotericin B; hematopoietic disorders. Monitor VS q15-30 min during 1st infus'n. Monitor fluid intake/output ratio. **Administer:** Reconstitute IV solut'n acc. to manufacturer's instruct'ns, using sterile distilled water without bacteriostatic agent. Add to IV solut'n of 500 mL D5W for administrat'n; infuse over 6 h using in-line filter and distal vein. Keep solut'n covered w. paper bag or Al foil during infus'n; discard unused reconstituted solut'ns after 24 h if stored in a dark place or 1 week if refrigerated. **Evaluate:** For redness, swelling, indurat'n, pain at infus'n site; muscle weakness (hypokalemia); reduced fluid intake/output ratio, oliguria, hematuria; allergic react'ns; renal toxicity, ototoxicity.

Generic Name (Trade Name)	Use (Dose)	Action	Adverse Effects	Drug Interactions	Nursing Process
Flucytosine (Ancotil, Ancobon)	Tx of serious infect'ns caused by susceptible strains of candida and/or cryptococcus. Septicemia, endocarditis and urinary tract infect'ns due to candida have been treated effectively. Meningitis and pulmonary infect'ns caused by cryptococcus have also responded to tx **(Oral:** Us. dosage is 50-150 mg/kg/day in 4 divided doses. Nausea and vomiting may be avoided if drug is given over 15-min interval at each dosing period. Reduce dose in pts w. renal impairment acc. to manufacturer's instruct'ns)	Structural analog of cytosine. By serving as antimetabolite of cytosine and blocking thymidylate synthetase, flucytosine prevents format'n of RNA in sensitive fungi.	Bone marrow depress'n (anemia, leukopenia, thrombocytopenia, neutropenia); GI distress (nausea, vomiting, diarrhea); hepatotoxicity (elevat'n of hepatic enzymes, lactate dehydrogenase, bilirubin); nephrotoxicity (elevat'n of BUN, creatinine); neurologic effects (confus'n, hallucinat'ns, sedat'n, vertigo); rash.	**Drugs known to reduce renal funct'n** (diuretics, aminoglycoside antibiotics, amphotericin B): Should be used carefully because flucytosine is excreted primarily by kidneys. Reduced renal funct'n can lead to drug accumulat'n in body. **Drugs that depress bone marrow:** Can interact w. flucytosine. Pts taking flucytosine may be prone to bone marrow depress'n if they are being treated w. drugs that depress bone marrow, or have a hx of tx w. such drugs.	**Assess:** For hx liver/kidney disease, hematopoietic disorders; concurrent tx of malignancy using radiat'n or chemotx; collect lab. specimens for culture and sensitivity. **Administer:** Capsules slowly during 20-min period. **Evaluate:** Initiate CBC q3days; for confus'n, hallucinat'ns, headache, vertigo, elevated BUN and SGOT, jaundice. **Teach:** Warn pt that long-term (poss. 1-2 months) tx may be needed to clear infect'n.
Ketoconazole (Nizoral)	Tx of serious life-threatening systemic fungal infect'ns in normal, predisposed or immunocompromised pts in whom alternate tx is inappropriate or has been unsuccessful **(Oral:** Adults - 200 mg od. Pts who fail to respond and have inadequate blood levels [< 1 μg/mL] may receive 400 mg. Children - ≤ 20 kg - 50 mg od; 20-40 kg - 100 mg od; > 40 kg - 200 mg od)	Disrupts plasma membrane of susceptible fungi by interfering w. ergosterol biosynthesis. Absorpt'n improved if ingested ac. Effective in many mucocutaneous and systemic fungal infect'ns.	Nausea, pruritus, headache, dizziness, abd. pain, constipat'n, diarrhea, somnolence, nervousness, poss. hepatotoxicity.	**Antacids; anticholinergics; H₂ blockers; omeprazole:** Should be avoided or given not < 2 h after ketoconazole, because bioavailability of ketoconazole depends on gastric acidity. **Anticoagulants, oral:** May have incr. effects if ketoconazole is taken. **Cyclosporin:** Blood levels may be incr. by ketoconazole. **Hypoglycemics, oral:** May produce severe hypoglycemia if ketoconazole is taken. **Phenytoin:** And ketoconazole, may affect each other's rates of metabolism. **Rifampin; INH:** Can reduce blood levels of ketoconazole.	**Assess:** Review hx for liver disease; ensure that lab. specimens for culture and sensitivity are taken before 1st dose. **Administration:** ac w. citrus or other acidic juice; avoid substances that raise stomach pH. **Teach:** To avoid driving, using power tools or heavy machinery till response to drug is determined; to continue drug in prescribed manner until lab. and clinical tests indicate absence of fungal infect'n. Warn pts to avoid antacids, OTC drugs and alkaline products.

| Miconazole nitrate (Monistat IV) | Effective in tx of paracoccidioidomycosis. May have some benefit in coccidioidomycosis (**IV:** Adults - *For paracoccidioidomycosis* - 200-1200 mg/day. *For coccidioidomycosis* - 1.8-3.6 g/day. Dose is divided into 2-3 infus'ns given in 200 mL normal saline or D5W over 60-120 min. Children - 20-40 mg/kg/day; no single infus'n > 15 mg/kg) | Disrupts plasma membranes of sensitive fungi. | Thrombophlebitis, pruritus, rash, nausea, anorexia, tachypnea, tachycardia, ventr. tachycardia. | **Administer:** IV in at least 200 mL of 0.9% NaCl or D5W during 1-2 h period. **Evaluate:** For erythema, stinging, blistering, localized edema, peeling, itching, urticaria at site of applicat'n or administrat'n. Monitor test dose, then be alert for systemic allergic react'ns during infus'n. |

CHAPTER 68

Antiviral Drugs

Teaching Objectives

Following completion of this chapter, the reader should be able to:

1. List the steps in the development of a viral infection in a human.
2. Define and discuss the term retrovirus.
3. List two approaches to the treatment of AIDS.
4. Describe briefly the mechanism of action of AZT in the treatment of AIDS, its place in therapy, adverse effects, and nursing process.
5. Describe briefly the use of ddI, rifabutin and ribavirin in the treatment of AIDS.
6. Discuss the actions, uses, adverse effects and nursing processes for ganciclovir, pentamidine isethionate and fluconazole when these drugs are used as supportive therapy for AIDS.
7. Discuss the mechanism of action, therapeutic uses, adverse effects and nursing process for acyclovir.
8. Describe briefly the mechanism of action, therapeutic uses, adverse effects and nursing process for amantadine.
9. Describe the mechanism of action, therapeutic uses, adverse effects and nursing process for idoxuridine.
10. Discuss the mechanism of action and therapeutic uses of ribavirin in the treatment of respiratory synctial virus, as well as its adverse effects and nursing process.
11. Describe the mechanism of action, therapeutic uses, adverse effects and nursing process for trifluridine.
12. Discuss the mechanism of action and therapeutic uses of vidarabine, together with its adverse effects and nursing process.

General Information

With the development of an increasing number of antibiotics, capable of eradicating many bacterial diseases, attention is switching to antiviral drugs. The general public is increasingly alarmed about viral diseases, particularly as they relate to the sexually transmitted infections herpes genitalis and acquired immunodeficiency syndrome (AIDS). Publicity given to these problems has overshadowed the fact that the great majority of viral infections occur without any accompanying illness. If this were not the case, respiratory viruses belonging to hundreds of serotypes would immobilize humankind. When a viral infection does produce sickness, the illness is usually self-limited and of short duration, and results in long-term immunity to the virus involved.

Notwithstanding these comments, new antiviral drugs must be developed. At present the treatment of viral disorders is almost entirely of a preventative nature. Because of effective programs, humans have been immunized against many viral disorders. Vaccines for the prevention of poliomyelitis, measles, rubella, mumps and yellow fever are very effective. Immunization procedures have also been developed against influenza and rabies.

Immunization, however, has two major shortcomings. It is of prophylactic value only and of no benefit once the individual has contracted the disease. Furthermore, scientists have been unable to develop specific immunization procedures for many viral disorders. Therefore, it is important to develop drugs capable of eradicating contracted viral infections.

Viruses are divided into two classes, depending on whether their nucleic acid is deoxyribonucleic acid (DNA) or ribonucleic acid (RNA). The nucleic acid core, referred to as the **genome,** is surrounded by a protein-containing shell. Viruses reproduce only inside living cells. The larger and more complex the virus, the greater the likelihood that a drug can interrupt its activity. Most viruses causing human disease are very small RNA viruses. Up to the present time they have remained largely refractive to drug treatment. Prior to discussing individual drugs used to treat viral disorders, we will spend a short time describing the multiplication cycle of viruses so that the reader will be better prepared to understand the means by which drugs can interfere with the life cycle of the virus.

A virus initially attaches to specific receptor sites on the cell membrane of the host before subsequently penetrating the cell. Once encapsulated in the host's cell, the protein coat of the virus is dissolved by the host's enzymes, freeing either DNA or RNA. The DNA or RNA genome of the virus then duplicates, and viral proteins are synthesized. Subsequently, the components assemble to form a mature virus particle, and the genome usually becomes encapsulated by viral proteins. The virus is released from the host cell, which may be lysed and die. Thereafter, the virus is free to attach to the membrane of another host cell and begin the procedure once again.

Antiviral drugs may inhibit the penetration of a virus into the host cell, impair the uncoating of the viral nucleic acid molecule, or prevent viral replication.

This chapter will be divided into two parts: drugs for the treatment of AIDS and drugs for the treatment of other viral diseases. The importance given to the treatment of AIDS, together with the rapid expansion of research into anti-AIDS drugs, makes mandatory a separate section in this chapter for drugs used in the treatment of AIDS.

Drugs for the Treatment of AIDS

Retroviruses form a subgroup of RNA viruses which, in order to replicate, must first "reverse transcribe" the RNA of the genome into DNA ("transcription" conventionally describes the synthesis of RNA from DNA). Once in the form of DNA, the viral genome is incorporated into the host cell genome, allowing it to take full advantage of the host cell's transcription/translation machinery for the purpose of replication. Once incorporated, the viral DNA is virtually indistinguishable from the host's DNA and, in this state, the virus may persist for as long as the cell lives. As it is virtually invulnerable to attack in this form, any treatment must be directed at another state of the life cycle and must necessarily continue until all virus-carrying cells have died.

AIDS is caused by a species of retrovirus, the **human immunodeficiency virus (HIV).** It is important to understand this relationship, as HIV and AIDS are often used synonymously. Treatment directed against the HIV should reduce the progression of AIDS. It is hoped that eventually drug therapy will be developed either to prevent the HIV from attacking humans or to kill the virus once it has been found in the host. Only then can we provide patients with adequate therapy for AIDS.

Drugs are currently used to combat the virus or to treat infections that have arisen as result of the host's reduced immune response. The two groups of agents will be discussed separately.

Anti-HIV Drugs

Therapeutic advances against the HIV have been unprecedented, compared with those against other viral diseases. Because of the rapidly expanding nature of this field of research, comments made in this text will probably be out of date by the time of publication.

It will also be noted that the doses and drug interactions for most anti-AIDS drugs are not presented here because at the time of preparing this text only zidovudine and ribavirin had been cleared for sale in North America.

Zidovudine, AZT, Azidothymidine (Retrovir)

It is generally assumed that the mechanism of action of zidovudine lies in its selective capacity to be incorporated by the retroviral reverse transcriptase, rather than by the host cell polymerase, causing premature chain elongation termination. There appears to be little doubt the zidovudine delays the fall in T4 cells in patients infected with the HIV. The standard recommended dose of zidovudine was originally 200 mg every four hours (1200 mg/day) for patients with advanced AIDS-related complex (ARC) or AIDS. However, data have shown at least equal effectiveness and much less hematological toxicity with an initial dose of 200 mg every four hours (1200 mg/day) for the first month, followed by 100 mg every four hours (600 mg/day). At the time of publication, that was the recommended dosage. Some experts contend that the initial 1200 mg/day dose for one month is unnecessary.

Most patients develop nausea and headache over the first couple of weeks of treatment with zidovudine, but these effects are usually transient. Some develop insomnia, myalgia, fever, asthenia, diarrhea and abdominal pain. Although the symptoms are common they rarely cause withdrawal of the drug. Bone marrow depression is a far more worrying consideration. In one study, forty-five per cent of patients receiving zidovudine developed grade 3 bone marrow depression (hemoglobin < 7.5 g/dL, neutrophils < 750/dL, or white cells < 1500/dL). Other studies have also reported instances of severe bone marrow depression. There is interesting evidence to suggest that using the drug earlier in the disease, in lower doses, reduces the rate of fall of T4 lymphocytes and decreases the incidence of toxicity. Only time will tell if this protocol will engender resistance to the drug on the part of the HIV.

Nursing Process

The nursing process for zidovudine is presently being developed as more is learned about the drug and patient reactions. Nurses administering the drug are advised to read the manufacturer's package insert carefully and to seek advice from the pharmacist. The following nursing process observations are advised.

Assessment
Nurses should check blood studies clearly every two weeks and watch for decreasing granulocytes and hemoglobin. If blood counts fall too low, it may be necessary to stop the drug and give a blood transfusion.

Administration
Zidovudine capsules are stored in a cool place, protected from light, and administered by mouth. Patients should be advised to swallow them whole. Anti-infective drugs may be ordered concomitantly to prevent opportunistic infections.

Evaluation
Nurses should observe patients for signs of blood dyscrasias, bruising, fatigue, bleeding and poor healing.

Teaching
Nurses must first explain that the drug is not a cure but will help control symptoms. Zidovudine must be taken every four hours, around the clock. Patients must be told to call the nurse or physician if adverse effects occur, such as swollen lymph nodes, malaise, fever or other infections. Nurses must warn patients that serious drug interactions may occur if over-the-counter medications are taken. Patients must be taught that other anti-infective drugs may be necessary to control other infections.

Nurses should also warn the patient that treatment with zidovudine does not prevent the possibility of infecting others with the HIV. Caution patients that followup visits must be continued to monitor blood counts and drug toxicity.

Dideoxyinosine, ddI

Several $2^1,3^1$-dideoxynucleosides inhibit HIV replication. The dideoxynucleosides are DNA chain terminators. Dideoxyinosine is converted to dideoxyadenosine monophosphate via dideoxyinosine monophosphate. Studies of ddI are currently taking place throughout the world. The main advantage of ddI appears to be its minimal toxicity to bone marrow. With low doses, the most frequent adverse effects are headache, insomnia and increased serum uric acid concentrations. Higher doses of the drug can produce sensory neuropathy (especially foot pain) and pancreatitis.

Rifabutin (Ansamycin)

Concentrations of rifabutin between 0.1 – 0.8 mg/L will inhibit HIV replication in vitro. The mechanism of action is thought to be inhibition of the DNA-dependent RNA transcriptase. HIV replication in human peripheral blood lymphocytes in vitro can be inhibited, presumably by the binding of rifabutin to reverse transcriptase. The anti-HIV activity of a combination of rifabutin with heparin or dideoxycytidine (ddC) has been claimed to be greater than either drug alone, with no signs of in vitro toxicity.

Ribavirin (Virazole)

Ribavirin is marketed as an aerosol treatment for infants with respiratory viral infections (see below). The drug has also been tested for its anti-HIV effects. Its mechanism of action is thought to involve alterations of the intracellular guanosine pool and the guanylation step required for 5^1-capping of viral messenger RNA. Ribavirin has caused suppression of HIV replication in continuous cell lines and human peripheral blood leukocytes. Unfortunately, initial clinical trials with ribavirin have yielded equivocal results.

Supportive Therapy for AIDS Patients

People living with AIDS are susceptible to infections that would not normally be found in most patients with normal host defense mechanisms. The appropriate use of antibiotics, antifungals and antivirals can significantly prolong life in the HIV-infected individual. Many of the drugs used in these conditions have previously been described in earlier chapters. At this point, it is appropriate to review only those drugs that have not yet been discussed.

Ganciclovir Sodium (Cytovene)

Ganciclovir is a synthetic nucleoside analog that inhibits the replication of herpes viruses both in vitro and in vivo. The drug is indicated for the treatment of cytomegalovirus (CMV) retinitis in immunocompromised individuals, such as patients with AIDS, iatrogenic immunosuppression secondary to organ transplantation, or those undergoing chemotherapy for neoplasia. The emergence of clinically significant viral resistance to ganciclovir has been reported.

During clinical trials, ganciclovir treatment was withdrawn or interrupted in approximately thirty-two per cent of the patients because of adverse effects. The most frequent adverse events involved the hematopoietic system. Neutropenia occurred in thirty-eight per cent and thrombocytopenia in nineteen per cent of patients.

Nursing Process

The following comments relate to the use of ddI, rifabutin, ribavirin and ganciclovir. The nursing process for these drugs is similar to that for zidovudine (AZT). Nurses are advised to check the manufacturer's insert and consult the pharmacist for directions and *current* information before administering these drugs. If these drugs are given concurrently with other antivirals or medications, check each drug closely for possible interactions.

Pentamidine Isethionate (Pentacarinat, NebuPent, Pneumopent)

Pneumocystis carinii pneumonia (PCP) occurs in approximately eighty per cent of AIDS patients, and is an important cause of death. Most initial episodes of PCP in HIV-positive patients occur when the blood CD4+ lymphocyte count is less than 200 cells/mm^3, or less than twenty per cent of total lymphocytes. A recurrence rate has been reported of up to sixty per cent within one year after the initial episode of PCP. Aerosolized pentamidine isethionate (NebuPent, Pneumopent) once a month is effective in preventing recurrence of PCP in AIDS patients and probably effective in preventing first episodes. Pentamidine isethionate powder (Pentacarinat), approved for intravenous or intramuscular injection, can also be aerosolized and inhaled by patients with AIDS.

Pentacarinat should be used only in a hospital setting with facilities to monitor blood glucose, blood count, and renal and hepatic functions. Fatalities due to severe hypotension, hypoglycemia and cardiac arrhythmias have been reported in patients treated with Pentacarinat. Profound severe hypotension may result after a single dose.

Nursing Process

Nurses are advised to consult the nursing process for zidovudine (AZT) closely and add the following observations for pentamidine.

Assessment

Nurses should note the fluid intake and output ratios and report imbalances, proteinuria or oliguria. It is important also to review the patient's history for liver or renal disease and the electrocardiogram for abnormalities. Blood pressure must be monitored for abnormalities.

Evaluation

Nurses should evaluate the injection site for pain or abnormalities when parenteral pentamidine is administered. The respiratory status of the patient should also be monitored for rate, wheezing or dyspnea.

Fluconazole (Diflucan)

Fluconazole is a broad-spectrum antifungal drug that can be employed as supportive therapy in AIDS patients. The fungistatic activity of fluconazole is exhibited in vitro against *Cryptococcus neoformans* and candida species. Fluconazole is well absorbed when taken orally and can also be administered parenterally. Currently the drug is indicated for the treatment of oropharyngeal and esophageal candidiasis, as well as for serious systemic candidal infections, including urinary tract infections, peritonitis and pneumonia. Fluconazole is also indicated for cryptococcal meningitis.

Fluconazole diffuses well throughout the body and its volume of distribution is approximately that of total body water. The drug crosses the blood-brain barrier well. Fluconazole is cleared primarily by renal excretion. There is an inverse relationship between the elimination half-life and creatinine clearance.

The adverse effects of fluconazole may include hepatic reactions and exfoliative skin disorders, including Stevens-Johnson syndrome. Because most of the patients experiencing these effects were receiving multiple medications, including many known to be hepatotoxic or associated with exfoliative skin disorders, the causal association of these reactions with fluconazole therapy is not clear. Nevertheless, patients who develop abnormal liver function tests during fluconazole therapy should be monitored for the development of severe hepatic injury. If clinical signs and symptoms consistent with liver disease develop that may be attributable to fluconazole, the drug should be stopped. Immunocompromised patient who develop rashes during treatment with fluconazole should be monitored closely and the drug discontinued if the lesions progress. Other adverse effects of fluconazole include nausea, headache, skin rash, vomiting, abdominal pain and diarrhea.

Nursing Process

Nurses are advised to consult the nursing process for zidovudine (AZT) closely if the patient is receiving fluconazole. Add the following observations for fluconazole.

Assessment

Nurses must monitor vital signs closely during the first infusion and be alert for changes in pulse and blood pressure. Fluid intake and output ratios must be watched for decreased fluid output. Nurses must also be alert for changes in specific gravity of urine. Patients must be watched for development of edema or weight gain.

Evaluation

If fluconazole is administered intravenously, the infusion site must be evaluated for tissue damage. It is recommended that a distal vein be selected for infusion purposes. Nurses must monitor patients for possible renal or liver toxicity.

Drugs for the Treatment of Other Viral Infections

Acyclovir (Zovirax)

Mechanism of Action and Therapeutic Uses

Acyclovir is metabolized to acyclovir triphosphate, which inhibits DNA polymerase and viral multiplication in herpes simplex types 1 and 2, varicella-zoster, herpes simiae (B virus) and Epstein-Barr virus. Acyclovir is available in parenteral, oral and topical formulation. When injected, it is indicated for the treatment of initial and recurrent mucosal and cutaneous herpes simplex infections in immunocompromised adults and children. The parenteral form is also approved for severe initial episodes of herpes simplex infections in patients who may not be immunocompromised. Oral acyclovir may be indicated in the treatment of initial episodes of herpes genitalis and the suppression of unusually frequent recurrences of herpes genitalis. Acyclovir applied topically is used for the management of initial episodes of genital herpes simplex infections. It is also indicated in the management of nonlife-threatening cutaneous herpes simplex virus infections in immunocompromised patients.

Adverse Effects

Acyclovir appears to be a relatively safe drug, but a few patients have experienced delirium. Although it cannot be established that this was a result of acyclovir treatment, it must be borne in mind. Other adverse effects mentioned for the drug include inflammation and/or phlebitis (13.8%) at the injection site, and diaphoresis, hematuria, hypotension, headache and nausea, each of which occurred in 1.6% of patients treated. Hives have been reported in 4.7% of patients on parenteral acyclovir. Nausea and vomiting may be encountered with oral acyclovir. Other adverse effects include headache, diarrhea, skin rash, vertigo and arthralgia. When applying the topical preparation, patients may experience discomfort.

Nursing Process

Nursing actions related to the intravenous use of acyclovir involve evaluation of the patient during and following administration of the drug. Patients must be closely observed for behavioral changes, indicating impending central nervous system toxicity, and for redness, induration, swelling and pain at the infusion site, reflecting thrombophlebitis. Nurses should also be alert for signs of renal or liver toxicity, or changes in blood studies. Patients and partners need to realize that acyclovir is not a cure for infection, and that herpes can passed on during drug therapy.

Amantadine (Symmetrel)

Mechanism of Action and Therapeutic Uses

Amantadine may inhibit penetration of influenza A viruses into the host cell or reduce the uncoating of those viruses that do penetrate the cell.
Amantadine is indicated in the prevention and treatment of respiratory infections caused by influenza A virus strains. Amantadine may have its greatest value in patients at high risk of developing influenza because of underlying disease, such as the elderly in hospitals or nursing homes. The drug does not interfere with immunization, and patients may receive amantadine while waiting for the effects of immunization to appear. If used to treat an influenza A virus infection, amantadine must be started within forty-eight hours of the onset of symptoms.

Adverse Effects

Amantadine is generally well tolerated. High doses are more likely to produce adverse effects. Amantadine is excreted unchanged by the kidneys, and patients with compromised renal function may experience drug-related toxicities with normal doses. The more important adverse effects of amantadine are orthostatic hypotensive episodes, congestive heart failure, depression, psychosis and urinary retention. Other adverse effects of amantadine include acute neurotoxicity consisting of tremors, hallucinations and abnormal behavior. Some patients experience depression, confusion, detachment, lethargy, nervousness and dizziness. Occasionally, physical manifestations of central nervous system toxicity occur, including nausea, vomiting, ataxia, slurred speech and livedo reticularis.

Nursing Process

Nursing processes related to the use of amantadine were presented in Chapter 52 and are summarized in Table 102.

Idoxuridine (Herplex, Stoxil)

Mechanism of Action and Therapeutic Uses

Idoxuridine is incorporated into viral DNA, destabilizing the nucleic acid and altering viral protein synthesis. Ophthalmic idoxuridine is used topically in the treatment of herpes simplex keratitis only. Epithelial infections, especially initial attacks, characterized by the presence of a dendritic figure, are highly responsive to idoxuridine. Infections located in the stroma have shown a less favorable response. In recurrent cases, idoxuridine will often control the current episode of the viral infections, but scarring that resulted from previous attacks will not be corrected.

Adverse Effects

Idoxuridine can cause clouding of the cornea and small defects in the corneal epithelium. It may also cause local irritation, itching, mild edema and photophobia.

Nursing Process

Administration
Idoxuridine should be administered from a refrigerated container. The cleanliness of the dropper should be maintained during instillation of drops in the eye by preventing contact with the eyelid or

lashes. Nurses are advised to use careful asepsis, hand washing and careful cleansing of the eye before applying idoxuridine.

Teaching
Patients should be taught the proper technique for administering idoxuridine drops. They should also be advised of the importance of completing the prescribed course of therapy in order to ensure against reinfection.

Ribavirin (Virazole)

Mechanism of Action and Therapeutic Uses

Ribavirin is active against respiratory syncytial (RS) virus. Its mechanism of action is not known. Ribavirin is indicated only for lower respiratory tract infections due to RS virus. Ribavirin aerosol treatment must be accompanied by (and does not replace) standard supportive respiratory and fluid management for infants and children with severe respiratory tract infections.

Adverse Effects

Serious adverse events that have occurred during ribavirin therapy have included worsening of respiratory status, bacterial pneumonia and pneumothorax. It is not clear whether these effects are related to the use of ribavirin.

Nursing Process

Nurses are advised to follow the nursing process outlined previously in this chapter.

Trifluridine (Viroptic)

Mechanism of Action and Therapeutic Uses

Trifluridine is phosphorylated by a cellular thymidine kinase to its nucleotide monophosphate. Trifluridine monophosphate is an inhibitor of thymidylate synthetase, the target enzyme for the action of the monofluorinated pyrimidines. Trifluridine monophosphate is further phosphorylated by cellular enzymes to the triphosphate that is incorporated into DNA by competitively inhibiting the incorporation of the natural nucleotide, thymidine triphosphate.

Trifluridine is active against the following DNA viruses: herpes simplex types 1 and 2, varicella zoster, adenovirus and vaccinia virus. Trifluridine is indicated for the treatment of primary keratocon-

junctivitis and recurrent epithelial keratitis due to herpes simplex viruses, types 1 and 2.

Adverse Effects

The most common adverse effect is burning upon instillation and superficial punctate keratitis.

Nursing Process

The nursing process for trifluridine includes the following observations.

Administration
The nurse is advised to use careful asepsis, hand washing and cleansing of crusts or discharge from the eyes before application.

Teaching
The patient should be taught to use the drug exactly as prescribed. Nurses must also tell patients not to use eye makeup, eye cleansing materials, or face cloths or towels of others to prevent the spread of the infection. Patients should be taught to report allergic reactions, itching, redness and burning immediately.

Vidarabine (Vira-A)

Mechanism of Action and Therapeutic Uses

Vidarabine is adenine arabinoside. The drug probably impairs the initial steps in the synthesis of viral DNA. Vidarabine, infused intravenously for the treatment of herpes simplex virus encephalitis, appears to slow the process of neurologic deterioration but cannot reverse existing damage. Maximum benefits, involving alterations in morbidity and the prevention of serious neurologic sequelae, depend on early diagnosis and treatment. Controlled studies indicate that vidarabine therapy reduces the mortality rate from seventy to twenty-eight per cent.

Intravenous vidarabine may also be effective in decreasing both the mortality and morbidity of neonatal herpes simplex infections, particularly milder forms of the disease. It has prevented severe ocular and neurologic sequelae in neonates with only localized skin, eye or mouth infections. In neonates with central nervous system and disseminated disease, the drug has reduced both morbidity and mortality.

Intravenous vidarabine has proven beneficial in the treatment of immunocompromised adults and children with localized zoster and chicken pox infections, respectively.

Vidarabine may also be applied in the eye for the treatment of herpes keratoconjunctivitis manifested by dendritic keratitis or geographic corneal ulcers. It may also be indicated in patients who have developed toxic or allergic manifestations to idoxuridine.

Adverse Effects

Intravenous vidarabine produces nausea, vomiting, diarrhea and anorexia. Its effects on the central nervous system can also include dizziness, hallucinations, ataxia and psychosis. When applied topically in the form of an ophthalmic preparation, the most common adverse effects are burning, irritation, lacrimation, pain and photophobia.

Nursing Process

Assessment

A patient whose nursing assessment reveals a previous allergic response to vidarabine, a current pregnancy, or kidney or liver disease should not receive the drug parenterally.

Administration

Intravenous infusion is the only parenteral route of administration that provides adequate therapeutic concentrations of the drug. Vidarabine is diluted in approximately one liter of any intravenous solution, except blood or blood fractions, and infused slowly over twelve hours.

Evaluation

Patients should be observed for evidence of circulatory fluid overload, liver or renal toxicity.

Teaching

Individuals using ophthalmic preparations of vidarabine should be instructed in the proper technique of drug administration and the importance of completing the entire course of therapy.

Further Reading

Aerosol pentamidine (1989). Health & Welfare Canada: Health Protection Branch Issues [July 10].

Byram, D.A. (1989). Future expectations for critical care: Competence in immunotherapy. *Critical Care Nursing Clinics of North America 1* (4) :787-806. Drugs for HIV infection (1990). *The Medical Letter 32* :11-13.

Drugs for the treatment of AIDS (1989). Health & Welfare Canada: Health Protection Branch Issues [February 8].

Ganciclovir (1989). *The Medical Letter 31* :79-90.

Goa, K.L. and Campoli-Richards, D.M. (1987). Pentamidine isethionate. A review of its antiprotozoal activity, pharmacokinetic properties and therapeutic uses in *Pneumocystis carinii* pneumonia. *Drugs 33* : 242-258.

Impact of AZT study on Canadians with AIDS (1989). Health & Welfare Canada: Health Protection Branch Issues [August 10].

Jackson, J.B., Kwok, S.Y., Sninsky, J.J., Hopsicker, J.S., Sannderud, K.J. et al. (1990). Human immunodeficiency virus type 1 detected in all seropositive symptomatic and asymptomatic individuals. *J. Clin. Microbiol. 28* :16-19.

Luce, J.M. and Hopewell, P.C. (1989). Aerosolized pentamidine for *Pneumocystis carinii* pneumonia. *Chest 96* :713-714.

Pentamidine aerosol to prevent *Pneumocystis carinii* pneumonia (1989). *The Medical Letter 31* :91-92.

Prevention of *Pneumocystis carinii* pneumonia (1988). *The Medical Letter 30* :94-95.

Ribavirin (Virazole) (1986). *The Medical Letter 28* :46-47.

Sandstrom, E. (1989). Antiviral therapy in human immunodeficiency virus infection. *Drugs 38* :417-450.

Tauzon, C.U. and Labriola, A.M. (1987). Management of infectious and immunological complications of acquired immunodeficiency syndrome (AIDS). Current and future prospects. *Drugs 33* :66-84.

Treatment of sexually transmitted diseases (1990). *The Medical Letter 32* :5-10.

Table 102
Antiviral drugs.

Generic Name (Trade Name)	Use (Dose)	Action	Adverse Effects	Drug Interactions	Nursing Process
Pharmacologic Classification: Anti-HIV Drugs					
Zidovudine, AZT, azidothymidine (Retrovir)	Anti-HIV drug (**Oral:** Dose still under discuss'n. Dose at time of publicat'n - 200 mg q4h for 1st month, followed by 100 mg q4h)	Selectively incorporated by retroviral reverse transcriptase, causing premature chain elongat'n terminat'n. Delays fall in T4 cells in pts infected w. HIV.	Bone marrow depress'n is major concern. Other adv. effects incl. nausea, headache, myalgia, fever, asthenia, diarrhea and abd. pain.		**Assess:** Blood studies q2weeks for decr. granulocytes and Hgb. If blood counts fall too low, consider discontinuing drug and giving blood transfus'ns. **Administer:** Give orally; advise pt to swallow capsule whole. Store caps in cool place, protected from light. **Evaluate:** Pt for s/s of blood dyscrasias, bruising, fatigue, bleeding, poor healing. Monitor concurrent need for other anti-infective drugs to prevent opportunistic infect'n. **Teach:** That drug is not a cure, but will help control symptoms; that virus can still be passed on during tx; importance of taking drug q4h ATC; that followup visits must be continued to monitor blood counts and drug toxicity. Ensure pt understands adv. effects and importance of reporting s/s immediately. Warn that serious drug interact'ns can occur if OTC drugs are taken without advice from physician.
Ganciclovir (Cytovene)	Tx of CMV retinitis in immuno-compromised pts (**IV:** Initially, 5 mg/kg q12h for 14-21 days, given as constant infus'n over 1 h. After induct'n tx, recomm. dose is 5 mg/kg given as IV infus'n over 1 h od for 7 days/week, or 6 mg/kg od for 5 days/week)	Synthetic nucleoside analogue that inhibits replicat'n of herpes virus.	Most frequent involve hematopoietic system; neutropenia occurred in 38% and thrombocytopenia in 19% of pts treated w. ganciclovir.	**AZT:** And ganciclovir produce neutropenia. It is recomm. that AZT not be given concomitantly during ganciclovir induct'n phase. **Imipenem + cilastatin (Primaxin):** And ganciclovir given together, have been reported to produce gen'lized seizures. The 2 agents should be used concomitantly only after careful considerat'n of risk involved.	*The Nsg Process is sim. to that for zidovudine (AZT). Nurses are advised to check current manufacturer's and pharmacist's informat'n before administering this drug.*

Generic Name (Trade Name)	Use (Dose)	Action	Adverse Effects	Drug Interactions	Nursing Process
Pentamidine isethionate (Pentacarinat, NebuPent, Pneumopent)	Prevent'n of PCP in HIV-infected pts who have recovered from at least 1 previous episode of PCP (Inhalat'n: Recomm. dose specific to device for delivery. Recomm. dose for Pneumopent when given using FISONEB Ultrasonic Nebuliser is 1 dose of 60 mg on 5 days during 1st 2 weeks as loading-dose regimen [doses to be given not < 24 h and not > 72 h apart], followed by maint. regimen of 60 mg q2weeks. **IV/IM:** Adults - 4 mg/kg od for 14-21 days. *Pts w. renal failure* [CrCl < 35 mL/min] - *For life-threatening infect'ns* - 4 mg/kg od for 7-10 days; then 4 mg/kg qod to complete course of 14 days. *For less severe infect'ns* - 4 mg/kg qod for 14 doses)	Mechanism of action not fully understood. Several poss. biochemical mechanisms have been proposed. Of these, inhibit'n of oxidative phosphorylat'n by *Pneumocystis carinii* is most widely accepted at this time.	Rare instances of acute pancreatitis or renal insufficiency and acute renal failure have been observed w. pentamidine. Adv. effects that have occurred w. IV/IM administrat'n incl. GI bleeding, renal insufficiency, hypotens'n, syncope, local allergic react'ns, myonecrosis, urticaria, rash, spasticity, loss of consciousness and tinnitus. Adv. effects noted w. aerosolized drug incl. cough, bronchospasm, taste pervers'n, chest pain, dyspnea, headache, fatigue, fever, paresthesias and diarrhea.		*As for zidovudine (AZT), with the following addit'ns:* **Assess:** Observe fluid intake/output ratio and report imbalances; hematuria; oliguria. Check pt hx for liver/renal disease; review ECG for abnormalities; check for BP abnormalities. **Evaluate:** Inject'n site for pain or abnormalities. Respiratory status for rate, wheezing, dyspnea.
Fluconazole (Diflucan)	Broad-spectrum antifungal that can be employed as supportive tx in AIDS pts (**Oral/IV:** *Oropharyngeal candidiasis* - 200 mg on day 1, followed by 100 mg od. Tx should continue for at least 2 weeks. *Esophageal candidiasis* - 200 mg on day 1, followed by 100 mg od. Doses up to 400 mg/day may be used prn. Tx should continue for min. 3 weeks and for at least 2 weeks following resolut'n of symptoms. *Systemic candidiasis* - 400 mg on day 1,	Fungistatic activity exhibited against *Cryptococcus neoformans* and candida spp. Well absorbed when taken orally; can also be administered parenterally. Drug diffuses well throughout body and crosses blood-brain barrier well. Fluconazole is cleared primarily by renal excret'n, w. inverse relat'nship bet. eliminat'n half-life	Hepatic react'ns, exfoliative dermatitis, Stevens-Johnson syndrome, nausea, headache, skin rash, vomiting, abd. pain, diarrhea.	**Cimetidine:** Can reduce area under curve (AUC) and max. plasma concentrat'n (C-max) of orally admin. fluconazole. **Cyclosporine:** Plasma concentrat'ns have been infrequently incr. in pts. given fluconazole. **Hydrochlorothiazide:** Has incr. both C-max and AUC of orally admin. fluconazole. **Hypoglycemics** (oral tolbutamide, glyburide, glipizide): Fluconazole can reduce their metabolism and incr. their plasma concentrat'ns and effects. **Phenytoin:** Plasma concentrat'ns	Nurses are advised to consult the Nsg Process for zidovudine, if given concurrently, and add the following: **Assess:** If given IV, monitor VS during 1st infus'n for changes in pulse, BP. Monitor fluid intake/output ratio for decr. output, change in specific gravity, weight gain, edema. **Evaluate:** If given IV, check infus'n site for tissue problems. Use distal vein. Monitor for renal/liver toxicity.

followed by 200 mg od. Tx should continue for min. 4 weeks and for at least 2 weeks after resolut'n of symptoms. *Cryptococcal meningitis* - 400 mg on day 1, followed by 200 mg od. Dosage of 400 mg od may be used prn. Continue initial tx for 10-12 weeks after CSF becomes culture-neg. Dosage for suppress'n of relapse of cryptococcal meningitis in pts w. AIDS is 200 mg od. *For pts w. impaired renal funct'n, consult product monograph*)

of fluconazole and creatinine clearance.

can be incr. by fluconazole. **Rifampin:** Can incr. metabolism of concurrently admin. fluconazole. **Warfarin:** And fluconazole, should be given tog. cautiously. Fluconazole can incr. prothrombin time after warfarin administrat'n.

Pharmacologic Classification: Antiviral Drugs

Acyclovir (Zovirax)

Systemic and topical tx of various herpes infect'ns (**IV:** Adults - 5 mg/kg infused at constant rate over 1-h period q8h [15 mg/kg/day] in pts w. normal renal funct'n for 7 days. Children < 12 years - 250 mg/m² infused at constant rate over 1-h period q8h [750 mg/m²/day] for 7 days. *For pts w. renal failure - Consult product monograph.* **Oral:** *Tx of initial infect'n* - 200 mg q4h while awake, for total of 1 g/day for 10 days. *Suppressive tx for recurrent disease* - 200 mg tid; incr. if breakthrough occurs to 200 mg 5x/day. If nec., 400 mg bid may be considered. Tx may continue for up to 12 months. *Pts w. CrCl < 10 mL/min/1.73 m²* - 200 mg q12h. **Topical:** Apply 5% ointment liberally to affected area 4-6x/day for 10 days)

Acyclovir is metabolized within host to acyclovir triphosphate, which inhibits DNA polymerase and viral multiplicat'n in herpes simplex types 1 and 2, varicella zoster, herpes simiae (B virus) and Epstein-Barr virus.

After systemic administrat'n - Elevat'ns in BUN and serum creatinine concentrat'ns; phlebitis at inject'n site. *Upon topical applicat'n* - Pts may experience discomfort.

Evaluate: For behavioral changes; redness, indurat'n, swelling, pain at infus'n site, other adv. effects. Monitor for s/s renal or liver toxicity or changes in blood studies.
Teach: Pts and partners that drug is not a cure and that herpes can be passed on during drug tx.

Generic Name (Trade Name)	Use (Dose)	Action	Adverse Effects	Drug Interactions	Nursing Process
Amantadine HCl (Symmetrel)	Prevent'n and tx of respiratory infect'n caused by influenza A virus strains, esp. for high-risk pts, close household or hospital contacts of index cases, and those w. severe influenza A virus infect'ns. Can be used chemoprophylactically in conjunct'n w. inactivated influenza A virus vaccine until protective antibody responses develop **(Oral:** Adults - 200 mg/day. If CNS effects develop on 1x/day dosage, give drug in doses of 100 mg bid. Children 9-12 years - 100 mg bid. Children 1-9 years - 4.5-9 mg/kg/day [not > 150 mg/day] in 2-3 equal port'ns)	Inhibits penetrat'n of influenza A virus into host cell and/or reduces uncoating of those viruses that do penetrate cell.	Most important adv. react'ns are orthostatic hypotensive episodes, CHF, depress'n, psychoses and urinary retent'n.	*For Drug Interact'ns w. amantadine, refer to Table 75.*	**Assess:** For hx of parkinsonism 2⁰ to use of antipsychotic drugs; dementia, memory loss, confus'n, hallucinat'ns, paranoia; postural hypotens'n; endocrine, renal or hepatic impairment; glaucoma; malignant melanoma; tachycardia, ventr. fibrillat'n; diabetes; hypothermia; for concurrent use of pyridoxine, MAOIs, antipsychotics or TCAs. Establish baseline BP (standing/reclining), pulses (apical/radial), color/temp. of extremities. **Administer:** W. food. **Evaluate:** For sympathomimetic effects: BP, pulses, color/temp. of extremities, urinary output; mental'n, psych. behavior; for tx effect (reduct'n in s/s of infect'n). **Teach:** To change posit'ns slowly; that urine, perspirat'n may darken in color.
Idoxuridine (Herplex, Stoxil)	*For tx of herpes simplex keratitis, consult Table 57.*	*See Table 57.*	*See Table 57.*	*See Table 57.*	**Administer:** Use careful asepsis, good hand washing, and cleansing of eye. Administer from refrigerated container; avoid dropper contact w. eyelids or lashes. **Teach:** Pt proper technique for administering medicat'n. Advise careful use of eye makeup, face cloths, towels to avoid spread of infect'n. Caution pt to complete prescribed course of tx.
Ribavirin (Virazole)	Indicated only for lower respiratory tract infect'ns due to respiratory syncytial (RS) virus (For doses, consult manufacturer's informat'n)	Active against RS virus. Mechanism of action not known.	Worsening of respiratory status, bacterial pneumonia, pneumothorax.		*The Nsg Process is sim. to that for zidovudine (AZT). Nurses are advised to check current manufacturer's and pharmacist's informat'n before administering ribavirin.*

Drug	Use	Action	Side Effects / Interactions	Nursing Considerations
Trifluridine (Viroptic)	For tx of herpes simplex infect'n of conjunctiva and cornea, consult Table 57.	See Table 57.	See Table 57.	**Administer:** Use careful asepsis, handwashing, cleansing of crust/discharge from eyes before applying drug. **Teach:** Pt to use drug exactly as prescribed; not to use eye makeup or eye cleansing materials, face cloths or towels of others to prevent spread of infect'n. Report allergic react'n, itching, redness, burning stat.
Vidarabine (Vira-A)	IV vidarabine is useful in tx of herpes simplex encephalitis. May also be effective for other severe herpes infect'ns. IV vidarabine has also been used in tx of localized zoster and chicken pox infect'ns in immunocompromised adults and children, respectively. Applied to eye in tx of herpes keratoconjunctivitis manifested by dendritic ketatitis or geographic corneal ulcers (**IV:** *For herpes simplex encephalitis* - 15 mg/kg/day for 10 days. **Topical:** 1.5 cm of ointment in conjunctival sac 5x/day until corneal re-epithelializat'n has occurred. Continue tx for an addit'nal 7 days at reduced dosage [such as bid] to prevent recurrences)	Impairs synthesis of viral DNA.	Given IV, vidarabine has minimal toxicity. Most commonly pts experience mild GI dusturbances. Occasionally, CNS disturbances have been noted such as tremors, dizziness, confus'n, hallucinat'ns, ataxia and psychoses. Applied locally in eye, pts may experience lacrimat'n, foreign-body sensat'n, burning, irritat'n, superficial punctate keratitis, pain, photophobia, punctal occlus'n, sensitivity. **Corticosteroids:** Are us. contraindicated in tx of herpes simplex keratoconjunctivitis. If vidarabine tx is combined w. topical corticosteroid tx for associated condit'ns, hazards of customary corticosteroid-induced ocular abnormalities must be considered. These incl. corticosteroid-induced glaucoma or cataract format'n and progress'n of bacterial infect'ns.	**Assess:** For previous allergy to this drug; pregnancy, kidney/liver disease. **Administer:** IV infus'n over 12 h. Dilute in approx. 1 L of IV fluid (*not* blood). **Evaluate:** For fluid overload of circulatory system; liver/renal toxicity. **Teach:** Importance of completing entire course of tx. When using ophthal. preparat'ns, teach proper technique.

CHAPTER 69

Antimalarial Drugs

Teaching Objectives
Following completion of this chapter, the reader should be able to :
1. List the forms of plasmodia responsible for malaria in humans.
2. Describe the life cycle of the malarial parasite.
3. Discuss the rationale behind the use of drugs in the treatment of malaria.
4. Describe the mechanism of action, therapeutic uses and adverse effects of chloroquine and hydroxychloroquine, and the nursing process related to their use.
5. Discuss the mechanism of action, therapeutic uses and adverse effects of quinine, and the nursing process associated with its administration.
6. Describe the mechanism of action, therapeutic uses and adverse effects of primaquine, together with the nursing process related to its use.
7. Discuss the mechanism of action, therapeutic uses and adverse effects of pyrimethamine, and the nursing process associated with its use.

Malaria

Malaria remains one of the major health problems of the world. Because of this disease, as many as three million lives may be lost annually in Africa, India, Southeast Asia, and Central and South America. Malaria is a result of infection with protozoa of the genus plasmodium. Spread by the bite of the female anopheles mosquito, it has largely been eradicated in the United States by insecticide spraying programs.

Malaria produces paroxysms of severe chills, fever and profuse sweating that vary in severity depending on the species of plasmodium involved. Of the more than forty species of this genus, only four — *Plasmodium vivax, Plasmodium falciparum, Plasmodium malariae,* and *Plasmodium ovale* — affect humans, and all are transmitted in the saliva of the anopheles mosquito. *P. vivax* causes the most common form of malaria, characterized by fever spells that occur every other day. *P. falciparum* causes the most severe and second most common form of the disease: malignant malaria characterized by irregular paroxysms of fever and chills of longer duration. *P. malariae*-induced malaria is generally characterized by fever spikes every seventy-two hours.

The Life Cycle of the Malarial Parasite

The life cycle of the malarial parasite is presented in Figure 30. The female anopheles mosquito is the vector for malaria. By taking its pound of flesh, and a little blood as well, from a human carrying the male and female sexual forms of the parasite, it becomes the carrier of the plasmodium. Once in the

Figure 30
Schematic diagram of the life cycle of the malarial parasite.

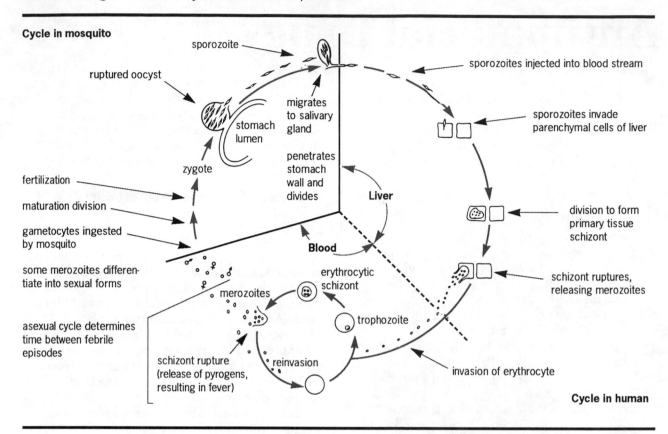

Cycle in mosquito

sporozoite

ruptured oocyst

migrates to salivary gland

stomach lumen

penetrates stomach wall and divides

zygote

fertilization

maturation division

gametocytes ingested by mosquito

some merozoites differentiate into sexual forms

asexual cycle determines time between febrile episodes

schizont rupture (release of pyrogens, resulting in fever)

merozoites

reinvasion

erythrocytic schizont

trophozoite

Liver

Blood

sporozoites injected into blood stream

sporozoites invade parenchymal cells of liver

division to form primary tissue schizont

schizont ruptures, releasing merozoites

invasion of erythrocyte

Cycle in human

From: W.B. Pratt (1977), *Chemotherapy of Infection.* New York: Oxford Press. Reproduced with permission.

stomach of the mosquito, the male gametocyte fertilizes the female to form a zygote, which then penetrates the stomach wall, forming a cyst on its outer surface. Numerous cell divisions take place to produce an oocyst, containing thousands of sporozoites. Rupture of the cysts results in the release of sporozoites, which are carried to the mosquito's salivary glands. When the mosquito subsequently goes on a hunting foray, she may bite an unfortunate human, injecting sporozoites into the blood of the new host.

Once injected into the host's blood, the sporozoites accumulate within liver parenchymal cells, where they divide to form a hepatic schizont, containing numerous merozoites. This is referred to as the **exo-erythrocytic phase** of malaria. Merozoites require six to twelve days to develop, after which time they leave the liver and invade the host's erythrocytes to produce the **erythrocytic phase** of malaria or erythrocytic schizogony. Schizonts formed in the red blood cells grow and eventually rupture the erythrocytes, releasing merozoites, lytic materials and parasitic toxins into

the blood. The recurrent chills and fever experienced by patients are due to the release of the latter two materials.

Merozoites released from the red blood cells may either reinvade erythrocytes, producing the same series of events just described, or undergo sexual division in blood to form male and female gametocytes. It is these promiscuous little rogues that are ingested by the passing mosquito. All of which brings us back to the point where we started this trip through the stomach, stinger and saliva of the mosquito, and liver and erythrocytes of the human.

Rationale Behind the Use of Drugs in the Treatment of Malaria

Ideally, it would be best to treat the mosquito rather than the human. By adopting this approach only the purveyors of the plasmodium would be exposed to the adverse effects of pharmacotherapy. Alas, however, this is not possible with the current state of knowledge. There is no drug for the bug. Our only approach is to spray copious amounts of insecticides in its general vicinity.

True, in the northern United States and Canada, we can always claim smugly that we could freeze her stinger for at least nine months of the year. However, this approach is more academic than practical because the little anopheles is more prudent than humans and refuses to take up residence in such inhospitable surroundings.

Returning to spraying, no one would question the success of the program. However, mosquito resistance to insecticides is a constant problem and explains, in part, the continued presence of malaria. It is therefore necessary to administer drugs capable of treating the disease in humans.

Transferring our attention from mosquitos to humans, it would obviously be best if we could prevent viable plasmodia from reaching the liver. However, here again we fail. At present there are no drugs that stand between the bite of the mosquito and the liver of the human. As a result, we are left with treating the infection within the liver or erythrocyte.

Because the fever and chills of malaria result from the release of lytic materials and parasitic toxins from the ruptured erythrocyte, drugs that prevent plasmodia from prospering in red blood cells may make the patient asymptomatic. However, they do not eradicate *P .vivax* and *P. ovale* because when therapy is stopped, merozoites harbored in the liver return to the blood and reinfect erythrocytes. *P. vivax* and *P. ovale* can be eliminated only by drugs that attack the hepatic forms of plasmodia. This approach is reasonable in areas such as Canada and the United States, where malaria is not endemic. In endemic areas, however, continual reinfection is likely and drug therapy is usually aimed only at suppressing the symptoms of malaria by treating the erythrocytic stage.

The preceding comments pertain only to the treatment of *P. vivax* and *P. ovale*. When the liver schizont containing *P. falciparum* ruptures, spilling merozoites into the blood, these latter organisms do not reinfect the liver. As a result, the successful treatment of the initial malarial attack usually results in complete eradication of the plasmodium from the body. It is also likely that *P. malariae* does not have exo-erythrocytic forms.

Drugs work within the liver or erythrocytes. They are given for the purpose of (1) suppressive therapy, (2) treating an acute attack (clinical cure), and (3) producing a radical cure.

Suppressive therapy is exactly as the name indicates. It suppresses malaria but does not cure it. Suppressive therapy involves the use of drugs to prevent or restrict the erythrocytic asexual stage of the disease. Chloroquine is usually the drug of choice. Chloroquine-resistant *P. falciparum* is treated with pyrimethamine plus sulfadoxine (Fansidar). Suppressive therapy may be curative if used for years, such that the life of the patient exceeds (it is hoped) the life of the parasite. Usually, however, malarial attacks can recur if suppressive therapy is stopped. Suppressive therapy is recommended during periods of exposure to the mosquito and for several weeks after leaving a malarious zone of the world. Short-term suppressive treatment may also be of value in patients with a history of malaria who are undergoing severely stressful situations.

Acute attacks of malaria likewise are treated with drugs that are effective against the erythrocytic stage of the plasmodium. The drug of choice for *P. vivax, P. malariae* and *P. ovale* is chloroquine. Many strains of *P. falciparum* have developed resistance to chloroquine and require treatment with alternate agents such as quinine sulfate, pyrimethamine and sulfadiazine.

Radical cure implies the elimination of the hepatic forms of *P. vivax* and *P. ovale*. This is usually attempted after the initial acute attack is treated. Primaquine is often employed for this purpose.

Drugs Effective against Erythrocytic Forms of the Plasmodium

Chloroquine (Aralen) and Hydroxychloroquine (Plaquenil)

Mechanism of Action and Therapeutic Uses

Chloroquine and hydroxychloroquine are concentrated within the parasitized erythrocyte, where they may act by inhibiting nucleic acid synthesis by the plasmodium.

Both drugs are effective against all four types of malaria, with the exception of chloroquine-resistant falciparum. They destroy the erythrocytic stages of the infection and are used both to prevent and to treat attacks. Chloroquine is the drug of choice for treatment of acute attacks. Neither chloroquine nor hydroxychloroquine will eradicate plasmodia from the liver. If this is desired, these drugs should be followed by primaquine therapy. Chloroquine resistance should be considered if a good response is not noted in two to three days.

Adverse Effects

Adverse reactions to chloroquine include dizziness, headache, itching, skin rash, vomiting and blurring of vision. In low suppressive doses, these effects are minor. They are seen more frequently, and with greater intensity, if higher doses are given. Nausea and vomiting can occur with either drug. This can be reduced by taking the drugs with food. Higher doses may also cause an exacerbation of lupus erythematosus. Chloroquine and hydroxychloroquine concentrate in melanin-containing areas of the body. Prolonged administration of high doses can produce corneal deposits, leading to blindness. Neither drug should be used in patients with retinal or visual field defects.

Nursing Process

Assessment
Before administering the initial dose of chloroquine, nurses should assure themselves that the patient has no history of renal or hepatic disorders and no retinal or visual field defects. Nurses should also review the patient's cardiac function.

Administration
Chloroquine is administered with meals to reduce the gastric irritation that often accompanies its use. The drug should be given at the same time each day to maintain blood levels.

Evaluation
Nursing responsibilities related to patient evaluation during long-term therapy include initiating ophthalmological examinations at regular intervals and eliciting information from the patient regarding the occurrence of blurred vision, blind spots or night blindness. Nurses should monitor patients for allergic reactions, blood dyscrasias and ototoxicity.

Teaching
Nurses must teach patients who are self-administering this drug on an outpatient basis to self-evaluate for adverse effects and notify their physician immediately should any occur. Patients must be warned to use sunglasses in bright sunlight.

Quinine

Mechanism of Action and Therapeutic Uses

Quinine's mechanism of action in the treatment of malaria is not known. It may reduce the ability of the parasite to feed within the erythrocyte.

Although quinine is effective in both suppressing and treating malarial attacks, its use in malaria would probably be of historical interest only, had resistance not developed in *P. falciparum* to chloroquine and hydroxychloroquine. When used against *P. falciparum,* quinine is usually combined with pyrimethamine and a sulfonamide, such as sulfadiazine. Alternatively, uncomplicated attacks can be treated with quinine, plus tetracycline or clindamycin.

Adverse Effects

Quinine often causes cinchonism. This term is derived from the fact that quinine is obtained from the bark of the cinchona tree. Cinchonism symptoms are similar to those produced by high doses of aspirin (salicylism) and include nausea, vomiting, diarrhea, sweating, blurred vision, ringing in the ears and impaired hearing. In addition, patients may rarely experience leukopenia and agranulocytosis. High concentrations of quinine can cause hypotension and depress myocardial function.

Nursing Process

Assessment
A patient whose nursing assessment reveals a history of cardiac, liver or renal disease should be subject to increased vigilance following the administration of quinine.

Administration
Ingesting the drug with food will alleviate some of the gastric irritation that accompanies its use, as well as disguising its bitter taste. Quinine should be given at the same time each day to maintain blood levels.

Evaluation
Nurses should check for nausea, blurred vision, tinnitus, headache and difficulty focusing the eyes.

Teaching
Patients should be taught to self-evaluate for adverse effects as identified in the previous section. Nurses should warn patients to avoid over-the-counter preparations and tonic water.

Drug Treatment of Exo-Erythrocytic Forms of the Plasmodium

Primaquine

Mechanism of Action and Therapeutic Uses

The mechanism of action of primaquine may be related to the fact that it causes the mitochondria of the exo-erythrocytic (hepatic) forms of plasmodia to swell and become vacuolated.

Primaquine is effective only against the exo-erythrocytic stage of the plasmodium. Primaquine is important because it is the only agent effective against the liver forms of the plasmodium. It is used to provide a radical cure of malaria caused by *P. vivax* and *P. ovale*. Primaquine is similarly taken to prevent an attack after departure from areas where *P. vivax* and *P. ovale* are endemic. Because primaquine will also kill the sexual forms in the blood, it can be given to eradicate gametocytes in patients recovering from falciparum malaria.

Adverse Effects

Primaquine is a relatively safe drug. It can produce occasional gastrointestinal distress, nausea, headache, pruritus and leukopenia. Agranulocytosis may occur very rarely. Five to ten per cent of black males, dark-skinned Caucasians (such as Indians), Asians, and people from Mediterranean areas demonstrate a primaquine sensitivity that can result in acute hemolytic anemia. Extensive investigations into primaquine sensitivity has determined that these subjects have a genetically determined deficiency in the erythrocytic enzyme glucose-6-phosphate dehydrogenase. Without pursuing the biochemical aberrations that occur in these patients, it is enough to say that the deficiency in the enzyme enables primaquine to produce hemolysis. In addition to hemolysis, patients who are deficient in glucose-6-phosphate dehydrogenase may also develop methemoglobinemia when treated with primaquine.

Nursing Process

Assessment

Nursing assessment should emphasize a review of the patient's history for evidence of renal or hematopoietic disorders. Patients with these conditions require more rigorous nursing evaluation during therapy because of increased risk of adverse effects.

Administration

Administer primaquine with meals to reduce gastric distress. Give the drug at the same time each day to maintain blood levels.

Evaluation

Nursing evaluation following primaquine administration must stress early detection of adverse effects as identified in the preceding section.

Teaching

Patient teaching should emphasize self-evaluation for adverse effects and stress the importance of keeping regularly scheduled appointments for laboratory blood studies to detect potentially fatal hematopoietic effects.

Drugs That Inhibit Both the Erythrocytic and Exo-Erythrocytic Forms of the Plasmodium

Pyrimethamine (Daraprim)

Mechanism of Action and Therapeutic Uses

Pyrimethamine inhibits the enzyme dihydrofolic acid reductase, preventing the activation of folic acid. The reduction of folic acid by dihydrofolic acid reductase is essential to humans as well as plasmodia. Pyrimethamine has selective toxicity for the parasite because it binds very strongly to the dihydrofolic acid reductase from plasmodia and very weakly to the human enzyme.

Pyrimethamine is used prophylactically against

all susceptible strains of plasmodia. Because of the widespread existence and rapid development of resistance to pyrimethamine by *P. falciparum,* it should never be used alone in the treatment of malaria. It has, however, been used successfully in combination with other agents. The drug is often used in combination with sulfadoxine to treat chloroquine-resistant *P. falciparum.* The combination product containing both pyrimethamine and sulfadoxine carries the trade name Fansidar. Sulfadoxine reduces the formation of folic acid by plasmodia, and pyrimethamine inhibits the activation of any folic acid that is formed by the malarial parasite. The combination increases the activities of both drugs many times, decreases the number of resistant strains, and delays the development of resistance. The addition of quinine to pyrimethamine and a sulfonamide assists in controlling symptoms during the initial stages of an acute attack by chloroquine-resistant *P. falciparum.*

Pyrimethamine is also combined with mefloquine and sulfadoxine. Mefloquine is an effective blood schizonticide against *P. falciparum, P. vivax* and *P. malariae.* It destroys the early asexual blood stages and therefore acts earlier than pyrimethamine/sulfadoxine. It is not an effective tissue schizonticide.

Adverse Effects

Pyrimethamine is a relatively safe drug, and few adverse effects are associated with normal doses. Signs of toxicity at higher doses, such as those used in the treatment of toxoplasmosis, include anorexia, vomiting, anemia, leukopenia and thrombocytopenia. In addition, atrophic glossitis has been reported. These effects reflect the inhibition of human dihydrofolate reductase. An acute dose of pyrimethamine can produce central nervous system stimulation, including convulsions.

Multiple-dose regimens of pyrimethamine/sulfadoxine (Fansidar) are associated with severe cutaneous adverse reactions. Toxic epidermal necrolysis, Stevens-Johnson syndrome, or erythema multiforme can occur. Other adverse effects attributed to the combination of pyrimethamine plus sulfadoxine include agranulocytosis, aplastic anemia, thrombocytopenia, leukopenia, neutropenia, hemolytic anemia, purpura, hypoprothrombinemia, methemoglobinemia and eosinophilia. Gastrointestinal adverse effects include glossitis, stomatitis, gastritis, dyspepsia, dry mouth, black tongue, gastroenteritis, anorexia, nausea, vomiting, abdominal pains, diarrhea, pancreatitis and pseudomembranous enterocolitis. Abnormal liver function tests have also been observed (elevated SGPT, SGOT, alkaline phosphatase and bilirubin).

The toxic effects of mefloquine are usual mild and include nausea, diarrhea, dizziness, vomiting and abdominal pain. When taken in combination with pyrimethamine and sulfadoxine, the most common adverse effects reported were vertigo and vomiting.

Nursing Process

Assessment
A patient whose nursing assessment reveals a history of seizure disorders should be subjected to particularly rigorous nursing evaluation during the course of therapy with pyrimethamine. Blood studies should be reviewed for evidence of dyscrasias and abnormalities.

Administration
This drug should be taken with meals to reduce its effects on the gastrointestinal tract. It should be taken at regular intervals either on the same day each week when used as an antimalarial or at the same time each day when used to treat toxoplasmosis.

Evaluation
Nurses should observe the patient for sore tongue, fever, rash or diarrhea. These adverse effects are more likely to occur at the high doses associated with daily administration of the medication.

Further Reading

Advice for the travelers (1990). *The Medical Letter 32* :33-36.

Drugs for parasitic infections (1990). *The Medical Letter 30* :15-24.

Drugs for parasitic infections (1986). *The Medical Letter 28 :9-18.*

Keystone, J.S. (1990). Prevention of malaria. *Drugs 39* :337-354.

Mefloquine for malaria (1990). *The Medical Letter 32* :13-14.

Panisko, D.M. and Keystone, J.S. (1990). Treatment of malaria. *Drugs 39* :160-189.

Table 103
Antimalarial drugs.

Generic Name (Trade Name)	Use (Dose)	Action	Adverse Effects	Drug Interactions	Nursing Process
Pharmacologic Classification: Drugs Effective against Erythrocytic Forms of the Plasmodium					
Chloroquine phosphate (Aralen Phosphate for oral use); chloroquine HCl (Aralen for parenteral use)	Suppressive tx in acute attacks of malaria due to P. vivax, P. malariae, P. ovale and susceptible strains of P. falciparum. All doses expressed as chloroquine base (*For tx of clinical attacks of malaria -* **Oral:** Adults - 600 mg, followed by 300 mg in 6 h and 300 mg/day for next 2 days. Children - 10 mg/kg initially, followed by 5 mg/kg in 6 h and 5 mg/kg/day for next 2 days. **IM:** Adults - 3 mg/kg initially; repeat prn q6h. Max. dose, 1 g/24 h. Us. dose, 200-250 mg q6h for 3 days. Use oral dose asap. Infants/children - Use IM only when absolutely nec. because of potential for local irritat'n and necroses. Sugg. dose, 6.25 mg/kg initially; repeat in 6 h prn. Dosage must not > 12.5 mg/kg/24 h. **IV:** Adults - 200 mg or 3 mg/kg, infused over not < 1 h, while monitoring CV status to detect hypotens'n or arrhythmias; then 3 mg/kg q6h. Max. dose, 1 g/day. *For prophylaxis of malaria -* **Oral:** Adults - 300 mg 1x/week on same day each week. Children - 5 mg/kg 1x/week on same day each week. Start 1-2 weeks before entering malarious area and continue for 6 weeks after leaving area. Primaquine may be added to regimen immediately after leaving endemic area)	Concentrates in erythrocytes and poss. inhibits nucleic acid synthesis to kill plasmodia.	Mild and transient headache, pruritus, GI complaints, psychic stimulat'n. Occ. hypotens'n, ECG changes.		**Assess:** For hx renal/hepatic disease, retinal/visual field defects. Review cardiac funct'n. **Administer:** W. meals. Give at same time each day to maintain blood levels. **Evaluate:** Initiate ophthalmic exams. at regular intervals during long-term tx. Check for blurred vision, blind spots, night blindness; also allergic react'ns, blood dyscrasias, ototoxicity. **Teach:** Self-evaluat'n for adv. effects. Warn pt to use sunglasses in bright sunlight.

Generic Name (Trade Name)	Use (Dose)	Action	Adverse Effects	Drug Interactions	Nursing Process
Quinine	For condit'n as follows [all doses expressed as quinine base] (*For chloroquine-sensitive malaria [quinine sulfate]* - **Oral:** Adults - 650 mg [or 10 mg/kg] q8h for 7-10 days. Children - 25 mg/kg/day in divided doses q8h for 7-10 days. *For chloroquine-resistant P. falciparum malaria* - Adults - Use same dose as for chloroquine-sensitive malaria. *For severe malaria. For severe infect'ns* - Adults - Loading dose of 20 mg/kg of quinine. Pyrimethamine 25 mg bid is added for 1st 3 days, and sulfadiazine 500 mg qid is given for 5 days. In place of pyrimethamine + sulfadizine, 2-3 tabs of Fansidar/day may be added to regimen for 3 days. Alternatively, quinine may be given for 3-5 days and tetracycline [1 g/day] may be given in divided doses q6h for 7-10 days. Children - 25 mg/kg/day of quinine given in divided doses q8h for 3 days; pyrimethamine 0.5-1 mg/kg/day in divided doses q12h for 3 days [supplemental folic acid]; and sulfadiazine 120-150 mg/kg/day [max., 2 g/day] in divided doses q6h for 5 days. In place of pyrimethamine + sulfadizine, Fansidar can be given. *For severe malaria [quinine dihydrochloride]* - **IV:** Adults - 600 mg [or 10 mg/kg] in 300 mL of 0.9% NaCl solut'n infused over not < 1 h or pref. a 4-h period. Repeat dose in 6-8 h. Max. daily dose, 1.8 g. CV	Unknown, but may reduce ability of plasmodium to feed within erythrocyte.	Mild to moderate cinchonism (tinnitus, headache, altered auditory acuity, nausea, blurred vision); disturbances in vision. Toxic doses produce CNS react'ns such as severe headache, apprehens'n, excitement, confus'n and delirium. GI react'ns incl. gastric and intestinal irritat'n.	**Anticoagulants:** May have incr. effect as quinine can depress prothrombin format'n.	**Assess:** For hx cardiac, liver or renal disease. **Administer:** W. food to reduce GI symptoms, bitter taste. **Evaluate:** For nausea, vomiting, diarrhea, sweating, blurred vision, tinnitus, hearing deficiency. **Teach:** Pts to be aware of adv. effects; to avoid OTC drugs, cold preparat'ns and tonic water.

status should be monitored to detect hypotens'n or arrhythmias. After clinical response has occurred, quinine sulfate should be given orally as soon as practical. Infants/children - 12.5 mg/kg infused over not ≤ 1 h or preferably 4 h; repeat in 6-8 h if oral dose cannot be tolerated. Max. dose, 25 mg/kg/day. If infect'n is caused by chloroquine-resistant *P. falciparum*, pyrimethamine + sulfonamide or tetracycline should be added, as described earlier)

Pharmacologic Classification: Drug Effective against Exo-Erythrocytic Forms of the Plasmodium

| Primaquine phosphate | For condit'ns as follows **(Oral:** *For malaria [radical cure] due to P. vivax and P. ovale, or to prevent relapses in travelers after their return from malarious areas and prolonged exposure to P. vivax and P. ovale* - Adults - 15 mg/day. Children - 0.3 mg/kg/day. Both adults'/children's doses should be given daily for 14 days, pref. consecutively w. chloroquine or other tx, which is given on 1st 3 days of acute attack) | Unknown, but may be rel to fact that it causes mitochondria in hepatic forms of plasmodia to swell and become vacuolated. | **GI effects:** Nausea, vomiting, epigastric distress and abd. cramps. **Hematologic:** Leukopenia, hemolytic anemia in G-6-PD deficient pts, and methemoglobinemia in NADH methemoglobin reductase deficient pts. | **Quinacrine:** Appears to potentiate primaquine; thus, concomitant use contraindicated. In fact, primaquine should not be administered to pts who have received quinacrine recently, owing to incr. toxicity. | **Assess:** For hx renal/hematopoietic disorders. **Administer:** W. meals at same time each day to maintain blood levels. **Evaluate:** For decr. urine output, dark or red urine, chills, fever, cyanosis. **Teach:** Self-evaluat'n for adv. effects; importance of regular lab. studies of blood. |

Pharmacologic Classification: Drugs That Inhibit Erythrocytic and Exo-Erythrocytic Forms of the Plasmodium

| Pyrimethamine (Daraprim) | For condit'ns as follows **(Oral:** *For prophylaxis of malaria* - Doses are given on same day of week. Adults and children > 10 years - 25 mg; 3-10 years - 12.5-25 mg; ≤ 2 years - 6.25-12.5 mg. Strongly recomm. that pyrimethamine be given w. sulfonamide for prophylaxis and | Blocks dihydrofolic acid reductase, preventing activat'n of folic acid. Pyrimethamine binds very strongly to plasmodial dihydrofolic acid reductase and very weakly to | Anorexia, vomiting, megaloblastic anemia, leukopenia, thrombocytopenia, pancytopenia and atrophic glossitis. These effects us. occur w. large doses of **drug.** Acute intoxi- | **Lorazepam:** Admin. concurrently w. pyrimethamine, may induce hepatotoxicity. **Myelosuppressive agents:** Interact w. pyrimethamine, which may cause exacerbat'n of myelosuppressive effects of cytostatic agents, esp. those of antifolate methotrexate. Convuls'ns have | **Assess:** For hx seizure disorders. **Administer:** W. meals, on same day each week, when used as antimalarial; or at same time each day when used to treat toxoplasmosis. **Evaluate:** For fever, sore tongue, rash, diarrhea. Initiate biweekly blood studies during tx of toxoplasmosis. |

Generic Name (Trade Name)	Use (Dose)	Action	Adverse Effects	Drug Interactions	Nursing Process
	tx of chloroquine-resistant strains of *P. falciparum* malaria)	human form of this enzyme. This accounts for its selective toxicity against plasmodia.	cat'n following ingest'n of excess. am'ts may involve CNS stimulat'n, e.g., convuls'ns.	occurred after concurrent administrat'n of methotrexate and pyrimethamine to children w. CNS leukemia; cases of fatal bone marrow aplasia have been assoc. w. administrat'n of daunorubicin, cytosine arabinoside and pyrimethamine to pts w. acute myeloid leukemia.	
Pyrimethamine + sulfadoxine (Fansidar)	[Fansidar tabs containing 25 mg pyrimethamine + 500 mg sulfadoxine] (*For acute attack of chloroquine-resistant P. falciparum malaria* - **Oral:** Take single dose acc. to following schedule: Adults - 2-3 tabs. Children 9-14 years - 2 tabs; 4-8 years - 1 tab; < 4 years - $\frac{1}{2}$ tab. *For prophylaxis of malaria* [if Fansidar is to be given rather than held as single dose for self-tx] - Adults - 1 tab weekly 1-2 weeks before, during and for 6 weeks after last exposure in endemic area. Children 9-14 years - $\frac{3}{4}$ tab weekly; 4-8 years - $\frac{1}{2}$ tab weekly; 1-3 years - $\frac{1}{4}$ tab weekly; 6-11 *months* - $\frac{1}{8}$ *tab weekly*)	Sulfadoxine and pyrimethamine inhibit sequential steps in biosynthesis of tetrahydrofolic acid by sensitive protozoa. This depletes folic acid, an essential cofactor in biosynthesis of nucleic acids, resulting in interference w. protozoal nucleic acid and protein production.	Fansidar has been assoc. w. severe cutaneous adv. react'ns (erythema multiforme, Stevens-Johnson syndrome or toxic epidermal necrolysis). Blood dyscrasias incl. agranulocytosis, aplastic anemia, thrombocytopenia, leukopenia, neutropenia, hemolytic anemia, purpura, hypoprothrombinemia, methemoglobinemia and eosinophilia. GI adv. effects incl. glossitis, stomatitis, gastritis, dyspepsia, dry mouth, black tongue, gastroenteritis, anorexia, nausea, vomiting, abd. pain, diarrhea, pancreatitis and pseudomembranous enterocolitis. Abnormal liver funct'n tests have also been observed (elevated SGPT, SGOT, alkaline phosphatase and bilirubin). For other adv. effects., consult product monograph.		

CHAPTER 70

Antiprotozoal Drugs

Teaching Objectives

Following completion of this chapter, the reader should be able to:

1. Describe the life cycle of *Entamœba histolytica*.
2. Discuss the mechanism of action, therapeutic uses and adverse effects of metronidazole, emetine and dehydroemetine when used to treat amebiasis, as well as the nursing process related to their use.
3. Discuss the mechanism of action, therapeutic uses and adverse effects of iodoquinol, and the nursing process for this drug.
4. Explain the role of paromomycin in the treatment of amebiasis.
5. Discuss the etiology of giardiasis and describe briefly the roles of metronidazole, quinacrine and furazolidone in the treatment of giardiasis.
6. Explain the cause of pneumocystosis and the roles of pentamidine and trimethoprim plus sulfamethoxazole in its treatment.
7. Discuss briefly the etiology of toxoplasmosis and its treatment.
8. Describe briefly the cause of trichomoniasis and its treatment.

The preceding chapter dealt with the treatment of malaria. As mentioned at that time, malaria is a protozoal disease caused by the genus plasmodium. Strictly speaking, it should be discussed along with all other protozoal diseases. We did not take this approach because of the serious nature of malaria and its prevalence in the world. The present chapter continues our discussion on the treatment of protozoal diseases and concentrates on amebiasis, giardiasis, pneumocystosis, toxoplasmosis and trichomoniasis, conditions that also present health hazards.

Amebiasis

Amebiasis is caused by infection with the protozoan *Entamœba histolytica*. It occurs in all parts of North America and throughout the world. Patients become infected when they ingest mature cysts (Figure 31). Once in the small bowel the cysts disintegrate, releasing four amebae, which in turn divide to form eight trophozoites. The trophozoites are carried into the large intestine, where they may live and multiply for a time in the crypts of the bowel. Some trophozoites invade the intestinal epithelium, where they form cysts and produce ulceration. Although diarrhea often occurs at this point, ulceration does not usually result in prolonged diarrhea or abdominal pain. Cysts formed from the trophozoites on the colonic surface and subsequently passed in formed feces can lead to spread of the disease. Patients with diarrhea, on the other hand, do not spread the disease because the trophozoites are not allowed sufficient time in the bowel to mature into active cysts before they are eliminated.

Figure 31
Life cycle of *Entamœba histolytica*.

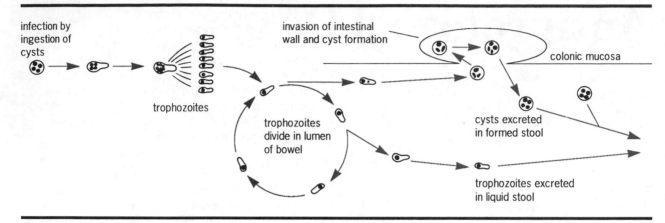

From: W.B. Pratt (1977), Chemotherapy of Infection. New York: Oxford Press. Reproduced with permission.

Amebiasis is not always limited to the bowel. If trophozoites are absorbed through the ulcerated intestinal mucosa, they can locate in the liver. Amebicides can be divided into drugs that are effective against either the intestinal or the extraintestinal form of the disease.

Metronidazole (Flagyl, Protostat)

Mechanism of Action and Therapeutic Uses

Metronidazole is well absorbed following oral administration. High levels of the drug are found in plasma and cerebrospinal fluid. Metronidazole is metabolized in the liver and has a half-life of eight to nine hours. Metronidazole is concentrated within *E. histolytica,* where it inhibits hydrogen production, thereby blocking the ability of the parasite to synthesize chemicals vital to its survival. The drug has little activity on the metabolic processes of humans because it is not retained in high concentrations in mammalian cells.

Because most of an oral dose of metronidazole is absorbed, it is given with another luminal amebicide (usually iodoquinol) to eradicate organisms in the intestine and avoid relapse. The combination of 750 mg of metronidazole three times daily for ten days followed by 650 mg iodoquinol three times daily for twenty days is considered first-line therapy for mild to moderate and severe intestinal disease, as well as for hepatic abscesses.

Adverse Effects

Nausea, vomiting, epigastric distress, diarrhea and headache are the most common adverse effects of the drug. Metronidazole can also produce a metallic taste and discolor the urine, which can be alarming signs to patients if they are not forewarned. More rarely, reversible leukopenia can occur. Central nervous system toxicity, in the form of weakness, paresthesias, vertigo and ataxia, has been observed. Metronidazole has a disulfiram (Antabuse)-like effect. Patients receiving metronidazole who embrace the joyous juices of hops or other libacious liquids may experience intense flushing, tachycardia, nausea, vomiting and circulatory collapse.

Metronidazole is carcinogenic in rats and mutagenic in bacteria; however, no evidence has been found that metronidazole is carcinogenic in humans. Furthermore, it has been used in pregnant patients without evidence that it produces fetal malformation. Despite these comments, many authorities recommend that metronidazole not be used during the first trimester of pregnancy and be avoided, if possible, during the next six months.

Nursing Process

Assessment
Nursing assessment prior to metronidazole administration should emphasize review of the patient's history for evidence of alcohol abuse or hematopoietic disorders. These predict the development of metronidazole-induced adverse effects. Because of questions related to the mutagenicity of metronidazole, it should be given to pregnant women only when absolutely necessary.

Administration
Administering metronidazole with food may alleviate some of its gastric distress.

Evaluation
Nursing evaluation of patients taking metronidazole should emphasize detection of numbness, tremor, ataxia, paresthesias, decreased sensation, weakness, vertigo and headache, indicators of central nervous system toxicity. Sore throat, fatigue and increased bleeding tendencies suggest leukopenia. Stools are examined during the entire treatment. They should be clear at the end of therapy and remain clear for one year before the patient is considered cured.

Teaching
Patients for whom metronidazole has been prescribed should be advised that the drug will cause a metallic taste in the mouth and discolor the urine. They should also be warned about the disulfiram-like reaction that occurs when alcohol and metronidazole are consumed concurrently. Finally, because metronidazole is usually self-administered on an outpatient basis, patients should be taught the indicators of adverse effects so that they can self-evaluate during therapy. Nurses should teach the patient to use proper hygiene after bowel movements, to use condoms, and to comply with the dosage schedule.

Emetine and Dehydroemetine

Mechanism of Action and Therapeutic Uses

Emetine and dehydroemetine are injected subcutaneously or intramuscularly to circumvent the nausea and vomiting produced by oral administration and the severe cardiotoxicities of intravenous treatment. The drugs block protein synthesis in both parasitic and mammalian cells but are more toxic to the protozoa. Both agents are amebicidal in the intestinal lumen against trophozoites of *E. histolytica* but are not active against cysts.

Emetine or dehydroemetine may be combined with iodoquinol as alternative therapy to metronidazole plus iodoquinol in the treatment of severe intestinal disease.

Adverse Effects

Emetine and dehydroemetine can produce serious local and systemic reactions. The drugs cause pain, tenderness and muscular weakness at the injection site. Stimulation of intestinal smooth muscle is common. Patients may complain of diarrhea, cramps and vomiting.

Severe cardiovascular adverse reactions, including hypotension, tachycardia, chest pain, shortness of breath and changes in the electrocardiogram (prolongation in the P-R and Q-T intervals, as well as a flattening of the T-waves) can occur. Careful monitoring of the patient is essential. Patients should be hospitalized and kept in bed during treatment. It is essential to follow the patient closely, including frequent electrocardiograms, to prevent lasting heart damage.

Nursing Process

Assessment
Nursing assessment of patients for whom emetine or dehydroemetine has been prescribed should establish baseline measurements of blood pressure, as well as apical and radial pulse rates. The patient's history should be reviewed for evidence of any previous cardiac or renal disease. As these drugs are excreted through the kidneys, patients with renal disease are at increased risk. Because of their cardiotoxicity, use of these drugs in patients with pre-existing cardiac disease can prove fatal.

Administration
Subcutaneous or intramuscular injections of emetine or dehydroemetine must include careful aspiration to avoid inadvertent intravenous administration. The drugs should be injected slowly to reduce pain. Because localized muscle weakness at the injection site results from the irritating effects of these drugs, patients must refrain from all exercise and exertion during therapy and for ten days following.

Evaluation
Patients must be monitored at least four times per day for cardiotoxicity as indicated by increased pulse rates or decreased blood pressure. Complete bed rest is essential for the prevention of cardiac complications. Fluid intake and output should also be monitored. Stools should be examined throughout therapy and should be clear at the end of the treatment period. Vision should be checked by ophthalmologic examination during and after therapy to detect any possible effects of drug therapy.

Teaching
Nurses must caution patients not to allow these drugs to contact their eyes or mucous membranes. Patients must also understand the importance of proper hygiene following a bowel movement.

Iodoquinol (Diodoquin, Yodoxin)

Mechanism of Action and Therapeutic Uses

Iodoquinol blocks several important parasitic enzymes. It is the drug of choice for the treatment of asymptomatic amebiasis. Metronidazole plus iodoquinol is first-choice therapy for mild to moderate or severe intestinal disease and for hepatic abscess therapy. Iodoquinol plus either emetine or dehydroemetine represents second-line treatment for severe intestinal disease. Emetine, or dehydroemetine, combined with iodoquinol plus chloroquine is considered alternate therapy to metronidazole plus iodoquinol for hepatic amebic abscesses.

Adverse Effects

Headaches, diarrhea, nausea, vomiting, anal pruritus and skin rashes are seen occasionally following use of iodoquinol. Because it contains iodine, iodoquinol can cause occasional enlargement of the thyroid. It should not be given to patients with known iodine sensitivity or to persons with pre-existing optic neuropathy. The latter contraindication can be explained by the fact that iodoquinol has caused subacute myeloptic neuropathy when used in high doses. Patients so afflicted experience weakness, dyasthesia, peripheral neuropathy and sometimes blindness. Iodoquinol is also contraindicated in patients with hepatic damage.

Nursing Process

Assessment
Nursing assessment for iodine sensitivity and for the existence of current pregnancy or lactation is essential prior to the administration of iodoquinol. Individuals who are hypersensitive to iodine are liable to experience severe allergic responses to the drug. The consequences of administering it to pregnant women must be weighed against the severity of the illness. Stool examinations are taken during treatment and should be clear at the end of therapy.

Evaluation
Nursing evaluation of patients receiving iodoquinol should emphasize detection of adverse effects, especially myeloptic neuropathy and allergic reactions.

Paromomycin Sulfate (Humatin)

Paromomycin is an aminoglycoside antibiotic. The pharmacology of this group of drugs is presented in Chapter 63. It is an alternative to iodoquinol for asymptomatic amebiasis. Paromomycin may also be used as second-line therapy to metronidazole plus iodoquinol for mild to moderate amebic intestinal disease. The nursing process related to the use of paromomycin sulfate is the same as that discussed in Chapter 63 for the other aminoglycoside antibiotics. Readers should refer to that material for detailed information.

Giardiasis

Giardiasis is an intestinal infection by *Giardia lamblia*. The disease may be transmitted by beavers (beaver fever) who contaminate waters in mountainous watersheds. Once ingested, the motile trophozoite of *G. lamblia* attaches to the intestinal mucosa, where it can cause a foul diarrhea and/or flatulence, abdominal distention, pain and vomiting. Giardiasis may also be associated with other parasitic or bacterial infections of the intestine.

Metronidazole is replacing quinacrine (Atabrine) in the treatment of giardiasis because it is more active and less toxic. However, quinacrine may be preferred for initial therapy in adults, especially those with severe infection. Children do not tolerate quinacrine well; therefore, metronidazole or furazolidone (Furoxone) are more commonly prescribed for them. The pharmacology of metronidazole is presented earlier in this chapter. The effects of quinacrine are described in Chapter 71. Only furazolidone is not discussed elsewhere in this text.

Furazolidone is an alternative to quinacrine for the treatment of giardiasis. It is claimed to be effective in more than ninety per cent of cases. The most common adverse effects of furazolidone are nausea, vomiting and a vesicular or morbilliform pruritic rash. Furazolidone can also cause agranulocytosis. Patients with glucose-6-phosphate dehydrogenase deficiency can experience acute hemolysis. Similar to metronidazole, furazolidone can cause a disulfiram-like reaction after alcohol consumption.

Nursing Process

The nursing process of giardiasis is similar to that given for the preceding drugs in this chapter. Nurses are advised to follow the nursing process outlined for metronidazole.

Pneumocytosis

Pneumocystosis is caused by *Pneumocystis carinii,* an opportunistic parasite that infects mainly children and patients receiving immunosuppressive drugs. *P. carinii* pneumonia is also prevalent in patients with acquired immunodeficiency syndrome (AIDS; see Chapter 68). Patients often appear pale and experience a dry cough, dyspnea, tachypnea and chest discomfort. Infants have difficulty feeding, fail to gain weight, and sometimes have foamy saliva. The treatment of pneumocystosis with pentamidine is presented in Chapter 68. Trimethoprim plus sulfamethoxazole (Bactrim, Septra) is an alternative agent for the treatment of pneumocystosis. The pharmacology of this combination is presented in Chapter 64.

Toxoplasmosis

Toxoplasmosis is caused by the nonfacultative intracellular protozoon *Toxoplasma gondii.* Cats are hosts for both the enteric sexual and extraintestinal asexual forms. Humans contract toxoplasmosis by ingesting cysts, often from poorly cooked or raw meat, or oocysts from cat feces. The symptoms of toxoplasmosis range from none to encephalitis and death. The most common are retinochoroiditis, lymphadenopathy, fever, and on occasion a rash on the soles and palms. Toxoplasmosis is treated with pyrimethamine (Daraprim) plus trisulfapyrimidines.

Trichomoniasis

Trichomoniasis vaginalis infections are seen most frequently during the sexually active years. Recurrent infections may result from the presence of flagellae in the urethra. Metronidazole (Flagyl, Protostat) is the drug of choice for the treatment of trichomoniasis.

Further Reading

Drugs for parasitic infections (1990). *The Medical Letter 32* :23-30.

Drugs for parasitic infections (1988). *The Medical Letter 30* :15-24.

Drugs for parasitic infections (1986). *The Medical Letter 28* :9-18.

Table 104
Antiprotozoal drugs.

Generic Name (Trade Name)	Use (Dose)	Action	Adverse Effects	Drug Interactions	Nursing Process
Pharmacologic Classification: Antiamebic Drugs					
Metronidazole (Flagyl, Protostat)	Tx of hepatic and intestinal amebiasis, giardiasis. Eradicat'n of trichomonal infect'ns **(Oral:** *For amebiasis [intestinal disease or tissue abscess]* - Adults - 750 mg tid for 10 days, followed by 650 mg of iodoquinol tid for 20 days. Max. dose, 2 g/day. Children - 35-50 mg/kg/day in 3 divided doses for 10 days, followed by iodoquinol 30-40 mg/kg/day in 3 doses for 20 days. Max. dose, 2 g/day)	Enters protozoon, inhibiting H+ product'n essential to its survival.	GI: Diarrhea, nausea, vomiting, anorexia, epigastric distress, dyspepsia, constipat'n. Mouth: Furred tongue, dry mouth, unpleasant metallic taste. Hematopoietic: Transient eosinophilia or leukopenia. Dermatologic: Rash, pruritus. CV: Palpitat'ns, chest pain. CNS: Convulsive seizures, peripheral neuropathy, transient ataxia, dizziness, drowsiness, confus'n, insomnia, headache. Other: Proliferat'n of C. albicans in vagina; vaginal dryness, burning; dysuria; occ. flushing and headaches, esp. w. concomitant ingest'n of alcohol; altered taste of alcoholic beverages.	**Alcohol:** Interacts w. metronidazole, which has a disulfiram (Antabuse)-like effect. Warn pts receiving metronidazole not to drink alcohol for fear of precipitating such a react'n. **Anticoagulants:** Such as warfarin, may have incr. effects if given w. metronidazole. **Disulfiram:** And metronidazole, have been reported to produce psychotic episodes and confus'nal states in some pts.	**Assess:** For hx alcohol abuse, pregnancy, hematopoietic disorders. **Evaluate:** For numbness, tremor, ataxia, paresthesias, decr. sensat'n, weakness, vertigo, incr. bleeding tendencies. Stools are examined throughout and should be clear at end of tx. **Teach:** To expect metallic taste and discolorat'n of urine; to avoid use of alcohol; self-evaluat'n for adv. effects. Pt to use proper hygiene after BMs, to use condoms, to comply w. dosage schedule.
Iodoquinol (Diodoquin, Yodoxin)	Drug of choice for tx of asymptomatic amebiasis. Metronidazole + iodoquinol is 1st-choice tx for mild to moderate or severe intestinal disease, or hepatic abscess. Iodoquinol + either emetine or dehydroemetine represents	Organic iodine compound acts against amebae in intestine. Can be used alone in tx of asymptomatic intestinal amebiasis or combined w. other	Rash, acne, slight enlargement of thyroid gland, nausea, diarrhea, cramps, anal pruritus, rarely atopic atrophy, loss of vision after prolonged use (i.e., months) in high doses.		**Assess:** For iodine hypersensitivity, pregnancy, lactat'n. **Evaluate:** For weakness, dyasthesia, peripheral neuropathy, loss of visual acuity; pruritus, urticaria, chills, fever. Stools are examined throughout and should be clear at end of tx.

Drug	Uses/Dosage	Action	Adverse effects	Nursing process
	2nd-line tx for severe intestinal disease. Emetine, or dehydroemetine, combined w. iodoquinol + chloroquine is alternative tx to metronidazole + iodoquinol for hepatic amebic abscesses (**Oral:** *For asymptomatic amebiasis [cyst-carrier state]* - Adults - 650 mg tid for 20 days. Max. dose, 2 g/day. Children - 30-40 mg/kg/day in 2-3 doses for 20 days. Max. dose, 2 g/day. Refer also to dosage instruct'ns for adults and children under metronidazole)	drugs in other common forms of amebiasis.		**Assess:** Establish baseline measures of BP, apical/radial pulse rates; hx of cardiac/renal disorders. **Administer:** Aspirate carefully; inject slowly. **Evaluate:** Qid for cardiotoxicities, incr. pulse rates, decr. BP. Monitor fluid intake/output, localized muscle weakness at inject'n sites. Examine stools throughout; should be clear at end of tx. Test vision during and after tx. **Teach:** To avoid exert'n or exercise. Caution pts not to get drug in eyes or on mucous membranes; to use proper hygiene after BMs.
Emetine	Used tog. w. iodoquinol as alternative tx for severe intestinal amebiasis. Administered before chloroquine phosphate and iodoquinol as alternative tx for hepatic amebic abscesses (**IM:** *For amebiasis - Emetine -* Adults - 1 mg/kg/day [max., 60 mg/day] for 5 days, followed by 650 mg of iodoquinol PO tid for 20 days. Children - Not > 0.5 mg/kg bid for 5 days, followed by 30-40 mg/kg/day of iodoquinol PO in 2-3 doses for 20 days. Max., 2 g/day.	Blocks protein synthesis in protozoon.	Cardiac arrhythmias, precordial pain, muscle weakness, cellulitis at site of inject'n, diarrhea, vomiting, peripheral neuropathy, heart failure	
Dehydroemetine	**IM:** *Dehydroemetine* - Adults - 1-1.5 mg/kg/day for 5 days. Max. dose, 90 mg/day, followed by 650 mg of iodoquinol PO tid for 20 days. Max., 2 g/day. Children - Not > 1-1.5 mg/kg/day in 2 doses for 5 days, followed by 30-40 mg/kg/day of iodoquinol PO in 3 doses for 20 days. Max., 2 g/day)	As for emetine	As for emetine	

Generic Name (Trade Name)	Use (Dose)	Action	Adverse Effects	Drug Interactions	Nursing Process
Paramomycin sulfate (Humatin)	Alternative tx to iodoquinol for asymptomatic amebiasis. Alternative tx to metronidazole + iodoquinol for mild to moderate intestinal amebiasis (**Oral:** *Asymptomatic amebiasis (cyst-carrier state)* - Adults/children 25-30 mg/kg/day in 3 divided doses w. meals for 7-10 days. *Mild to moderate intestinal amebiasis* - 25-35 mg/kg/day in 3 doses w. meals for 7-10 days, plus: Adults - 650 mg iodoquinol tid for 20 days. Children - 30-40 mg/kg/day in 2-3 doses for 20 days. Max., 2 g/day)	Aminoglycoside antibiotic. Mechanism of action in amebiasis unknown. Active against amebae in intestinal lumen.	Diarrhea, abd. pain, alterat'n of normal colonic bacterial flora	As for aminoglycosyde antibiotics, Table 96	As for aminoglycoside antibiotics, Table 96.

Pharmacologic Classification: Antigiardiasis Drugs

Generic Name (Trade Name)	Use (Dose)	Action	Adverse Effects	Drug Interactions	Nursing Process
Quinacrine HCl (Atabrine)	Drug of choice for tx of giardiasis (**Oral:** Adults - 100 mg tid pc for 5 days. Children - 2 mg/kg tid pc for 5 days. Max., 300 mg/day)	Mechanism of action not known.	Nausea, vomiting, headache, dizziness, toxic psychosis, anemia, exfoliative dermatitis, yellowish discolorat'n of skin	*For Drug Interact'ns involving hepatotoxic drugs and primaquine, see Table 103.*	**Administer:** Following 2-day low-fat diet and 18-h fast. Immed. before and 1 h after administrat'n, purge pt w. saline enema. Give w. 600 mg NaHCO₃ in 200 mL water. **Evaluate:** As for niclosamide (Chapter 71). **Teach:** As for niclosamide (Chapter 71).
Metronidazole (Flagyl, Protostat)	Metronidazole is replacing quinacrine for tx of giardiasis as it is more active and less toxic (**Oral:** Adults - 250-500 mg tid for 5-7 days or 2 g/day as single dose for 3 days. Children - 5 mg/kg tid for 5-7 days)	Enters protozoon, inhibiting H⁺ product'n essential to its survival.	*See informat'n presented earlier in this table.*	*See informat'n presented earlier in this table.*	*See informat'n presented earlier in this table.*

Furazolidone (Furoxone)	Alternative to quinacrine in tx of giardiasis **(Oral:** Adults - 100 mg qid for 7-10 days. Children - 6 mg/kg/day divided into 4 equal doses, w. meals for 7-10 days. *Do not give to children <* 1 month of age)	One of the more potent, effective agents employed in tx of giardiasis.	Nausea, vomiting, allergic react'ns, headache, pulmonary infiltrat'n, orthostatic hypotens'n, hypoglycemia, polyneuritis, urticaria, fever, vascular or morbilliform pruritus	**Adrenergic drugs:** *Can interact w. furazolidone. A metabolite of furazolidone inhibits MAO. If furazolidone is given w. adrenergic agents, TCAs or similar compounds, or food containing tyramine, it can cause hypertensive react'n.* **Alcohol:** *Can interact w. furazolidone, which produces a disulfiram (Antabuse)-type react'n in some pts after consuming ethanol.*	**Assess:** Hx for diabetes, previous hypersensitivity to MAOIs, alcohol abuse; check current drug regimen for concurrent use of antihistamines, MAOIs, sedatives, indirect-acting sympathomimetics, ephedrine, phenylephrine or tyramine. **Evaluate:** For drug efficacy (reduct'n in number and liquid consistency of stools); for hypersensitivity react'ns; diabetics for incr. hypoglycemia. **Teach:** To avoid foods containing tyramine; to abstain from alcohol for at least 4 days after stopping drug. Caution that urine may turn brown.

Pharmacologic Classification: Antipneumocystosis Drugs

Pentamidine isethionate	Tx of choice for *Pneumocystis carinii* infect'ns. See Chapter 68, Table 102.	See Table 102	See Table 102	See Table 102	See Table 102
Trimethoprim + sulfamethoxazole (Bactrim, Septra)	Alternative to pentamidine (see Table 102) for pneumocystosis **(Oral:** Adults/children - 5 mg trimethoprim/kg + 25 mg sulfamethoxazole/kg qid for at least 14 days)	Sulfamethoxazole inhibits folic acid format'n in parasite; trimethoprim blocks activat'n of any folic acid that is formed.	Nausea, vomiting, rash, hemolysis in G-6-PD deficiency, acute megaloblastic anemia, granulocytopenia, thrombocytopenia, pseudomembranous colitis, kernicterus in newborn	*For sulfonamide Drug Interact'ns involving local anesthetics, oral anticoagulants, antidiabetics, diuretics, PABA and phenytoin, see Table 98.*	See Table 98

Pharmacologic Classification: Antitoxoplasmosis Drugs

Generic Name (Trade Name)	Use (Dose)	Action	Adverse Effects	Drug Interactions	Nursing Process
Pyrimethamine (Daraprim)	Tx of toxoplasmosis (**Oral: Adults** - Initially, 50-100 mg/day for 1-3 days, followed by 25 mg/day for 3-4 weeks; plus trisulfapyrimidines, 2-6 g/day in 4-6 divided doses for 3-4 weeks. Sulfadiazine may be used in place of trisulfapyrimidines [initially, 2-4 g, followed by 1 g q4-6h for 3-4 weeks]. **Children** - 2 mg/kg/day of pyrimethamine for 3 days [max., 25 mg/day]; then 1 mg/kg/day for 4 weeks. Give w. 100-200 mg/kg/day of trisulfapyrimidines in 4-6 divided doses for 3-4 weeks. **Infants** - 2 mg/kg/day pyrimethamine for 3 days, then 1 mg/kg/day q2-3 days for 4 weeks)	Sulfonamide and pyrimethamine have synergistic effects and alter folic acid cycle of toxoplasma. Sulfonamides block format'n of folic acid and pyrimethamine interferes w. folic acid use.	*Consult Table 98 for Adverse Effects of sulfonamides and Table 103 for Adverse Effects of pyrimethamine.*	*For Drug Interact'ns involving local anesthetics, oral anticoagulants, oral antidiabetics, diuretics, PABA and phenytoin, see Table 98.*	*Refer to Table 98 for Nsg. Process rel. to sulfonamides and Table 103 for Nsg. Process rel. to pyrimethamine.*
Metronidazole (Flagyl, Prostat)	Drug of choice in tx of trichomoniasis. Individualize dose to improve compliance, minimize reinfect'n (**Oral: Adults** - 1-day tx - 2g as single dose [preferred] or in 2 equal doses; 7 consecutive days' tx - 250 mg tid).	Enters protozoon, inhibiting H+ product'n essential for its survival.	*See informat'n presented earlier in this table.*	*See informat'n presented earlier in this table.*	*See informat'n presented earlier in this table.*

CHAPTER 71

Anthelmintic Drugs

Teaching Objectives

Following completion of this chapter, the reader should be able to:

1. Divide worms into the three major groups that plague humans.
2. Identify the two major tapeworms that infect humans.
3. Discuss the mechanism of action, therapeutic uses and adverse effects of niclosamide, as well as the nursing process related to its use.
4. Explain the roles of paromomycin and quinacrine in the treatment of tapeworm infections.
5. List the more common nematodes.
6. Describe the life cycle and effects of *A. lumbricoides*.
7. Discuss the mechanisms of action, therapeutic uses and adverse effects of pyrantel pamoate, mebendazole and piperazine, as well as the nursing process associated with their use.
8. Describe the life cycle and effects of *E. vermicularis*.
9. Discuss the mechanism of action, therapeutic uses and adverse effects of pyrvinium pamoate, and the nursing process associated with its use.
10. Describe the use of thiabendazole in the treatment of *S. stercoralis*, including its adverse effects and nursing process.
11. List the drugs used to eradicate *T. trichiura*.
12. Describe the life cycle and effects of *N. americanus* and *A. duodenale*.
13. Discuss the mechanism of action and use of bephenium hydroxynaphthoate in the treatment of hookworm, together with its adverse effects and nursing process.
14. List the trematodes that infect humans and describe the manner in which they are contracted, their sites of infection and their effects.

Worms

Worms, or **helminths,** have plagued humankind since the beginning of time. In spite of recent developments in drug therapy, they continue to extract a tremendous cost in human suffering. Even today, approximately fifty per cent of humans are infected with worms. It has been estimated that the number of worm infections harbored by humans exceeds the world's population; meaning, of course, that at this moment millions of people are providing nice, warm hostels for more than one type of worm.

Helminths can be divided into cestodes (flatworms), nematodes (roundworms) and trematodes (flukes) (Table 105). Worms can also be classified according to parts of the body infected. Some infect only the gastrointestinal tract. Others live in body tissues.

Table 105
Classification of human helminths.

Biological Classification	Examples
Cestodes (flatworms or tapeworms)	*Tænia saginata* and *Tænia solium*
Nematodes (roundworms)	*Ascaris lumbricoides* (roundworm) *Enterobius vermicularis* (pinworm) *Necator americanus* and *Ancylostoma duodenale* (hookworms)
Trematodes (flukes)	Schistosomes

Cestodes (Tapeworms)

Tapeworm infections occur when humans eat uncooked meat or fish containing encysted larvae. The tapeworm is segmented and flat, with a small sucker on its head (scolex). Once larvae are ingested, the sucker attaches to the small intestine, and the worm grows by producing one segment after another. The extent to which the worm can grow is illustrated by the fact that the fish tapeworm (*Diphyllobothrium latum*) can reach a length of ten meters and contain three to four thousand segments.

It is not surprising that patients with tapeworms neatly encased within the lumen of their intestinal tracts may experience symptoms. What is remarkable is that many individuals show few effects. The symptoms of tapeworm infection may include vague abdominal discomfort and pain, weakness, weight loss, epigastric fullness and anemia.

Tænia saginata and *Tænia solium* are the two chief tapeworms infecting humans. Improperly cooked beef is the source of *T. saginata* (beef tapeworm). Although the tapeworm can grow to ten meters in humans, it cannot propagate in the intestines. The fertilized eggs of *T. saginata* can form larvae only in the gastrointestinal tract of cattle. *T. solium* differs from the beef tapeworm in two respects. First, it is obtained from uncooked pork (pork tapeworm), and second, it can propagate in the gastrointestinal tract of humans. If this happens, larvae hatched in the gastrointestinal tract are carried into the blood and spread throughout the body, developing into space-occupying masses in the orbit of the eye, brain, muscle, liver and other organs.

Niclosamide (Niclocide, Yomesan)

Mechanism of Action, Therapeutic Uses and Adverse Effects

Tapeworms derive most of their energy in the intestine from anaerobic metabolism, and niclosamide inhibits anaerobic metabolism in the helminth. As a result, the scolex releases its hold on the intestinal wall and the worm is passed in the feces.

Niclosamide is administered orally to treat both beef and pork tapeworms. Because niclosamide is not absorbed from the gastrointestinal tract, tapeworms are exposed to high concentrations of the drug. In the case of *T. solium,* viable eggs may be released when segments of the worm are destroyed. Therefore, a laxative is usually administered one or two hours after the drug to prevent cysticercosis. The drug is also given to eradicate fish tapeworm (*Diphyllobothrium latum*) and dwarf tapeworm (*Hymenolepis nana*).

Niclosamide produces few adverse effects. Some patients may complain of abdominal pain and others may experience diarrhea.

Nursing Process

The nursing process for niclosamide includes general considerations to be followed for all anthelmintic drugs.

Assessment

Stool specimens are examined throughout treatment and for one to three months after therapy. Specimens must be sent to the laboratory while still warm.

Administration

Niclosamide tablets may be crushed and mixed with water if the patient is unable to swallow the chewed tablet. Laxatives may be used if the patient is constipated, but are not necessary for drug effectiveness.

Evaluation

Nurses should evaluate patients for the therapeutic effectiveness of niclosamide by inspecting feces for the head of the worm. Three negative stool cultures are needed after completion of treatment. Patients should be monitored for allergic reactions, a rash or itching in the anal area. Nurses should also watch for diarrhea during the expulsion of the worm. Other family members should be evaluated for infection, because person-to-person infection is common.

Teaching

Nurses should teach patients to use proper hygiene following bowel movements, to sleep alone, to change bed linen every day and to wash bed linen daily. Patients should be advised to cook meat thoroughly in order to avoid recurrent infections.

Quinacrine, Mepacrine (Atabrine)

Quinacrine, also known by the alternate generic name of mepacrine, continues to be a popular drug in many parts of the world for tapeworm infections. In North America it has largely been replaced by niclosamide. When taken orally, quinacrine often causes nausea and vomiting. In the treatment of tapeworm infections it is often given via a duodenal tube to reduce the incidence of nausea and vomiting. Quinacrine's other adverse effects include headache, dizziness, toxic psychosis, anemia, exfoliative dermatitis and a yellowish discoloration of the skin.

Nursing Process

Administration

Prior to the administration of quinacrine, patients are subjected to a two-day low-fat diet, followed by an eighteen-hour fast. Immediately preceding and one hour following administration of this drug, the patient is purged with saline enemas. If a duodenal tube is not used to administer the quinacrine, the drug is administered orally in four doses of 200 mg each at ten-minute intervals. The administration of 600 mg of sodium bicarbonate in 200 mL of water with each dose of quinacrine may reduce the nausea and vomiting associated with use of this drug.

Evaluation and Teaching

Nursing evaluation and patient teaching in relation to the use of quinacrine are the same as those identified in relation to niclosamide.

Nematodes (Roundworms)

Nematodes, or roundworms, are the most common helminths bothering humans. Depending on the actual worm involved, they may be found within the gastrointestinal tract or in the tissues of the body. The next few pages will discuss the main characteristics of the more common roundworm infections and the drugs used to treat them.

Ascaris lumbricoides (Roundworm)

Ascaris lumbricoides is the most common human parasite. It is found in about one-third of the world's population — about one billion people. Although ascaris is commonly called a roundworm, it should be understood that it is only one member of the general classification of roundworms (nematodes). Infection with *Ascaris lumbricoides* is more prevalent in warmer areas of the world, but is also seen in colder climates.

Humans become infected with roundworms when they ingest embryonated eggs. Children playing in sandboxes provide an excellent example of how this can happen. The larvae hatch in the duodenum and are absorbed into the blood. Carried to the alveoli, they ascend the airways to reach the epiglottis and are swallowed. Upon their return to the small intestines, the larvae develop into male and female roundworms. At this stage patients may be asymptomatic or experience abdominal distress (epigastric pain, nausea, vomiting and anorexia). More serious problems are created if the worms migrate into the pancreatic and bile ducts, gall bladder or liver, or if they completely obstruct the appendix or intestinal lumen.

Pyrantel Pamoate (Antiminth, Combantrin)

Pyrantel pamoate is poorly absorbed from the gastrointestinal tract. Administered orally, it paralyzes roundworms. A single oral dose of pyrantel pamoate is the drug of choice for the treatment of *Ascaris lumbricoides*. Pyrantel pamoate is also indicated for the treatment of pinworms (enterobiasis) and hookworms (*Ancylostoma duodenale, Necator americanus*). It is not recommended for pregnant patients or for children under one year of age. Sufficient drug may be absorbed to produce headache, irritability, insomnia, dizziness and drowsiness. Abdominal cramps have also been reported.

Nursing Process

Pyrantel pamoate is metabolized in the liver. Patients whose nursing assessment reveals a history of hepatic disease, age of less than one year, or a current pregnancy should not be given this drug. Patient teaching related to the use of pyrantel pamoate should stress the importance of personal hygiene and hand washing in achieving a complete cure.

Mebendazole (Vermox)

Mebendazole is also poorly absorbed from the gastrointestinal tract. It inhibits glucose uptake by *Ascaris lumbricoides,* depletes the worm's supply of glycogen, and lowers adenosine triphosphate (ATP) synthesis. In addition to *Ascaris lumbricoides,* mebendazole is used to eradicate *Enterobius vermicularis* (pinworm) and *Trichuris trichiura* (whipworm). Hookworm infections caused by *A. duodenale* or *N. americanus* may also be treated with mebendazole. It has also been used to treat infections caused by *T. solium* (pork tapeworm).

Patients treated with mebendazole may suffer diarrhea, vomiting and/or abdominal pain. Other adverse effects reported include drowsiness, itching, headache and dizziness. Special attention should be given to patients with intestinal pathology (e.g., Crohn's ileitis, ulcerative colitis).

Nursing Process

The nursing process for roundworm treatment is similar to that previously described for tapeworms. Nurses are advised to follow the nursing process of niclosamide.

The major advantage of mebendazole is that it may be administered in any manner the patient finds acceptable. The fact that it can be chewed, buried in a tablespoonful of jam and swallowed whole, or crushed and mixed with food is a particular asset when dealing with children, who are often the primary victims of these worms. An additional advantage is that patients are also spared the indignity of purging. Again, in patient teaching, nurses must stress the importance of personal asepsis and hand washing in effecting a complete cure.

Piperazine Citrate (Antepar) and Piperazine Adipate (Entacyl)

Piperazine produces a flaccid paralysis in the worm, which is eliminated in the feces. Piperazine is well absorbed from the gastrointestinal tract. Most of the drug is eliminated in urine within twenty-four hours. Piperazine is effective against *Ascaris lumbricoides* and *Enterobius vermicularis* (pinworm). Given as either the citrate, phosphate or adipate salts, it cures more than eighty per cent of ascaris infections when given for two days. Piperazine is generally well tolerated. Its adverse reactions include gastrointestinal upset, urticaria and dizziness. It can also cause neurologic symptoms that include hypotonia and ataxia — the

so-called "worm-wobble" effect. Visual disturbances and exacerbations of epilepsy can also occur. Piperazine is contraindicated in patients with impaired renal or hepatic function, convulsive disorders, or a history of hypersensitivity reactions to piperazine or its salts.

Nursing Process

The nursing process for piperazine is similar to that for niclosamide. Nurses are advised to follow the process given earlier in the chapter, with the following additions for piperazine.

Assessment
Because piperazine can produce central nervous system toxicity, patients should undergo nursing assessment of their histories for evidence of seizure disorders. Piperazine is eliminated by the kidney. Therefore, nursing assessment should include an attempt to determine any history of undisclosed renal disease.

Administration
Piperazine should be administered in precisely the prescribed amounts to avoid serious adverse effects due to overdose.

Evaluation
Nursing evaluation of the patient should emphasize early identification of central nervous system toxicity as indicated by dizziness, hypotonia, ataxia, visual disturbances or seizures.

Teaching
Nurses should teach the patient the hygiene precautions described earlier for niclosamide.

Enterobius vermicularis (Pinworm)

Enterobius vermicularis, also called oxyuris, is the infamous pinworm, the most common human helminth in the United States and Canada. As any parent with young children will readily attest, this little fellow can make life very difficult around the house. Not content to torment children, it can also weigh heavily on the minds of men and women of all walks of life. Its ability to tickle the seats of the mighty has led to the development of many drugs, all capable of giving this parasite a well-deserved shellacking.

Pruritus in the perianal and perineal regions is the most common consequence of pinworm infections. Scratching may lead to infection. In female patients the worms may migrate to the genital tract. Because pinworm infections are often found in several members of the same family, it is appropriate to treat the entire family and close friends of an infected child.

Pinworms are treated with mebendazole, pyrantel pamoate, piperazine and pyrvinium. All but the last drug were discussed previously.

Pyrvinium Pamoate (Povan, Vanquin)

The mechanism of action of pyrvinium is not known. Given orally, it is not well absorbed. Pyrvinium pamoate is considered an alternative drug to pyrantel pamoate or mebendazole for the treatment of *E. vermicularis*. Pyrvinium is given in a single dose, but the treatment is repeated in two weeks to clear any worms that have matured from the remaining eggs. The drug has few adverse effects. Patients should be warned that feces will be stained a harmless, bright red. Pyrvinium may occasionally cause a photosensitive skin rash.

Nursing Process

Assessment
Nursing assessment should attempt to determine whether the patient has any pre-existing salicylate allergy because there appears to be a cross-sensitivity between salicylates and the tartrazine dye that coats pyrvinium tablets.

Administration
The tablets should be swallowed whole to avoid staining the teeth.

Teaching
Patients and their parents should be prepared for the fact that pyrvinium pamoate will color gastric contents, vomitus and feces red. Nurses should emphasize the importance of personal hygiene in achieving and maintaining a worm-free state. Patients should be taught the hygiene precautions given before for niclosamide.

Strongyloides stercoralis (Threadworm)

Stronglyoides stercoralis (threadworm) is encountered frequently in the tropics. It can also be common in the southern United States. Threadworm infections are often found in conjunc-

tion with other worm infestations. Thiabendazole is the drug of choice; pyrvinium pamoate is a back-up agent.

Thiabendazole (Mintezol)

Thiabendazole is rapidly absorbed from the gastrointestinal tract and metabolized in the liver. Its mechanism of action is not known. Nematodes sensitive to this drug include *Ascaris lumbricoides* (roundworm), *Enterobius vermicularis* (pinworm), *Trichuris trichiura* (whipworm), *Nector americanus* and *Anyclostoma duodenale* (hookworm). The adverse effects of thiabendazole limit it as a drug of first choice to the treatment of *Strongyloides stercoralis*. About one-third of patients taking the drug experience anorexia, nausea, vomiting, drowsiness or vertigo. Pruritus, rash, diarrhea, hallucinations, crystalluria and leukopenia occur less frequently.

Nursing Process
Thiabendazole is metabolized in the liver and excreted by the kidneys. Patients whose nursing assessment reveals a history of either renal or hepatic disease are at increased risk of developing adverse effects due to the accumulation of toxic levels of the drug. Nurses identifying these conditions should withhold administration of this drug pending further consultation with the physician. Nurses must evaluate patients for the previously described adverse effects of thiabendazole, and teach the hygiene precautions given previously for niclosamide.

Trichuris trichiura (Whipworm)

Whipworm infections are found throughout the world. They are more prevalent in warm, humid climates. *Trichuris trichiura* is often found in patients suffering from roundworm and hookworm infections. Usually whipworm infections do not cause major problems, except in severely infected children.

Mebendazole is the drug of first choice for the treatment of whipworms. Thiabendazole is the back-up drug. Both agents were discussed earlier in this chapter.

Necator americanus and Ancylostoma duodenale (Hookworm)

Hookworms burrow through the skin of humans and are transported via blood to the alveoli. After ascending the respiratory tree to the epiglottis they are swallowed, after which they reach the intestinal lumen. Within the intestine, hookworms attach to the mucosa and cause ulcerations, abdominal fullness and epigastric pain. Because hookworms can suck blood from the intestinal mucosa, patients may demonstrate progressive hypochromic, microcytic anemia of the nutritional-deficiency type. Other problems created by hookworms are localized erythema and severe itching at the point where larvae penetrate the skin. The passage of large numbers of larvae through the lungs can cause pneumonitis.

Mebendazole, pyrantel pamoate, thiabendazole and bephenium hydroxynaphthoate are recommended for the treatment of hookworms. Except for the last drug, all others have been discussed previously.

Bephenium Hydroxynaphthoate (Alcopar)

Administered orally, bephenium hydroxynaphthoate is poorly absorbed from the gastrointestinal tract. It causes an initial contraction of the worm muscle followed by muscular paralysis. The worm is eliminated in the feces. The availability of mebendazole has reduced the use of bephenium hydroxynaphthoate. However, the drug is effective against hookworm infections and is still used for this indication. The major adverse effects of the drug are nausea, vomiting and diarrhea, usually not of serious proportions. Because of the very limited availability of bephenium hydroxynaphthoate in North America, its dosage will not be presented in this book.

Nursing Process

Bephenium hydroxynaphthoate is most effective when administered first thing in the morning (assuming that the patient has not eaten during the night), followed by a further two-hour fast. The patient can usually tolerate the very bitter taste of this product if it is mixed with a syrup. Nurses should teach the patient the hygiene precautions previously described for niclosamide.

Trematodes (Flukes)

Trematodes are nonsegmented flattened worms. Usually, they have two suckers — one at the mouth and the other located on the ventral surface. Trematode larvae are acquired by humans through food (aquatic vegetation, fish, crayfish) and by direct penetration of the skin. Most trematodes mature in the intestinal tract (intestinal flukes); others migrate and mature in the liver and bile duct (liver flukes), whereas still others penetrate the intestinal wall and are carried to the lung (lung flukes).

The symptoms vary, depending on the location of the flukes. Diarrhea, abdominal pain and anorexia are often seen, regardless of the infection site. Lung flukes cause coughs, chest pain and hemoptysis. Liver flukes can block the bile duct, enlarge the liver and produce right-quadrant pain and diarrhea.

It is beyond the scope of this book to discuss the use of niradazole (Ambilhar) to treat *Schistosoma hematobium* and *Schistosoma mansoni* infections, or stibophen for infections caused by *Schistosoma mansoni*. By the same token, space limitations prevent a discussion of the use of antimony potassium tartrate for the treatment of *Schistosoma japonicium* infections, biothionol as the drug of first choice in the treatment of infections caused by *Paragonimus westermani* (lung fluke) and *Fasciola hepatica* (sheep liver fluke), or chloroquine phosphate as the drug of first choice in the treatment of *Clonorchis sinensis* (liver fluke) infections. Nurses requiring the use of these drugs should consult reference texts, such as the *AMA Drug Evaluations,* 6th ed. (Chicago: American Medical Association, 1986).

Further Reading

Drugs for parasitic infections (1990). *The Medical Letter 32* :23-30.

Drugs for parasitic infections (1986). *The Medical Letter 28* :9-18.

Katz, M. (1986). Anthelmintics: Current concepts in the treatment of helminthic infections. *Drugs 32* :358-371.

Table 106
Anthelmintic drugs.

Pharmacologic Classification: Drugs for the Treatment of Cestodes

Generic Name (Trade Name)	Use (Dose)	Action	Adverse Effects	Drug Interactions	Nursing Process
Niclosamide (Nicloside, Yomesan)	Preferred agent for tx of tapeworm infect'ns (**Oral:** Adults - 2 g as single dose. Children > 34 kg - 1.5 g as single dose; 11-34 kg - 1 g as single dose. If treating *H. nana* infect'ns, give for 5 successive days. Omit breakfast on day of tx. Chew tabs thoroughly and swallow w. a little water. Pt may eat 2 h after taking drug)	Inhibits anaerobic metabolism in worm, causing it to release hold on intestinal wall.	No serious adv. react'ns. Pts may experience malaise, mild abd. pain and nausea.		**Assess:** Stool specimens throughout tx and for 1-3 months thereafter. Specimens must to sent to lab. while still warm. **Administer:** Tabs may be crushed and mixed w. water. Laxatives may be used but are not nec. for tx. **Evaluate:** Tx efficacy by inspecting feces for head of worm. 3 neg. stool cultures are needed after tx. Monitor pt for allergic react'ns, rash, itching in anal area. Check family members for infect'n. **Teach:** Pt to use proper hygiene following BMs, to sleep alone, to change bed linen daily and to clean toilet daily w. disinfectant.
Quinacrine HCl, mepacrine HCl (Atabrine HCl)	For condit'ns as follows (**Oral:** *Beef, pork and fish tapeworm* - Bland nonfat diet, or milk, on day before medicat'n, w. fasting following evening meal. Saline purge and cleansing enema before tx if desired. Adults - 4 doses of 200 mg 10 min apart [total dose, 800 mg]. NaHCO₃ 600 mg is given w. each dose to reduce tendency to nausea and vomiting. Children 5-10 years - Total dose, 400 mg; 11-14 years - Total dose, 600 mg, divided into 3-4 doses given 10 min apart. NaHCO₃ 300 mg is given w. each dose. Saline purge 1-2 h later. Expelled worm is stained yellow for identificat'n of scolex. For	Mechanism of action not known. Continues to be a popular drug in many parts of the world.	Nausea, vomiting, headache, dizziness, toxic psychosis, anemia, exfoliative dermatitis and yellowish discolorat'n of skin.	**Hepatotoxic drugs:** May interact w. quinacrine, which concentrates in liver. It should be used w. caution in pts w. hepatic disease or alcoholism or in conjunct'n w. known hepatotoxic drugs. **Primaquine:** Quinacrine incr. primaquine's toxicity; thus, concomitant use is contraindicated.	**Administer:** Following 2-day low-fat diet and 18-h fast. Immed. preceding and 1 h following administrat'n, purge pt w. saline enemas; give 600 mL water. **Evaluate:** As for niclosamide. **Teach:** As for niclosamide.

Generic Name (Trade Name)	Use (Dose)	Action	Adverse Effects	Drug Interactions	Nursing Process
	dwarf tapeworm - Adults - Hs before medicat'n, give 1 tablespoon Na$_2$SO$_4$. On day 1, give 900 mg quinacrine on an empty stomach, in 3 doses 20 min apart, w. Na$_2$SO$_4$ purge 90 min later. On following 3 days, 100 mg tid. Children - Hs before medicat'n, $^1/_2$ tablespoon Na$_2$SO$_4$; *4-8 years* - Initial dose 200 mg, followed by 100 mg after breakfast for 3 days; *8-10 years* - Initial dose 300 mg, followed by 100 mg bid for 3 days; *11-14 years* - Initial dose 400 mg, followed by 100 mg tid for 3 days)				

Pharmacologic Classification: Drugs for the Treatment of Nematodes — (A) Ascaris lumbricoides (Roundworms)

Generic Name (Trade Name)	Use (Dose)	Action	Adverse Effects	Drug Interactions	Nursing Process
Pyrantel pamoate (Antiminth, Combantrin)	Drug of choice for tx of ascariasis. Also effective in tx of pinworms [enterobiasis] and hookworms [*N. americanus*] (**Oral:** *Pinworms and roundworms* - Administered in single dose on basis of body mass. For pts 12-23 kg - 125-250 mg; 24-45 kg - 250-500 mg; 46-68 kg - 500-750 mg; > 68 kg - 1 g. Do not exceed recomm. dose. *Hookworms* - Same doses as for pinworms and roundworms, but give od for 3 days)	Poorly absorbed. Paralyzes worms, allowing them to be expelled in feces.	Headache, irritability, insomnia, dizziness, drowsiness, abd. cramps.		**Assess:** For pregnancy, age < 1 year, hepatic disease. **Teach:** Importance of personal hygiene as outlined previously for niclosamide.
Mebendazole (Vermox)	Tx of single or mixed helminthic infestat'ns. Effective in tx of roundworms [*A. lumbricoides*], pinworms [*E. vermicularis*], whipworms [*T. trichiura*] and	Inhibits glucose uptake in nematode and thereby inhibits ATP synthesis.	Diarrhea, vomiting and/or abd. pain, drowsiness, itching, headache, dizziness. Incr. SGOT, SPGT,		**Administer:** Tabs in any manner acceptable to pt (chewing, swallowing whole, crushed and mixed w. food). **Teach:** Importance of personal hygiene as outlined previously for niclosamide.

hookworms [A. duodenale and N. americanus]. Also used in tx of infect'ns due to large tapeworms [T. solium] (**Oral:** Children > 2 years/adults - Control of trichuriasis, ascariasis, ancylostomiasis, strongyloidiasis, taeniasis and mixed infect'ns - 100 mg q m. et n. for 3 consec. days. For enterobiasis - 100 mg only. Chew tabs. If not cured 3 weeks after tx, 2nd course is advised)				alkaline phosphatase and BUN.
Piperazine citrate syrup and tablets (Antepar)	Tx of roundworm or pinworm infestat'ns (**Oral:** Ascariasis - Children/adults - 75 mg/kg [max, 3.5 g] od for 2 consec. days. Enterobiasis - 65 mg/kg [max, 2.5 g] od for 7 consec. days. Should be repeated after 1 week)	Produces flaccid paralysis in nematode, which is eliminated in feces.	GI effects: Nausea, vomiting, abd. cramps, diarrhea. CNS [rarely and us. in pts w. neurologic disturbances or in overdose]: Headache, vertigo, ataxia, tremors, choreiform movement, muscular weakness, hyporeflexia. Hypersensitivity: Urticaria, erythema multiforme, purpura, fever, arthralgia.	**Phenothiazines:** And piperazine, may exaggerate phenothiazine-induced extrapyramidal effects. Concomitant tx should be undertaken w. caution.	**Assess:** Hx of seizure disorders, kidney disease. **Administer:** Precisely the prescribed dose. **Evaluate:** For dizziness, hypotonia, ataxia, visual disturbances, seizures. **Teach:** Importance of personal hygiene as outlined previously for niclosamide.
Piperazine adipate suspension (Entacyl); piperazine adipate granule packets containing 2 g piperazine adipate (Entacyl)	Tx of roundworm or pinworm infestat'ns (**Oral:** Ascariasis and enterobiasis - Suspens'n: 1-day tx. Children < 2 years - 0.6 g tid; 2-8 years - 1.2 g bid; > 8 years /Adults - 1.8 g tid. Repeat dosage given over 12-h period in 2 weeks. **Granules:** 1-day tx. Children 2-8 years [13.6-27.3 kg] - 1 packet; 8-14 years [27.3-40.9 kg] - 1 packet bid; > 14 years /Adults [> 40.9 kg] - 1 packet tid. Dose is given in 57 mL water, milk or juice. Repeat dosage given over 12-h period in 2 weeks)	As for piperazine citrate	As for piperazine citrate	As for piperazine citrate	As for piperazine citrate

Generic Name (Trade Name)	Use [Dose]	Action	Adverse Effects	Drug Interactions	Nursing Process

Pharmacologic Classification: Drugs for the Treatment of Nematodes — (B) Enterobius vermicularis (Pinworms)

Pyrantel pamoate and mebendazole are usually considered drugs of choice. Piperazine may also be used. Informat'n on these drugs is provided above in this table. Pyrinium pamoate is an alternative drug for enterobiasis.

Generic Name (Trade Name)	Use [Dose]	Action	Adverse Effects	Drug Interactions	Nursing Process
Pyrvinium pamoate (Povan, Vanquin)	Tx of pinworms **(Oral:** Single dose of 50 mg/10 kg. Take immed. pc. Repeat in 2 weeks)	Mechanism of action unknown.	In rare cases, nausea, vomiting and/or diarrhea		**Assess:** For salicylate allergy. **Administer:** Tabs whole. **Teach:** That drug will cause gastric contents to be stained red; importance of personal hygiene as presented previously for niclosamide.

Pharmacologic Classification: Drugs for the Treatment of Nematodes — (C) Strongyloides stercoralis (Threadworms)

Thiabendazole is the drug of choice. Pyrvinium pamoate may be considered a backup drug. Informat'n on its use can be found above in this table.

Generic Name (Trade Name)	Use [Dose]	Action	Adverse Effects	Drug Interactions	Nursing Process
Thiabendazole (Mintezol)	Drug of 1st choice in tx of S. stercoralis infect'ns. Also effective in A. lumbricoides, E. vermicularis, T. trichiura, N. americanus, and A. duodenale infect'ns **(Oral:** Strongyloidiasis - Adults/children - 25 mg/kg bid for 2 days. Max., 3 g/day for at least 5 days in disseminated infect'ns [i.e., hyperinfect'n syndrome]. Occurs primarily in immunocompromised pts. For trichuriasis - 25 mg/kg bid. Max., 3 g/day for 2-4 days)	Mechanism of action unknown.	Frequent: Anorexia, nausea, vomiting and dizziness. Less frequent: Diarrhea, epigastric distress, pruritus, weariness, drowsiness, giddiness, headache. For rare adv. effects, consult manufacturer's literature.		**Assess:** For hepatic/renal disease. **Evaluate:** For adv. effects. **Teach:** Importance of personal hygiene as previously outlined for niclosamide.

Pharmacologic Classification: Drugs for the Treatment of Nematodes — (D) Trichuris trichiura (Whipworms)

Mebendazole is the drug of first choice; thiabendazole the drug of second choice. Informat'n on these drugs is provided above in this table.

Pharmacologic Classification: Drugs for the Treatment of Nematodes — (E) Necator americanus and Ancylostoma duodenale (Hookworms)

Mebendazole is the drug of first choice. Pyrantel pamoate, thiobendazole and bephenium hydroxynaphthoate are alternate choices. With the except'n of bephenium hydroxynaphthoate, inform-at'n on these drugs is provided above in this table.

CHAPTER 72

Antineoplastic Drugs

Teaching Objectives

Following completion of this chapter, the reader should be able to:

1. List and discuss the three common characteristics of malignant cells.
2. Name the types of therapy available for the treatment of cancer.
3. Discuss the relationship of the growth fraction of cancer cells to the use of chemotherapy.
4. Define the expressions cell-cycle-independent, cell-cycle-dependent and phase-dependent antineoplastics.
5. Provide justification for the use of more than one drug in the treatment of cancer.
6. List the groups of antineoplastics currently in use, based on their mechanisms of action, and explain why these drugs are effective against neoplasms.
7. Discuss the adverse effects of antineoplastic drugs.
8. Discuss the implications for nursing care associated with the prescription and use of antineoplastic drugs.

Cancers and Their Treatment

This chapter will review drugs used in the treatment of cancer. They are called either anticancer or antineoplastic drugs. We will not discuss in detail their mechanisms of action or their precise therapeutic applications because of the complexity of the subject and the inability to do complete justice to it in only one chapter. Instead, our approach will be to concentrate on the general principles that guide the use of antineoplastic agents and the adverse effects common to most anticancer drugs. It must also be emphasized that although the treatment of cancers in general will be discussed, nurses should be aware that the term cancer refers to many different disorders and not to a single disease entity.

Perhaps no word strikes fear into the hearts of men and women so much as cancer. This is understandable because as mortality from infectious disease has declined, as a result of the development of new antibacterials, cancer has emerged as a leading cause of death. The number of deaths due to cancer in the United States is second only to those caused by heart failure. In women between thirty and fifty-four and children aged three to fourteen, cancer leads all other causes of mortality.

Cancer, or **neoplasia,** arises from transformed cells. It is characterized by an uncontrolled cellular proliferation that takes place at the expense of the host. Neoplastic cells have three common characteristics: persistent proliferation, invasive growth and the formation of metastases. **Persistent proliferation** refers to the ability of cancer cells to undergo unrestrained growth and division, and is the most distinguishing aspect of malignant cells.

This is in marked contrast to normal cells, whose proliferation is carefully controlled. Persistent proliferation in cancer is due to the fact that malignant cells are unresponsive to the feedback mechanisms that regulate cellular proliferation in healthy tissue. Thus, cancer cells are able to continue multiplying under conditions that would suppress further growth and division of normal cells. As a result of persistent proliferation cancerous tissues will continue to grow, unless intervention is instituted, until they cause death.

Invasive growth refers to ability of cancer cells to move into territory normally belonging to cells of a different type. Under normal conditions, the various types of cells that compose a tissue remain segregated from each other. That is to say, cells of one type do not invade areas in the body that are the normal habitat of cells of a different type. Malignant cells are not fettered by these constraints and, as a result, cells of a solid tumor can penetrate adjacent tissues.

Cancer cells can also form **metastases,** or secondary tumors that appear at other locations in the body. They result from malignant cells breaking away from the original tumor and migrating via the lymphatic or circulatory systems to other parts of the body, where they produce a new tumor.

Cancer may be treated by surgery, irradiation and drug therapy (chemotherapy). Surgery or radiation therapy, or both, are preferred for most solid tumors. These forms of treatment can often cure or control tumors locally. However, because of the ability of tumors to metastasize, many patients eventually die because of metastases in distant sites. Therefore, effective systemic therapy with drugs is needed to cure most cancers.

Relationship of Growth Fraction to Chemotherapy

Figure 32 presents the cell cycle. Every cell that divides passes through specific phases before undergoing mitosis. During the S phase, lasting from six to fifty hours, DNA synthesis increases and chromosomal material doubles. Thereafter the cell proceeds through the G_2 phase, lasting about six hours, during which time a series of biochemical

events occur that prepare the cell for mitosis. After mitosis, new cells enter the G_1 phase. Depending on the cells involved, G_1 may last minutes or years. Cells progressing through G_1, S, G_2 and mitosis are said to be "in cycle." Cells not actively dividing are said to be in G_0 phase.

Figure 32
The cell cycle.

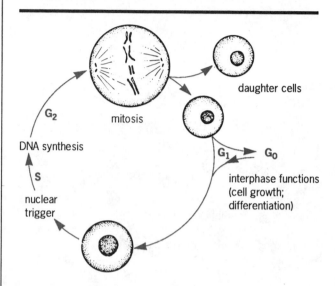

Every tissue, whether normal or neoplastic, has a portion of its cells that are not actively dividing. They can be found side-by-side with dividing cells. The number of cells in cycle divided by the total number of cells in the tissue is the **growth fraction.** The growth fraction does not remain constant. Larger tumors have smaller growth fractions. If the size of the tumor is reduced, either by surgery, radiotherapy or antineoplastic drugs, more resting cells begin to cycle.

Cells in cycle $\rightleftharpoons$ Resting cells

Anticancer drugs are more effective against proliferating cells than cells in G_0 because antineoplastic agents usually kill cells by disrupting either DNA synthesis or mitosis, functions that occur only in proliferating cells. Thus as a general rule, antineoplastic drugs are much more toxic to tissues that have a high growth fraction than to tissues whose growth fraction is low. Solid tumors, e.g., solid tumors of the lung, breast, stomach, colon and rectum, have a low growth fraction and often respond poorly to anticancer drugs. Disseminated tumors, e.g., leukemias and lymphomas, have a high growth fraction and generally respond well to antineoplastic drugs.

Chemotherapy against cancer that employs a combination of drugs is considerably more effective than therapy with just one drug. The benefits of **combination therapy** are (a) suppression of drug resistance, (b) enhancement of therapeutic effects and (c) reduced injury to normal cells. If several drugs are selected, with different mechanisms of action, drug resistance occurs less frequently and more malignant cells are killed. Furthermore, so long as drugs are selected that do not have overlapping toxicities, oncologists can extend anticancer action beyond that which might be safely achieved using any one of the chemicals alone.

Classification of Antineoplastic Drugs Based on the Cell Cycle

Antineoplastics are characterized as **cell-cycle-independent** if they affect cells during any phase of the cycle, including resting or G_0 cells, or **cell-cycle-dependent,** if they affect only cells that are actively cycling at the time of exposure to drugs. Anticancer drugs may also be **phase-dependent** if one specific phase of the cycle is the principal site of drug action. For example, vincristine and vinblastine block mitosis and are considered phase-dependent drugs.

Classification of Antineoplastic Drugs Based on Mechanism of Action

Although it useful to classify drugs in relation to the cell cycle, it is more practical to categorize them in terms of their mechanisms of action. This system for the classification is described below.

Alkylating Agents

Alkylating agents are a heterogeneous group of drugs. They include nitrogen mustard, melphalan, cyclophosphamide, chlorambucil, busulphan, bischloroethyl nitrosourea (BCNU), chloroethyl-cyclohexyl nitrosourea (CCNU), methyl-CCNU and cisplatin. These drugs contain chloroalkyl groups (CH_2Ch_2Cl) that combine with a variety of biologically important molecules. Their most important targets are the pyrimidine and purine bases in DNA. By attaching to components of DNA molecules, alkylating agents inhibit separation or produce abnormal separation of DNA during cell division, leading to cell death.

Antimetabolites

Methotrexate, 5-fluorouracil (5-FU), cytosine arabinoside, 6-mercaptopurine (6-MP), 6-thioguanine and hydroxyurea are synthetic drugs that act as inhibitors of critical biochemical pathways in the formation of DNA, or as abnormal substitutes for naturally occurring nucleic acid bases, resulting in the formation of abnormal DNA. These drugs are usually cycle-dependent and affect both tumor cells and rapidly dividing normal cells. Exactly why these drugs are called antimetabolites can best be illustrated by referring to the actions of just one of the agents. Methotrexate is similar in structure to folic acid. It is an antimetabolite of folic acid and competes with dihydrofolate (a naturally occurring folate) for binding to the enzyme dihydrofolate reductase. This enzyme plays a pivotal role in the transfer of single-carbon units that are necessary in DNA and purine biosynthesis. Because methotrexate replaces dihydrofolate on dihydrofolate reductase, it competitively inhibits this enzyme, stops DNA synthesis and decreases purine biosynthesis.

Antitumor Antibiotics

Doxorubicin, daunorubicin, bleomycin, mitomycin-C and actinomycin-D are cytotoxic compounds produced by micro-organisms. All of these drugs were originally isolated from strains of streptomyces. In all cases, the antitumor antibiotics produce their cytotoxic effects through direct interaction with DNA.

Mitotic Inhibitors

Vinblastine (Velben) and vincristine (Oncovin), vinca alkaloids derived from the *Vinca rosea* plant (periwinkle), disorganize the mitotic spindle and arrest cell division. Obviously, these drugs are phase-dependent agents.

Hormones

Estrogens, progestins, androgens and corticosteroids are used in the treatment of various cancers. Estrogens are employed in the treatment of prostatic cancer and in the management of five-year postmenopausal breast tumors. Androgens are sometimes given to premenopausal patients with mammary cancer. Progestins are used on occasion to treat kidney and endometrial carcinomas. Corticosteroids, particularly prednisone, are administered in high doses to patients with lymphomas and some other cancers.

The rationale behind the use of these drugs is the belief that some cancers are hormone dependent. If, for example, a prostatic cancer is androgen dependent, treatment with estrogens, together with castration, is reasonable. The converse is also true. If breast cancer in premenopausal patients is estrogen dependent, the use of androgens makes sense. Corticosteroids induce a regression of lymphoid tissue by causing a breakdown of existing lymphocytes and inhibiting the production of new lymphocytes. The biochemical mechanism behind these actions is not clear.

Tamoxifen (Nolvadex) competitively blocks estrogen receptors. Certain forms of cancer, notably breast cancer in premenopausal women, often depend on endogenous estrogens for growth. When given in high doses, tamoxifen prevents endogenous estrogens from stimulating their receptors and significantly reduces cancer growth.

Leuprolide (Lupron) is a synthetic derivative of gonadotropin-releasing hormone (GnRH). It is used to treat advanced carcinoma of the prostate. For patients with prostatic cancer, leuprolide is an alternative to castration or estrogen therapy. Although the drug does not alter the course of the disease, leuprolide does offer palliation.

Goserelin acetate (Zoladex) is also a synthetic analog of GnRH. Administered chronically, goserelin inhibits gonadotropin production, resulting in gonadal and accessory sex organ regression. Goserelin is indicated for the palliative treatment of patients with hormone-dependent advanced carcinoma of the prostate.

Miscellaneous Antineoplastics

Asparaginase (Elspar, Kidrolase) is an enzyme extracted from cultures of *Escherichia coli*. It converts asparagine to aspartic acid. Certain cancers are unable to make asparagine and are dependent on the blood bringing them adequate amounts. In the absence of asparagine, because of its hydrolysis to aspartic acid, they cannot proliferate. Asparaginase is not toxic to normal cells, which have the ability to synthesize asparagine. Asparaginase appears to act selectively during the G_1 phase of the cell cycle.

Procarbazine (Matulane, Natulan) is converted to its active metabolite in the liver of the patient. Following activation, it can cause chromosomal damage and suppress DNA, RNA and protein synthesis.

Adverse Effects of Antineoplastic Drugs

Antineoplastic drugs are cellular poisons. They kill both malignant and normal cells. The selective toxicity seen with antibiotics, antifungals, antivirals and anthelmintics, in which the drug attacks preferentially the microbe, fungus, virus or worm, leaving the host cells largely unaffected, is not seen with antineoplastics. For example, a drug that blocks DNA or RNA synthesis and/or function will damage both normal and malignant cells. This is particularly true for cell-cycle-independent drugs. Cell-cycle-dependent drugs will also damage both normal and neoplastic tissue, but these agents show a selectivity for tissues with the highest percentage of cells "in cycle." This means that they can kill both cancer cells and normal cells (e.g., bone marrow, gastrointestinal tract, hair) with a rapid turnover rate. They also damage the immune system of the body, with the consequence that the production of both T- and B-lymphocytes falls.

The hematopoietic system is particularly at risk when antineoplastic drugs are administered. Patients often show pancytopenia as the production of red cells, white cells and platelets falls. The decrease in platelets predisposes patients to hemorrhage. A decrease in neutrophils, together with the fall in B- and T-lymphocytes, places patients at risk with respect to infections.

The mucosal cells of hollow organs normally have a rapid rate of turnover. By inhibiting cell duplication, antineoplastics damage the gastrointestinal and genitourinary tracts. This can lead to ulceration and bleeding.

Antineoplastic treatment is perhaps most obvious when one looks at the hair and nails of patients receiving therapy. Alopecia and baldness are common adverse effects.

Antineoplastics increase tissue breakdown, raising both the purine load and the production of uric acid. If the uric acid concentration increases above 12 mg/100 mL (750 μmol/L) of blood, kidney damage can occur. Allopurinol (Zyloprim) blocks xanthine oxidase, thereby decreasing uric acid production. It is often administered to patients receiving antineoplastics to decrease uric acid formation. Care must be taken when it is used together with 6-mercaptopurine, because this latter drug is metabolized by xanthine oxidase. Lower doses of 6-mercaptopurine must be used to compensate for the reduced rate of inactivation.

Vinca alkaloids interfere with the microtubular structures important in nerve cell function. As a result, they can produce significant nerve damage. Some drugs, notably busulphan, can cause pulmonary fibrosis.

Nausea and vomiting are often experienced by patients receiving anticancer drugs. It is particularly pronounced with cisplatin (Platinol). Phenothiazines, usually effective as antinauseants, are often of little value in treating antineoplastic-induced emesis. Metoclopramide (Maxeran, Reglan) increases gastric emptying and is often very helpful in reducing nausea and vomiting due to anticancer drugs.

Doxorubicin (Adriamycin) and daunomycin (Cerubidine) can cause dose-dependent cardiac arrhythmias and, eventually, heart failure. This danger is minimized by reducing their dosages. These drugs are red dyes and can produce red urine. To prevent alarm, patients should be informed of this fact.

Procarbazine (Natulan) is metabolized to a monoamine oxidase inhibitor. It can produce a variety of central nervous system effects. Patients should be warned to refrain from eating or drinking foods containing tyramine. The toxicities of monoamine oxidase inhibitors are explained in Chapter 45.

Caution should be taken in the intravenous administration of dactinomycin (Cosmegen), cytosine arabinoside (Cytosar), nitrogen mustards and vinca alkaloids. Extravasation of these drugs can cause tissue damage.

Nursing Process

It is beyond the scope of this text to discuss in detail the complete nursing care for cancer patients. This section deals only with the nursing process related to the use of antineoplastic drugs. Readers are referred to a medical-surgical or oncological nursing text for a comprehensive discussion of other aspects of oncological nursing care.

Assessment

Nursing assessment of patients prior to the administration of antineoplastic agents should include a review with the patient of the complete treatment regimen. Nurses should ask the patient to specify his or her learning needs and then provide appropriate written information regarding the management of adverse effects.

Administration

Administration of these drugs must occur in compliance with local policies and procedures designed to promote patient and staff safety. In many institutions, this means that only physicians or chemotherapy-certified nurses administer these medications, particularly those given intravenously. Intravenous antineoplastics must be prepared in a laminar flow hood or according to Workers Compensation Board standards.

Administration of antineoplastics should be accompanied by a daily fluid intake of 2 – 3 L of fluid to prevent dehydration due to vomiting, promote adequate urinary output for excretion of the drug, and prevent adverse renal effects such as hyperuricemia. Providing a small amount of bland food in advance of the oral administration of these drugs may alleviate some of the nausea and gastric irritation and prevent vomiting. Prophylactic use of antiemetics or a regular schedule of antiemetics is recommended for a period of twenty-four to forty-eight hours post-treatment.

Evaluation

Nurses caring for patients receiving these drugs should be alert for vomiting shortly after the administration of oral preparations. Emesis should be inspected to determine the approximate amount of unabsorbed medication.

Intravenous infusions should be monitored for swelling, induration, redness, pain or burning at the infusion site. These observations indicate extravasation of the infusion and should result in immediate discontinuation of the infusion and restarting at another site.

Patients should report any fever to their nurse or physician as soon as possible. Alteration in the patient's fluid intake/output ratio may indicate adverse renal effects. Observation of sore throat, fatigue, fever, petechiae, bruising or bleeding gums suggest hematologic effects. Cough and dyspnea in association with fever suggest pulmonary fibrosis. Joint pain in the lower extremities indicates hyperuricemia. Jaundice, manifested by yellowing of the skin and sclera, enlarged liver, tea-colored urine, clay-colored stools, abdominal pain and pruritus is characteristic of hepatotoxicity. Headache, dizziness, fatigue, disorientation, parasthesias and slurred speech suggest central nervous system toxicity. Loss of sensation or tingling of the face or extremities and loss of taste are associated with peripheral neuropathy. A rash indicates the development of allergic dermatitis. Patients who develop hematemesis or tarry stools are suspected of having ulceration of the gastrointestinal tract.

Teaching
Patient teaching by nurses is aimed at assisting the individual to tolerate the course of therapy. Patients should be instructed in modifications to oral hygiene and diet to reduce discomfort. These include the use of a soft-bristled toothbrush or a water pic, a mild antiseptic mouthwash for rinsing the mouth at regular intervals and a soft bland diet. This diet will prevent mechanical trauma and irritation often caused by the ingestion of spicy, acidic or abrasive foods. In addition, it may diminish nausea and vomiting often associated with antineoplastic chemotherapy.

Patients should be reassured that alopecia and baldness resulting from therapy is temporary and that hair will regrow following termination of treatment. Nurses should also advise patients that the effects of these drugs linger for several weeks following the end of chemotherapy treatment. Also, during this period they should seek medical advice before using any over-the-counter medications. Nurses should ensure that their patients are prepared for the eventuality that treatment with antineoplastics may result in permanent sterility.

Further Reading

Antineoplastic agents (1986). *AMA Drug Evaluations,* 6th ed. Chicago: American Medical Association, pp. 1167-1224.

Camp-Sorrell, D. (1991). Controlling the adverse effects of chemotherapy. *Nursing 21* (4):34-41.

Crawley, M.M. (1990). Recent advances in chemotherapy: Administration and nursing implications. *Nursing Clinics of North America 25* (2):377-391.

Creaton, E., Leonard, F.E. and Day, A.L. (1991). A hospital-based chemotherapy education and training program. *Cancer Nursing 14* (2):79-90.

Drugs of choice for cancer chemotherapy (1991). *The Medical Letter 33* :21-28.

Erlichman C. (1987). The pharmacology of anticancer drugs. In: Tarnock, I.F. and Hill, R.P., eds., *The Basic Science of Oncology.* Toronto: Pergamon Press, pp. 292-307.

Holland, J.F. and Frei, E. III (1982). *Cancer Medicine,* 2nd ed. Philadelphia: Lea and Febiger.

Nursing, Pharmacology and the Law

The use of drugs is strictly controlled by law. In this, our last section of the book, we present an overview of the laws controlling the prescribing and handling of drugs. We are most fortunate in having Dr. A.J. Remillard as the author of Chapter 73. Dr. Remillard is an Associate Professor in Clinical Pharmacy in the College of Pharmacy, University of Saskatchewan. His extensive professional experience in both the United States and Canada ideally suits him to write this most important chapter dealing with the legal responsibilities of nurses in the handling and control of drugs.

CHAPTER 73

Legal Implications Related to the Pharmacologic Aspects of Nursing Practice

by A.J. Remillard, Pharm. D.

A drug is defined as "any substance used in the diagnosis, treatment, mitigation, or prevention of a disease, disorder, or abnormal physical state and in restoring, correcting, or modifying organic function in man or animal" (1).

By this definition, it is quite clear that drugs are potent chemicals, capable of causing as much harm as good. Their use must therefore be controlled. The availability of drugs is governed by their safety and efficacy, their potential for abuse and the amount of professional consultation required for their appropriate use.

Drugs are a very diverse group of compounds. At one end of the spectrum, aspirin or acetylsalicylic acid (ASA) can provide relief of minor pain and be purchased over the counter. At the other is lysergic acid diethylamide (LSD), a substance with no known medicinal use and available only to research institutions on authorization from the Food and Drug Administration in the United States or the Health Protection Branch in Canada.

Physicians, pharmacists and nurses are important in controlling and monitoring drug use. The extent of their involvement depends on the safety of the products concerned. Safe drugs are widely available and require minimal supervision. Drugs with a greater potential for abuse are usually available only on prescription, and require the assistance of a health professional to ensure their safe and effective use.

Federal laws in both Canada and the United States regulate the availability of drugs. Provincial or state laws may supplement federal laws and further restrict the distribution of a drug. For example, federal laws in Canada do not classify digoxin as a prescription product. However, various provincial acts have placed digoxin on the prescription list within their respective provincial borders. Provincial or state laws may not remove a drug from the prescription list if it has been placed there by federal authority.

In general, there are two categories of medications: those that require and those that do not require a prescription. The latter group is referred to as nonprescription or over-the-counter drugs. Prescription drugs themselves represent a diversified group, ranging from those prescribed and refilled over the telephone (e.g., antihypertensive drugs) to those requiring a written prescription with no allowance for refills (e.g., potent narcotics).

Canadian Drug Regulations

Drug Laws

Drug laws evolved for the purpose of ensuring the safe and effective use of drugs. They control both the quality of drugs placed on the market and their use in the community. In Canada, the Food and Drug Act and the Narcotic Control Act form the basis of drug laws. The Health Protection Branch, which is part of the Department of National Health and Welfare, is responsible for administering these acts.

The Inland Revenue Act of 1875 was the first drug act introduced in Canada. It dealt specifically with the adulteration of alcohol. In 1953, after many revisions, the Food and Drug Act became law. This act presently controls the manufacture, distribution and sale of all drugs except narcotics.

The Opium Act of 1908 prohibited the unauthorized importation and possession of gum and smoking of opium. This was the first act of the present-day Narcotic Control Act (1961) which controls the manufacture, distribution and sale of narcotic drugs.

Nonprescription Drugs

Nonprescription drugs can be obtained without a medical prescription. In Canada there are three groups of nonprescription medications.

The first group includes **proprietary medicines** and may be purchased in any retail outlet. They are effective for the treatment of self-limited minor illness, injury or discomfort. Generally, the directions for proper use are clearly indicated on the package, and the advice of a health professional is not required. Examples of proprietary medicines are some minor pain relievers, medicated shampoos, and cough drops.

The second group of drugs includes those available mainly in pharmacies and commonly referred to as **over-the-counter medications.** These agents are also intended for the treatment of self-limiting problems but may require the advice of a health professional to ensure their proper use. Examples of such drugs include laxatives, cough and cold medicines, and vitamins.

The third group is the smallest. It consists of **medications available only in the pharmacy** and to be used only upon the advice and recommendation of a physician. Insulin, nitroglycerin and muscle relaxants are examples of such medicines. Also included in this category are medications that can be purchased only if the pharmacist dispenses the drug personally after consulting with the patient. These drugs must be placed so as to limit public access. Examples include analgesic compounds containing low doses of codeine (e.g., 222s).

Prescription Drugs (Schedule F)

Many drugs require a prescription. A prescription is an order given by a practitioner directing that a stated amount of a drug be dispensed for the person named in the order. Drugs for humans are available on prescription if the conditions they treat require the diagnosis and medical management of a physician or dentist.

All prescription drugs are listed in Schedule F of the Food and Drug Regulation and must be identified by the symbol **Pr** on their labels. More than two hundred drugs, representing a wide diver-

sity of classes including antibiotics, antihypertensives, hormones and psychotropic medications, are listed in this schedule. Schedule F is frequently revised as new drugs are discovered. Nonprescription drugs may be transferred to Schedule F if new hazards are uncovered.

Controlled Drugs (Schedule G)

Controlled drugs are listed in Schedule G of the Food and Drug Act. Controlled drugs have mood-modifying effects and can be habit forming. Like drugs listed in Schedule F, chemicals placed in Schedule G also require a prescription. However, greater control is exercised over their use because of their abuse potential. The symbol ⊘ must appear on labels and all professional advertisements. Schedule G includes some narcotic analgesics (nalbuphine, butorphanol), amphetamines and related stimulants, and barbiturates (e.g., phenobarbital, ambobarbital, secobarbital). Anxiolytics, such as the benzodiazepines, have a lower potential for abuse and are not controlled drugs. They are found in Schedule F.

Narcotic Drugs

Narcotic drugs are controlled by the Narcotic Control Act and Regulations. This schedule includes derivatives of the coca leaf (cocaine), opiates and opium derivatives (morphine, codeine, hydromorphone, methadone and meperidine), phencyclidine, and cannabis (marijuana). Drugs classified legally as narcotics have potent psychotropic and addictive properties. This has led to stringent restrictions on their availability. The letter **N** must appear on all labels and professional advertisements.

Among the narcotics, only codeine can be purchased without a prescription. To qualify for nonprescription status, codeine must be combined with at least two additional drugs and contain no more than 8 mg of codeine per tablet, or 20 mg per 28 mL of oral solution. These codeine-containing products are known as **narcotic preparations.**

Restricted Drugs (Schedule H)

These substances have no recognized medicinal properties, have hallucinogenic properties and are dangerous. There are about twenty-three chemicals listed in Schedule H of the Food and Drug Act. Examples include LSD, peyote and mescaline.

Distribution of Drugs

As one progresses from nonprescription drugs to narcotic drugs, the distribution of these agents becomes more restrictive. Schedule F medications (prescription drugs) can be obtained by written or oral (i.e., verbal telephone order) prescription and may be refilled as often as indicated by the physician. Schedule G drugs (controlled drugs) can also be prescribed in written or oral format, but may be refilled only if indicated on a written prescription. Narcotic agents can be dispensed only according to a written prescription and cannot be refilled (i.e., they require a new written prescription every time).

Hospital and retail pharmacies are required by law to keep records of all narcotics received and dispensed. Although there are some federal regulations on the distribution of controlled drugs, the provinces dictate how much record keeping is necessary.

United States Drug Regulations

The Food, Drug and Cosmetic Act contains the basic laws relating to food and drugs in the United States and is enforced by the Food and Drug Administration. The Controlled Substances Act is enforced by the Drug Enforcement Administration, which is part of the United States Justice Department.

Drug Laws

The Import Drugs Act of 1848 was the first federal statute enacted to ensure drug quality. The act was initiated when adulterated quinine from Mexico was administered to American army troops suffering from malaria. The Food and Drug Act of 1906 required that drugs marketed for interstate commerce meet minimal standards of strength, purity, quality and proper labeling.

Revision of the act in 1938 was precipitated by the death of many patients who had used elixir of sulfanilamide containing toxic ethylene glycol. The Federal Food, Drug and Cosmetic Act required that drugs entering interstate commerce and sold in the United States must also meet standards of safety for human use.

The Durham-Humphrey Amendment of 1951 determined whether a drug should be available as a prescription or nonprescription product. The Kefauver-Harris Amendment of 1962 required that products need proof of safety and efficacy. This applied to all products entering the market after 1938. This amendment also enforced tighter control, testing and marketing of new drugs.

The Comprehensive Drug Abuse Prevention and Control Act of 1970 regulates the manufacture, distribution and dispensing of controlled substances.

Nonprescription Drugs

Nonprescription or over-the-counter (OTC) medicines must be safe and effective. Safety is defined as a low potential for adverse drug effects causing harm which may result from abuse under conditions of widespread availability. Efficacy implies reasonable expectation of clinically significant relief in the majority of the population.

All nonprescription drugs in the United States can be purchased at any retail outlet. At present there are no categories of OTC that are restricted to pharmacy-only sales. For many years there have been attempts to create a "third class of drugs" that could be sold only in a pharmacy without the prescriber's order. However, the authority to create such a class of agents would require amendments to the Food, Drug and Cosmetic Act by Congress. In 1985 the State of Florida took the initiative and found a way to overcome the federal law restriction. Pharmacists in that state may, after extensive consultation with the consumer, dispense medications from a limited formulary. The formulary lists medications previously requiring a prescription. Some examples include antihistamines, lindane, keratolytics and anthelmintics.

Prescription Drugs

As a result of the Durham-Humphrey Amendment, a class of agents was developed requiring the use of a prescription. A drug is placed on the prescription list if it is (1) habit-forming, (2) not safe for self-medication because of its toxicity, potential for harmful effects or method of administration, or (3) a "new drug" that has not been shown to be safe and is restricted to prescription-only status by the FDA when it issues the New Drug Application.

The purpose of these restrictions is to ensure safe use by the general public and adequate supervision by a licensed practitioner. Prescription drugs, also known as "legend drugs," require that their label bear the following statement: "Caution — Federal law prohibits dispensing without a prescription." Examples of legend or prescription drugs include antibiotics, antihypertensives and steroid medications.

Controlled Drugs

The Controlled Substances Act of 1971 supersedes most previous narcotic and drug abuse control laws. The act categorizes drugs into five schedules according to their potential for abuse.

Schedule I

Drugs in this schedule have a high potential for abuse and for the most part no accepted medical use in the United States. Schedule I contains certain opiates and opium derivatives, such as heroin. It also contains the hallucinogens LSD, cannabis, peyote and mescaline. The FDA has authorized the use of marijuana for treatment of glaucoma, and vomiting secondary to cancer chemotherapy.

Controlled substances require symbols located in the upper right-hand corner of the label. Schedule I drugs are identified by the symbols Ⓒ or I.

Schedule II

Drugs in this category also have a high potential for abuse. In contradistinction to the chemicals listed in Schedule I, drugs in Schedule II have a currently accepted medical use. These are agents that, if abused, may lead to severe psychological or physical dependence. Schedule II includes opiates and opium derivatives (morphine, codeine, methadone and meperidine), derivatives of coca leaves (cocaine), and certain central nervous system stimulants (amphetamines, methylphenidate). All drugs in this class are labeled Ⓒ or II.

Schedule III

Drugs in Schedule III have an accepted medical use and perhaps a lower potential for abuse than those in Schedules I or II. This category contains narcotic and non-narcotic drugs not listed in other schedules. Examples are glutethimide and nalorphine. Schedule III agents are labeled Ⓒ or III.

Schedule IV

Schedule IV drugs have a lower potential for abuse than those of Schedule III. However, abuse of these agents may still lead to limited physical or psychological dependence. This group includes long-acting barbiturates (phenobarbital), certain hypnotics (chloral hydrate) and minor tranquilizers (all benzodiazepines and meprobamate). All are labeled Ⓒ or IV.

Schedule V

Drugs in Schedule V have the lowest potential for abuse of all controlled substances. They include preparations containing limited quantities of certain narcotics for antitussive and antidiarrheal purposes. Although some items in Schedule V are considered OTC but restricted to pharmacies only, most states have placed these drugs on the prescription list.

Distribution

All prescription or legend drugs can be dispensed by oral (i.e., telephone) or written prescription with no restriction on the number of refills or repeats. Many states include Schedule V drugs under the same regulations. Schedule III and IV drugs can be obtained by written or oral prescription. The prescription cannot be filled or refilled six months after the date of issue, and the maximum number of repeats allowed is six. Schedule II agents can be dispensed only with a written prescription and no refills are allowed.

Nursing Practice and the Drug Laws

We have reviewed the many drug acts and regulations that constitute the drug laws in Canada and the United States. The next issue is how these apply to nursing practice. Nursing practice is regulated not only by drug standards and legislation, but also by individual state or provincial nursing practice acts. The three areas deserving review are drug prescribing, drug administration and drug distribution.

Drug Prescribing

Kinkela summarized drug laws best: the physician prescribes, the pharmacist dispenses and the nurse administers (2). Prescribing of medications is exclusively a medical function. However, in remote areas where there is a shortage of physicians, some provinces or states may permit limited prescribing by nurse practitioners.

Although it is common for community nurses to authorize refilling prescriptions, this practice is illegal by most state and provincial statutes, even if the nurse is acting on direct orders of the physician. This method of relaying the message to the pharmacist constitutes "prescribing" by the nurse, and only licensed practitioners can prescribe.

Drug Administration

Drug administration is an accepted role for the nurse. Three conditions must be met before a nurse may legally administer medication. These are: (1) the medication order must be valid, (2) the physician and nurse must be licensed, and (3) the nurse must know the purpose, actions, effects and major side effects of the drug.

A valid order leaves no room for doubt. It must include the name of the medication, its dose, the route of administration and the prescriber's signature. The law requires that a nurse check a drug order only with the prescribing physician when faced with a question, doubt or apparent error in the order. The nurse has a moral, ethical and legal responsibility to ensure that the order is appropriate for the patient. It is the right of a nurse to refuse to give a medication if he or she feels it is inappropriate. The physician assumes full responsibility if he or she administers the medication personally.

The following case illustrates the importance of a valid order. A nursing supervisor helped her busy nursing staff by administering some medications. An order for 3 mL of digoxin was prescribed for a three-month-old baby. Since the supervisor was familiar with only the injectable formulations, she questioned the high dose with other nurses and finally with a physician consultant, who stated that if that was what the doctor ordered that was what he meant to give. She then proceeded to give the child 3 mL of injectable digoxin instead of the elixir, resulting in a digoxin dose about five times that intended. An hour later the baby died, and the family successfully recovered damages from the nurse and doctor.

Administration of Intravenous Medication

The function of giving medications directly into the vein has been primarily reserved for the physician. Although nurses have been given the freedom to administer large-volume intravenous infusions, the administration of small-volume, undiluted medications by direct intravenous push or into intravenous tubing places the nurse in a tenuous legal position. Since such procedures are potentially more risky, policies should be drawn up jointly by the administration of the hospital and nursing representatives. These policy statements must carefully delineate the roles of nurses and physicians, and present guidelines for their procedure. They should include a list of drugs and routes of administration to be used only by physicians and a list of criteria for permitting nurses to give medicines intravenously. In a life-threatening situation, any drug can be administered intravenously under physician supervision.

Once the policy for administering intravenous medications has been approved, the nurse must know the following information about the drug prior to proceeding with the order: dose and route of administration including rate, desired therapeutic effect, possible side effects, incompatibilities and patient allergies.

Drug Dispensing

In the hospital, the nurse must be careful to differentiate between drug administration and drug dispensing to avoid violation of the Pharmacy Practice Act. The act states that dispensing of medication is a function of a licensed pharmacist. It is generally agreed that it is legal for a nurse to take one dose of a drug for a particular patient from a pharmacy-prepackaged, properly labeled medication container at the nurses' station, since this constitutes drug administration. On the other hand, it is not legal for a nurse to fill or refill a container from the nurses' station, or any other container, with the drug specified because such an act is dispensing and may be performed legally only by a pharmacist.

The following acts are specifically *prohibited* by federal laws and apply to the nurse's handling of all prescription drugs.
1. Compounding or dispensing the designated drugs except by authorized parties for legal distribution and administration.
2. Distributing the drugs to any person who is not licensed or authorized by law to receive them.

Although the Pharmacy Act is clear in defining who is authorized to dispense, any experienced nurse who has worked in remote areas or where pharmacy service is limited can testify to the lack of adequate provisions for the act. Most will agree that in a situation where a pharmacist is not immediately available, a nurse may provide sufficient medications as ordered by the physician to cover such time that the services of a pharmacist are not available.

Consistent with the drug laws and Kinkela's summary on drug distribution, the physician may prescribe, dispense and administer ad lib. When a nurse is faced with a situation where he or she has to dispense a limited quantity of medication, it would seem reasonable to have the prescribing physician check that the proper drug has been given out and that the dose and instruction on the label are correct. This procedure would not contravene the Pharmacy Act. If this situation occurred frequently, it would be in the best interest of the nurse to become familiar with the basic aspects of pharmacy distribution, such as dispensing and labeling.

In remote areas, a registered nurse may have to assume responsibility for the pharmacy. In such cases, written policies need to be developed by administration, nursing and medical representatives of the institution for legal protection of the nurse and patient. It may be advisable to have these policies approved by the respective provincial or state professional associations in nursing and pharmacy. Once the policies have been adopted, the nurse should receive additional preparation and education in pharmacy practice, such as inventory and storage control, method of labeling drugs, and method of narcotic control. A periodic visit by a licensed pharmacist is recommended to ensure that all procedures and operations accord with accepted standards of practice.

Controlled and Narcotic Substances

Every practising nurse encounters situations that require knowledge of, or familiarity with, controlled or narcotic substances. Federal and provincial or state laws dealing with those substances are complex, but it is important for each nurse to know his or her responsibilities and limitations under the regulation.

The Narcotic Control Act in Canada and the Controlled Substances Act in the United States were enacted to improve the administration and regulation of the manufacturing, distribution and dispensing of these substances. They provide a closed system of distribution for legitimate handling of the drugs. The purpose of this system is to reduce the widespread diversion of these drugs from legitimate channels to the illicit market.

Only authorized persons can be in possession of a narcotic or controlled substance. Legal possession by a nurse is limited to the following situations:
1. When a drug is administered to a patient on the order of a physician. The nurse is then acting as an agent for the practitioner.
2. When the nurse is acting as the official custodian of narcotics in the hospital or clinic.
3. When the nurse is a patient for whom a physician has prescribed narcotics.

Federal and provincial or state laws make the possession of controlled or narcotic substances a crime except for the above specified cases. The laws make no distinction between professional and practical nurses in regard to possession of controlled drugs. Violating or failure to comply with the act is punishable by fine, imprisonment, or both.

Nursing Procedure and Controlled Substances

Unlike simple prescription drugs, certain rules for controlled drugs have been accepted in most hospitals. A **p.r.n. order** (*pro re nata,* or "as required") for narcotics must be rewritten every seventy-two hours. A **standing order** (i.e,. drug dose administered by the nurse for the physician without first obtaining a signed order) is not permitted for narcotic drugs. In an emergency situation, a **verbal order** is permitted if the nurse documents the nature of the emergency in the chart and the physician validates the order within twenty-four hours.

When a narcotic drug is administered to a patient the nurse must record the date, time of administration, patient's name, physician's name, and signature of the nurse. When a dose of a narcotic is refused by the patient, it should be placed in the sewage system in the presence of a witness. If a dose of the drug is contaminated or wasted, the nurse should make an entry in the records book explaining how the dose was disposed of, and the entry should be signed by a witness.

All controlled substances stored at nursing stations must be kept in locked cabinets so that only authorized personnel have access to them.

Sources of Drug Errors

Many drug distribution systems have been developed to minimize drug errors. However, in a busy hospital that may be short staffed, drug errors are not uncommon. Errors are minimized when the order is written by the physician. In this situation, the nurse acts as a safeguard as he or she interprets the order. If it does not look right or is incomplete, it can be corrected by contacting the physician. The most common sources of drug errors are telephone orders and transcribing orders.

Telephone Orders

Telephone orders constitute a real problem for nurses in a number of situations. The nurse accepting the telephone order often may not read it back to the physician to make sure it is correct after writing it down. The nurse must ensure that the physician signs the order the next day. Telephone orders should be limited to emergencies. The use of telephone orders in nonemergency situations acts as a substitute for the physician examining the patient. This can lead to serious errors and may border on malpractice.

Transcribing Orders

In many hospitals, ward secretaries or clerks transcribe orders. It is important that these staff be thoroughly instructed in transcribing the order as it is written by the physician. Although ward clerks are liable for their own errors, there is a common requirement that the transcribed order be countersigned by a professional nurse. If the nurse countersigns an order incorrectly transcribed, he or she is liable for error along with the clerk.

Product Liability

Although manufacturers are liable for injury caused by defects in their products, nurses should be alert to defects in the drugs they administer. Detection of chemical defects is beyond the nurse's responsibility, but detection of observable physical defects is not. Nurses should be keenly aware of the proper physical characteristics of drugs they administer. Discoloration or improper consistency of tablets, capsules, liquids, or precipitates or foreign bodies in parenteral fluids, should be considered suspect and be referred to the pharmacist.

Drug Information Sources

Many good reference books provide excellent drug information. They are helpful for double-checking doses, rates of administration, drug interactions and side effects. They can be used to clarify orders and avoid drug errors. However, they should never be used as a substitute for contacting the prescribing physician. The most popular texts are the *American Hospital Formulary Service* (*AHFS*), the *United States Pharmacopeial Drug Information* (*USP DI*), and the *Physician's Desk Reference* (*PDR*) in the United States, and the *Compendium of Pharmaceuticals and Specialties* (*CPS*) in Canada. All of these reference sources are continually being reviewed and revised on an annual basis.

The *AHFS* is published by the American Society of Hospital Pharmacy and it is updated with four supplements yearly. The volume contains monographs on every drug available in the United States. The *USP DI*, published by the United States Pharmacopeial Convention Inc., comprises drug monographs from both the United States and Canada. It also is updated throughout the year with supplements.

The *PDR* and *CPS* are very similar and contain a list of drug monographs. Both contain a limited product-recognition section with colored illustrations of medications for identification purposes. The *PDR* is published by the Medical Economics Co. Inc. and is intended primarily for physicians, although it is available at most public book stores. The *CPS* is compiled and produced by the Canadian Pharmaceutical Association for the benefit of all health professionals. It can be purchased only through the Association or at health-professional book stores.

Conclusion

The nursing profession is a challenging and interesting career. Along with the responsibilities of providing safe and effective medical care, the nurse also has a major responsibility in the administration of medications. The nurse must be familiar not only with the ethical and moral issues surrounding the administration of drugs, but the legal issues as well.

References

1. *Health Protection and Drug Laws* (1983). Ottawa: Health and Welfare Canada, Canadian Government Publishing Centre.
2. Gulysassy-Kinkely, G. and Kinkela, R.V. (1973). Dispensing drugs: A professional nurse's responsibility? *J. Nurs. Admin.* 7 (1).

Further Reading

Angorn, R. and McCormick, W. (1986). The pharmacist as a limited prescriber: The liability factor. *U.S. Pharmacist 11* :30.

Creighton, H. (1981). *Law Every Nurse Should Know,* 4th ed. Philadelphia: W.B. Saunders.

Fink, J. and Simonsmeler, L. (1985). Laws governing pharmacy. Chapter 107 in: A. Gennaro, ed., *Remington's Pharmaceutical Sciences,* 17th ed. Easton, PA: Mack.

Strauss, S. and Sherman, M. (1985). A capsulated history of drug laws in the U.S. *U.S. Pharmacist 10* :11.

United States Pharmacopeia, 21st rev. Rockville, MD: U.S. Pharmacopeial Convention.

Table 107
Drug schedules.

United States Category	Symbol on Labels	Canada Category	Symbol on Labels	Examples	
Prescription (Legend)	*	Schedule F (Food & Drug Regulations)	Pr	Antibiotics Antihypertensives Hormonal products	Can. only: Benzodiazepines U.S. only: Nalbuphine Butorphanol
† Schedule I	Ⓘ or I	Schedule H (Food & Drug Act)	—	Peyote LSD Mescaline	U.S. only: Heroin Cannabis
Schedule II	Ⓘ or II	Narcotics (Narcotic Act)	N	Morphine Codeine Methadone	Can. only: Heroin Cannabis Pentazocine U.S. only: Amphetamine Short-acting barbiturates
Schedule III	Ⓘ or III	Control (Schedule G, Food & Drug Act)	Ⓒ	Butalbital preparations Chlorphentermine	Can. only: Amphetamine All barbiturates Nalbuphine Butorphanol
Schedule IV	Ⓘ or IV	—	—	Benzodiazepines Phenobarbital Pentazocine	
Schedule V	Ⓥ or V	Mostly OTC restricted to pharmacy	—	Low-dose codeine preparations	

* All labels must bear the warning, "Caution: Federal law prohibits dispensing without a prescription."
† Comprehensive Drug Abuse Prevention and Control Act.

Commonly Used Equivalencies Among the Two Systems of Measurement

Reprinted from: Miller and Keane (1983), *Encyclopedia and Dictionary of Medicine, Nursing and Allied Health*, 3rd ed.

Metric Doses with Approximate Apothecary Equivalents*– Liquid Measure

These approximate dose equivalents represent the quantiles usually prescribed, under identical conditions, by physicians trained, respectively, in the metric or in the apothecary system of weights and measures. In labelling dosage forms in both the metric and the apothecary systems, if one is the approximate equivalent of the other, the approximate figure shall be enclosed in parentheses.

When prepared dosage forms such as tablets, capsules, pills, etc. are prescribed in the metric system, the pharmacist may dispense the corresponding approximate equivalent in the apothecary system, and vice versa, as indicated in the following table.

Caution: For the conversion of specific quantities in a prescription that requires compounding, or in converting a pharmaceutical formula from one system of weights or measures to the other, exact equivalents must be used.

Metric (mL)	Approx. Apothecary Equivalents	
1000	1	quart
750	1.5	pints
500	1	pint
250	8	fluid ounces
200	7	fluid ounces
100	3.5	fluid ounces
50	1.75	fluid ounces
30	1	fluid ounce
15	4	fluid drams
10	2.5	fluid drams
8	2	fluid drams
5	1.25	fluid drams
4	1	fluid dram
3	45	minims
2	30	minims
1	15	minims
0.75	12	minims
0.6	10	minims
0.5	8	minims
0.3	5	minims
0.25	4	minims
0.2	3	minims
0.1	1.5	minims
0.06	1	minim
0.05	0.75	minim
0.03	0.5	minim

Note: A milliliter (mL) is the approximate equivalent of a cubic centimeter (cc).
* Adopted by the latest Pharmacopeia, National Formulary, and New and Nonofficial Remedies, and approved by the Federal Food and Drug Administration.

Metric Doses with Approximate Apothecary Equivalents*– Weight

These approximate dose equivalents represent the quantiles usually prescribed, under identical conditions, by physicians trained, respectively, in the metric or in the apothecary system of weights and measures. In labelling dosage forms in both the metric and the apothecary systems, if one is the approximate equivalent of the other, the approximate figure shall be enclosed in parentheses.

When prepared dosage forms such as tablets, capsules, pills, etc. are prescribed in the metric system, the pharmacist may dispense the corresponding approximate equivalent in the apothecary system, and vice versa, as indicated in the following table.

Caution: For the conversion of specific quantities in a prescription that requires compounding, or in converting a pharmaceutical formula from one system of weights or measures to the other, exact equivalents must be used.

Metric	Approx. Apothecary Equivalents		Metric	Approx. Apothecary Equivalents		Metric	Approx. Apothecary Equivalents	
30 g	1	ounce	75 mg	1.25	grains	0.5 mg	0.008	grain
15 g	4	drams	60 mg	1	grain	0.4 mg	0.007	grain
10 g	2.5	drams	50 mg	0.75	grain	0.3 mg	0.005	grain
7.5 g	2	drams	40 mg	0.67	grain	0.25 mg	0.004	grain
6 g	90	grains	30 mg	0.5	grain	0.2 mg	0.003	grain
5 g	75	grains	25 mg	0.375	grain	0.15 mg	0.0025	grain
4 g	60	grains	20 mg	0.33	grain	0.12 mg	0.002	grain
3 g	45	grains	15 mg	0.25	grain	0.1 mg	0.0017	grain
2 g	30	grains	12 mg	0.2	grain			
1.5 g	22	grains	10 mg	0.17	grain			
1 g	15	grains	8 mg	0.125	grain			
0.75 g	12	grains	6 mg	0.1	grain			
0.6 g	10	grains	5 mg	0.08	grain			
0.5 g	7.5	grains	4 mg	0.07	grain			
0.4 g	6	grains	3 mg	0.05	grain			
0.3 g	5	grains	2 mg	0.03	grain			
0.25 g	4	grains	1.5 mg	0.025	grain			
0.2 g	3	grains	1.2 mg	0.02	grain			
0.15 g	2.5	grains	1 mg	0.016	grain			
0.12 g	2	grains	0.8 mg	0.0125	grain			
0.1 g	1.5	grains	0.6 mg	0.01	grain			

Note: A milliliter (mL) is the approximate equivalent of a cubic centimeter (cc).
* Adopted by the latest Pharmacopeia, National Formulary, and New and Nonofficial Remedies, and approved by the Federal Food and Drug Administration.

Index